# Nipple-Areolar Complex Reconstruction

Melvin A. Shiffman
Editor

# Nipple-Areolar Complex Reconstruction

## Principles and Clinical Techniques

Springer

*Editor*
Melvin A. Shiffman
Private Practice
Tustin, CA, USA

ISBN 978-3-319-60924-9    ISBN 978-3-319-60925-6 (eBook)
https://doi.org/10.1007/978-3-319-60925-6

Library of Congress Control Number: 2017959146



Printed on acid-free paper

This Springer imprint is published by Springer Nature
The registered company is Springer International Publishing AG
The registered company address is: Gewerbestrasse 11, 6330 Cham, Switzerland

# Foreword

*Nipple-Areolar Complex Reconstruction: Principles and Clinical Techniques* is a uniquely thorough analysis and overview of nipple-areola complex (NAC) reconstruction. Traditionally, such a review would be confined to a solitary journal publication or single chapter in a textbook on breast reconstruction, and a surgeon seeking more thorough analysis would be limited to shorter reviews (Boccola MA, Savage J, Rozen WM, Ashton MW, Milner C, Rahdon R, Whitaker IS. Surgical correction and reconstruction of the nipple-areola complex: current review of techniques. J Reconstr Microsurg. 2010;26(9):589–600). To this effect, the current book successfully brings together international experts to discuss various types of nipple malformations and provide relevant, up-to-date techniques of NAC reconstruction, and it comprehensively summarizes them in a stand-alone book.

The importance of NAC in body image perception, sexuality, and self-esteem in women and, subsequently, the significance of its reconstruction in nipple inversion, hypertrophy, or loss from oncological treatment are increasingly being recognized by clinicians. As a result, in conjunction with autologous breast reconstruction, NAC reconstruction forms an important component of the holistic treatment of patients affected by breast cancer.

The first reported NAC reconstruction was performed using a local flap by Berson in 1946, followed by skin graft by Adams in 1949. Since then, a plethora of local flap designs and hybrid methods using both local flaps and skin grafts have been reported, publishing variable rates of successful main tenance of nipple projection and pigmentation. Needless to say, the field is relatively new and the holy grail of NAC reconstruction (symmetry in NAC position, size, shape, texture, pigmentation, and permanent projection) still eludes many, leaving exciting potentials for novel developments in this field.

This book reviews the history of NAC reconstruction and the relevant anatomy in depth, before discussing various abnormalities and benign and malignant disorders of NAC. Subsequently, it provides an extensive list of surgical management options for the correction of nipple hypertrophy, inversion, and NAC reconstruction. Well-described NAC reconstruction local flap techniques, such as C-V flap, skate flap with purse-string sutures, doubleopposing flaps, spiral flaps made using scar tissue, Bell flap, Angel flap, and "cigar roll" flap; graft-based methods, such as rolled dermal graft support; and adjuncts, such as acellular dermal matrix onlay grafts and everted umbilicus, are revised. In addition, modifications of several notable techniques, such as V-to-Y technique in bilateral wise pattern mastectomy or reduction mammaplasty, dermal-fat flap with rolled auricular cartilage, arrow flap with rib cartilage graft, and top hat flap with banked costal cartilage graft, are reported. Encouragingly, the book also discusses the current role and the future potential of innovative technologies, such as 3D bioprinting and tissue engineering, that have been introduced in the last decade. The future in terms of clinical studies is touched upon, and certainly there is a role for future work on clinical trials, particularly in terms of quality of life studies between matched groups of patients having no NAC reconstruction versus having one or any of the available options. Robust evidence in this field is warranted.

It has been an honor to be invited to write this brief foreword to this book, edited by Dr. Melvin A. Shiffman, a well-respected and well-published stalwart in cosmetic and reconstructive breast surgery. His role as one of the key members of highly relevant societies in cosmetic surgery, such as American Academy of Cosmetic Surgery, and as an editor of critically acclaimed international journals, such as *American Journal of Cosmetic Surgery*, places him at a high esteem to edit such a pivotal book.

This book would be valuable for early-career surgeons who are keen to build their practice in cosmetic surgery and for plastic surgery trainees as a "go-to" textbook to learn about NAC reconstruction and pick up clinical pearls.

Frankston, VIC, Australia

Warren Matthew Rozen
Michael P. Chae
David J. Hunter-Smith

# Preface

I have always been intrigued with the many manifestations of breast surgery whether it be breast augmentation, mastopexy, breast reduction, or breast reconstruction. Since 1964 I have performed breast reconstruction with implants as the Cronin implant had recently been introduced (1962) and was extremely useful in breast augmentation. My training in my residency and in the years that followed included assisting Dr. Irving Rappaport in his reconstructive surgeries, and I found that there were better ways to reconstruct the breast using various skin and muscle flaps. The major problem was reconstructing the nipple-areolar complex (NAC) since breast cancers were being treated with radical surgical procedures. Despite many attempts with nippleareolar transplants from the opposite breast the problem of flattening of the nipple over time remained. This same problem occurred with transplanting the NAC from breasts that had cancers far enough from the complex and preserving them by transplanting them onto the abdominal wall slightly superior to the groin. After about 6 months the NAC was then transplanted to the reconstructed breast.

Over time, other procedures have been devised and used for NAC reconstruction. More recently I realized that there were no books available that concentrated on reconstructing the NAC, although there were often chapters in books that mostly concentrated on reconstruction of the breast.

This book on NAC reconstruction contains fairly detailed information on the medical literature available, thus enabling the reader to find almost any available technique, and also includes chapters on more recent types of procedures proposed by national and international experts. Their contributions to the book and willingness to spend their time and effort in producing detailed chapters dealing with their techniques are greatly appreciated.

There is information in the book on the history and development of NAC reconstruction that, in my opinion, will help surgeons to see and understand the struggles involved in repairing the damaged NAC as far back as the late 1800s. Those early surgeons did not have the technology that has been developed more recently to perform breast reconstruction, such as large flaps, tissue transfer with free flaps, angiographic studies, mammography, etc. We are fortunate to now be in a position to offer patients far better esthetic results.

Tustin, CA — Melvin A. Shiffman

# Contents

# Part I

# History

# History of Nipple-Areolar Complex Reconstruction

1

Melvin A. Shiffman

## 1.1 Introduction

The breast is an organ for infant feeding but is also a structure that exudes sexuality to most males. The physiological purpose of nipple-areolar complex (NAC) is to deliver milk produced by the mammary glands during lactation. The color of the areola can range from pink to red to dark brown or nearly black but generally tends to be paler among people with lighter skin tones and darker among people with darker skin tones. It has been suggested that a reason for the differing color is to make the nipple area more visible to the infant [1].

The size and shape of areolas are variable, with those of sexually mature women usually being larger than those of men and prepubescent girls. Human areolas are mostly circular in shape, but many women and some men have areolas that are noticeably elliptical. The average diameter of male areolas is around 25 mm (1 in.). Sexually mature women have an average of 38.1 mm (1.5 in.), but sizes range up to 100 mm (4 in.) or greater. Lactating women, or women with particularly large breasts, may have even larger areolas.

The nipple has several small openings arranged radially around the tip of the nipple (lactiferous ducts) from which milk is released during lactation. Other small openings in the areola are sebaceous glands called Montgomery's glands (or glands of Montgomery). These can be raised above the surface of the areola, giving the appearance of "gooseflesh" (Fig. 1.1). The NAC consists of numerous vessels, intermixed with plain muscular fibers, which are principally arranged in a circular manner around the base or even radiating from base to apex. The nipple-areolar complex also contains many sensory nerve endings, smooth muscle, and an abundant lymphatic system called subareolar plexus or Sappey's plexus. Nipple-areolar anatomy is variable in dimension, texture, and color depending on ethnic groups and also among individuals.

## 1.2 Ideal Breast

Mallucci and Branford [1] identified the aesthetic ideal of the breast by analyzing women who were models. The ideal breast had the proportion of the upper to the lower pole at a 45:55 ratio, the angulation of the nipple as upward at a mean angle of 20° from the nipple meridian, the upper pole slope as linear or slightly concave, and the lower pole as convex. Deviation from this pattern yields a less attractive breast—the greater the deviation, the less attractive the breast.

M.A. Shiffman, M.D., J.D.
Private Practice, 17501, Chatham Drive,
Tustin, CA 92780-2302, USA
e-mail: shiffmanmdjd@gmail.com



M.A. Shiffman (ed.), *Nipple-Areolar Complex Reconstruction*,
https://doi.org/10.1007/978-3-319-60925-6_1

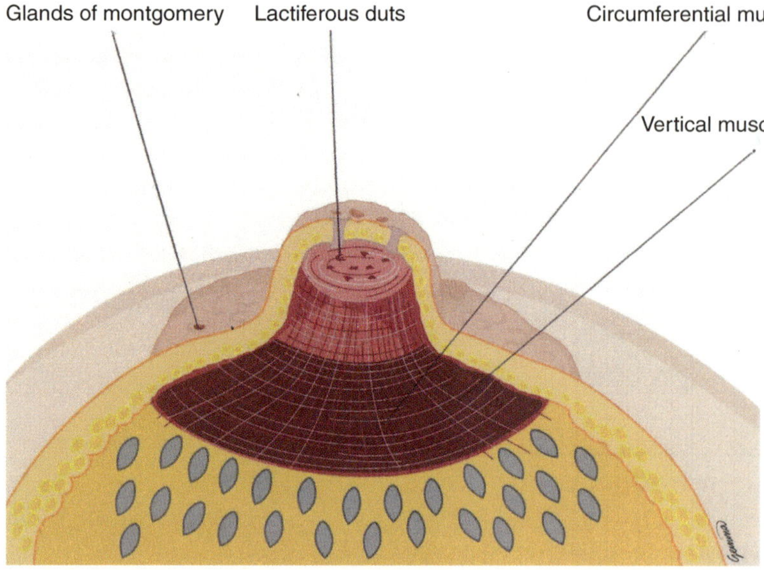


**Fig. 1.1** Anatomy of the nipple-areolar complex

## 1.3 Optimal Breast NAC Proportions

Jaimovich [2] stated that the normal nipple represents the apex of the breast and must keep a proportion 1:3 with the areola. The optimal NAC proportions were found by Hauben et al. [3] to be with the proportion of the upper to the lower pole as a 45:55 ratio, the angulation of the nipple as upward at a mean angle of 20° from the nipple meridian, the upper pole slope as linear or slightly concave, and the lower pole as convex. The areola-breast and nipple-areola proportions were 1:3.4 and 1:3, respectively. The natural nipple-areola-breast proportion is approximately 1:3. This provides a general guideline for plastic surgeons for planning breast surgery with optimal aesthetic results.

Beckenstein et al. [4] studied 100 males with ages ranging from 17 to 30 and reported that:

1. The average diameter of the areola was 2.8 cm with a range of 2.5–3.0 cm.
2. The average sternal notch to nipple distance was 20.12 cm with a range of 19–21 cm.
3. Average midclavicular line to nipple distance was 18.19 cm with a range of 19–21 cm.
4. The average nipple to nipple distance was 21.25 cm with a range of 20–22 cm.

## 1.4 Nipple-Areolar Complex Position

The nipple-areolar complex (NAC) is the center of the breast and as such contributes to the beauty of the breast by its symmetrical position. There are innumerable methods of determining the position of the NAC, and this supports the concept that the position of the NAC is not easy to determine.

Altchek [5] stated that placement of an artificial nipple on the mound greatly facilitates locating of the optimal nipple position by enabling both the surgeon and patient to "preview" the anticipated final appearance of the breast. The artificial nipple has a double-back adhesive disk that will adhere to the skin and allow the surgeon to move the nipple from one site to another until the desired position is found. A ballpoint pen is then inserted through a previously made hole in the nipple, and an imprint is made at the site. The imprinted site is circled using a 20% silver nitrate solution that will leave a stain on the skin for at least 1 week.

Kon and Sagi [6] proposed a simple, inexpensive aid for nipple-areola site determination is the disposable electrocardiographic electrode. Patients participate in positioning of the future nipple-areolar complex, and accurate localization can be checked even when the breast is covered with a brassiere.

The author (MAS), with the patient standing or sitting, utilizes a line from the midclavicular point (MC) to the mid-nipple (N). At the same time, a line is marked in the center of the chest wall from the center of the sternum superiorly to the mid-xiphoid process. The inframammary fold is palpated from underneath the breast inferiorly and the tip of the finger palpated superficially and marked on the MC to N line. Then a measurement is made from the marked point horizontally to the midline on each side and the lengths recorded. If one line is above the other, this distance is recorded. This will determine how different the center of the nipple is from each side, and a decision has to be made as to whether or not to correct this difference at the time of surgery with crescent excisions. The breast mound on each side should be made to coincide. The nipple should be at the most projecting part of the breast.

The reports in the medical literature show a variety of personal methods of determining the nipple position [7–35]. Using measurements that vary in length along any line as suggested by many authors is another way of saying, "guess where the point should be," since it varies with the height of the individual and depends on the physician's accuracy by visualization. Other authors place the nipple at a measured distance from some point on the chest.

## 1.5 Abnormalities of the NAC

One of the critical areas of breast reconstruction is the reconstruction of the nipple-areolar complex (NAC). Abnormalities in the position of the NAC or distortion of the shape of the NAC may very well result in patient dissatisfaction. Although the surgeon takes considerable time in performing reconstruction surgery of the breast and nipple-areolar complex (NAC) in order to get the best results, there is almost no possibility of getting complete symmetry of the breasts and NAC. Although at the time of surgery the breasts and NAC may appear symmetrical, healing and scarring of the tissues may result in distortion of the shape and position of the NAC.

To understand the complexity of the subject of reconstruction of the NAC, the variety of NAC problems and the techniques used to correct these problems will be described. Making use of the variety of techniques is a personal matter for the surgeon to decide according to the type of problem to be corrected. It is also necessary to understand how some of these NAC abnormalities originated in order to avoid problems in the future.

The nipple-areolar complex may be affected by many normal variations in embryologic development such as absent NAC from amastia (breast tissue, nipple, and areola are absent—either congenital or iatrogenic) or athelia (congenital absence of one or both nipples. It is a rare condition. It sometimes occurs on one side in children with the Poland sequence and on both sides in certain types of ectodermal dysplasia).

Benign processes that may affect the nipple-areolar complex include eczema, duct ectasia, periductal mastitis, adenomas, papillomas, leiomyomas, and abscesses. Malignant processes include Paget disease, lymphoma, and invasive and breast cancers. Patients may present with benign developmental variations such as inversion, retraction, or enlargement of the nipple, a palpable mass, nipple discharge, skin changes in and around the nipple, infection with resultant nipple changes or a subareolar mass, or abnormal findings at routine mammographic screening, many of which may have either a benign or a malignant cause.

Postsurgical loss of the NAC can occur from NAC composite transplant, breast reduction, breast reconstruction with a variety of flaps, and trauma.

## 1.6 Prevention of Nipple-Areolar Complex Loss or Deformity

The causes of loss of the nipple-areolar complex from breast reduction as described by Rapin [36] include:

1. Placing the nipple too high
2. Excessive torsion of the breast pedicle
3. Over-tightness of the "skin brassiere"
4. Hemorrhage
5. Imperfect or insufficient drainage

Other factors that may cause loss of NAC are smoking, breast reconstruction, trauma, congenital, and free transplanting of the NAC.

Minimizing the risks of avascular necrosis of the nipple-areolar complex following reduction mammaplasty according to McKissock [29] requires:

1. Keep within the size limits of safety of the operation.
   (a) The gigantic breast should be handled by free nipple graft.
   (b) Predetermine the overall length of the vertical bipedicle flap. Inframammary fold to superior point of the keyhole pattern should not exceed 35 cm.
   (c) Consider the likely vascular qualities of the parenchyma. In older or obese patients with fatty breasts and atrophic skin, reduce the acceptable limits.
2. Do not thin the pedicle excessively.
   (a) Superior pedicle should not be thinner than 1.5 cm.
   (b) Inferior pedicle should not be thinner than 5.0 cm.
3. Do not undermine the areola. The resection beneath the superior pedicle ends at the upper edge of the areola.

Various techniques are described in the literature to prevent problems when performing breast reduction or mastectomy [37–45]. Hallock and Altobelli [46] and Ayhan et al. [47] described methods to prevent the teardrop areola following mammaplasty.

The author (MAS) uses the 6 s rule for venous refill. If the NAC becomes cyanotic, press on the NAC firmly and then release. If refill (loss of blanching) is less than 6 s, then watch and wait for the dark area to slough superficially. This may result in some areas of hypopigmentation that can be treated by tattooing. The pigment should be slightly darker than the remaining areola since the pigment color will almost always get slightly lighter. If refill is 6 s or over, then the NAC is excised and replanted in the abdominal wall just above the groin. This NAC can be replanted following complete healing of the wound and then a delay of at least 3 more months.

## 1.7 Correcting Improper Nipple-Areolar Complex Position

Improperly placed nipples that are excessively high are difficult to correct. The resulting scar may exceed the benefits derived from lowering the nipple. When the nipple is too low, elevation without additional scarring is easily achieved. Other forms of NAC malposition require corrections that may leave a trailing scar. In some the nipple-areolar complex can be left attached to the gland mass and, after rather extensive undermining of the surrounding skin, can be repositioned through a properly located areola opening. When the malposition is significant, the secondary defect may be closed horizontally as described by Millard et al. [48]. This avoids the trailing scar and the superior extension of the scar.

When malposition is associated with significant relaxation of the skin envelope, a full ellipse should be resected, either with or without a horizontal inframammary excision. In cases where the nipple is less than half the diameter of the areola, an acceptable correction may result from an inferior crescent excision. Also, the inclusion of a small, highly placed prosthesis (if the patient will accept it) may help create the illusion of a properly located nipple. A nipple-areolar complex placed too far medially may be corrected with a lateral crescent excision and if too far lateral then a medial crescent excision.

Pseudomalposition of the nipple due to late descent of a gland mass below the level of the properly located nipple does not involve repositioning of the nipple for correction. Raising the breast gland into the correct position will resolve the problem. The author (MAS) uses silk suture to fix the breast tissue to the underlying pectoralis fascia. Silk causes more fibrous tissue than other types of suture.

## 1.8 Correcting the High-Riding Nipple-Areolar Complex

The high-riding nipple-areolar complex is the most difficult disorder to correct since lowering the NAC almost always results in a visible scar above the NAC.

The high-riding nipple was classified by Colwell et al. [49]:

Grade 1: Pseudoelevation—inferior pole descent or bottoming out.

Lower pole remodeling.

Grade 2: Mild elevation— the nipple is mildly superiorly displaced.

Requires a combination of techniques including scar revision, skin excision, and inferior pole remodeling.

Grade 3: Severe elevation—moderate to severe nipple elevation.

Spear et al. [50] proposed a similar classification.

Reports indicate a variety of techniques. Raffel [51] recommended tissue expander followed by an implant, while Elsahy [52] excised tissue superior to the inframammary fold. A double apposing flap was utilized by Mohmand and Naasan [53] and Frenkiel [54]. There were other reports for correcting the high-riding nipple [55–57].

## 1.9 Nipple-Areola Sharing

Vincenz Czerny transplanted the nipple following a simple mastectomy to preserve the natural breast according to Gilman [58] and Purohit [59]. Thorek [60] was the first to advocate free nipple grafting in cases of pronounced macromastia. Nipple-areolar complex sharing is one simple method of replacing an absent nipple. The normal nipple can be transected transversely in height for transfer [61–63], be halved vertically, have a V-shaped transverse excision, have areola skin removed from the normal NAC, or other techniques [64–90].

## 1.10 Nipple-Areolar Body Grafts

The areas of the body where grafts are taken to reconstruct the NAC vary. However, the best areas are those that have pigmentation similar to the nipple-areolar area. Grafts have been taken from the auricle, banked cartilage, buttock, costal cartilage, groin, hallux, labia, retroauricular, oral mucosa, rima ani, suprapubic, inner upper thigh, vaginal mucosa, or vulva.

The early cases used pedicles from the abdomen and axilla. Rapin [36] and Gruber [67] described the use of an axillary tubed pedicle, and Gillies [91] and Gruber [67] described the use of an abdominal flap pedicle.

Other reports of grafts from portions of the body include auricular graft [92–96], banked cartilage [97], buttock [98, 99], costal cartilage graft [100, 101], groin [102], hallux pulp composite graft [99], labia [67, 70, 99, 102–107], oral mucosa [67], retroauricular skin graft [67], rima ani [108], suprapubic skin graft [67], upper inner thigh graft [67, 109–115], vaginal mucosa [102], and vulva [116].

## 1.11 Nipple Inversion

Inverted nipples can be acquired or congenital. The most common causes of acquired nipple inversion include:

1. Born with the problem.
2. Breastfeeding.
3. Trauma which can be caused by conditions such as fat necrosis and scars or it may be a result of surgery.
4. Breast sagging, drooping, or ptosis.
5. Breast cancer including breast carcinoma, Paget's disease, and inflammatory breast cancer.
6. Large, pendulous breasts.
7. Breast infections or inflammations such as mammary duct ectasia, periductal abscess, and mastitis.
8. The inferior pyramidal dermal pedicle flap breast reduction can have nipple inversion when insufficient breast tissue is left inferior to the nipple-areolar complex [23]. "This problem cannot be corrected once the breast tissue has been resected and prevention can only be attained by leaving sufficient bulk at the nipple base at the time of the initial resection."

### 1.11.1 Congenital Causes of Nipple Inversion

An arrest of the ductal system at an early stage of growth causing tension on the nipple is thought to cause nipple inversion [117]. The accumulation of subcutaneous fat makes it more prominent.

A Jewish Sephardic family was reported by Shafir et al. [118] in which 16 members are affected (15 females and 1 male) with inverted nipples. The one affected male and his brother also have gynecomastia. Under the assumption that this trait is transmitted as an autosomal dominant, linkage studies were done but were not revealing. Further family and investigative studies are needed in this disorder to understand better its pathogenesis and precise mode of genetic transmission.

#### 1.11.1.1 Chromosome 2q Deletion Syndrome [119]

Deletion of the long arm of chromosome 2 with a highly variable phenotype marked mainly by low birth weight, delayed somatic and mental development, craniofacial defects (relative small facial features with eye, ear, and nose abnormalities), small head, short neck, finger deformities, heart and lung congenital defects, inverted nipples, brachydactyly, syndactyly, and cleft lip or palate.

#### 1.11.1.2 Congenital Disorder of Glycosylation Type Ia (CDG-Ia) [120]

Congenital disorder of glycosylation type Ia (CDG-Ia), also known as phosphomannomutase 2 deficiency, is an inherited condition that affects many parts of the body. The type and severity of problems associated with CDG-Ia vary widely among affected individuals, sometimes even among members of the same family. Symptoms include retracted (inverted) nipples, hypotonia, strabismus, failure to thrive, high forehead, a triangular face, large ears, a thin upper lip, seizures, moderate intellectual disability, kyphoscoliosis, hypergonadotropic hypogonadism, retinitis pigmentosa, and other symptoms.

#### 1.11.1.3 Congenital Disorder of Glycosylation Type 1L [121]

The signs and symptoms include inverted nipples, lipodystrophy, brain atrophy, psychomotor retardation, mental retardation, very large head, unusual facial appearance, central hypotonia, seizures, esotropia (a squint), and other symptoms.

Hereditary Lymphedema-Distichiasis Syndrome

Mutations in FOXC2 (MFH-1) are responsible for the syndrome that includes widely spaced and inverted nipples [122, 123].

#### 1.11.1.4 Kennerknecht-Sorgo-Oberhoffer Syndrome [124, 125]

This syndrome is mainly characterized by the absence of testicles in case of men and ovaries in case of women. Other associated features include underdevelopment of the right-side portions of the heart, lungs, and some blood vessels, dextrocardia, omphalocele, small head, dysplastic hips, scoliosis, mental retardation, partial toe webbing, and short neck. Inversion of the nipples is also noticed in individuals affected by this syndrome along with other features such as unusual facial structure, short neck, and webbing of the toes.

#### 1.11.1.5 MR/MCA Syndrome (Fryns-Aftimos Syndrome) [126, 127]

Symptoms of the syndrome include hypoplastic inverted nipples, underdeveloped nipples, epilepsy, pachygyria (malformation of the cerebral hemisphere), mental retardation, arched eyebrows, droopy eyelids, wide-set eyes, trigonocephaly, broad nose bridge and root, short neck, large mouth, and narrow upper chest.

#### 1.11.1.6 Weaver Syndrome

Weaver syndrome is characterized by a wide variety of features that include large size of the baby at birth; faster growth and maturation; abnormalities of the hands and legs, head and facial region, and nervous system; and other abnormalities such as loose skin, low-pitched voice, and inverted nipples [128].

### 1.11.2 Classification of Inverted Nipples

In 1946, Waller [129] described a protractility test that is still widely used. Classifications of inverted nipples have been devised using the nipple's protractility [130–133]. Han and Hong's [130] classification appears to be the most useful since it also includes pathology.

Grade I: The nipple can be easily pulled out manually and maintains its projection quite well without traction. It is believed to have minimal or no fibrosis. The lactiferous ducts should be normal without any retraction.

Grade II: The nipple can be pulled out manually, but not as easily as in grade I. The nipple has difficulty maintaining its position and tends to retract. There is a moderate degree of fibrosis, and the lactiferous ducts are mildly retracted but do not need to be cut for release of the fibrosis. There is a rich collagenous stroma with numerous bundles of smooth muscle.

Grade III: The nipple is severely inverted and retracted. It is difficult to pull out manually. It promptly retracts. A traction suture is needed to hold these nipples protruded. The fibrosis is marked and lactiferous ducts are short and severely retracted. There are atrophic terminal duct lobular units and severe fibrosis.

Terrill and Stapleton [134] studied patients who had and did not have the lactiferous ducts divided. They found that there were similar rates of failure for umbilicated nipples whether the ducts were divided (27%) or not (25%). Invaginated nipples showed an increased tendency to reinvert postoperatively if the ducts were not divided (80%) than if they were (42%). Permanent loss of nipple sensation was noted in 20% of cases when the lactiferous ducts were divided. Postoperatively 2 women out of 26 were able to breastfeed despite complete division of their lactiferous ducts. They concluded that correction of the umbilicated nipple can usually be successfully performed and function maintained without dividing the ducts. Correction of the invaginated nipple requires duct division.

Axford [135] appears to have been the first to treat inverted nipples. This was followed by Kehrer [136], Basch [137], and Williams [138]. Since then there are many articles on the treatment of inverted nipples [28, 95, 105, 117, 139–229].

## 1.12 Nipple Hypertrophy

Jaimovich [229] stated that the normal nipple represents the apex of the breast and must keep a proportion 1:3 with the areola. Knowledge of this proportion should be used when correcting the abnormal nipple.

Pitanguy [230] performed a horizontal incision and another vertical to the nipple base keeping a small flap on this area and resecting the inferior hemisphere of the nipple. The remaining flap is folded and sutured to the base diminishing the nipple height. Sperli [231] marked six equidistant points on the circumference of the base of the nipple. A 5.0 mm circle was outlined on the end of the nipple. Three wedge-shaped areas, each of which base lies between 2 of the equidistant points and whose apex is at the 5.0 mm circle, were excised. On each of the three remaining columns, a rectangular area large enough to reduce the remaining nipple tissue to a normal size was excised. Resulting is a pole with three flaps remaining. All the wounds are closed. This reduced the height and the diameter of the nipple.

The author (MAS) prefers the simple method of nipple circumcision reported by Regnault [232]. This consists of a circular incision, avoiding injury to the lactiferous ducts, near the top of the nipple. Then measuring upward 8 mm from the nipple base, another circular incision is performed. The skin is removed between the two incisions. The nipple skin is closed with 5-0 nylon suture.

There are other reports of the treatment of the hypertrophic nipple [2, 28, 233–250].

## 1.13 Nipple-Areolar Complex Reconstruction with Flap Methods

Erwin Payr [251], chief surgeon at the University of Greifswald, reported an operation for a less-extensive skin defect, after mastectomy, in individuals with ample subcutaneous fat. He reconstructed a breast by using a large, superior-medial-based, sickle-shaped skin flap from the medial side of the defect. Based superiorly, this flap was rotated laterally into the defect with primary closure of the donor site, causing a twisting of the center that mimicked a nipple. The medial design of this flap limited its use, and future use of flaps depended on a more lateral origin, of which numerous kinds were designed.

There are various reports of NAC reconstruction with flaps in the medical literature [36, 67, 70, 73, 79, 91, 94, 97, 100, 101, 106, 110–112, 114, 183, 252–295]:

Berson [252]: Triple flap for nipple reconstruction.

Rapin [36]: Tubed axillary pedicle.

Gillies H, Millard [91]: Abdominal tubed pedicle.

DiPirro [106]: Construction of the nipple by infolding and suturing the local skin.

Snyder et al. [253]: V-Y advancement flap.

Gruber [67]: Axillary tubed pedicle and abdominal flap pedicle,

V-Y flap, and cartwheel for flaps.

Dubin [254]: Central core technique.

Barton [110]: Latissimus dermal-epidermal nipple reconstruction. Blunted Maltese-cross pattern to allow spherical closure of areola.

Asplund and Korloff [255]: Mushroom plasty.

Serafin and Georgiade [256]: Extended central core technique.

Asplund [111]: Epidermis lifted circumferentially leaving central nipple core (mushroom cap). The outer border of the cap is sutured to the base of the stalk to form the nipple.

Little et al. [257]: Quadrapod flap.

Silversmith [258]: Simplified quadrapod flap.

Chang [259]: Local skin T flap.

Bosch and Ramirez [112]: Single U-flap dermal pedicle to reconstruct the nipple.

Kon [260]: Latissimus dorsi three-flap nipple reconstruction.

Little [261]: Quadrapod flap and fortified quadrapod flap.

Hartrampf and Culbertson [262]: Dermal-fat flap.

Kon [263]: T- and three-flap nipple reconstruction.

Georgiade et al. [70]: Deepithelialized U-flap.

Cohen et al. [113]: Pinwheel flap nipple and barrier areola graft reconstruction.

Smith and Nelson [114]: Mushroom-shaped pedicle.

Mukherjee et al. [264]: Buried dermal hammock technique.

Anton and Hartrampf [265]: Star flap.

Nohira et al. [266]: Skate flap.

Anton et al. [267]: Star and wrap flaps.

Eskenazi [268]: Modified star flap.

Hallock and Altobelli [269]: Cylindrical H-flap.

Hugo et al. [270]: Used double-opposing flaps (called pennant flaps).

Wong et al. [271]: Star flap.

Cederna [272]: Star flap.

Jones and Bostwick [73]: Skate flap and C-V flap.

Teimourian and Duda [273]: Propeller flap.

Thomas et al. [274]: Cylinder from rectangle and circle.

Tanabe et al. [94]: Dermal-fat flap and rolled auricular cartilage.

Ramakrishnan et al. [183]: Twin flap technique for nipple reconstruction.

Kroll et al. [275]: Modified double-opposing tab and star flaps.

Yamamoto and Sugihara [276]: Star flap.

Hamori and LaRossa [277]: Top hat flap.

Kroll [278]: Double-opposing tab flap.

Kroll [279]: Rectangular wraparound flap.

Few et al. [280]: Modified star flap.

Yamamoto et al. [281]: Innovations of star flap technique.

Shestak et al. [282]: Bell flap, star flap, and skate flap.

Bogue et al. [283]: Skate flap.

Cheng et al. [97]: Modified top hat flap.

Kolberg et al. [79]: Skate flap preferred after augmentation. Star-shaped flap, mushroom flap, or modified Hartrampf nipple preferred after breast reconstruction.

Motamed and Davami [284]: Modified star flap.

Farhadi et al. [285]: Described centrally based local flaps, centrally based three flaps, V-Y advancement flaps, centrally based four flaps, inverted dermal flap, central core technique, buried dermal hammock, extended central core technique, modified quadrapod flap, simplified quadrapod flap, pinwheel flap, H-flap, single dermal pedicle flap, deepithelialized U-flap, skate flap, star flap, cylindrical flap, Hartrampf nipple, double U-shaped flap, S-flap, and twin flap.

Beckenstein [101]: The "penny flap" design.

Cheng et al. [100]: Modified top hat flap.

Fitoussi et al. [286]: F- and Z-flaps.

Foustanos [287]: Double flap technique.

Grotting [288]: Modified fishtail flap.

Gullo et al. [289]: Star flap enhanced by scar tissue.

Sierakowski and Niranjan [290]: Star flap with a dermal platform.

Katerinaki et al. [291]: C-V flap.

Gurunluoglu et al. [292]: Star flap.

Wong et al. [293]: The angel flap.

Chun et al. [294]: Skate flap, bell flap, star flap, spiral flap, double-opposing flap, and trapeze flap (modified Thomas technique).

Mu et al. [295]: Circular flap.

## 1.14 Tattooing

The word "tattoo" is derived from the Polynesian word "ta" ("to strike"), which describes the sound of a tattooing spike being knocked on the skin. The first recorded references to the word "tattoo" are in the papers of Joseph Banks (1743–1820), a naturalist aboard Captain Cook's ship. Before Captain Cook brought the word to Europe, tattoos in the West were known as "prics" or "marks" [296].

Levites et al. [297] stated that "the decline in qualitative color and shape score agrees with clinical experience of tattoo quality declining over time. The color qualities of the tattoo approach those of the patient's skin over time, ultimately reaching a plateau." However, tattooing is utilized to obtain a facsimile of the normal nipple-areolar complex and will usually require repeat tattooing to maintain the color. Many patients are satisfied with the initial tattooing and prefer not returning for further tattooing.

The skin to be utilized for replacing the areola can be tattooed prior to surgery or following the surgical procedure on skin grafting. Some areas of the body have some darker skin that can be used to replace an absent areola. When tattooing to simulate the nipple, the patient should be comfortable with the lack of projection.

There are possible complications with the use of tattooing. These include:

1. Allergic reaction to dye
2. Asymmetry of color
3. Bleeding
4. Cellulitis
5. Fading of dye

6. Infection
7. Inflammation
8. Photoallergic dermatitis
9. Pyoderma
10. Rejection of the dye (color not taking)
11. Uneven color of pigment on the areola

Becker [298] uses a Permark surgical pigmenting pen (Permark Corp., Glenpointe Centre East, Teaneck, NJ). The oxide pigments are mixed to the appropriate color. The color should be slightly darker than that of the opposite breast. A multiple needle-type brush is used for the tattooing procedure. Approximately 25% of patients had to have touch-up tattoos or retattoos in order to improve the color match. Masser et al. [299] were the first to use pigment particles that have been suspended in a gel rather than adsorbed on an opaque mineral. Using this new method, a third of the patients achieved a completely natural appearance and two-thirds were judged to be intermediate.

Rees [300] performed intradermal tattooing and then transferred the tattooed area to replace the absent areola. Since then there have been reports of tattooing as part of breast reconstruction [73, 75, 79, 102, 115, 271–273, 275, 283, 286, 288, 299, 301–314].

## 1.15 Examples of Nipple-Areolar Complex Reconstruction

### 1.15.1 Nipple Inversion

Hinderer et al. [166] performed surgery for nipple inversion and asymmetry using two flaps attached in the midline and pulled through a tunnel to the opposite side to hold the nipple everted (Fig. 1.2). Yamamoto and Sugahara [276] used a modified star flap for inverted nipples. They raised three flaps and lifted the middle larger flap while wrapping the other two flaps (wings) to close the defect of the larger flap after releasing the lactiferous ducts (Fig. 1.3). Huang [194] reported the use of three diamond-shaped flaps to pass through tunnels under the nipple while the nipple was retracted and the lactiferous ducts and fibrous tissue were transected (Fig. 1.4). Yamada et al. [200] utilized splitting and stretching of the tissue under the nipple while the nipple had traction (Fig. 1.5). Then artificial dermis (TERUDERMIS) was shaped and placed into the defects under the nipple through tunnels.

### 1.15.2 Nipple Hypertrophy

Hypertrophic nipples were treated by Vecchione [234] by taking a thin split-thickness graft from the tip of the nipple and then resected a 9 mm core of the nipple to match the contralateral side (Fig. 1.6). The graft was sutured to the remaining stump of the nipple. For reducing the diameter of the hypertrophic nipple, van Wingerden [237] resected a wedge from the nipple using a mathematical analysis of the ideal ratio of nipple to areolar diameter (Fig. 1.7). A circular flap on the nipple was raised by Mu et al. [295] and the tissue excised from the nipple base (Fig. 1.8). A purse-string suture was placed at the nipple base to reduce the base to 0.3 to 0.4 cm in diameter. The flap was then closed.

### 1.15.3 NAC Reconstruction

Kon in 1984 [260] reported the use of three flaps on a central disk for reconstructing a neo-nipple-areolar complex (Fig. 1.9). The central flap was raised and the two side wings wrapped around the central core of fat and flaps sutured together. The deepithelialized area was grafted to form the areola.

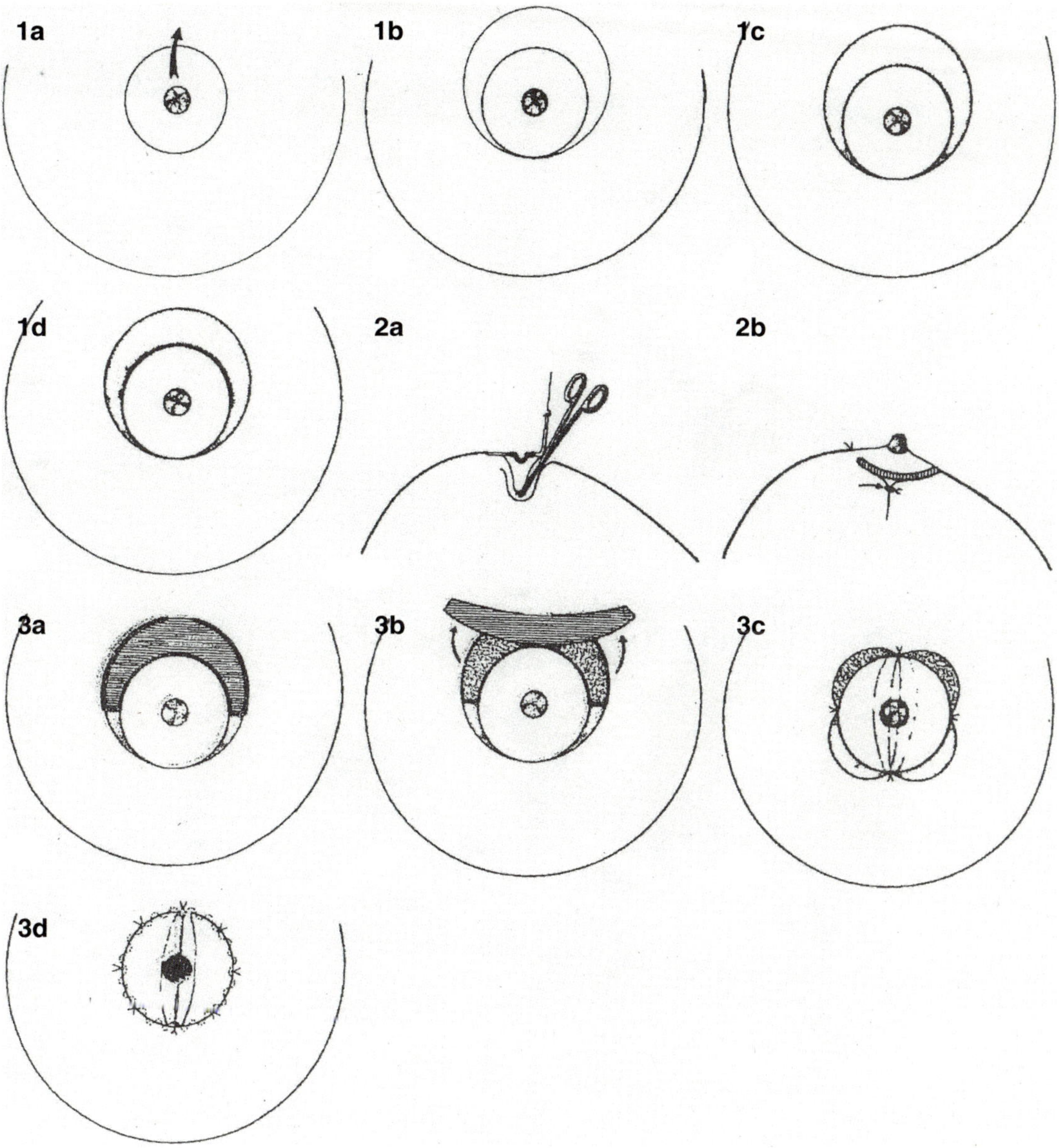


**Fig. 1.2** Hinderer et al. [166]. Nipple inversion and asymmetry. (1**a**, **b**) The ideal symmetric location of the areola is marked as well as for the new areola position (in patient with low position). (1**c**) The skin between both circular is deepithelialized but remains attached to the dermis in at least half its circumference. (1**d**) The incision in the upper half of the areola is deepened. (2**a**, **b**) In the deepened incision, the underlying tissues are undermined and retaining structures severed until complete eversion of the nipple. (3**a**) Another incision into the full depth of the dermis is made in the outer circle except for a 10 mm bridge at its furthest point (*left uncut*). (3**b**) Two straight cuts join the full-depth incision to form a "horn." (3**c**) The "horns" are lifted and pulled and pulled below the nipple to the opposite side and then sutured in position. (3**d**) The areola and external incisions are sutured. Reprinted with permission of Springer

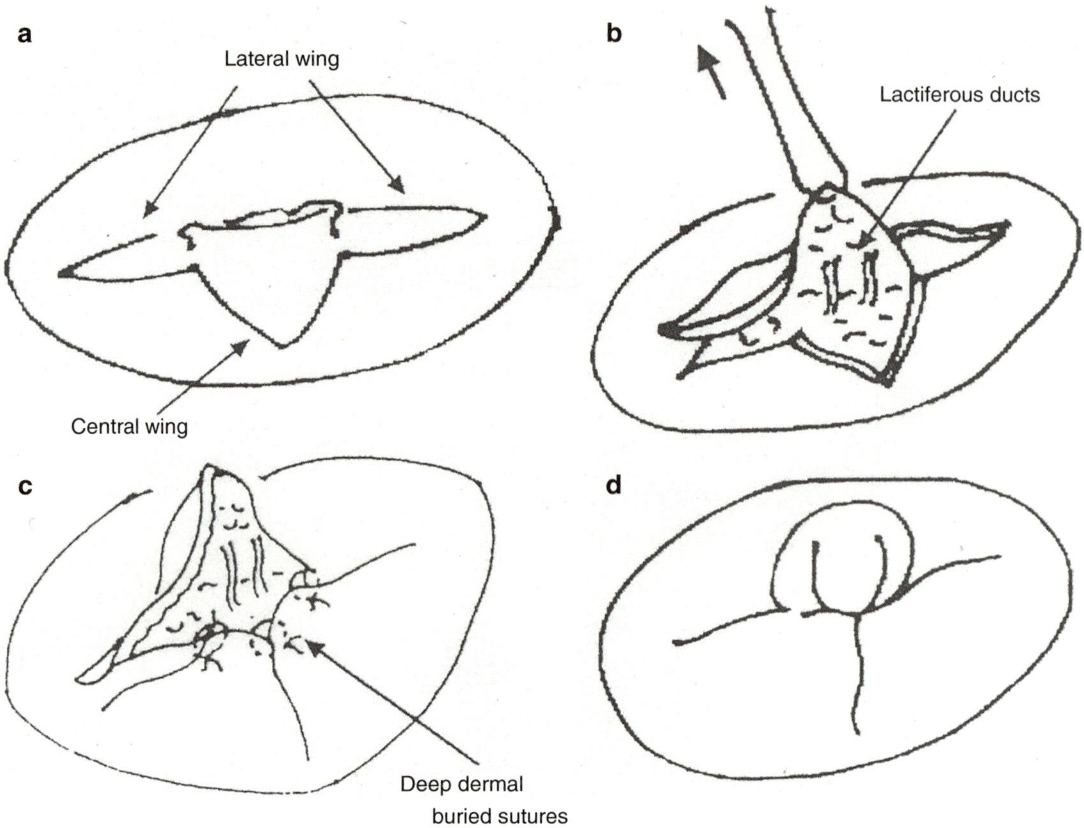


**Fig. 1.3** Yamamoto and Sugahara [276]. Modified star flap technique for inverted nipple. (**a**) Three wings of the flap are marked. The central wing is vertical to the longitudinal axis. The width of the central wing base is equal to the length of the longitudinal axis of the inverted nipple. (**b**) The three wings of the flap are elevated with a small amount of subcutaneous fat and getting thicker toward the nipple base. The lactiferous ducts are identified and released from the surrounding fibrous tissue. Myotomy of the areolar mammillary bundles is performed. (**c**) The nipple is everted and the three donor sites are closed. Deep dermal buried sutures are inserted. (**d**) The three wings of the flap are sutured in place covering the raw surface. Reprinted with permission of Springer

## 1.16 Discussion

The author has attempted many methods of neo-nipple-areolar reconstruction, nipple inversion, nipple hypertrophy, and areolar irregularities. The problems I have encountered center around nipple flattening. Reconstructing the nipple is not complicated, but there is no support offered to prevent flattening. Placing the neo-nipple over fat or breast tissue does not keep the nipple adequately projected for more than a year. Using cartilage or foreign materials to support the nipple allows projection for a longer period of time but is still not completely

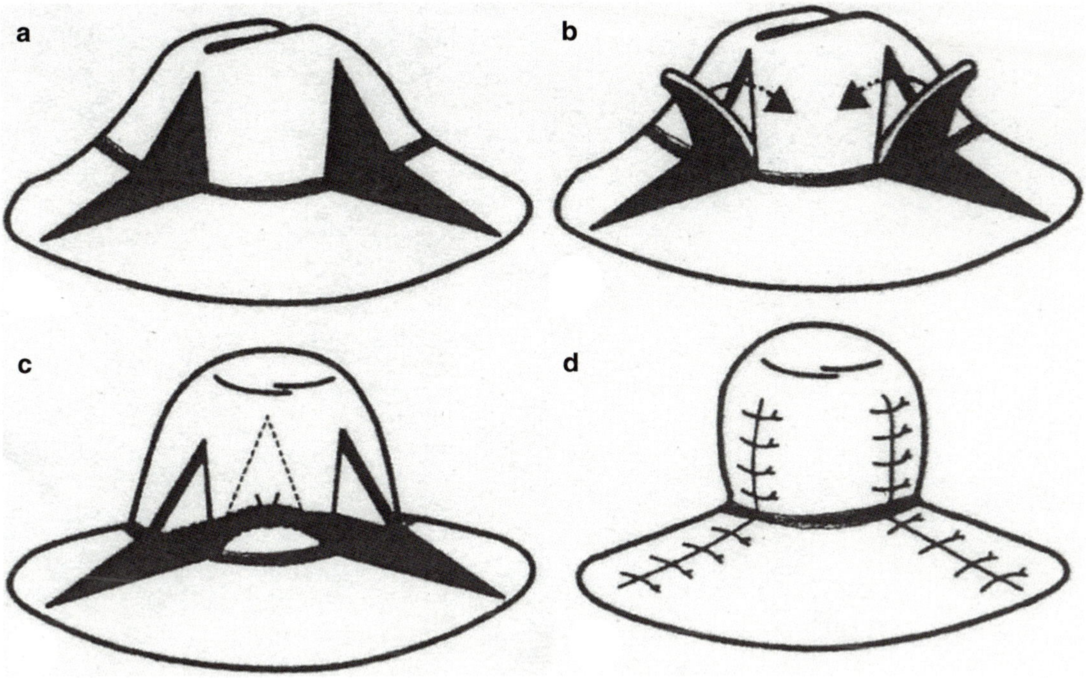


**Fig. 1.4** Huang [194]. Inverted nipple. The nipple is everted using traction suture. The dome margin and root of the nipple are marked as two concentric circles. The height of the nipple will be the radius discrepancy of the circles (5 mm or longer). Three *diamond*-shaped areas are marked at the 2, 6, and 10 o'clock positions. (**a**) The *diamond*-shaped areas are deepithelialized. (**b**) The nipple parts of the diamond are elevated with the areolomammary muscle and periductal dermofibrous tissue. The areolar parts are undermined subcutaneously to facilitate closure. The fibrous and retracting ducts are released under the nipple from the three sides until the nipple can stay everted without traction. (**c**) The dermofibrous flaps are turned down through the tunnels and sutured together to fill the dead space under the nipple. (**d**) The *diamond*-shaped areas are sutured in two layers closing the wounds. Reprinted with permission of Springer

satisfying and has complications of their own. Flaps that are pulled through tunnels under the nipple act as a hammock and seem to be the most satisfying technique.

Tattooing in my patients has not been satisfactory for a long period of time. The color over time does not match the contralateral areola and nipple. Repeat tattooing has occurred in almost 100% of my patients and even that tends to fade. Some patients do not want any more surgery and can be satisfied with tattooing as the simplest procedure despite its problems. These patients usually are not interested in repeat tattooing despite the loss of color. I am certainly happy to see a patient who can be satisfied with minimal procedures and do not expect perfect results.

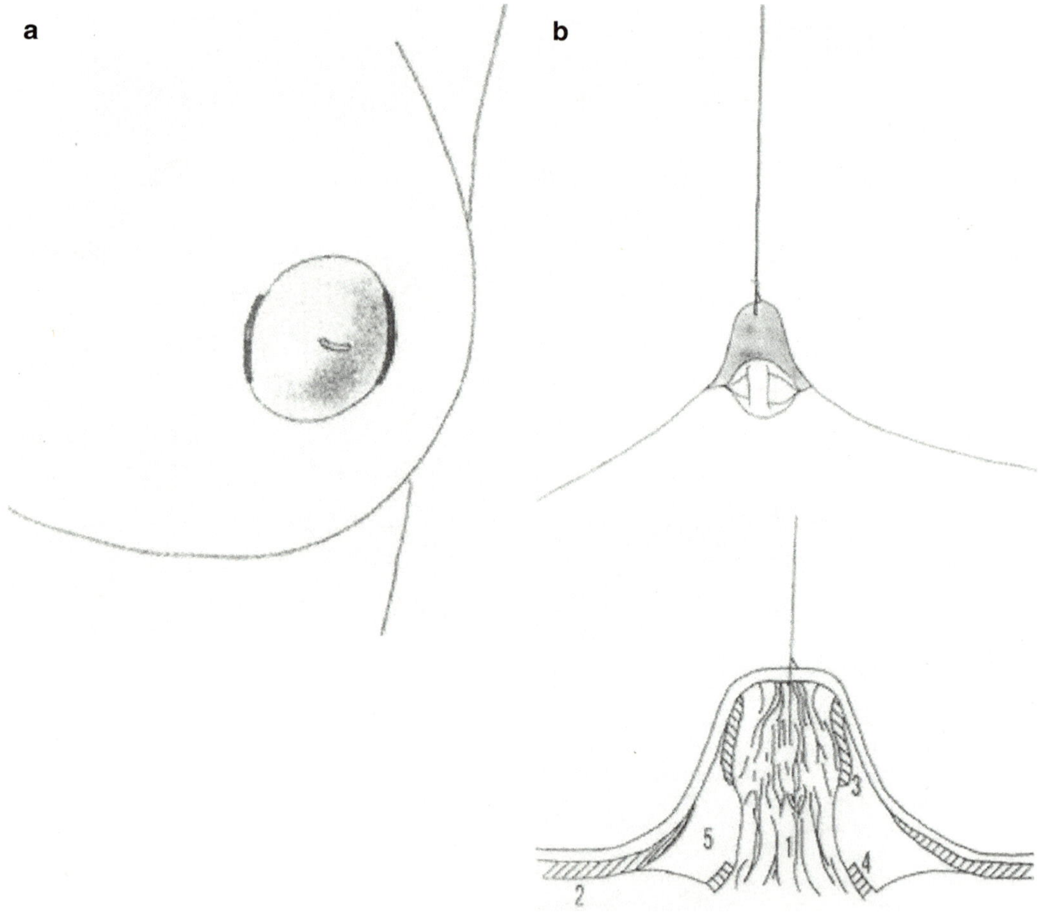


**Fig. 1.5** Yamada et al. [200]. Artificial dermis for inverted nipple. (**a**) Two 1.5 cm incisions are made at the 3 and 9 o'clock positions at the edge of the areola. (**b** *Top*) Traction is applied to the nipple, and a subcutaneous tunnel is made with sharp splitting and stretching maneuvers until the nipple is everted. (**b** *Bottom*) (1) Lactiferous ducts. (2) Areolomammillary muscle. (3) Distal portion of lacerated fibrofatty tissue and periductal fibrous tissue. (4) Proximal portion of lacerated fibrofatty tissue and periductal fibrous tissue. (5) Soft tissue deficiency. Artificial dermis (TERUDERMIS) is shaped to fit the soft tissue defect and inserted through the subcutaneous tunnel and secured to the lactiferous ducts. The incisions are then closed. Reprinted with permission of Springer

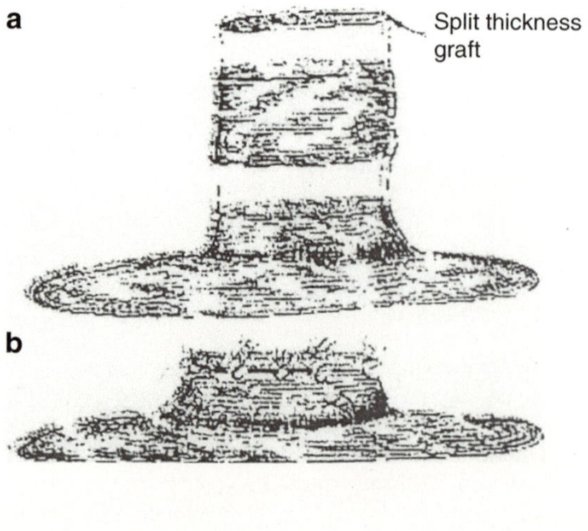


**Fig. 1.6** Vecchione [234]. Hypertrophic nipple. (**a**) A thin split-thickness graft is extracted from the nipple tip. A 9 mm core of the nipple is resected (should match the height of the contralateral nipple). (**b**) The graft is sutured to the raw nipple stump. Reprinted with permission of Springer

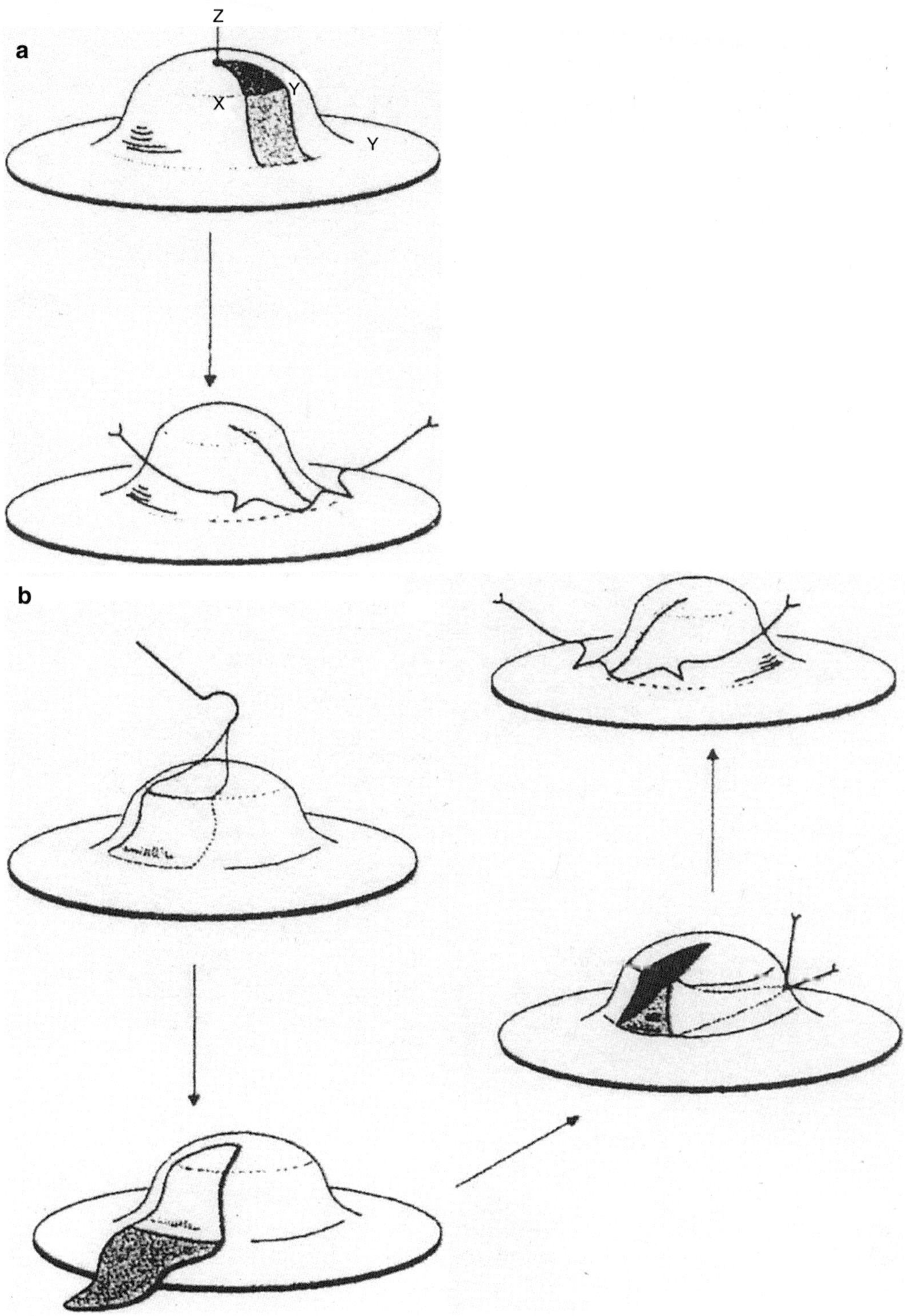


**Fig. 1.7** van Wingerden [237]. Wedge resection for diameter hypertrophy. Determining the width of the wedge to be resected to obtain an aesthetically pleasing ratio between nipple and areolar diameter: (1) Measure present nipple radius ($xz = r_1$). (2) $2\pi r_1$ = present nipple circumference = $A$. (3) Measure areolar diameter (mm). (4) Divide by 3.6 = ideal nipple diameter = 2 × ideal nipple radius ($r_2$). (5) $2\pi r_2$ = ideal nipple circumference = $B$. (6) $A-B=xy$ = wedge base width (mm). (**a**) (*Top*) The wedge is excised from the center of the hypertrophic nipple to the base of the nipple. (**b**) (*Bottom*) The wounds are closed and the two small dog-ears excised. Reprinted with permission of Springer

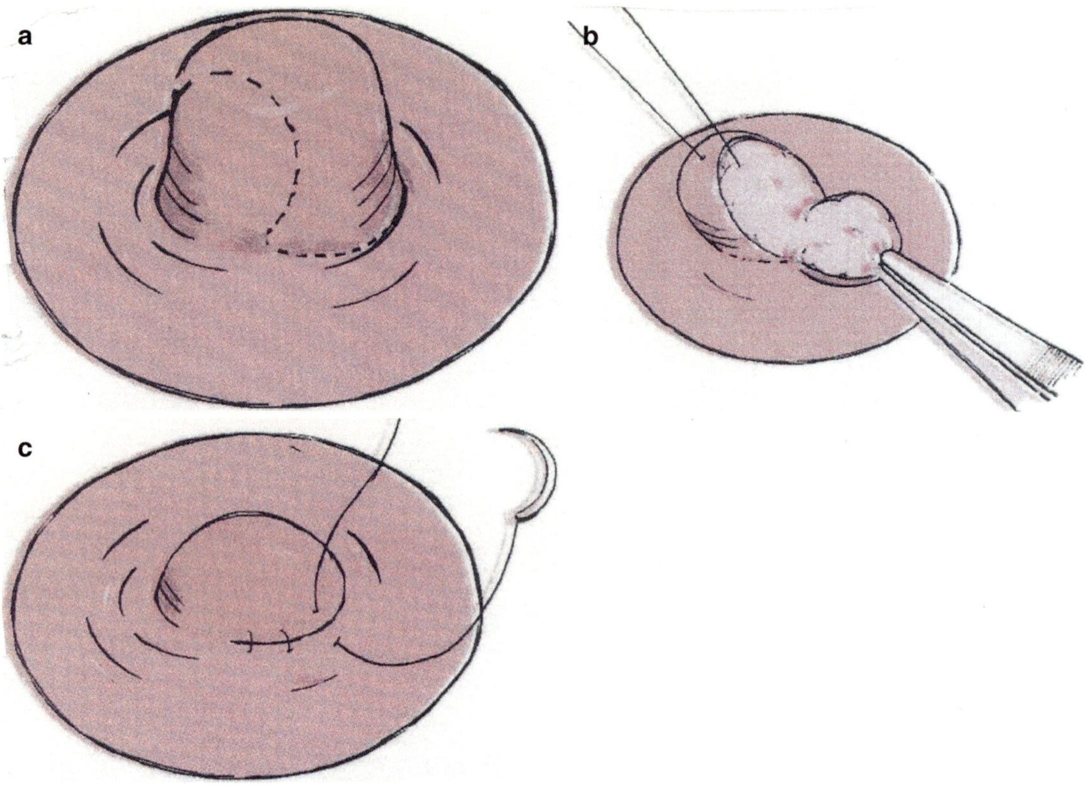


**Fig. 1.8** Mu et al. [296]. Circular flap for nipple reduction. (**a**) A 0.4–0.5 cm circular flap is marked at the 12 o'clock position of the base of the nipple. The pedicle base is not less than one-third of the flap width to ensure flap blood supply. (**b**) The flap is incised and elevated leaving an attachment at the base of the nipple. The flap is not less than 0.2 cm in thickness. The nipple tissue is excised from the nipple base without disturbing the flap. (**c**) A purse-string suture is placed at the nipple base reducing the base to approximately 0.3–0.4 cm in diameter. The flap is then sutured to the defect. Reprinted with permission of Oxford University Press

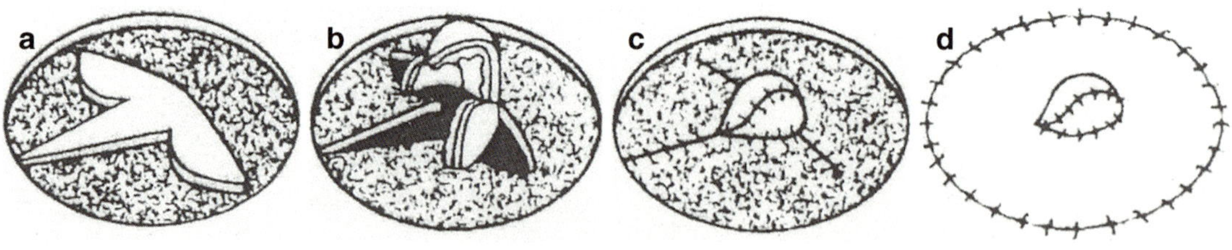


**Fig. 1.9** Kon [260]. Nipple reconstruction. Three flaps are marked based on a central disk with the middle flap twice the size as the two side wings. (**a**) The tissue around the flaps is deepithelialized. (**b**) The flaps are elevated at the dermal-subcutis level with some fat for bulk. (**c**) The middle flap is advanced upward and the two side wings rotated to close the bare sides. The donor defects are sutured closed. (**d**) The deepithelialized area is grafted. Reprinted with permission of Springer

Beware of patients who expect excellent results, without complications, since you will never satisfy them despite forewarnings of possible poor results. These patients can become litigious and be a thorn in your side for years.

## References


1. Mallucci P, Branford OA. Concepts in aesthetic breast dimensions: analysis of the ideal breast. J Plast Reconstr Aesthet Surg. 2012;65(1):8–16.
2. Jaimovich CA. mamilo hipertrófico contribuição ao estudo de sua reparação cirŭrgica a tecnica em "W". Rev Bras Cir. 1983;72(2):123–30.
3. Hauben DJ, Adler N, Silfen R, Regev D. Breast-areola-nipple proportion. Ann Plast Surg. 2003;50(5):510–3.
4. Beckenstein MS, Windle BH, Stroup RT Jr. Anatomical parameters for nipple position and areolar diameter in males. Ann Plast Surg. 1996;36(1):33–6.
5. Altchek ED. A method for accurate determination of the site of nipple areola reconstruction. Plast Reconstr Surg. 1982;70(3):405.
6. Kon M, Sagi A. A simple aid for determination of nipple-areola position. Ann Plast Surg. 1985;15(2):180–1.
7. Schwarzmann E. Die technic der mammaplastik. Der Chir. 1930;2:932–44.
8. Aufricht G. Mammaplasty for pendulous breasts; empiric and geometric planning. Plast Reconstr Surg (1946). 1949;4(1):13–29.
9. Maliniac JW. Evaluation of principal mammaplastic procedures. Plast Reconstr Surg (1946). 1949;4(4):359–73.
10. Gillies H, Millard DR Jr. Reduction and aesthetic surgery. In: Gillies H, Millard Jr DR, editors. The principles and art of plastic surgery. Boston: Little, Brown and Company; 1957. p. 390–429.
11. McIndoe AH, Rees TD. Mammaplasty indications, technique, and complications. Br J Plast Surg. 1957;10:307–20.
12. Strombeck JO. Mammaplasty: report of a new technique based on the two-pedicle procedure. Br J Plast Surg. 1960;13:79–90.
13. Tamerin JA. The Lexer-Kraske mammaplasty: a reaffirmation. Plast Reconstr Surg. 1963;31:442–4.
14. Regnault P. The hypoplastic and ptotic breast: a combined operation with prosthetic augmentation. Plast Reconstr Surg. 1966;37(1):31–7.
15. Pennisi VR, Klabunde EH, Pletsch ME. The location of the nipple in breast reconstruction. Plast Reconstr Surg. 1969;43(6):612–7.
16. Strombeck JO. Reduction mammaplasty. In: Grabb WC, Smith JW, editors. Plastic surgery: a precise guide to clinical practice. Boston: Little, Brown and Co.; 1973. p. 958–9.
17. Courtiss EH, Goldwyn RM. Reduction mammaplasty by the inferior pedicle technique. Plast Reconstr Surg. 1977;59(4):500–7.
18. Fredricks S. Skeletal and postural relations in augmentation mammaplasty. Ann Plast Surg. 1978;1(1):44–7.
19. Aston SJ, Rees TD. Breast reduction and mastopexy. In: Rees TD, editor. Aesthetic plastic surgery. Philadelphia: WB Saunders Co; 1980. p. 903–53.
20. Galvao MSL. Reduction mammoplasty with preservation of the superior, medial, lateral, and inferior pedicles. In: Georgiade NG, editor. Aesthetic breast surgery. Baltimore: Williams & Wilkins; 1983. p. 175–85.
21. Peterson RA. The McKissock vertical dermal pedicle: an adaptable operation for mammary reduction, mastopexy, and subcutaneous mastectomy. In: Georgiade NG, editor. Aesthetic breast surgery. Baltimore: Williams & Wilkins; 1983. p. 186–95.
22. Pitanguy I. Breast reduction and ptosis. In: Georgiade NG, editor. Aesthetic breast surgery. Baltimore: Williams & Wilkins; 1983. p. 247–59.
23. Georgiade NG, Georgiade GS. Reduction mammoplasty utilizing the inferio pyramidal dermal pedicle flap. In: Georgiade NG, editor. Aesthetic breast surgery. Baltimore: Williams & Wilkins; 1983. p. 291–9.
24. Rubin LR. The surgical treatment of the massive hypertrophic breast. In: Georgiade NG, editor. Aesthetic breast surgery. Baltimore: Williams & Wilkins; 1983. p. 322–3.
25. Goldwyn RM, Courtiss EH. Inferior pedicle technique. In: Regnault P, Daniel RK, editors. Aesthetic plastic surgery: principles and techniques. Boston: Little Brown and Co.; 1984. p. 522–38.
26. Regnault P, Daniel RK. Breast reduction. In: Regnault P, Daniel RK, editors. Aesthetic plastic surgery: principles and techniques. Boston: Little, Brown and Co.; 1984. p. 499–538.
27. Smith DJ Jr, Palin WE Jr, Katch VL, Bennett JE. Breast volume and anthropomorphic measurements: normal values. Plast Reconstr Surg. 1986;78(3):331–5.
28. Georgiade NG, Georgiade GS, Riefkohl R. Aesthetic breast surgery. In: McCarthy JG, editor. Plastic surgery. Philadelphia: WB Saunders Co.; 1990. p. 3839–96.
29. McKissock PK. Reduction mammaplasty. In: McKissock PK, editor. Color atlas of mammaplasty. New York: Thieme Medical Publishers; 1991. p. 3–46.
30. Matarasso A, Pitanguy I. The keel resection/Pitanguy reduction mammaplasty. Oper Tech Plast Reconstr Surg. 1996;3(3):156–69.
31. White DJ, Maxwell GP. Breast reduction. In: Achauer BM, Eriksson E, Guyuron B, Coleman III JJ, Russell RC, Vander Kolk CA, editors. Plastic surgery: indications, operations, and outcomes. St. Louis: Mosby; 2000. p. 2705–41.

32. Shulman O, Badani E, Wolf Y, Hauben DJ. Appropriate location of the nipple-areola complex in males. Plast Reconstr Surg. 2001;108(2):348–51.
33. Hall-Findlay EJ. Reduction mammaplasty. In: Nahai F, editor. The art of aesthetic surgery: principles and techniques. St. Louis, MO: Quality Medical Publishing, Inc; 2005. p. 1951–2043.
34. Khan HA, Bayat A. A geometric method for nipple localization. Can J Plast Surg. 2008;16(1):45–7.
35. Tebbetts JB. A process for quantifying aesthetic and functional breast surgery: I. Quantifying optimal nipple position and vertical and horizontal skin excess for mastopexy and breast reduction. Plast Reconstr Surg. 2013;132(1):65–73.
36. Rapin M. Reconstruction of the nipple. Br J Plast Surg. 1955;7(4):372–5.
37. Strombeck JO. Reduction mammaplasty by upper and lower glandular resections. In: Goldwyn H, editor. Plastic and reconstructive surgery of the breast. Boston: Little, Brown and Co.; 1976. p. 195.
38. Smith JW, Gillen FJ. Repairing errors of Nipple-areolar placement following reduction mammoplasty. Aesthetic Plast Surg. 1980;4(1):179–87.
39. Wray RC, Luce EA. Treatment of impending nipple necrosis following reduction mammaplasty. Plast Reconstr Surg. 1981;68(2):242–4.
40. Singer R, Krant SM. Intravenous fluorescein for evaluating the dusky nipple-areola during reduction mammaplasty. Plast Reconstr Surg. 1981;67(4):534–5.
41. Hallock GG. Prediction of nipple viability following reduction mammoplasty using laser Doppler flowmetry. Ann Plast Surg. 1992;29(5):457–60.
42. Chang P, Shaaban AF, Canady JW, Ricciardelli EJ, Cram AE. Reduction mammaplasty: the results of avoiding nipple-areolar amputation in cases of extreme hypertrophy. Ann Plast Surg. 1996;37(6):585–91.
43. Sterodimas A, Pineda EF, Meirelles V, Pitanguy I. Maximizing nipple graft survival after performing free nipple-areolar complex reduction mammaplasty. J Plast Reconstr Aesthet Surg. 2008;61(8):971–2.
44. Jensen JA, Lin JH, Kapoor N, Giuliano AE. Surgical delay of the nipple-areolar complex: a powerful technique to maximize nipple viability following nipple-sparing mastectomy. Ann Surg Oncol. 2012;19(10):3171–6.
45. Carlson GW, Chu CK, Moyer HR, Duggal C, Losken A. Predictors of nipple ischemia after nipple sparing mastectomy. Breast J. 2014;20(1):69–73.
46. Hallock GG, Altobelli JA. Prevention of the inverted teardrop areola following mammaplasty. In: Shiffman MA, editor. Mastopexy and breast reduction: principles and practice. Berlin: Springer; 2009. p. 621–4.
47. Ayhan M, Görgu M, Edoğan B, Sevýn Z. Prevention of teardrop areola and increasing areola projection in inferior pedicle reduction mammoplasty. In: Shiffman MA, editor. Mastopexy and breast reduction: principles and practice. Berlin: Springer; 2009. p. 625–7.
48. Millard DR, Mullin WR, Lasavoy MA. Secondary correction of the too-high areala and nipple after a mammaplasty. Plast Reconstr Surg. 1976;58(5):568–72.
49. Colwell AS, May JW Jr, Slavin SA. Lowering the postoperative high-riding nipple. Plast Reconstr Surg. 2007;120:596–9.
50. Spear SL, Albino FP, Al-Attar A. Repairing the high-riding nipple with reciprocal transposition flaps. Plast Reconstr Surg. 2013;131(4):687–9.
51. Raffel B. Technique for correction of areola misplacement with no new scars. Plast Reconstr Surg. 1991;88(5):895–7.
52. Elsahy NI. Correction of abnormally high nipples after reduction mammaplasty. Aesthetic Plast Surg. 1990;14(1):21–6.
53. Mohmand H, Naasan A. Double U-plasty for correction of geometric malposition of the nipple-areola complex. Plast Reconstr Surg. 2002;109(6):2019–22.
54. Frenkiel BA, Pacifico MD, Ritz M, Southwick G. A solution to the high-riding nipple-areola complex. Aesthetic Plast Surg. 2010;34:525–7.
55. Swanson E. Defining nipple displacement, and the prevention and treatment of the high-riding nipple. Plast Reconstr Surg. 2014;133(1):64e–6e.
56. Bovill ES, Macadam SA, Lennox PA. Repairing the high-riding nipple with reciprocal transposition flaps; and classification and management of the postoperative, high-riding nipple. Plast Reconstr Surg. 2014;133(1):57e–8e.
57. Small K, Kelly KM, Swistel A, Dent BL, Taylor EM, Talmor M. Surgical treatment of nipple malposition in nipple-sparing mastectomy device-based reconstruction. Plast Reconstr Surg. 2014;133(5):1053–62.
58. Gilman SL. Making the body beautiful. Princeton and Oxford: Princeton University Press; 2001.
59. Purohit S. Reduction mammoplasty. Indian J Plast Surg. 2008;41(Suppl):S64–79.
60. Thorek M. Possibilities in the reconstruction of the human form. N Y Med J. 1922;116:572.
61. Millard DR Jr. Nipple and areola reconstruction by split-skin graft from the normal side. Plast Reconstr Surg. 1972;50(4):350–3.
62. Wexler MR, Oneal RM. Areolar sharing to reconstruct the absent nipple. Plast Reconstr Surg. 1973;51(2):176–8.
63. Guida CA, Picchi A, Inzirillo S. Areola and nipple reconstruction. Plast Reconstr Surg. 1975;56(4):454–5.
64. Klein D. Correction of loss of the areola mammae. Plast Reconstr Surg (1946). 1952;10(6):469–72.
65. De Cholnoky T. Late adverse results following breast reconstruction. Plast Reconstr Surg. 1963;31:445–52.
66. Lewis JR. Atlas of aesthetic plastic surgery. Boston: Little, Brown & Co; 1973. p. 246.
67. Gruber RP. Nipple-areola reconstruction: a review of techniques. Clin Plast Surg. 1979;6(1):71–83.

68. Eder H, Lejour M. Reconstruction of the nipple-areolar complex after radical mastectomy. Acta Chir Belg. 1980;79(2):147–53.
69. Rintaia AE. Modified subtotal mastectomy and free nipple graft in the treatment of severe mammary hypertrophy and ptosis. Ann Chir Gynaecol. 1983;72(1):9–12.
70. Georgiade GS, Riefkohl R, Georgiade N. To share or not to share. Ann Plast Surg. 1985;14:180.
71. Ishikawa H, Kawahara H, Hidaka M, Mizoguchi Y, Tokunaga H, Yoshimatsu H, Tokunaga S. Autotransplantation of nipple-areolar complex in a modified radical mastectomy--indications and three-stage breast reconstruction. Nihon Geka Gakkai Zasshi. 1988;89(11):1879–85.
72. Thorek M. Possibilities in the reconstruction of the human form 1922. Aesthetic Plast Surg. 1989;13:55–8.
73. Jones G, Bostwick III. Nipple-areolar reconstruction. Oper Tech Plast Reconstr Surg. 1994;1(1):35–8.
74. Bardot J, Samson P, Aubert JP, Magalon G. Reduction mammaplasty with free nipple. Apropos of 5 cases. Ann Chir Plast Esthet. 1995;40(1):77–82.
75. Bhatty MA, Berry RB. Nipple-areola reconstruction by tattooing and nipple sharing. Br J Surg. 1997;50(5):331–4.
76. Jabor MA, Shayani P, Collins DR Jr, Karas T, Cohen BE. Nipple-areolar reconstruction: satisfaction and clinical determinants. Plas Reconstr Surg. 2002;110(2):457–63.
77. Little JW. Discussion: cryopreserved autologous nipple-areola complex transfer to the reconstructed breast. Plast Reconstr Surg. 2003;111(1):148–9.
78. Nakagawa T, Yano K, Hosokawa K. Cryopreserved autologous nipple-areola complex transfer to the reconstructed breast. Plast Reconstr Surg. 2003;111(1):141–7.
79. Kolberg HC, Friedrich M, Schmolling J, Golz N, Diedrich K. Techniken zur Rekonstruktion des Mamillen-Areola-Komplexes. Der Gynäkologe. 2005;38(3):230–5.
80. Wraight WM, Davison JA. Nipple sharing for nipple-areolar complex reconstruction: still a useful technique. J Plast Reconstr Aesthet Surg. 2006;59(12):1471–2.
81. Mess SA, Gradinger GP, Spear SL. Breast reduction with the free-nipple technique. In: Spear AL, editor. Surgery of the breast: principles and art. 2nd ed. Philadelphia, PA: Lippincott Williams and Wilkins; 2006. p. 1172–88.
82. Gorgu M, Ayhan M, Aytug Z, Aksungur E, Demirdover C. Maximizing breast projection with combined free nipple graft reduction mammaplasty and back-folded dermaglandular inferior pedicle. Breast J. 2007;13:226–32.
83. Zenn MR, Garofalo JA. Unilateral nipple reconstruction with nipple sharing. Time for a second look. Plast Reconstr Surg. 2009;123:1648–53.
84. Güven E, Aydin H, Başaran K, Aydin U, Kuvat SV. Reduction mammaplasty using bipedicled dermoglandular flaps and free-nipple transplantation. Aesthetic Plast Surg. 2010;34:738–44.
85. Karsidag S, Akcal A, Karsidag T, Yesiloglu N, Yesilada AK, Ugurlu K. Reduction mammaplasty using the free-nipple-graft vertical technique for severe breast hypertrophy: improved outcomes with the superior dermaglandular flap. Aesthetic Plast Surg. 2011;35(2):254–61.
86. Firat C, Gurlek A, Erbatur S, Aytekin AH. An autoprosthesis technique for better breast projection in free nipple graft reduction mammaplasty. Aesthetic Plast Surg. 2012;36:1340–6.
87. Rietjens M, De Lorenzi F, Andrea M, Chirappapha P, Martella S, Barbieri B, Gottardi A, Giuseppe L, Hamza A, Petit JY, Lohsiriwat V. Free nipple graft technique to correct nipple and areola malposition after breast procedures. Plast Reconstr Surg Glob Open. 2013;1(8):e69.
88. Basaran K, Saydam FA, Ersin I, Yazar M, Aygit AC. The free-nipple breast-reduction technique performed with transfer of the nipple-areola complex over the superior or superomedial pedicles. Aesthetic Plast Surg. 2014;38(4):718–26.
89. Kudva A, Hemavathi U, Patil BR. Regrafting of nipple areolar complex during pectoralis major myocutaneous flap reconstruction. J Maxillofac Oral Surg. 2014;13(2):211–2.
90. King IC, Harvey JR, Bhaskar P. One-stage breast reconstruction using the inferior dermal flap, implant, and free nipple graft. Aesthetic Plast Surg. 2014;38(2):358–64.
91. Gillies H, Millard DR. The principles and art of plastic surgery. Boston: Little, Brown and Company; 1957. p. 286–301.
92. Brent B, Bostwick J. Nipple-areola reconstruction with auricular tissues. Plast Reconstr Surg. 1977;60(3):353–61.
93. Rose EH. Nipple reconstruction with four-lobe composite auricular graft. Ann Plast Surg. 1985;15(1):78–81.
94. Tanabe HY, Tai Y, Kiyokawa K, Yamauchi T. Nipple-areola reconstruction with a dermal-fat flap and rolled auricular cartilage. Plast Reconstr Surg. 1997;100(2):431–8.
95. Pribaz JJ, Pousti T. Correction of recurrent nipple inversion with cartilage graft. Ann Plast Surg. 1998;40(1):14–7.
96. Yanaga H. Nipple-areola reconstruction with a dermal-fat flap: technical improvement from rolled auricular cartilage to artificial bone. Plast Reconstr Surg. 2003;112:1863–9.
97. Cheng MH, Ho-Asjoe M, Wei FC, Chuang DC. Nipple reconstruction in Asian females using banked cartilage graft and modified top hat flap. Br J Plast Surg. 2003;56(7):692–4.
98. Fujino T, Harasina T, Aoyagi F. Reconstruction for aplasia of the breast and pectoral region by microvascular transfer of a free flap from the buttock. Plast Reconstr Surg. 1975;56(2):178–81.

99. Amarante JT, Santa-Comba A, Reis J, Malheiro E. Halux pulp composite graft in nipple reconstruction. Aesthetic Plast Surg. 1994;18(3):299–300.
100. Cheng MH, Rodriguez ED, Smartt JM, Cardenas-Mejia A. Nipple reconstruction using the modified top hat flap with banked costal cartilage graft: long-term follow-up in 58 patients. Ann Plast Surg. 2007;59(6):621–8.
101. Beckenstein MS. Nipple reconstruction. In: Thorne CH, editor. Grabb and Smith's plastic surgery. 6th ed. Philadelphia: Lippincott Williams & Wilkins; 2007. p. 657–61.
102. Kargül G, Deutinger M. Reconstruction of the breast areola complex. Comparison of different techniques. Handchir Mikrochir Plast Chir. 2001;33(2):133–7.
103. Spina V. Inverted nipple. Plast Reconstr Surg. 1957;19:63.
104. Adams WM. Labial transplant for correction of loss of the nipple. Plast Reconstr Surg (1946). 1949;4(3):295–8.
105. Silsby JJ. Nipple reconstruction. Plast Reconstr Surg. 1976;57(5):667–8.
106. DiPirro ME. Reconstruction of the nipple and areola after a burn. Case report. Plast Reconstr Surg. 1970;46(3):299–300.
107. Snyderman RK, Guthrie RH. Reconstruction of the female breast following radical mastectomy. Plast Reconstr Surg. 1971;47(6):565–7.
108. Di Benedetto G, Sperti V, Pierangeli M, Bertani A. A simple and reliable method of nipple reconstruction using a spiral flap made of residual scar tissue. Plast Reconstr Surg. 2004;114(1):158–61.
109. Broadbent T. Restoring the mammary areola by a skin graft from the upper inner thigh. Br J Plast Surg. 1977;30(3):230–3.
110. Barton FE Jr. Latissimus dermal-epidermal nipple reconstruction. Plast Reconstr Surg. 1982;70(2):234–7.
111. Asplund O. Nipple and areola reconstruction. Scand J Plast Reconstr Surg. 1983;17(3):234–9.
112. Bosch G, Ramirez M. Reconstruction of the nipple: a new technique. Plast Reconstr Surg. 1984;73(6):977–81.
113. Cohen IK, Ward JA, Chandrasekhar B. The pinwheel flap nipple and barrier areola graft reconstruction. Plast Reconstr Surg. 1986;77(6):995–9.
114. Smith JW, Nelson R. Construction of the nipple with a mushroom-shaped pedicle. Plast Reconstr Surg. 1986;78(5):684–7.
115. Weiss J, Herman O, Rosenberg L, Shafir R. The S nipple-areola reconstruction. Plast Reconstr Surg. 1989;83(5):904–6.
116. Rubin LR. The burned female breast. N Y State J Med. 1975;75(6):865–9.
117. Lee KY, Cho BC. Surgical correction of inverted nipples using the modified Namba or Teimourian technique. Plast Reconstr Surg. 2004;113(1):328–36.
118. Shafir R, Bonne-Tamir B, Ashbel S, Tsur H, Goodman RM. Genetic studies in a family with inverted nipples (mammillae invertita). Clin Genet. 1979;15(4):346–50.
119. Chromosome 2q Deletion Syndrome. http://www.rightdiagnosis.com/2q_deletion/symptoms.htm. Accessed 20 July 2014.
120. Congenital Disorder of Glycosylation Type 1. http://ghr.nlm.nih.gov/comditions/congenital-disorder-of-glyosylation-type-ia. Accessed 17 July 2014.
121. Congenital Disorder of Glycosylation Type 1L. http://www.rightdiagnosis.com/c/congenital_disorder_of_glycosylation_type_1l/symptoms. Accessed 20 July 2014.
122. Northup KA, Witte MH, Witte CL. Syndromic classification of hereditary lymphedema. Lymphology. 2003;36(4):162–89.
123. Fang J, Dagenais SL, Erickson RP, Arlt MF, Glynn MW, Gorski JL, Seaver LH, Glover TW. Mutations in FOXC2 (MFH-1), a forkhead family transcription factor, are responsible for the hereditary lymphedema-distichiasis syndrome. Am J Hum Genet. 2000;67(6):1382–8.
124. Kennerknecht-Sorgo-Oberhoffer Syndrome. http://www.rightdiagnosis.com/k/kennerknecht_sorgo_oberhoffer_syndrome_symptoms.htm. Accessed 17 July 2014.
125. Kennerknecht-Sorgo-Oberhoffer Syndrome. http://www.checkorphan.org/disdeases/kennerknecht-sorgo-oberhoffer-syndrome. Accessed 20 Jan 2015.
126. Fryns JP, Aftimos S. New MR/MCA syndrome with distinct facial appearance and general habitus, broad and webbed neck, hypoplastic inverted nipples, epilepsy, and pachygyria of the frontal lobes. J Med Genet. 2000;37(6):460–2.
127. Fryns-Aftimos Syndrome. http://www.rightdiagnosis.com/f/fryns_aftimos_syndrome/intro.htm. Accessed 20 July 2014.
128. Weaver Syndrome. www.rarediseases.org/rare-disease-information/rare-diseases/byID/817/printFullReport. Accessed 20 Jan 2015.
129. Waller H. The early failure of breastfeeding. A clinical study of its causes and their prevention. Arch Dis Child. 1946;21(105):1–12.
130. Han S, Hong YG. The inverted nipple: its grading and surgical correction. Plast Reconstr Surg. 1999;104(2):389–95.
131. Sakai S, Sakai Y, Izawa H. A new surgical procedure for the very severe inverted nipple. Aesthetic Plast Surg. 1999;23(2):139–43.
132. Scholten E. The classification of inverted nipples. Plast Reconstr Surg. 2000;106(3):737–8.
133. Inverted nipple. Wikipedia http://en.wikipedia.org/wiki/Inverted_nipple. Accessed 8 Aug 14.
134. Terrill PJ, Stapleton MJ. The inverted nipple: to cut the ducts or not? Br J Plast Surg. 1991;44(5):372–7.
135. Axford WL. Mamillaplasty. Ann Surg. 1889;9:278.
136. Kehrer FA. Uber excision des warzenhofs bei hohlwerzen. Beitr Exper Geburtshulfe Gynaek Gizessen 1879–1890. 1890;43:170.

137. Basch KS. Zur anatomie und physiologie der brustwarze. Arch Gynaekol. 1890;43:170.
138. Williams WR. Diseases of the breast. London: J. Bale and Son; 1894.
139. Selheim H. Brust warzen plastik bei hohlwarzen. Zentrabl Gynäk. 1917;41:305.
140. Grodsky M. Reconstruction des mamelons deformes. Rev Chir Struct. 1937;15:126–36.
141. DuFourmental L. Chirurgie Reparatrice et Corrective des Teguments et des Formes. 2nd ed. Masson: Partis; 1950. p. 370–2.
142. Hoffman JB. A suggested treatment for inverted nipples. Am J Obstet Gynecol. 1953;66(2):346–8.
143. Skoog T. An operation for inverted nipples. Br J Plast Surg. 1952;5:65.
144. Skoog T. Una operación para pezones umbilicados. Anal Argentin Med. 1957;2:31.
145. Skoog T. Surgical correction of inverted nipple. J Am Med Womens Assoc. 1965;20(10):931–5.
146. Namba K, Itoh T. Some devices for surgical repair of inverted nipple. Jpn J Plast Surg. 1966;9:93.
147. Julliard A. Un traitment de l'obilication du mamelon. Ann Chir Plast. 1967;12(3):251–3.
148. Lamont E. Congenital inversion of the nipple in identical twins. Brit J Plast Surg. 1973;26:178.
149. Schwager RG, Smith JW, Gray GF, Goulian D Jr. Inversion of the human female nipple, with a simple method of treatment. Plast Reconstr Surg. 1974;54(5):564–9.
150. Marino. Report of the Seventh International Congress of Surgery. Buenos Aires; 1974.
151. Skoog T. Inverted nipples: a method of correction. In: Skoog T, editor. Plastic surgery: new methods and refinements. Philadelphia: WB Saunders; 1974. p. 383–90.
152. Hartrampe CR Jr, Schneider WJ. A simple direct method for correction of inversion of the nipple. Plast Reconstr Surg. 1976;58(6):678–9.
153. Broadbent TR, Woolf RM. Benign inverted nipple: trans-nipple-areolar correction. Plast Reconstr Surg. 1976;58(6):673–7.
154. Elsahy NI. An alternative operation for inverted nipple. Plast Reconstr Surg. 1976;57(4):438–91.
155. D'Assumpção EA, Rosa MS. Correcting the inverted nipple. Br J Plast Surg. 1977;30(4):249–50.
156. Wolfort FG, Marshall KA, Cochran TC. Correction of the inverted nipple. Ann Plast Surg. 1978;1(3):294–7.
157. Gangal HT, Gangal MH. Suction method for correcting flat nipples or inverted nipples. Plast Reconstr Surg. 1978;61(2):294–6.
158. Teimourian B, Adham MN. Simple technique for correction of inverted nipple. Past Reconstr Surg. 1980;65(4):504–6.
159. Scatafassi S, Genzini G. Correzione dei capezzoli introflessi: una nuovo metodica operatoria. Rev Ital Chir Plast. 1980;12:27.
160. Rayner CR. The correction of permanently inverted nipples. Br J Plast Surg. 1980;33(4):413–7.
161. Hamilton JM. Inverted nipples. Plast Reconstr Surg. 1980;65(4):507–9.
162. deLima GR, DeFreitas V, Netto JG, Stávale JN, Grabert H, Miyada CC, DeSouza AZ. Surgical technic for correction of inverted nipples. Rev Paul Med. 1981;97(1–3):17–20.
163. Carramenha e Costa MA. Tecnica cirurgica para correcao de mamilos invaginados. Rev Paul Med. 1981;97(1/3):17–20.
164. Hauben DJ, Mahler D. A simple method for the correction of the inverted nipple. Plast Reconstr Surg. 1983;71(4):556–9.
165. Pitanguy I. Breast reduction and ptosis. In: Georgiade NG, editor. Aesthetic breast surgery. Baltimore: Williams & Wilkins Co.; 1983. p. 247.
166. Hinderer UT, del Rio JL. Treatment of the postoperative inverted nipple with or without asymmetry of the areola. Aesthetic Plast Surg. 1983;7(3):139–44.
167. Haeseker B. The application of de-epithelialised "turn-over" flaps to the treatment of inverted nipples. Br J Plast Surg. 1984;37(2):253–5.
168. Yanai A, Okabe K, Tanaka H. Correction of the inverted nipple. Aesthetic Plast Surg. 1986;10(1):51–3.
169. Nakajima T, Yoshimura Y, Kami T. The subcutaneous pedicle flap: widening of its application. Ann Plast Surg. 1987;19(2):103–16.
170. Hauben DJ. Correction of the inverted nipple. Plast Reconstr Surg. 1988;80(3):470–1.
171. Hyakusoku H, Okubo M, Fumiiri M. Combination of the square flap method and the dermal sling to correct flat or inverted nipples. Aesthetic Plast Surg. 1988;12(2):107–9.
172. Kami T, Wong AC, Kim IG. A simple method for the treatment of the inverted nipple. Ann Plast Surg. 1988;21(4):316–21.
173. Crestinu JM. Inverted nipple: the new method of correction. Aesthetic Plast Surg. 1989;13(3):189–97.
174. Kurihara K, Maezawa N, Yanagawa H, Imai T. Surgical correction of the inverted nipple with a tendon graft: hammock procedure. Plast Reconstr Surg. 1990;86(5):999–1003.
175. Chandler PJ Jr, Hill SD. A direct surgical approach to correct the inverted nipple. Plast Reconstr Surg. 1990;86(2):352–4.
176. Aiache A. Surgical repair of the inverted nipple. Ann Plast Surg. 1990;25(6):457–60.
177. Megumi Y. Correction of inverted nipple with periductal fibrous flaps. Plast Reconstr Surg. 1991;88(2):342–6.
178. Kesaree N. Treatment of inverted nipples using disposable syringe. Indian Pediatr. 1993;30(3):429–30.
179. Kesaree N, Banapurmath CR, Banapurmath S, Shamanur K. Treatment of inverted nipples using a disposable syringe. J Hum Lact. 1993;9(1):27–9.
180. Bracaglia R. La correzione chirurgica del capezzollo introflesso: nostra esperienza. Riv Ital Chir Plast. 1993;25:167.

181. McGeorge DD. The "Niplette": an instrument for the non-surgical correction of inverted nipples. Br J Plast Surg. 1994;47(1):46–9.
182. el Sharkawy AG. A method for correction of congenitally inverted nipple with preservation of the ducts. Plast Reconstr Surg. 1995;95(6):1111–4.
183. Ramakrishnan VV, Mohan D, Villafane O, Krishna A. Twin flap technique for nipple reconstruction. Ann Plast Surg. 1997;39(3):241–4.
184. Arsenault G. Using a disposable syringe to treat inverted nipples. Can Fam Physician. 1997;43:1517–8.
185. Oh YW, Lew DH, Park C, Park BY. Correction of inverted nipple using two rotational dermal flaps. J Korean Soc Aesthetic Plast Surg. 1997;3(1):74–80.
186. Lee HJ. Results of treatments for inverted nipples and chronic subareolar abscesses. J Korean Surg Soc. 1997;53(5):635–8.
187. Lee HB, Roh TS, Chung YK, Kim SW, Kim JB, Shin KS. Correction of inverted nipple using strut reinforcement with deepithelialized triangular flaps. Plast Reconstr Surg. 1998;102(4):1253–8.
188. Peled IJ. Purse-string suture for nipple projection. Plast Reconstr Surg. 1999;103(5):1480–2.
189. Pompei S, Tedesco M. A new surgical technique for the correction of the inverted nipple. Aesthetic Plast Surg. 1999;23(5):371–4.
190. Crestinu JM. The correction of inverted nipples without scars: 17 years' experience, 452 operations. Aesthetic Plast Surg. 2000;24(1):52–7.
191. Scholten E. A contemporary correction of inverted nipples. Plast Reconst Surg. 2001;107(2):511–3.
192. Pereira Filho OJ, Bins-Ely J, Granemann AS, Bertelli JA, Abdalla SC. Closed inverted nipple treatment through a microincision procedure. Plast Reconstr Surg. 2001;108(4):1000–5.
193. Tal MG. Correction of inverted nipple using piercing. Plast Reconstr Surg. 2003;112(4):1178–9.
194. Huang WC. A new method for correction of inverted nipple with three periductal dermofibrous flaps. Aesthetic Plast Surg. 2003;27(4):301–4.
195. Kim DY, Jeong EC, Eo SR, Kim KS, Lee SY, Cho BH. Correction of inverted nipple: an alternative method using two triangular areolar dermal flaps. Ann Plast Surg. 2003;51(6):636–40.
196. Lee MJ, DePoli PA, Casas LA. Aesthetic and predictable correction of the inverted nipple. Aesthet Surg J. 2003;23(5):353–6.
197. Lee TJ, Kim WR. Nipple suspension using biopsy bottle after surgical correction for inverted nipple. J Korean Soc Aesthetic Plast Surg. 2004;10(2):115–7.
198. Stevens WG, Fellows DR, Vath SD, Stoker DA. An integrated approach to the repair of inverted nipples. Aesthet Surg J. 2004;24(3):211–5.
199. Serra-Renom J, Fontdevila J, Monner J. Correction of the inverted nipple with an internal 5-point star suture. Ann Plast Surg. 2004;53(3):293–6.
200. Yamada N, Kakibuchi M, Kitayoshi H, Kurokawa M, Hosokawa K, Hashimoto K. A method for correcting an inverted nipple with an artificial dermis. Aesthetic Plast Surg. 2004;28(4):233–8.
201. Park SS, Park JM, Ha JS, Lee KC, Kim SK, Park SH. The correction of inverted nipple by modified Elsahy and Broadbent-Woolf methods. J Korean Soc Aesthetic Plast Surg. 2005;11(2):201–6.
202. Teng L, Wu GP, Sun XM, Lu JJ, Ding B, Ren M, Ji Y, Jin XL. Correction of inverted nipple: an alternative method using continuous elastic outside distraction. Ann Plast Surg. 2005;54(2):120–3.
203. Ritz M, Silfen R, Morgan D, Southwick G. Simple technique for inverted nipple correction. Aesthetic Plast Surg. 2005;29(1):24–7.
204. Yoon IM, Yoo JS, Lee DL, Lim JK. Inverted nipple correction through modified Broadbent-Woolf method. J Korean Soc Aesthetic Plast Surg. 2006;12(2):177–80.
205. Lee HM, Na YC. Simple traction device for inverted nipple correction. J Korean Soc Plast Reconstr Surg. 2006;33(6):789–91.
206. Kim JT, Lim YS, Oh JG. Correction of inverted nipples with twisting and locking principles. Plast Reconstr Surg. 2006;118(7):1526–31.
207. Ağaoğlu G, Manavbaşi I, Külahçi Y, Erol O. Inverte meme ucu: lieratürün gözden geçirilmesi. Turk Polast Rekonstr Est Cer Derg. 2006;14(22):125–8.
208. Kim JK, Yu SC. Convenient nipple suspension method using Aquaplast Thermoplastic (Optimold) Splint after surgical correction of inverted nipple. J Korean Soc Aesthetic Plast Surg. 2007;13(1):89–91.
209. Bosch G, De los Ríos G, Giachero V. Nipple invagination: the umbrella effect. Aesthet Plast Surg. 2007;31(1):76–84.
210. Chen SH, Gedebou T, Chen PH. The endoscope as an adjunct to correction of nipple inversion deformity. Plast Reconstr Surg. 2007;119(4):1178–82.
211. Burm JS, Kim YW. Correction of inverted nipples by strong suspension with areola-based dermal flaps. Plast Reconstr Surg. 2007;120(6):1483–6.
212. Wu HL, Huang X, Zheng SS. A new procedure for correction of severe inverted nipple with two triangular areolar dermofibrous flaps. Aesthetic Plast Surg. 2008;32(4):641–4.
213. Yoon SY, Kang MG. The correction of severe inverted nipple: using under skin dermal flaps, through-and-through suture and purse-string sutures. J Korean Soc Plast Reconstr Surg. 2009;36(3):322–6.
214. Karacaoglu E. Correction of recurrent grade III inverted nipple with antenna dermoadipose flap: case report. Aesthetic Plast Surg. 2009;33(6):843–8.
215. Kolker AR, Torina PJ. Minimally invasive correction of inverted nipples: a safe and simple technique for reliable, sustainable projection. Ann Plast Surg. 2009;62(5):549–53.
216. Peeters G, Decloedt J, Nagels H, Cambier B. Treatment of the severe or recurrent inverted nipple by interposition of a resorbable polydioxanone sheet. J Plast Reconstr Aesthetic Surg. 2010;63(2):e175–e6.

217. Min KH, Park SS, Heo CY, Min KW. Scar-free technique for inverted-nipple correction. Aesthetic Plast Surg. 2010;334(1):116–9.
218. Cabalag MS, Kong Chui CH, Tan B. Correction of nipple inversion using a micro-knife and transverse to longitudinal skin closure. J Plast Reconstr Aesthet Surg. 2010;63(8):e627–e30.
219. Shiau JP, Chin CC, Lin MH, Hsiao CW. Correction of severely inverted nipple with telescope method. Aesthetic Plast Surg. 2011;35(6):1137–42.
220. Moretti EA, Gallo S, Huck W. Tratmiento del pezón invertado: comparación de los ténicas. Chir Plast Iberolatinam. 2011;37(1):55–61.
221. McG Taylor D, Lahiri A, Laitung JK. Correction of the severely inverted nipple: areola-based dermoglandular rhomboid advancement. J Plast Reconstr Aesthet Surg. 2011;64(12):e297–302.
222. Bracaglia R, Tambasco D, Gentileschi S, D'Ettorre M. Recurrent inverted nipple: a reliable technique for the most difficult cases. Ann Plast Surg. 2012;69(1):24–6.
223. Lee J, Lee S, Bae Y. Trans-nipple double Z-plasty for benign periareolar disease with inverted nipple. Aesthetic Plast Surg. 2013;37(2):327–31.
224. Pagkalos VA, Ghali S, Hedén P. Nipple elevation using loupes magnification and a double-layer purse-string suture. Aesthetic Plast Surg. 2013;37(2):354–8.
225. Basurto AM, Cano EG. Pezón invertido: una técnica más. Cir Plast. 2013;23(2):97–101.
226. Durgun M, Ozakpinar HR, Selçuk CT, Sarici M, Ceran C, Seven E. Inverted nipple correction with dermal flaps and traction. Aesthetic Plast Surg. 2014;38(3):533–9.
227. Gould DJ, Nadeau MH, Macias LH, Stevens WG. Inverted nipple repair revisited: a 7-year experience. Aesthet Surg J. 2015;35(2):156–64.
228. Tunsel U, Turan A, Aytac S, Kanturk R, Aydin U, Kostakoglu N. Inverted nipple: contemporary techniques. Gaziosmanpaşa Üniversitesi Tıp Fakültesi Dergisi. tipder.gop.edu.tr/indir.aspx?id=493&dergi=3&dil=tr. Accessed 4 May 2015.
229. Isac C, Isac A. Inverted nipples. In: Mugea T, Shiffman MA, editors. Aesthetic Surgery of the Breast. Berlin: Springer; 2015. p. 1009–15.
230. Pitanguy I, Cansancao A. Reduçãcao do mamilo. Rev Bras Cir. 1970;61:73–6.
231. Sperli AE. Cosmetic reduction of the nipple with functional preservation. Br J Plast Surg. 1974;27(1):42–3.
232. Regnault P. Nipple hypertrophy. A physiologic reduction by circumcision. Clin Plast Surg. 1975;2(3):391–6.
233. Marshall KA, Wolfort FG, Cochran TC. Surgical correction of nipple hypertrophy in male gynecomastia: case report. Reconstr Surg. 1977;60(2):277–9.
234. Vecchione TR. The reduction of the hypertrophic nipple. Aesthetic Plast Surg. 1979;3(1):343–5.
235. Ferreira LM, Neto MS, Okamoto RH, Andrews JM. Surgical correction of nipple hypertrophy. Plast Reconstr Surg. 1995;95(4):753–4.
236. Lai YL, Wu WC. Nipple reduction with a modified circumcision technique. Br J Plast Surg. 1996;49(5):307–9.
237. van Wingerden JJ. Nummular nipple hypertrophy and repair as part of an aesthetic nipple-areola unit. Aesthetic Plast Surg. 1997;21(6):408–11.
238. DeBono R, Rao GS. A simple technique for correction of male nipple hypertrophy: the "sinusoidal" nipple reduction. Plast Reconstr Surg. 1997;100(7):1890–2.
239. Cheng MH, Smartt JM, Rodriguez ED, Ulusal BG. Nipple reduction using the modified top hat flap. Plast Reconstr Surg. 2006;118(7):1517–25.
240. Chang YC. Aesthetic surgery for hypertrophic nipple: a simple technique. Rev Soc Bras Cir Plast. 2007;22(1):30–3.
241. Basile FV, Chang YC. The triple-flap nipple-reduction technique. Ann Plast Surg. 2007;59(3):260–2.
242. Fanous N, Tawile C, Fanous A. Nipple reduction – An adjunct to augmentation mammaplasty. Can J Plast Surg. 2009;17(3):81–8.
243. Kerr-Valentic MA, Agarwal JP. Reduction of the hypertrophic nipple following total skin sparing mastectomy. J Plast Reconstr Aesthet Surg. 2009;62(12):e652–3.
244. Tuncer S, Eryilmaz T, Atabay K. Correction of nipple hypertrophy: nipple circumcision technique revisited. Plast Reconstr Aesthet Surg. 2010;63(9):1575–6.
245. van den Berg W, van der Lei B. Ying-Yang flap technique for correction of male nipple hypertrophy: a case report and a review of the English-language literature. J Plast Reconstr Aesthet Surg. 2010;63(12):2194–6.
246. Ren M, Wang Y, Wang B. Nipple reduction using a three-dimensional z-shaped incision technique. Plast Reconstr Aesthet Surg. 2013;66(6):770–5.
247. Jin US, Lee HK. Nipple reduction using circumcision and wedge excision technique. Ann Plast Surg. 2013;70(2):154–7.
248. Moliver C, Kargel J, Sullivan M. Treatment of nipple hypertrophy by a simplified reduction technique. Aesthet Surg J. 2013;33(1):77–83.
249. Lee EI, Withers EH. Geometric nipple reduction technique: an approach to management of nipple hypertrophy. J Plast Reconstr Aesthet Surg. 2014;67(9):1301–3.
250. LaBove G, Davison SP. Combined base imbrication and top hat nipple reduction. Plast Reconstr Surg. 2014;134(6):997e–8e.
251. Payr E. Beitrage aur plastischen Deckung der Hautdefekte nach brustdrusen-exstirpation. Dtsch Z Chir. 1906;81:361.
252. Berson NL. Construction of pseudoareola. Surgery. 1946;20(6):808.
253. Snyder C, Pickens JE, Slater TB. Surgery of the areola-nipple complex. In: Master FW, Lewis Jr JR,

editors. Symposium on aesthetic surgery of the face. Mosby, St. Louis: Eyelid and Breast; 1972. p. 192.
254. Dubin DB. A new simplified method for nipple reconstruction. New Orleans: Annual Meeting of American Society of Plastic and Reconstructive Surgeons; 1980.
255. Asplund O, Korloff B. Reconstruction of mamma with submuscular prosthesis. A preliminary report. In: Bohmert H, editor. Breast cancer and breast reconstruction. Stuttgart: Thieme Verlag; 1982.
256. Serafin D, Georgiade N. Nipple-areola reconstruction after mastectomy. Ann Plast Surg. 1982;8(1):29–34.
257. Little JW 3rd, Munasifi T, McCulloch DT. One-stage reconstruction of a projecting nipple: the quadrapod flap. Plast Reconstr Surg. 1983;71(1):126–33.
258. Silversmith PE. Nipple reconstruction by quadrapod flaps. Plast Reconstr Surg. 1983;72(3):422.
259. Chang WH. Nipple reconstruction with a T flap. Plast Reconstr Surg. 1984;73(1):140–3.
260. Kon M. Latissimus dorsi three-flap nipple reconstruction. Aesthetic Plast Surg. 1984;8(4):243–5.
261. Little JW 3rd. Nipple-areola reconstruction. Clin Plast Surg. 1984;11(2):351–64.
262. Hartrampf CR Jr, Culbertson JH. A dermal-fat flap for nipple reconstruction. Plast Reconstr Surg. 1984;73(6):982–6.
263. Kon M. T- and three-flap nipple reconstruction. Plast Reconstr Surg. 1985;75(2):284–5.
264. Mukherjee RP, Gottlieb V, Hacker L. Nipple-areolar reconstruction with buried dermal hammock technique. Ann Plast Surg. 1987;19(5):421–3.
265. Anton MA, Hartrampf CR Jr. Nipple reconstruction with star flap. Plast Surg Forum. 1990;13:100–3.
266. Nohira K, Shintomi Y, Ohura T. Nipple-areola reconstruction using a skate flap and an intradermal tattoo. Jpn J Plast Reconstr Surg. 1991;34:67–72.
267. Anton MA, Eskenazi LB, Hartrampf CR Jr. Nipple reconstruction with local flaps: star and wrap flaps. Persp Plast Surg. 1991;5(1):67–78.
268. Eskenazi L. A one-stage nipple reconstruction with the "modified star" flap and immediate tattoo: a review of 100 cases. Plast Reconstr Surg. 1993;92(4):671–80.
269. Hallock GG, Altobelli JA. Cylindrical nipple reconstruction using an H flap. Ann Plast Surg. 1993;30(1):23–6.
270. Hugo NE, Sultan MR, Hardy SP. Nipple-areola reconstruction with intradermal tattoo and double-opposing pennant flaps. Ann Plast Surg. 1993;30(6):510–3.
271. Wong RK, Banducci DR, Feldman S, Kahler SH, Manders EK. Pre-reconstruction tattooing eliminates the need for skin grafting in nipple areolar reconstruction. Plast Reconstr Surg. 1993;92(3):547–9.
272. Cederna JP. A simplified two-step approach to nipple-areola reconstruction. Plast Reconstr Surg. 1994;93(5):1105–6.
273. Teimourian B, Duda G. The propeller flap: a one-stage procedure for nipple-areola reconstruction. Aesthetic Plast Surg. 1994;18(1):81–4.
274. Thomas SV, Gellis MB, Pool R. Nipple reconstruction with a new local tissue flap. Plast Reconstr Surg. 1996;97(5):1053–6.
275. Kroll SS, Reece GP, Miller MJ, Evans GR, Robb GL, Baldwin BJ, Wang BG, Schusterman MA. Comparison of nipple projection with the modified double-opposing tab and star flaps. Plast Reconstr Surg. 1997;99(6):1602–5.
276. Yamamoto Y, Sugihara T. Correction of inverted nipple with modified star flap technique. Aesthetic Plast Surg. 1997;21(3):193–5.
277. Hamori CA, LaRossa D. The top hat flap: for one stage reconstruction of a prominent nipple. Aesthetic Plast Surg. 1998;22(2):142–4.
278. Kroll SS. Nipple reconstruction with the double-opposing tab flap. Plast Reconstr Surg. 1999;104(2):511–4.
279. Kroll SS. Integrated breast mound reduction and nipple reconstruction with the wraparound flap. Plast Reconstr Surg. 1999;104(3):687–93.
280. Few JW, Marcus JR, Casas LA, Aitken ME, Redding J. Long-term predictable nipple projection following reconstruction. Plast Reconstr Surg. 1999;104(5):1321–4.
281. Yamamoto Y, Furukawa H, Oyama A, Horiuchi K, Funayama E, Tsutsumida A, Sugihara T, Nohira K. Two innovations of the star-flap technique for nipple reconstruction. Br J Plast Surg. 2001;54(8):723–6.
282. Shestak KC, Gabriel A, Landecker A, Peters S, Shestak A, Kim J. Assessment of long-term nipple projection: a comparison of three techniques. Plast Reconstr Surg. 2002;110(3):780–6.
283. Bogue DP, Mungara AK, Thompson M, Cederna PS. Modified technique for nipple-areola reconstruction: a case series. Plast Reconstr Surg. 2003;112(5):1274–8.
284. Motamed S, Davami B. Postburn reconstruction of nipple-areola complex. Burns. 2005;31(8):1020–4.
285. Farhadi J, Maksvytyte GK, Schaefer DJ, Pierer G, Scheufler O. Reconstruction of the nipple-areola complex: an update. J Plast Reconstr Aesthet Surg. 2006;59(1):40–53.
286. Fitoussi AD, Pollet AG, Couturaud B, Laki F, Salmon RJ. Nipple and areola reconstruction by tattooing, "F" and "Z" flaps. Ann Chir Plast Esthet. 2008;53(4):348–57.
287. Foustanos A. Double flap technique: an alternative mastopexy approach. In: Shiffman MA, editor. Mastopexy and breast reduction. Berlin: Springer; 2009. p. 97–102.
288. Grotting JC. Reoperation following free flap breast reconstruction. In: Grotting JC, editor. Aesthetic & reconstructive plastic surgery. St. Louis, MO: Quality Medical Publishing, Inc; 2009. p. 1411–79.
289. Gullo P, Buccheri EM, Pozzi M, De Vita R. Nipple reconstruction using a star flap enhanced by scar tissue: the Regina Elena Cancer Institute experience. Aesthetic Plast Surg. 2011;35(5):731–7.

290. Sierakowski A, Niranjan N. Star flap with a dermal platform for nipple reconstruction. J Plast Reconstr Aesthet Surg. 2011;64(2):e55–6.
291. Katerinaki E, Sircar T, Sterne GD. The C-V flap for nipple reconstruction after previous skin-sparing mastectomy and immediate breast reconstruction: refinements of donor-site closure. Aesthetic Plast Surg. 2011;35(4):624–7.
292. Gurunluoglu R, Shafighi M, Williams SA, Kimm GE. Incorporation of a preexisting scar in the star-flap technique for nipple reconstruction. Ann Plast Surg. 2012;68(1):17–21.
293. Wong WW, Hiersche MA, Martin MC. The angel flap for nipple reconstruction. Can J Plast Surg. 2013;21(1):e1–4.
294. Chun YS, Long JN, Orgill DP, Tiwari P, Talavera F, Slenkovich NG. Nipple-areola reconstruction. http://emedicine.medscape.com/article/1274411-overview updated 2013. Accessed 15 May 2014.
295. Mu D, Luan J, Guo X, Xu BD. Male nipple reduction with a simple circular-flap technique. Aesthetic Surg J. 2015;36(1):113–6.
296. Bailey D. Tattoo art around the world. New York, NY: Rosen Publishing Group; 2012.
297. Levites HA, Fourman MS, Phillips BT, Fromm IM, Khan SU, Dagum AB, Bui DT. Modeling fade patterns of nipple areola complex tattoos following breast reconstruction. Ann Plast Surg. 2014;73(Suppl 2):S153–6.
298. Becker H. The use of intradermal tattoo to enhance the final result of nipple-areola reconstruction. Plast Reconstr Surg. 1986;77(4):673–6.
299. Masser MR, Di Meo L, Hobby JA. Tattooing in reconstruction of the nipple and areola: a new method. Plast Reconstr Surg. 1989;84(4):677–81.
300. Rees TD. Reconstruction of the breast areola by intradermal tattooing and transfer. Case report. Plast Reconstr Surg. 1975;55(5):620–1.
301. Pensler JM, Haab RL, Parry SW. Reconstruction of the burned nipple-areola complex. Plast Reconstr Surg. 1986;78(4):480–5.
302. Spear SL, Little JW, Convit R. Intradermal tattoo as an adjunct to nipple–areola reconstruction. Plast Reconstr Surg. 1989;83(5):907–11.
303. Little JW. Nipple-areola reconstruction. In: Cohen M, editor. Mastery of plastic and reconstructive surgery. Boston: Little, Brown and Co.; 1994.
304. Bernard RW. Prereconstruction tattooing eliminates the need for skin grafting in nipple-areola reconstruction. Plast Reconstr Surg. 1994;93(7):1531.
305. Spear SL, Arias J. Long-term experience with nipple-areola tattooing. Ann Plast Surg. 1995;35(3):232–6.
306. Eng JS. Bell flap nipple reconstruction--a new wrinkle. Ann Plast Surg. 1996;36(5):485–8.
307. Henseler H, Cheong V, Weiler-Mithoff EM, MacKay IR, Webster MH. The use of Munsell colour charts in nipple-areola tattooing. Br J Plast Surg. 2001;54(4):338–40.
308. Guerra AB, Khoobehi K, Metzinger SE, Allen RJ. New technique for nipple areola reconstruction: arrow flap and rib cartilage graft for long-lasting nipple projection. Ann Plast Surg. 2003;50(1):31–7.
309. Hoffman S, Mikell A. Nipple-areola tattooing as part of breast reconstruction. Plast Surg Nurs. 2004;24(4):155–7.
310. Chen SG, Chiu TF, Su WF, Chou TD, Chen TM, Wang HJ. Nipple-areola complex reconstruction using badge flap and intradermal tattooing. Br J Surg. 2005;92(4):435–7.
311. El-Ali K, Dalal M, Kat CC. Tattooing of the nipple-areola complex: review of outcome in 40 patients. J Plast Reconstr Aesthet Surg. 2006;59(10):1052–7.
312. Valdatta L, Montemurro P, Tamborini F, Fidanza C, Gottardi A, Scamoni S. Our experience of nipple reconstruction using the C-V flap technique: 1 year evaluation. J Plast Reconstr Aesthet Surg. 2009;62:1293–8.
313. Goh SC, Martin NA, Pandya AN, Cutress RI. Patient satisfaction following nipple-areolar complex reconstruction and tattooing. J Plast Reconstr Aesthet Surg. 2011;64(3):360–3.
314. Halvorson EG, Cormican M, West ME, Myers V. Three-dimensional nipple-areola tattooing: a new technique with superior results. Plast Reconstr Surg. 2014;133(5):1073–5.
315. Penn J. Breast reduction. Br J Plast Surg. 1955;7(4):357–71.
316. Oh SH, Woo JS, Lee SR, Kim JR. The correction of inverted nipple using modified purse-string suture. J Korean Soc Plast Reconstr Surg. 2008;35(6):687–91.

# Part II

# Anatomy and Embryology

# 2 Congenital Malformations and Developmental Changes of the Breast: A Dysmorphological View

Paul Merlob

## 2.1 Introduction

A congenital malformation is a morphologic defect (error of morphogenesis) of an organ, part of an organ, or larger region of the body that is present at the time of birth and is the result of an intrinsically abnormal developmental process [1, 2]. That is, the abnormality is present already in the primordium, or the group of cells in the embryo that represents the first trace of an organ, so that the potential for development of a normal form or structure is nil to begin with.

In the breast, congenital malformations may involve the breast gland or the nipple-areolar complex. Though already existing at birth, some may become visibly apparent only in puberty. The classification of breast malformations used in this review (Table 2.1) was based on the accepted nomenclature in the medical literature [3] and on the method of examination used in our neonatal department [4] called the PPSSAC system ("psac" means "decision" in Hebrew), wherein every organ in the body is rated for six features: presence, position, size, shape, adjacent area, and components.

In this review, congenital malformations of the breast and nipple-areolar complex are described from a clinical and dysmorphological point of view.

**Table 2.1** Classification of breast malformations

| | Breast | Nipple and areola |
|---|---|---|
| Presence and number | Amastia | Athelia (absence of nipple) |
| | Amazia | |
| | Polymastia | Polythelia (supernumerary nipples) |
| | Aberrant mammary tissue | Supernumerary areolas |
| Position | Low-set breast | Widely spaced nipples |
| | | Short internipple distance |
| | | Low-set nipples |
| | Symmastia | |
| Size | Micromastia, hypoplasia, aplasia | Small nipples (hypoplastic) |
| | Macromastia, hyperplasia | Large nipples (hyperplastic) |
| | Asymmetry of breasts | Asymmetric nipples |
| Shape | Shape variations | Inverted nipple |
| | Tuberous breasts | |
| Adjacent area | Skin tag | Skin tag of the nipple |
| | Inclusion cyst | Inclusion cyst of the nipple |
| | Breast masses | |

P. Merlob, M.D.
Department of Neonatology, Schneider Children's Medical Center and Rabin Medical Center, Tetach Tikva, Israel

Tel-Aviv University, Tel-Aviv, Israel
e-mail: merlobp@post.tau.ac.il


M.A. Shiffman (ed.), *Nipple-Areolar Complex Reconstruction*,
https://doi.org/10.1007/978-3-319-60925-6_2

## 2.2 Developmental Changes of the Breast

The mammary glands are highly modified sweat glands that originate from surface epithelium growing down into the underlying mesenchyme [5]. The human breast consists of the parenchyma and stroma. The parenchyma forms a system of branching ducts eventually leading to secretory acini development [5, 6]. The stroma consists mainly of adipose tissue, providing the environment for the development of the parenchyma. The process of development of the ductal system and acini is termed "branching morphogenesis" [6].

At term, approximately 15–20 lobes of glandular tissue have formed, each containing a lactiferous duct that opens onto the breast surface through the mammary pit. The breast bud becomes palpable at 34 weeks' gestation, measuring approximately 3 mm at 36 weeks' gestation and 4–10 mm in a 40-week full-term infant [7]. A palpable breast of 7 mm or more is one of the maturational signs for determining the gestational age of a full-term newborn.

Shortly after birth, the nipples become everted from proliferation of the underlying mesoderm, and the areolae increase in pigmentation [5–7]. The development of erectile tissue in the nipple-areolar complex causes the nipple to protrude even further upon stimulation.

During the first days after birth, the level of maternal estrogens in the newborn blood falls, which stimulates the neonatal pituitary to produce prolactin. This results in breast enlargement and/or transient secretion of milk in as many as 70% of term neonates [8]. This physiologic "gynecomastia" typically regresses within a few weeks or months after birth. Preterm infants do not develop breast enlargement or secrete milk after birth, which indicates that the intrauterine environment is essential for breast development [6].

At approximately 3–4 months postnatally, the infant breast undergoes stimulation through a surge of the infant's own reproductive hormones, including estradiol [9]. Breast tissue in female infants persists longer than in male infants due to higher estradiol levels in infancy in girls [9].

The first 2 years of life are a critical period for some aspects of breast maturation [6, 8]. The most well-accepted morphological and functional maturation stages from birth to 2 years have been described by Anbazhagan et al. [8]. The morphological changes of the breast are depicted by the degree of glandular differentiation (branching, formation of acini, and well-developed lobular system). After 2 years of age, the infant breast remains quiescent until puberty with no developmental changes.

## 2.3 Malformations of the Breast

### 2.3.1 Amastia

Amastia is defined by the complete absence of the breast tissue, nipple, and areola and can be unilateral or bilateral. It is a result of complete failure of mammary line development at about 6 weeks in utero [5].

Amastia is a very rare malformation, with a male-to-female ratio of 1:5. Trier [10] found only 43 reported cases over a period of 126 years, for a worldwide prevalence of one patient every 3 years. The oldest documentation of amastia appears in the Song of Solomon (VIII:8): "We have a little sister, and she hath no breasts: What shall we do for our sister in the day when she shall be spoken for?" [11].

At birth, amastia is characterized by the absence of the breast and the nipple-areolar complex. At puberty, there is a lack of breast development, but other secondary sexual characteristics and fertility are normal.

Amastia should be differentiated from amazia, wherein the breast tissue is absent but the nipple is present, and from athelia, where only the nipple is absent but the breast tissue is present.

Unilateral amastia is frequently associated with the absence of the pectoralis major muscle (Poland sequence); this was true in 18 of the 20 patients with unilateral amastia described by Trier [10]. At clinical examination, these two conditions may be easily confused unless thoracic ultrasound is performed to identify the presence or absence of the pectoralis muscle [12].

Amastia may be isolated, associated, syndromic, and embryopathic. All these types can be unilateral or bilateral. Isolated congenital amastia is a rare condition in that the pectoralis muscles and rib cage are usually normal (OMiM113700) [13]. Isolated congenital bilateral amastia in otherwise normal patients (with no other malformations) was described in the literature only four times [14]. About 40% of all cases of bilateral amastia are associated with other congenital malformations:

1. Skeletal: absence of ulna, lobster-claw malformation of the hands and feet, absence of fingers, syndactyly, clinodactyly, and cubitus valgus
2. Facial: cleft palate, high-arched palate, hypertelorism, macrostomia, low-set ears, hearing defect, and multiple whorls
3. Renal: ureteral triplication, malrotated kidneys, and chronic renal disease
4. Genital: hypoplasia of the labia majora

The syndromes described with amastia are as follows [13, 15]:

1. Congenital (anhydrotic) ectodermal dysplasia (tricho-odonto-onychial type)
2. AREDYLD: **a**cro**re**nal, **e**ctodermal **d**ysplasia, **l**ipoatrophy, **d**iabetes
3. Ulnar-mammary syndrome (UMS)
4. Scalp-ear-nipple syndrome (Finlay-Marks syndrome)
5. Amastia, polywhorls, and webbed fingers
6. Amastia with vaginal atresia and de novo translocation
7. Ureteral triplication with hydronephrosis, brachydactyly, patent ductus, and facial anomalies

Embryopathic amastia has been described in connection with dehydroepiandrosterone or methimazole treatment during pregnancy [4]. With regard to its inheritance, amastia may be sporadic or familial. In familial amastia, both autosomal dominant and autosomal recessive inheritance have been reported [11, 13, 15].

The treatment of amastia requires total breast reconstruction.

### 2.3.2 Amazia

Amazia is a congenital malformation of the breast, defined by the absence of glandular mammary tissue with the presence of a normal or abnormal nipple-areolar complex. Amazia should be differentiated from amastia (absence of mammary tissue and nipple-areolar complex), athelia (absence of nipple and areola only), and breast hypoplasia (deficiency of mammary tissue only). Up until now, only four cases of amazia have been published in the medical literature: bilateral amazia in three [16–18] and isolated unilateral amazia in one [19].

Ozsoy et al. [16] described a 17-year-old girl with bilateral amazia. Nipples were normal on palpation, whereas both of the areolas were hypoplastic. This patient presented also with midface anomalies: nasomaxillary retrusion, a short and recessed nose, and a long upper lip. Some skeletal anomalies were observed: bilateral camptodactyly, scoliosis, and thoracic vertebral anomalies. The karyotype was normal, and there were no major chromosomal abnormalities in the family. Before operation (augmentation of the breasts), random biopsies were taken which showed the absence of glandular tissue, thus confirming the diagnosis of amazia.

Papadimitriou et al. [17] presented a 13.5-year-old girl with bilateral amazia associated with bilateral choanal atresia. On physical examination, the authors found bilateral absence of mammary glands and hypoplastic areolas. However, both nipples were normal in size and shape. No other malformations were present.

Dreifuss et al. [18] observed a 13-year-old girl with bilateral congenital absence of the breast (amazia) but low-set nipple-areolar complex. In addition, an accessory nipple on the left abdomen was observed as well as axillary fullness that felt like fatty tissue.

Amazia in this patient was associated with:

1. Limb anomalies: right foot postaxial polydactyly and bilateral syndactyly of the second and third toes.
2. Facial anomalies: left ptosis and amblyopia, frontal upsweep of the hairline, and low-set, posteriorly rotated ears. The karyotype was normal. No syndrome was identified.

Nso-Roca et al. [19] found one isolated case of unilateral amazia in a 13-year-old girl consisting of the absence of the mammary gland with normal nipple-areolar complex.

In their systematic review of the literature regarding congenital breast anomalies, Dreifuss et al. [18] concluded that the data presented are rarely complete. There is a great confusion in diagnosis of amazia, amastia, and hypoplastic breast because only a clinical diagnosis was used to verify the presence or absence of breast tissue. Complementary testing essential for diagnosis such as ultrasound or mammography was rarely performed, making the diagnosis inaccurate.

### 2.3.3 Polymastia (Supernumerary Breast)

Polymastia (poly = many + mastos = breast) is a congenital malformation characterized by the presence of more than two breasts. Traditionally, there are two general patterns: supernumerary breast (SNB) and aberrant (accessory) mammary tissue (AMT) [20]. Though usually distinguishable, in some clinical situations, the differentiation of the two types is arbitrary [20]. Of the various types of SNB, a normal-size, complete breast (true polymastia) is a very rare finding, fewer than 1% of all the cases in a large series [21].

Complete SNBs have all components of normal breasts (well-formed nipple, areola, and ductal system). Incomplete polymastia will have a ductal system but may lack nipple and areola [22].

Polymastia may occur along the milk line or outside of it (ectopic breast) [22, 23]. The first is explained by the failure of the embryonic mammary ridge to undergo normal regression [5, 22]. The reason for its occurrence outside the mammary line remains unclear. Some authors hypothesize that it is due to displacement of the embryonic crests [21, 22]. Others suggested that because the breasts are modified apocrine sweat glands, polymastia can occur anywhere apocrine sweat glands are found [23].

Clinically, the great majority of SNBs occur along the milk line, either unilaterally (left more than right) or bilaterally, above or below the normal mammae. The most frequent locations are the axilla and inguinal (vulvar) region. When located above the normal breast, SNBs are usually lateral, well formed, and of considerable size and can lactate [22]. When situated below the normal breast, they are medial, small, imperfectly developed, and incapable of lactation [22]. Single SNBs are more common than multiple ones, although patient with eight or more SNBs have been described. Although SNBs are present at birth, they do not become prominent until influenced by female sex hormones at puberty, pregnancy, or lactation. Like the normal breast, they undergo cyclic changes in size and density and are subject to the same diseases, including carcinoma [24]. The diagnosis of polymastia should be based on triple investigations: ultrasound scan, mammography, and fine-needle biopsy [25–27] The ultrasound scan confirms the presence of mammary gland tissue (hyperechogenic); the other two show the breast parenchyma and exclude the possibility of malignancy [26, 27].

Polymastia usually occurs sporadically, but familial cases have been reported with probable autosomal dominant transmission [28, 29]. Polymastia may be either isolated or associated with other anomalies or syndromic. Associated anomalies include urogenital malformations (obstructive urinary tract, unilateral renal agenesis), chest wall deformity [30] (agenesis and fusion of ribs), absence of part of the lung, epilepsy, and malignancy [22, 23]. Syndromes with polymastia include mammo-renal syndrome, mandibular-facial-digital-nipple syndrome, and chromosomal abnormalities (trisomy 8, partial 3p trisomy, translocations 3 and 8).

Possible problems associated with polymastia are discomfort (pain, tenderness, secretion), psychological and esthetic embarrassment, and complications like mastitis, fibrocystic modifications, fibroadenomas, or adenocarcinoma [22, 24]. As a result, excision is recommended, not only for cosmetic purposes.

### 2.3.4 Aberrant (Accessory) Mammary Tissue (AMT)

AMT is defined as mammary glandular parenchyma not located in the usual place of mammary

**Table 2.2** Modern classification of accessory mammary tissue (AMT)

| | |
|---|---|
| *Type 1* | AMT with glandular parenchyma |
| *Type 2* | AMT without evidence of glandular parenchyma |
| Subtype 2a | Polythelia (nipple only) |
| Subtype 2b | Supernumerary areola (areola only) |
| Subtype 2c | Mixed (nipple with areola = pseudomamma) |
| *Type 3* | Intra-areolar polythelia |
| Subtype 3a | AMT arises from areola (paired or dysplastic divided nipples) |
| Subtype 3b | AMT arises from primary nipple ("nipple nevus") |

breasts (Table 2.2) [20]. Ducts and lobules that make up AMT are structurally normal but are not so well organized as in normal or supernumerary breasts [20].

AMT develops usually along the mammary ("milk") line which runs bilaterally from the axilla to growing ventrally and from mid-shoulder to mid-scapula dorsally [31] but also outside the milk line (ectopic). In normal breast development, the mammary ridge recedes, leaving only bilateral mammary tissue at the fourth intercostal space [5, 22]. Partial regression of this tissue will lead to AMT that may reveal itself as structures varying from rudimentary to full-grown breast tissue [31].

The modern classification of AMT, proposed by Urbani and Betti [32] and modified by Lewis et al. [33], is presented in Table 2.2. This classification emphasizes the wide spectrum of AMT, which entails many entities based on the presence of glandular tissue, nipple, areola, or any combination of these [31–33]. However, the terminology pertaining to AMT and its different types constitutes a great source of confusion in the literature. Most publications refer to different types of AMT (especially polymastia and polythelia) as the same entity.

AMT is often asymptomatic and becomes noticeable only after hormonal stimulation usually during puberty and pregnancy [20, 31]. As a result, AMT should be differentiated from lipoma, lymphadenopathy, sebaceous cyst, vascular malformation, and malignancy [6, 34]. The diagnosis of AMT may be confirmed by using imaging evaluation (ultrasonography and/or mammography) [34]. Magnetic resonance imaging of the breast is occasionally performed in challenging atypical cases. Definitive diagnosis can be established by fine-needle aspiration [27, 34].

In whites, AMT usually occurs below the normal breast, while in Japanese women, it appears above [22]. The left-sided location is the more relevant clinical feature in familial AMT; in sporadic forms, the right side is involved [20]. In the familial cases, the two most common inheritances are autosomal dominant with incomplete penetration and X-linked dominance [35].

Patients with AMT should have an ultrasound of the kidneys because of the possibility of associated nephrourinary malformations [36]. A broad spectrum of renal malformations was described in AMT: adult polycystic kidney disease, unilateral renal agenesis, cystic renal dysplasia, familial renal cysts, and hydronephrosis due to pyeloureteral junction stenosis [36].

### 2.3.5 Micromastia/Hypoplasia/Aplasia

This congenital malformation is the result of failure of breast growth despite the presence of mammary gland tissue [37]. It ranges from a small breast (micromastia) to complete breast underdevelopment (aplasia).

The breast tissue in micromastia consists of fibrous stroma and ductal structures without acinar differentiation [20]. There is no definitive explanation for this entity. Some authors suggest that it is caused by nonresponse to the circulating estrogens (defect in end-organ response). Sun et al. [38] found a significant ($p < 0.05$) lower estrogen receptor protein level in the 13 patients with micromastia versus 13 women with mammary hypertrophy. Other authors attribute this malformation to a defect in the formation of the primitive breast tissue during embryonic development [37].

Micromastia may be unilateral or bilateral. A diagnosis of unilateral hypoplasia/aplasia may be made if there is a substantial difference in breast size that far exceeds the mild asymmetry commonly seen, and there is no evidence of macromastia of the unilateral breast [20]. Occasionally, the supporting structures are also inadequate, and there is a considerable degree of ptosis, giving the breast a sagging or flattened appearance [37].

Congenital micromastia/hypoplasia/aplasia may be isolated, associated, or syndromic. Ipsilateral mammary hypoplasia has been reported in association with Becker's nevus, chest wall anomalies (pectus excavatum, pectus carinatum, or anterior thoracic hypoplasia) [39], Jeune syndrome (asphyxiating thoracic dystrophy), and Poland sequence.

Bilateral hypoplasia/aplasia was found in ulnar-mammary syndrome (autosomal dominant inheritance), Turner's syndrome, congenital adrenal hyperplasia, and incontinentia pigmenti [13, 15]. Plastic surgery for breast hypoplasia/aplasia is performed in the late teenage years when appearance becomes of paramount importance.

### 2.3.6 Macromastia/Hyperplasia/Hypertrophy

Breast size varies according to birth weight and gestational age. Infants who are large for gestational age have larger breast nodules than those who are appropriate or small for gestational age. There is little appreciable difference in breast size between female and male infants of the same weights, although measured diameters are larger in females (8.5 ± 2 mm vs 7.8 ± 2.1 mm) [40].

Physiologic "gynecomastia" (transient neonatal breast hypertrophy) develops in up to 70% of term neonates of both sexes a few days after birth and lasts a few weeks to several months (maximum 4–6 months). In general, there is mild to moderate swelling with prominence of the breast, which is tender but without erythema or warmth (Fig. 2.1). In rare cases, the engorgement is quite marked, and in a small percentage of cases, there may be a discharge of clear or cloudy fluid from the nipples ("witch's milk") due to stimulation of prolactin production by the newborn pituitary gland in response to the estrogen withdrawal at birth [8]. The quantity of "witch's milk" is directly proportional to the size of the breast nodule, and it increases if the breasts are massaged (not recommended). The discharge usually disappears spontaneously within a few days and requires no intervention. In some newborns, breast hypertrophy may be associated with vaginal withdrawal bleeding or testicular enlargement.

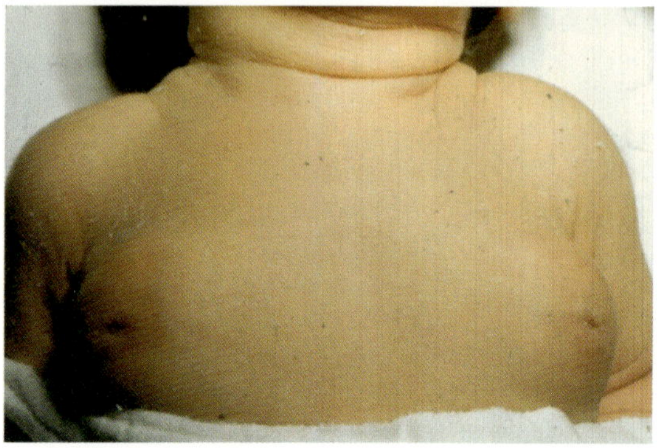

**Fig. 2.1** Transient neonatal breast hypertrophy (physiologic gynecomastia)

In a prenatal ultrasound study, Bezzi et al. [41] described prominent fetal breasts at gestational age 17–20 weeks, appearing as bilateral and symmetric bulges on the anterior wall, of 3–4 mm in thickness with a hypoechoic echotexture, characteristic of a homogeneous tissue without prominent fibrous stroma. These findings were transient and disappeared after 2–3 months. At birth, the anterior chest wall appeared normal. The authors suggested that transient hypertrophy of the fetal breast could be a result of physiological changes in the maternal fetal hormonal pool (balance) [41].

Prepubertal macromastia has been described only twice in the world medical literature. Mick et al. [42] observed a 6-month-old female who presented with severe idiopathic macromastia. The breast enlargement began at 2 months of age, and subtotal mastectomies were necessary at 23 months. Extensive hormonal evaluation prior to surgery revealed no evidence of estrogenization or precocious puberty. There was no galactorrhea. This girl presented an idiopathic degenerative neurologic condition characterized by psychomotor delay, ataxia, and seizures. This neurologic dysfunction and increased gonadotropins suggest that central nervous system factors were etiologic [42].

Zinn et al. [43] reported macromastia in a newborn with Alagille syndrome (arteriohepatic dysplasia). This autosomal dominant disorder seems to be unrelated to the neonatal macromastia, although the authors hypothesized that it may be related to severe liver disease and abnormal metabolism of estrogens [43].

Pubertal, gravid, and drug-induced (penicillamine, indinavir) breast growth have been described as forms of macromastia [20]. Other developmental abnormalities occur later in childhood and at puberty and include premature menarche, precocious puberty, and tuberous breast abnormality.

### 2.3.7 Asymmetry of the Breasts

Asymmetry of the breasts is a common finding, especially in girls in the early stages of breast development. Since each breast arises from an individual anlage (primordium) [5, 37], it is not surprising that one breast bud will appear before its counterpart responds to the hormonal stimulus and either begin to develop sooner or grow at a more rapid rate [37]. Indeed, the breast dimensions of normal persons are rarely found to be truly equal if they are accurately measured [37], though the asymmetry is usually mild and of insignificant cosmetic importance [44]. Most individuals remain unaware of it [45].

When the irregularities of breast shape, size, and position are more pronounced, the asymmetry becomes an esthetic and psychological problem. Significant asymmetry of the breasts has been observed in 5.2% of women treated with mammoplasty [45]. Asymmetry may be the result of unilateral hypoplasia or hyperplasia or an association of the two. It should be differentiated from pseudoasymmetry in which an illusion of inequality is due to scoliosis or a rib cage abnormality [44]. Asymmetry of the breast should be carefully documented using objective measurements, photography, and three-dimensional simulations [46].

Asymmetry of the breasts is usually an isolated finding, though it may sometimes be associated with mitral valve prolapse or connective tissue disease. It may also occur as part of a syndrome, such as cranio-fronto-nasal syndrome or Simpson-Golabi-Behmel syndrome. In only a few cases is this malformation so severe that it requires surgical intervention in late adolescence.

### 2.3.8 Breast Shape Variations

The general shape of the breast varies from woman to woman, just like body build and facial characteristics [47]. Changes occur with age and physiological condition of the woman, from dome-shaped or conical in adolescence to more hemispheric in adulthood and pendulous in parous women. Shape also varies by race (discoidal, hemispheric, pear-shaped, conical) and body construction.

The definitions of congenital breast shape changes are very descriptive. Anomalies of breast shape have been described under a variety of names, although all share the same breast base anomaly (tuberous breasts) with various degrees of clinical severity. Breast shape anomalies first appear at puberty when the breasts develop; no such anomaly is visible in the newborn or during childhood.

## 2.4 Malformations of the Nipple and Areola

### 2.4.1 Athelia

Athelia, or congenital absence of the nipple, is the rarest of the breast anomalies [37]. It may be unilateral or bilateral, and it is not necessarily associated with the absence of breast tissue. Athelia may be isolated (without other malformations), associated with other malformations, syndromic, or embryopathic.

Dermoid cysts [48], pectus excavation, choanal atresia posterior, jejunal atresia the appropriate renal tubular dysgenesis were described in association with athelia.

Unilateral syndromic athelia has been observed in Poland sequence (Fig. 2.2). Bilateral syndromic athelia was reported in ectodermal dysplasias [49], limb-mammary syndrome, scalp-ear-nipple syndrome [50], and Al-Awadi/Raas-Rothschild syndrome [51]. Teratogenic defects caused by maternal use of antithyroid drugs during pregnancy (methimazole/carbimazole embryopathy) include athelia together with bilateral choanal atresia, esophageal atresia, facial dysmorphy, and other abnormalities [52, 53].

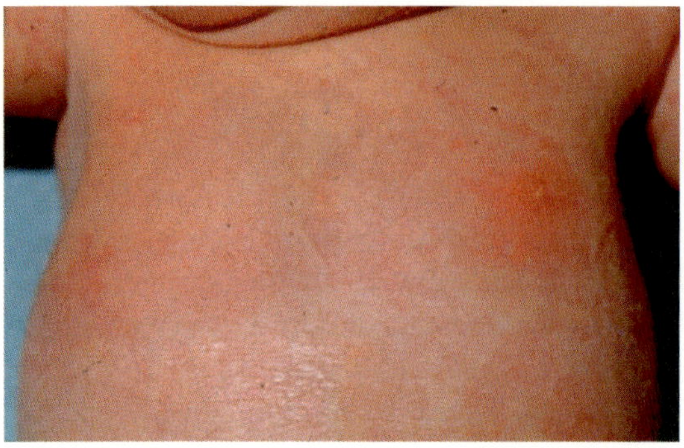

Fig. 2.2 Right athelia in Poland sequence

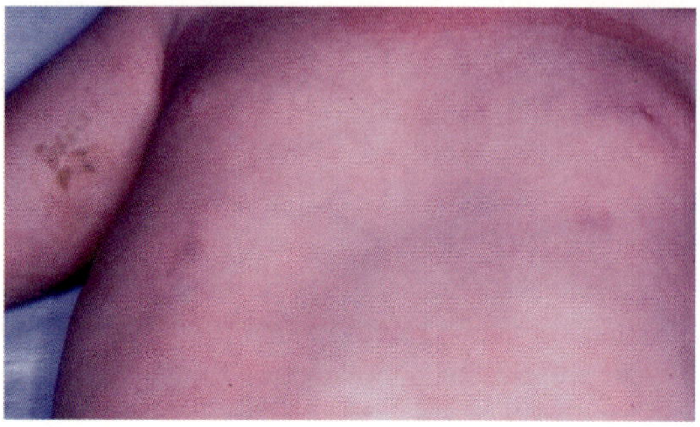

Fig. 2.3 Supernumerary nipples

Athelia might be explained as a failure of the development of the lower cervical and upper thoracic somites, so that the overlying mammary base cannot grow [5, 47]. Parathyroid hormone-related protein (PHRP) produced by the epithelium mammary bud can be implicated in the genesis of the nipple [54]. As a result, athelia might be caused by a failure in PHRP production [49]. Borck et al. [55] found that a disruption of one allele of protein tyrosine phosphatase receptor type F (PTPRF) by a balanced translocation plays a key role in the development of the nipple-areola region.

### 2.4.2 Polythelia (Hyperthelia or Supernumerary Nipples)

Polythelia (many nipples) is a minor congenital malformation (error of morphogenesis) and is characterized by the occurrence of a supernumerary nipple (SNN), in addition to the two normally appearing nipples (Fig. 2.3). Every SNN has an areola, although not every supernumerary areola has a nipple [56]. Histologically, the SNNs have all the characteristics of the normal nipple, including hyperpigmentation, epidermal thickening, pilosebaceous structures, smooth muscle, and, in some cases, mammary glands [57].

The reported prevalence of SNNs varies from 0.22% in a Hungarian population to 1.63% in Black American neonates, 2.5% in Israeli neonates [58], 4.7% in Israeli-Arab children [59], and 5.6% in German children [56]; the highest frequency was found in a Native American population in Chile (11–16%) [60]. These variations are attributed, at least in part, to differences in ethnicity, geographic regions, methods of physical examination, and age of the sample populations [60].

Some authors consider polythelia an atavistic or reversionary manifestation wherein a remote ancestral characteristic unexpectedly appears for unknown reasons [56, 61]. Using transgenic animal models, researchers have produced atavistic features by over- or underexpression of individual genes, especially the Hox genes [62]. The ectopic expression of many Hox genes changes spatial information and is associated with the development of structures out of place and time.

Clinically, SNNs appear as a small pigmented or pearl-colored mark or concave spot with a diameter of only 2–3 mm [58–61]. They vary sharply in size, shape, color, and location, particularly when they occur outside the embryonic mammary line. Breast tissue and areola may or may not be present. They usually appear as a single lesion; a finding of two or more SNNs is rare. SNNs may be unilateral or bilateral, and they are usually located along the mammary line (Fig. 2.4). Eighty-seven percent are found below the normal nipple and 13% above it [58]. About 5% are ectopic and are situated on the back, shoulder, vulva, thigh, limbs, face, and neck [58, 60, 61]. In 75% of patients, the SNNs measure no more than 30% of the diameter of the normal nipple [60]. In the other 25% of patients, they are of medium size, as large as 50% of the normal nipple [60]. Only rarely are they as large as a normal nipple [56].

The male-to-female ratio differs in various studies, but most report a male predominance (1.7:1).

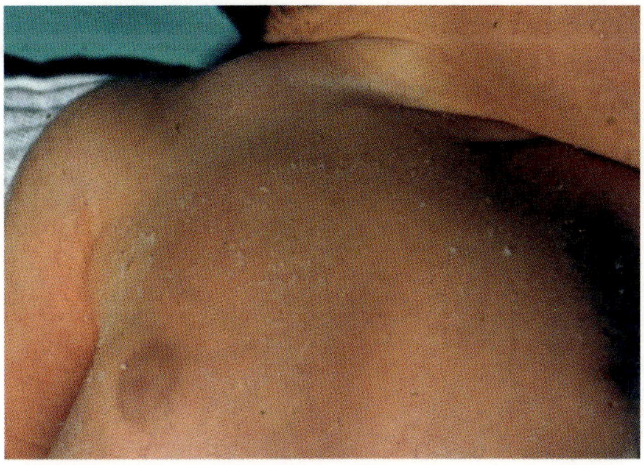

**Fig. 2.4** Inverted nipple left side

**Table 2.3** Differential diagnosis of supernumerary nipples

| | |
|---|---|
| 1. | Macule |
| 2. | Pigmented nevus |
| 3. | Skin tag |
| 4. | Wart |
| 5. | Fibroma |
| 6. | Neurofibroma |
| 7. | Monitoring scar |
| 8. | Amniocentesis scar |
| 9. | Lipoma |
| 10. | Lymphangioma |
| 11. | Lymphadenitis |
| 12. | Hidradenitis suppurativa |

If breast tissue is present, the SNN may show any of the pathological changes exhibited in normally situated breasts, including abscesses, fibrocystic disease, fibroadenoma, and carcinoma. Although malignant changes occur, it is not established whether carcinoma arises with greater frequency in ectopic than in normally situated nipples.

To detect SNN, a wet gauze pad is passed along the mammary line from the axillary region to the upper anterior part of the thigh on each side [58]. This technique is particularly helpful in the dry and desquamating skin of full-term and post-term infants [58]. When the suspected lesion is concave, folding it between the fingers yields a typical wrinkling [60]. The differential diagnosis of SNN is presented in Table 2.3 [60].

SNN may be an isolated finding, associated with other congenital malformations and diseases or syndromic. Table 2.4 presents the various congenital malformations and diseases described in connection with polythelia.

The reported prevalence of SNN with kidney and urinary tract malformations and malignancies ranges from a high 40% to 0%. Hersh et al. [63] suggested a combined SNN-renal field defect in accordance with numerous publications claiming a close association, but many other studies failed to provide supportive evidence. Therefore, the need for full urinary tract investigation in every newborn with SNN remains controversial. Based on critical evaluation of the literature on SNNs and the wide range of renal defects observed in these studies (Table 2.4), most authors today believe that otherwise morphologically normal infants and children can be spared a thorough radiographic and ultrasonographic evaluation. An isolated and sporadic SNN does not typically present an indication for a thorough workup [59]. However, when an SNN is associated with other mild errors of morphogenesis or a major malformation, and in cases of a prominent ectopic SNN or established familial SNN, a complete renal investigation should be done, bearing in mind that pathological urinary findings can be present but remain dormant [60].

Syndromic polythelia has been reported in chromosomal aberrations (Turner's syndrome, chromosome 8 trisomy, partial chromosome 3p trisomy), cutaneous lesions (ectodermal dysplasia, aplasia cutis with syndactyly, scalp defect, microcephaly, and developmental delay), and other syndromes (Table 2.5).

Polythelia may be sporadic or familial. Most cases are sporadic [61], although familial occurrence has been recognized (in 40% of all patients, one of the parents confirmed the presence of an SNN) [56]. The mode of inheritance of familial polythelia seems to be heterogeneous, since three modes have been suggested: autosomal dominant with variable penetration [56], X-linked dominant [61], and autosomal recessive [64]. The most frequently observed polythelia in familial series was pseudomamma (72% of patients) [65]. Polythelia (nipple only) was the most frequent in the sporadic forms of accessory mammary tissue (60% of patients) [65].

The management of patients with SNN is also controversial. In infants and children, it appears to be a benign finding which requires no treatment. Later in life, as a genodermatosis with

**Table 2.4** Associated congenital malformations and diseases with polythelia

| | Congenital malformations | Diseases |
|---|---|---|
| Central nervous system | Neural tube defects | Epilepsy |
| | Intracranial aneurysm | Migraine |
| | | Neurosis |
| | | Familial alcoholism |
| Cardiac | Patent ductus arteriosus | Conduction defects |
| | Atrial septal defect | Bundle branch block |
| | Ventricular septal defect | Essential hypertension |
| Ear, nose, and throat | Ear abnormalities | – |
| | Laryngeal web | |
| | Bifid mandibular condyle | |
| Gastrointestinal | Pyloric stenosis | Peptic ulcer |
| Renal | Hydronephrosis | Wilm's tumor |
| | Ureteropelvic junction stenosis | Renal adenocarcinoma |
| | Ureteral duplication | Fibroadenoma |
| | Unilateral renal agenesis | Carcinoma (bladder, testicular) |
| | Multicystic dysplastic kidney | Membranoproliferative glomerulonephritis |
| | Polycystic kidneys | Familial nephritis |
| | Solitary renal cysts | Nephrosclerosis |
| | Ectopic kidneys | |
| | Horse shoe kidneys | |
| | Supernumerary kidneys | |
| | Vesicoureteral reflux | |
| | Megaureter | |
| | Bladder neck obstruction | |
| | Ureterocele | |
| | Urethral cyst | |
| Skeletal | Coronal suture synostosis | |
| | Vertebral anomaly | |
| | Absence of rib | |
| | Hand malformation | |
| | Hemihypertrophy | |
| | Arthrogryposis | |

**Table 2.5** Syndromic polythelia[a]

| |
|---|
| Adams-Oliver syndrome |
| Ankyloblepharon-ectodermal defect-cleft lip/palate (AEC) |
| Bannayan-Riley-Ruvalcaba syndrome (BRRS) |
| Branchio-oculo-facial syndrome (BOFS) |
| Bohring-Opitz syndrome (BOPS) |
| Char syndrome |
| Incontinentia pigmenti |
| Pallister-Killian syndrome (PKS) |
| Postaxial acrofacial dysostosis syndrome (POADS) |
| Simpson-Golabi-Behmel syndrome (SGBS) |

[a]In these syndromes, polythelia is a part of the clinical phenotype but not a cardinal feature

malignant potential, some authors recommend surgical removal. Surgical treatment may also be indicated for cosmetic reasons or for a protruding SNN that causes embarrassment.

### 2.4.3 Intra-areolar Polythelia

Intra-areolar polythelia (IAP) is a special type of polythelia characterized by the occurrence of a supernumerary nipple within the areola [66]. It is also called "paired nipples" or "dysplastic divided nipples." IAP must be classified as different from supernumerary nipples, in which the nipples are along the mammary line and not within the areola [29].

Although polythelia is common, IAP is an extremely rare congenital malformation [67, 68]. IAP may be a sporadic minor congenital malformation [66], although familial cases were also published [69]. IAP is usually bilateral (two nipples in each breast) in the sporadic cases, but unilateral (two nipples on one areola) type has also been observed [68].

The embryological background of IAP is different from that of polythelia. IAP is due to an intrauterine dichotomy of the developing nipple or the incomplete development or disruption of the epithelial pit or mammillary anlage.

Intra-areolar nipples are well structured, without dysmorphic changes, soft in consistency and asymptomatic, located within a normal areola. The breasts and nipple-areola complex are usually morphologically normal. There is no lateral displacement of the nipple. IAP may produce esthetic discomfort and a mild psychological embarrassment. For these reasons, surgical excision is recommended.

### 2.4.4 Supernumerary Areola (Polyareolae)

Supernumerary areola (SNA) is a very rare form of aberrant breast tissues, a mild error of morphogenesis, characterized by the presence of more than one areola (areola only). It has also been called "polythelia areolaris," but this is an inaccurate and contradictory terminology [70] because polythelia means "many nipples" and not many areolae. Therefore, supernumerary areolae or polyareolae are more adequate terms.

Clinically, SNAs appear as a pigmented "wrinkled" macule located on the mammary line or ectopic to it (shoulder, pubis, etc.). They are no known to be associated with systemic diseases. However, if glandular tissue is present, carcinomatous change—though very rare—can occur [70]. One of the most characteristic histopathological features of areolar tissue is the presence of a large number of smooth muscle bundles. Lack of lactiferous ducts and the glands of Montgomery are also constant features. Surgery is usually performed for cosmetic reasons.

### 2.4.5 Abnormal Nipple Position

The clinical impression of nipple position may be misleading, and accurate measurement of the internipple distance is required [71]. Newborns between 25 and 40 weeks' gestation showed progressive increase in the internipple distance with increasing gestational age [72]. The ratio of internipple distance to chest circumference is called internipple index, and it is constant during various gestational ages [71, 72]. In healthy Chinese children aged from birth to 18 years, Leung et al. [73] found an increase of internipple distance with age. However, the internipple index, highest in the neonatal period, decreased steadily until the age of 4 years and thereafter was relatively constant through age 18 years in males and age 11 years in females. In females, the internipple index decreased gradually from the age of 11 to 18 years [73]. Leung et al. [73] found also ethnic differences in the internipple index.

Widely spaced nipples in newborns are defined by a long internipple distance of more than +2SD in relation to birth weight and gestational age [71]. Another diagnostic criterion is an internipple index greater than 0.28, independent of gestation age [71].

Widely spaced nipples rarely occur in newborns or children with a normal chest configuration. They have been observed in some chromosomal anomalies (Turner's syndrome; trisomies 4, 8, 18, and 20; and deletion of 8p, 9p, 18p−, 18q−, and 4p+), after drug intake (fetal hydantoin embryopathy), and in association with facial defects (cerebro-oculo-facio-skeletal syndrome and cryptophthalmos syndrome) or other syndromes (Juberg-Hayward, Bartsocas-Papas, Fryns, scalp-ear-nipple, acrocallosal, and velocardiofacial syndrome).

A short internipple distance has been observed in Jeune syndrome (asphyxiating thoracic dystrophy) and cerebro-costo-mandibular syndrome. Fleischer [74] described lateral displacement of the nipple as a sign of bilateral renal hypoplasia.

### 2.4.6 Abnormal Nipple Size

Nipple size at birth depends on gestational age, measuring 7 mm or more in diameter in full-term infants and 6 mm or less in preterm infants (36 weeks = 6 mm; 28 weeks = 1 mm). Nipple size anomalies are expressed clinically as small, large, or asymmetric nipples.

Microthelia is defined as a small or hypoplastic nipple, usually poorly pigmented, with a narrow or absent areolar zone and little palpable breast tissue. Both sides are equally affected. The nipples may be somewhat widely spaced as well.

Hypoplastic nipple is described as part of a phenotype of some syndromes— ablepharon-macrostomia, Poland, Robinow, scalp-ear-nipple, and ulnar-mammary syndrome—and in some chromosomal aberrations: 10q26 deletion and monosomy 21.

Macrothelia is defined as a hypertrophic nipple, forming a large, bulbous, rather flabby mass atop the areola, rather than a firm, erectile papilla [37]. It is a rare anomaly that is usually asymptomatic; its possible effect on breast feeding is not known [37].

### 2.4.7 Inverted Nipple

Inverted nipples do not extend beyond the breast surface at birth; they usually become everted within a few days/weeks postpartum. There are two types of inverted nipples—umbilicated and invaginated. Umbilicated nipples can be pulled out from their depressed position beneath the alveolar surface, whereas invaginated nipples cannot (Fig. 2.4).

In adults, inverted nipples are divided into three groups on the basis of clinical findings, histology, and predictable response to invasive surgery [75]. The appropriate grading is confirmed with operative findings:

1. Grade I: The nipple can be easily pulled out manually and the projection is maintained without traction; there is no or minimal fibrosis.
2. Grade II: The nipple can be pulled out manually but with difficulty, and it tends to retract; there is a moderate degree of fibrosis.
3. Grade III: The nipple is severely inverted and retracted. It is very difficult to pull it out manually, and it promptly retracts. The fibrosis is remarkable, and the lactiferous ducts are short and severely retracted.

The prevalence of inverted nipples varies in different populations from 1.77% [76] to 3.26% [77] in unmarried women aged 19–26 years. In the latter subgroups, Park et al. [77] reported bilaterality in 86.7% of cases and unilaterality in 13.2%. The umbilicated type was much more common: 96.23% in one study [77] and 73% in another [78].

Congenital inverted nipples may result from a failure of the underlying mesenchyme to proliferate and push the nipple out of its normal depressed position. According to one histological analysis [76], the primary cause is a lack of bulk in the dense connective tissue, so that nipple retraction by the muscle and fibrous elements lying parallel to large ducts is prevented. However, many authors currently believe that the major pathophysiological basis for inverted nipples is shortened, underdeveloped breast ducts combined with resistant collagen fibers.

Inverted nipples are usually an isolated and sporadic occurrence. However, they may be familial with a possible autosomal dominant transmission [79] or syndromic (Robinow syndrome, ulnar-mammary syndrome, chromosome 2q37 deletion, and congenital disorders of glycosylation I).

Besides being a cosmetic/psychological problem, inverted nipples are prone to infection unless excellent hygiene is practiced assiduously [44]. Congenital inverted nipples may also induce nursing difficulties, chronic mastitis, and other functional problems during lactation [77].

There are many techniques for the treatment of inverted nipples [76, 78, 80, 81], some of which involve major surgery and others, simpler ingenious methods, used even during the third trimester of pregnancy [80]. The results of a 7-year experience demonstrate the safety and efficacy of the authors' technique to correct inverted nipples [81].

## Conclusions

The author reviews the available data on congenital malformations of the breast from the aspect of neonatologic dysmorphology. Early diagnosis and proper treatment of congenital breast malformations are essential, especially in today's breast-conscious society.

A wide spectrum of malformations of the breast, nipple, and areola has been described. Their classification, however, is still confusing, at least for some traits. Except for amastia, polymastia, and polythelia, which have received much attention, the data for many other breast malformations are sparse. Case-control studies or even case series are rare, and good evidence is often lacking. The discovery of multigene families which play a critical role in mammary gland development and in producing congenital breast malformations will contribute substantially to our understanding and clinical approach in the future.

## References


1. Spranger J, Benirschke K, Hall JG, Lenz W, Lowry RB, Opitz JM, Pinsky L, Schwarzacher HG, Smith DW. Errors of morphogenesis: concepts and terms. Recommendations of an international working group. J Pediatr. 1983;100(1):160–5.
2. Hennekam RC, Biesecker LG, Allanson JE, Hall JG, Opitz JM, Temple IK, Carey JC, Elements of Morphology Consortium. Elements of morphology: general terms for congenital anomalies. Am J Med Genet A. 2013;161A(11):2726–33.
3. Letterman G, Schurter M. Suggested nomenclature for aesthetic and reconstructive surgery of the breasts: IV. Congenital anomalies of the breast. Aesthetic Plast Surg. 1989;13(1):59–61.
4. Merlob P. Congenital malformations and developmental changes of the breast: a neonatological view. J Pediatr Endocrinol Metab. 2003;16(4):471–85.
5. Moore KL. The developing human: clinically oriented embryology. 4th ed. Philadelphia: WB Saunders Co.; 1988. p. 426–8.
6. Javed A, Lteif A. Development of the human breast. Semin Plast Surg. 2013;27(1):5–2.
7. Shermak MA. Congenital and abnormalities of the breast. In: Jatoi I, Kaufmann M, editors. Management of breast diseases. Berlin, Heidelberg: Springer-Verlag; 2010. p. 37–51.
8. Anbazhagan R, Bartek J, Monaghan P, Gusterson BA. Growth and development of the human infant breast. Am J Anat. 1991;192(4):407–17.
9. Schmidt IM, Chellakooty M, Haavisto AM, Boisen KA, Damgaard IN, Steendahl U, Toppari J, Skakkebaek NE, Main KM. Gender difference in breast tissue size in infancy: correlation with serum estradiol. Pediatr Res. 2002;52(5):682–6.
10. Trier WC. Complete breast absence: case report and review of the literature. Plast Reconstr Surg. 1965;36(4):431–9.
11. Tawil HM, Najjar SS. Congenital absence of the breasts. J Pediatr. 1968;73(5):751–3.
12. Bianca S, Licciardello M, Barrano B, Ettore G. Isolated congenital amastia: a subclavian artery supply disruption sequence? Am J Med Genet A. 2010;152A(3):792–4.
13. Hamosh A, Scott AF, Amberger J, Bocchini C, Valle D, McKusick VA. Online Mendelian Inheritance in Man (OMIM), a knowledgebase of human genes and genetic disorders. Nucleic Acids Res. 2002;30(1):52–5.
14. Patil LG, Shivanna NH, Benakappa N, Ravindranath H, Bhat R. Congenital amastia. Indian J Pediatr. 2013;80(10):870–1.
15. Jones KL. Smith's recognizable patterns of human malformations. 5th ed. Philadelphia: WB Saunders Co.; 1997.
16. Ozsoy Z, Gozu A, Ozyigit MT, Genc B. Amazia with midface anomaly: case report. Aesthet Plast Surg. 2007;31(4):392–4.
17. Papadimitriou A, Karapanou O, Papadopoulou A, Nicolaidou P, Fretzayas A. Congenital bilateral amazia associated with bilateral choanal atresia. Am J Med Genet A. 2009;149A(7):1529–31.
18. Dreifuss SE, MacIsaac ZM, Grunwaldt LJ. Bilateral congenital amazia: a case report and systematic review of the literature. J Plast Reconstr Aesthet Surg. 2014;67(1):27–33.
19. Nso-Roca AP, Aquirre-Balsalobre FJ, Juste RM. Isolated unilateral amazia: an exceptional breast anomaly. J Pediatr Adolesc Gynecol. 2012;25(6):e147–8.
20. Rosen PP. Rosen's breast pathology. 2nd ed. Philadelphia: Lippincott Williams & Wilkins; 2001. p. 23–9.
21. Hanson E, Segovia J. Dorsal supernumerary breasts. Plast Reconstr Surg. 1978;61(3):441–5.
22. Buyse ML, editor. Birth defects encyclopedia: the comprehensive, systematic, illustrated reference source for the diagnosis, delineation, etiology, biodynamics, occurrence, prevention, and treatment of human anomalies of clinical relevance. Dover, MA: Blackwell Scientific Publications; 1990. p. 246–7.
23. Leung W, Heaton JPW, Morales A. An uncommon urologic presentation of a supernumerary breast. Urology. 1997;50(1):122–4.
24. Giron GL, Friedman I, Feldman S. Lobular carcinoma in ectopic axillary breast tissue. Am Surg. 2004;70(4):312–5.
25. Patel RV, Govani D, Patel R, Bhayani B. Adolescent right axillary accessory breast with galactorrhoea. BMJ Case Rep. 2014;2014. pii: bcr2014204215.
26. Hiremath B, Subramaniam N, Chandrashekhar N. Giant accessory breast: a rare occurrence reported,

with a review of the literature. BMJ Case Rep. 2015;2015. pii: bcr2015210918.
27. Velanovich V. Fine needle aspiration cytology in the diagnosis and management of ectopic breast tissue. Am Surg. 1995;61(3):277–8.
28. Weinberg SK, Motulksy AG. Aberrant axillary breast tissue: a report of a family with six affected women in two generations. Clin Genet. 1976;10(6):325–8.
29. Cellini A, Offidani A. Familial supernumerary nipples and breasts. Dermatology. 1992;185(1):56–8.
30. Deshpande SN, Jagtap SR, Thatte RL. An unusual case of congenital wall deformity with polymastia and absence of part of the lung. Br J Plast Surg. 1989;42(4):484–6.
31. Ghosn SH, Khatri KA, Bhawan J. Bilateral aberrant axillary breast tissue mimicking lipomas: report of a case and review of the literature. J Cutan Pathol. 2007;34(Suppl 1):9–13.
32. Urbani CE, Betti R. Accessory mammary tissue in clinical practice. Milan: McGraw-Hill; 1996. p. 35–56.
33. Lewis EJ, Crutchfield CE, Ebertz MJ, Prawer SE. Report of a nipple nevus and an overview of accessory mammary tissue. Cutis. 1998;62(5):243–6.
34. DeFilippis EM, Arleo EK. The ABCs of accessory breast tissue: basic information every radiologist should know. AJR Am J Roentgenol. 2014;202(5):1157–62.
35. Urbani CE, Betti R. Familial aberrant mammary tissue – a clinico-epidermiological survey of 18 cases. Dermatology. 1995;190(3):207–9.
36. Urbani CE, Betti R. Accessory mammary tissue associated with congenital and hereditary nephrourinary malformations. Int J Dermatol. 1996;35(5):349–52.
37. Huffman JW, Dewhurst CJ, Caprano VJ. The gynecology of childhood and adolescence. 2nd ed. Philadelphia, PA: WB Saunders Co.; 1981. p. 542–59.
38. Sun J, Qiao Q, Qi K. The difference in estrogen receptor protein level between breast hypertrophy and micromastia. Plast Reconstr Surg. 2004;113(7):2241–2.
39. Spear SL, Pelletiere CV, Lee ES, Grotting JC. Anterior thoracic hypoplasia: a separate entity from Poland syndrome. Plast Reconstr Surg. 2004;113(1):69–77.
40. Francis GL, Hoffman WH, Gala RR, McPherson JCD, Zadinsky J. A relationship between neonatal breast size and cord blood testosterone level. Ann Clin Lab Sci. 1990;20(4):239–44.
41. Bezzi M, Mitchell DG, Kurtz AB, Ronkin SL, Goldberg BB. Prominent fetal breasts. A normal variant. J Ultrasound Med. 1987;6(11):655–8.
42. Mick GJ, McCormick KL, Wakimoto H. Massive breast enlargement in an infant girl with central nervous system dysfunction. Eur J Pediatr. 1991;150(3):154–7.
43. Zinn HL, Haller JO, Kedia S. Macromastia in a newborn with Alagille syndrome. Pediatr Radiol. 1999;29(5):331–3.
44. Greydanus DE, Parks DS, Farrell EG. Breast disorders in children and adolescents. Pediatr Clin N Am. 1989;36(3):601–38.
45. Gliosci A, Presutti F. Asymmetry of the breast: some uncommon cases. Aesthet Plast Surg. 1994; 18(4):399–403.
46. Glicksman CA, Ferenz SE. The etiologies of chest wall and breast asymmetry and improvement in breast augmentation. Clin Plast Surg. 2015;42(4):519–30.
47. Lawrence RA, Lawrence RM. Breastfeeding: a guide for the medical profession. 5th ed. St. Louis: Mosby; 1999. p. 35–57.
48. Hosokawa K, Hata Y, Yano K, Susuki T, Kikui T, Tahara S. Unilateral athelia with a subcutaneous dermoid cyst. Plast Reconstr Surg. 1987;80(5):732–4.
49. Ishida LH, Alves HR, Munhoz AM, Kaimoto C, Ishida LC, Saito FL, Gemperlli R, Ferreira MC. Athelia: case report and review of the literature. Br J Plast Surg. 2005;58(6):833–7.
50. Baris H, Tan WH, Kimonis VE. Hypothelia, syndactyly, and ear malformation--a variant of the scalp-ear-nipple syndrome?: Case report and review of the literature. Am J Med Genet A. 2005;134A(2):220–2.
51. Mollica F, Mazzone D, Cimino G, Opitz JM. Severe case of Al Awadi/Raas-Rothschild syndrome or new, possibly autosomal recessive facio-skeleto-genital syndrome. Am J Med Genet. 1995;56(2):168–72.
52. Greenberg F. Choanal atresia and athelia: methimazole teratogenicity or a new syndrome? Am J Med Genet. 1987;28(4):931–4.
53. Douchement D, Rakza T, Holder M, Bonne NX, Fayoux P. Choanal atresia associated with tracheoesophageal fistula: the spectrum of carbimazole embryopathy. Pediatrics. 2011;128(3):e703–6.
54. Foley J, Dann P, Hong J, Cosgrove J, Dreyer B, Rimm D, Dunbar M, Philbrick W, Wysolmerski J. Parathyroid hormone-related protein maintains mammary epithelial fate and triggers nipple skin differentiation during embryonic breast development. Development. 2001;128(4):513–25.
55. Borck G, de Vries L, Wu HJ, Smirin-Yosef P, Nürnberg G, Lagovsky I, Ishida LH, Thierry P, Wieczorek D, Nürnberg P, Foley J, Kubisch C, Basel-Vanagaite L. Homozygous truncating PTPRF mutation causes athelia. Hum Genet. 2014;133(8):1041–7.
56. Schmidt H. Supernumerary nipples: prevalence, size, sex and side predilection -- a prospective clinical study. Eur J Pediatr. 1998;157(10):821–3.
57. Mehregan AH. Supernumerary nipple. A histologic study. J Cutan Pathol. 1981;8(2):96–104.
58. Mimouni F, Merlob P, Reisner SH. Occurrence of supernumerary nipples in newborns. Am J Dis Child. 1983;137(10):952–3.
59. Jaber L, Merlob P. The prevalence of supernumerary nipples in Arab infants and children. Eur J Pediatr. 1988;147(4):443.
60. Metzker A. Supernumerary nipple. www.emedicine.com/derm/topic 735.htm. Accessed 7 May 2015.
61. Leung AKC, Robson LM. Polythelia. Int J Dermatol. 1989;28(7):429–33.
62. Hall BK. Atavismus and atavistic mutations. Nat Genet. 1995;10(2):126–7.
63. Hersh JH, Bloom AS, Cromer AO, Harrison HL, Weisskopf B. Does a supernumerary nipple/renal field defect exist? Am J Dis Child. 1987;141(9): 989–91.

64. Toumbis-Joannou E, Cohen PR. Familial polythelia. J Am Acad Dermatol. 1994;30(4):667–8.
65. Urbani CE, Betti R. The significance of familial polythelia. J Am Acad Dermatol. 1995;32(4):687–8.
66. Urbani CE, Betti R. Sporadic unilateral intra-areolar polythelia. Acta Derm Venerol. 1996;76(2):156.
67. Arranz López JL, García L, Elena E, Benito P, De Juan A. Unilateral dichotomy of nipple (intraareolar polythelia) and areola: report of a case and surgical correction. Aesthet Plast Surg. 2006;30(4):494–6.
68. Jain M, Jain S, Roy S. Intra-areolar polythelia in pregnancy: a rare anomaly. J Obstet Gynaecol. 2013;33(8):626–32.
69. Rintala A, Norio R. Familial intra-areolar polythelia with mammary hypoplasia. Scand J Plast Reconstr Surg. 1982;16(3):287–91.
70. Shewmake SW, Izuno GT. Supernumerary areolae. Arch Dermatol. 1977;113(6):823–5.
71. Sivan Y, Merlob P, Reisner SH. Sternum length, torso length and internipple distance in newborn infants. Pediatrics. 1983;72(4):523–5.
72. Hassan Z, Karna P, Dolanski EA. Intermamillary indices in premature infants. Am J Perinatol. 1988;5(1):54–6.
73. Leung AK, Kao CP, Sauve RS, Fang JH, Leong AG, Liu EK. Internipple distance and internipple index. J Natl Med Assoc. 2004;96(8):1092–6.
74. Fleisher DS. Lateral displacement of the nipple, a sign of bilateral renal hypoplasia. J Pediatr. 1966;69(5):806–9.
75. Han S, Hong YG. The inverted nipple: its grading and surgical correction. Plast Reconstr Surg. 1999;104(2):384–95.
76. Schwager RG, Smith JW, Gray GF, Goulian DJ. Inversion of the human female nipple, with a simple method of treatment. Plast Reconstr Surg. 1974;54(5):564–9.
77. Park HS, Yoon CH, Kim HJ. The prevalence of congenital inverted nipples. Aesthet Plast Surg. 1999;23(2):144–6.
78. Crestinu JM. Inverted nipple: the new method of correction. Aesthet Plast Surg. 1989;13(3):189–97.
79. Shafir R, Bonne-Tamir B, Ashbel S, Tsur H, Goodman RM. Genetic studies in a family with inverted nipples (mammillae invertita). Clin Genet. 1979;15(4):346–50.
80. Scholten E. A contemporary correction of inverted nipples. Plast Reconstr Surg. 2001;107(2):511–3.
81. Gould DJ, Nadeau MH, Macias LH, Stevens WG. Inverted nipple repair revisited: a 7-year experience. Aesthet Surg J. 2015;35(2):156–64.

# Men's Nipple-Areola Complex

# 3

Richard Vaucher and Raphael Sinna

## 3.1 Introduction

The chest wall for women and for men ends unavoidably with the nipple-areola complex (NAC) constituted by the areola and the nipple. The NAC is an essential component of the aesthetic of the breast and the anterior chest wall.

The areola is constituted by protuberances associated with several types of glands: Montgomery's tubers (similar to the sweat glands), allowing the evacuation of the sweat, which are around 30 per nipple, and sebaceous glands without hairy follicles, situated around the areola. The areola, just like the nipple, is protected by a hyperpigmented thin skin including dermal clusters.

From an anatomical and physiopathological point of view, the mammary gland exists in nor mal man, but it is of an infantile type reduced to a simple mammary bud and often considered as a vestige of sexual differentiation.

The surgical approach of gynecomastia, the sexual reassignment surgery in female-to-male transsexuals, and the increase number of post-bariatric patients wishing to turn to plastic surgery led us to deepen the anatomical knowledge of the nipple-areola complex (NAC) in men, which is poorly dealt with in the literature. The aesthetic aspect for men, which has in the past been neglected, takes on quite another social dimension today.

## 3.2 Where Is the NAC in Men?

The most important stage and certainly the most difficult to define the NAC position and dimension is its localization on the men's thorax. A mistaken position, as in women, can lead to an unaesthetic result. Various measurements can be necessary to analyze the position (Figs. 3.1 and 3.2):

Internipple distance (Em): distance between the middle of both areolas

Thoracic length (Lt): distance from interaxillary line, the arm against the body via the internipple line

Sternal notch (internipple line (Sm)): distance between the sternal notch and the middle of the internipple line

Thoracic circumference (Cf): distance of the thoracic circumference passing by the axillary hollow

Umbilicus-sternal notch (Os): distance between the upper pole of the navel and the middle of the upper pole sternal notch

Sternal notch-areola (Sa): distance between the middle of the upper pole of the sternal notch and the middle of the areola

Nipple diameter (Dm)

R. Vaucher, M.D. (✉) • R. Sinna
Department of Plastic, Reconstructive and Aesthetic Surgery, Amiens University Hospital,
Site Sud, Amiens Cedex 1 80054, France
e-mail: richardvaucher@gmail.com


M.A. Shiffman (ed.), *Nipple-Areolar Complex Reconstruction*,
https://doi.org/10.1007/978-3-319-60925-6_3

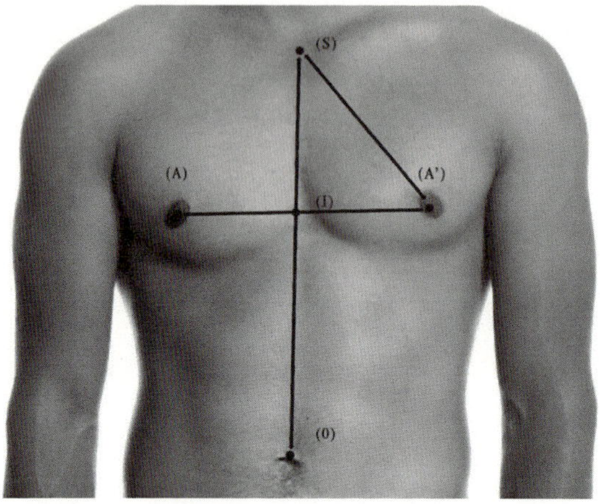


**Fig. 3.1** Measurements. (AA′) Internipple distance. (SO) Distance between sternal notch and the upper side of the umbilicus. (SA′ = SA) Distance between the sternal notch and the middle of the nipple. (*I*) Intersection between the internipple line and the medio-sternal line

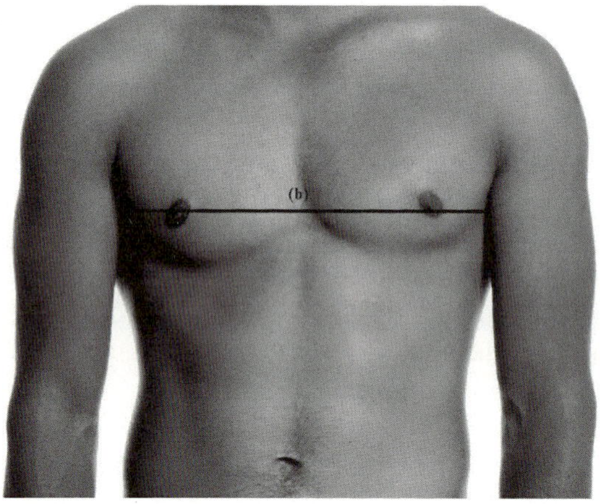


**Fig. 3.2** Landmarks. (b) Interaxillary line

Areola diameter (Da)
Horizontal position of the nipple (Em/Lt)
Vertical position of the nipple (Sm/Os)

The subjective character of the positioning and the size of the NAC are linked to the differences of the size and weight of the subject. There is no one size and diameter of the areola and the nipple; everything is a question of proportionality. If it is advisable to define the position of the NAC, it is then necessary to establish it according to the weight (body mass index (BMI)) and to the size of the subject.

During surgery for post-bariatric sequela management or for gynecomastia, the repositioning of the nipple is not as frequent as in mastectomies for sex reassignment where the repositioning is almost systematic. However, the positioning/decrease of size of the NAC, after an upper body lift, is an important stage for the outcome and a harmonious result. Drawings can be done in the preoperative stage according to the new circumference and the thoracic amplitude predefined in order to position the NAC harmoniously.

As a result of our work [1], we ended up defining a more lateral position subjects presenting a high IMC and a lower vertical position for tall people. For a person presenting a BMI in the standard (defined by the World Health Organization) 22.7 ± 1.4 kg/m$^2$, the position of the nipple retained should be the intersection of the internipple line and the vertical axis of the sternal notch, and the umbilicus should be in 16.1 ± 2.5 cm of the sternal notch (Sm). The distance between the middle of the sternal notch and the middle of the nipple (Sa) is 18.1 ± 2.8 cm, the internipple distance (Em) of 21.7 ± 1.3 cm, the areola diameter (Da) of 2.9 ± 0.5 cm, and the nipple diameter (Dm) of 0.5 ± 0.15 cm.

For an overweight person presenting with a BMI in the standard (defined by the World Health Organization) of 28.2 ± 1.9 kg/m$^2$ (BMI), there will be a distance (Sm) of 1.8 ± 3.1 cm, a distance (Sa) of 21 ± 4 cm, an internipple distance (Em) of 26.5 ± 3.5 cm, one diameter (Da) of 3.4 ± 0.6 cm, and one diameter (Dm) of 0.6 ± 0.2 cm.

For Shulman et al. [2], the positioning of the NAC can be defined by the relation between three correlations:

The height of the PAM (standing patient: distance between the ground and the middle of the areola) = (0.668 × height) 9.491.

Ratio of the internipple distance (Em) - thoracic circumference (Cf) = (0.190 × thoracic circumference) + 2.192.

Ratio of the distance between the middle of the sternal notch and middle of the areola and the size of the patient = (0.120 × height) −2.782.

The first two parameters allow the surgeon to position the NAC and the third to verify the right

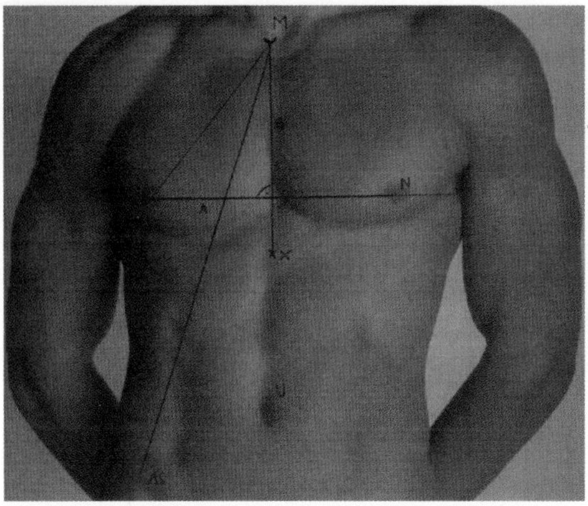

**Fig. 3.3** Beer et al. [3] measurements. *M* sternal notch, *U* umbilicus, *AC* acromioclavicular joint, *AS* anterosuperior iliac spine. *Horizontal line*: circumference of the thorax. Line A and B intersection (*S*) determines the nipple-areola complex localization

correlation. This method has been defined for patients who are not obese.

For Beer et al. [3], the position of the NAC can be defined as the combination of two measures: the thoracic circumference and the height of the sternal notch (distance between the middle of the upper pole of the sternal notch and the xiphoid). So by the means of the following algorithms, they define the horizontal position of the NAC (A) cm = 2.4 + (0.09 × thoracic circumference) and its vertical position (B) cm = 1.2 + (0.28 × sternal height) + (0.1 × thoracic circumference) (Fig. 3.3).

**Conclusions**

Finally, these measurements that different authors tried to find in order to improve their surgical results are just landmarks to help us during surgery. Just as most of plastic surgery which relies more of a subjective assessment, and then scientific measurements, the positioning of the NAC is often realized depending on the appreciation and the experience of the surgeon. The unique anatomical character of each patient will never allow the surgeon only to use measurements. However, the opinion and especially the experience of the surgeon in the positioning of the PAM could be supported by standardized measurement tools and most particularly at the beginning of the new surgeon's training.

## References

1. Vaucher R, Dast S, Assaf N, Sinna R. Men's nipple areola complex. Ann Chir Plast Esthet. 2016;61(3):206–11.
2. Shulman O, Badani E, Wolf Y, Hauben DJ. Appropriate location of the nipple-areola complex in males. Plast Reconstr Surg. 2001;108(2):348–51.
3. Beer GM, Budi S, Seifert B, Morgenthaler W, Infanger M, Meyer VE. Configuration and localization of the nipple-areola complex in men. Plast Reconstr Surg. 2001;108(7):1947–52.

# Vascular Anatomy of the Breast and Nipple-Areola Complex

4

Petrus van Deventer

## 4.1 Introduction

Cooper [1] and Manchot [2] were the pioneers in describing the blood supply of the breast.

Since then, a paucity in research studies followed. These included research of Würinger [3], van Deventer [4], Marcus [5], O'Dey [6], Salmon [7], Nakajima [8], Anson and Wright [9], le Roux et al. [10] and Seitz et al. [11].

The study by Palmer and Taylor [12] was not specifically aimed on the blood supply of the breast but on the vascular architecture of the thoracic wall which has improved our understanding of the anastomoses between the major vessels and the location of their perforating branches, some of which supply the breast.

## 4.2 Main Sources

### 4.2.1 Internal Thoracic Artery

#### 4.2.1.1 Nomenclature

The internal thoracic artery is commonly referred to in textbooks as the internal mammary artery. Although this artery is the most important blood supplier of the breast, it also supplies the thoracic wall with its intercostal branches, the upper abdominal wall with its superior epigastric branch and the diaphragm with its musculophrenic branch. Therefore, the term internal thoracic is more appropriate for this artery.

The perforating branches 1–4 of the internal thoracic artery are the most reliable sources of blood supply to the nipple-areola complex (NAC) [4, 11, 13, 14]. The pattern of supply is a basic horizontal segmental one with the branches taking a meandering course laterally passing above and below the NAC to anastomose with branches of the lateral thoracic artery (Fig. 4.1). Most frequently found was the third perforator, followed by the second, the first and the least the fourth. If the development of the branches from the lateral thoracic artery is deficient or absent, the horizontal pattern can change into a variety of different patterns. Therefore, a ring anastomosis encircling the NAC can be found or even an oblique vertical pattern due to anastomoses between the perforators of the internal thoracic artery with branches of the anterior intercostal arteries (Fig. 4.2).

P. van Deventer, M.B.Ch.B., M.Med.Sc., M.Med. (✉)
Division of Plastic and Reconstructive Surgery, University of Stellenbosch, Tygerberg 7505, South Africa

Faculty of Health Sciences, University of Stellenbosch, Tygerberg 7505, South Africa
e-mail: peetvandeventer@telkomsa.net, pvvandeventer@gmail.com


M.A. Shiffman (ed.), *Nipple-Areolar Complex Reconstruction*,
https://doi.org/10.1007/978-3-319-60925-6_4

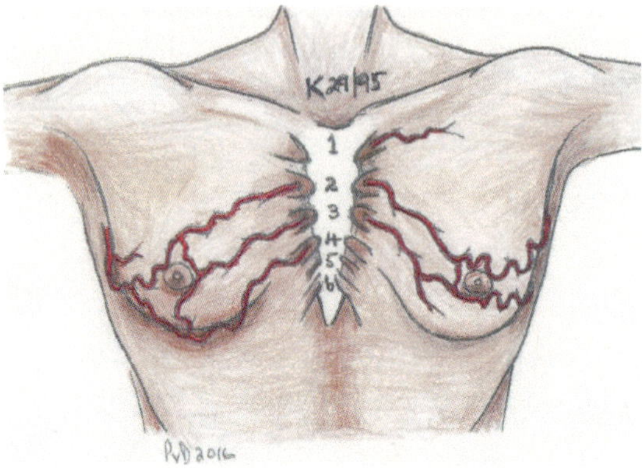


**Fig. 4.1** The basic horizontal segmental blood supply to the NAC. Note the absence of branches from the anterior intercostal arteries to supply the nipple in the left breast

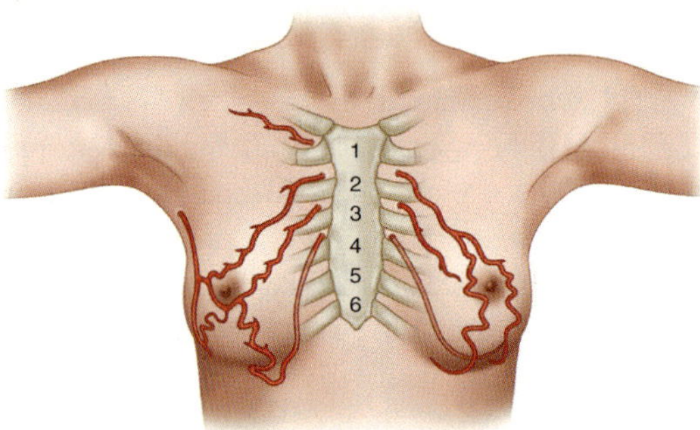


**Fig. 4.2** In the left breast, an oblique vertical pattern of blood supply to the NAC is seen due to the absence of the lateral thoracic artery and anastomoses between the perforators of the internal thoracic artery and branches from the anterior intercostal arteries

### 4.2.2 Lateral Thoracic Artery

This artery is a branch of the axillary artery, but it may arise from the acromio-thoracic artery [15]. It runs along the lateral border of the pectoralis minor muscle on the lateral thoracic wall.

The lateral thoracic artery supplies the NAC with two and sometimes three branches, most frequently anastomosing with the perforators of the internal thoracic artery above and below the nipple (Figs. 4.1 and 4.3). It is one of the major sources of supply to the NAC but not as reliable as the internal thoracic artery because studies have demonstrated complete absence of this artery in some instances [4, 15].

### 4.2.3 Anterior Intercostal Arteries

Branches from the fourth to the sixth anterior intercostal arteries supply the NAC inferiorly (Figs. 4.2 and 4.3). Sometimes more than one branch from the same intercostal artery. It is also a major source of blood supply to the NAC but may be absent in certain individuals (Fig. 4.1) [4].

### 4.2.4 Acromio-thoracic Artery (Thoracoacromial Artery)

The acromio-thoracic artery is a branch of the axillary artery which after piercing the clavipectoral fascia divides in four branches. The pectoral branch running inferiorly between the pectoral muscles reaching on the inferior border of pectoralis major muscle sends off superficial branches to the skin. The contribution to the blood supply of the nipple is debatable, but it is an important main source of blood supply to the breast due to the fact that the lateral thoracic artery frequently arises from it [15].

## 4.3 Other Sources of Blood Supply

The superficial thoracic artery described by Manchot, posterior intercostal artery and superior intercostal artery are not frequently present to supply the breast and NAC.

### 4.3.1 Anastomoses and Different Patterns of Supply to the NAC

Most frequent anastomoses are found between the internal thoracic perforators and branches from the lateral thoracic arteries resulting in segmental loops in a horizontal pattern [4].

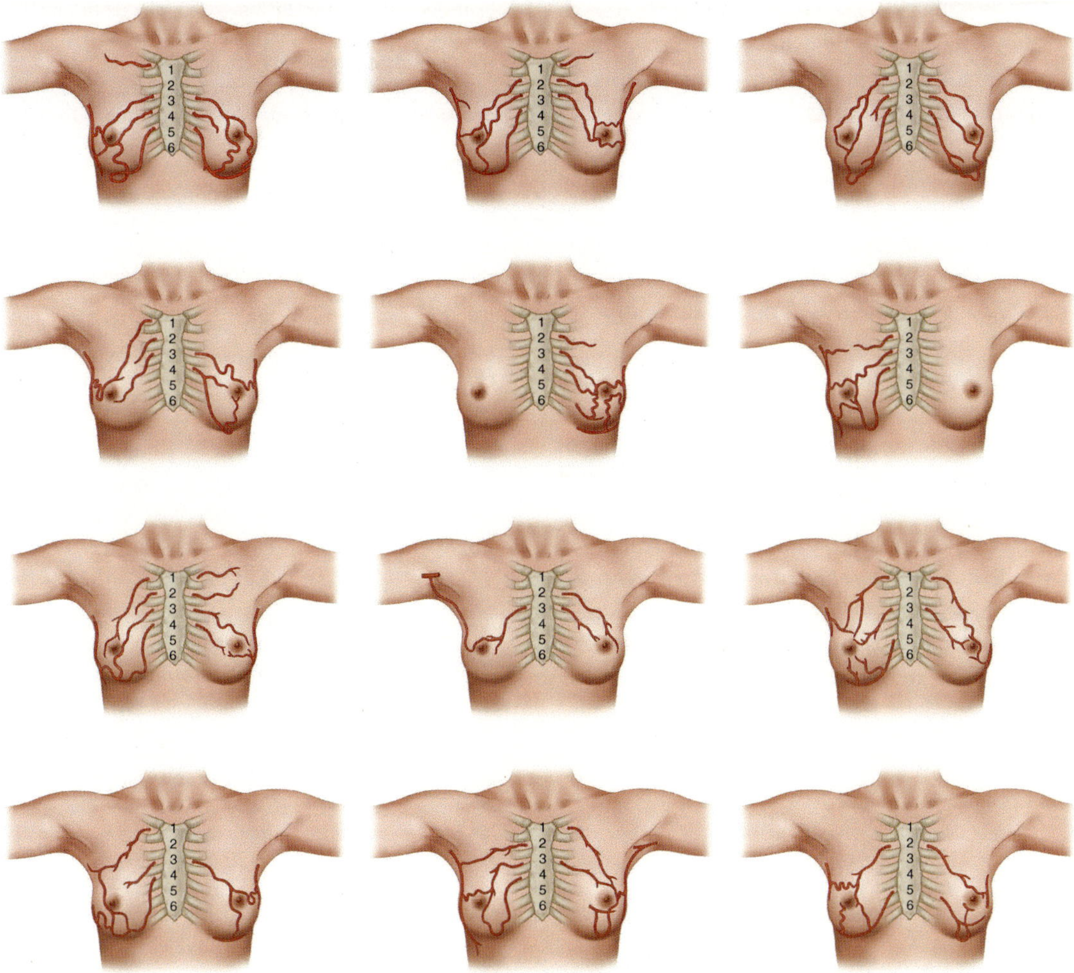

**Fig. 4.3** Dissections of female cadaver breasts demonstrating the variety of different patterns of blood supply to the NAC

If a main source is underdeveloped or absent, the supply to the NAC is usually enhanced by additional branches from remaining main sources resulting in change of the basic segmental pattern. A radial pattern of supply (Fig. 4.4) is seen in some instances but unfortunately not frequently, according to Marcus with an incidence of only 6%.

Many other patterns of supply do exist (Fig. 4.3) [4], but if cognisance of the location of the main sources and the basic horizontal segmental pattern is realised, it is easier to understand the blood supply to the breast.

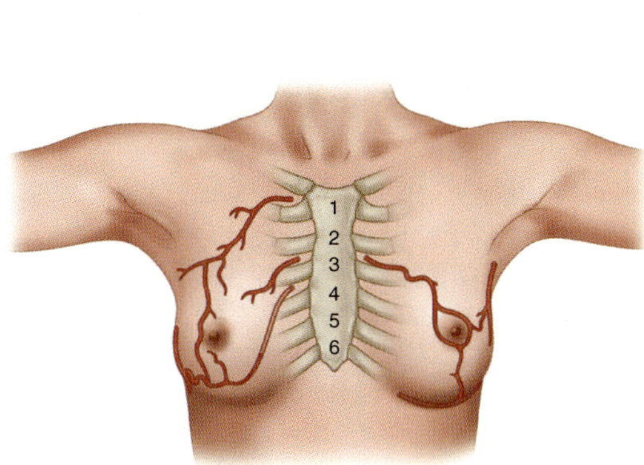


**Fig. 4.4** In the left breast, a radial pattern of blood supply to the NAC can be seen with branches from the internal thoracic, lateral thoracic and anterior intercostal arteries. Note that, in the right breast, the first and fourth perforators from the internal thoracic artery supply the NAC with the absence of the second and third perforators. A narrow-based supero-medial pedicle in that breast will therefore not be arterialised

## Conclusions

Due to the embryonic development, a basic horizontal segmental pattern similar to that of the thoracic wall exists.

The main sources are the internal thoracic, lateral thoracic, anterior intercostal and acromio-thoracic arteries. Branches from the main sources have fixed areas where they originate on the thoracic wall, but there can be a considerable variation in the pattern of blood supply to the NAC.

In some instances branches from a main source may be underdeveloped or absent, and their function is then taken over by branches of the other main sources changing the pattern of supply.

The most reliable source is the perforators of the internal thoracic artery. However, some of the perforators may be absent, and it is advisable to try and include the upper four perforators in the pedicle to ensure adequate blood supply to the NAC (Fig. 4.3).

## References


1. Cooper AP. Volume 1: On the anatomy of the breast. Pascal Brooke Bland: Longman, Orme, Green, Brown & Longmans, London, Harrison & Co printers; 1840. pp. 32–4, 74–8.
2. Manchot C. Die Haut Arterien des Menslichen Korpers. Leipzig: Vogel F.C.W. Erstes Capitel; 1899. p. 8–11.
3. Würinger E, Mader N, Posch E, Holle J. Nerve and vessel supplying ligamentous suspension of the mammary gland. Plast Reconstr Surg. 1998;101:1486–93.
4. Van Deventer PV. The blood supply to the nipple-areola complex of the human mammary gland. Aesthet Plast Surg. 2004;28:393–8.
5. Marcus GH. Unter suchungen uber die arterielle blutversorgung der mamilla. Arch Klin Chir. 1934;179:361–9.
6. O'Dey DM, Pallua N, Perscher A. Vascular reliability of nipple-areola complex bearing pedicles: an anatomical microdissection study. Plast Reconstr Surg. 2006;119:1167–77.
7. Salmon M. Les artères de la glande mammaire. Ann Anat Pathol. 1939;16:477–500.
8. Nakajima H, Imanishi N, Aiso S. Arterial anatomy of the nipple-areola complex. Plast Reconstr Surg. 1995;96:843–5.
9. Anson BJ, Wright RR, Wolfer JH. Blood supply of the mammary gland. Surg Gynecol Obstet. 1939;69:468–73.
10. Le Roux CM, Birgitte JK, Wei-Ren P, Warren MR, Mark WA. Preserving the neurovascular supply in the Hall-Findlay superomedial pedicle breast reduction: an anatomical study. JPRAS. 2009;63:655–62.
11. Seitz IA, Nixon AT, Friedewald SM, Rimler JC, Schechter LS. "NACsomes": a new classification system of the blood supply to the nipple areola complex (NAC) based on diagnostic breast MRI exams. JPRAS. 2015;68(6):792–9.
12. Palmer JH, Taylor GI. The vascular territories of the anterior chest wall. Br J Plast Surg. 1986;39:287–99.
13. Van Deventer PV, Page BJ, Graewe FR. The safety of pedicles in breast reduction and mastopexy procedures. Aesthet Plast Surg. 2008;32:307–12.
14. Loukas M, du Plessis M, Owens DG, Kinsella CR Jr, Litchfield CR, Nacar A, Lu O, Tubbs RS. The lateral thoracic artery revisited. Surg Radiol Anat. 2014;36(6):543–9.
15. Van Deventer PV, Graewe FR. Enhancing pedicle safety in mastopexy and breast reduction procedures: the posteroinferomedial pedicle, retaining the medial vertical ligament of Würinger. Plast Reconstr Surg. 2010;126:786–93.

# Blood Supply to the Nipple–Areola Complex and Intraoperative Imaging of Nipple Perfusion Patterns

**5**

Mingsha Zhou, Irene Wapnir and David Kahn

## 5.1 Introduction

The anatomy of the blood supply to the breast was first studied by Cooper and Manchot in the nineteenth century. They described a radial pattern of blood supply to the nipple–areola complex (NAC). More recent studies show a segmental pattern of blood supply, from four main arterial sources. A better understanding of the blood supply to the NAC allows more informed designs of pedicled flaps and soft tissue resection. New technologies used in intraoperative imaging permit direct visualization of blood flow to the NAC during breast surgery and complement clinical judgment in tissue resection and preservation.

M. Zhou, M.D., C.M.
Université de Montréal, CP 6128, Succ. Centre-ville, Pavillon Roger-Gaudry - Local S-716, 2900 Edouard Montpetit Blvd, Montréal, QC H3C 3J7, Canada
e-mail: mingsha.zhou@umontreal.ca

I. Wapnir, M.D.
Stanford Womens Cancer Center, 900 Blake Wilbur, Stanford, CA 94305, USA
e-mail: wapnir@stanford.edu

D. Kahn, M.D.
Department of Plastic Surgery, Stanford University, 1000 Welch Road, Suite 100, MC 5348, Palo Alto, CA 94304, USA
e-mail: David.Kahn@Stanford.edu

## 5.2 Anatomy

Blood supply to the breast comes primarily from the internal thoracic, lateral thoracic, anterior intercostal, and acromiothoracic arteries [1]. Studies have shown considerable variation in the contribution of branches of these arteries to the NAC.

The internal thoracic artery is the most reliable vascular supply of the breast, via its perforators from the four upper intercostal spaces, of which one or more supply the NAC. These intercostal perforators anastomose with branches of the lateral thoracic artery. Perforators of the third intercostal space are usually the dominant blood supply to the breast and the most reliable supply of the NAC. The most frequent variations are, in order, the second, the first, and the fourth intercostal space perforators. The depth of the perforators is approximately 10.3 mm at the NAC boundary and 14.2 mm at 3 cm medial to the NAC [2].

The lateral thoracic artery gives off one to three branches which anastomose with branches of the internal thoracic artery above and below the NAC. The lateral thoracic artery can originate from the axillary artery or the thoracoacromial artery. The anterior intercostal arteries supply the NAC with branches from the fourth to sixth intercostal spaces. The posterior intercostal, superficial thoracic, superior intercostal (highest intercostal), and highest thoracic arteries occasionally also supply blood to the breast. Anastomoses between the internal thoracic and


M.A. Shiffman (ed.), *Nipple-Areolar Complex Reconstruction*,
https://doi.org/10.1007/978-3-319-60925-6_5

lateral thoracic arteries exist in 50% of cadaver dissections and follow the segmental pattern of blood supply to the breast.

Hypervascular zones, where major cutaneous perforators emerge, fall along the medial, lateral, and inferior perimeter of the breast. They coincide with fixed skin areas, around the perimeter of the pectoralis major muscle, the costal margin, and the lateral chest wall overlying the interdigitations of the serratus anterior muscle. The hypovascular plane of the breast is the anterior surface of the pectoralis major muscle.

## 5.3 Clinical Application

The variation in blood supply to the NAC implies that a surgeon cannot know the exact vascular pattern of a NAC being operated on, short of direct visualization. Therefore, including branches from more than one main source is safer. In inferior pedicle techniques, preserving the horizontal septum retains branches of the anterior intercostal arteries, and preserving the medial vertical ligament retains perforators of the internal thoracic artery, assuring a dual blood supply. Dual blood supply from the lateral thoracic and anterior intercostal arteries can be created by preserving the lateral vertical ligament with the horizontal septum. In superomedial pedicle techniques, preserving the upper four perforators of the internal thoracic artery with a wide-based pedicle ensures adequate blood supply to the NAC.

## 5.4 Imaging for NSM

During the past decade, nipple-sparing mastectomies (NSM) have gained acceptance in the field of breast surgical oncology and are offered today to a continuously growing number of breast cancer patients [1–5]. Its use is being extended to women who present with multicentric lesions, tumors in closer proximity to the NAC, or following neoadjuvant chemotherapy [6–8]. Inadequate skin perfusion to the NAC is the Achilles heel of this operation, as illustrated in Fig. 5.1, of a woman who experienced significant ischemia after a NSM via an inframammary fold (IMF) incision. Acute or subacute ischemia can lead to wound infection, wound dehiscence, or implant exposure. Less severe complications such as superficial eschar formation or epidermolysis are much more common, ~30%, and impact negatively on the long-term appearance of the NAC [3].

Studies from 2011 to 2012 have reported a higher rate of perfusion deficit with incisions that combine circumareolar and radial approaches and lowest rates with vertical infra-areolar incisions [4, 5]. Carlson et al.'s study [6] on 71 NSM with immediate reconstruction has reported that inframammary fold incisions have the lowest rate of NAC necrosis (19%), followed by radial incision (33%), while periareolar (60%) and vertical incisions (50%) have the highest rate of NAC necrosis. Inframammary fold incisions have been associated with higher rates of tumor-involved margins however [7].

### 5.4.1 Fluorescein Dye Angiography

Perfusion to the NAC is imaged intraoperatively most commonly by fluorescein dye angiography or near-infrared (NIR) imaging. Fluorescein dye angiography is an older technique, first used to assess skin perfusion in the 1940s and first applied to mastectomy skin flap perfusion imaging around 1970 [8]. Fluorescein's injection to optimal imaging time is 15 min. It extravasates into extravascular space. Its half-life of 5 h only permits single use during an operation [9]. Intraoperative perfusion imaging-guided excisions decreased tissue necrosis and flap failure [10]. However, fluorescein dye angiography does not help predict the changes in perfusion in the hours following surgery. Causes of poor perfusion on fluorescein dye angiography cannot be differentiated into reversible, such as acute arterial constriction and vasospasm of skin vasculature, or irreversible, such as inadequate arterial supply to the NAC or venous blockage. For this reason, fluorescein overpredicts nonviability and could result in excessive

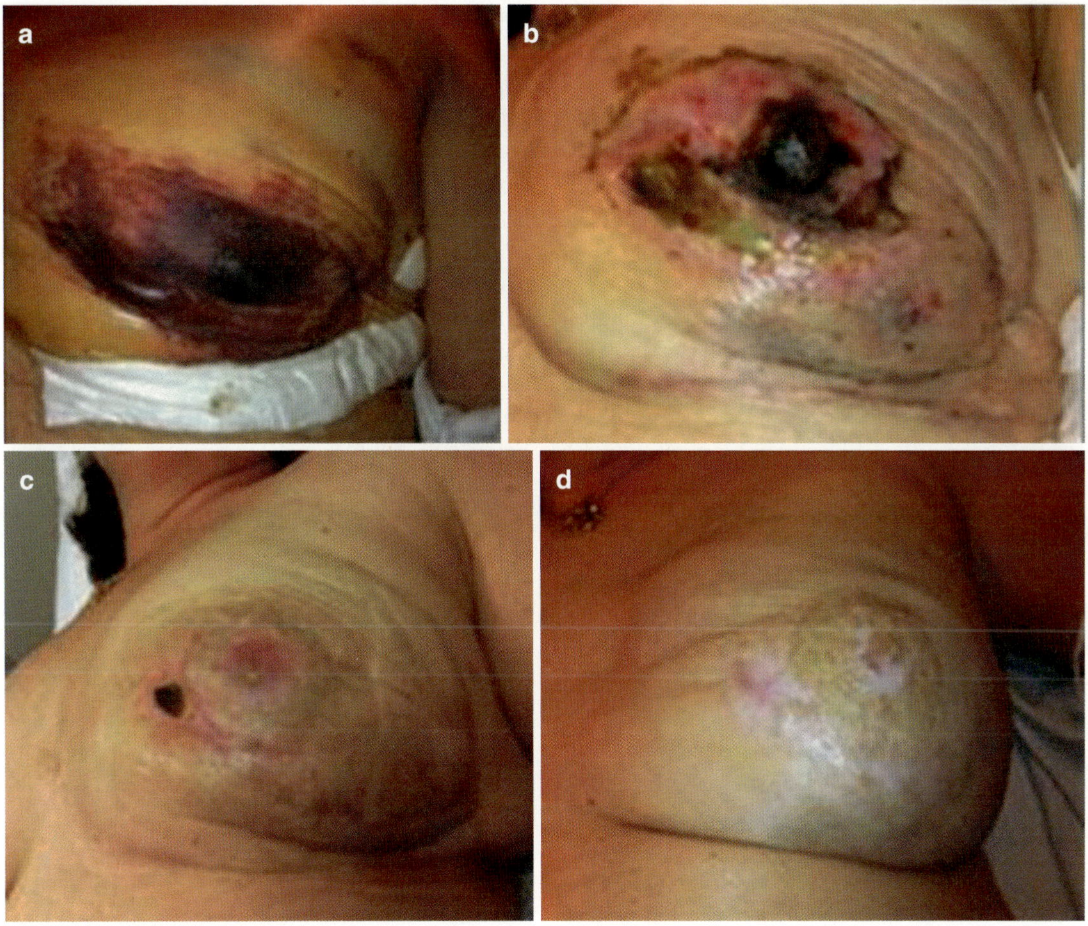

**Fig. 5.1** Long-term consequences of mastectomy flap ischemia. Nipple-sparing mastectomy via an inframammary fold without perfusion-guided surgery. (**a**) 7 days. (**b**) 17 days. (**c**) 8 weeks. (**d**) 1 year. Springer Annals of Surgical Oncology, Intraoperative Imaging of Nipple Perfusion Patterns and Ischemic Complications in Nipple-Sparing Mastectomies, 21, 2013, Supplementary material 1, Wapnir I, Dua M, Kieryn A, Paro J, Morrison D, Kahn D, Meyer S, Gurtner G., © Society of Surgical Oncology 2013, "With permission of Springer"

excision of tissue that otherwise can recover perfusion postoperatively and survive.

Losken et al. [9] used intravenous fluorescein dye on 50 consecutive periareolar incision skin-sparing mastectomy (SSM) flaps with autologous reconstruction. Fluorescein was found to be a sensitive test for ischemia but underpredicted survival. For areas of poor fluorescence, location on the skin flap, size, and history of radiation therapy can be used to determine likelihood of survival. Areas of nonfluorescence <4 $cm^2$ typically survive, except in the irradiated breast. Any area of nonfluorescence >4 $cm^2$ typically does not survive, except when located more proximally on the flap.

### 5.4.2 Near-Infrared Imaging

Near-infrared (NIR) imaging uses the deep photon penetration of NIR light into living tissue to image endogenous or exogenous contrast at <1 cm from the skin surface [11]. The three types of possible light sources for excitation of NIR fluorophores are filtered broadband sources, light-emitting diodes (LEDs), and laser diodes. Filtered broadband sources are the least efficient, with most photons discarded to filter excitation light to a narrow band and only a small fraction of the optical power propagating toward the surgical field. LEDs provide good power, spectral confinement, efficiency, and cost, but heat dissipation remains a challenge, and excitation filters must be used to reduce spectrum, collimators to reduce solid angle, and lenses to concentrate optical power. Laser diodes are the most efficient spatially and spectrally, but are subject to safety concerns related to maximum permissible exposure (MPE) and protective equipment, and require precise control in current and in temperature. LEDs are fit for local lighting, with the light source placed immediately above the patient, while laser diodes are the only practical option for remote lighting with a light guide. Excitation fluence rates are chosen based on the depth of the fluorophore, the f-number (f/#) of the collection optics, and the sensitivity of the charge-coupled device (CCD) camera. For simultaneous imaging of color video and NIR fluorescence emission, "white light" must be filtered to 400–650 nm, to isolate the color video channel from NIR fluorescence channels.

All currently available NIR imaging systems use laser diodes (SPY and Fluobeam) or LEDs (PDE, FLARE, and Mini-FLARE). SPY and PDE use 8-bit CCD cameras, and FLARE™, Mini-FLARE™, and Fluobeam use 12-bit cameras. Zeiss INFRARED 800 (Oberkochen, Germany) and Leica FL800 (Heerbrugg, Switzerland) are two surgical microscopes equipped with NIR fluorescence modules. They use broadband sources which are optimized for superficial tissue imaging and are used in neurosurgical applications.

NIR absorption and emission require double bonds in fluorophores. Seven to ten double bonds reach wavelengths of ~700 nm (methylene blue), and nine to twelve double bonds reach wavelengths of ~800 nm (indocyanine green (ICG)). Each double bond increases molecular weight and hydrophobicity of the fluorophore, which translates into poor aqueous solubility. Compact chemical structures have been developed, however, which permit NIR fluorescence and in vivo imaging. There are also various NIR fluorescent nanoparticles in preclinical development [12].

### 5.4.3 ICG Angiography

ICG angiography has both been described as infrared and near-infrared imaging. It has become the most common form of intraoperative imaging for mastectomy and breast reconstructions. ICG is a water-soluble tricarbocyanine dye with a peak spectral absorption at 800–810 nm when dissolved in blood. It rapidly binds to plasma proteins and remains in the intravascular space. It has a very fast clearance from tissues, which allows it to be used multiple times during the same procedure. It is excreted into bile unchanged. Persistent fluorescence indicative of plasma-bound ICG trapped within the perfusion zone suggests venous congestion [13]. Adequate intraoperative perfusion on ICG angiography correlates highly with reduced postoperative tissue necrosis and flap loss. Arterial-arteriolar filling is observed 20–30 seconds after ICG injection (Fig. 5.2). Diffuse skin fluorescence follows for a few seconds before there is filling of veins at approximately 30–45 s. After resection of underlying breast tissue, imaging sequences typically show slower filling and decreased overall fluorescence in the skin flaps. Adverse reactions are similar to fluorescein: nausea, vomiting, and vasovagal episodes, but less common, occurring in less than 0.2% of patients. A contraindication is iodine allergy due to its iodide content.

One specialized infrared camera-computer system that images ICG is the SPY Elite™ imaging system (Novadaq Technologies, Inc., Toronto, Canada; distributed in North America by LifeCell Corp., Branchburg, NJ). Perfusion imaging is performed after induction of general anesthesia and before mastectomy incision. 3 mL of ICG (2.5 g/mL) are injected intravenously followed by a 10 mL saline flush. Video recording begins immediately after injection and continues over 180 s [3]. Fluorescence or light colors represent blood flow on the infrared camera screen. Dark gray or black represents no blood flow.

Wapnir et al. [3] classified NAC perfusion into three circulatory patterns based on whether the arterial-arteriolar filling originated predominantly from the underlying breast tissue (V1), the surrounding skin (V2), or a combination of breast

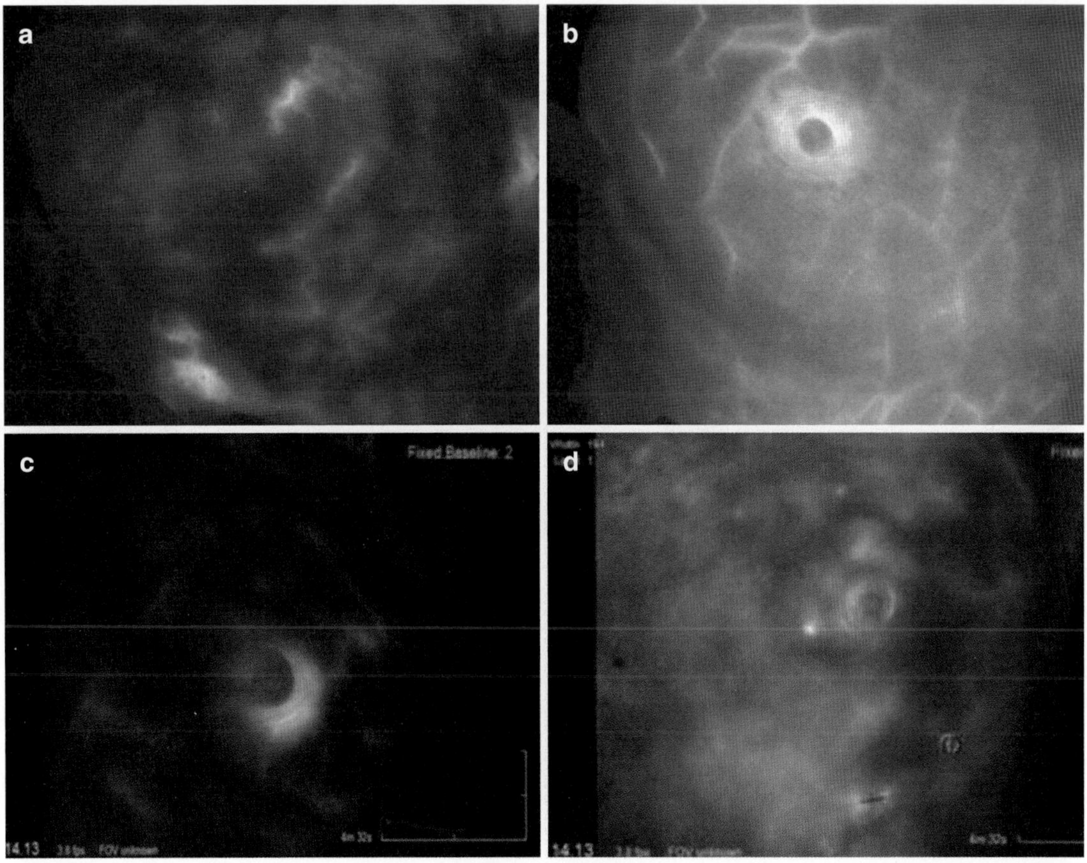


**Fig. 5.2** Physiologic blood flow to nipple–areola complex and nipple perfusion patterns. Blood supply to the nipple–areola complex was judged on the distribution of fluorescence captured in the initial frames during the baseline studies. (**a**) Normal arterial blood flow phase demonstrating V2 pattern, inflow from surrounding skin into nipple–areola complex; (**b**) venous phase; (**c**) V1 inflow predominantly from underlying breast tissue; (**d**) V3 inflow mixed pattern, combination of V1 and V2. Springer Annals of Surgical Oncology, Intraoperative Imaging of Nipple Perfusion Patterns and Ischemic Complications in Nipple-Sparing Mastectomies, 21, 2013, 100-106, Irene Wapnir, Monica Dua, Anne Kieryn, John Paro, Douglas Morrison, David Kahn, Shannon Meyer, and Geoffrey Gurtner, © Society of Surgical Oncology 2013, "With permission of Springer"

and surrounding skin (V3). They compared post-mastectomy skin perfusion to baseline assessments using the SPY Elite™ software to analyze the relative skin fluorescence in four or five regions of interests (ROIs). The ROIs were set at the nipple, right and left areolar edge, along the sternal border, and one additional selected location. ROIs did not overlie a vessel trajectory. Thirty-nine breasts in 24 patients underwent intraoperative ICG angiography during NSM and immediate reconstruction. Eighteen percent of breasts were found to have a V1 perfusion pattern from the underlying breast tissue, 46% of breasts have a V2 pattern from the surrounding skin, and 36% have a V3 pattern from both the surrounding skin and the underlying breast tissue (Table 5.1). One third of bilateral breast studies had discordant patterns between breasts, involving V2 and V3 patterns. ICG dye angiography identified severe ischemia in seven NACs and, when correlated with clinical judgment, led to the removal of six NACs intraoperatively and one 15 days later (Table 5.1).

The V1–V3 classification is useful for stratifying risk of NAC loss. V1 perfusion, from the underlying breast tissue, places a NAC at the highest risk of ischemia in NSM. Seventy-one percent of V1 perfusion patterns of NACs were removed intraoperatively for ischemia based on the absence of fluorescence and clinical

**Table 5.1** Perfusion pattern and outcome. Springer Annals of Surgical Oncology, Intraoperative Imaging of Nipple Perfusion Patterns and Ischemic Complications in Nipple-Sparing Mastectomies, 21, 2013, 103, Wapnir I, Dua M, Kieryn A, Paro J, Morrison D, Kahn D, Meyer S, Gurtner G., © Society of Surgical Oncology 2013, "With permission of Springer"

| Perfusion pattern baseline | Intraoperative post-Mx SPY imaging of NAC | | Incisions | | | Breast RT | Intraoperative resection of nipple | Postoperative < 45 days | | Outcome deficits |
|---|---|---|---|---|---|---|---|---|---|---|
| *N* (%) | Ischemia | Deficit | Periareolar ± radial extension | Radial | IMF | | *N* (%) | Epidermolysis/ partial skin flap necrosis | Necrosis NAC/ delayed removal | |
| V1 7 (18) | 5 | 2 | 3 | 4 | 0 | 1 | 5 (71) | 2 | 0 | |
| V2 18 (46) | 2 | 8 | 5 | 7 | 6 | 2[a] | 1 (11) | 4 | 1 | 3 Hypopigmentation |
| V3 14 (36) | 0 | 4 | 1 | 6 | 7 | 1[a] | 0 | 4 | 0 | 4 Hypopigmentation |

*Mx* mastectomy, *IMF* inframammary fold, *NAC* nipple-areolar complex
[a]Patient with bilateral breast cancer

judgment. The other two NACs with a V1 perfusion in this study also demonstrated epidermolysis of part of the NAC that resolved with conservative management. In contrast, V2 and V3 patterns of NACs had 11% and zero resection, respectively. Figures 5.3, 5.4, and 5.5 depict preincision and postmastectomy skin fluorescence. Wapnir et al. [3] have shown that ICG intraoperative imaging decreases postoperative complications by identifying ischemic areas.

Another ICG image capturing system is FLARE™ (Beth Israel Deaconess Medical Center, Boston, MA). Ashitate et al. [14] evalu-

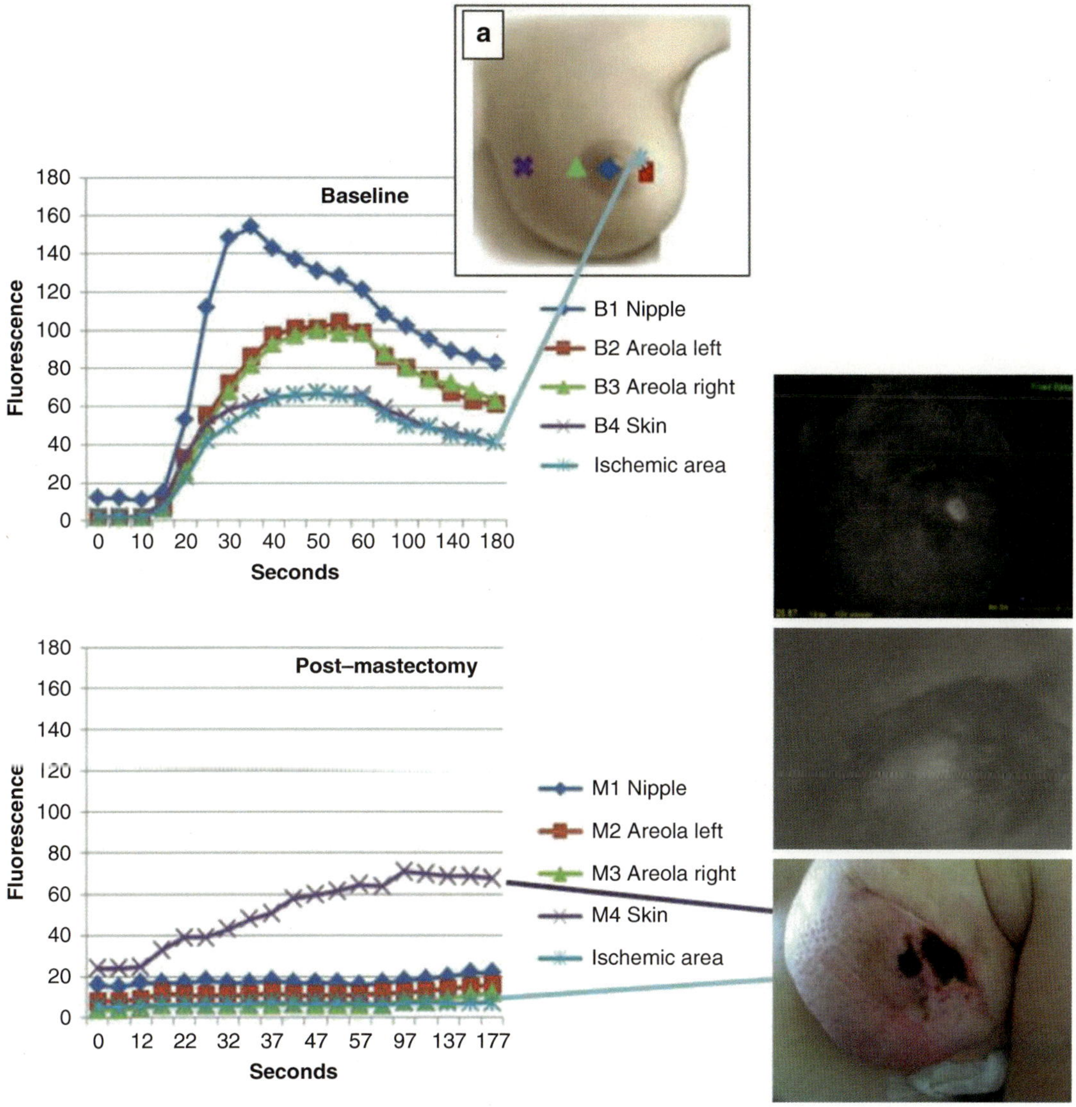


**Fig. 5.3** V3 perfusion pattern with ischemic area. Premenopausal patient who failed attempt at breast-conserving surgery. Mastectomy was performed by extending laterally upper-central quadrant lumpectomy incision. (**a**) Relative skin fluorescence was measured sequentially at points indicated in the picture: B1, nipple; B2, left areolar edge; B3, right areolar edge; and B4, parasternal skin. The corresponding areas in postmastectomy imaging are referred to as M1–M4. Decreased blood flow is noted in the NAC (*M1*) and ischemic area zone (*aqua line*) resulted in eschar formation, infection, and loss of tissue expander. Again, a slight increase in fluorescence is registered in parasternal ROI after mastectomy. Springer Annals of Surgical Oncology, Intraoperative Imaging of Nipple Perfusion Patterns and Ischemic Complications in Nipple-Sparing Mastectomies, 21, 2013, 103, Wapnir I, Dua M, Kieryn A, Paro J, Morrison D, Kahn D, Meyer S, Gurtner G., © Society of Surgical Oncology 2013, "With permission of Springer"

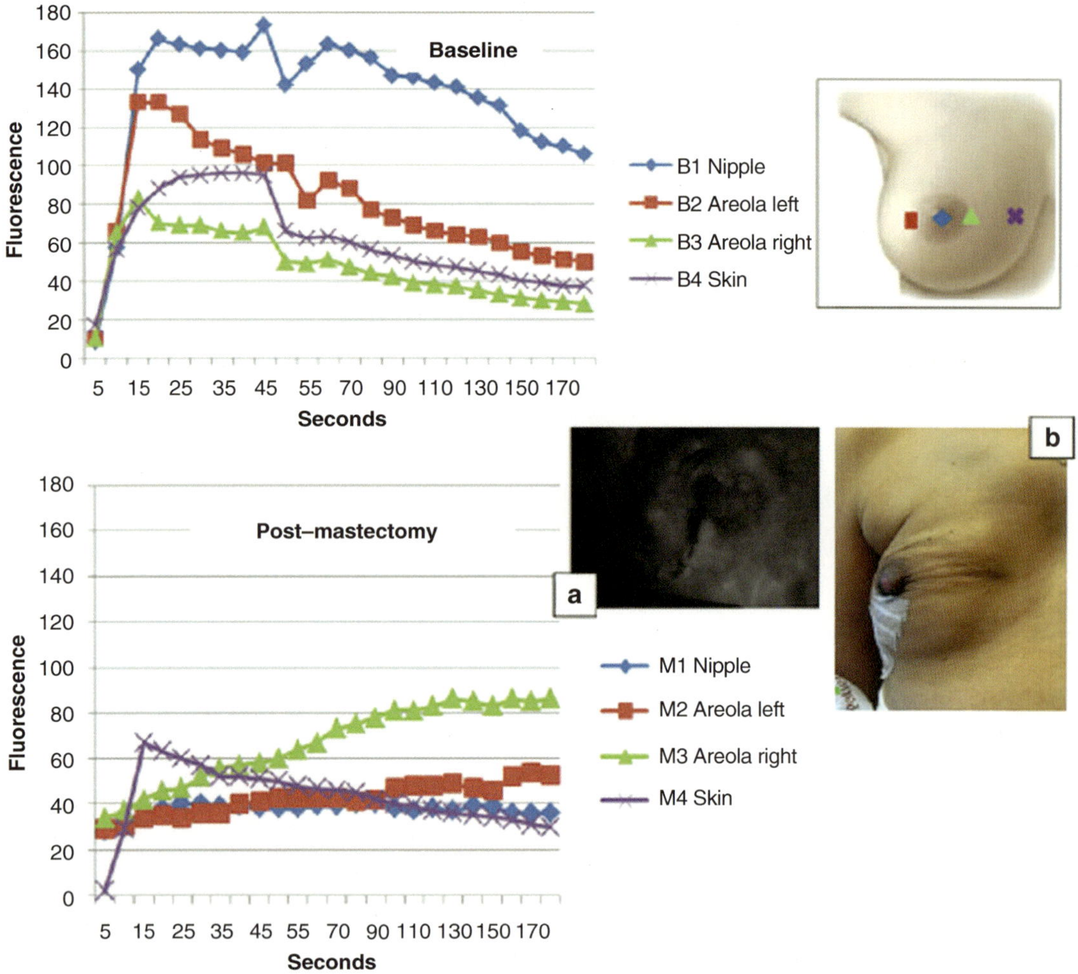


**Fig. 5.4** V2 perfusion pattern. Nipple-sparing mastectomy performed via a radial incision on a patient who underwent neoadjuvant chemotherapy. Postmastectomy imaging (**a**) indicated a compensatory increase in blood flow in right periareolar ROI compared to baseline study. The parasternal skin suffered the least amount of change in perfusion after mastectomy, while perfusion to the tip of the nipple exhibited the most dramatic decrease in blood flow. In spite of these changes, 3-week postoperative picture (**b**) shows slight superficial epidermolysis and overall good appearance of skin flaps. Springer Annals of Surgical Oncology, Intraoperative Imaging of Nipple Perfusion Patterns and Ischemic Complications in Nipple-Sparing Mastectomies, 21, 2013, 104, Wapnir I, Dua M, Kieryn A, Paro J, Morrison D, Kahn D, Meyer S, Gurtner G., © Society of Surgical Oncology 2013, "With permission of Springer"

ated two NSM incision models using NIR fluorescence to assess perfusion quantitatively in a porcine model. Periareolar and radial incisions were compared using FLARE™ and ICG and methylene blue, two NIR fluorophores with different distributions and half-lives. Methylene blue is extracted by many cell types and fluoresces for a longer duration than ICG. FLARE imaging's advantage over other NIR imaging systems is its two channels of NIR fluorescence which capture ICG and methylene blue's signal simultaneously. The authors found a circumareolar incision with no undermining to have the same perfusion as a nonoperated control. Periareolar and radial incisions both showed a decrease in fluorescence intensity with partial recovery postoperatively. The radial incision model had a higher perfusion than the periareolar incision at 72 h postoperative. ICG shows more variance than methylene blue due to its shorter NIR fluorescence signal.

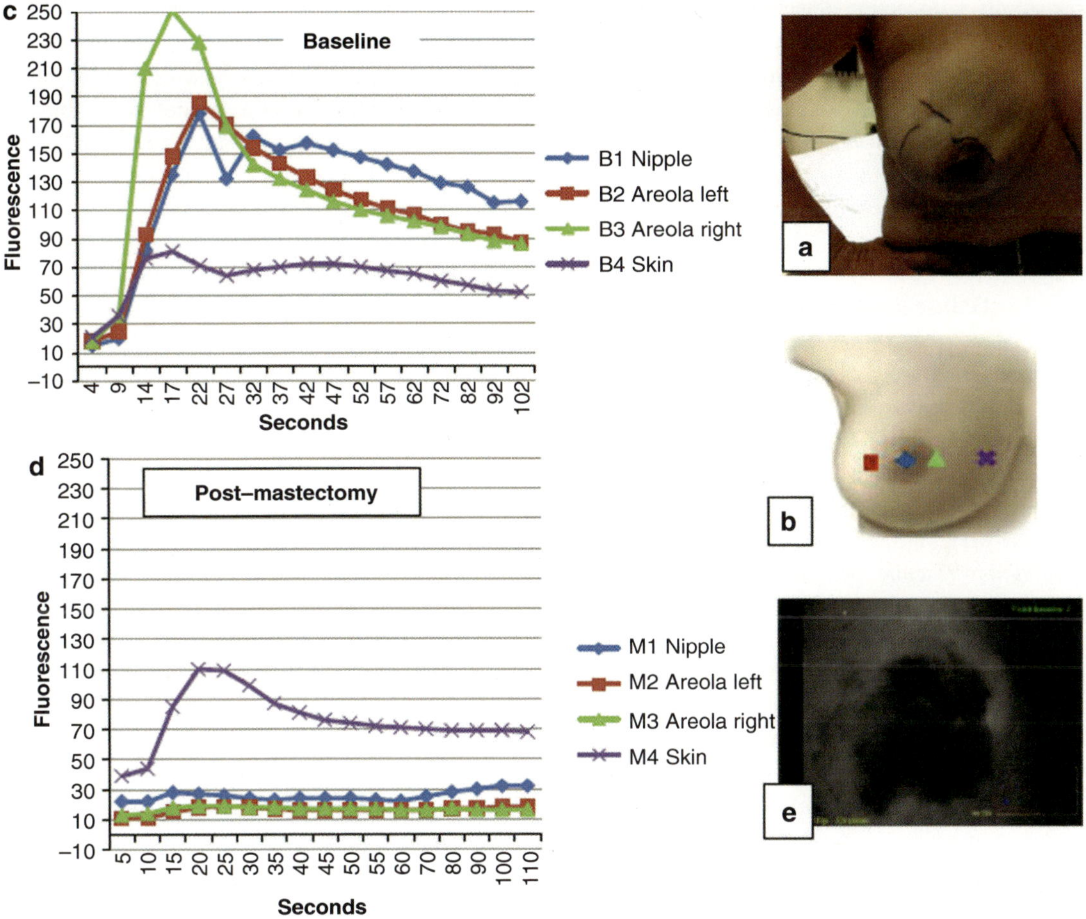


**Fig. 5.5** V1 perfusion pattern in a patient with multiple prior biopsy scars. Intraoperative imaging identifies central skin flap ischemia involving nipple–areola complex and surrounding skin. (**a**) Preoperative photograph depicting multiple preexisting surgical scars. A periareolar incision with radial extension was used for attempted nipple-sparing mastectomy. (**b**) Relative skin fluorescence was measured sequentially at points indicated in the picture. (**c**) Pre-mastectomy or baseline values are shown in graph and designated as B1, B2, B3, and B4. (**d**) Post nipple-sparing mastectomy values are graphed and designated as M1, M2, M3, and M4. (**e**) Corresponding postmastectomy perfusion deficit of NAC shown in a still photograph at approximately 120 s post ICG administration administration. Springer Annals of Surgical Oncology, Intraoperative Imaging of Nipple Perfusion Patterns and Ischemic Complications in Nipple-Sparing Mastectomies, 21, 2013, 105, Wapnir I, Dua M, Kieryn A, Paro J, Morrison D, Kahn D, Meyer S, Gurtner G., © Society of Surgical Oncology 2013, "With permission of Springer"

The cost-effectiveness of ICG fluorescence angiography in breast reconstruction after skin-sparing mastectomy was examined by Duggal et al. [15]. They compared 184 patients who underwent breast reconstruction before the introduction of ICG angiography and 184 patients who had ICG angiography intraoperatively. The use of ICG angiography was calculated to save $614 per patient.

ICG can also be used for sentinel lymph node detection and excision, alone or with methylene blue. Chi et al. [16] used a prototype surgical navigation system with a LED light source and two animal models, mice and rabbits, to demonstrate feasibility of lymph node detection with ICG. Following success in the animal studies, ICG angiography in 22 patients allowed detection of 59 lymph nodes, 8 of which contained metastases. Axillary dissection detected and removed 361 lymph nodes, 27 of which contained metastases. No side effects from ICG were reported. Chi's study confirms the safety of ICG use in axillary lymph node detection, but sensitivity is low, and much progress is still needed before ICG angiography becomes clinically reliable in metastasis detection.

### 5.4.4 Other Imaging Techniques

Doppler sonography can be used to monitor free flaps to the breast. A major limitation for intraoperative use is the need for a radiologist, as recipient vessels may be mistaken for the flap pedicle. The implantable Doppler system consists of an implantable 20-MHz ultrasonic probe that is wrapped around the vascular pedicle (either the artery or vein) and fixed to itself by micro-clips, sutures, or fibrin sealant. This system measures blood flow across microvascular anastomoses [17]. Its main limitations are the need for another surgery to remove the ultrasound probe, and arterial and venous flow cannot be evaluated simultaneously.

Laser Doppler flowmetry is a noninvasive monitoring method. A fiber-optic cable illuminates the tissue with coherent laser light. The light is scattered in tissues, some of it is collected and analyzed by the captor system. Density of the shifted light is a linear function of the average velocity of the cells moving within the tissue, and this principle is used to calculate the blood flow in the flap.

Tissue spectrophotometry and near-infrared spectroscopy (NIRS) measure relative changes in tissue concentrations of oxygenated, deoxygenated, and total hemoglobin. Hemoglobin, myoglobin, and cytochrome C oxidase are chromophores, molecules which change their optical properties when binding to oxygen. Oxygenated and deoxygenated hemoglobins have different absorption spectra and thus different optical signals. NIRS devices emit selected wavelengths of light and then collect and analyze the optical signals exiting the tissue. Changes in emitted light mirror changes in oxyhemoglobin and deoxyhemoglobin concentration in the tissue. NIRS measures hemoglobin content and oxygenation in small vessels (arterioles, venules, and capillaries). Larger diameter vessels absorb the light completely. Therefore, NIRS is specific for assessment of microcirculation. The most common model is InSpectra (Hutchinson Technology Inc., BioMeasurement Division, Hutchinson, MN, USA) [18].

**Conclusions**

In this chapter, we reviewed blood supply to the NAC and methods of intraoperative imaging of perfusion. Blood supply to the NAC comes primarily from the internal thoracic, lateral thoracic, anterior intercostal, and acromiothoracic arteries, with considerable variation in the branches from the main sources supplying the NAC. Determining the extent to which a particular NAC's blood supply comes from the breast tissue beneath the NAC or the surrounding dermis helps predict the risk of nipple ischemia in NSM. ICG angiography has demonstrated that radial incisions place a NAC at lower risk of ischemia than periareolar incisions. Intraoperative ICG dye angiography, since FDA approval, has rapidly become a popular means of visualizing blood flow to the NAC to guide flap design and tissue excision. Fluorescein angiography, methylene blue NIR imaging, Doppler sonography, tissue spectrophotometry, and NIRS are other means of monitoring perfusion to the breast.

## References

1. van Deventer PV, Graewe FR. The blood supply of the breast revisited. Plast Reconstr Surg. 2016;137(5):1388–97.
2. Michelle le Roux C, Kiil BJ, Pan WR, Rozen WM, Ashton MW. Preserving the neurovascular supply in the Hall-Findlay superomedial pedicle breast reduction: an anatomical study. J Plast Reconstr Aesthet Surg. 2010;63(4):655–62.
3. Wapnir I, Dua M, Kieryn A, Paro J, Morrison D, Kahn D, Meyer S, Gurtner G. Intraoperative imaging of nipple perfusion patterns and ischemic complications in nipple-sparing mastectomies. Ann Surg Oncol. 2014;21(1):100–6.
4. Boneti C, Yuen J, Santiago C, Diaz Z, Robertson Y, Korourian S, et al. Oncologic safety of nipple skin-sparing or total skin-sparing mastectomies with immediate reconstruction. J Am Coll Surg. 2011;212(4):686–93.

5. Moyer HR, Ghazi B, Daniel JR, Gasgarth R, Carlson GW. Nipple-sparing mastectomy: technical aspects and aesthetic outcomes. Ann Plast Surg. 2012;68(5):446–50.
6. Carlson GW, Chu CK, Moyer HR, Duggal C, Losken A. Predictors of nipple ischemia after nipple sparing mastectomy. Breast J. 2014;20(1):69–73.
7. Donovan CA, Harit AP, Chung A, Bao J, Giuliano AE, Amersi F. Oncological and surgical outcomes after nipple-sparing mastectomy: do incisions matter? Ann Surg Oncol. 2016;23(10):3226–31.
8. Phillips B, Khan S. Mastectomy skin flap perfusion. In: Shiffman M, editor. Breast reconstruction: art, science, and new clinical techniques. Berlin: Springer; 2016. p. 1548–9.
9. Losken A, Styblo TM, Schaefer TG, Carlson GW. The use of fluorescein dye as a predictor of mastectomy skin flap viability following autologous tissue reconstruction. Ann Plast Surg. 2008;61(1):24–9.
10. Myers MB, Brock D, Cohn I Jr. Prevention of skin slough after radical mastectomy by the use of a vital dye to delineate devascularized skin. Ann Surg. 1971;173(6):920–4.
11. Gioux S, Choi HS, Frangioni JV. Image-guided surgery using invisible near-infrared light: fundamentals of clinical translation. Mol Imaging. 2010;9(5):237–55.
12. Choi HS, Frangioni JV. Nanoparticles for biomedical imaging: fundamentals of clinical translation. Mol Imaging. 2010;9(6):291–310.
13. Piper M, Sbitany H. Strategies for recognizing and managing intraoperative venous congestion in abdominally based autologous breast reconstruction. In: Shiffman M, editor. Breast reconstruction: art, Science, and new clinical techniques. Berlin: Springer; 2016. p. 1449.
14. Ashitate Y, Lee BT, Ngo LH, Laurence RG, Hutteman M, Oketokoun R, et al. Quantitative assessment of nipple perfusion with near-infrared fluorescence imaging. Ann Plast Surg. 2013;70(2):149–53.
15. Duggal CS, Madni T, Losken A. An outcome analysis of intraoperative angiography for post-mastectomy breast reconstruction. Aesthet Surg J. 2014;34(1):61–5.
16. Chi C, Ye J, Ding H, He D, Huang W, Zhang GJ, et al. Use of indocyanine green for detecting the sentinel lymph node in breast cancer patients: from preclinical evaluation to clinical validation. PLoS One. 2013;8(12):e83927.
17. Swartz WM, Jones NF, Cherup L, Klein A. Direct monitoring of microvascular anastomoses with the 20-MHz ultrasonic Doppler probe: an experimental and clinical study. Plast Reconstr Surg. 1988;81(2):149–61.
18. Martellani L, Arnez T, Papa G, Arnez Z. The use of near infrared spectroscopy (nirs) for monitoring of free flaps. In: Shiffman M, editor. Breast reconstruction: art, science, and new clinical techniques. Berlin: Springer; 2016. p. 611.

# Nipple-Areola Complex Relies Solely on the Dermal Plexus

# 6

Yoav Barnea

## 6.1 Introduction

The nipple-areola complex (NAC) is the focus of the breast and a key component in breast surgery. Since the 1950s, numerous publications have introduced various dermal and breast parenchyma pedicles in breast reduction and mastopexy procedures, presenting different techniques in optimizing surgical outcome and NAC viability [1–25]. These articles were based on earlier publications of the blood supply to the breast [26–32].

Nakajima et al. [33] first described the arterial anatomy of the NAC using injections of lead oxide into fresh cadavers, and they concluded that branches of the internal and external mammary arteries provide the primary blood supply to that complex. They observed that those branches travel in the subcutaneous tissue, communicating with each other above and below the areola and sending small branches to the base of the nipple. These also noted that the intercostal and thoracoacromial arteries supplement the blood supply (Fig. 6.1), but the dermal and subdermal plexuses were not found to be especially vascular and did not anastomose widely with the plexus in the NAC. Transposition of the NAC that is based on a dermal pedicle preserves the blood supply. An arterial pathway to the NAC is maintained because the nutrient vessels of the NAC run in the subcutaneous tissue. In breast reduction by means of the inferior pedicle technique, the blood supply relies on cutaneous perforators of the fourth and/or the fifth intercostal arteries, which are relatively large. Later studies that examined the blood supply to the NAC supported these findings [34–37] and described the vascular variability that is present in each breast.

## 6.2 Case Report

This is a report of a patient that previously underwent total sternectomy due to chronic sternal osteomyelitis and reconstruction by means of a right pectoralis major turnover muscle flap [38]. The undermining of the chest skin and the turnover of the right pectoralis muscle resulted in disruption of the parenchymal branches to the right breast, specifically, the mammary arteries (internal and external) and the intercostal perforators of the right chest (Fig. 6.1). The right NAC now relied solely on the dermal and subdermal

Y. Barnea, M.D.
Breast Reconstruction Unit, Department of Plastic and Reconstructive Surgery, Tel-Aviv Sourasky Medical Center, Sackler Faculty of Medicine, Tel-Aviv University,
6 Weizmann Street, Tel-Aviv 6423906, Israel
e-mail: ybarnea@gmail.com


M.A. Shiffman (ed.), *Nipple-Areolar Complex Reconstruction*,
https://doi.org/10.1007/978-3-319-60925-6_6

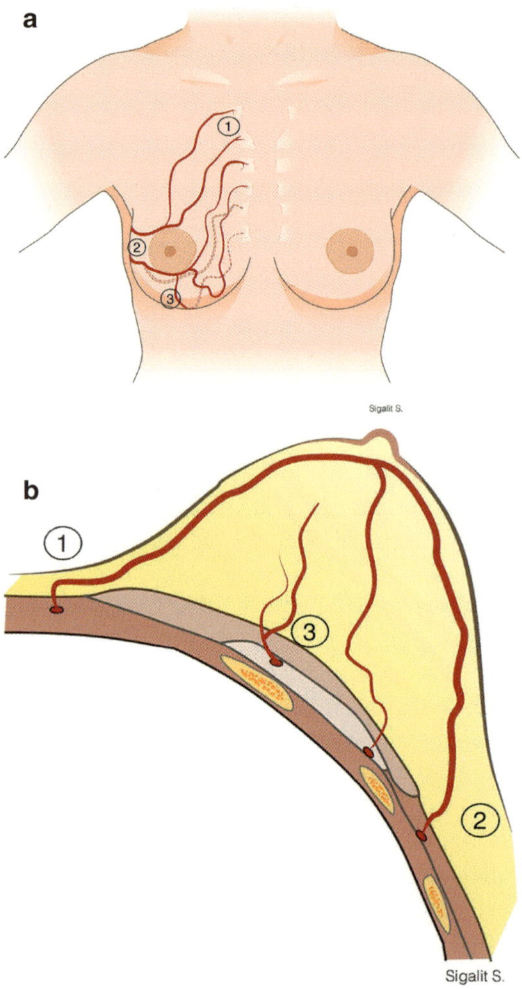


**Fig. 6.1** (**a**, **b**) The main blood supply to the nipple-areola complex of the breast. (*1*) Internal mammary arteries. (*2*) external mammary arteries. (*3*) intercostal perforator arteries

plexuses. Two years later, she underwent bilateral breast reduction, to alleviate the severe discomfort caused by her breast hypertrophy (Fig. 6.2). The reduction technique was based on the inferior pedicle, leaving a wide dermal pedicle on both breasts. Immediately following the procedure, the right NAC developed cyanosis that progressed to complete nipple necrosis (Fig. 6.2).

The complete necrosis of the right NAC supports the contention that the dermal and subdermal plexuses play a minor role in supplying the NAC. Deepithelialization of the inferior pedicle is probably important for keeping the integrity of the flap, but it plays a relatively negligible part in NAC survival.

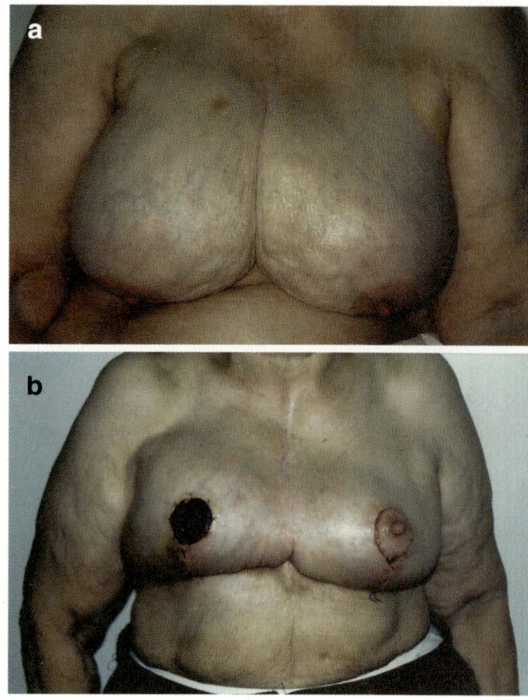


**Fig. 6.2** (**a**) An 82-year-old patient with hypertrophic breasts after sternal reconstruction by means of a right pectoralis major turnover flap. (**b**) Postoperative showing complete right nipple-areolar necrosis

## References


1. Wise RJ. A preliminary report of a method of planning the mammaplasty. Plast Reconstr Surg. 1956;17(5):367–75.
2. Strombeck JO. Mammaplasty: report of a new technique based on the two-pedicle procedure. Br J Plast Surg. 1960;13:79–90.
3. Dufourmentel C, Mouly R. Plastie mammaire par la methode oblique. Ann Chir Plast. 1961;6:45–58.
4. Skoog T. A technique of breast reduction: transposition of the nipple on a cutaneous vascular pedicle. Acta Chir Scand. 1963;126:453–65.
5. Robertson DC. The technique of inferior flap mammaplasty. Plast Reconstr Surg. 1967;40(4):372–7.

6. Pitanguy I. Surgical treatment of breast hypertrophy. Br J Plast Surg. 1967;20(1):78–85.
7. Lassus C. A technique for breast reduction. Int Surg. 1970;53(1):69–72.
8. McKissock PK. Reduction mammaplasty with a vertical dermal flap. Plast Reconstr Surg. 1972;49(3):245–52.
9. Weiner DL, Aiache AE, Silver L, Tittiranonda T. A single dermal pedicle for nipple transposition in subcutaneous mastectomy, reduction mammaplasty, or mastopexy. Plast Reconstr Surg. 1973;51(2):115–20.
10. Regnault P. Reduction mammaplasty by the "B" technique. Plast Reconstr Surg. 1974;53(1):19–24.
11. Ribeiro L. A new technique for reduction mammaplasty. Plast Reconstr Surg. 1975;55(3):330–4.
12. Robbins TH. A reduction mammoplasty with the areola-nipple based on an inferior dermal pedicle. Plast Reconstr Surg. 1977;59(1):64–7.
13. Courtiss E, Goldwyn R. Reduction mammaplasty by the inferior pedicle technique. Plast Reconstr Surg. 1977;59(4):500–7.
14. Marchac D, de Olarte G. Reduction mammaplasty and correction of ptosis with a short inframammary scar. Plast Reconstr Surg. 1982;69(1):45–55.
15. Peixoto G. Reduction mammaplasty: a personal technique. Plast Reconstr Surg. 1980;65(2):217–26.
16. Balch CR. The central mound technique for reduction mammaplasty. Plast Reconstr Surg. 1981;67(3):305–11.
17. Hester TR Jr, Bostwick J III, Miller L, Cunningham SJ. Breast reduction utilizing the maximally vascularized central breast pedicle. Plast Reconstr Surg. 1985;76(6):890–900.
18. Lejour M, Abboud M, Declety A, Kertesz P. Reduction of mammaplasty scars: from a short inframammary scar to a vertical scar (in French). Ann Chir Plast Esthet. 1990;35(5):369–79.
19. Benelli L. A new periareolar mammaplasty: the "round block" technique. Aesthet Plast Surg. 1990;14(2):93–100.
20. Aiache AE. Arch reduction mammaplasty. Plast Reconstr Surg. 1999;103:862–8.
21. Hammond DC. Short scar periareolar inferior pedicle reduction (SPAIR) mammaplasty. Plast Reconstr Surg. 1999;103(3):890–1.
22. Hall-Findlay EJ. A simplified vertical reduction mammaplasty: shortening the learning curve. Plast Reconstr Surg. 1999;104(3):748–59.
23. Sampaio Goes JC. Periareolar mammaplasty: double skin technique with application of mesh support. Clin Plast Surg. 2002;29(3):349–64.
24. Blondeel PN, Hamdi M, Van de Sijpe KA, Van Landuyt KH, Thiessen FE, Monstrey SJ. The latero-central glandular pedicle technique for breast reduction. Br J Plast Surg. 2003;56(4):348–59.
25. Corduff N, Taylor GI. Subglandular breast reduction: the evolution of a minimal scar approach to breast reduction. Plast Reconstr Surg. 2004;113(1):175–84.
26. Anson BJ, Wright RR, Wolfer JH. Blood supply of the mammary gland. Surg Gynecol Obstet. 1939;69:468–73.
27. Salmon M. Les artères de la glande mammaire. Ann Anat Pathol. 1939;16:477–500.
28. Maliniac JW. Arterial blood supply of the breast. Arch Surg. 1943;47:329–43.
29. Carr BW, Bishop WE, Anson BJ. Mammary arteries. Q Bull Northwest U Med School. 1942;16:150–4.
30. Cunningham L. The anatomy of the arteries and veins of the breast. J Surg Oncol. 1977;9(1):71–85.
31. Palmer JH, Taylor GI. The vascular territories of the anterior chest wall. Br J Plast Surg. 1986;39(3):287–99.
32. Würinger E, Mader N, Posch E, Holle J. Nerve and vessel supplying ligamentous suspension of the mammary gland. Plast Reconstr Surg. 1998;101(6):1486–93.
33. Nakajima H, Imanishi N, Aiso S. Arterial anatomy of the nipple-areola complex. Plast Reconstr Surg. 1995;96(4):843–5.
34. van Deventer PV. The blood supply to the nipple-areola complex of the human mammary gland. Aesthet Plast Surg. 2004;28(6):393–8.
35. O'Dey DM, Prescher A, Pallua N. Vascular reliability of nipple-areola complex-bearing pedicles: an anatomical micro-dissection study. Plast Reconstr Surg. 2007;119(4):1167–77.
36. van Deventer PV, Page BJ, Graewe FR. The safety of pedicles in breast reduction and mastopexy procedures. Aesthet Plast Surg. 2008;32(2):307–12.
37. Taylor GI, Corlett RJ, Dhar SC, Ashton MW. The anatomical (angiosome) and clinical territories of cutaneous perforating arteries: development of the concept and designing safe flaps. Plast Reconstr Surg. 2011;127(4):1447–59.
38. Barnea Y, Cohen M, Weiss J, Shafir R. Clinical confirmation that the nipple areola complex relies solely on the dermal plexus. Plast Reconstr Surg. 1998;101(7):2009–10.

# 7 Smooth Muscle Morphology in the Nipple-Areola Complex

Murat Tezer

## 7.1 Introduction

Nipples serve as the points of access to milk for infants. The nipple functions by transmitting stimulation from suction into an induction of the milk ejection reflex due to intense sensory innervation, preventing the leakage of milk between breast-feeding episodes and erection to facilitate breast-feeding and during sexual arousal. Additionally, the nipple can be erected with cold and other tactile stimulations [1–10].

## 7.2 Anatomy

The nipple-areola complex (NAC) is a specialized skin structure covered by hairless skin, including connective tissue (formed by elastic fibers and smooth vascular and nonvascular muscles), ducts, glands, vascular structures, and nerve fibers.

The NAC smooth musculature is divided into outer, intermediate, and inner layers from the areola to the nipple. The inner part of the smooth musculature surrounds the infundibular region of the mammillary milk ducts in a basketlike manner. The inner muscular fibers continue into the stronger intermediate layer, which is covered by an outer layer of smooth musculature situated around the ducts of the Montgomery glands [11]. Muscle fibers in the NAC extended vertically (longitudinally) or horizontally relative to the nipple base, in the form of thin, fusiform fibers or bundles (Fig. 7.1) [1, 2, 4, 12, 13]. The muscle fibers may branch or change direction throughout their progression, and longitudinal and horizontal muscles may extend separately or be found intermixed with one another [13]. Some of the muscle fibers orient vertically toward the epidermis with one of their edges, and some extend parallel to the epidermis (Fig. 7.1) [2, 13].

Smooth muscles are also closely associated with blood vessels, and some of the smooth muscles extend to surround the blood vessels (Fig. 7.1) [5, 12, 13]

Some muscle fibers are associated with the lactiferous ducts. Although particularly prominent proximal to ducts, longitudinal muscles extending parallel to the ducts are also found in the distal, sphincter-like horizontal muscles (Fig. 7.2). These muscles prevent milk leakage between breast-feeding episodes [1, 5, 13].

NAC smooth muscles function to support nipple erection with the vascular system. The nipple rises and becomes prominent; as wrinkles form in the areola, the surface area of the areola decreases; hyperemia and local venous stasis also occur during nipple erection [1, 2, 4, 14–18].

Sympathetic adrenergic nerve fibers [5, 15, 19] and cholinergic nerve fibers [19–22]

M. Tezer, M.D.
Department of Urology, Esenyurt State Hospital,
Istanbul, Esenyurt 34517, Turkey
e-mail: dr_murat3@hotmail.com


M.A. Shiffman (ed.), *Nipple-Areolar Complex Reconstruction*,
https://doi.org/10.1007/978-3-319-60925-6_7

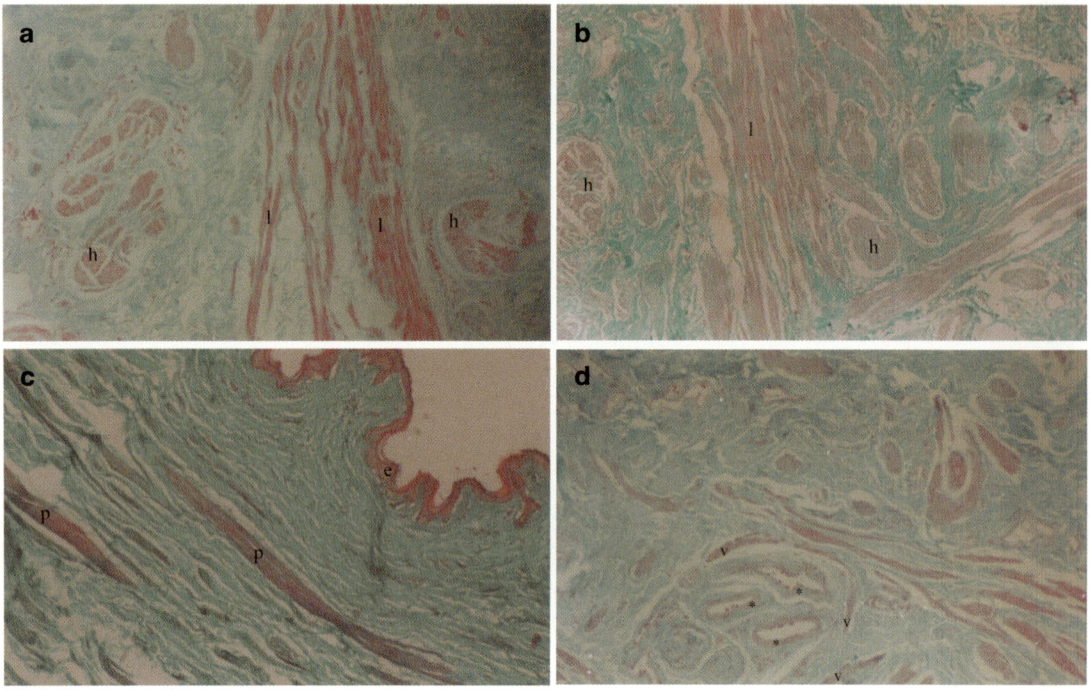


**Fig. 7.1** (**a**, **b**) Longitudinally (*l*) and horizontally (*h*) extended muscles. (**c**) Parallel muscles (*p*) extended to the epidermis (*e*). (**d**) Smooth muscles (*v*) closely associated with blood vessels (*asterisk*) and extended to surround them

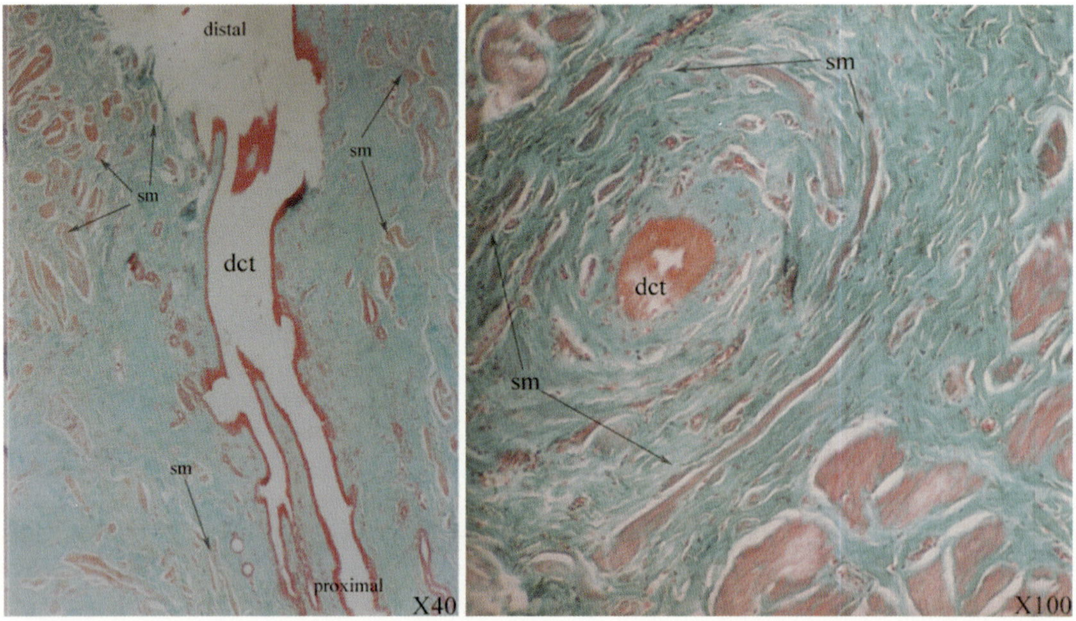


**Fig. 7.2** (*Left*) Smooth muscles (*sm*) are closely associated with the lactiferous ducts (*dct*). (*Right*) In the distal of ducts, sphincter-like horizontal muscles

reaching the NAC enable the control of the NAC vascular and nonvascular smooth muscles.

In molecular studies, peptides (TH (tyrosine hydroxylase), VIP (vasoactive intestinal polypeptide), PHI (peptide histidine isoleucine), NPY (neuropeptide Y), galanin, and somatostatin) identified in the nerves innervating the NAC affect the functions of vascular and nonvascular smooth muscles [5, 15, 19, 23]. Apart from these peptides, nitric oxide synthase expression, which synthesizes nitric oxide to affect smooth muscle functions, is also found in the NAC [10].

## References


1. Giacometti L, Montagna W. The nipple and the areola of the human female breast. Anat Rec. 1962;144:191–7.
2. Montagna W. Histology and cytochemistry of human skin XXXV. The nipple and areola. Br J Dermatol. 1970;83(Suppl):2–13.
3. Cowie AT. Overview of the mammary gland. J Invest Dermatol. 1974;63:2–9.
4. Montagna W, Macpherson E. Some neglected aspects of the anatomy of human breast. J Invest Dermatol. 1974;63:10–6.
5. Eriksson M, Lindh B, Uvnäs-moberg K, Hökfelt T. Distribution and origin of peptide-containing nerve fibres in the rat and human mammary gland. Neuroscience. 1996;70(1):227–45.
6. Munarriz R, Kim NN, Goldstein I, Traish AM. Biology of female sexual function. Urol Clin North Am. 2002;29(3):685–93.
7. Shepherd JE. Therapeutic options in female sexual dysfunction. J Am Pharm Assoc. 2002;42(3):479–87.
8. Levin RJ. The breast/nipple/areola complex and human sexuality. Sex Relationship Ther. 2006;21(2):237–49.
9. Levin R, Meston C. Nipple/breast stimulation and sexual arousal in young men and women. J Sex Med. 2006;3:450–4.
10. Tezer M, Özlük Y, Şanlı Ö, Asoğlu O, Kadıoğlu A. Nitric oxide may mediate nipple erection. J Androl. 2012;33(5):805–10.
11. Dabelow A. Die milchdrüse. In: Bargmann W, editor. Haut und Sinnesorgane, Handbuch der Mikroskopischen Anatomiedes Menschen, vol. 3, part 3. Berlin: Springer-Verlag; 1957. p. 277–485.
12. Gairns FW, Garven HS. The smooth muscle cell types and their associated elastic fibers in the female nipple. J Physiol. 1949;110(1–2):18.
13. Tezer M, Bakkaloğlu H, Ergüven M, Bilir A, Kadıoğlu A. Smooth muscle morphology in the nipple-areola complex. J Morphol Sci. 2011;28(3):171–5.
14. McCarty KS, Nath M. Breast. In: Sternberg SS, editor. Histology for pathologist. 2nd ed. Philadelphia: Lippincott-Raven; 1997. p. 71–82.
15. Uvnäs-Moberg K, Eriksson M. Breast feeding: physiological, endocrine and behavioural adaptations caused by oxytocin and local neurogenic activity in the nipple and mammary gland. Acta Paediatr. 1996;85(5):525–30.
16. Eriksson M, Lundeberg T, Uvnas-Moberg K. Studies on cutaneous blood flow in the mammary gland of lactating rats. Acta Physiol Scand. 1996;158:1–6.
17. Perez-aparicio FJ, Dantzer V, Navarro M, Carretero A, Ruberte J. Vascular architecture of the lactating and non-lactating teat of the bitch: a scanning electron and light microscope study. Scanning Microsc. 1995;9:1255–64.
18. Vorherr H. The breast: morphology, physiology, and lactation. New York: Academic Press; 1974. p. 1–70.
19. Franke-radowiecka A, Kaleczyc J, Klimczuk M, Lakomy M. Noradrenergic and peptidergic innervation of the mammary gland in the immature pig. Folia Histochem Cytobiol. 2002;40(1):17–25.
20. Ballantyne B, Bunch GA. The neurohistology of quiescent mammary tissue in Lepus albus. J Comp Neur. 1966;127:471–87.
21. Hebb CO, Linzell JL. A histological study of the innervation of the mammary gland. J Physiol. 1966;186:82–3.
22. Franke-Radowiecka A, Wasowicz K. Adrenergic and cholinergic innervation of the mammary gland in the pig. Anat Histol Embryol. 2002;31:3–7.
23. Pinho MS, Gulbenkian S. Innervation of the canine mammary gland: an immunohistochemical study. Histol Histopathol. 2007;22:1175–84.

# Part III

# Abnormalities of the Nipple-Areolar Complex

# 8 The Nipple-Areolar Complex: A Pictorial Review of Common and Uncommon Conditions

Kyu Soon Kim

## 8.1 Introduction

The nipple-areolar complex is a specialized region of the mammary gland. It is a major anatomic landmark of the breast, serves to drain and express breast milk during lactation, and contains specialized cells for the function [1, 2]. The nipple contains many sensory nerve ending and smooth muscle bundles. The latter perform an erectile function to facilitate nursing. The pigmented tissues of the areola contain numerous apocrine sweat glands and sebaceous glands, as well as hair follicles. The skin of the areola is thicker than the rest of the skin of the breast, tapering down toward the limbus of the areola. The surface of the nipple itself is irregular and contains numerous crevices. The mammary duct orifices are at the bottom of these crevices [1]. The nipple-areolar complex may be affected by a broad spectrum of disease [2–4].

K.S. Kim, M.D. (✉)
Department of Radiology, Eulji University Hospital, Dunsan-dong, Seo-gu, Daejeon 35233, Republic of Korea
e-mail: kskim@eulji.ac.kr

## 8.2 Normal Appearance and Normal Variants

### 8.2.1 Montgomery Tubercles

The pigmented tissues of the areola include numerous apocrine sweat glands and sebaceous glands, as well as hair follicles. The glands help lubricate the nipple-areolar surface. The nipple-areolar complex contains raised structures on the surface of the areola known as Montgomery tubercles (Fig. 8.1) [2–4].

### 8.2.2 Nipple Retraction or Inversion

The terms retraction and inversion are used interchangeably, but that is incorrect usage. Nipple inversion should only be used when the entire nipple is pulled inward, whereas retraction should be used when the nipple only has an inward slit-like area [2].

Nipple retraction and inversion are either congenital or acquired and either unilateral or bilateral [2, 3]. Nipple inversions typically occur during puberty. Nipple inversions are normal variants of the nipple position or result from the development of fibrous tissue between the nipple and the subareolar parenchyma. This


M.A. Shiffman (ed.), *Nipple-Areolar Complex Reconstruction*,
https://doi.org/10.1007/978-3-319-60925-6_8

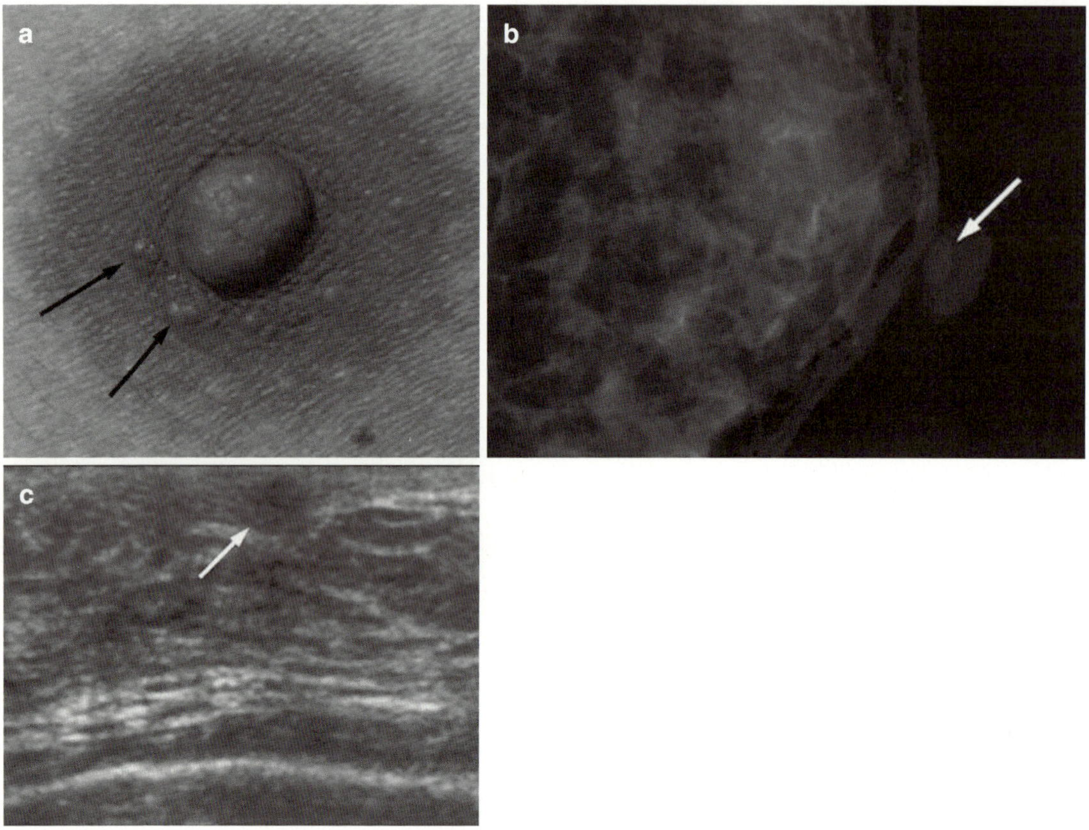


**Fig. 8.1** Montgomery tubercle in a 54-year-old woman. (**a**) Small round elevations on the surface of the areola. (**b**) Left mediolateral oblique mammogram showing well-defined small round areolar nodule (*arrow*). (**c**) Sonogram showing prominent isoechoic areolar nodule (*arrow*)

condition hinders breast-feeding and predisposes to mastitis and abscess formation (Fig. 8.2) [5].

### 8.2.3 Accessory Nipples

Accessory nipples most commonly occur in the anterosuperior abdominal wall below the breast, but they may develop anywhere along the course of the embryologic mammary ridge, the so-called milk line, which extends bilaterally from the axilla to the inguinal area. The most inferior location of the accessory nipples has been in the proximal thigh. Accessory nipples may be confused with moles because they are pigmented [2–4].

## 8.3 Benign Processes

Benign lesions that affect the nipple-areolar complex are varied. These lesions include benign calcifications, inflammation, duct dilatations, intraductal papillomas (IDPs), fibroadenomas, neurofibromatosis, and dermatosis of the nipple.

### 8.3.1 Benign Calcifications

Nipple calcifications are rare [3, 6]; however, the glands and hair follicles of the nipple-areolar complex contain calcifications [3, 4]. Lucent-centered, spherical, or polygonal calcifications are generally benign calcifications, including the

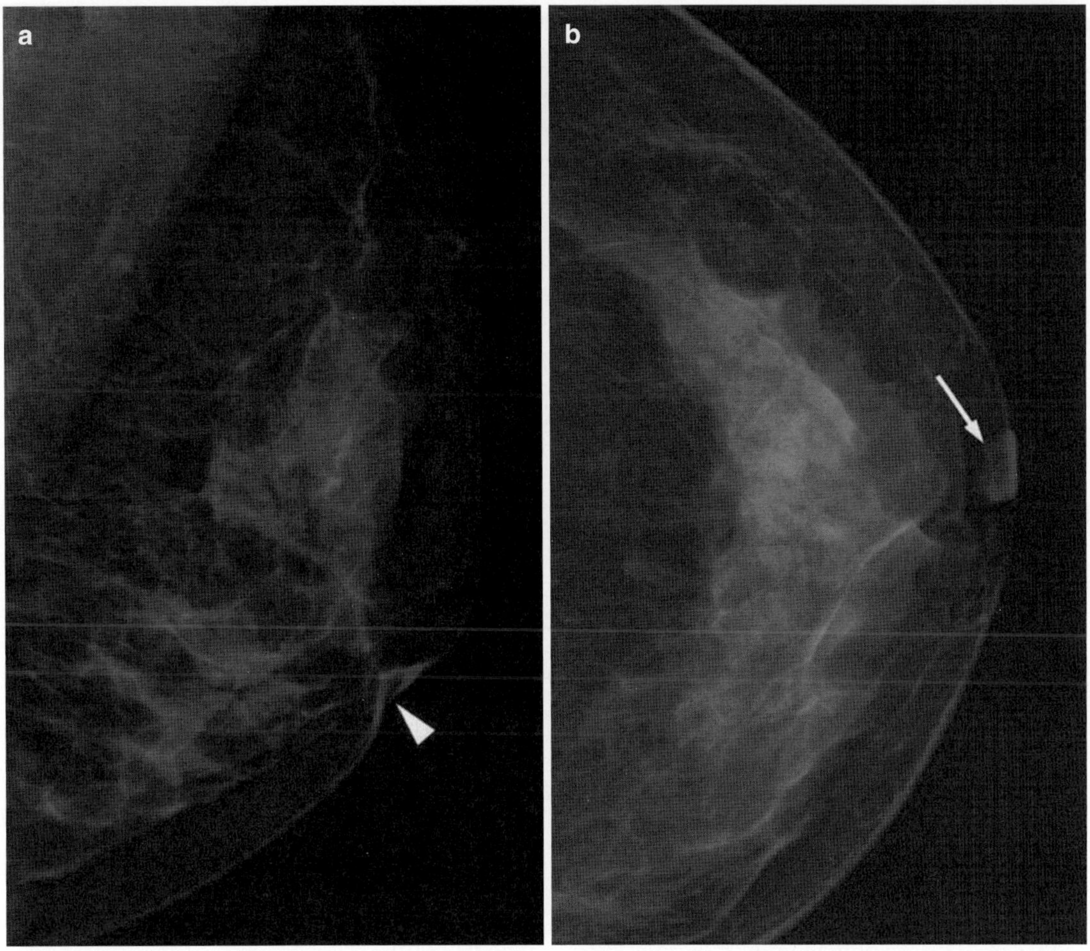


**Fig. 8.2** Nipple inversion in a 49-year-old woman. (**a**) Right craniocaudal mammogram showing subareolar pseudo-mass (*arrow*) representing mammographically inverted nipple. (**b**) Right mediolateral oblique mammogram showing gross inversion

calcified debris in ducts, fat necrosis, and skin calcifications. Skin calcifications are usually scattered widely over the breast (Fig. 8.3). Multiple benign dermal calcifications often develop in a classic pattern within the periareolar surgical scars after breast reduction. Occasionally, they can project as intramammary deposits, but this problem can be solved by using tangential views [6].

### 8.3.2 Inflammation

Periductal mastitis is a suppurative inflammatory disease of the mammary gland and results from the obstruction of a small duct beneath the areola. Occasionally, an abscess (a collection of pus) may develop. A subareolar abscess is unusual. Most cases of mastitis and breast abscesses occur during lactation, whereas subareolar abscesses mostly occur in non-lactating young and middle-aged women [3, 7].

Abscesses appear as irregular, poorly defined, or spiculated hyperdense masses caused by edema and inflammation on a mammography and cystic masses with low-level internal echoes, which are difficult to differentiate from intracystic neoplasm, on sonography (Fig. 8.4). When an abscess is suspected and associated with a mammographically suspicious finding, follow-up imaging in

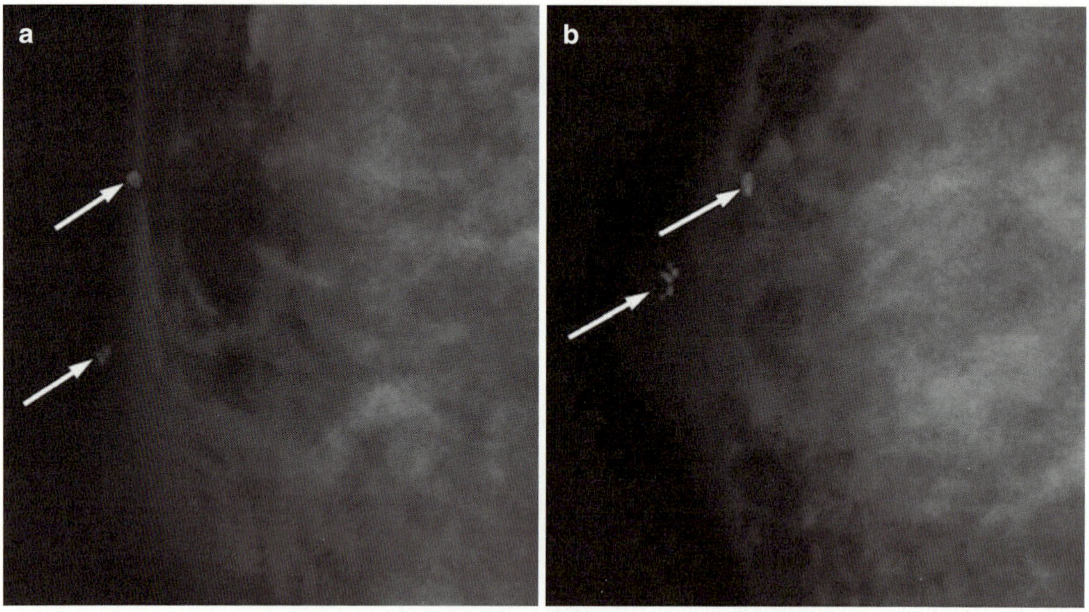


**Fig. 8.3** Benign skin calcifications in a 36-year-old woman. (**a**) Right mediolateral oblique and (**b**) right craniocaudal digital mammograms showing multiple calcifications with central lucency diagnostic of benign skin calcifications (*arrow*) in the right nipple and subareolar region

4–6 weeks is recommended to ensure resolution of the suspicious mammographic findings.

A history of fever, breast pain and response to antibiotics help differentiate an abscess from a neoplasm. Because of the presence of breast pain and tenderness, clinical and mammographic examinations are often inadequate. Therefore, sonography is optimal imaging modality for assessment of mastitis or abscess of the breast [2, 3, 7, 8].

### 8.3.3 Mammary Duct Ectasia

Duct ectasia presents with a nipple discharge, nipple retraction, pain, or tenderness [3, 8]. Tubular or branching structures that converge toward the nipple are characteristic mammographic features of duct ectasia. Tubular or branching structures are most commonly seen in the subareolar area. Bilateral symmetric subareolar ductal dilatation is common in postmenopausal women but has no clinical importance [9]. However, if asymmetric subareolar duct dilatation is detected on mammograms, spot magnification views plus sonography may prove helpful in evaluating for an underlying mass, such as IDP or carcinoma [3, 9].

On sonography, dilated ducts are filled with fluid, and concentrated secretions and debris are visible as intraductal echoes, which are difficult to differentiate from intraductal tumors (Fig. 8.5) [3, 8, 9]. Movement of echogenic materials on real-time sonography may be a diagnostic feature of ductal ectasia [3].

### 8.3.4 Intraductal Papilloma (IDP)

Intraductal papillomas are relatively common benign neoplasm originating from proximal ducts or retroareolar mammary ducts [10]. Papillomas are known to occur anywhere within the ductal system and are classified into central and peripheral types. Central types tend to be single and located in the subareolar region within

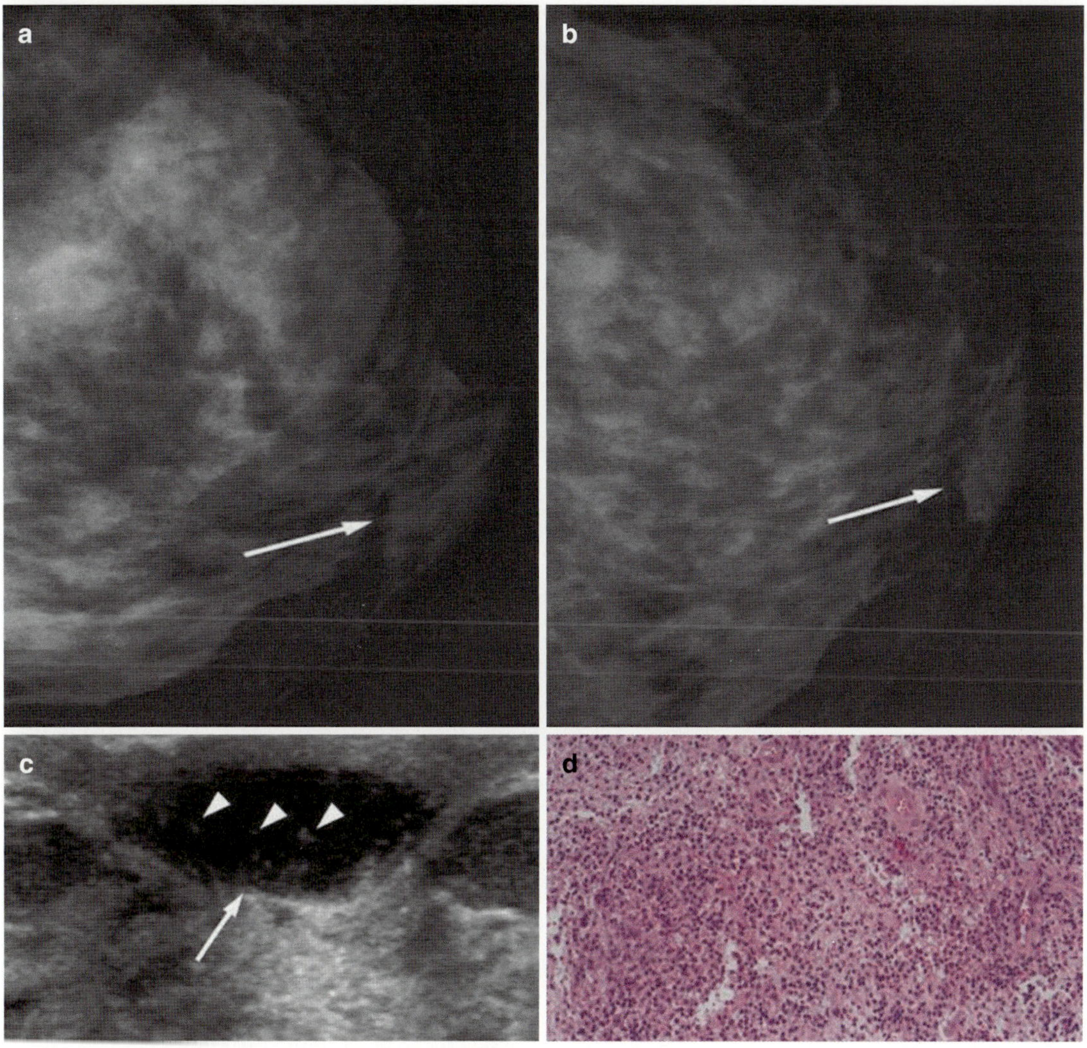


**Fig. 8.4** Subareolar abscess in a 43-year-old woman. (**a**) Left mediolateral oblique and (**b**) left craniocaudal mammograms showing isodense ovoid subareolar focal asymmetry (*arrow*). (**c**) Sonogram showing a hypoechoic mass (*arrow*) with focally thick irregular microcalcification walls and mobile internal echogenic debris (*arrowheads*). (**d**) Excisional biopsy specimen showing congestion with a chronic inflammatory infiltrate consisting of lymphocytes, plasma cells, histiocytes, and Langhans type of giant cells (hematoxylin-eosin, original magnification ×200)

major ducts, whereas peripheral types are commonly multiple within the terminal ductal-lobular unit. Peripheral duct types have an increased risk of carcinoma, which is directly related to the degree of cellular atypia. Histologically, papillomas reveal hyperplastic proliferation of the ductal epithelium, having a frond-like growth pattern with a branching fibromuscular core of myoepithelial and epithelial cells [11].

The sonographic features of IDP have three basic patterns: (1) an intraductal mass with or without duct dilatation, (2) an intracystic mass, and (3) a predominantly solid pattern with an intraductal mass totally filling the duct (Fig. 8.6). Dilated ducts or cysts with an intraductal or intracystic solid mass are the hallmark of IDP [11].

Small IDPs are often mammographically occult. A moderately dilated duct may be observed as pro-

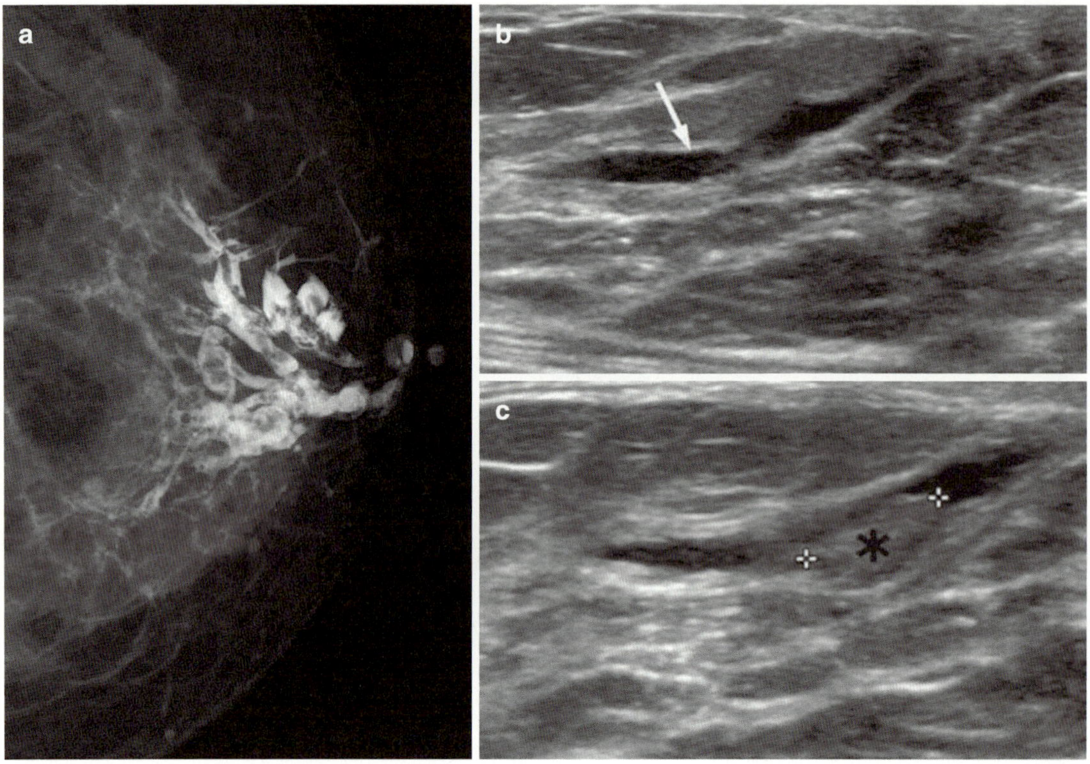


**Fig. 8.5** Mammary duct dilatation in a 49-year-old woman. (**a**) Left craniocaudal galactogram showing multifocal filling defects in the dilated ducts. (**b**, **c**) Sonograms showing fluid-filled structures (**b**, *arrow*) behind the nipple with echogenic sludge (**c**, *asterisk*)

gressively tapering band-like density that converges toward the nipple. Large IDPs may show a focal, well-circumscribed hyperdense mass [12].

### 8.3.5 Fibroadenomas

Fibroadenomas are the most common benign tumor of the breast. They are composed of epithelium and stroma of the terminal ductal-lobular units. Gross pathologic specimens of fibroadenomas usually show round, oval, or lobulated shapes, which are sharply defined by a pseudocapsule of compressed parenchyma. Therefore, fibroadenomas are typically well-circumscribed, round, or oval solid masses associated with smooth contours and homogeneous internal echoes on sonography [13, 14]. However, some fibroadenomas have atypical sonographic findings, such as poorly defined margin or irregular shape with heterogeneous internal echoes or posterior shadowing (Fig. 8.7) [15]. A poorly defined margin or an irregular shape is associated with interdigitation of the surrounding parenchyma with a mass [15, 16]. Other atypical sonographic findings, such as a heterogeneous internal echo texture and posterior shadowing, are related to dilated ducts, phyllodes, collagen bundles, adenosis, and microcalcifications [15–19].

### 8.3.6 Neurofibromas

Neurofibromas are common benign tumors that arise from the peripheral nervous system. Most neurofibromas occur in the skin of the trunk. However, breast involvement is very rare. However, these lesions are frequently seen in patients with neurofibromatosis and are most common in the areolar area [7, 20, 21].

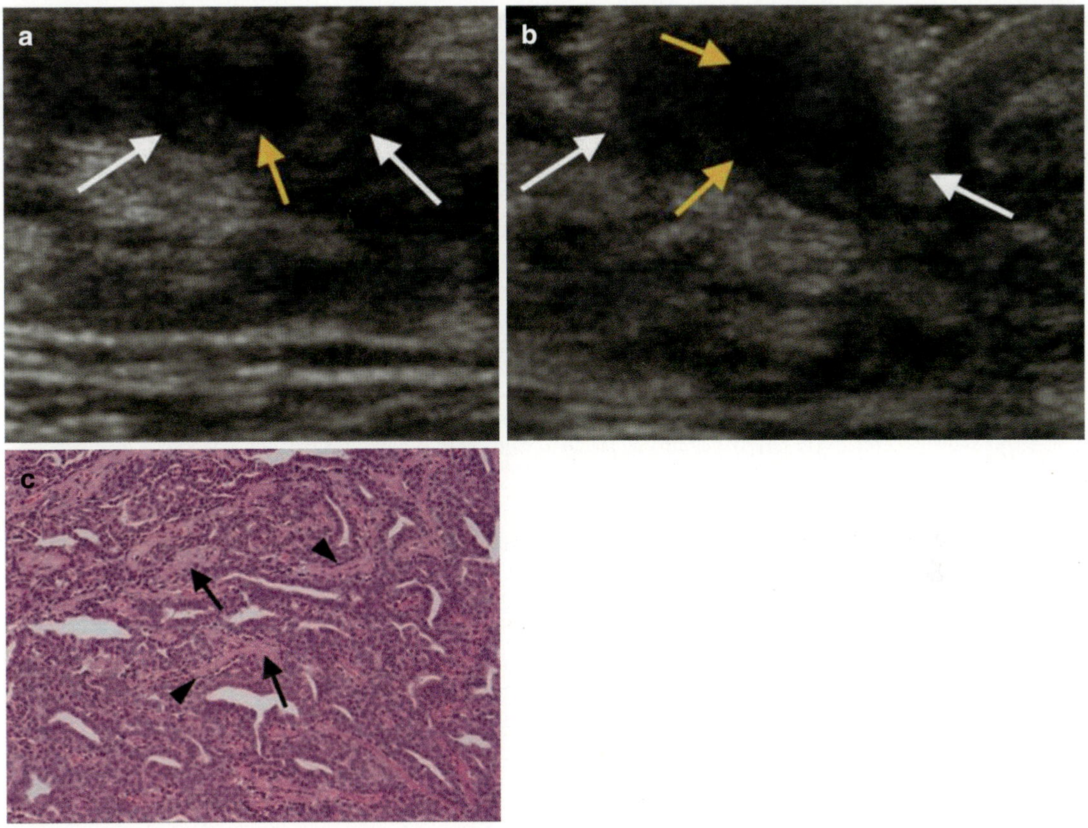

**Fig. 8.6** Intraductal papilloma (IDP) in a 39-year-old woman. (**a**, **b**) Sonograms showing well-defined hypoechoic nodule (*yellow arrows*) in the left nipple (*white arrows*). (**c**) Microductectomy specimen showing prominent fibrovascular cores (*arrows*), lined by a benign myoepithelial cell layer (hematoxylin-eosin, original magnification ×200)

Neurofibromas are oval or round with a well-circumscribed margin on mammography and sonography (Fig. 8.8). On sonography, they have hypoechoic nodules with a posterior acoustic enhancement, resembling cysts. This effect has been described with other solid tumors of uniform cellularity, such as a lymphoma [21–23].

### 8.3.7 Dermatoses of the Nipple and Areola

Dermatosis of the nipple and areola is rare. Neoplastic dermatoses can be underestimated because early dermatoses are scaly and erythematous and can be misdiagnosed as eczema or an inflammatory skin disorder. The most common neoplastic dermatosis is Paget's disease, which presents as a well-demarcated erythematous area, sometimes erosive, oozing, or hyperkeratotic. In 98.5–100% of cases, Paget's disease is associated with underlying breast carcinoma. Other neoplastic dermatoses of the nipple include nipple adenomas, soft fibroma (Fig. 8.9), epidermal cyst, and cellular blue nevi. Infectious dermatoses (viral warts (Fig. 8.10), molluscum contagiosum, and scabies) are accompanied by lesions in other sites [24–26].

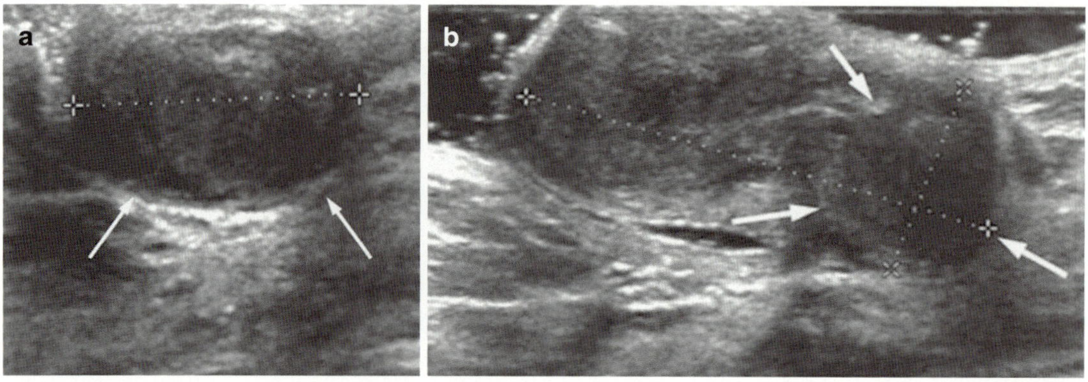


**Fig. 8.7** Fibroadenoma in a 33-year-old woman. (**a**, **b**) Sonograms showing a relatively poorly marginated round mass (*arrows*) with a heterogeneous internal echo and posterior enhancement beneath the nipple. The long set of calipers in B measures the nipple and mass together

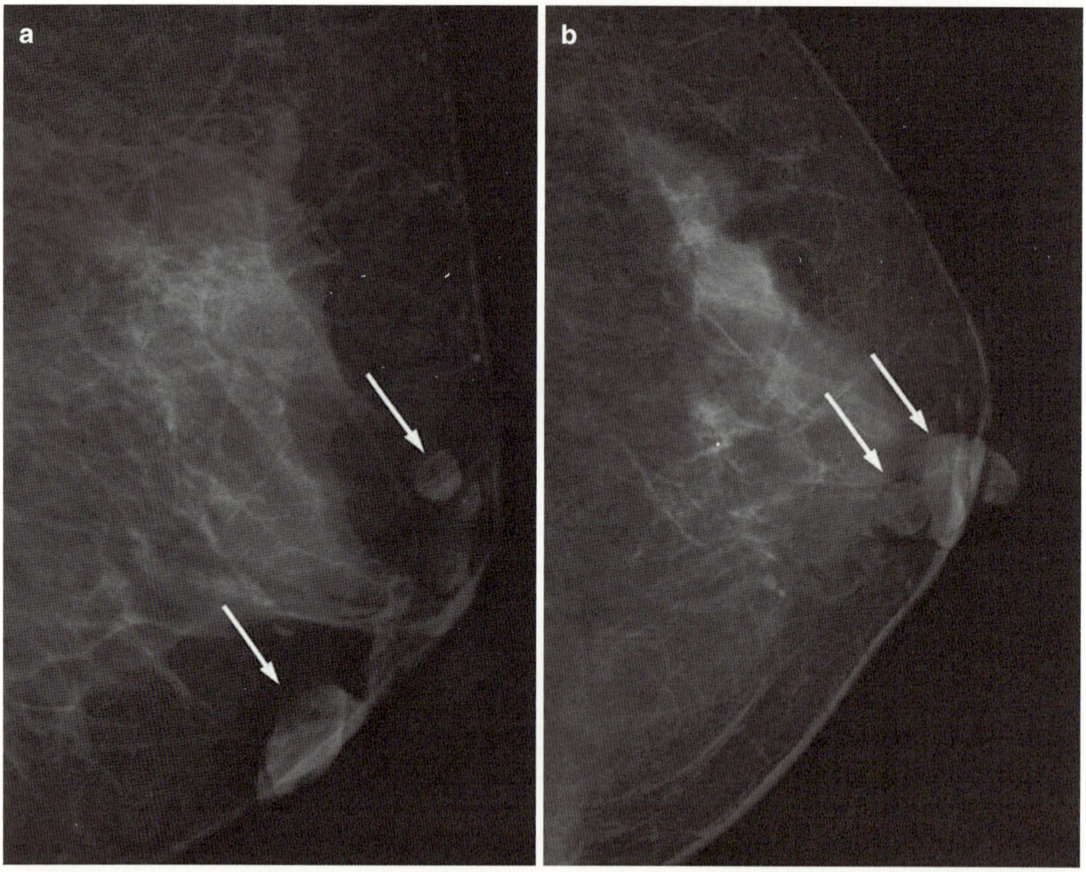


**Fig. 8.8** Neurofibromas in a 33-year-old woman. (**a**) Left mediolateral and (**b**) left craniocaudal mammograms showing several round and oval well-circumscribed isodense skin nodules (*arrows*) in the periareolar region. (**c**, **d**) Sonograms showing well-circumscribed, smooth-marginated, hypoechoic masses (*arrows*) located intracutaneously. *NI* indicates nipple. (**e**) Excisional biopsy specimen showing spindle cells with fibrillar cystoplasm and elongated nuclei (hematoxylin-eosin, original magnification ×200)

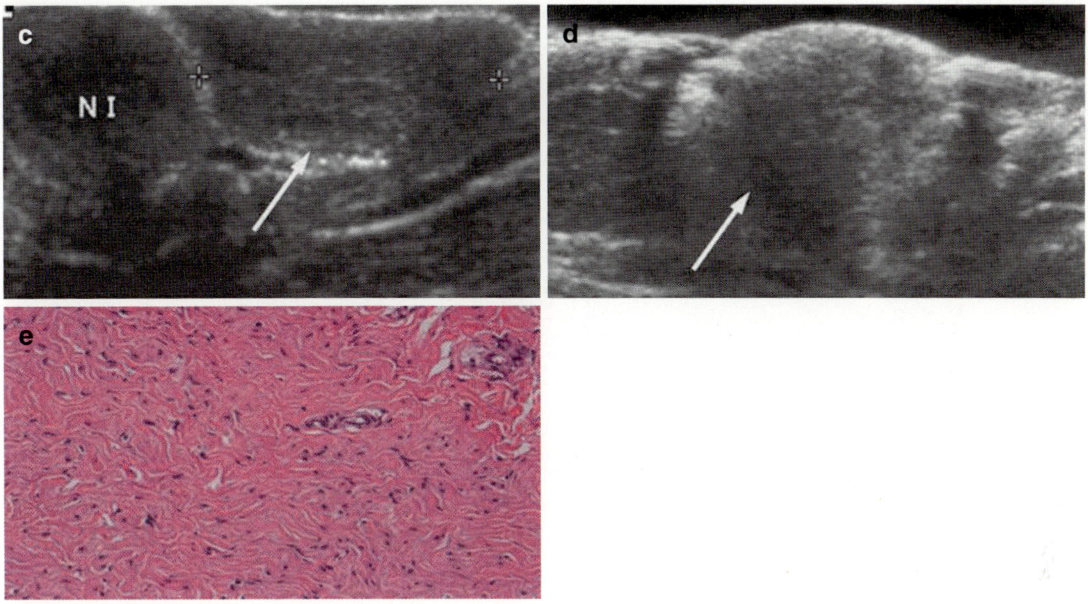


**Fig. 8.8** (continued)

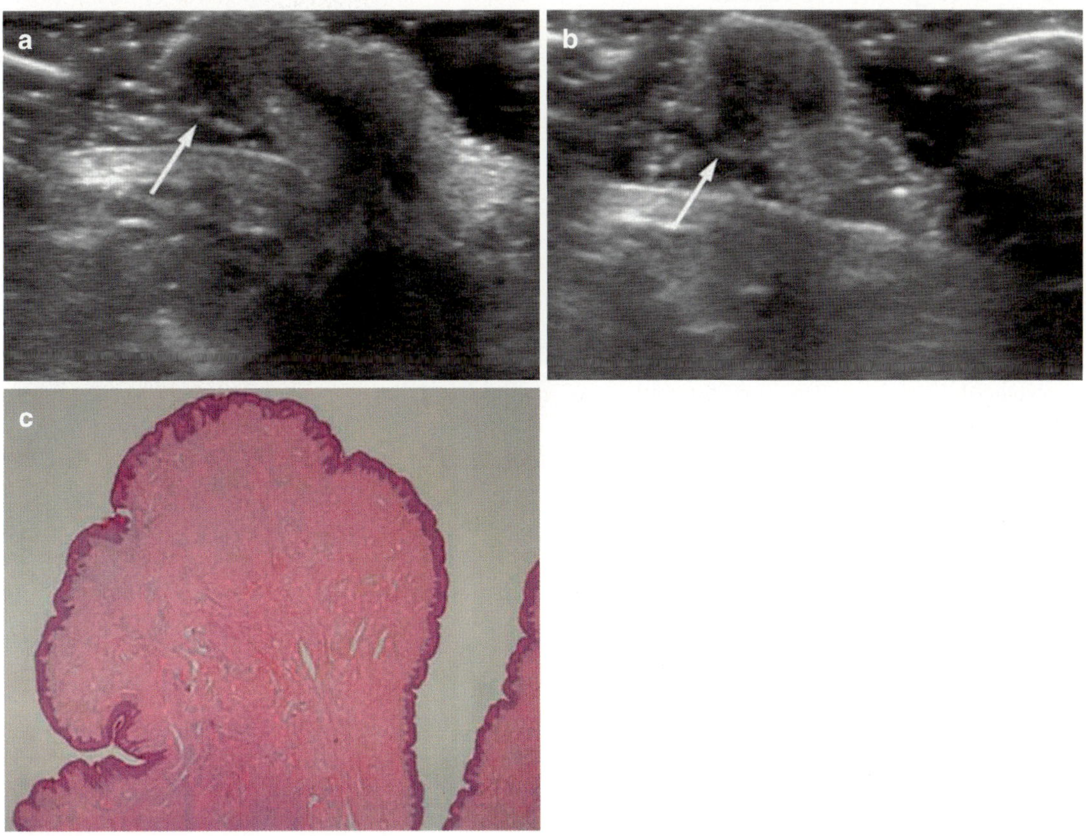


**Fig. 8.9** Soft fibroma in a 23-year-old woman. (**a**, **b**) Sonograms showing a hypoechoic mass (*arrows*) arising from the tip of the left nipple. (**c**) Excisional biopsy specimen showing the epidermis raised in a papilliform shape and underlying loose collagenous stroma with scattered spindle cells and dilated capillaries (hematoxylin-eosin, original magnification ×200)

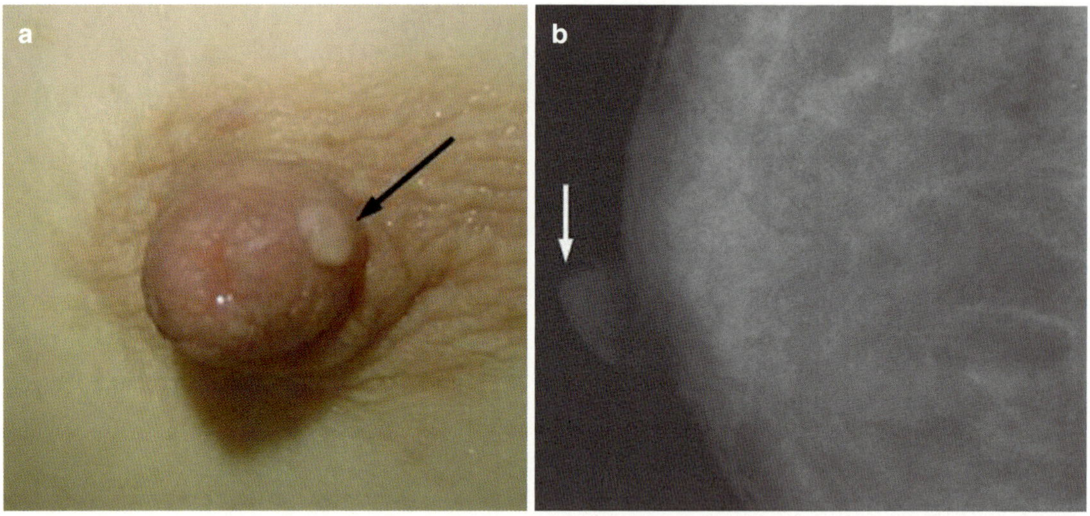


**Fig. 8.10** Nipple wart in a 34-year-old woman. (**a**) Exophytic cutaneous nodular lesion (*arrow*). (**b**) Right mediolateral oblique mammogram showing a benign-looking nodule in superior portion of the nipple (*arrow*)

## 8.4 Malignant Processes

### 8.4.1 Paget's Disease

Paget's disease of the breast is a rare disorder of the nipple-areolar complex, constituting 0.5–5% of all breast cancer, and is often associated with an underlying in situ or invasive carcinoma [27].

Eczematoid change and soreness, burning, and an itching sensation of the nipple-areolar complex are common and early symptoms. The later stages of Paget's disease of the breast are characterized by ulceration, crusting, and serous or bloody discharge [28].

Paget's disease of the breast shows malignant calcifications at the level of the nipple or elsewhere in the breast, skin thickening, nipple retraction, and a discrete mass or masses on mammography. However, mammographic findings are normal in half of patients with Paget's disease of the breast [3].

Magnetic resonance imaging (MRI) is useful to diagnose Paget's disease of the breast and plays an important role in the selection of patients with Paget's disease for breast-conserving surgery without clinical or mammographic evidence of breast carcinoma. Magnetic resonance images show abnormal nipple enhancement and linear clumped enhancement indicative of ductal carcinoma in situ in association with Paget's disease (Fig. 8.11) [3, 27, 29].

### 8.4.2 Carcinoma

Malignant masses of the nipple-areolar complex may be more difficult to diagnose than cancers elsewhere in the breast, because subareolar masses can be easily confused with normal nipple structures on mammography. Therefore, additional diagnostic mammographic views (spot compression with or without magnification) may be used to improve the visibility of subareolar masses. On sonography, subareolar masses or intraductal lesions may be more easily identified than on mammography [1, 3]. Contrast-enhanced MR imaging is useful when mammographic and sonographic findings are inconclusive (Figs. 8.12 and 8.13) [3].

Underlying cancer may originate immediately deep to the nipple or extend XEfrom another location in the breast to the nipple-areolar complex [1–3]. Nipple retraction and ulceration XEare secondary signs of malignancy and may occur with the extension of advanced breast cancer to the skin surface [3, 4].

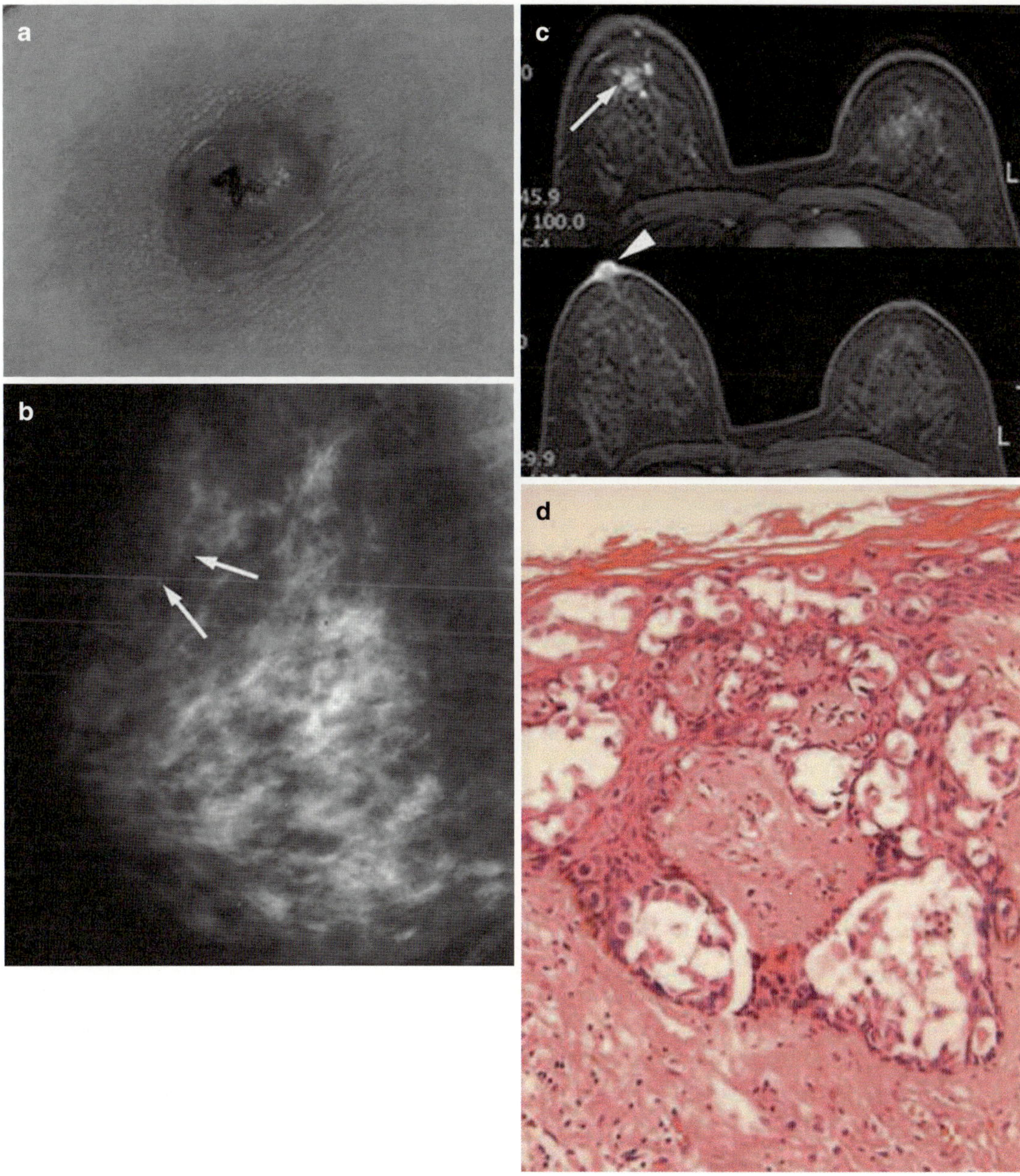


**Fig. 8.11** Paget's disease in 46-year-old women. (**a**) Ulceration, crusting, and eczema at the nipple. (**b**) Right mediolateral oblique mammogram showing multiple microcalcifications in the upper portion (*arrows*). (**c**) Axial contrast-enhanced MRI showing multiple nodular enhancement in the upper portion of the right breast (*arrow*) and enhancement of ipsilateral nipple-areolar complex (*arrowhead*). (**d**) Mastectomy specimen showing nests of malignant Paget cells predominantly involving the lower layers of the epidermis. The cytoplasm of the tumor cells contains abundant pale-staining granular mucinous material (hematoxylin-eosin, original magnification ×200)

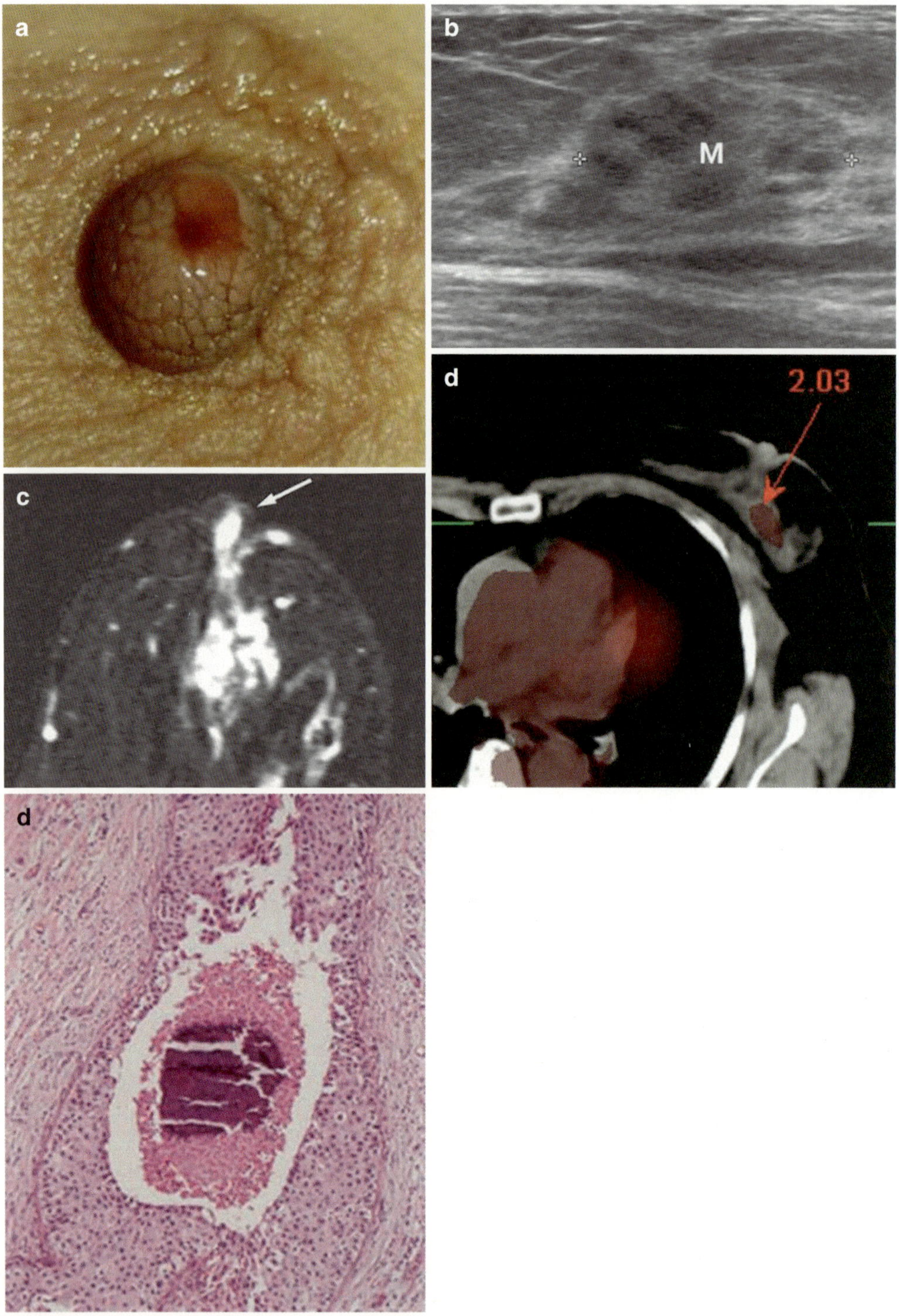


**Fig. 8.12** Ductal carcinoma in situ in a 51-year-old woman. (**a**) Bloody nipple discharge. (**b**) Sonogram showing a lobulated hypoechoic lesion (*M*), a finding suggestive of malignancy. (**c**) Axial contrast-enhanced substraction MRI showing a nodular clumped linearly enhanced lesion with direct invasion of the nipple (*arrow*). (**d**) Positron emission tomogram showing a hypermetabolic subareolar lesion (*arrow*; maximum standardized uptake value, 2.03) in the left breast. (**e**) Mastectomy specimen showing central necrosis, calcification, and a high nuclear grade, findings suggestive of ductal carcinoma in situ (hematoxylin-eosin, original magnification ×200)

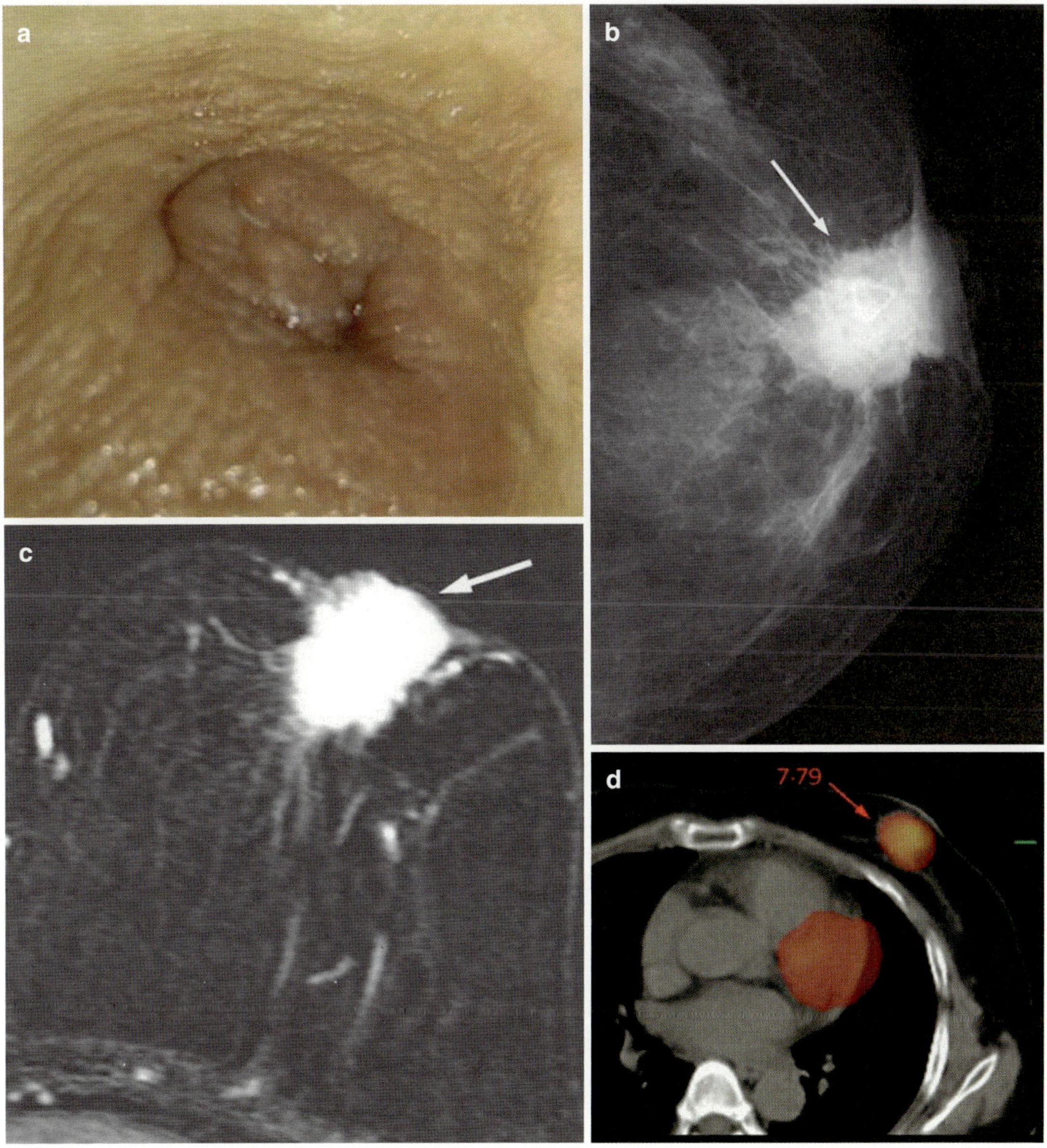


**Fig. 8.13** Invasive ductal carcinoma in a 61-year-old woman. (**a**) Retracted nipple. (**b**) Left craniocaudal mammogram showing a large irregularly shaped dense subareolar mass (*arrow*) with speculated margin and associated nipple retraction. (**c**) Axial contrast-enhanced substraction MRI showing a large irregularly shaped speculated subareolar mass extending to the nipple (*arrow*). (**d**) Positron emission tomogram showing a hypermetabolic subareolar mass (*arrow*; maximum standardized uptake value, 7.79) in the left breast. (**e**) Mastectomy specimen showing invasive ductal carcinoma (hematoxylin-eosin, original magnification ×200)

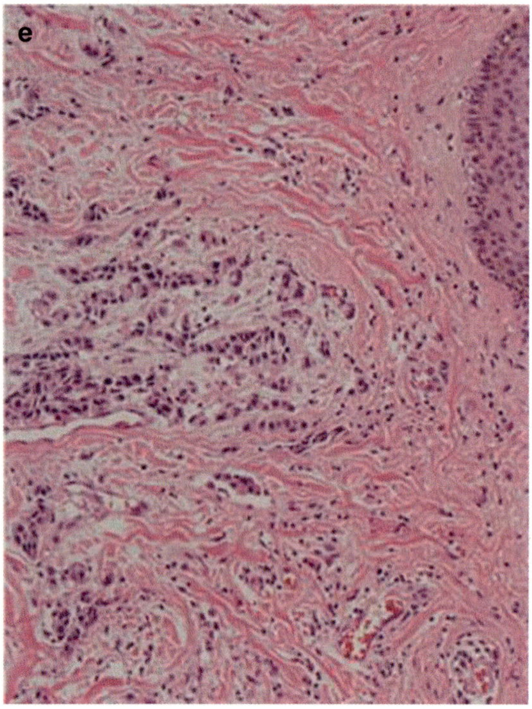


Fig. 8.13 (continued)

## Conclusions

The nipple-areolar complex is affected by various diseases, which have unique and various clinical findings of this region of the breast. Clinical history and physical examination are most particularly important, and a tailored image evaluation with multiple modalities often is necessary to accurately diagnose an underlying abnormality of the nipple-areolar complex.

## References

1. Kopans DB. Anatomy, histology, physiology, and pathology. In: Kopans DB, editor. Breast imaging. 3rd ed. Philadelphia: Lippincott Williams & Wilkins; 2007. p. 3–27.
2. Nicholson BT, Harvey JA, Cohen MA. Nipple-areolar complex: normal anatomy and benign and malignant processes. Radiographics. 2009;29(2):509–23.
3. Da Costa D, Taddese A, Cure ML, Gerson D, Poppiti R Jr, Esserman LE. Common and unusual diseases of the nipple-areolar complex. Radiographics. 2007;27(Suppl 1):S65–77.
4. Kopans DB. Breast anatomy and basic histology, physiology, and pathology. In: Kopans DB, editor. Breast imaging. 3rd ed. Philadelphia: Lippincott Williams & Wilkins; 2007. p. 7–43.
5. Kalbhen CL, Kezdi-Rogus PC, Dowling MP, Flisak ME. Mammography in the evaluation of nipple inversion. Am J Roentgenol. 1998;170(1):117–21.
6. Kopans DB. Interpreting the mammogram. In: Kopans DB, editor. Breast imaging. 3rd ed. Philadelphia: Lippincott Williams & Wilkins; 2007. p. 365–479.
7. Kim HS, Cha ES, Kim HH, Yoo JY. Spectrum of sonographic findings in superficial breast masses. J Ultrasound Med. 2005;24(5):663–80.
8. Kopans DB. Breast ultrasound. In: Kopans DB, editor. Breast imaging. 3rd ed. Philadelphia: Lippincott Williams & Wilkins; 2007. p. 555–605.
9. Huynh PT, Parellada JA, de Paredes ES, Harvey J, Smith D, Holley L, Maxin M. Dilated duct pattern at mammography. Radiology. 1997;204(1):137–41.
10. Cilotti A, Bagnolesi P, Napoli V, Lencioni R, Bartolozzi C. Solitary intraductal papilloma of the breast. An echographic study of 12 cases. Radiol Med. 1991;82(5):617–20.
11. Ganesan S, Karthik G, Joshi M, Damodaran V. Ultrasound spectrum in intraductal papillary neoplasms of breast. Br J Radiol. 2006;79(946):843–9.
12. Boonjunwetwat D, Prathombutr A. Imaging of benign papillary neoplasm of the breast: mammographic, galactographic and sonographic findings. J Med Assoc Thail. 2000;83(8):832–8.
13. Cole-Beuglet C, Soriano RZ, Kurtz AB, Goldberg BB. Fibroadenoma of the breast: sonomammography correlated with pathology in 122 patients. Am J Roentgenol. 1983;140(2):369–75.
14. Harper AP, Kelly-Fry E, Noe JS, Bies JR, Jackson VP. Ultrasound in the evaluation of solid breast masses. Radiology. 1983;146(3):731–6.
15. Jackson VP, Rothschild PA, Kreipke DL, Mail JT, Holden RW. The spectrum of sonographic findings of fibroadenoma of the breast. Investig Radiol. 1986;21(1):34–40.
16. Tohno E, Cosgrove DO, Sloane JP. Benign processes-tumors. In: Tohno E, editor. Ultrasound diagnosis of breast diseases. 1st ed. Edinburgh; New York: Churchill Livingstone; 1994. p. 76–91.
17. Fornage BD, Lorigan JG, Andry E. Fibroadenoma of the breast: sonographic appearance. Radiology. 1989;172(3):671–5.
18. Adler DD. Ultrasound of benign breast conditions. Semin Ultrasound CT MR. 1989;10(2):106–18.
19. Guyer PB, Dewbury KC, Rubin CM, Butcher C, Royle GT, Theaker J. Ultrasonic attenuation in fibroadenoma of the breast. Clin Radiol. 1992;45(3):175–8.
20. Murat A, Kansiz F, Kabakus N, Kazez A, Ozercan R. Neurofibroma of the breast in a boy with neurofibromatosis type 1. Clin Imaging. 2004;28(6):415–7.
21. Gokalp G, Hakyemez B, Kizilkaya E, Haholu A. Myxoidneurofibromas of the breast: mammo-

graphical, sonographical and MRI appearances. Br J Radiol. 2007;80(958):e234–7.
22. Reynolds DL Jr, Jacobson JA, Inampudi P, et al. Sonographic characteristics of peripheral nerve sheath tumors. Am J Roentgenol. 2004;182(3):741–4.
23. Lin J, Martel W. Cross-sectional imaging of peripheral nerve sheath tumors: characteristic signs on CT, MR imaging, and sonography. Am J Roentgenol. 2001;176(1):75–82.
24. Cordoliani F, Rybojad M, Verola O, Espié M. Dermatoses of the nipple and the areola. Arch Anat Cytol Pathol. 1995;43(1–2):82–7.
25. Parlakgumus A, Yildirim S, Bolat FA, Caliskan K, Ezer A, Colakoglu T, Moray G. Dermatoses of the nipple. Can J Surg. 2009;52(2):160–1.
26. Iancu D, Nochomovitz LE. Pseudoangiomatous stromal hyperplasia: presentation as a mass in the female nipple. Breast J. 2001;7(4):263–5.
27. Amamo G, Yajima M, Moroboshi Y, Kuriya Y, Ohuchi N. MRI accurately depicts underlying DCIS in a patient with Paget's disease of the breast without palpable mass and mammography findings. Jpn J Clin Oncol. 2005;35:149–53.
28. Lloyd J, Flanagan AM. Mammary and extramammary Paget's disease. J Clin Pathol. 2000;53:742–9.
29. Capobianco G, Spaliviero B, Dessole S, Cherchi PL, Marras V, Ambrosini G, Meloni F, Meloni GB. Paget's disease of the nipple diagnosed by MRI. Arch Gynecol Obstet. 2006;274:316–8.

# 9 Origin of Nipple-Areolar Complex Irregularities

Melvin A. Shiffman

## 9.1 Introduction

In order to repair abnormalities of the nipple-areolar complex, the surgeon should understand the origins of the deformity. Prevention of the irregularity can then be determined and further surgery avoided. Reconstruction depends on proper preoperative measurements, blood supply, and familiarity with the variety of techniques available.

## 9.2 Irregularities

Asymmetry of the nipple-areolar complex (NAC) may be caused by the surgeon's error in producing areola diameter, size, and contour differences through inadequate planning of breast reduction or mastopexy. There may be significant differences preoperatively between the sides such as the level of the inframammary fold, amount of ptosis, position, and/or height of the NAC. When there is a preoperative discrepancy of the NAC position, the surgeon should consider elevating the level of the lower NAC during the surgery or bringing the NAC medially or laterally during surgery depending on the differences in NAC position. Laterally the lower NAC will leave no scar above the NAC, whereas lowering the high NAC is more difficult in preventing excessive scarring. McKissock [1] has stated that "Improperly placed nipples that are excessively high are difficult to correct. The resulting scar may exceed the benefits derived from lowering the nipple. On the other hand, in those rare cases where the nipple is too low, elevation without additional scarring is easily achieved." He also said that "Other forms of nipple malposition require corrections that necessarily leave a trailing scar. In some the nipple-areola can be left attached to the gland mass and, after rather extensive undermining of the surrounding skin, can be repositioned through a properly located areola window. When the malposition is significantly greater than the diameter of the areola, a wide bridge of skin separates the past and future areola windows." In such a case, the secondary defect may be closed horizontally as described by Millard et al. [2]. This avoids the trailing scar and the superior extension of the scar.

A tethered or comma-shaped areola may be seen at the time of closure following reduction mammaplasty. "…usually caused by tugging on the areola by the folded dermal flap and is correctable by cautiously relaxing incisions at the time of surgery. When the areola deformity is obliquely oval, it usually does not self-correct. It is usually due to the asymmetrical tension resulting when the vertical closure does not correspond to the midline. It may also result when the cutout for the areola does not become circular when closed. It is best managed by a secondary surgery, which usually results in some asymmetry" [1].

M.A. Shiffman, M.D., J.D.
Private Practice, 17501 Chatham Drive, Tustin, CA 92780-2302, USA
e-mail: shiffmanmdjd@gmail.com





M.A. Shiffman (ed.), *Nipple-Areolar Complex Reconstruction*,
https://doi.org/10.1007/978-3-319-60925-6_9

Designing the procedure for breast reduction with the patient sitting or standing allows the inframammary fold position to be designated on the chest wall along the midclavicular line with the fingers under the breast. However, the most common error is in the patient with very large or gigantic breasts where the selection of the level of the inframammary fold is the site for the nipple, when in fact the nipple position should be estimated lower by 1 or 2 cm.

## 9.3 Discussion

No matter how hard one tries to achieve bilateral NAC symmetry, there is great difficulty in achieving equality. There always is slight asymmetry even in the normal unoperated breast.

Changes in areola diameter affect the appearance of symmetry to a greater degree than changes in NAC position or pigmentation. The most meaningful assessment belongs to the woman who has undergone the surgery [3].

## References

1. McKissock PK. Reduction mammaplasty. In: Courtiss EH, editor. Aesthetic surgery trouble: how to avoid it and how to treat it. Saint Louis: C.V. Mosby Company; 1978. p. 189–203.
2. Millard DR, Mullin WR, Lasavoy MA. Secondary correction of the too-high areola and nipple after a mammaplasty. Plast Reconstr Surg. 1976;58(5):568–72.
3. Brown MH, Semple JL, Neligan PC. Variables affecting symmetry of the nipple-areola complex. Plast Reconstr Surg. 1995;96(4):846–51.

# Part IV

# Malposition

# Double U-Plasty for the Correction of Nipple-Areola Complex Malposition

# 10

Christopher C. West and Anas Naasan

## 10.1 Introduction

The normal appearance of the breast includes symmetry of the nipple-areola complex (NAC), and variations from this can have significant influence on a patient's overall satisfaction. Variations in the position of the NAC can arise due to the natural changes to a breast associated with aging, but also due to other factors including aesthetic and reconstructive surgery, radiotherapy, and trauma including burns [1].

While many successful techniques to elevate an inferiorly positioned NAC have been described [2, 3], repositioning a NAC that is too high or deviated laterally is a significant challenge to the surgeon. This is a particular problem when trying to minimize scarring in the upper quadrants of the breast, when trying to relocate the NAC without making alterations to the size and shape of the breast, and when the quality of the surrounding tissue has been affected by previous surgery, radiotherapy, or trauma such as burns or skin grafts [4, 5]. With the increasing incidence of oncoplastic breast surgery, the challenge of repositioning a NAC is likely to be more frequently encountered in surgical practice [6].

In addition to the aesthetic appearance of the breast, the principal function is that of lactation during the breastfeeding and also as a secondary sexual organ. Therefore techniques that aim to reposition the NAC should also aim to preserve these functions.

The authors describe the double U-plasty to correct malposition of the NAC. In our original article describing the technique, we used it to correct malposition in a post-burn patient [4]; however, its utility is wide reaching. We give a detailed description of the technique and compare and contrast the potential advantages and disadvantages of this method with other published methods to correct malposition.

## 10.2 Technique

Patients should be marked standing. We prefer to carry out the surgery under general anesthesia (GA) although it can be done as a local anesthetic (LA) procedure.

The first marking is that of the new nipple-areola complex (NAC) which is drawn with reference to the dimensions of the contralateral, undistorted and normally positioned, side. The

C.C. West, M.B., Ch.B., B.Med.Sci., Ph.D.
A. Naasan, M.B., Ch.B., FRCS FRCS(Plast) (✉)
The Department of Plastic and Reconstructive Surgery, Ninewells Hospital, Dundee DD1 9SY, UK
e-mail: c.c.west@doctors.net.uk; anaasan@doctors.org.uk


M.A. Shiffman (ed.), *Nipple-Areolar Complex Reconstruction*,
https://doi.org/10.1007/978-3-319-60925-6_10

first "U" is marked as a semicircle around the new NAC (flap A). The second "U" is marked at the proposed site of the NAC (flap B), taking care to match this to the inner positions of NAC of the contralateral breast. The limbs of the two "U"s are joined to form an "S" (Fig. 10.1). Flap A is raised with minimal dissection of the glandular tissue to minimize the disruption to the ductal system of the NAC. Flap B is then raised thinner than flap A. Following thorough and meticulous hemostasis, the flaps are transposed delivering flap A and the NAC to the desired position on the breast. Due to the thicker flap and the underlying ductal tissue, projection of the NAC is also achieved. The skin is closed with interrupted deep dermal 3-0 and a continuous subcuticular 4-0 monofilament absorbable suture (Monocryl®) and dressed with Steri-Strips and a shower-proof dressing. Subsequent procedures such as tattooing of the NAC are possible and should be performed once satisfactory healing has been achieved (Figs. 10.2, 10.3, and 10.4).

In the original description of this technique based upon a single case, the orientation of this "U" was from the 4 o'clock position to the 10 o'clock position (Fig. 10.1a–c); however, in reality the geometric position of the "U" can be orientated in an indefinite number of ways according to the required transposition of the NAC (Fig. 10.1d). Consideration to the orientation of the pedicles should also be made to ensure the avoidance of any previous scars that might compromise the vascularity and preservation of sensation to the NAC.

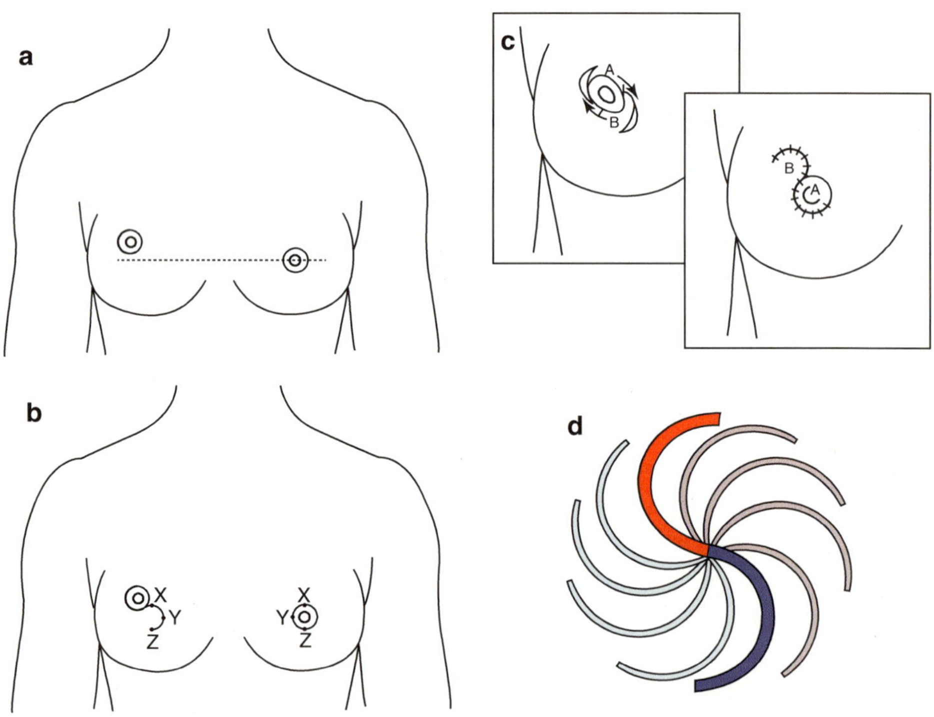


**Fig. 10.1** (**a–d**) Marking of the U flaps and the double U-plasty

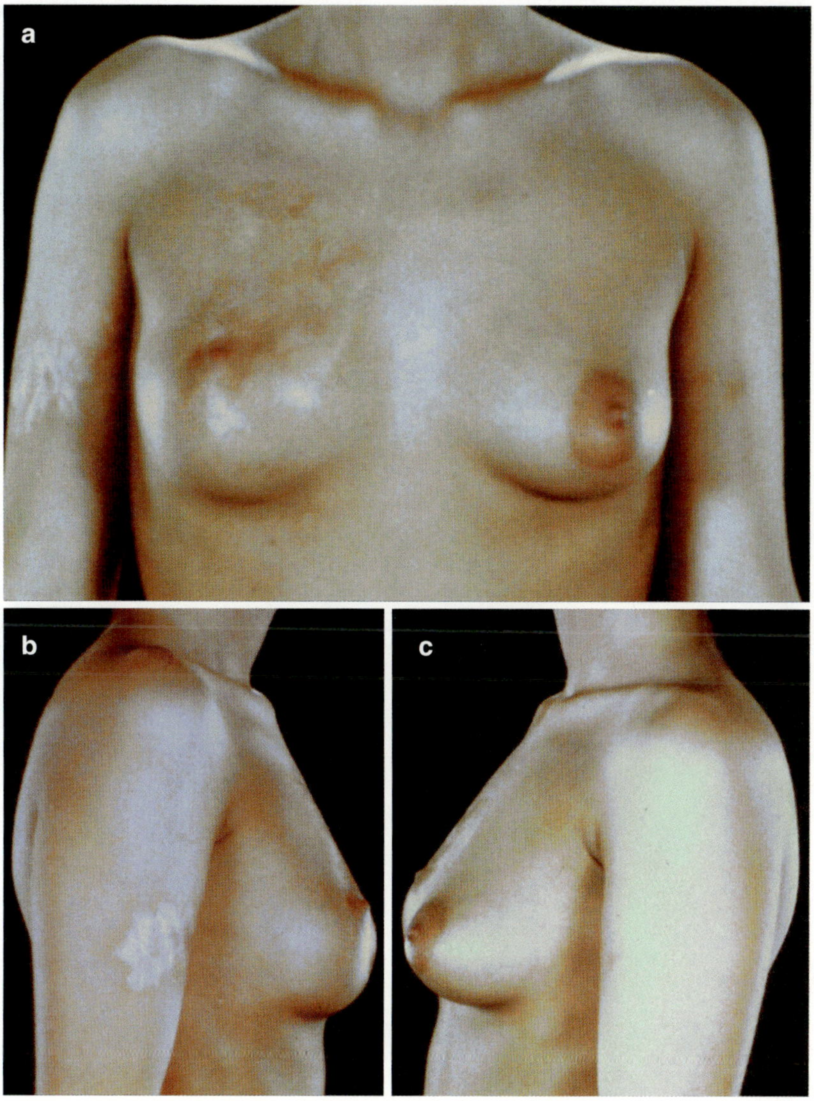


**Fig. 10.2** (**a–c**) Preoperative patient

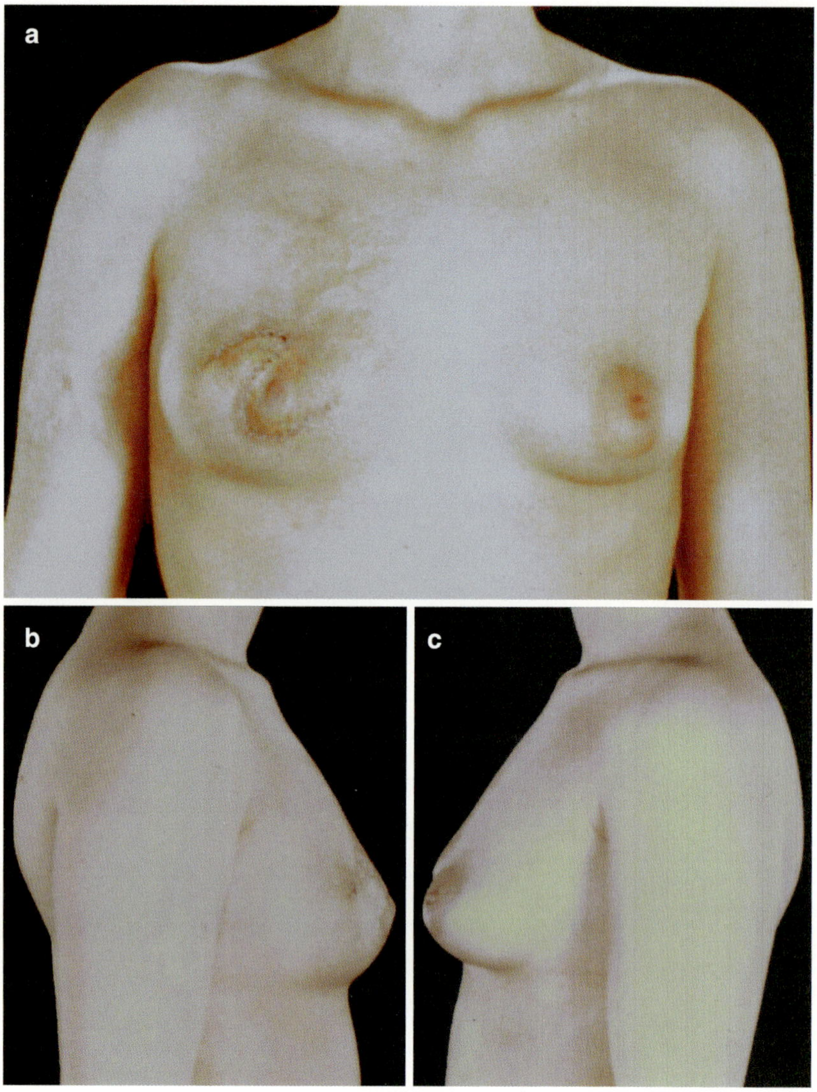

**Fig. 10.3** (**a–c**) Early postoperative

**Fig. 10.4** (**a–c**) Eighteen months postoperative. (**d**) (*1*) Close up to corrected NAC eighteen months post surgery. (*2*) Close up to normal NAC of the other side

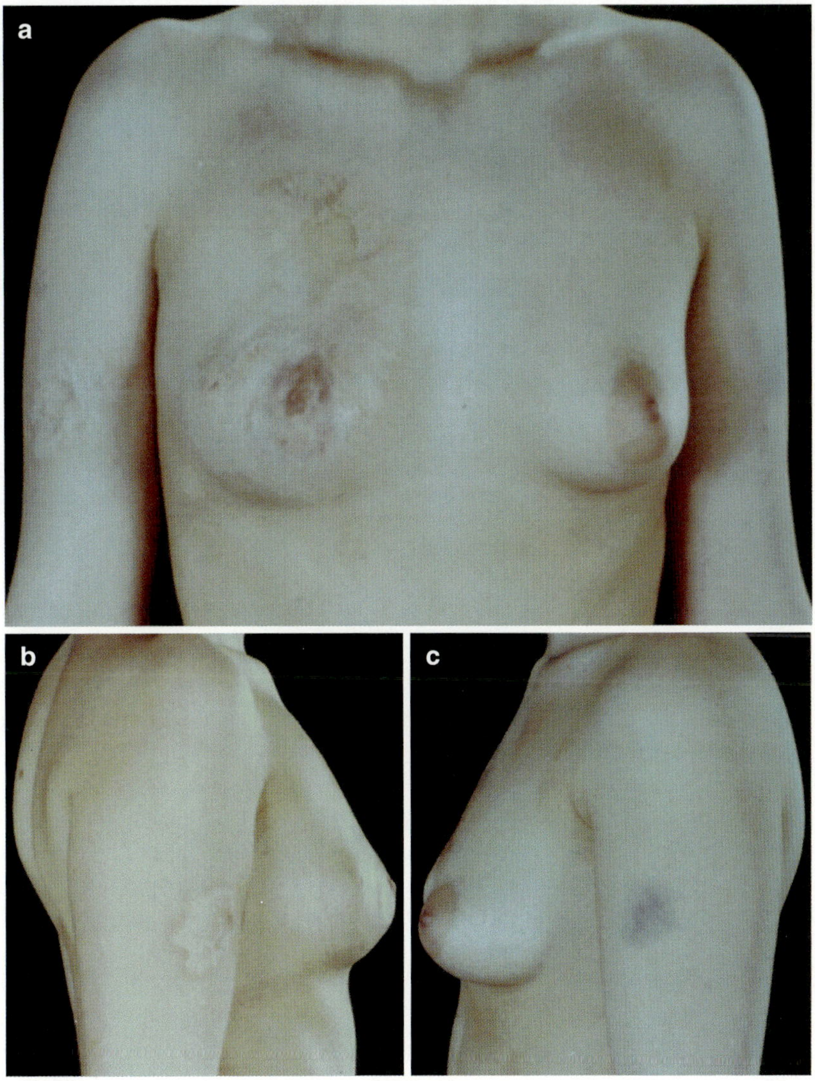

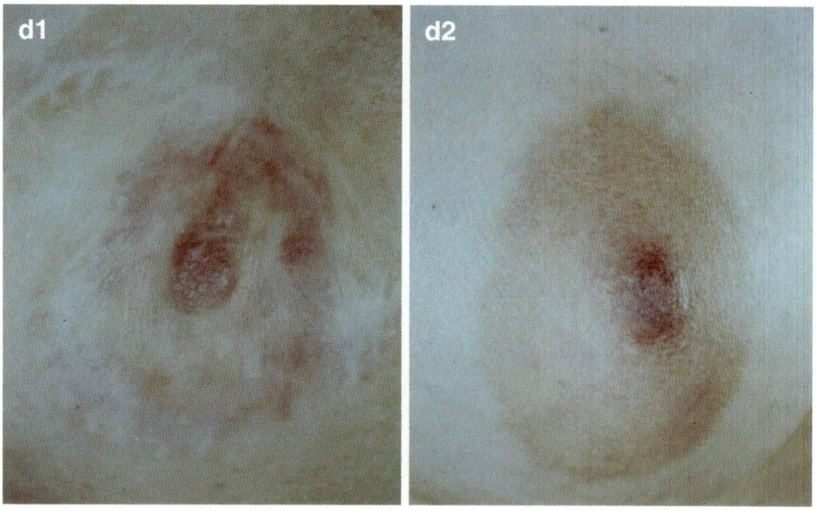


**Fig 10.4** (continued)

## 10.3 Discussion

Malposition of the NAC is a commonly encountered problem. Low NAC is most frequently associated with breast ptosis due to the natural effects of aging on the breast, and many different mastopexy techniques have been described to address this [2, 3, 7]. A NAC that is geometrically malpositioned either too high or deviating medially or laterally from the breast meridian is a less frequently encountered problem but poses a much greater challenge to the surgeon [8]. This is due to the fixed distance between the sternal notch and the NAC, difficulty in recruiting tissue to relocate the NAC, and a desire to minimize scarring in the upper and medial parts of the breast [6]. Common causes of malposition include oncological resection, reconstruction, reduction, mastopexy, radiotherapy, and trauma including burns [8–10].

In trying to address the issue of a malpositioned nipple, many different techniques have been described including V-Y advancement flaps, skin grafts, tissue expansion, breast resection, and volume addition [1]. While these techniques might be suitable for some patients, they will also produce changes to the overall shape of the breast that may be undesirable, or necessitate the need for contralateral procedures. For patients who have otherwise symmetrical and aesthetically acceptable breasts, there are limited techniques that allow for repositioning of the NAC without significant readjustment of the breast itself.

A method of reciprocal skin grafts has been described by two different authors. The principle is similar to that described in the double U-plasty; however, instead of raising two flaps, full thickness grafts are harvested that include the NAC and the skin overlying the site of the new NAC before being rotated and replaced [8, 9]. The advantage of this technique, similar to the double U-plasty, is that it can be performed under local anesthetic. However, as a result of the grafting, both the NAC and the skin graft will be insensate, have the inherent risk of graft loss, and are at a greater risk of contracture and subsequent distortion. In addition the ductal system to the NAC will be irreversibly disrupted.

The use of pedicled flaps to transpose the NAC—as described in this chapter—has also been described by other authors. Van Straalen et al. [5] report the use of two subcutaneous pedicled flaps to treat post-burn malposition of the NAC in 15 patients. In this method, two subcutaneous flaps were raised, one incorporating the NAC and the second the skin of the recipient site of the NAC. In some patients they were able to perform this technique under local anesthetic. Average follow-up was 4 years and all patients reported satisfactory outcome. The principal advantages of this technique reported by the authors were the ability to manipulate the NAC with minimal change to the breast itself, improved vascularity of the flaps by maintaining underlying attachments, and the preservation of sensation and ductal function. This supports the theory and findings of our technique.

A more recent study described the use of reciprocal transposition flaps in the treatment of high-riding nipple on five breasts in four patients [6]. Once again the principles of the technique are similar to that described in this chapter whereby two flaps are raised to incorporate the NAC and the intended site of the new NAC. The significant difference between this technique and ours is that the flaps are raised in the deep subcutaneous plane, just superficial to the implant capsule if one is present. This is a much deeper plane than the one we described and the one described by van Straalen [4, 5]. The implications of this more extensive dissection may be a reduction in the sensation to the nipple and the function of the ductal system; however, neither of these outcomes is mentioned in the paper [6]. One of the patients in this case series experienced transient flap ischemia that was successfully treated with hyperbaric oxygen therapy that may be a consequence of the more extensive dissection and undermining.

**Conclusions**

The double U-plasty is a simple and elegant procedure for repositioning of the NAC and can be utilized to reposition the NAC in any direction. With careful planning and attention to precise surgical technique, the sensation to the nipple and function of the ductal system can also be preserved. The original description of this technique was employed by the senior author (AN) to address a malpositioned nipple as a result of burn scarring [4]. Subsequently this technique and variations based upon it have been described by multiple other authors and used to reposition NAC due to multiple causes with great success [5, 6]. The double U-plasty is therefore a useful and reliable technique that can be used to produce excellent results in a variety of carefully selected patients, with preservation of nipple sensation and breast function.

## References

1. Spear SL, Albino FP, Al-Attar A. Classification and management of the postoperative, high-riding nipple. Plast Reconstr Surg. 2013;131(6):1413–21.
2. Lassus C. Reduction mammaplasty with short inframammary scars. Plast Reconstr Surg. 1986;77(4):680–1.
3. Lejour M. Vertical mammaplasty. Plast Reconstr Surg. 1993;92(5):985–6.
4. Mohmand H, Naasan A. Double U-plasty for correction of geometric malposition of the nipple-areola complex. Plast Reconstr Surg. 2002;109(6):2019–22.
5. van Straalen WR, van Trier AJ, Groenevelt F. Correction of the post-burn malpositioned nipple-areola complex by transposition of two subcutaneous pedicled flaps. Br J Plast Surg. 2000;53(5):406–9.
6. Spear SL, Albino FP, Al-Attar A. Repairing the high-riding nipple with reciprocal transposition flaps. Plast Reconstr Surg. 2013;131(4):687–9.
7. Marchac D, de Olarte G. Reduction mammaplasty and correction of ptosis with a short inframammary scar. Plast Reconstr Surg. 1982;69(1):45–55.
8. Spear SL, Hoffman S. Relocation of the displaced nipple-areola by reciprocal skin grafts. Plast Reconstr Surg. 1998;101(5):1355–8.
9. Ali S, Jaffe W, Howcroft A. A simple method of resiting the malpositioned nipple. Br J Plast Surg. 1997;50(6):470.
10. Frenkiel BA, Pacifico MD, Ritz M, Southwick G. A solution to the high-riding nipple-areola complex. Aesthet Plast Surg. 2010;34(4):525–7.

# 11 Free Nipple Graft Technique for Correcting a Malpositioned Nipple After Breast Procedures

Prakasit Chirappapha and Mario Rietjens

## 11.1 Introduction

The malpositioned nipple-areolar complex (NAC) can occur after several breast procedures. Dislocation of NAC after breast-conserving surgery (BCS) can occur in patients with large tumors in whom large volumes of breast tissue must be removed and are exacerbated by radiation. The NAC can also retract high above or laterally after nipple-sparing mastectomy (NSM) procedures. Management of the malpositioned NAC is a challenge in these patients. Several techniques have been described for treating malpositioned NAC including transposition of NAC on a pedicle [1, 2], lowering of NAC with implants [3, 4], expanding the skin superior to the NAC, and elevating the inframammary fold with breast parenchyma. Free nipple grafts have been reported for reduction mammoplasty [5–9]. Spear and Hoffman [10] corrected NAC displacement following NSM by using the reciprocal transposition flaps. Frenkiel et al. [11] reported a case of successful correction of a high-riding nipple using a Z-plasty technique. Thus, currently there are no generally accepted surgical techniques for managing NAC malposition. We present an alternative approach to relocate the NAC between both breasts by using free NAC grafts combined with lipofilling. By using lipofilling, symmetry between both NACs can be restored in terms of contour, size, and site.

P. Chirappapha, M.D. (✉)
Department of Surgery, Faculty of Medicine
Ramathibodi Hospital, Mahidol University,
270 Rama VI Road, Ratchathewi, Bangkok 10400,
Thailand
e-mail: onco.prakasit@gmail.com

M. Rietjens, M.D.
Department of Plastic and Reconstructive Surgery,
European Institute of Oncology,
Via Ripamonti, 435, 20141 Milan, Italy
e-mail: mario.rietjens@ieo.it

## 11.2 Technique

Patients in our series had NAC that was superior to and/or lateral to the correct location. The malposition was quite obvious on both lateral and frontal views when compared with the normal side (Fig. 11.1).

### 11.2.1 Preoperative Evaluation and Surgical Planning

Physical examination was performed for all patients by oncologic or plastic surgeons both preoperatively and postoperatively. Midsternal and midclavicular lines were marked before surgery with the patient in the standing position. The area of parenchymal defect and the new NAC location were marked on the breast. The new


M.A. Shiffman (ed.), *Nipple-Areolar Complex Reconstruction*,
https://doi.org/10.1007/978-3-319-60925-6_11

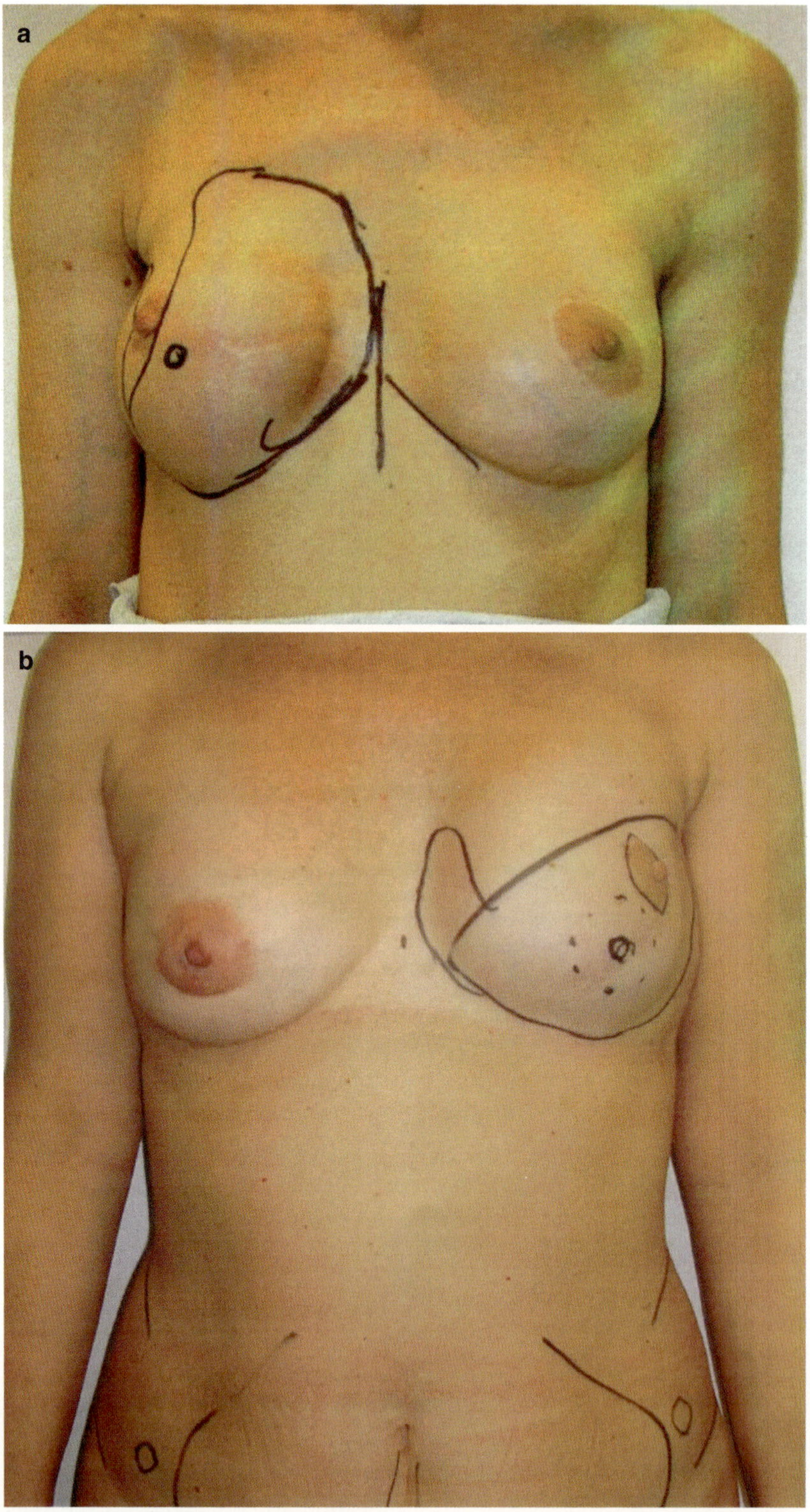


**Fig. 11.1** (**a**) Preoperative planning showing the area of new NAC design at the right breast. (**b**) Preoperative patient with the NAC retracted high above and laterally after NSM procedures. (**c**) Preoperative patient with NAC that was in superior location

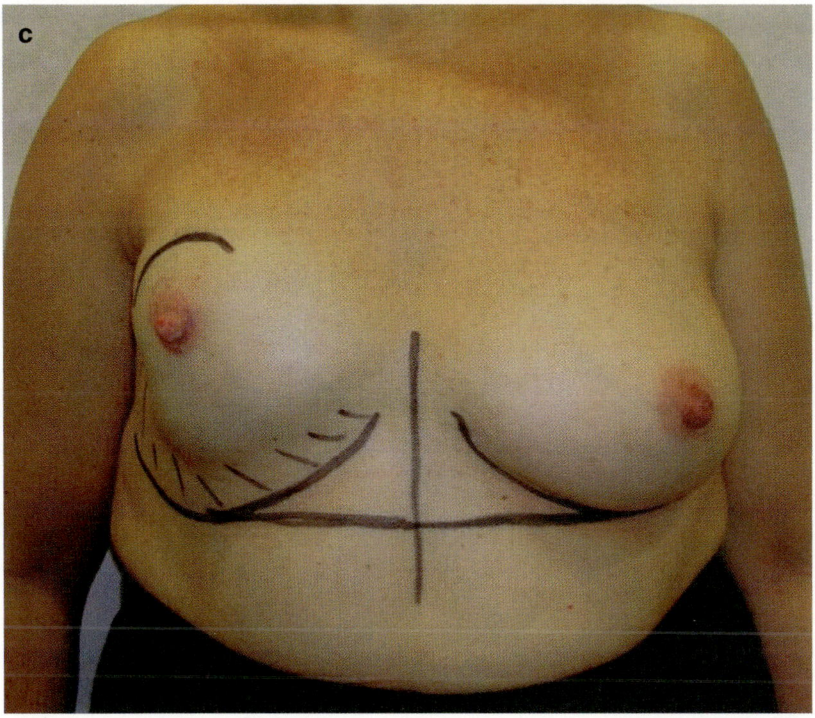


**Fig. 11.1** (continued)

position of NAC was planned to be 21–23 cm from the suprasternal notch. This new NAC location was designed to be approximately at the level of the contralateral NAC position with the patient's arm at her side (Fig. 11.1).

### 11.2.2 Operative Technique

With the patient standing, the new NAC area was marked corresponding to the size of the existing NAC (Figs. 11.1 and 11.2). The NAC was harvested as a full-thickness graft with a scalpel at the level of the subdermis (Fig. 11.2), preserving the complete thickness of the dermis layer while ensuring that all subcutaneous tissue had been trimmed. The graft was then placed in normal saline solution for later use. The new NAC area was carefully deepithelialized with a number-10 blade. The patient was moved to a seated position and the new NAC location was determined. The NAC graft was then placed on the deepithelialized bed and fixed with interrupted subcuticular 4-0 Monocryl around the edge of NAC area. A key point is that horizontal mattress sutures be used. The bolus tie-over dressing gauze was applied on NAC graft and was secured with 4-0 nylon sutured above both the graft and the skin edge at six circumferential points. Emekli et al. [12] reported an alternative syringe stent-assisted bolus tie-over dressing method to secure NAC grafts. The procedure of lipofilling was performed according to Coleman's technique after completion of a free nipple graft procedure [13]. The fat graft was injected into the defect area through a blunt Coleman cannula. We estimated the amount of fatty tissue injected in each individual case, based on shape and size of the defect. The patients were followed at the outpatient department, and the free nipple graft was examined on postoperative days 5–7 (Fig. 11.3).

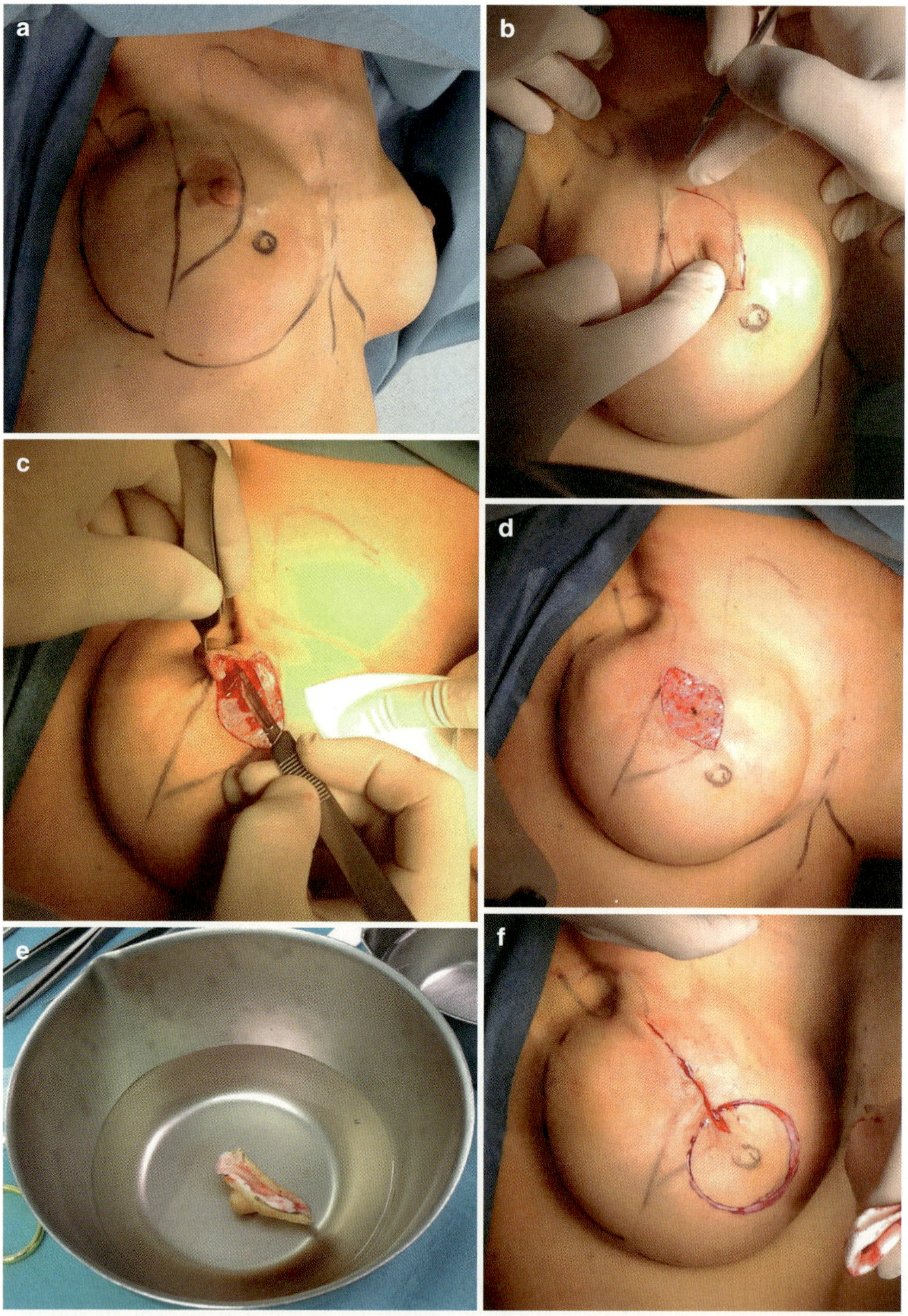


**Fig. 11.2** (**a**) Preoperative marking of the new NAC area. (**b**) The NAC was excised with a scalpel at the level of the subdermis. (**c**) The NAC was excised as a full-thickness graft. (**d**) Intraoperative showing deepithelialized area after harvesting NAC. (**e**) The NAC graft is removed and saved in normal saline solution. (**f**) The new NAC area was deepithelialized after closing the harvesting NAC site. (**g**) Recipient site after deepithelialization. (**h**) The NAC was placed in the deepithelialized bed. (**i**) Four points were fixed with interrupted sutures. (**j**) Correction of parenchyma defect with lipofilling technique. (**k**) Using horizontal mattress suture technique, we fixed with interrupted subcuticular 4-0 Monocryl around the edge of NAC area. (**l**) The free nipple graft has been positioned and the bolus will be placed to ensure immobilization

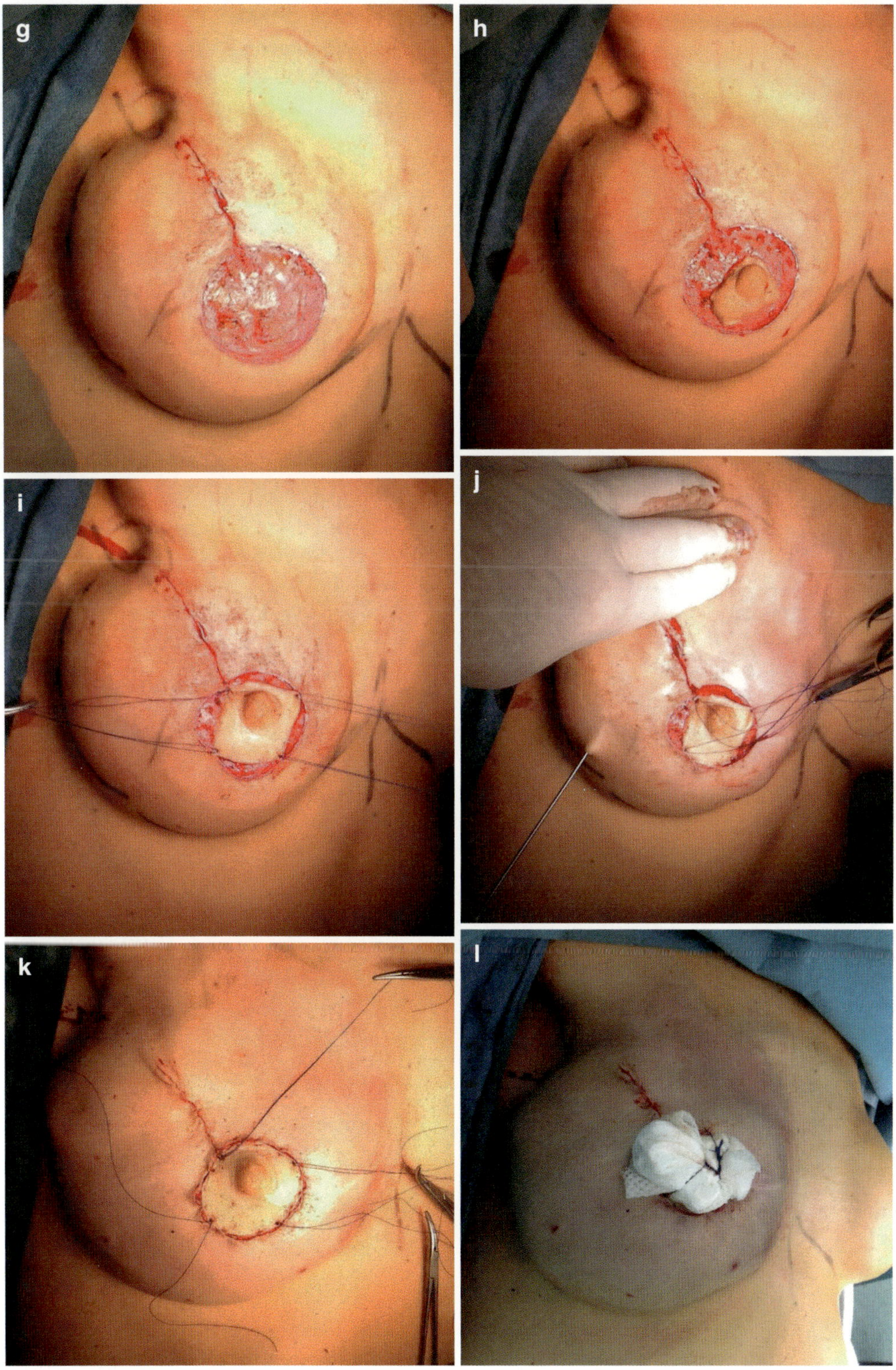


**Fig. 11.2** (continued)

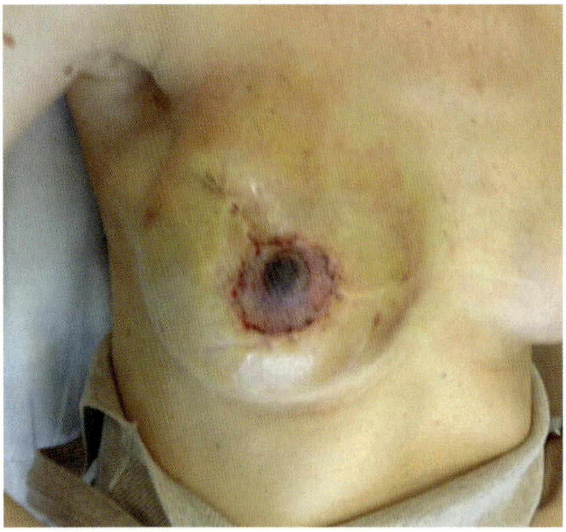

**Fig. 11.3** Early postoperative, day 5. The areola shows signs of vascularization; a superficial eschar on the nipple was seen as a sign of partial NAC necrosis

## 11.3 Discussion

Abnormally high location of NAC after reduction mammoplasty and breast deformity with a malpositioned NAC after BCS or NSM are devastating problems with few surgical solutions. Several studies demonstrated the value of free nipple transplantation in reduction mammoplasty [6–8, 14]. A few reports in the literature described using the NAC as a free graft at a new NAC location for correcting NAC malposition [10, 15]. A free NAC graft used to correct the NAC malposition after performing previous breast surgery in our series is a simple and reliable technique, even though some of our patients had a background of previous radiotherapy that could affect wound healing and might cause graft failure. We also used a lipofilling technique with the patient's own fat tissue for maintenance of the breast fullness in our series. The authors believe that this combined method has an advantage over other techniques because the parenchymal defect and malpositioned NAC can be simultaneously corrected and could preserve the fullness of breast in the long term.

Important technical points of our technique are that the surgeon must carefully and precisely dissect the NAC graft to ensure that all subcutaneous tissue has been trimmed and the graft is not too thin because nipple projection and erectility will be severely compromised or absent [5]. Horizontal mattress suturing of the NAC graft to the deepithelialized bed is another key feature. Meticulous preparation of the NAC graft and recipient bed with adequate postoperative immobilization of the graft should minimize the risk of NAC graft failure. The main disadvantages of the novel technique described here are the persistent scar at harvested NAC site and pigmentation change of the NAC. Depigmentation can be corrected with tattooing.

Three patients in the present series developed partial NAC necrosis due to insufficient tie-over dressing, with consequent decrease in the contact between the NAC graft and the recipient's bed. Partial necrosis of NAC was seen as a superficial eschar on the nipple. No NAC loss was observed in the present series. Necrotic complications were managed by conservative dressing of the NAC, which healed in all cases. Wound dehiscence, infection, and fat necrosis were not observed at all [16]. The excellent results seen in our series, however, may be due to the individual surgeon's technique, as the patients were operated on by one surgeon. Limitations of our study include the practice of only one surgeon as well as the small sample size. Indeed, other authors have published case reports describing several techniques that successfully moved the NAC to a more appropriate location (Table 11.1). However, the present series is the largest for this type of surgery with good operative results comparable to those reported in the studies listed in Table 11.1. Further comparative studies with larger sample sizes are required. In conclusion, a simple and effective technique of the free nipple graft is presented, in combination with lipofilling. This combined method allows correction of a malpositioned NAC and fat necrosis after BCS or NSM in all axes with acceptable results.

**Table 11.1** Comparison of different techniques and outcomes

| Author | Years | Number of cases | Preoperative diagnosis | Operative technique | Complication |
|---|---|---|---|---|---|
| Ali [15] | 1997 | 1 | Malposition of reconstructed NAC after NSM with a pedicled LD flap | Rotating the figure eight-shaped NAC graft | None |
| Spear [10] | 1998 | 2 | Displaced NAC after NSM with implant, augmentation with infection | Reciprocal full-thickness skin grafts | None |
| Mohmand [1] | 2002 | 1 | Distortion NAC after burn | Double U-plasty | None |
| Colwell [4] | 2007 | 3 | High position of nipples after reduction, augmentation/mastopexy | Infraclavicular subcutaneous tissue expansion | None |
| Frenkiel [11] | 2010 | 1 | High-riding nipple after NSM with implant and WBR | Z-plasty transposition | None |
| Takayanagi [17] | 2010 | 2 | Malpositioned nipple after NSM | Two subcutaneous pedicles and the purse-string suture | None |
| Taneda [18] | 2011 | 1 | Malpositioned nipple after NSM | Rotation flap and an advancement flap | None |
| Staley [19] | 2014 | 1 | Malpositioned nipple after wide local excision | Transposition flap and skin graft | None |
| Spear [20] | 2013 | 4 | High-riding nipple after NSM with implant and WBR, mastopexy | Reciprocal transposition flap | Transient flap ischemia one case |
| Rietjens [16] | 2013 | 16 | Malpositioned nipple after NSM, BCS with WBR | Free NAC graft | Partial necrosis of NAC three cases |

*LD* latissimus dorsi, *WBR* whole breast radiation, *NAC* nipple-areolar complex, *NSM* nipple-sparing mastectomy, *BCS* breast-conserving surgery

## References


1. Mohmand H, Naasan A. Double U-plasty for correction of geometric malposition of the nipple–areola complex. Plast Reconstr Surg. 2002;109:2019–22.
2. van Straalen WR, van Trier AJM, Groenevelt F. Correction of the post-burn malpositioned nipple–areola complex by transposition of two subcutaneous pedicled flaps. Br J Plast Surg. 2000;53:406–9.
3. Millard DR Jr, Mullin WR, Lesavoy MA. Secondary correction of the too-high areola and nipple after mammaplasty. Plast Reconstr Surg. 1976;58:568–72.
4. Colwell AS, May JW Jr, Slavin SA. Lowering the postoperative high-riding nipple. Plast Reconstr Surg. 2007;120:596–9.
5. Mess SA, Gradinger GP, Spear SL. Breast reduction with the free-nipple technique. In: Spear AL, editor. Surgery of the breast: principles and art. 2nd ed. Philadelphia, PA: Lippincott Williams and Wilkins; 2006. p. 1172–88.
6. Gorgu M, Ayhan M, Aytug Z, Aksungur E, Demirdover C. Maximizing breast projection with combined free-nipple graft reduction mammoplasty and back-folded dermaglandular inferior pedicle. Breast J. 2007;13:226–32.
7. Güven E, Aydin H, Başaran K, Aydin U, Kuvat SV. Reduction mammaplasty using bipedicled dermoglandular flaps and free-nipple transplantation. Aesthet Plast Surg. 2010;34:738–44
8. Fırat C, Gurlek A, Erbatur S, Aytekin AH. An autoprosthesis technique for better breast projection in free nipple graft reduction mammaplasty. Aesthet Plast Surg. 2012;36(6):1340.
9. Thorek M. Possibilities in the reconstruction of the human form 1922. Aesthet Plast Surg. 1989;13:55–8.
10. Spear SL, Hoffman S. Relocation of the displaced nipple–areola by reciprocal skin grafts. Plast Reconstr Surg. 1998;101:1355–8.
11. Frenkiel BA, Pacifico MD, Ritz M, Southwick G. A solution to the high-riding nipple-areola complex. Aesthet Plast Surg. 2010;34:525–7.
12. Emekli U, Güven E, Ozden BC, Kesim SN. A practical dressing method after nipple areola reconstruction. Eur J Plast Surg. 2004;27:99–100.
13. Coleman SR. Long-term survival of fat transplants: controlled demonstrations. Aesthet Plast Surg. 1995;19(5):421.

14. Misirlioglu A, Akoz T. Familial severe gigantomastia and reduction with the free-nipple-graft vertical mammoplasty technique: report of two cases. Aesthet Plast Surg. 2005;29:205–9.
15. Ali S, Jaffe W, Howcroft A. A simple method of resiting the malpositioned nipple. Br J Plast Surg. 1997;50:470–1.
16. Rietjens M, De Lorenzi F, Andrea M, Chirappapha P, Martella S, Barbieri B, Gottardi A, Giuseppe L, Hamza A, Petit JY, Lohsiriwat V. Free nipple graft technique to correct nipple and areola malposition after breast procedures. Plast Reconstr Surg Glob Open. 2013;1(8):e69.
17. Takayanagi S. Transposition of the malpositioned nipple-areola complex in breast reconstruction with implants. Aesthet Plast Surg. 2010;34:52–8.
18. Taneda H, Sakai S. Transposition technique for correction of a malpositioned nipple-areola complex after reconstruction following a nipple-sparing mastectomy: a case report. Ann Plast Surg. 2011;67:579–82.
19. Staley H, Serra MP. A technique to correct a malpositioned nipple within the confines of a well-placed areola. Ann Plast Surg. 2014;72:279–80.
20. Spear SL, Albino FP, Al-Attar A. Repairing the high-riding nipple with reciprocal transposition flaps. Plast Reconstr Surg. 2013;131:687–9.

# Part V

# Benign and Malignant Disorders of the Nipple-Areolar Complex

# Introduction to Benign and Malignant Disorders of the Nipple-Areolar Complex

**12**

Melvin A. Shiffman

## 12.1 Introduction

The nipple-areolar complex (NAC) may be affected by a variety of disorders that are benign and malignant. These can include skin changes in and around the nipple and areola, infection, benign tumors, and malignant tumors. Diagnostic imaging may be necessary such as mammography, ultrasonography, galactography, and/or magnetic resonance imaging (MRI). The physician may have to decide whether or not local treatment will suffice or whether more radical surgery may be needed.

## 12.2 Abscess

With lactation and suckling, the nipple can get irritated and appear red and swollen. A subareolar abscess may develop, but the more likely cause would be jewelry piercing of the nipple [1–3]. Nipples can become irritated, sore, or even cracked due to friction. Running and sexual activity are sometimes causes of temporary nipple problems due to vigorous rubbing.

Phlegmon (diffuse inflammation) of the areola was observed by Chalot [4]. Winkle [5] reported seeing inflammation of Montgomery glands with furuncular (irritative) prominence and pain as well as follicular abscess.

## 12.3 Adenoma

Adenoma of the nipple can present various histological features. The symptoms include erosion of the nipple, nipple discharge, induration, and tumor formation at the nipple [6, 7]. Gross [8] stated that cystic adenoma was hard to tell from fibroma. Cystic adenoma may have keratin cysts or focal necrosis within proliferating ducts. Galloway et al. [9] reported on a patient with adenoid cystic carcinoma.

Syringomatous adenoma has haphazard proliferation of oval/elongated ductules and tubules composed of small basophilic cells infiltrating dermis of the skin, nipple stroma, and nipple smooth muscle bundles, resembling cutaneous syringoma [10, 11]. The ducts have teardrop, comma-like tail (tadpole appearance), or branching shapes with open lumens, and there is fibrous stroma. There are solid nests and strands of basaloid cells that may be present in the dermis and variable squamous metaplasia with keratinizing cysts and calcification. Perineural invasion is common. In the clear cell variant the ducts are lined by epithelial cells with pale or clear

M.A. Shiffman, M.D., J.D.
Private Practice, 17501 Chatham Drive, Tustin, CA 92780-2302, USA
e-mail: shiffmanmdjd@gmail.com


M.A. Shiffman (ed.), *Nipple-Areolar Complex Reconstruction*, https://doi.org/10.1007/978-3-319-60925-6_12

cytoplasm. The infiltrating syringomatous adenoma of the nipple occurs almost exclusively in women of all ages and is cured by simple excision [12]. There are reports of syringomatous adenoma [13–29].

There are several articles on adenoma of the nipple [30–40], papillary adenoma of the nipple (florid papillomatosis, adenoma, adenomatosis) [41, 42], papillomatosis [43–48], and erosive adenomatosis [49–72].

Adenoma of the nipple is an uncommon lesion that is often mistaken clinically for Paget's disease and misinterpreted pathologically as ductal carcinoma [73, 74].

Brownstein et al. [41] stated that papillary adenoma may have erosion that can clinically mimic Paget's disease. A few have a nodule in the nipple with retraction, simulating invasive carcinoma. It is also important for pathologists to be familiar with this lesion since it can be mistaken for a well-differentiated adenocarcinoma both on frozen and permanent sections.

Montemarano et al. [45] reported that superficial papillary adenomatosis of the nipple is a benign tumor of the ductal epithelium that clinically resembles Paget's disease. Histologically, the tumor is characterized by proliferating ductal structures lined by a double layer of columnar epithelium. Keratin cysts and apical intraluminal projections are commonly found.

Gros et al. [49] called the condition of florid papillomatosis "erosive adenomatosis" because of the erosive nature of the lesion. Erosive adenomatosis of the nipple, according to Higginbotham and Mikhail [57], is a benign lesion that clinically mimics Paget's disease of the nipple but has the histological features of syringocystadenoma papilliferum. Some cases have been mistaken for intraductal papilloma or well-differentiated adenocarcinoma, and unnecessary mastectomies have been performed. Recognition of this lesion is important because it is benign and conservative excision is curative. All forms of this lesion are thought by Diaz et al. [61] to be composed of two apparent cell types: epithelial luminal cells and basal myoepithelial cells. Keratin cysts and apical intraluminal projections are commonly found according to Adant et al. [64]. Ku et al. [70] found that erosive adenomatosis is a complex proliferation of the lactiferous ducts that affects primarily middle-aged women.

## 12.4 Basal Cell Carcinoma

Basal cell carcinoma of the nipple is an erythematous lesion, scaling, ulceration, eczema, subareolar mass, plaques, papules, eczematous lesion, nodular mass, or crusty ulcer considered more aggressive in the NAC than in other areas. Ferguson et al. [75] reported on 34 cases of BCC of the nipple, areola, or both that were identified in the literature, mostly affecting middle-aged men. The majority of patients were treated with tissue-sparing surgery. There was a metastatic rate of 9.1%, and one patient died from the disease (3.0%). Kurokawa et al. [76] described a case of basal cell carcinoma of nipple and areola that had intraductal spread, while Kacerovska et al. [77] described basal cell carcinoma extending into the lactiferous duct.

Breast cancer can masquerade as a basal cell carcinoma [78]. Wang et al. [79] established predictors of nipple-areolar complex involvement by breast carcinoma.

Basal cell carcinoma of the nipple has many reports in the literature [80–112, 380].

## 12.5 Cysts

Cases of sebaceous cysts of areola and of nipple were described by Bryant [113].

Pèraire [114] reported a case of a cyst with polypoid excrescences of the nipple.

## 12.6 Eczema

Eczema of the nipple is an atopic dermatitis that has pruritis, soreness, and dry skin that may be scaly and red and can be crusting and bleeding that can get worse over time.

Treatment includes short, warm showers; mild soap and moisturizer, prescription-strength moisturizers such as Hylatopic Plus, Mimyx, and

Epiceram; hydrocortisone cream or ointment; antihistamines such as Benadryl; immunosupressants such as cyclosporine, azathioprine, or methotrexate; and immunomodulators such as Elidel and Protopic. (The FDA has issued its strongest "black box" warning on the packaging of Elidel and Protopic. The warning advises doctors to prescribe short-term use of Elidel and Protopic only after other eczema treatments have failed in adults and children over age 2.)

Many reports of eczema of the nipple are in the literature from 1877 to 2015 [115–129].

## 12.7 Epithelioma

Epitheliomas are classified according to the specific type of epithelial cells that are affected. The most common epitheliomas are basal cell carcinoma and squamous cell carcinoma (skin cancers). Epitheliomas may rise from any of the common dermatoses such as senile keratoses, warts, seborrheic keratoses, leukoplakia, psoriasis, papillomas, or cutaneous horns. Epitheliomas of the nipple have been reported in the literature.

Duhn [130] saw the disease in a 49-year-old man, the new growth having lasted 7 months without ulceration, beginning near the nipple. Czerny [131] added one more case of true epithelioma of the mamma meaning thereby a deeper form of epithelioma than that known as Paget's disease of the nipple.

Only seven references could be found with epithelioma of the nipple [130–136].

## 12.8 Fibroma

Fibroma is a benign soft tissue lesion with thick, haphazard collagen and bland fibroblasts that entrap adjacent tissue. Ninety percent are associated with familial adenomatous polyposis (FAP), Gardner's syndrome that is FAP with soft and/or hard tissue tumors and adenomatous polyposis coli (APC) germline mutation.

Curtis [137] stated that Pilz reports a case in which a fibroma developed in the nipple, becoming pedunculated, and was removed after 4 years of growth, having reached the size of a walnut. Higaki et al. [138] reported a case of soft fibroma on the nipple that was accompanied by a blister. Histologically, a subepidermal blister was overlying the tumor, and degeneration of the lower part of the epidermis was observed.

Other cases have been reported of fibroma of the nipple [139–152].

## 12.9 Fibrous Histiocytoma

The only report of fibrous histiocytoma of the nipple was by Castillo et al. [153] who stated that it is usually benign. The painless papule is tan brown, pink to red, or blue. May be pedunculated and may dimple when lateral compression is applied. Malignant fibrous histiocytoma implies that the tumor cells are of fibroblastic and histiocytic origin.

## 12.10 Hyperkeratosis

In hyperkeratosis microscopically there are variable orthokeratotic hyperkeratosis, slight acanthosis, and marked papillomatosis changes as well as mild dermal lymphocytic perivascular inflammation and epidermal spongiosis with microabscesses. Treatment includes lactic acid 12% cream, salicylic acid gel 6%, topical tretinoin (retin-A), topical calcipotriol (vitamin D), low-dose acitretin (second-generation retinoid), cryotherapy, shave of lesion, excision of involved portion, excision of areola with skin graft reconstruction, carbon dioxide laser, radiofrequency surgery, and curettage.

There are multiple reports of hyperkeratosis of the nipple in the literature [154–177].

## 12.11 Ichthyosis Circumscripta (Scaling of the Skin)

The only report of ichthyosis circumscripta involving the nipple was described by Friolet in 1905 [178]. This was a 28-year-old female with bilateral areolas covered by brownish-black excrescences. Deep furrows separated the excrescences the one from the other. Treated by soaking in olive oil and in 2 days, the excrescences were easily removed.

## 12.12 Leiomyoma

Bulman [179] reported a case of a 52-year-old female who had a "pedunculated tumour of the left nipple…The nipple was replaced by a firm slightly lobulated tumour 1I in. (3.8 cm.) across. The tumour did not extend into the pedicle." Three patients with leiomyoma of the nipple are described by Nascimiento et al. [180]. The tumors all appeared to have arisen from the muscularis mamillae and areolae. One lesion recurred 9 years after incomplete excision. Two of the tumors were clinically apparent painful nodules, while the third was an asymptomatic, incidental microscopic finding in a mastectomy performed for carcinoma. As in these cases and others described in the literature, patients with leiomyoma of the nipple or areola often present with a painful, ill-defined mass. Complete excision is indicated to prevent recurrence.

There are a number of other reports of leiomyoma of the nipple [181–199, 381].

## 12.13 Leiomyosarcoma

A case of leiomyosarcoma of the breast in a 53-year-old man originating in the erectile musculature of the nipple was described by Hernandez [200]. The tumor assumed roughly the conical configuration of the nipple musculature and was limited to the mammary gland. Ultrastructural study of the tumor revealed neoplastic smooth muscle cells with typical myofilaments.

Luh et al. [201] describe a 52-year-old female presenting with a 1.5 × 1.1 × 0.7 cm nodular lesion over her left nipple that on pathology was leiomyosarcoma. Positron emitted tomogram (PET) revealed no abnormal signal other than the primary site. Microscopically, this poorly circumscribed tumor was composed of interlacing bundles of smooth muscle cells with bizarre and pleomorphic nuclei, as well as prominent nucleoli. Its mitotic count was up to seven mitoses per ten high-power fields (HPF). Immunohistochemical study of tumor cells revealed positive stain for α-smooth muscle actin and vimentin, and negative for cytokeratin, CD34, and S-100. Left simple mastectomy was undertaken, and no residual mass lesion was noted on the resected specimen.

There are other reports of leiomyosarcoma of the nipple [202–208].

## 12.14 Melanoma

The intraepidermal component contains junctional nests of melanocytes uniform in size, distributed at the tips of the rete ridges [209]. The dermal component has three morphologies:

1. Type A morphology
   (a) In superficial dermis
   (b) Pigmented epithelioid cells with well-defined cell boundaries
   (c) Abundant eosinophilic to amphophilic cytoplasm containing coarse melanin granules
   (d) Uniform round/oval nuclei slightly smaller than that of adjacent keratinocytes
   (e) Finely dispersed chromatin
   (f) Delicate nuclear membrane
   (g) No small distinct eosinophilic nucleoli
2. Type B morphology
   (a) In intermediate dermis
   (b) Cells more lymphoid than epithelioid
   (c) Decreased cytoplasm with no melanin
   (d) Smaller and slightly hyperchromatic nuclei with dispersed chromatin and no nucleoli
3. Type C morphology
   (a) In deep dermis
   (b) Spindled, fibroblast-like or Schwannian cells with oval nuclei and bland chromatin
   (c) Single cell infiltration of superficial reticular collagen

Papachristou [210] reported 14 primary melanomas arising in the nipple and areola of the breast that were treated by mastectomy and axillary dissection. Four patients had axillary lymph node metastases, and all were dead within 3 years of their operation, while the ten patients with no axillary node involvement were free from recurrent disease 5 years after their operation. On the basis of clinical and anatomical studies, it is suggested that a wide local excision without mastectomy is adequate for the treatment of nipple and areola melanomas.

Kinoshita et al. [211] described a case of a 42-year-old housewife who had a small dark-brown nevus on her left nipple for about 30 years without any changes. Six months before her initial visit, it had begun to enlarge and rapidly changed from dark brown to black. A small bleeding ulcer was also present in the center of the lesion. Excisional biopsy was performed to differentiate between mammary Paget's disease and malignant melanoma. The histopathological examination revealed malignant melanoma, about 4 mm in thickness. She then underwent wide excision with axillary lymph node dissection. The surgical margin was made in a 3 cm radius around the biopsy site. The excision included the nipple, areola, and part of the underlying breast parenchyma, adipose tissue, and corresponding superficial layer of fascia. Microscopy showed metastasis in one of 13 axillary lymph nodes. After the operation, the patient received adjuvant DAV-Ferron therapy.

More cases of melanoma of the nipple have been reported [212–222].

## 12.15 Melanosis

Folberg and McLean [223] stated that primary acquired melanosis with atypia including epithelioid melanocytes and the distribution of melanocytes in a pattern other than basilar can lead to melanoma.

Isbary et al. [224] had five women aged between 26 and 34 years who presented with pigmentation of the areola and/or nipple. Considering this, benign condition on clinical and dermoscopic features should lead to biopsy rather than excision to confirm the diagnosis.

A few cases of melanosis of the nipple have been reported [225–228].

## 12.16 Molluscum Contagiosum

Molluscum contagiosum is a common cutaneous infection caused by a double strand.

DNA poxvirus. Skin lesions classically present as small, flesh-colored papules with central umbilication [229].

Treatment includes currettage, cryosurgery with liquid nitrogen, cantharidin (potent vesicant or blistering agent), and topical retinoic acid (retin-A).

The literature contains other cases of molluscum contagiosum involving the nipple [148, 230–235].

## 12.17 Neuroma and Neurofibromatosis (von Recklinghausen Disease)

Friedrich and Hage [236] stated that in their patients, tumors arising in the areola and nipple area and mimicking an accessory nipple were all neurofibromas. Local excision of neurofibromas was adequate to relief patients from an often unsightly appearance.

According to Zhou et al. [237], patients with NF1 belong to a high-risk population of possible breast cancer patients who should receive early screening. Breast lumps in patients with NF1 might be mistaken for neurofibroma or may be covered by an enlarged nipple with neurofibroma appendices. We advocate that careful physical examination and multiple screening imaging modalities be used in the screening procedure for patients with NF1.

Other cases of neuroma and neurofibromatosis have been reported [238–250].

## 12.18 Nevus

A rare case of a 13-year-old female patient with epidermal verrucous nevus on the right areola was reported by Cunha Filho et al. [251].

According to the Levy-Franckel classification, this variant is a type I nipple and areola hyperkeratosis, when associated to verrucous nevus. Histopathological examination showed papillomatosis, acanthosis, and hyperkeratosis. Cryotherapy yielded unsatisfactory results after two sessions. A good result was obtained with shaving and electrocauterization.

The types of nevoid hyperkeratosis are:

1. Type I—hyperkeratosis of the nipple and/or areola due to the extension of an epidermal nevus
2. Type II—hyperkeratosis of the nipple and/or areola in conjunction with disseminated dermatoses
3. Type III—Nevoid hyperkeratosis of the nipple and/or areola

There are multiple articles that discuss nevus of the nipple [155, 208, 252–261].

## 12.19 Nodular Mucinosis

The nodular mucinous mass is poorly circumscribed, subareolar, myxoid mass, slow-growing, soft, non-tender, and lobulated in the subareolar region. It is a multinodular myxoid lesion containing scattered capillaries and histiocytes but void of epithelial components. There are myxoid dermal deposits and lobular arrangement, and there may be an infiltrate of spindle cells within the mucinous pool.

Sanati et al. [262] describe a 21-year-old white woman who presented with a mass in the left breast of 6 months' duration. She had never been pregnant or had any history of breastfeeding, surgery, trauma, or use of exogenous hormones or a family history of breast cancer. Clinical breast examination demonstrated a 1 cm "rubbery" mass directly under and continuous with the left nipple. The skin that covered the mass had an edematous and irregular appearance without erythema or drainage from the nipple. Ultrasonography demonstrated a 1 cm, nonintraductal, circumscribed, homogeneous, isoechoic mass that was continuous or part of the base of the left nipple. The mass was smooth, with a thin echogenic rim. Doppler flow showed some vascularity. The patient desired excision of the lesion. Gross examination revealed a nodular, rubbery-firm, ovoid, pink, polypoid mass that measured 1.5 × 0.9 × 0.8 cm. Microscopic examination showed a well-circumscribed tumor with a nodular appearance, which consisted of an accumulation of pink myxoid tissue and contained spindle cells with bland-appearing nuclei, no mitosis, and mild cellularity. The pink myxoid tissue was stained with Hale colloidal iron and Alcian blue. The Alcian blue stain was removed by pretreatment with hyaluronidase. The spindle cells are stained with vimentin and smooth muscle actin; however, they did not express smooth muscle myosin or cytokeratin.

Kempf et al. [263] discussed a patient who had a 2–3 month history of a solitary, round, translucent, asymptomatic white exophytic nodule with a bluish hue on the right areola. The lesion measured 1.2 cm in diameter. He had worn a nipple ring piercing for 3 years only on the right side. He decided to remove it because of relapsing episodes of infectious dermatitis that had been treated with topical antibiotics. The lesion started a couple of weeks after the ring piercing had been removed with progressive enlargement. The lesion was totally excised. Histopathology showed a polypoid, dome-shaped dermal nodule with abundant mucin filling the dermis, not extending into the subcutis.

There are further reports of nodular mucinous of the nipple in the literature [264–268].

## 12.20 Paget's Disease

Paget's disease consists of cancer cells collect in or around the nipple. The cancer usually affects the ducts of the nipple first, then spreads to the nipple surface and the areola. The nipple and areola often become scaly, red, crusted, itchy, tingling, burning, irritated, and painful. More than 97% of people with Paget's disease also have cancer, either DCIS or invasive cancer, somewhere else in the breast.

Treatment consists of lumpectomy or mastectomy to surgically remove the tumor. Chemotherapy and/or radiotherapy may be necessary.

Paget [269] described a disorder that was ultimately termed Paget's disease. There are many reports of Paget's disease of the nipple in the literature [270–329].

## 12.21 Papilloma

Dennis et al. [330] stated that papilloma excision with percutaneous biopsy allows safe and accurate tissue analysis and a high probability of terminating the symptomatic nipple discharge.

Cases of nipple papilloma are in the medical literature [331–345].

## 12.22 Sarcoma

Reports of sarcoma of the nipple include large cell sarcoma [346], medullary sarcoma [347], primitive sarcoma [348], and reticulum cell sarcoma [349].

## 12.23 Seborrheic Keratosis

Shamsadini et al. [350] reported the case of a patient with Paget's disease of the nipple and intraductal carcinoma who presented with ipsilateral, eruptive grouped seborrheic keratoses of the areola and nipple of the breast and called this combination the Leser-Trélat sign. The sign of Leser-Trélat is defined as the sudden eruption of multiple seborrheic keratoses caused by a malignancy [351]. Leser [352] reported the combination of seborrheic keratoses and cancer in 1901. However, according to Hollander [353], Trélat apparently never wrote down his observation that bright red spots (cherry spots) can occur with malignancy, but one of his students introduced the term "Trélat's sign" years before 1901. However, "de Morgan spots" were described in Campbell de Morgan's treatise in 1871 [354] that stated "I have noticed and it has been verified by the observation of others, that concurrently with, or following on, the development of cancer, small outgrowths of warty or vascular or dermoid structure are frequent."

Narsimha et al. [355] reported a case of a 43-year-old female patient who complained of pigmented nodule over the nipple on the left breast for 2 months. Examination showed a hard, pigmented nodule on the left nipple measuring 1.5 cm across. This histologically was a seborrheic keratosis (melanoacanthoma). A seborrheic keratosis with melanin pigmentation associated with proliferation of intraepidermal melanocytes. There are further reports on eruptive seborrheic keratosis of the nipple [356, 357].

## 12.24 Squamous Cell Carcinoma

Mandry [358] reported a case of a patient who had an injury to the left breast 2 years previously that developed a flat, bloody ulcer of the nipple that extended into the areola. The breast was removed, and pathology showed a primary squamous cell carcinoma of the nipple.

Loveland-Jones et al. [359] noted that radiation-induced nonmelanoma skin cancer was first reported 7 years after the discovery of X-rays but has received relatively little consideration in the literature. They reported the case of a 66-year-old African-American woman presented to the hospital with a non-healing ulcer of the right nipple. Her past medical history was significant for right breast ductal carcinoma in situ for which she had undergone lumpectomy and whole breast radiation therapy 9 years previously. Mammography and magnetic resonance imaging studies were negative for recurrent breast cancer. However, the latter demonstrated abnormal enhancement in the nipple-areolar region. An incisional biopsy of the lesion demonstrated invasive squamous cell carcinoma. Subsequently, the patient underwent wide excision of the nipple-areolar complex. Sentinel lymph node biopsy was offered but our patient declined. She was considered to have a local disease, and hence no further treatment was recommended.

Upasham et al. [360] reported a case of an 87-year-old female who presented with an ulcerating and a fungating growth over the left-sided nipple-areola complex. There was no evidence of nipple discharge; previous history for any other risk factor related to this squamous cell carcinoma was negative.

Squamous cell carcinoma of the nipple has further reports in the literature [361–379].

## References


1. Bengualid V, Singh V, Singh H, Berger J. Mycobacterium fortuitum and anaerobic breast abscess following nipple piercing: case presentation and review of the literature. J Adolesc Health. 2008;42(5):530–2.
2. Leibman AJ, Misra M, Castaldi M. Breast abscess after nipple piercing: sonographic findings with clinical correlation. J Ultrasound Med. 2011;30(9):1303–8.
3. Abbass K, Adnan MK, Markert RJ, Emig M, Khan NA. Mycobacterium fortuitum breast abscess after nipple piercing. Can Fam Physician. 2014;60(1):51–2.
4. Chalot. Gaz. Hebd. d. sc. Méd de Montpellier. 1881;III:253. In: Deaver JB, McFarland J, Herman L, editors. The breast: its anomalies, its diseases, and their treatment. Philadelphia: P. Blakiston's Son & Co.; 1917. p. 671–702.
5. Winckle. Lehrbuch der Frauenkrankheiten 1886:741. In: Deaver JB, McFarland J, Herman L, editors. The breast: its anomalies, its diseases, and their treatment. Philadelphia: P. Blakiston's Son & Co.; 1917. p. 671–702.
6. Miyahara M, Saito T, Kaketani K, Suzuki K, Kuwahara A, Shimoda K, Kobayashi M. Adenoma of the nipple. Surg Today. 1992;22(4):368–70.
7. Tsushimi T, Enoki T, Takemoto Y, Harada E, Hayashi M, Furuya T, Hamano K. Adenoma of the nipple, focusing on the contrast-enhanced magnetic resonance imaging findings: report of a case. Surg Today. 2011;41(8):1138–41.
8. Gross SW. On the diagnosis of tumours of the mamma. In: Braithwaite W, Braithwaite J, Trevelyen EF, editors. The retrospect of practical medicine. New York: W.A. Townsend; 1881. p. 198–200.
9. Galloway JR, Woolner LB, Clagget OT. Adenoid cystic carcinoma. Surg Gynecol Obstet. 1966;122:1289–94.
10. Patterson JW, Wick MR. Nonmelanotic tumors of the skin. AFIP atlas of tumor pathology, fourth series, Fascicle 4. Washington, DC: Armed Forces Institute of Pathology; 2006. pp. 158–61.
11. Roy S. Pathology of nipple adenoma (erosive adenomatosis or florid papillomatosis). http://www.histopathology-india.net/niad.html
12. Sarma DP, Stevens T. Infiltrating syringomatous eccrine adenoma of the nipple: a case report. Cases J. 2009;2:9118.
13. Rosen PP. Syringomatous adenoma of the nipple. Am J Surg Pathol. 1983;7(8):739–45.
14. Hwang TS, Ham EK, Kim JP. Syringomatous adenoma of nipple—a case report. J Korean Med Sci. 1987;2(4):263–5.
15. Jones MW, Norris HJ, Snyder RC. Infiltrating syringomatous adenoma of the nipple: a clinical and pathological study of 11 cases. Am J Surg Pathol. 1989;13(3):197–201.
16. Suster S, Moran CA, Hurt MA. Syringomatous squamous tumors of the breast. Cancer. 1991;67(9):2350–5.
17. Slaughter MS, Pomerantz RA, Murad T, Hines JR. Infiltrating syringomatous adenoma of the nipple. Surgery. 1992;111(6):711–3.
18. Coulthard A, Liston J, Young JR. Case report: infiltrating syringomatous adenoma of the breast appearances on mammography and ultrasonography. Clin Radiol. 1993;47:6244.
19. Toyoshima O, Kanou M, Kintaka N, Miyashita M, Shigematsu S, Sano J. Syringomatous adenoma of the nipple: report of a case. Surg Today. 1998;28(11):1196–9.
20. Wadhwa N, Mishra K, Agarwal S. Syringomatous adenoma of the nipple: a case report. Pathology. 2003;35(3):271–2.
21. Chang CK, Jacobs IA, Calilao G, Salti GI. Metastatic infiltrating syringomatous adenoma of the breast. Arch Pathol Lab Med. 2003;127:e155–6.
22. Healy CE, Dijkstra B, Walsh M, Hill AD, Murphy J. Nipple adenoma: a differential diagnosis for Paget's disease. Breast J. 2003;9(4):325–6.
23. Ku J, Bennett RD, Chong KD, Bennett IC. Syringomatous adenoma of the nipple. Breast. 2004;13(5):412–5.
24. Kubo M, Tsuji H, Kunitomo T, Taguchi K. Syringomatous adenoma of the nipple: a case report. Breast Cancer. 2004;11(2):214–6.
25. Carter E, Dyess DL. Infiltrating syringomatous adenoma of the nipple: a case report and 20-year retrospective review. Breast J. 2004;10(5):443–7.
26. Kijima Y, Matsukita S, Yoshinaka H, Owaki T, Aikou T. Adenoma of the nipple: report of a case. Breast Cancer. 2006;13(1):95–9.
27. Kono S, Kurosumi M, Simooka H, Kawanowa K, Takei H, Suemasu K. Nipple adenoma found in a mastectomy specimen: report of a case with special regard to the proliferation pattern. Breast Cancer. 2007;14(2):234–8.
28. Oliva VL, Little JV, Carlson GW. Syringomatous adenoma of the nipple—treatment by central mound resection and oncoplastic reconstruction. Breast J. 2008;14(1):102–5.
29. Oo KZ, Xiao PQ. Infiltrating syringomatous adenoma of the nipple clinical presentation and literature review. Arch Pathol Lab Med. 2009;133:1487–9.
30. Healy CE, Dijkstra B, Walsh M, Hill AD, Murphy J. Nipple adenoma: a differential diagnosis for Paget's disease. Breast J. 2003;9(4):325–6.

31. Kijima Y, Matsukita S, Yoshinaka H, Owaki T, Aikou T. Adenoma of the nipple: report of a case. Breast Cancer. 2006;13(1):95–9.
32. Kono S, Kurosumi M, Simooka H, Kawanowa K, Takei H, Suemasu K. Nipple adenoma found in a mastectomy specimen: report of a case with special regard to the proliferation pattern. Breast Cancer. 2007;14(2):234–8.
33. Clune JE, Kozakewich HP, Van Beek CA, Labow BI, Greene AK. Nipple adenoma in infancy. J Pediatr Surg. 2009;44(11):2219–22.
34. Kazakov DV, Kacerovska D, Michal M. Lactation adenoma in a supernumerary nipple. J Cutan Pathol. 2011;38(6):532–3.
35. Tao W, Kai F, Yue HL. Nipple adenoma in an adolescent. Pediatr Dermatol. 2010;27(4):399–401.
36. Rao P, Shousha S. Male nipple adenoma with DCIS followed 9 years later by invasive carcinoma. Breast J. 2010;16(3):317–8.
37. Kazakov DV, Kacerovska D, Michal M. Lactation adenoma in a supernumerary nipple. J Cutan Pathol. 2011;38(6):532–3.
38. Shioi Y, Nakamura S, Kawamura S, Kasami M. Nipple adenoma arising from axillary accessory breast: a case report. Diagn Pathol. 2012;7:162.
39. Fujii T, Yajima R, Morita H, Yamaguchi S, Tsutsumi S, Asao T, Kuwano H. Adenoma of the nipple projecting out of the nipple: curative resection without excision of the nipple. World J Surg Oncol. 2014;12:91.
40. Di Bonito M, Cantile M, Collina F, D'Aiuto M, Liguori G, De Cecio R, Botti G. Adenoma of the nipple: a clinicopathological report of 13 cases. Oncol Lett. 2014;7(6):1839–42.
41. Brownstein MH, Phelps RG, Magnin PH. Papillary adenoma of the nipple: analysis of fifteen new cases. J Am Acad Dermatol. 1985;12(4):707–15.
42. Perzin KH, Lattes R. 1972. Papillary adenoma of the nipple (florid papillomatosis, adenoma, adenomatosis). A clinicopathologic study. Cancer. 29 996–1009. https://www.researchgate.net/publication/227771224_Papillary_adenoma_of_the_nipple_florid_papillomatosis_adenoma_adenomatosis_A_clinicopathologic_study. Accessed 31 Mar 2016.
43. Jones DB. Florid papillomatosis of the nipple ducts. Cancer. 1955;8(2):315–9.
44. Doctor VM, Sirsat MV. Florid papillomatosis (adenoma) and other benign tumours of the nipple and areola. Br J Cancer. 1971;25(1):1–9.
45. Montemarano AD, Sau P, James WD. Superficial papillary adenomatosis of the nipple: a case report and review of the literature. J Am Acad Dermatol. 1995;33(5 Pt 2):871–5.
46. Perzin KH, Lattes R. Papillary adenoma of the nipple (florid papillomatosis, adenoma, adenomatosis). A clinicopathologic study. Cancer. 1972;29(4):996–1009.
47. Tuveri M, Cald PG, Mocci C, Nicolosi A. Florid papillomatosis of the male nipple. Am J Surg. 2010;3:e39–40.
48. Perzin KH, Lattes R. Papillary adenoma of the nipple (florid papillomatosis, adenoma, adenomatosis). A clinicopathologic study. Cancer. https://www.researchgate.net/publication/227771224_Papillary_adenoma_of_the_nipple_florid_papillomatosis_adenoma_adenomatosis_A_clinicopathologic_study. Accessed 31 Mar 2016.
49. Gros CM, Le Gal Y, Bader P. Erosive adenomatosis of the nipple. Presse Med. 1959;67(15):615–6.
50. Le Gal Y, Gros CM, Bader P. Erosive adenomatosis of the nipple. Ann Anat Pathol (Paris). 1959;4(2):292–304.
51. Peloux Y, Franco R. Erosive adenomatosis of the nipple. Apropos of a case observed in New Caledonia. Med Trop (Mars). 1965;25:71–5.
52. Pratt-Thomas HR. Erosive adenomatosis of the nipple. J S C Med Assoc. 1968;64(2):37–40.
53. Smith EJ, Kron SD, Gross PR. Erosive adenomatosis of the nipple. Arch Dermatol. 1970;102(3):330–2.
54. Smith NP, Jones EW. Erosive adenomatosis of the nipple. Clin Exp Dermatol. 1977;2(1):79–84.
55. Civatte J, Restout S, Delomenie DC. Erosive adenomatosis of a supernumerary nipple. Ann Dermatol Venereol. 1977;104(11):777–9.
56. Palermo A, Urso C. Adenoma (erosive adenomatosis) of the nipple. G Ital Dermatol Venereol. 1985;120(2):145–7.
57. Higginbotham LH, Mikhail GR. Erosive adenomatosis of the nipple. J Dermatol Surg Oncol. 1986;12(5):514–6.
58. Piérard G. Paget's disease or erosive adenomatosis of the nipple? Dermatologica. 1990;180(1):55.
59. Moulin G, Darbon P, Balme B, Frappart L. Erosive adenomatosis of the nipple. Report of 10 cases with immunohistochemistry. Ann Dermatol Venereol. 1990;117(8):537–45.
60. Bourlond J, Bourlond-Reinert L. Erosive adenomatosis of the nipple. Dermatology. 1992;185(4):319–24.
61. Diaz NM, Palmer JO, Wick MR. Erosive adenomatosis of the nipple: histology, immunohistology, and differential diagnosis. Mod Pathol. 1992;5(2):179–84.
62. Ward KA, Burton JL. Dermatologic diseases of the breast in young women. Clin Dermatol. 1997;15:45–52.
63. Moulin G. Superficial papillary adenomatosis of the nipple (with reply). J Am Acad Dermatol. 1997;36:133.
64. Adant JP, Paquet P, Bluth F, Nelissen X, Pierard G. Erosive adenomatosis of the nipple. Report of 2 cases. Ann Chir Plast Esthet. 1997;42(6):638–41.
65. Miller L, Tyler W, Maroon M, Miller OF 3rd. Erosive adenomatosis of the nipple: a benign imitator of malignant breast disease. Cutis. 1997;59(2):91–2.
66. Kuflik EG. Erosive adenomatosis of the nipple treated with cryosurgery. J Am Acad Dermatol. 1998;38:270–1.
67. Van Mierlo PL, Geelen GM, Neumann HA. Mohs micrographic surgery for an erosive adenomatosis of the nipple. Dermatol Surg. 1998;24(6):681–3.
68. Albers SE, Barnard M, Thorner P, Krafchik BR. Erosive adenomatosis of the nipple in an eight-year-old girl. J Am Acad Dermatol. 1999;40(5 Pt 2):834–7.

69. Lee HJ, Chug KY. Erosive adenomatosis of the nipple: conservation of the nipple by Mohs micrographic surgery. J Am Acad Dermatol. 2002;47:578–80.
70. Ku BS, Kwon OE, Kim DC, Song KH, Lee CW, Kim KH. A cade of erosive adeno matosis of the nipple treated with total excision using purse-string suture. Dernatol Surg. 2006;32:1093–6.
71. Cosechen MS, Wojcik AS, Piva FM, Werner B, Serafini SZ. Erosive adenomatosis of the nipple. An Bras Dermatol, 2011. 86(4 Suppl 1):S17–20.
72. Kumar PK, Thomas J. Erosive adenomatosis of the nipple masquerading as Paget's disease. Indian Dermatol Online J. 2013;4(3):239–40.
73. Handley RS, Thackray AC. Adenoma of the nipple. Br J Cancer. 1962;16:187–94.
74. Goldman RL, Cooperman H. Adenoma of the nipple: a benign lesion simulating carcinoma clinically and pathologically. Am J Surg. 1970;119(3):322–5.
75. Ferguson MS, Nouraei SA, Davies BJ, McLean NR. Basal cell carcinoma of the nipple-areola complex. Dermatol Surg. 2009;35:1771–5.
76. Kurokawa E, Kikkawa N, Taniguchi H. A case of basal cell carcinoma of the nipple and areola with intraductal spread. Breast Cancer. 2001;8(3):229–33.
77. Kacerovska D, Michal M, Kazakov DV. Basal cell carcinoma of the nipple extending into the lactiferous duct. Int J Surg Pathol. 2011;19(6):779–80.
78. Moennich J, Ort R, High W, Brown M. Breast carcinoma masquerading as basal cell carcinoma of the nipple. JAAD Case Rep. 2015;1(6):361–3.
79. Wang J, Xiao X, Wang J, Iqbal N, Baxter L, Skinner KA, Hicks DG, Hajdu SI, Tang P. Predictors of nipple-areolar complex involvement by breast carcinoma: histopathologic analysis of 787 consecutive therapeutic mastectomy specimens. Ann Surg Oncol. 2012;19(4):1174–80.
80. Robinson HB. Rodent ulcer of the male breast. Trans Pathol Soc Lond. 1893;44:147–8.
81. Farrow JH. Benign and malignant lesions of the nipple. CA Cancer J Clin. 1958;8(1):16–9.
82. Bleehen SS. Pigmented basal cell epithelioma. Light and electron microscopic studies on tumours and cell cultures. Br J Dermatol. 1975;93:361–70.
83. Davis AB, Patchefsky AS. Basal cell carcinoma of the nipple: case report and review of the literature. Cancer. 1977;40:1780–1.
84. Tezuka T, Ohkuma M, Hirose I. Melanosomes of pigmented basal cell epithelioma. Dermatologica. 1977;154:14–22.
85. Lupton GP, Goeffe DK. Basal cell carcinoma of the nipple. Arch Dermatol. 1978;114:1845.
86. Sauven P, Roberts A. Basal cell carcinoma of the nipple. J R Soc Med. 1983;76:699–701.
87. Bruce S, Tschen JA, Goldberg LH. Basal cell carcinoma of the nipple. J Dermatol Surg Oncol. 1985;11:434–5.
88. Shertz WT, Balogh K. Metastasizing basal cell carcinoma of the nipple. Arch Pathol Lab Med. 1986;110:761–2.
89. Nirodi NS, Mudd DG. Basal cell carcinoma of the male nipple. J R Coll Surg Edinb. 1986;31:121–3.
90. Cain RI, Sau P, Benson PM. Basal cell carcinoma of the nipple. Report of two cases. J Am Acad Dermatol. 1990;22:207–10.
91. Benharroch D, Geffen DB, Peiser J, Rosenberg L. Basal cell carcinoma of the male nipple: case report and review of the literature. J Dermatol Surg Oncol. 1993;19(2):137–9.
92. Cooper RA, Eilers DB. Mammographic findings in basal cell carcinoma of the male nipple. Am J Roentgenol. 2000;175(4):1065–6.
93. Sánchez-Carpintero I, Redondo P, Solano T. Basal cell carcinoma affecting the areola-nipple complex. Plast Reconstr Surg. 2000;105(4):1573.
94. Yamamoto H, Ito Y, Hayashi T, Urano N, Kato T, Kimura Y, Tanigawa T, Endo W, Kurokawa E, Kikkawa N, Taniguchi H. A case of basal cell carcinoma of the nipple and areola with intraductal spread. Breast Cancer. 2001;8(3):229–33.
95. Zhu YI, Ratner D. Basal cell carcinoma of the nipple: a case report and review of the literature. Dermatol Surg. 2001;27(11):971–4.
96. Betti R, Martino P, Moneghini L, Vergani R, Tolomio E, Crosti C. Basal cell carcinomas of the areola-nipple complex: case reports and review of the literature. J Dermatol. 2003;30:822–6.
97. Gupta C, Sheth D, Snower DP. Primary basal carcinoma of the nipple. Arch Pathol Lab Med. 2004;128:792–3.
98. Huang CW, Pan CK, Juan CC, Shih TF, Tsai CC, Juan CC, Ker CG. Basal cell carcinoma of the nipple-areola complex: a case report. Kaohsiung J Med Sci. 2005;21(10):480–3.
99. Rosen N, Muhn CY, Bernstein SC. A common tumor, an uncommon location: basal cell carcinoma of the nipple and areola in a 49-year-old woman. Dermatol Surg. 2005;31(4):480–3.
100. Chu PY, Teng TH, Lee CC. Primary superficial basal cell carcinoma of the nipple. Ann Saudi Med. 2007;27(4):296–7.
101. Avci O, Pabuççuoĝlu U, Koçdor MA, Unlü M, Akin C, Soyal C, Canda T. Basal cell carcinoma of the nipple—an unusual location in a male patient. J German Soc Dermatol. 2008;6(2):130–2.
102. Ferguson MS, Nouraei SA, Davies BJ, McLean NR. Basal cell carcinoma of the nipple-areola complex. Dermatol Surg. 2009;35:1771–5.
103. Oram Y, Demirkesen C, Akkaya AD, Koyuncu E. Basal cell carcinoma of the nipple: an uncommon but ever-increasing location: case reports. Dermatol Med. 2011;2011:81891.
104. Kacerovska D, Michal M, Kazakov DV. Basal cell carcinoma of the nipple extending into the lactiferous duct. Int J Surg Pathol. 2011;19(6):779–80.
105. Jung HJ, Jun JH, Kim HK, Lee SJ, Kim DW, Lee WJ, Jung JH. Pigmented basal cell carcinoma of the nipple-areola complex in an elderly woman. Ann Dermatol. 2011;23(Suppl 2):S201–S4.

106. Sinha AJ, Langtry AA. Secondary intention healing following mohs micrographic surgery for basal cell carcinoma of the nipple and areola. Acta Derm Venereol. 2011;91(1):78–9.
107. Kwasniak LA, Garcia-Zuazaga J. Basal cell carcinoma: evidence-based medicine and review of treatment modalities. Int J Dermatol. 2011;50(6):645–58.
108. Sharma A, Tambat RM, Singh A, Dayananda S, Bhalig DS. Basal cell carcinoma of the nipple areola complex. J Midlife Health. 2011;2(2):89–90.
109. Trignano E, Manzo MJ, Paliogiannis P, Madonia M, Marongiu F, Lissia A, Campus GV. Basal cell carcinoma of the nipple-areola complex: report of a case and literature review. Ann Ital Chir. 2013;84. (ePub) Published online 2013. http://www.academia.edu/8359931/Basal_cell_carcinoma_of_the_nipple-areola_complex
110. Kalvani R, Vani BR, Srinivasm MV, Veda P. Pigmented basal cell carcinoma of nipple and areola in a male breast. Int J Biomed Sci. 2014;10(1):69–72.
111. Akizuki S, Kamei M, Suehiro S, Yamashita S, Kawahara K. Basal cell carcinoma of the nipple in male patients with gastric cancer recurrence: report of a case. Breast Cancer. 2014;21(1):102–7.
112. Dewan K, Jash PK, Chattopadhyay D, Saraf A, Np S, Gupta S. Basal cell carcinoma of the nipple: a rare case report. J Dental Med Sci. 2014;13(6):71–2.
113. Bryant T. Diseases of the breast, London 1887:332. In: Deaver JB, McFarland J, Herman L, editors. The breast: its anomalies, its diseases, and their treatment. Philadelphia: P. Blakiston's Son & Co.; 1917. p. 671–702.
114. Pèraire. Bull et Mém Soc D'Anat de Paris. 1910;LXXV:931. In: Deaver JB, McFarland J, Herman L, editors. The breast: its anomalies, its diseases, and their treatment. Philadelphia: P. Blakiston's Son & Co.; 1917. p. 671–702.
115. Butlin HT. On the minute anatomy of two cases of carcinoma of the breast preceded by eczema of the nipple and areola. Med Chir Trans. 1877;60:153–160.1.
116. Morris H. On two cases of carcinoma of the breast, preceded by so-called eczema of the nipple and areola. Med Chir Trans. 1880;63:37–50.3.
117. Koretsky L. A case for diagnosis (eczema? carcinoma simplex of the nipple?). Arch Dermatol Syphilol. 1947;55(5):711.
118. Ah S, El-Nasr HS. A clinical study of eczema of the nipple and areola, and its treatment with oestrogenic hormone. Br J Dermatol Syph. 1949;61(6):216–21.
119. Farrow JH. Benign and malignant lesions of the nipple. CA Cancer J Clin. 1958;8(1):16–9.
120. Graham DF. Eczema of the nipple. Trans St Johns Hosp Dermatol Soc. 1972;58(1):98–9.
121. Brackett VH. Eczema of the nipple/areola area. J Hum Lact. 1988;4(4):167–9.
122. Amir L. Eczema of the nipple and breast: a case report. J Hum Lact. 1993;9(3):173–5.
123. Roumen RM, Haas FD. Eczema of the nipple: cancer or not? Ned Tijdschr Geneeskd. 1997;141(36):1721–4.
124. Kim DH, Kim CW, Kang SJ, Kim TY. A case of clear cell acanthoma presenting as nipple eczema. Br J Dermatol. 1999;141(5):950–1.
125. Barankin B, Gross MS. Nipple and areolar eczema in the breastfeeding woman. J Cutan Med Surg. 2004;8(2):126–30.
126. Tougeron D, Wierzbicka-Hainaut E, Osdoit S, Chagneau-Derrode C, Yacoub M, Silvain C. Hyperkeratotic eczema of the nipple and areola associated with sorafenib treatment. Eur J Dermatol. 2010;20(6):854–6.
127. Kim SK, Won YH, Kim SJ. Nipple eczema: a diagnostic challenge of allergic contact dermatitis. Ann Dermatol. 2014;26(3):413–4.
128. Song HS, Jung SE, Kim YC, Lee ES. Nipple eczema, an indicative manifestation of atopic dermatitis? A clinical, histological, and immunohistochemical study. Am J Dermatopathol. 2015;37(4):284–8.
129. Jenkins D, Cooper SM, McPherson T. Unilateral nipple eczema in children: report of five cases and literature review. Pediatr Dermatol. 2015;32(5):718–22.
130. Duhn. J Cutaneous Venereal Dis 1886;IV:5. In: Ashhurst J, editor. The international encyclopedia of surgery: a systematic treatise on the theory and practice of surgery. New York: William Wood & Company; 1895. p. 276.
131. Czerny. Epithelioma of breast. Centralblatt f. Chirurgie 1886 Beilage S. 38. In: Ashhurst J, editor. The international encyclopedia of surgery: a systematic treatise on the theory and practice of surgery. New York: William Wood & Company; 1895. p. 276.
132. Curtis BF. Tumors. In: Ashhurst J, editor. The international encyclopedia of surgery: a systematic treatise on the theory and practice of surgery. New York: William Wood & Company; 1895. p. 276.
133. Dennis FS. Diseases of the female breast. In: Dennis FS, Billings JS (eds), System of surgery: tumor, hernia, surgery of the alimentary canal, appendicitis, surgery of the liver and biliary passages, of the uterus, of the ovary and tubes, gynecological surgery, symphysiotomy, surgery of the thyroid, surgical peculiarities of the negro, surgery of the female breast, use of the Röntgen rays in surgery, New York: Lea Brothers & Co.; 1896. p. 871–946.
134. Battle WH, Maybury BC. Primary epithelioma of the nipple in a girl aged eleven. Lancet. 1913;181(4683):1521–2.
135. Farrow JH. Benign and malignant lesions of the nipple. CA Cancer J Clin. 1958;8(1):16–9.
136. Périn L, Bourdon R, Desprez-Curely JP, Chomé J, Ripault J. Paget's disease of the nipple and mammary epithelioma. Importance of mammography in diagnosis. Bull Soc Fr Dermatol Syphiligr. 1967;74(3):355–8.
137. Curtis BF. Tumors. In: Ashhurst J, editor. The international encyclopedia of surgery: a systematic treatise on the theory and practice of surgery. New York: William Wood & Company; 1895. p. 247.

138. Higaki Y, Yoshinaga Y, Kawashima M. Blister formation over a soft fibroma of the nipple. J Dermatol. 1993;20(7):447–8.
139. Gross SW. On the diagnosis of tumours of the mamma. In: Braithwaite W, Braithwaite J, Trevelyen EF, editors. The retrospect of practical medicine. New York: W.A. Townsend; 1881. p. 198–200.
140. Bidder. Fibroma pendulum mammillae. Deutsche Med Wocheschrift. 1884;X:40. In: Deaver JB, McFarland J, Herman L, editors. The breast: its anomalies, its diseases, and their treatment. Philadelphia: P. Blakiston's Son & Co.; 1917. p. 671–702.
141. Kalischer. Fibroma pendulum mammillae. Berliner Klin Wochenscrrift. 1884;XXI:44. In: Deaver JB, McFarland J, Herman L, editors. The breast: its anomalies, its diseases, and their treatment. Philadelphia: P. Blakiston's Son & Co.; 1917. p. 671–702.
142. Winckel. Lehrbuch der Freuenkrankheit. 1886:740. In: Deaver JB, McFarland J, Herman L, editors. The breast: its anomalies, its diseases, and their treatment. Philadelphia: P. Blakiston's Son & Co.; 1917. p. 671–702.
143. Green GD. Lobulated fibroma of the nipple. Trans Path Soc, Londo. 1897–98;XLIX:308. In: Deaver JB, McFarland J, Herman L, editors. The breast: its anomalies, its diseases, and their treatment. Philadelphia: P. Blakiston's Son & Co.; 1917. p. 671–702.
144. Sheild AM. Pedunculated fibroma of the nipple. Br Med J. 1896;I:1499. In: Deaver JB, McFarland J, Herman L, editors. The breast: its anomalies, its diseases, and their treatment. Philadelphia: P. Blakiston's Son & Co.; 1917. p. 671–702.
145. Doctor VM, Sirsat MV. Florid papillomatosis (adenoma) and other benign tumours of the nipple and areola. Br J Cancer. 1971;25(1):1–9.
146. Prasad M, Pradhan PK, Bisarya BN. Pedunculated fibroma of nipple. J Indian Med Assoc. 1973;61(12):517.
147. Nakayama H, Mihara M. Giant pendulous fibroma arising on the areola. Acta Derm Venereol. 1998;78(2):152.
148. Parlakgumus A, Yildirim S, Bolat FA, Caliskan K, Ezer A, Colakoglu T, Moray G. Dermatoses of the nipple. Can J Surg. 2009;52(2):160–1.
149. Seo BF, Jung SN. Fibroma of the nipple. Breast J. 2012;18(5):494–5.
150. You HS, Park SM, Cho HH, Kim WJ, Mun JH, Song M, Kim HS, Ko HC, Kim MB, Kim BS. A case of soft fibroma of the nipple with a cauliflower-like appearance. Ann Dermatol. 2015;27(1):102–3.
151. You HS, Park SM, Cho HH, Kim WJ, Mun JH, Song M, Kim HS, Ko HC, Kim MB, Kim BS. A case of soft fibroma of the nipple with a cauliflower-like appearance. Ann Dermatol. 2015;27(1):102–3.
152. Baratelli GM. Pedunculated fibroma of the nipple. http://radiopaedia.org/cases/pedunculated-fibroma-of-the-nipple. Accessed 27 Mar 2016.
153. Castillo M, Sanjuán A, Pérez N, Zanón G, Bons N, Vilanova M, Vanrell JA, Merino MJ, Fernández PL. Fibrous histiocytoma-like spindle-cell proliferation in the nipple after body-piercing. Int J Surg Pathol. 2006;14:89–93.
154. Moncorps C. Generalisierte (diffuse) regionare (flachenhafte) und zirkumskripte (solitar, gruppiert oder disseminiert auftretenden) Keratosen. In: Jadassohn J, editor. Handbuch der Haut- und Geschlechtskrankheiten, vol. VIII/2. Berlin: Julius Springer; 1931. p. 281–499.
155. Levy-Frankel A. Les hyperkeratoses de l'areole et du mamelon. Paris Med. 1938;28:63–6.
156. Halter K. Isoliert mamilläre hyperkeratosis follicularis et parafollicularis in cutem penetrans (Kyrle). Arch Derm Syph (Berl). 1938;176:689–93.
157. Oberste-Lehn H. Hyperkeratosen im Beireich von mamille und areola. Z Haut Geschlechtskr. 1950;8:388–93.
158. Mehregan AH, Rahbari H. Hyperkeratosis of nipple and areola. Arch Dermatol. 1977;113(12):1691–2.
159. Schwartz RA. Hyperkeratosis of nipple and areola. Arch Dermatol. 1978;114(12):1844–5.
160. Kim KJ, Cho KH, Kim WS. Hyperkeratosis of nipple and areola: a case report. Korean J Dermatol. 1978;16(6):465–6.
161. Mold DE, Jegasothy BV. Estrogen-induced hyperkeratosis of the nipple. Cutis. 1980;26(1):95–6.
162. Soden CE. Hyperkeratosis of the nipple and areola. Cutis. 1983;32(1):69–71, 74.
163. Kuhlman DS, Hodge SJ, Owen LG. Hyperkeratosis of the nipple and areola. J Am Acad Dermatol. 1985;13(4):596–8.
164. Vestey JP, Bunney MH. Unilateral hyperkeratosis of the nipple: the response to cryotherapy. Arch Dermatol. 1986;122(12):1360–1.
165. Allegue F, Soria C, Rocamora A, Fraile G, Ledo A. Hyperkeratosis of the nipple and areola in a patient with cutaneous T-cell lymphoma. Int J Dermatol. 1990;29(7):519–20.
166. Perez-Izquierdo JM, Vilata JJ, Sanchez JL, Gargallo E, Millan F, Aliaga A. Retinoic acid treatment of nipple hyperkeratosis. Arch Dermatol. 1990;126:687–9.
167. Ahn SK, Chung J, Soo Lee W, Kim SC, Lee SH. Hyperkeratosis of the nipple and areola simultaneously developing with cutaneous T-cell lymphoma. J Am Acad Dermatol. 1995;32(1):124–5.
168. Alpsoy E, Yilmaz E, Aykol A. Hyperkeratosis of the nipple: report of two cases. J Dermatol. 1997;24(1):43–5.
169. Obayashi H, Tsuchida T, Ikeda S. Hyperkeratosis of the nipple and areola. Rinsho Dermatol. 1998;40:147–50.
170. Mehanna A, Malak JA, Kibbi AG. Hyperkeratosis of the nipple and areola. Arch Dermatol. 2001;137:1327–8.
171. Lambiris AG, McCormick F. Unilateral hyperkeratosis of nipple and areola associated with androgen insensitivity and oestrogen replacement therapy. J Eur Acad Dermatol Venereol. 2001;15(4):376–7.

172. Lee HW, Suh HS, Choi JC, et al. Hyperkeratosis of the nipple and areola as a sign of malignant acanthosis nigricans. Clin Exp Dermatol. 2005;30(6):721–2.
173. Kavak A, Parlak AH, Aydogan I, Alper M. Hyperkeratosis of the nipple and areola in a patient with chronic mucocutaneous candidiasis. J Dermatol. 2006;33(7):510–1.
174. Samimi M, Maitre F, Esteve E. Hyperkeratotic lesion of the nipple revealing cutaneous leiomyoma. Ann Dermatol Venereol. 2008;135(8–9):571–4.
175. Kartal Durmazlar SP, Eskioglu F, Bodur Z. Hyperkeratosis of the nipple and areola: 2 years of remission with low-dose acitretin and topical calcipotriol therapy. J Dermatolog Treat. 2008;19(6):337–40.
176. Higgins HW, Jenkins J, Horn TD, Kroumpouzos G. Pregnancy-associated hyperkeratosis of the nipple: a report of 25 cases. JAMA Dermatol. 2013;14(6):722–6.
177. Martinez-Garcia E, Taibjee S, Koch D, Osborne R. Vemurafenib-induced hyperkeratosis of the areola treated with topical adapalene. Clin Exp Dermatol. 2015;41(2):148–51.
178. Friolet H. Ichthyosis Circumscripta of the areola mammae. Münch Med Wochenschr. 1905;LII:1818.
179. Bulman JFH. Leiomyoma of nipple. Br Med J. 1951;2(4737):975. In: Deaver JB, McFarland J, Herman L, editors. The breast: its anomalies, its diseases, and their treatment. Philadelphia: P. Blakiston's Son & Co.; 1917. p. 671–702.
180. Nascimento AG, Karas M, Rosen PP, Caron AG. Leiomyoma of the nipple. Am J Surg Pathol. 1979;3(2):151–4.
181. Virchow R. Uber cavernose (erektile) Geschwulste und Teleangiektasien. Virchows Arch Pathol Anat. 1854;6:525–4. In: Deaver JB, McFarland J, Herman L, editors. The breast: its anomalies, its diseases, and their treatment. Philadelphia: P. Blakiston's Son & Co.; 1917. p. 671–702.
182. Klob. Path Anat der Weiblichen Sexorgane 1864. In: Deaver JB, McFarland J, Herman L, editors. The breast: its anomalies, its diseases, and their treatment. Philadelphia: P. Blakiston's Son & Co.; 1917. p. 671–702.
183. Solokov. Virchow's Archiv. 1873;LVIII:336. In: Deaver JB, McFarland J, Herman L, editors. The breast: its anomalies, its diseases, and their treatment. Philadelphia: P. Blakiston's Son & Co.; 1917. p. 671–702.
184. Tsujioka K, Klashihara M, Imamura S. Cutaneous leiomyoma of the male nipple. Dermatologica. 1985;170:98–100.
185. Allison JG, Dodds HM. Leiomyoma of the male nipple. A case report and literature review. Am Surg. 1989;55(8):501–2.
186. Pujol RM, Fernandez MT. A solitary papule on the nipple. Arch Dermatol. 1991;127:571–6.
187. Velasco M, Ubeda B, Antonell F, Serra C. Leiomyoma of the male areola infiltrating the breast tissue. Am J Roentgenol. 1995;164(22):511–2.
188. Kaufman HL, Hirsch EF. Leiomyoma of the breast. J Surg Oncol. 1996;62:62–4.
189. Haier J, Haensch W, Schon M. Leiomyoma as a rare differential diagnosis of Paget's disease of the nipple. Act Obstet Gynecolog Scaand. 1997;76(5):490–1.
190. Roustan G, Sanchez E, Ruiz P, Simon A. Leiomioma de la areola mamaria. Presentación de dos casos. Actas Dermosifiliogr. 2001;92:35–7.
191. Chaudhary KS, Shousha S. Leiomyoma of the nipple, and normal subareolar muscle fibres, are oestrogen and progesterone receptor positive. Histopathology. 2004;44(6):626–8.
192. Khachemoune A, Rodriguez C, Lyle S, Jiang SB. Genital leiomyoma: surgical excision for both diagnosis and treatment of a unilateral leiomyoma of the male nipple. Dermatol Online J. 2005;11(1):20.
193. Ku J, Campbell C, Bennett I. Leiomyoma of the nipple. Breast J. 2006;12(4):377–80.
194. Shibata S, Imafuky S, Tashiro A, Gondo CH, Toyoshima S, Furue M. Leiomyoma of the male nipple. J Dermatol. 2011;38:727–9.
195. Leaño CD, María Garritano MV, Tobares N, Rafti P, Pianzola H. Leiomioma solitario en el complejo areola pezón. A propósito de un caso. Revisión de la literatura. Arch Argent Dermatol. 2011;61:203–8.
196. Cho HJI, Km SH, Kang BJ, Kim H, Song BJ, Lee AW. Leiomyoma of the nipple diagnosed by MRI. Acta Radiolog Short Rep. 2012;1(9):4.
197. Nakamura S, Hashimoto Y, Takeda K, Nishi K, Ishida-Yamamoto A, Mizumoto T, Lizuka H. Two cases of male nipple leiomyoma: idiopathic leiomyoma and gynecomastia-associated leiomyoma. Am J Dermatopathol. 2012;34(3):287–91.
198. Lòpez V, Lòpez I, Alcaccer J, Ricart JM. Successful treatment of leiomyoma of the nipple with carbon dioxide laser. Acta Dermosifilogr. 2013;104(10):928–30.
199. Pavlidis L, Vakirlis E, Spyropoulou GA, Pramateftakis MG, Dionyssiou D, Demiri E. A 35-year-old woman presenting with an unusual post-traumatic leiomyoma of the nipple. J Med Case Rep. 2013;7:49.
200. Hernandez FJ. Leiomyosarcoma of male breast originating in the nipple. Am J Surg Pathol. 1978;2(3):299–304.
201. Luh SP, Wong LC, Huang PC, Luh SP, Huang CS. Primary leiomyosarcoma of the nipple-areola complex: report of a case and review of literature. J Zhejiang Univ Sci B. 2008;9(2):109–13.
202. Lonsdale RN, Widdison A. Leiomyosarcoma of the nipple. Histopathology. 1992;20(6):537–9.
203. Liang WC, Sickle-Santanello BJ, Nims TA, Accetta PA. Primary leiomyosarcoma of the breast: a case report with review of the literature. Breast J. 2003;9(6)(6):494.
204. Samimi M, Maître F, Estève E. Hyperkeratotic lesion of the nipple revealing cutaneous leiomyoma. Ann Dermatol Venereol. 2008;135(8–9):571–4.
205. Wong LC, Huang PC, Luh SP, Huang CS. Primary leiomyosarcoma of the nipple-areola complex:

report of a case and review of literature. J Zhejiang Univ Sci B. 2008;9(2):109–13.
206. Kamio T, Nishizawa M, Aoyama K, Ohchi T, Nishikawa T, Kobayashi M, Kameoka S. Primary leiomyosarcoma of the breast treated by partial resection of the breast including nipple and areola: report of a case. Surg Today. 2010;40(11):1063–7.
207. Deveci U, Kapakli MSX, Altintoprak F, Cayirci MX, Manukyan MN, Kebudi A. Bilateral nipple leiomyomas. Case Rep Surg. 2013;2013(2013):475215.
208. Guedes X, Matarde M, Parra T, Martinez MJ, de Caralt E, Serra C. Primary leiomyosarcoma of the nipple-areola complex with an unusual clinical presentation: a case report. IJCRI. 2014;5(1):66–70.
209. Skin-melanocytic tumor. http://pathologyoutlines.com/topic/skintumormelanocteicsuperpage.html. Accessed 4 Apr 2016.
210. Papachristou DN, Kinne D, Ashikari R, Fortner JG. Melanoma of the nipple and areola. Br J Surq. 1979;66(4):287–8.
211. Kinoshita S, Yoshimoto K, Kyoda S, Hirano A, Shioya H, Kobayashi S, Ishiji T, Komine K, Takeyama H, Uchida K, Morikawa T, Sakamoto G. Malignant melanoma originating on the female nipple: a case report. Breast Cancer. 2007;14(1):105–8.
212. Jensen AK. Melanoma of the nipple. Arch Dermatol Syphilol. 1947;56(1):113.
213. Farrow JH. Benign and malignant lesions of the nipple. CA Cancer J Clin. 1958;8(1):16–9.
214. Kuten A, Cohen Y, Kerner V. Malignant melanoma of the nipple with autoamputation of the breast. Harefuah. 1976;90(7):321–2.
215. D'Aiuto G, Del Vecchio S, Mansi L, D'Aprile M, Botti G, Salvatore M. Malignant melanoma of the nipple: a case studied with radiolabeled monoclonal antibody. Tumori. 1991;77(5):449–51.
216. Carmichael AR, McIntyre M, Chetty U. Malignant melanoma in accessory nipple in a male. J Coll Physicians Surg Pak. 2006;16(12):799–800.
217. Lin CH, Lee HS, Yul JC. Melanoma of the nipple mimicking Paget's disease. Dermatol Online J. 2007;13(2):18.
218. Mourmouras V, Ambrosio MR, Onorati M, Rocca BJ, Di Mari N, De Luca F, Miracco C. Melanoma of the nipple. An additional case. Pathologica. 2011;103(1):25–6.
219. Srikanth S, Anandam G. Malignant melanoma of male breast with nodal metastasis. Case report. Med J Dr DY Patil Univ. 2014;7(2):192–4.
220. He Y, Mou JH, Luo D, Gao B, Wen Y. Primary malignant melanoma of the breast: a case report and review of the literature. Oncol Lett. 2014;8(1):238–40.
221. Shiga K, Oiso N, Narita T, Kimura M, Kawada A. Dermoscopy for malignant melanoma of the nipple and the areola. J Dermatol. 2015;42(3):339–41.
222. Sills M, Norton S, Landers R, O'Donoghue G. Malignant melanoma of the breast: a case report. J Cancer Biol Res. 2016;4(1):1075.
223. Folberg R, McLean IW. Primary aquired melanosis and melanoma of the conjunctive: terminology, classificaion, and biologic behavior. Mod Pathol. 1986;17:652–4.
224. Isbary G, Coras-Stepanek B, Stolz W. Pigmented lesion of the left nipple in a 49-year-old woman. J Dtsch Dermatol Ges. 2013;11(12):1206–8.
225. Sceppa JA, Smith BL, Marghoob AA, Gottlieb GJ. Melanosis of the areola and nipple. J Am Acad Dermatol. 2008;59(2 Suppl 1):S33–4.
226. Huerta-Brogeras M, Garrido-Ríos A, Borbujo J, Tardío JC. Unilateral hyperpigmented lesion of the breast in a young woman. Melanosis of the areola and nipple. JAMA Dermatol. 2013;149(3):357–63.
227. Isbary G, Coras-Stepanek B, Dyall-Smith D, Guther S, Tillmann A, Stolz W. Five patients with melanosis of the nipple and areola clinically mimicking melanoma. J Eur Acad Dermatol Venereol. 2014;28(9):1251–4.
228. Antonov NK, Bosenberg MW, Halasz CL. Melanosis of the areola and nipple with an atypical pigment network. Int J Dermatol. 2015;55:811–3.
229. Hoyt BS, Tschen JA, Cohen PR. Molluscum contagiosum of the areola and nipple: case report and literature review. Dermatol Online J. 2013;19(7):18965.
230. Heath. Lancet, London. 1872;i:603. In: Deaver JB, McFarland J, Herman L, editors. The breast: its anomalies, its diseases, and their treatment. Philadelphia: P. Blakiston's Son & Co.; 1917. p. 671–702.
231. Klauber. Prager Med Wochenschrift. 1904;XXIX,65:663. In: Deaver JB, McFarland J, Herman L, editors. The breast: its anomalies, its diseases, and their treatment. Philadelphia: P. Blakiston's Son & Co.; 1917. p. 671–702.
232. Carvalho G. Molluscum contagiosum in a lesion adjacent to the nipple. Report of a case. Acta Cytol. 1974;18(6):532–4.
233. Kumar N, Okiro P, Wasike R. Cytological diagnosis of molluscum contagiosum with an unusual clinical presentation at an unusual site. J Dermatol Case Rep. 2010;4(4):63–5.
234. Likhar KS, Hazari RA, Gupta SG, Patle Y. Isolated molluscum contagiosum of nipple: a rare case study. J Evolution Med Dental Sci. 2014;3(28):7696–700.
235. Caroppo D, Natella V, Scalvenzi M, Vetrani A, Cozzolino I. Molluscum contagiosum diagnosis on nipple scraping sample. Breast J. 2016;22(1):120–1.
236. Friedrich RE, Hage C. Appendices of the nipple and areola of the breast in neurofibromatosis type 1 patients are neurofibroma. Anticancer Res. 2010;30(5):1815–7.
237. Zhou Y, Pan B, Mao F, Zhu Q, Huo Z, Wang H, Cai F, Liang Z, Wang C, Zhang Y, Sun Q. A hidden breast lump covered by nipple appendices in a patient with von Recklinghausen disease: a case report and review of the literature. Clinl Breast Cancer. 2012;12(1):71–5.
238. Sherman JE, Smith JW. Neurofibromas of the breast and nipple-areolar area. Ann Plast Surg. 1981;7(4):302–7.

239. Lima RO, Stefenon CC. Neurofibroma de mama. Rev Bras Mastol. 2000;10(2):100–2.
240. Lannon DA, Harris PA, Butler PE. Treatment of severe neurofibromatosis of the nipple-areola complex. Plast Reconstr Surg. 2003;111(2):952–3.
241. Murat A, Kansiz F, Kabakus N, Kazez A, Ozercan R. Neurofibroma of the breast in a boy with neurofibromatosis type 1. Clin Imaging. 2004;28:415–7.
242. Millman SL, Mercado CL. An unusual presentation of neurofibromatosis of the breast. Breast J. 2004;10(1):45–7.
243. Posada JG, Chakmakjian CG. Images in clinical medicine. Von Recklinghausen's disease and breast cancer. N Engl J Med. 2005;352(17):1799.
244. Gokalp G, Hakyemez B, Kizilkaya E, Haholu A. Myxoid neurofibromas of the breast: mammographical, sonographical and MRI appearances. Br J Radiol. 2007;80:e234–7.
245. Tostes RO, Chagas LN, Guedes JCC, Quinsan MP, Avellán LJV, Costa JM. Nipple-areolar complex neurofibromas: case report. Rev Bras Cirurg Plast. 2007;22(2):122–5.
246. An HY, Kim KY, Yu IK, Kim KW, Kim HH. The nipple-areolar complex: a pictorial review of common and uncommon conditions. J Ultrasound Med. 2010;29:949–62.
247. Friedrich RE, Hage C. Appendices of the nipple and areola of the breast in neurofibromatosis type 1 patients are neurofibroma. Anticancer Res. 2010;30(5):1815–7.
248. Bongiorno MR, Doukaki S, Aricò M. Neurofibromatosis of the nipple-areolar area: a case series. J Med Case Rep. 2010;4:22.
249. Goksugur N, Gurel S. Neurofibromatosis of nipple-areola complex. Breast J. 2011;17(4):424.
250. Spyropoulou GA, Pavlidis L, Trakatelli M, Athanasiou E, Pazarli E, Sotiriadis D, Demiri E. Rare benign tumours of the nipple. J Eur Acad Dermatol Venereol. 2015;29(1):7–13.
251. Cunha Filho RR, Almeida HLJ, Cartell A. Verrucous epidermal nevus manifesting as nipple and areola hyperkeratosis. An Bras Dermatol. 2006;81(4):377–9.
252. Urbani CE, Betti R. Supernumerary nipple in association with Becker nevus vs. Becker nevus syndrome: a semantic problem only. Am J Med Genet. 1998;77(1):76–7.
253. Lewis EJ, Crutchfield CE 3rd, Ebertz MJ, Prawer SE. Report of a nipple nevus and an overview of accessory mammary tissue. Cutis. 1998;62(5):243–6.
254. Xifra M, Lagodin C, Wright D, Abbruzzese M, Woscoff A. Nevoid keratosis of the nipple. J Am Acad Dermatol. 1999;41:325–6.
255. Mehanna A, Malak JA, Kibbi A-G, Büyükbabani N, Kavak A, Murat A. Nevoid hyperkeratosis of nipple and areola: a distinct entity. J Am Acad Dermatol. 2002;46:414–8.
256. Krishnan RS, Angel TA, Roark TR, Hsu S. Nevoid hyper keratosis of the nipple and/or areola: a report of two cases and a review of the literature. Int J Dermatol. 2002;41:775–7.
257. Baykal C, Biiyiikbabani N, Kavak A, Alper M. Nevoid hyperkeratosis of the nipple and areola: a distinct entity. Am Acad Dermatol. 2002;46(3):414–8.
258. Baz K, Kokturk A, Kaya TI, Ikizoglu G, Düsmez D, Koca A. A case of hyperkeratosis of the nipple and areola resulting from organoid nevus. Int J Dermatol. 2003;42:318–20.
259. Pastar Z, Massone C, Ahlgrimm-Siess V, Koller S, Mofarrah R, Hofmann-Wellenhof R. Dermoscopy and in vivo reflectance confocal microscopy of a congenital nevus of the nipple. Dermatology. 2010;221(2):127–30.
260. Verma P, Pandhi D, Yadav P. Unilateral nevoid/primary hyperkeratosis of nipple and areola successfully treated with radiofrequency ablation. Cutan Aesthet Surg. 2011;4(3):214–5.
261. Yikilmaz ŞR, Wilson-Clay B. Successful breastfeeding outcome of a woman with a nevus of the nipple: a case study. J Hum Lact. 2016;32:361–3.
262. Sanati S, Leonard M, Khamapirad T, Eltorky MA. Nodular mucinosis of the breast: a case report with pathologic, ultrasonographic, and clinical findings and review of the literature. Arch Pathol Lab Med. 2005;129(3):e58–61.
263. Kempf W, von Stumberg B, Denisjuk N, Bode B, Rongioletti F. Trauma-induced cutaneous focal mucinosis of the mammary areola: an unusual presentation. Dermatopathology. 2014;1:24–8.
264. Vázquez-Doval FJ, Sola MA. Mucinosis of the mammary areolae and mycosis fungoides. Clin Exp Dermatol. 1996;21:374–6.
265. Michal M, Ludvikova M, Zamecnik M. Nodular mucinosis of the breast: report of three cases. Pathol Int. 1998;48:542–4.
266. Koide N, Akashi-Tanaka S, Fukutomi T, Nanasawa T, Hasegawa T. Nodular mucinosis of the breast: a case report with clinical and imaging findings. Breast Cancer. 2002;9:261–4.
267. Manglik N, Berlingeri-Ramos AC, Boroumand N, Eltorky M. Nodular mucinosis of the breast in a supernumerary nipple: case report and review of the literature. J Cutan Pathol. 2010;37(11):1178–81.
268. Fernández-Figueras MT, Kazakov DV, López Martos R, Ojanguren I, Vila J, Ariza A. Nodular mucinosis of the breast in a male: reassessment of diagnostic criteria and proposal for its classification as a soft tissue tumor in the myofibroblastoma and spindle cell lipoma spectrum. Dermatopathology. 2014;1:47–54.
269. Paget JY. St. Barttholew's Hosp Rep., London. 1874;X:87–9. In: Deaver JB, McFarland J, Herman L, editors. The breast: its anomalies, its diseases, and their treatment. Philadelphia: P. Blakiston's Son & Co.; 1917. p. 671–702.
270. Butlin. Medico-Chirurgical Transactions, London. 1876;IX:107. In: Deaver JB, McFarland J, Herman L, editors. The breast: its anomalies, its diseases, and their treatment. Philadelphia: P. Blakiston's Son & Co.; 1917. p. 671–702.

271. Thin. Trans Path Soc of London. 1881;XXXII:218. In: Deaver JB, McFarland J, Herman L, editors. The breast: its anomalies, its diseases, and their treatment. Philadelphia: P. Blakiston's Son & Co.; 1917. p. 671–702.
272. Duhring. Am J Med Sci. 1883;LXXXVI:116. In: Deaver JB, McFarland J, Herman L, editors. The breast: its anomalies, its diseases, and their treatment. Philadelphia: P. Blakiston's Son & Co.; 1917. p. 671–702.
273. Wile. Am J Med Sci. 1884;LXXXVIII:141. In: Deaver JB, McFarland J, Herman L, editors. The breast: its anomalies, its diseases, and their treatment. Philadelphia: P. Blakiston's Son & Co.; 1917. p. 671–702.
274. Bowlby. Medico-Chirurgical Transactions, London. 1890–91;LXXIV:341. In: Deaver JB, McFarland J, Herman L, editors. The breast: its anomalies, its diseases, and their treatment. Philadelphia: P. Blakiston's Son & Co.; 1917. p. 671–702.
275. Bowlby AA. Thirteen cases of Paget's disease of the nipple, with special reference to the causation of the malady by psorosperms. Med Chir Trans. 1891;74:341–366.1.
276. O'Neill H. Report of a case of Paget's disease of the right nipple. Br Med J. 1891;1(1581):846–8.
277. Karg. Deutsche Zeitschrift für Chirurgie. 1892;XXXIV. In: Deaver JB, McFarland J, Herman L, editors. The breast: its anomalies, its diseases, and their treatment. Philadelphia: P. Blakiston's Son & Co.; 1917. p. 671–702.
278. Evans W. Paget's disease. Proc R Soc Med. 1909;2(Dermatol Sect):162.
279. Davis H. Paget's disease of the nipple. Proc R Soc Med. 1913;6(Dermatol Sect):5.
280. Bunch JL. Paget's disease of the nipple. Proc R Soc Med. 1914;7(Dermatol Sect):255–7.
281. Jopson JH, Speese J. Paget's disease of the nipple and allied conditions. Ann Surg. 1915;62(2):212–37.
282. Sekiguchi S. Studies on Paget's disease of the nipple and its extramammary occurrence: reports of eighteen cases personally investigated. Ann Surg. 1917;65(2):175–98.
283. Gabriel WB. Case of Paget's disease. Proc R Soc Med. 1926;19(Surg Sect):14.
284. Little EG. Ulceration of nipple: Paget's disease. Proc R Soc Med. 1928;21(7):1177.
285. Cheatle L. Paget's disease of the nipple. Proc R Soc Med. 1930;23(4):550.
286. Gardham AJ. Early Paget's disease of the nipple, with an extensive carcinoma of the breast. Proc R Soc Med. 1931;24(6):779.
287. Barber HW. Paget's disease of the nipple associated with diffuse carcinomatosis of the chest wall. Proc R Soc Med. 1932;25(5):670–2.
288. Bamber G. Intra-epidermal carcinoma. Paget's disease of the nipple. Proc R Soc Med. 1933;26(7):841.
289. West JP, Nickel WF. Paget's disease of the nipple. Ann Surg. 1942;116(1):19–25.
290. Inglis K. Paget's disease of the nipple: with special reference to the changes in the ducts. Am J Pathol. 1946;22(1):1–33.
291. Costello MJ. Paget's disease of the nipple. Arch Dermatol Syphilol. 1946;54:110.
292. Allen H, Stout AP. Carcinoma of breast with Paget's disease. Mo Med. 1947;44(8):584.
293. Wagner M. Report of a case of Paget's disease in an 18 year old male, with a review of the literature. Wis Med J. 1947;46(11):1098–107.
294. Setala K. Paget's disease of the nipple with special reference to its relation of dermal gland carcinomata. Acta Pathol Microbiol Scand. 1949;26(2):207–22.
295. Marx R. Significance of ductal sclerosis in Paget's disease; regression of intraductal carcinoma. Arch Pathol (Chic). 1949;47(4):404–6.
296. Clymer JH, Halpert B, et al. Paget's disease of the nipple. J Okla State Med Assoc. 1949;42(9):393–6.
297. Tzanck. Paget's disease of the nipple. Ann Dermatol Syphiligr (Paris). 1950;10(5):opp 545.
298. Jonquieres EJ, Grillo A, Melamed AJ. Paget's disease of the nipple; therapeutic considerations. Sem Med. 1950;57(42):800–4.
299. Eisen MJ, Taft RH. Cytological diagnosis of mammary cancer associated with incipient Paget's disease of the nipple. Cancer. 1951;4(1):150–3.
300. Michalany J. Carcinoma of the breast and Paget's disease of the nipple. Hospital (Rio J). 1951;39(1):81–94.
301. Dockerty MB, Harrington SW. Preclinical Paget's disease of the nipple. Surg Gynecol Obstet. 1951;93(3):317–20.
302. Oddo R, Martin-Laval J. Degenerated Paget's disease of the nipple in pregnancy. Bull Fed Soc Gynecol Obstet Lang Fr. 1952;4(5):963–4.
303. Johnson N. Paget's disease of the nipple. Aust N Z J Surg. 1952;22(2):111–9.
304. Veronesi U, Rabotti G. Cytological diagnosis of Paget's disease of the nipple. Tumori. 1954;40(2):204–12.
305. Culberson JD, Horn RC Jr. Paget's disease of the nipple; review of twenty-five cases with special reference to melanin pigmentation of Paget cells. AMA Arch Surg. 1956;72(2):224–31.
306. Helman P, Kliman M. Paget's disease of the nipple; a clinical review of 27 cases. Br J Surg. 1956;43(181):481–8.
307. Devine JW, Devine JW Jr, Thornhill TM. Paget's disease of the nipple. Va Med Mon (1918). 1956;83(7):303–4.
308. Farrow JH. Benign and malignant lesions of the nipple. CA Cancer J Clin. 1958;8(1):16–9.
309. Wiman LG, Skogh M. Cytodiagnosis of Paget's disease of the nipple. Some reflections on a case with negative biopsy. Sven Lakartidn. 1960;57:3154–8 passim.
310. Toker C. Some observations on Paget's disease of the nipple. Cancer. 1961;14:653–72.

311. Carcassonne F, Temime P, Bonneau H. A case of Paget's disease strictly localized in the nipple. Cytological and histological study. Bull Soc Fr Dermatol Syphiligr. 1962;69:133–4.
312. Orr JW, Parish DJ. The nature of the nipple changes in Paget's disease. J Pathol Bacteriol. 1962;84:201–8.
313. Rogers J. Paget's disease of the nipple. Br J Clin Pract. 1962;16:813.
314. Aboumrad MH, Horn RC Jr, Fine G. Lipid-secreting mammary carcinoma. Report of a case associated with Paget's disease of the nipple. Cancer. 1963;16:521–5.
315. Greenwood SM, Minkowitz S. Paget's disease in metastatic breast carcinoma. Arch Dermatol. 1971;104(3):312–5.
316. Sugimoto M, Matsushima T, Ando M, Tsuda T, Ozaki T. Unusual pulmonary metastasis of mammary cancer: unilateral pulmonary fibrosis after mammary Paget's disease. Kumamoto Med J. 1974;27(3):176–82.
317. Dabski K, Stoll HL Jr. Paget's disease of the breast presenting as a cutaneous horn. J Surg Oncol. 1985;29:237–9.
318. Menon RS, van Geel AN. Cancer of the breast with nipple involvement. J Cancer. 1989;59(1):81–4.
319. Tousignant J, Grossin M, Crickx B, Belaïch S. Paget's disease of the nipple associated with epidermal basaloid hyperplasia simulating basal cell carcinoma. Ann Dermatol Venereol. 1991;118(3):211–4.
320. Roumen RM, Haas FD. Eczema of the nipple: cancer or not? Ned Tijdschr Geneeskd. 1997;141(36):1721–4.
321. Fu W, Mittel VK, Young SC. Paget disease of the breast: analysis of 41 patients. Am J Clin Oncol. 2001;24:397–400.
322. Frei KA, Bonel HM, Pelte MF, Hylton NM, Kinkel K. Paget disease of the breast: findings at magnetic resonance imaging and histopathologic correlation. Investig Radiol. 2005;40:363–7.
323. Amano G, Yajima M, Moroboshi Y, Kuriya Y, Ohuchi N. MRI accurately depicts underlying DCIS in a patient with Paget's disease of the breast without palpable mass and mammography findings. Jpn J Clin Oncol. 2005;35:149–53.
324. Mitchell ML, Napoletano J, Penman EJ. The MRI appearance of Paget's disease of the nipple: images from a single case. Del Med J. 2006;78:105–6.
325. Gunhan-Bilgen I, Oktay A. Paget's disease of the breast: clinical, mammographic, sonographic and pathologic findings in 52 cases. Eur J Radiol. 2006;60:256–63.
326. Betal D, Puri N, Roberts K, Kalra L, Rapisarda F, Bonomi R. Hyperpigmented Paget's disease of the nipple - a diagnostic dilemma. JRSM Short Rep. 2012;3(5):31.
327. Challa VR, Deshmane V. Challenges in diagnosis and management of Paget's disease of the breast—a retrospective study. Indian J Surg. 2015;77(Suppl 3):1083–7.
328. Akita M, Kusunoki N, Nakajima T, Takase S, Maekawa Y, Kajimoto K, Ohno M. Paget's disease of the male breast: a case report. Surg Case Rep. 2015;1(1):103.
329. Challa VR, Deshmane V. Challenges in diagnosis and management of paget's disease of the breast-a retrospective study. Indian J Surg. 2015;77(Suppl 3):1083–7.
330. Dennis MA, Parker S, Kaske TI, Stavros AT, Camp J. Incidental treatment of nipple discharge caused by benign intraductal papilloma through diagnostic mammotome biopsy. Am J Roentgenol. 2000;174(5):1263–8.
331. Reverdin. Tumeur papillaire pedunculée de l'areola du sein. Bull et Mém de la Soc d'Anat de Paris. 1867;XLII:540. In: Deaver JB, McFarland J, Herman L, editors. The breast: its anomalies, its diseases, and their treatment. Philadelphia: P. Blakiston's Son & Co.; 1917. p. 671–702.
332. Shaw. Tumor attached by a pedicle to the areola of the left breast. Trans Pathological Soc London. 1850–51;III:186. In: Deaver JB, McFarland J, Herman L, editors. The breast: its anomalies, its diseases, and their treatment. Philadelphia: P. Blakiston's Son & Co.; 1917. p. 671–702.
333. Porter FT. Erectile tumor of the nipple. Irish Hospital Gazette, Dublin. 1873;I:30. In: Deaver JB, McFarland J, Herman L, editors. The breast: its anomalies, its diseases, and their treatment. Philadelphia: P. Blakiston's Son & Co.; 1917. p. 671–702.
334. Pollard. Trans Path Soc Lond 1886;XXV. In: Deaver JB, McFarland J, Herman L, editors. The breast: its anomalies, its diseases, and their treatment. Philadelphia: P. Blakiston's Son & Co.; 1917. p. 671–702.
335. Robinson. Cystic papilloma of the nipple. Trans Path Soc., London. 1890;XLI. In: Deaver JB, McFarland J, Herman L, editors. The breast: its anomalies, its diseases, and their treatment. Philadelphia: P. Blakiston's Son & Co.; 1917. p. 671–702.
336. Linfors. Monatschrift für Geburtshülft Gynäkologie. 1900;XI:763. In: Deaver JB, McFarland J, Herman L, editors. The breast: its anomalies, its diseases, and their treatment. Philadelphia: P. Blakiston's Son & Co.; 1917. p. 671–702.
337. Salzac E. Papillomas cutanées de mamelon. Thèse Paris 1903. In: Deaver JB, McFarland J, Herman L, editors. The breast: its anomalies, its diseases, and their treatment. Philadelphia: P. Blakiston's Son & Co.; 1917. p. 671–702.
338. Negri L. Uncommon cases of mammary pathology. 1. Acute diffuse superficial phlegmon. 2. Papilloma of the male nipple. 3. Epidermoid cysts. 4. Infantile mammary fibroma. 5. Fibrosarcoma. Arch De Vecchi Anat Patol. 1951;16(3):1247–64.
339. Farrow JH. Benign and malignant lesions of the nipple. CA Cancer J Clin. 1958;8(1):16–9.
340. Ferlito A. On intraductal papilloma of the nipple in the male breast. Riv Anat Patol Oncol. 1969;35:339–44.

341. Innocenti P, Ucchino S, Cianchetti E, Basilico L, Angelone A. Papilloma of the nipple. General remarks and comment apropos of a personal case. Minerva Chir. 1976;31(19):1089–94.
342. Keswani NK, Gupta SC. Unusual case of squamous papilloma of nipple. J Indian Med Assoc. 1979;72(4):83–4.
343. Manavi M, Baghestanian M, Kucera E, Berger A, Schatten C, Pischinger K, Czerwenka K. Papilloma virus and c-erbB-2 expression in diseases of the mammary nipple. Anticancer Res. 2001;21(1B):797–801.
344. Wei H, Jiayi F, Qinping Z, Junyi S, Yuan S, Li L, Dongwei S, Liying Q. Ultrasound-guided vacuum-assisted breast biopsy system for diagnosis and minimally invasive excision of intraductal papilloma without nipple discharge. World J Surg. 2009;33(12):2579–81.
345. Singh A, Nigam JS, Misra V, Singh PA. Diagnosis of a nonpalpable intraductal papilloma without radiological abnormality by nipple discharge smear examination: a case report. Breast Cancer (Auckl). 2014;8:69–72.
346. Kleb. Handbuch der Pathologgisch Anatomie. 1876;I,2:1225. In: Deaver JB, McFarland J, Herman L, editors. The breast: its anomalies, its diseases, and their treatment. Philadelphia: P. Blakiston's Son & Co.; 1917. p. 671–702.
347. Gross SW. On the diagnosis of tumours of the mamma. In: Braithwaite W, Braithwaite J, Trevelyen EF, editors. The retrospect of practical medicine. New York: W.A. Townsend; 1881. p. 198–200.
348. Fruhling L, Le Gall Y. Six cases of genuine primitive sarcoma of the nipple. Bull Fed Soc Gynecol Obstet Lang Fr. 1952;4(3):565–6.
349. Kopacz A, Kucharski A, Cicholska A, Jaśkiewicz J. Reticulum cell sarcoma of the nipple. Nowotwory. 1979;29(2):121–3.
350. Shamsadini S, Wadji MB, Shamsadini A. Surrounding ipsilateral eruptive seborrheic keratosis as a warning sign of intraductal breast carcinoma and Paget's disease (Leser Trelat sign). Dermatol Online J. 2006;12:27.
351. Schwartz RA. Sign of Leser-Trélat. J Am Acad Dermatol. 1996;35(1):88–95.
352. Leser E. Ueber ein die Krebskrankheit beim Menschen haufig begleitendes, noch wenig gekanntes Symptom. Munchener Med Wochenschr. 1901;51:2035–6.
353. Hollander EV. Beitrage zur Fruhdiagnose des Darmcarcinomas (Hereditatsverhaltnisse und Hautveranderungen). Deutsche Medicinische Wochenschrift. 1900;26:483–5.
354. De Morgan C. On the origin of cancer. Lancet. 1871;II:6–7, 41–42.
355. Narasimha A, Harendra Kumar ML, Divyarani MN, Bhaskaran A. Pigmented seborrheic keratosis (melanoacanthoma) of nipple: a case report with review of literature. J Clin Biomed Sci. 2013;3(2):96–100.
356. Mckee PH, Calonje E, Grant SR. Pathology of skin with clinical correlation. 3rd ed. Philadelphia: Elsevier Mosby; 2005. p. 1158–63.
357. Mullikan JB. Capillary malformations, hyperkeratotic stains, telangiectasis, and miscellaneous vascular blots. In: Mulliken JB, Burrows PE, Fishman SJ, editors. Mulliken and Young's vascular anomalies: hemangiomas and malformations. Oxford: Oxford University Press; 2013. p. 508–61.
358. Mandry G. Primäres carcinom der Brustwartze. Beiträge zur Klinischen Chirurgie, Tübingen 1893;X:231. In: Deaver JB, McFarland J, Herman L, editors. The breast: its anomalies, its diseases, and their treatment. Philadelphia: P. Blakiston's Son & Co.; 1917. p. 671–702.
359. Loveland-Jones CE, Wang F, Bankhead RR, Huang Y, Reilly KJ. Squamous cell carcinoma of the nipple following radiation therapy for ductal carcinoma *in situ*: a case report. J Med Case Rep. 2010;4:186.
360. Upasham SP, VinodKiri M, Sudhamani S. One more common tumor in an uncommon location: Squamous cell carcinoma on nipple areola complex. Indian J Cancer. 2014;51(3):376–7.
361. Brodie B. Lecture on pathology and surgery, London 1846. In: Deaver JB, McFarland J, Herman L, editors. The breast: its anomalies, its diseases, and their treatment. Philadelphia: P. Blakiston's Son & Co.; 1917. p. 671–702.
362. Kroell H. Praktischer Arzt Wetzler. 1878;XIX, 25:40. In: Deaver JB, McFarland J, Herman L, editors. The breast: its anomalies, its diseases, and their treatment. Philadelphia: P. Blakiston's Son & Co.; 1917. p. 671–702.
363. D'Alger B. Bull et Mém Soc de Chirurgie de Paris. 1885. In: Deaver JB, McFarland J, Herman L, editors. The breast: its anomalies, its diseases, and their treatment. Philadelphia: P. Blakiston's Son & Co.; 1917. p. 671–702.
364. Weil J. Prage Med Wocheschrift 1893;XVIII:81. In: Deaver JB, McFarland J, Herman L, editors. The breast: its anomalies, its diseases, and their treatment. Philadelphia: P. Blakiston's Son & Co.; 1917. p. 671–702.
365. Morestin H. Bull et Mèm de la Soc de Paris. 1907:LXXXXII:608. In: Deaver JB, McFarland J, Herman L, editors. The breast: its anomalies, its diseases, and their treatment. Philadelphia: P. Blakiston's Son & Co.; 1917. p. 671–702.
366. Battle and Mayberry. Lancet, London. 1913;I:22. In: Deaver JB, McFarland J, Herman L, editors. The breast: its anomalies, its diseases, and their treatment. Philadelphia: P. Blakiston's Son & Co.; 1917. p. 671–702.
367. Edwards MJ, Hirsch RM, Broadwater JR, Netscher DT, Ames FC. Squamous cell carcinoma arising in previously burned or irradiated skin. Arch Surg. 1989;124:115–7.
368. Van Hoeven KH, Drudis T, Cranor ML, Erlandson RA, Rosen PP. Low-grade adenosquamous carci-

noma of the breast: a clinicopathologic study of 32 cases with ultrastructural analysis. Am J Surg Pathol. 1993;17(3):248–58.
369. Venkataseshan VS, Budd DC, Kim DU, Hutter RVP. Intraepidermal squamous carcinoma (Bowen's disease) of the nipple. Hum Pathol. 1994;25(12):1371–4.
370. Uzoaru I, Adeyanju M, Ray VH, Nadimpalli V. Primary squamous cell carcinoma of the breast presenting as a nipple discharge. Acta Cytol. 1994;38(1):112–3.
371. Brookes PT, Jhawar S, Hinton CP, Murdoch S, Usman T. Bowen's disease of the nipple—a new method of treatment. Breast. 2005;14(1):65–7.
372. Brookes PT, Jhawar S, Hinton CP, Murdoch S, Usman T. Bowen's disease of the nipple—a new method of treatment. Breast. 2005;14:65–7.
373. Sharma R, Iyer M. Bowen's disease of the nipple in a young man with AIDS: a case report. Clin Breast Cancer. 2009;9(1):53–5.
374. Chen CH, Rowlands C, Sengupta SK, George RL, Parulekar W, Thain K, O'Malley F, Isotalo PA. Primary basaloid carcinoma of the nipple with associated squamous cell carcinoma in situ. Breast J. 2009;15(4):409–13.
375. Hosaka N, Uesaka K, Takaki T, Zhang Y, Takasu K, Ikehara S. Poorly differentiated squamous cell carcinoma of the nipple: a unique case for marked exophytic growth, but little invasion with neuroendocrine differentiation. Med Mol Morphol. 2011;44(3):174–8.
376. King F, Kremer H. Squamous cell carcinoma of the nipple: an unusual location in a male patient. Am Surg. 2012;78(2):E101–E2.
377. Sofos SS, Tehrani H, Lymperopoulos N, Constantinides J, James MI. Primary squamous cell carcinoma of the nipple: a diagnosis of suspicion. J Plast Reconstr Aesthet Surg. 2013;66(11):e315–7.
378. Upasham SP, Vinodkiri M, Sudhamani S. One more common tumor in an uncommon location: squamous cell carcinoma on nipple areola complex. Indian J Cancer. 2014;51(3):376–7.
379. Pendse AA, O'Connor SM. Primary invasive squamous cell carcinoma of the nipple. Case Rep Pathol. 2015;2015:327487.
380. Congdon G, Dockerty M. Malignant lesions of the nipple exclusive of Paget's disease. Surg Gynecol Obstet. 1956;103:185–92.
381. Fernández-Jorge B, Yebra-Pimentel T. Nódulo solitario en la areola mamaria de un varón. Piel. 2007;22:353–4.

# 13 Pedunculated Fibroma of the Nipple

Ketan Vagholkar

## 13.1 Introduction

Tumours of the nipple-areola complex are uncommon. When diagnosed, malignancy always remains high on the list [1]. Dermatoses of the nipple are a spectrum of diseases ranging from malignant to benign lesions [2]. However arriving at a definitive diagnosis is pivotal to avert mismanagement.

## 13.2 Surgical Pathology

A wide spectrum of diseases is included in the collective terminology called dermatoses. These include Paget's disease, adenomas, molluscum contagiosum, fibromas, and nevi. Fibromas of the nipple are the rarest of the lot [2, 3]. Fibrous neoplasms range from fibromatosis to fibrosarcomas [4]. They display tendency to recur and even to metastasize in malignant forms. Pedunculated fibromas are an extreme rarity. These are benign lesions which have a very slow growth rate. Histologically, they exhibit typical spindle cells with thin-walled vasculature (Fig. 13.1). No atypia is seen [3]. Recurrence after complete removal is uncommon.

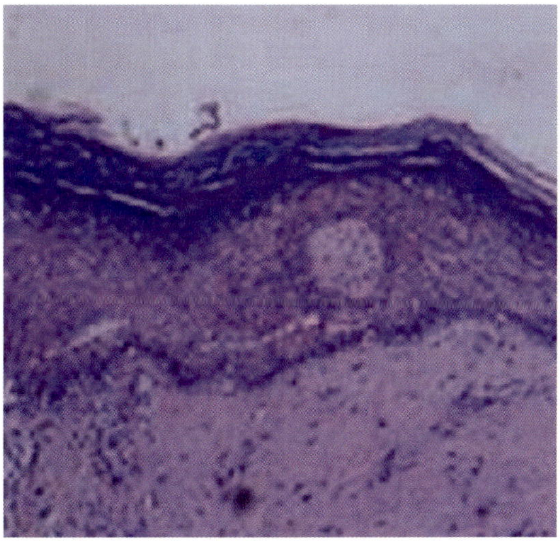

**Fig. 13.1** Spindle-shaped cells devoid of atypia with interspersed thin-walled vasculature

K. Vagholkar, M.S., D.N.B., F.R.C.S.
Department of Surgery, D.Y. Patil University School of Medicine, Navi Mumbai, Maharashtra 400706, India
e-mail: kvagholkar@yahoo.com


M.A. Shiffman (ed.), *Nipple-Areolar Complex Reconstruction*,
https://doi.org/10.1007/978-3-319-60925-6_13

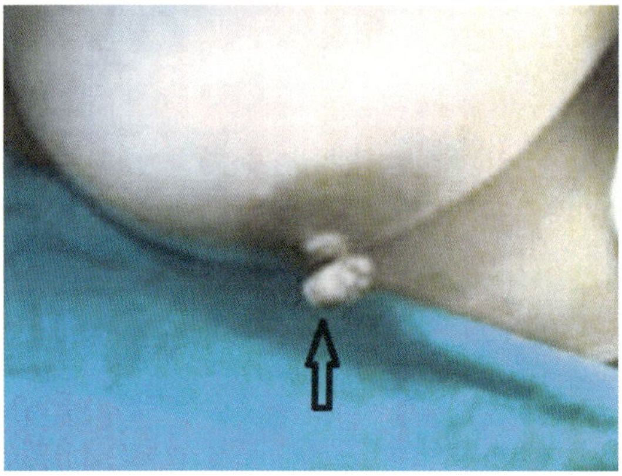

Fig. 13.2 Pedunculated fibroma arising from the nipple

## 13.3 Clinical Features

These tumours present as slow-growing lesions. The tumours go unnoticed due to their small size and absence of associated symptoms. Pedunculated lesions however are noticed early (Fig. 13.2). Pedunculated lesions are extremely rare. In certain cases ulceration of the pedunculated mass may be seen [5].

## 13.4 Management

Wide excision of the fibromas is the mainstay of treatment (Fig. 13.3). An elliptical incision made around the base of the stalk ensures ligation of the pedicle at the base. Histopathological examination of the excised lesion is confirmatory for diagnosis [1–3]. These tumours do not have any malignant potential. Recurrence is extremely uncommon [4].

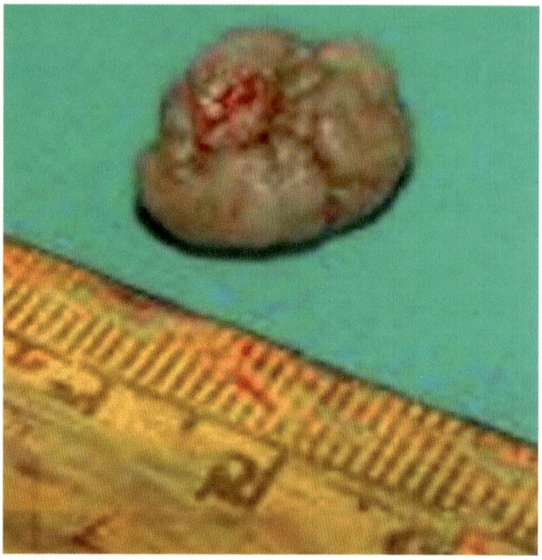

Fig. 13.3 Excised specimen

**Acknowledgements** I would like to thank Parth Vagholkar for his help in typesetting the manuscripts and editing the photographs.

## References

1. Vagholkar K, Nair S, Tople S, Gopinathan I. Pedunculated fibroma of the nipple: case report and review of literature. The Internet J of Oncol. 2013;9(1):1–3.
2. Parlakgumus A, Yildirim S, Bolat FA, Caliskan K, Ezer A, Colakglu T, Moray G. Dermatoses of the nipple. Can J Surg. 2009;52(2):160–1.
3. Prasad M, Pradhan PK, Bisarya BN. Pedunculated fibroma of nipple. J Indian Med Assoc. 1973;61(12):517.
4. Doctor VM, Sirsat MV. Florid papillomatosis (adenoma) and other benign tumours of the nipple and areola. Br J Cancer. 1971;25(1):1–9.
5. Higaki Y, Yoshinga Y, Kawashima M. Blister formation over a soft fibroma of the nipple. J Dermatol. 1993;20(7):447–8.

# Nipple Areola Complex Management and Reconstruction in Subareolar Breast Abscess

14

Giuseppe Falco, Daniele Bordoni, Cesare Magalotti, Saverio Coiro, Moira Ragazzi, Matteo Ornelli, Ariel Tessone, and Guglielmo Ferrari

## 14.1 Introduction

A breast abscess is defined as a localized infection represented by a fluid collection in breast tissue. Despite it is considered a benign condition, it is characterized by an elevated morbidity. Breast abscesses can be classified as puerperal and non-puerperal [1]. Puerperal breast abscess is defined as breast abscess associated with pregnancy, or during the first 3 months after labor without lactation, during lactation, or during the first 3 months after cessation of lactation [2–4].

Non-puerperal breast abscesses, first described in 1951 by Zuska et al. [5], represent 1–2% of all symptomatic breast processes [6] and are divided into subareolar breast abscesses, located in the subareolar area or within 1 cm from the areola, and non-subareolar breast abscesses that are located in different areas of the breast.

Subareolar breast abscesses have an elevated tendency to recur and to form extended fistulas. Knowledge of the pathogenesis of this disease is essential to better understand the different ways of treatment.

## 14.2 Pathogenesis

The breast is a modified sweat gland composed as shown in Fig. 14.1

1. Parenchymal part (16–18 lobules, each one characterized by a major lactiferous duct; they connect each lobule to an opening at the apex of the nipple).

G. Falco, M.D. (✉) • S. Coiro, M.D. • G. Ferrari, M.D.
Breast Surgery Unit, IRCCS- Santa Maria Nuova,
Via Risorgimento n°80, Reggio Emilia, 42124, Italy
e-mail: giuseppe.falco81@gmail.com;
coiro.saverio@asmn.re.it;
ferrari.guglielmo@asmn.re.it

D. Bordoni, M.D. • C. Magalotti, M.D.
Department of Senology, Ospedale Santa Maria della Misericordia Urbino, Asur Marche Area Vasta 1,
Fano, Urbino, Italy
e-mail: dottorbordoni@gmail.com;
cesare.magalotti@sanita.marche.it

M. Ragazzi, M.D.
Pathology Unit, IRCCS- Santa Maria Nuova,
Reggio Emilia, Italy
e-mail: ragazzi.moira@asmn.re.it

M. Ornelli, M.D.
Department of Plastic Surgery, Università Politecnica delle Marche, Ancona, Italy
e-mail: ornellimatteo@hotmail.com

A. Tessone, M.D.
Department of Plastic Surgery, The Talpiot Medical Leadership Program, Sheba Medical Center,
Tel-Hashomer, Israel
e-mail: tessonemd@icloud.com


M.A. Shiffman (ed.), *Nipple-Areolar Complex Reconstruction*,
https://doi.org/10.1007/978-3-319-60925-6_14

2. Adipose tissue that surrounds the parenchymal part
3. Fibrous connective tissue represented by Cooper's ligament that separates and sustains the breast gland

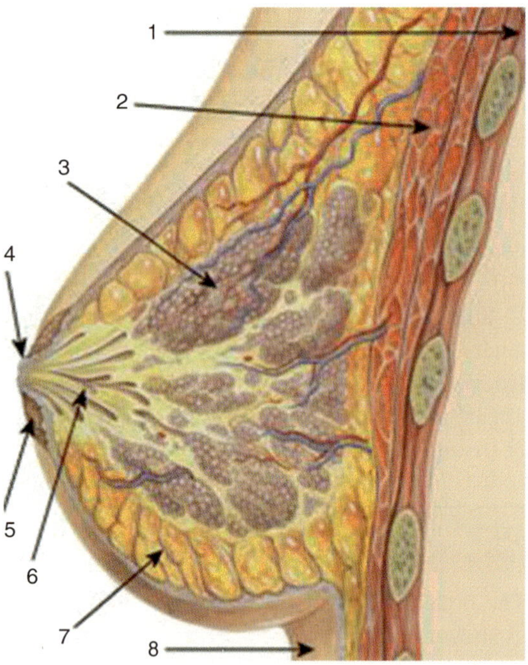


**Fig. 14.1** Breast normal anatomy cross section. (*1*) Chest wall, (*2*) pectoralis muscles, (*3*) lobules, (*4*) nipple surface, (*5*) areola, (*6*) lactiferous duct, (*7*) fat tissue, (*8*) breast skin. Patrick J. Lynch, medical illustrator

Lobules are composed of glandular tissue which contain the functional epithelial cells (acini cells) that produce milk.

At the base of the nipple, each major lactiferous duct dilates its lumen defining a space of collection of fluid called lactiferous ampulla or sinus. Each duct is lined by a double layer of cuboidal or low columnar epithelium supported by a prominent basement membrane, whereas the sinus and the last millimeters outward are lined by stratified squamous epithelium.

Tissue underlying areola is instead characterized by pilosebaceous follicles that appear on the areola skin like small bumps called protuberances of Montgomery.

The primary cause of the subareolar breast abscess is the transformation of the low columnar epithelium of the distant duct into squamous epithelium [7, 8]. Squamous metaplasia produces copious amounts of keratin. The aggregation of the keratin causes keratin plugs that obstruct the major duct. The obstruction of the ducts and the stasis of the acini secretions cause in the first period a dilatation of the ducts and successively a rupture of the epithelium with discharge of the keratin in the breast tissue. Macrophage and foreign-body giant cells try to remove the debris causing an inflammatory reaction leading, in case of bacteria invasion, to breast abscesses (Fig. 14.2).

Berná-Serna and Berná-Mestre [9] hypothesized a different pathogenesis for breast subareolar

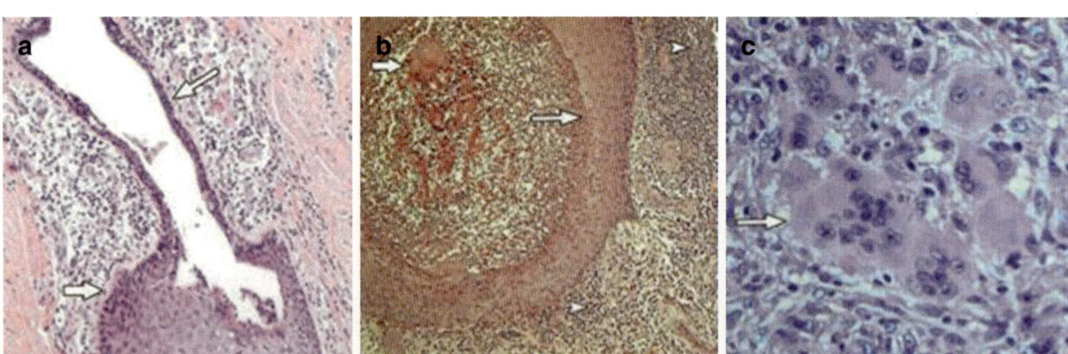


**Fig. 14.2** Non-puerperal subareolar breast abscess, histologic specimen. (**a**) Cuboidal epithelium (*thin arrow*) transitioning into region of hyperplastic squamous epithelium (*thick arrow*). (**b**) Metaplastic squamous cell lining duct (*thin arrow*) produces keratin plugs (*thick arrow*). Multiple small blue-staining monocytes (*arrowheads*) are present within lumen and outside duct and are responsible of the inflammation. (**c**) Multinuclear giant cell (*arrow*), which formed because of chronic inflammation and keratin debris [8]

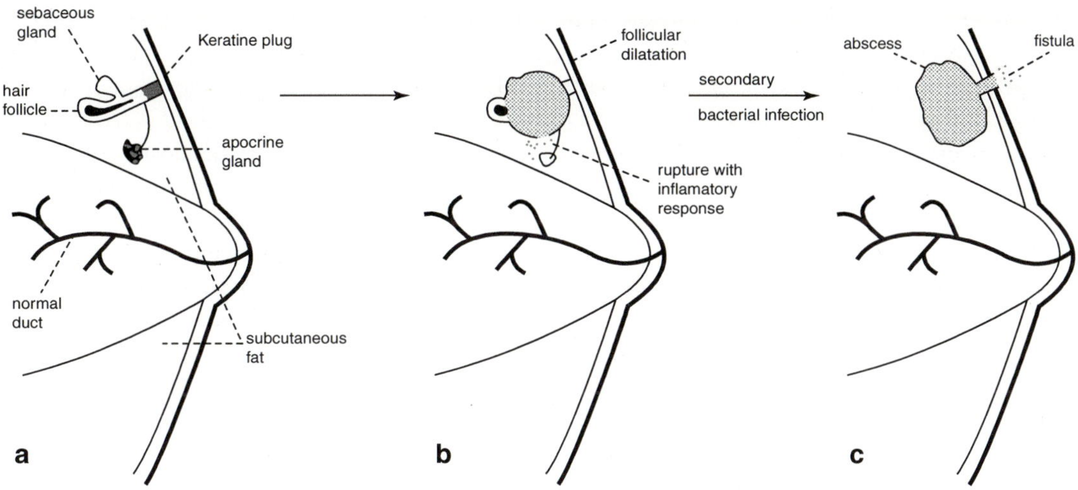


**Fig. 14.3** Follicular occlusion due to hyperkeratosis. (**a**) Follicular obstruction by keratin plugging. (**b**) Follicular dilatation with rupture and extravasation. (**c**) Secondary bacterial infection with abscess and fistula formation at the edge of the areola [9]

abscesses presenting with a skin fistula. In fact, they theorized that squamous metaplasia did not represent the cause of the breast abscess but only the response of the tissue to a chronic inflammatory process due to the occlusion of the pilosebaceous-apocrine unit located in the subareolar tissue (Fig. 14.3).

## 14.3 Clinical Presentation

Subareolar non-puerperal breast abscesses can be divided into acute abscesses characterized by early onset of palpable lump with erythema without skin ulceration and chronic abscesses when ulceration of the skin with a chronic fistula opening on the vermilion border of the areola is present (Fig. 14.4). In both cases, patients often have referred pain, and at the clinical examination, they could present with or without fever. Skin thickening and axillary adenopathy are usually evident. Palpably, the masses can be poorly defined and attached or not to the adjacent tissues. Also nipple retraction can be present.

In the majority of cases, puerperal abscess is caused by *Staphylococcus aureus* infection and characterized by a good response to antibiotic therapy with lower recurrence rate. Differently, non-puerperal breast abscess tends to have higher recurrence rate, and it is strongly associated to cigarette smoking [10]. *Staphylococcus aureus* is the most frequent microorganism isolated in primary breast abscesses, whereas anaerobic microorganisms are present in the majority of recurrent subareolar breast abscesses [11].

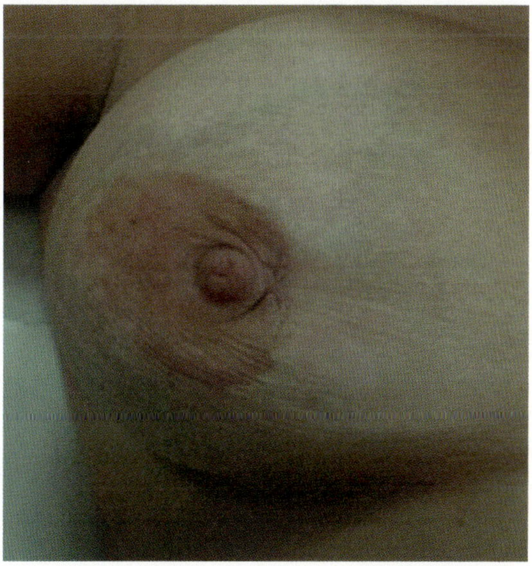

**Fig. 14.4** Recurrent subareolar breast abscess with skin retraction and ulceration opening on the vermilion border of the areola

Different from puerperal breast abscess, non-puerperal abscess affects people of all age with a highest peak of incidence around the fourth decade [12, 13].

The perception of pain is differently evaluated by patients: intense in younger patients and almost acceptable in older.

## 14.4 Radiological Features

Most patients with subareolar non-puerperal breast abscess usually present, in early stage, one or several breast masses without any other sign of inflammation. Ultrasonography (US), mammography, and also magnetic resonance imaging (MRI) will help to distinguish this benign disease from breast cancer.

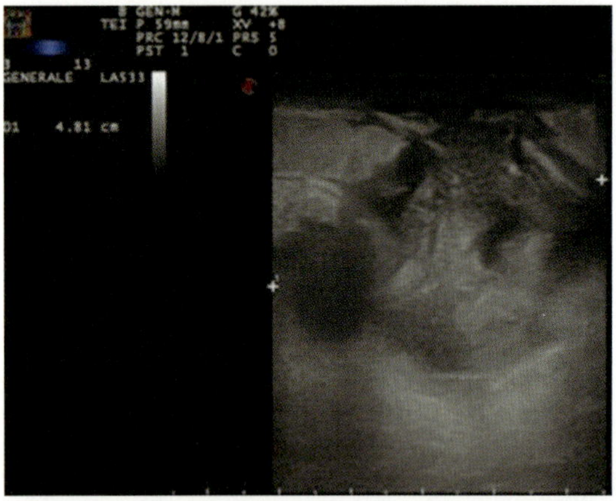

**Fig. 14.5** Longitudinal US image of a subareolar, not well-circumscribed, inhomogeneous, and hypoechoic breast abscess of 4.8 cm

At US examination, the diagnosis of subareolar abscess is confirmed by the presence of an irregular fluid collection (usually round or oval if located peripherally) characterized by homogeneous echogenicity with distal acoustic enhancement and no penetrating vessels at color Doppler examination (Fig. 14.5). The presence of penetrating vessels is suspicious for breast cancer.

Mammographic findings are considered non-specific, and in most cases the exam can result normal (above all young patients with dense breast parenchyma). Although Lequin et al. [14] first revealed the presence in the majority of the radiogram of non-circumscribed lesions, other authors have described multiple findings such as multiple small masses, irregular mass, focal asymmetric density, and architectural disorder [15, 16].

Conventional MRI cannot detect lesions less than a few millimeters in size. To overcome this limitation, Fu et al. [17] added to the standard technique a microscopy coil allowing a spatial resolution as high as 100 μm allowing the detection of features such as inverted nipples, abscess cavities, fistulas, dilated lactiferous ducts, and inflammatory signs around the abscesses (Fig. 14.6).

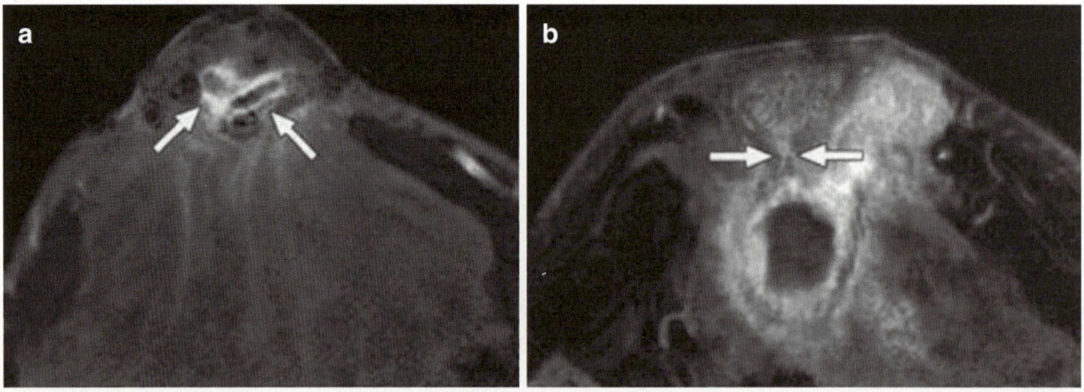


**Fig. 14.6** (**a**) Subareolar abscess with complex fistulas: contrast-enhanced T1-weighted image shows hartshorn-like complex fistulas with two orifices (*arrows*). (**b**) Subareolar abscess without skin ulceration. (**c**) Contrast-enhanced T1-weighted image shows hypointense tubular structure of dilated major lactiferous duct with enhanced wall (*arrows*) between inverted nipple and abscess cavity [17].

## 14.5 Treatment

Management of non-puerperal subareolar breast abscess is different for early and advanced manifestations and depends on the clinical-radiological features at the presentation. Early breast abscess in fact can be treated in different ways:

1. Antibiotics associated with anti-inflammatory therapy
2. Repeated ultrasound-guided aspiration
3. Ultrasound-guided percutaneous catheter drainage
4. Surgical treatment (in case of the failure of the above-described procedure)

Advanced breast abscess instead can be eradicated only with the surgical treatment.

### 14.5.1 Treatment of Early Subareolar Breast Abscess

With the term early, we mean a subareolar non-puerperal breast abscess that does not cause ulceration or fistula of vermilion border of the areola independently by its dimension. Each treatment starts with oral or endovenous antibiotic therapy associated with anti-inflammatory therapy, usually nonsteroidal anti-inflammatory drugs (NSAIDs).

If US shows a fluid collection smaller than 3 cm in diameter, we can attempt to discharge the abscesses with multiple needle punctures. Christensen et al. [18] showed a resolution rate of 93.7% in fluid collections <3 cm in diameter treated with multiple needle punctures (1 recurrence in 16 abscesses). Ulitzsch et al. [19] used the same technique on lactating women without finding any recurrences.

If US shows a fluid collection >3 cm, a percutaneous catheter drainage ultrasound-guided can be used (Fig. 14.7). Christensen et al. [18] performed this procedure and revealed a recurrence rate of 62.5% (5 recurrences in 8 abscesses treated).

Surgical intervention characterized by incision and drainage should be reserved for cases in which above-described procedures fail or cannot use (like the absence of a single cavity) in order to avoid prolonged healing time and the possibility of an unsatisfactory cosmetic result.

### 14.5.2 Treatment of Advanced Subareolar Breast Abscess

When ulceration or fistula is present on the vermilion border of the areola, surgery represents the treatment of choice. Meguid et al. [7] described an "en bloc" resection of all subareolar ampullae using a transverse incision from the

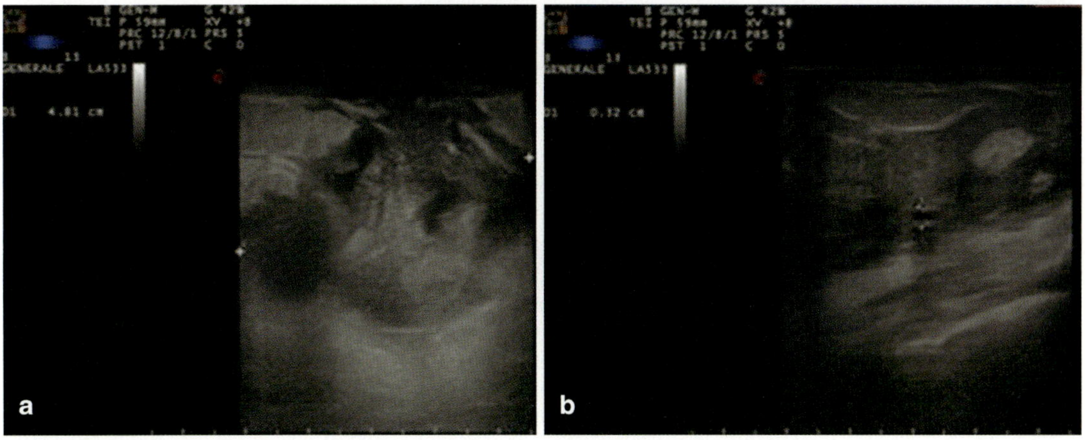


**Fig. 14.7** (**a**) Pretreatment: longitudinal US image of a subareolar breast abscess. (**b**) Immediate posttreatment: eight-French pigtail catheter walls (*white points*) after trocar removal and aspiration of 55 mL of pus

middle of the nipple to the border of the areola (Fig. 14.8). In patients with the inverted or retracted nipple (caused by previously drained chronic disease), the nipple was everted, and a fourth suture consisting of a purse-string was placed inside the base of the nipple to prevent the nipple from collapsing. In the Hadfield technique [20] in addition to the transverse incision of Meguid, a circumferential skin incision is made along the inferior margin of the areola with the removal of the fistula and the nipple duct allowing the nipple to be reflected away from the breast (Fig. 14.9). The described techniques require general anesthesia and a drain placement that is usually removed few days after the operation.

In our practice we observed a high resolution rate of a subareolar abscess with a fistula on vermilion border of the areola using the following technique. We insert a lacrimal probe into the cutaneous opening of the fistula to identify the extension of the abscess; in the majority of cases, it develops toward the base of the nipple. Successively, we draw an isosceles triangle with the apex (point A) at the base of the nipple. The base of the triangle is drawn along the areolar border from point B to point B1. Two equal sides are drawn from point A to B and B1 including in the triangle the cutaneous opening of the fistula.

Furthermore, as described in Meguid's technique, we perform a transverse incision of the nipple. Throughout a hinged opening of the nipple, we expose and remove "en bloc" the plugged lactiferous duct with its cutaneous fistula and the infected subcutaneous and glandular surrounding tissues if present. After multiple washes of the surgical wound with a mixture of sterile saltwater and a solution of hydrogen peroxide, we place an aspirative drain. It is preferable to place two layers of sutures for the glandular and subcutaneous tissue, respectively, with 2.0 and 4.0 absorbable sutures. Nonabsorbable interrupted 5.0 sutures are placed for skin closure.

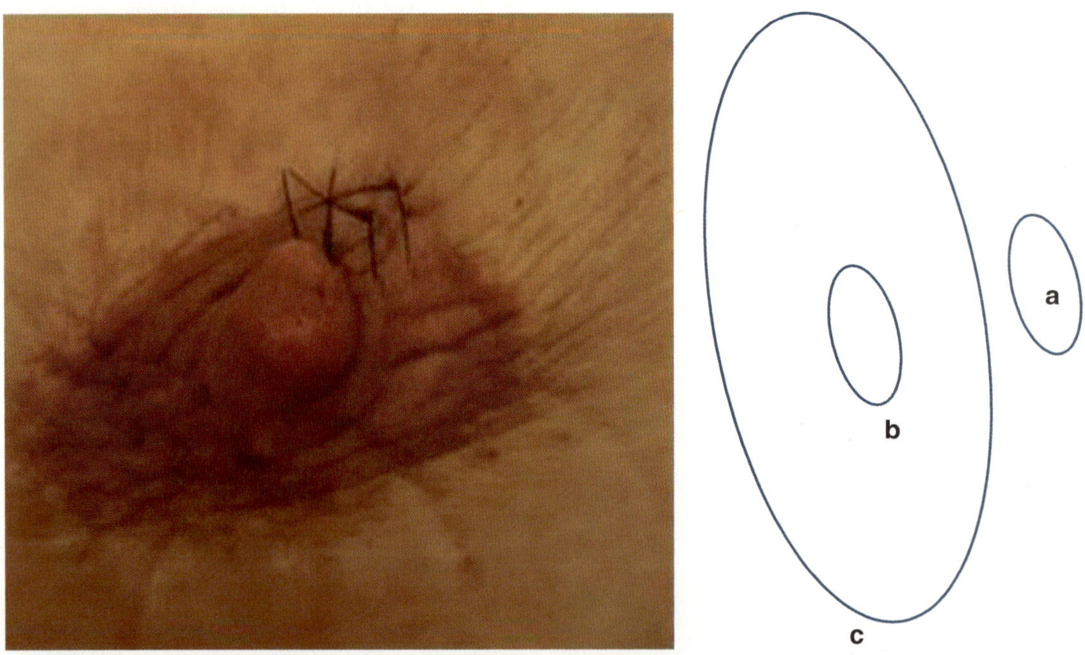


**Fig. 14.8** Meguid technique. After the transverse incision from the middle of the nipple to the areola and the removal of the fistula and part of the infected tissues under the skin, nipple is reconstructed by 40 absorbable sutures. Subcutaneous sutures were placed at three critical sites: (*a*) Approximating the circumferential edge of the apex of the nipple. (*b*) Approximating the base of the nipple. (*c*) Approximating the vermilion border of the areolas

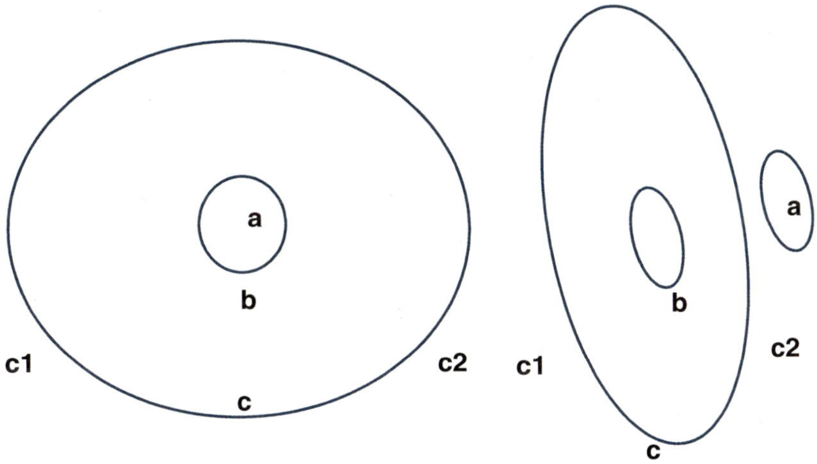


**Fig. 14.9** Hadfield technique. In addition to the transverse incision from point *a* (in the middle of the nipple) to point *c* (on the border of the areola through the point *b* (at the base of the nipple)), an ulterior incision from point *c1* to *c2* along the inferior margin of the vermilion border allows the removal of the fistula eventually present and the reflection of the nipple away from the breast

## 14.6 Discussion

Several hypotheses have been suggested concerning the process that causes the transition of the distal ductal epithelium into squamous metaplasia. Patey and Thackray [21] hypothesized that squamous metaplasia is caused by a congenital anomaly of the ductal system. Atkins [22] hypothesized that this condition is linked to nipple retraction, or a relative state of vitamin A deficiency [23]. Dixon et al. [10] postulated that smoking has a direct toxic effect on the retro-areolar lactiferous ducts. Irrespective of which is the mechanism at the basis of the breast abscess, a correct differential diagnosis not only from breast cancer but also into the different kinds of breast abscess is necessary to identify the most appropriate treatment. Clinical examination, radiological features, and in case of doubt percutaneous biopsy result indispensable to determine the adequate procedure to reduce morbidity of this disease and improve patient quality of life.

## References

1. Trop I, Dugas A, David J, El Khoury M, Boileau JF, Larouche N, Lalonde L. Breast abscesses: evidence-based algorithms for diagnosis, management, and follow-up. Radiographics. 2011;31:1683–99.
2. Cunningham FG, MacDonald PC, Leveno KJ, Gant NF, Gilstrap LC III, editors. Williams obstetrics. London: Prentice Hall International; 1993.
3. Larson BL, editor. Lactation: a comprehensive treatise. London: Academic Press; 1978. p. C5.
4. Lawrence RA, editor. Breastfeeding: a guide for the medical profession. St. Louis: Mosby; 1989.
5. Zuska JJ, Crile G Jr, Ayres WW. Fistulas of lactiferous ducts. Am J Surg. 1951;81:312–7.
6. Dixon JM. Periductal mastitis/duct ectasia. World J Surg. 1989;13:715–20.
7. Meguid MM, Oler A, Numann PJ, Khan S. Pathogenesis-based treatment subareolar breast abscesses. Surgery. 1995;118(4):775–82.
8. Kasales CJ, Han B, Smith JS Jr, Chetlen AL, Kaneda HJ, Shereef S. Nonpuerperal mastitis and subareolar abscess of the breast. Am J Roentgenol. 2014;202(2):W133–9.
9. Berná-Serna JD, Berná-Mestre JD. Follicular occlusion due to hyperkeratosis: a new hypothesis on the pathogenesis of mammillary fistula. Med Hypotheses. 2010;75(6):553–4.
10. Dixon JM, Ravisekar O, Chetty U, Anderson TH. Periductal mastitis and duct ectasia: different conditions with different aetiologies. Br J Surg. 1996;83:820–2.
11. Versluijs-Ossewaarde FN, Roumen RM, Goris RJ. Subareolar breast abscesses: characteristics and results of surgical treatment. Breast J. 2005;11(3):179–82.
12. Hanavadi S, Pereira G, Mansel RE. How mammillary fistulas should be managed. Breast J. 2005;11:254–6.
13. Lannin DR. Twenty-two year experience with recurring subareolar abscess and lactiferous duct fis-

tula treated by a single breast surgeon. Am J Surg. 2004;188:407–10.
14. Lequin MH, van Spengler J, van Pel R, van Eijck C, van Overhagen H. Mammographic and sonographic spectrum of non-puerperal mastitis. Eur J Radiol. 1995;21:138–42.
15. Han BK, Choe YH, Park JM, Moon WK, Ko YH, Yang JH, Nam SJ. Granulomatous mastitis: mammographic and sonographic appearances. Am J Roentgenol. 1999;173:317–20.
16. Yilmaz E, Lebe B, Usal C, Balci P. Mammographic and sonographic findings in the diagnosis of idiopathic granulomatous mastitis. Eur Radiol. 2001;11:2236–40.
17. Fu P, Kurihara Y, Kanemaki Y, Okamoto K, Nakajima Y, Fukuda M, Maeda I. High-resolution MRI in detecting subareolar breast abscess. Am J Roentgenol. 2007;188(6):1568–72.
18. Christensen AF, Al-Suliman N, Nielsen KR, Vejborg I, Severinsen N, Christensen H. Nielsen MB ultrasound-guided drainage of breast abscesses: results in 151 patients. Br J Radiol. 2005;78(927):186–8.
19. Ulitzsch D, Nyman MK, Carlson RA. Breast abscess in lactating women: US-guided treatment. Radiology. 2004;232(3):904–9.
20. Hadfield J. Excision of the major duct system for benign disease of the breast. Br J Surg. 1960;47:472–7.
21. Patey DH, Thackray AC. Pathology and treatment of mammary duct fistula. Lancet. 1958;2:871–3.
22. Atkins HJ. Mammillary fistula. Br Med J. 1955;2:1473–4.
23. Menkes MS, Comstock GW, Vuilleumier JP, Helsing KJ, Rider AA, Brookmeyer R. Serum beta-carotene, vitamins A and E, selenium, and their risk of lung cancer. N Engl J Med. 1986;13:1250–4.

# 15 Molluscum Contagiosum of the Nipple-Areola Complex

Tiffany Y. Loh, Brian S. Hoyt, Jaime A. Tschen, and Philip R. Cohen

## 15.1 Introduction

Viral infections of the skin are a common occurrence; sometimes, they can be localized to the nipple-areola complex (Table 15.1) [1–5]. Molluscum contagiosum, a poxvirus, has rarely been described to occur on either the areola or the nipple [4, 6–10]. This chapter summarizes the features of molluscum contagiosum and reviews the characteristics of women who develop this viral infection on the nipple-areola complex.

T.Y. Loh, M.D. (✉)
Memorial Sloan Kettering Cancer Center, New York, NY 10065, USA
e-mail: tiffany.yv.loh@gmail.com

B.S. Hoyt, M.D. (✉)
Dartmouth-Hitchcock Medical Center, Lebanon, NH, USA
e-mail: brianhoyt@gmail.com

J.A. Tschen, M.D. (✉)
St. Joseph Dermatopathology, Houston, TX 77030, USA
e-mail: jaimetschen@yahoo.com

P.R. Cohen, M.D. (✉)
Department of Dermatology, University of California San Diego, La Jolla, CA 92122, USA
e-mail: mitehead@gmail.com

**Table 15.1** Examples of viral infections that may occur in the nipple-areola complex

| |
|---|
| Condyloma acuminatum [1] |
| Herpes simplex virus [2] |
| Herpes zoster [3] |
| Molluscum contagiosum [4] |
| Viral wart (verruca vulgaris) [5] |

## 15.2 Molluscum Contagiosum: General Concepts

### 15.2.1 History

As a member of the poxvirus family, molluscum contagiosum virus is related to smallpox, but unlike smallpox, which can be severe and even fatal, molluscum contagiosum usually causes a self-limited, benign, localized infection of the skin [11, 12]. Molluscum contagiosum virus does not grow well in standard cell cultures; however, in the past decade, the 190,000 base pair genome of the virus has been sequenced. This has led to advancements in knowledge of the virus' replication cycle and how it defends itself against host immune mechanisms [13].

### 15.2.2 Epidemiology

Molluscum contagiosum most commonly affects two distinct populations—children and


M.A. Shiffman (ed.), *Nipple-Areolar Complex Reconstruction*,
https://doi.org/10.1007/978-3-319-60925-6_15

sexually active adults. In children, the viral infection usually represents a contagious but benign infection [14]. Due to the immaturity of their immune systems, children are easily infected by molluscum contagiosum, especially in environments with close contact, such as swimming pools or shared bathtubs [14, 15]. However, once they have cleared the infection, the virus usually does not present a problem later in life.

In adults, molluscum contagiosum infection may or may not be associated with sexually transmitted diseases (STDs) [12, 13, 15]. Therefore, in these individuals, histologic confirmation and screening for other STDs) such as human immunodeficiency virus (HIV), syphilis, gonorrhea, chlamydia, hepatitis B, and hepatitis C should be considered.

### 15.2.3 Clinical Presentation

Lesions of molluscum contagiosum present as dome-shaped papules with central umbilication [12, 13]. In children, these papules can occur anywhere on the body [14, 15]. If sexually transmitted, they are usually located in the genital area [12, 13, 15]. In addition, since molluscum contagiosum is capable of infecting the skin in any part of the body, this viral infection has also been observed to occasionally occur in uncommon locations (Table 15.2).

There is a variant of this lesion termed "giant molluscum." The lesions are characterized by large size. They are usually seen on the eyes and plantar surfaces of HIV-positive patients [24].

When molluscum contagiosum lesions are viewed under dermoscopy, orifices and specific vascular patterns (crown, radial, and punctiform) [25] may be observed.

**Table 15.2** Uncommon locations of molluscum contagiosum infection

| Location | References |
|---|---|
| Eyelid | [16, 17] |
| Mucous membrane | [18–21] |
| Conjunctiva | [18] |
| Oral mucosa | [19–21] |
| Nipple-areola complex | [4, 6–10] |
| Areola | [4, 6, 7] |
| Nipple | [8–10] |
| Plantar | [22] |
| Subungual | [23] |

### 15.2.4 Histology

Tissue biopsy of molluscum contagiosum reveals molluscum bodies. These are intracytoplasmic eosinophilic particles seen within epithelial cells. They are usually found in higher concentration in the stratum corneum [26]. Cytologic analysis of molluscum contagiosum samples may also demonstrate intracytoplasmic and extracytoplasmic molluscum bodies [26]. Under scanning electron microscopy, round viral structures with central umbilication are seen, along with subepidermal proliferation [27].

### 15.2.5 Clinical Differential Diagnosis

The differential diagnosis for lesions resembling molluscum contagiosum infection is listed in Table 15.3 [17, 28].

**Table 15.3** Differential diagnosis for lesions resembling molluscum contagiosum [17]

| |
|---|
| Aspergillosis |
| Basal cell carcinoma |
| Coccidiomycosis |
| Condyloma acuminatum |
| Cryptococcosis in HIV-positive patients |
| Cryptococcus |
| Eccrine poroma |
| Granuloma annulare |
| Histoplasmosis |
| Keratoacanthoma |
| Leiomyoma |
| Lichen planus |
| Paget's disease |
| Papilloma |
| Sebaceous hyperplasia |
| Syringoma |
| Verruca vulgaris |

### 15.2.6 Pathogenesis

Humans are the only known hosts for molluscum contagiosum [12, 13]. Like other poxviruses, molluscum contagiosum replicates intracellularly. It is spread by direct inoculation of the skin, which commonly occurs through direct skin-to-skin contact. Although it often presents in the genital region when associated with sexual transmission, molluscum contagiosum infection can occur in any part of the body, and autoinoculation frequently occurs in children when lesions are scratched [12, 13].

Characteristically, molluscum contagiosum virus proliferates within the cytoplasm of cells in the follicular epithelium. As viral particles steadily increase in number, the host cells gradually grow larger in size and the intracellular organelles are displaced until, eventually, the virus-filled cell ruptures. The released molluscum contagiosum virions can then infect other host cells, and the cycle begins anew [12].

### 15.2.7 Treatment

As molluscum contagiosum infection is usually self-limited, the decision to treat depends on transmission risk factors, patient demographics, as well as individual preference [29, 30]. In adults with molluscum contagiosum infections that may be associated with sexual transmission, treatment is usually recommended in order to prevent further spread of the infection to other individuals. In addition, infections in immunocompromised patients are treated early and aggressively, as infections in these individuals have the potential to progress to severe disease.

In immunocompetent children, treatment recommendations are less clear. Some studies have found that treated and untreated children have similar rates of molluscum contagiosum clearance. In some children, these infections self-resolve over time [30].

With regard to treatment, first-line options may include cantharidin, cryotherapy, electrodesiccation, and curettage, or podophyllotoxin. Other methods that may be considered include cidofovir, imiquimod, oral cimetidine, potassium hydroxide, and salicylic acid [29, 30].

## 15.3 Molluscum Contagiosum of the Nipple-Areola Complex

To the best of our knowledge, molluscum contagiosum of the nipple-areola complex has only been reported in six women. We present the reports and summarize the features of these infections (Table 15.4) [4, 6–10].

**Table 15.4** Six cases of molluscum contagiosum infection of the nipple-areola complex

| Case | Age | Location | Morphology | Symptoms | Ref. |
|---|---|---|---|---|---|
| 1 | 20 | R areola | Raised, flat, yellowish papule | Rapid growth | [6] |
| 2 | 22 | L areola | Small, superficial lesion with subsequent infection | Initially asymptomatic, then became infected and painful | [7] |
| 3 | 24 | L nipple | Small, flesh-colored, eczematous plaques | None | [10] |
| 4 | 28 | L areola | Flattened, flesh-colored papule | None | [4] |
| 5 | 45 | L nipple | Raised umbilicated nodule; ulceration after treatment with caustic pencil | Asymptomatic, then itchy and painful | [8] |
| 6 | ? | Nipple | Cutaneous bulging of nipple with firm mass | NR | [9] |

*NR* not reported, *Ref* reference

### 15.3.1 Case 1 [6]

A 20-year-old woman presented with a 3-week history of a growth on her right areola. She denied any injury or trauma to the region; there have been no previous lesions at the site. Her sexual history was noncontributory, and she had no other signs of skin infection. Other than rapid growth, the lesion exhibited no other significant symptoms.

Physical examination showed a flat, yellowish papule 4 × 5 mm with a central depression on the right areola. Dermoscopy revealed multiple aggregated yellowish lobules on the periphery. Histological examination showed intracytoplasmic eosinophilic inclusion bodies in the epidermis, establishing a diagnosis of molluscum contagiosum. Treponema pallidum hemagglutination assay (TPHA), Venereal Disease Research Laboratory (VDRL), and HIV-1 and HIV-2 serologies were negative.

### 15.3.2 Case 2 [7]

A 22-year-old G0P0 Caucasian woman was evaluated for a 0.6 cm lesion that had been present on the left areola of her breast for 9 months. The lesion had not bothered the patient until 3 days prior to presentation, when it became painful and infected. The patient was treated with a 5-day course of penicillin.

Cytological smears of the lesion were performed. Examination of the smears revealed marked inflammation, as well as cells with large vacuoles and eosinophilic cytoplasmic inclusions. The cytoplasm showed signs of degeneration, with peripherally located nuclei. Subsequently, the lesion was removed, and a diagnosis of molluscum contagiosum was confirmed with tissue sections.

### 15.3.3 Case 3 [10]

A 24-year old woman presented with a lesion on her left nipple which she noticed 4 weeks prior. Physical examination revealed small, flesh-colored, eczematous plaques, with no evidence of nipple discharge. A 4 mm dermatological curette was used to remove the lesion surface, and after crush-smearing the sample on two separate glass microscope slides, the specimen was stained with either the May-Grunwald-Giemsa or the Papanicolaou method. Cytological smears were highly cellular; molluscum bodies (eosinophilic bodies within single squamous cells) were identified among a background of inflammatory elements and anucleated squamous cells.

### 15.3.4 Case 4 [4]

A healthy 28-year-old woman presented with a 6 × 6 mm flat, flesh-colored papule on her left areola that had been present for about 3 months. The patient denied any pruritus, pain, recent trauma, oral or sexual contact with the area, or contact with any people who had similar symptoms (Fig. 15.1).

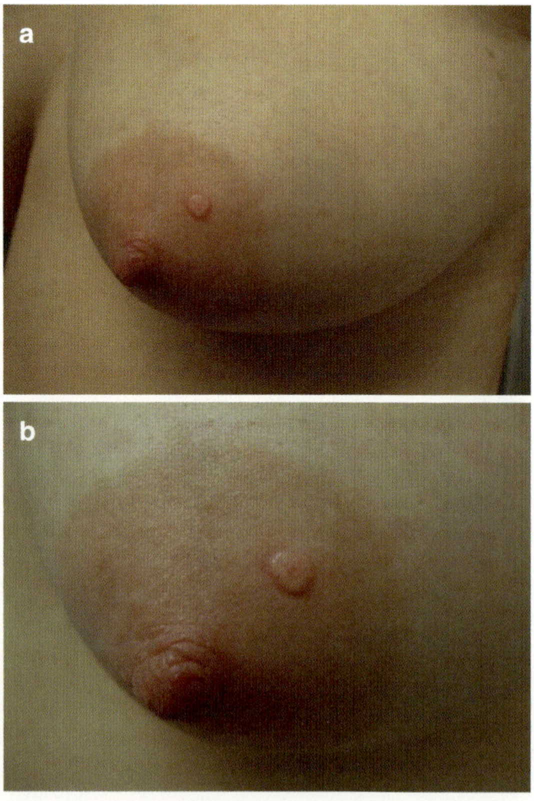


**Fig. 15.1** (**a**, **b**) Molluscum contagiosum lesions of the left areola in an immunocompetent, healthy 28-year-old woman [4]. Republished with permission

An 8 mm excisional biopsy demonstrated keratinocytes with ovoid, amorphous granules that were diagnosed as molluscum bodies. In addition, nuclei that had been displaced to the periphery of the cytoplasm were visualized. The papule was excised, and no recurrence was reported (Fig. 15.2).

### 15.3.5 Case 5 [8]

A 45-year-old woman presented for evaluation of a 0.3 × 0.2 cm ulcer on her left nipple, which she stated started as a small warty growth at the tip of her nipple 10 months earlier. The lesion became pruritic and painful, and she was given a caustic pencil by a pharmacist to burn it. However, treatment with the pencil resulted in ulceration of the lesion, which began to ooze cheesy material and blood.

Physical examination showed an ulcer with a pink base and ragged margins covered with hemorrhagic exudate. The patient had no other lesions on her breasts or any lymphadenopathy. Cytological smears of cheesy exudate expressed from the ulcer revealed dense, acute inflammatory exudate, as well as eosinophilic to basophilic round to oval dense bodies in the cytoplasm. These were identified as molluscum bodies, consistent with a diagnosis of molluscum contagiosum.

### 15.3.6 Case 6 [9]

A woman (unknown age) presented with cutaneous bulging of the nipple. Physical examination showed pearly, papular lesions with central umbilication. The patient was treated with local excision, as well as 5% imiquimod application

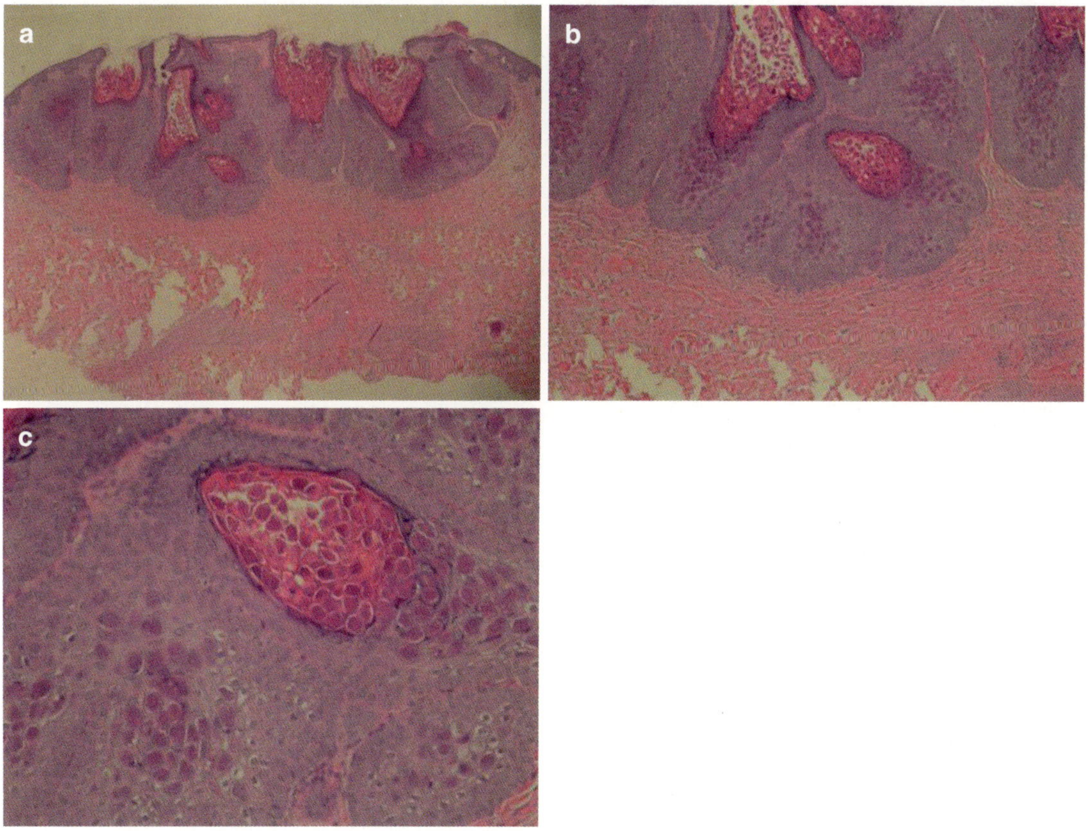


**Fig. 15.2** Biopsy sample from the molluscum contagiosum lesion of the left areola. Eosinophilic inclusion bodies (molluscum bodies) are visualized in the high magnification view. (**a**) Low magnification. (**b**) Medium magnification. (**c**) High magnification [4]. Republished with permission

three times a week for 2 months, with no recurrence noted.

### 15.3.7 Summary of Cases

Six women ranging from ages 20 to 45 presented with lesions on the breast that were diagnosed as molluscum contagiosum. Three were located on the nipple and three were on the areola. Three patients reported symptoms in association with these lesions, while the other three denied any associated symptoms. Molluscum contagiosum of the nipple-areola complex does not always present with the characteristic morphology of molluscum. While some patients presented with characteristic smooth, umbilicated papule(s), other lesions were described as flat yellowish lesions, warty growths, or ulcers.

The differential diagnosis of areola and nipple molluscum includes condyloma acuminatum, fungal infections, malignant tumors, and verruca vulgaris. The six women were diagnosed with one or more modalities: cytological smears (3 women, cases 2, 3, and 5), histological examination (3 women, cases 1, 2, and 3), and dermoscopy (1 woman, case 1). Treatment was described in four of the patients—excision (case 4) [4], curettage (case 3) [10], excision and imiquimod (case 6) [9], and removal with unspecified methods (case 2) [7]. No recurrences were noted in any of the cases.

**Conclusions**

Molluscum contagiosum is a poxvirus that is spread by direct skin-to-skin contact and can affect any area of the body. However, infection of the nipple or areola is rare. To the best of our knowledge, involvement of these areas has only been observed in six women.

The lesions ranged in size from 2 to 6 mm. Diagnosis was established with dermoscopy, cytology, histology, or a combination of these techniques. Excisional biopsy, curettage, and excision with subsequent imiquimod therapy were reported in three patients. Specific treatment methods and follow-up data were not described in other patients.

Although uncommon, solitary molluscum contagiosum of the nipple-areola complex, in the absence of involvement of other areas of the body, can occur. Therefore, this viral infection should be considered in the differential diagnosis of acquired lesions at this location.

## References

1. Wood C. Condyloma acuminatum of the nipple. J Cutan Pathol. 1978;5:88–9.
2. Mardi K, Gupta N, Sharma S, Gupta S. Cytodiagnosis of herpes simplex mastitis: report of a rare case. J Cytol. 2009;26:149–50.
3. Watanabe D, Kuhara T, Ishida N, Takama H, Tamada Y, Matsumoto Y. Herpes zoster of the nipple: rapid DNA-based diagnosis by the loop-mediated isothermal amplification method. Int J STD AIDS. 2010;21:66–7.
4. Hoyt BS, Tschen JA, Cohen PR. Molluscum contagiosum of the areola and nipple: case report and literature review. Dermatol Online J. 2013;19:18965.
5. Kiriyama N, Kato Y, Mitsuhashi Y, Tsuboi R. Viral wart on the nipple showing heightened FDG uptake. Eur J Dermatol. 2015;25:197–8.
6. Schmid-Wendtner MH, Rütten A, Blum A. Flat rapidly growing tumor in a 20-year-old woman. Hautarzt. 2008;59:838–40.
7. Carvalho G. Molluscum contagiosum in a lesion adjacent to the nipple. Report of a case. Acta Cytol. 1974;18:532–4.
8. Kumar N, Okiro P, Wasike R. Cytological diagnosis of molluscum contagiosum with an unusual clinical presentation at an unusual site. J Dermatol Case Rep. 2010;4:63–5.
9. Parlakgumus A, Yildirim S, Bolat FA, Caliskan K, Ezer A, Colakoglu T, Moray G. Dermatoses of the nipple. Can J Surg. 2009;52:160–1.
10. Caroppo D, Natella V, Scalvenzi M, Vetrani A, Cozzolino I. Molluscum contagiosum diagnosis on nipple scraping sample. Breast J. 2016;22(1):120.
11. Hanson D, Diven DG. Molluscum contagiosum. Dermatol Online J. 2003;9:2.
12. Chen X, Anstey AV, Bugert JJ. Molluscum contagiosum virus infection. Lancet Infect Dis. 2013;13:877–88.
13. Senkevich TG, Bugert JJ, Sisler JR, Koonin EV, Darai G, Moss B. Genome sequence of a human tumorigenic poxvirus: prediction of specific host response-evasion genes. Science. 1996;273:813.
14. Brown J, Janniger CK, Schwartz RA, Silverberg NB. Childhood molluscum contagiosum. Int J Dermatol. 2006;45:93–9.
15. Laxmisha C, Thappa DM, Jaisankar TJ. Clinical profile of molluscum contagiosum in children versus adults. Dermatol Online J. 2003;9:1.

16. Vardhan P, Goel S, Goyal G, Kumar N. Solitary giant molluscum contagiosum presenting as lid tumor in an immunocompetent child. Indian J Ophthalmol. 2010;58:236–8.
17. Beutler BD, Cohen PR. Molluscum contagiosum of the eyelid: case report in a man receiving methotrexate and literature review of molluscum contagiosum in patients who are immunosuppressed secondary to methotrexate or HIV infection. Dermatol Online J. 2016;22(3.) pii:13030/qt8vz669cj
18. Schornack MM, Siemsen DW, Bradley EA, Salomao DR, Lee HB. Ocular manifestations of molluscum contagiosum. Clin Exp Optom. 2006;89:390–3.
19. Laskaris G, Sklavounou A. Molluscum contagiosum of the oral mucosa. Oral Surg Oral Med Oral Pathol. 1984;58:688–91.
20. Scherer P, Fires J, Mischkowski A, Neugebauer J, Scheer M, Zöller JE. Intraoral molluscum contagiosum imitating a squamous-cell carcinoma in an immunocompetent person—case report and review of the literature. Int J Oral Maxillofac Surg. 2009;38: 802–5.
21. de Carvalho CH, de Andrade AL, de Oliveira DH, Ed L, da Silveira EJ, de Medeiros AM. Intraoral molluscum contagiosum in a young immunocompetent patient. Oral Surg Oral Med Oral Pathol Oral Radiol. 2012;14:e57–60.
22. Cohen PR, Tschen JA. Plantar molluscum contagiosum: a case report of mulluscum contagiosum occurring on the sole of the foot and a review of the world literature. Cutis. 2012;90:35–41.
23. Basaran YK, Turan E, Keklik B, Tarini EZ. A painful subungual lesion with a surprising diagnosis: molluscum contagiosum. Indian J Dermatol Venereol Leprol. 2013;80:278.
24. Vora RV, Pilani PA, Kota RK. Extensive giant molluscum contagiosum in an HIV positive patient. J Clin Diagn Res. 2015;9:WD01–2.
25. Ianhez M, Cestari Sda C, Enokihara MY, Seize MB. Dermoscopic patterns of molluscum contagiosum: a study of 211 lesions confirmed by histopathology. An Bras Dermatol. 2011;86:74–9.
26. Cribier B, Scrivener Y, Grosshans E. Molluscum contagiosum: histologic patterns and associated lesions: a study of 578 cases. Am J Dermatopathol. 2001;23:99–103.
27. Almeida HL Jr, Abuchaim MO, Schneider MA, Marques L, Castro LA. Scanning electron microscopy of molluscum contagiosum. An Bras Dermatol. 2013;88:90–3.
28. Hicks MJ, Flaitz CM, Cohen PR. Perioral and cutaneous umbilicated papular lesions in acquired immunodeficiency syndrome. Oral Surg Oral Med Oral Pathol Radiol Endod. 1997;83:189–91.
29. Guirguis-Blake J. Interventions for molluscum contagiosum. Am Fam Phyisican. 2006;74:1504.
30. Bikowski JB Jr. Molluscum contagiosum: the need for physician intervention and new treatment options. Cutis. 2004;73:202.

# 16 Utilizing Mohs Surgery for Tissue Preservation in Erosive Adenomatosis of the Nipple

Nikoleta Brankov and Tanya Nino

## 16.1 Introduction

Erosive adenomatosis of the nipple (EAN) is a benign condition characterized by a benign proliferation of lactiferous ducts within the breast tissue. Its incidence peaks in the fifth decade of life. EAN is often confused with malignancy such as mammary Paget's disease or ductal carcinoma due to its presentation with bloody nipple discharge, nipple erosion, erythema, or crusting [1]. Microscopically, it may be difficult to differentiate from syringocystadenoma papilliferum, hidradenoma papilliferum, or low-grade adenocarcinoma. Mohs micrographic surgery (MMS) is the treatment of choice for EAN because it conserves normal breast tissue while surgically removing the affected abnormal tissue [2].

N. Brankov, M.D.
Department of Medicine, Loma Linda University, Loma Linda, CA, USA
e-mail: Nikoleta.brankov@gmail.com

T. Nino, M.D. (✉)
Department of Dermatology and Mohs Surgery, St. Joseph Heritage Medical Group, 2501 E. Chapman Avenue, Suite 402, Orange, CA 92869, USA
e-mail: tanyanino@gmail.com

## 16.2 Technique

The clinically apparent tumor is carefully outlined prior to the infiltration of local anesthesia. The tumor is then narrowly excised with a #15 blade at a 45° angle to facilitate histopathologic tissue processing. Excision margins are 1–2 mm. The tumor is nicked, usually at the 12 o'clock margin, for precise tissue orientation. A map of the extirpated tissue is made for orientation, and the specimen is inked, horizontally sectioned on a cryostat, and stained with hematoxylin and eosin. The resulting microscope slides are examined for evidence of tumor. Additional tissue is excised as needed, corresponding specifically to the areas of residual tumor as seen on the processed tissue specimen.

## 16.3 Discussion

Mohs micrographic surgery is the treatment of choice for erosive adenomatosis of the nipple, because it preserves normal breast tissue while sacrificing predominantly the affected abnormal tissue. In contrast, women with this benign condition may unnecessarily undergo complete nipple removal, which is associated with additional morbidity, cosmetic disfigurement, and potential psychological sequelae.

Erosive adenomatosis of the nipple currently is also called adenoma of the nipple, florid


M.A. Shiffman (ed.), *Nipple-Areolar Complex Reconstruction*,
https://doi.org/10.1007/978-3-319-60925-6_16

papillomatosis of the nipple, and subareolar papillomatosis of the nipple [3]. It is important to recognize the differences in nomenclature to prevent misdiagnosis and unnecessary surgeries performed for this benign condition [3].

EAN was first described more than half a century ago, and treatment consisted of total excision of the nipple and areola with an underlying wedge of the breast. Similarly, the recommended treatment over the past several decades has been partial or total excision of the nipple [4]. Conversely, the first case of Mohs micrographic surgery performed for EAN was in 1998. In this case, the nipple and areola were completely removed in three stages with a final defect measuring 3.5 × 2.8 cm (total surface area of 9.8 $cm^2$) [2]. In 2002, a subsequent case of MMS for EAN was described, with final defect measuring 2.0 × 0.8 cm, with no postoperative recurrence [3]. The surgical case reported by Brankov et al. [5] describes an EAN excision by MMS, with the least amount of surface area sacrificed: a total of 1.1 $cm^2$. The tumor was cleared in three stages, and the defect was re-approximated primarily with interrupted 4-0 polydioxanone sutures in the deep tissue and 5-0 plain gut sutures for the cutaneous layer [5].

## Conclusions

It is important to recognize that this benign lesion of the breast may be misdiagnosed as a malignant entity, and thus tissue pathology and histological examination is essential for the diagnosis. Although MMS is usually performed for malignant tumors, this is an appropriate setting where MMS can be utilized for this benign entity.

## References

1. Ku BS, Kwon OE, Kim DC, Song KH, Lee CW, Kim KH. A case of erosive adenomatosis of nipple treated with total excision using purse-string suture. Dermatol Surg. 2006;32:1093–6.
2. Van Mierlo PL, Geelen GM, Neumann HA. Mohs micrographic surgery for an erosive adenomatosis of the nipple. Dermatol Surg. 1998;24:681–3.
3. Lee HJ, Chung KY. Erosive adenomatosis of the nipple: conservation of nipple by Mohs micrographic surgery. J Am Acad Dermatol. 2002;47:578–80.
4. Handley RS, Thackray AC. Adenoma of nipple. Br J Cancer. 1962;16:187–94.
5. Brankov N, Nino T, Hsiang D, Zeineh L. Utilizing Mohs surgery for tissue preservation in erosive adenomatosis of the nipple. Dermatol Surg. 2016;42(5): 684–6.

# Hyperkeratosis of the Nipple and Areola

17

Alireza Ghanadan

## 17.1 Introduction

Hyperkeratosis of the nipple and areola (HNA) is a rare, benign, and asymptomatic disorder of the nipple-areola complex (NAC) which is characterized by irregular and verrucous thickening of the nipple and areola with brownish discoloration and hyperpigmented plaques. The lesion is commonly bilateral and affects both women and men [1]. Approximately 80% of the cases are women, and usually men receiving hormonal therapy may be susceptible to this condition [2]. Levy-Frankel [3] classified HNA to three types in 1938: type 1 as an extension of an epidermal nevus; type 2 associated with ichthyosis, Darier's disease, acanthosis nigricans, or chronic eczema; and type 3 as an isolated nevoid form. Other than its cosmetic implications, the disease has an excellent prognosis. The condition may aggravate with pregnancy and may disturb breastfeeding [4].

A. Ghanadan, M.D.
Department of Dermatopathology and Faculty of Medicine, Razi Skin Hospital, Tehran University of Medical Sciences, Tehran, Iran

Department of Pathology and Faculty of Medicine, Cancer Institute, Tehran University of Medial Sciences, Imam Khomeini Hospital Complex, Tehran, Iran
e-mail: dermpath101@gmail.com; ghannadan@sina.tums.ac.ir

## 17.2 History and Classification

Hyperkeratosis of the nipple and areola (HNA) was first described in association with ichthyosis vulgaris by Tauber in 1923 (cited by Oberste-Lehn [5]). Levy-Frankel classified this condition into three categories in 1938 [3]. Type 1 HNA represents the extension of an epidermal nevus onto this area and occurs unilaterally in both genders. Type 2 HNA is associated with ichthyosis, ichthyosiform erythroderma, Darier's disease, acanthosis nigricans, and chronic dermatitis and affects both genders but tends to present bilaterally. Type 3 HNA is thought to represent an isolated nevoid form, called nevoid hyperkeratosis of the nipple and areola (NHNA) predominantly affecting women of childbearing age. The term "nevoid" is only used for this type because of "nevoid" character and is not associated with any disease or drug use [6, 7]. Perez-Izquierdo et al. [8] proposed an alternative classification of two types: (1) idiopathic or nevoid and (2) secondary to other dermatoses. Several authors have challenged the designation of "nevoid" for HNA type 3 and suggest that "idiopathic" should be used instead [9–11].

Some authors have disputed the inclusion of type 1 variant into the spectrum of HNA. In 2001, Mehanna et al. [9] expressed that epidermal nevus which involves the nipple and/or the areola in type 1 HNA should not be considered as hyperkeratosis of the nipple and areola. They also proposed an alternative classification including three variants:


M.A. Shiffman (ed.), *Nipple-Areolar Complex Reconstruction*,
https://doi.org/10.1007/978-3-319-60925-6_17

(1) primary HNA, occurring coincidentally with other skin diseases, namely, disorders of keratinization including ichthyosis, acanthosis nigricans, or Darier's disease; (2) secondary HNA, occurring secondary to hormonal changes, internal malignancies, or lymphoma; and (3) idiopathic HNA, occurring predominantly in women in the second and third decade of life for which no obvious cause can be detected. There are three subsets of idiopathic HNA according to the site of involvement: (a) idiopathic hyperkeratosis of the nipple and areola, (b) idiopathic hyperkeratosis of the nipple, and (c) idiopathic hyperkeratosis of the areola. In 2000, Kubota et al. [12] reviewed 45 cases of nevoid hyperkeratosis and found that both the nipple and the areola were involved in 58% of the cases, the nipple was involved in 17% of the cases, and the areola was involved in the remaining 25% of the cases.

## 17.3 Etiology and Pathogenesis

There is some evidence that HNA may be induced by changes in the estrogen level. For the first time, Mold and Jegasothy [13] suggested the hormonal etiology of HNA based on two patients who developed lesions after receiving diethylstilbestrol (DES) for adenocarcinoma of the prostate. Additional support for the hormonal etiology comes from the reports of patients whose lesions appeared with puberty [14] and pregnancy [2, 8, 9, 15–18] or converted from unilateral to become bilateral during pregnancy [8, 17, 19]. Further support for this theory is appearing acanthosis nigricans after DES therapy which is histologically similar to HNA [20]. In spite of the significant evidence supporting this theory, it fails to explain some cases of nevoid hyperkeratosis in men [12, 21–24] and in women who are not associated with hormonal changes.

## 17.4 Associations of HNA

### 17.4.1 An Association with MF

Mycosis fungoides (MF) rarely presents with verrucous and hyperkeratotic lesions on the distal extremities [25] but has been reported to involve the trunk [26]. Mycosis fungoides has been reported as solitary hyperkeratosis of the nipple and areola [27] or generalized skin eruptions simultaneously associated with verrucous hyperkeratotic lesions of the nipple [28].

There are two atypical cases of isolated NHNA characterized by histopathological features resembling MF but without any other MF lesions on the body, possibly indicating unilesional (solitary) MF in the nipple-areola complex [29, 30]. Rosman et al. [31] reported a case of HNA which they considered nevoid hyperkeratosis based on clinical presentation and the course of disease despite histopathologic features and immunophenotyping evidences of MF.

There is also a report of three cases of association of MF and NHNA; one of them represents specific histopathologic and immunohistochemistry features of MF, and two of them lack histopathological features of MF on the nipple-areola complex [32]. Given previous reports in the literature and these three novel cases, the authors suggested a hypothesis as follows: (1) association of MF in other parts of body with histopathologic features of MF involving nipple-areola complex and (2) MF in other parts of the body associated with hyperkeratosis of the nipple and areola without histopathologic features of MF.

### 17.4.2 Other Associations

One study reported hyperkeratosis of the nipple and areola in association with chronic mucocutaneous candidiasis which persisted despite the treatment of the infection, suggesting a distinct and prevailing etiologic factor in HNA. Also, graft versus host disease (GVHD) associated with HNA after allogeneic hematopoietic cell transplantation has been reported [33].

Syringocystadenoma papilliferum (SCAP) developing on hyperkeratosis of the nipple and areola has been reported in a pregnant woman. Given similar histopathologic features of HNA and epidermal nevus, it theoretically describes possible development of SCAP on the epidermal nevus (type 1 HNA), similar to what is seen in sebaceous nevus of Jadassohn [34].

### 17.4.3 Demographic Findings

Perez-Izquierdo et al. [8] reported that hyperkeratosis of the nipple-areola complex involved the nipple and areola in 72% and involved the nipple alone in 28% of the cases. Lesions often appear in women at menarche or during pregnancy or may worsen or become bilateral during pregnancy [8, 9, 15–19]. Obayashi et al. [35] reviewed 45 cases of hyperkeratosis of the nipple and areola reported in the literature and found that 80% were the idiopathic or nevoid variant, affecting predominantly females (80%) with a tendency to occur in the second or third decades of life.

### 17.4.4 HNA in Men

Hyperkeratosis of the nipple and areola is very rare in men and a medical history of estrogen therapy for prostatic adenocarcinoma has been postulated as an etiologic factor. Schwartz [36] in 1978 and Mold and Jegasothy [13] in 1980 reported two cases of prostatic adenocarcinoma treated with diethylstilbestrol which developed bilateral hyperkeratosis of the nipple and areola. However, Dupré et al. [22], Kuhlman et al. [23], and English and Coots [24] reported cases of HNA in men that were not associated with hormonal therapy or other underlying abnormalities. Therefore, HNA in men could be classified into two subtypes, the first affecting men receiving estrogen therapy and the second occurring in men with no underlying endocrinopathy or synthetic estrogenic drug treatment.

## 17.5 Clinical Presentation

Nevoid hyperkeratosis of the nipple and areola is a rare, sporadic, and asymptomatic disorder characterized by persistent verrucous thickening and brown pigmentation of the nipple and areola with no induration or discharge (Fig. 17.1). Physical examination usually reveals non-tender, darkly pigmented plaques with a velvety or filiform papular surface which partially or diffusely involves the nipple-areola complex. Hyperkeratosis of the nipple and areola is a diagnosis of exclusion and should be evaluated with inquiry, especially in men which is exceedingly uncommon.

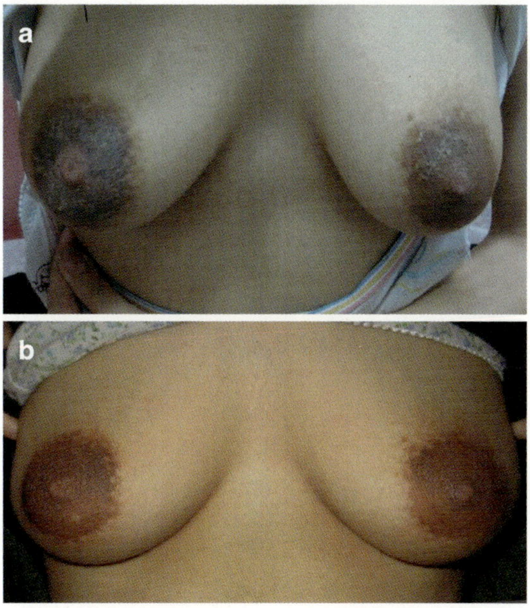

**Fig. 17.1** (**a**) Diffuse verrucous thickening of areolas with hyperpigmented plaques. (**b**) Acceptable improvement, 1 month after topical emollient and steroid therapy

## 17.6 Differential Diagnosis

The differential diagnosis of HNA includes acanthosis nigricans, epidermal nevus, Darier's disease, chronic eczema, verruca vulgaris, seborrheic keratosis, Paget's disease, superficial basal cell carcinoma, dermatophytosis, and Bowen's disease. These disorders can be distinguished from HNA by correlation of clinical and histological features.

A new entity proposed by Higgins et al. [37] is pregnancy-associated hyperkeratosis of the nipple (PAHN) which is different from HNA by a later onset during life, more involvement of the nipple, exclusive occurrence in pregnancy, and showing yellow-tan, hyperkeratotic warty lesions. The etiology of this entity is physiologic changes of pregnancy supported by its onset during pregnancy or immediately in the postpartum period and worsening during subsequent pregnancies. Along with these, typical histopathologic features of HNA such as ramifying epidermal hyperplasia with marked elongation of rete ridges, basal layer hyperpigmentation, irregular filiform acanthosis, and occasional keratotic plugging are not observed in PAHN.

## 17.7 Histopathologic Changes

Histopathologic findings of HNA are nonspecific but useful to help exclude conditions with more distinctive pathologic findings. Histologic examination shows orthokeratotic hyperkeratosis, filiform papillomatosis, and downward acanthosis with occasional keratin plugging (pseudohorn formation) in the epidermis. There is marked ramifying epidermal hyperplasia and anastomosing elongation of the rete ridges enclosing horn cysts with basal hyperpigmentation. In addition, papillary dermis is elongated by expansion of the collagen tissue composed of rather sclerotic collagen bundles and scant inflammatory cells infiltration (Fig. 17.2).

Similar histopathologic features may be seen in epidermal nevus and acanthosis nigricans such as varying degrees of acanthosis, hyperkeratosis, keratin plugging, papillomatosis, and hyperpigmentation. Although the above-mentioned conditions can mimic HNA histopathologically, some diagnostic histopathological clues in HNA such as striking filiform papillomatosis, downward acanthosis and anastomosing rete ridges can be used for differentiation [7, 38].

## 17.8 Treatment

There is no consensus on the treatment guideline because of the unknown pathogenesis and rarity of the lesion, but some medical and ablative modalities are available.

### 17.8.1 Medical Modalities

Treatment of this condition is usually unsatisfactory [29]. Topical agents including emollients, keratolytics, corticosteroids, retinoic acid, and calcipotriol all have been tried with varying degrees of success [2, 8, 12, 18, 23, 33, 38–44]. However, without therapy, HNA persists and response to treatment tends to be highly variable.

The excellent results achieved with topical calcipotriol suggest that this drug is a simple, inexpensive, and effective therapeutic agent for HNA, even when associated with acanthosis nigricans [42, 45]. Although the mechanism of action of topical calcipotriol in HNA is unclear, it may be its effects on keratinocyte differentiation and prolif-

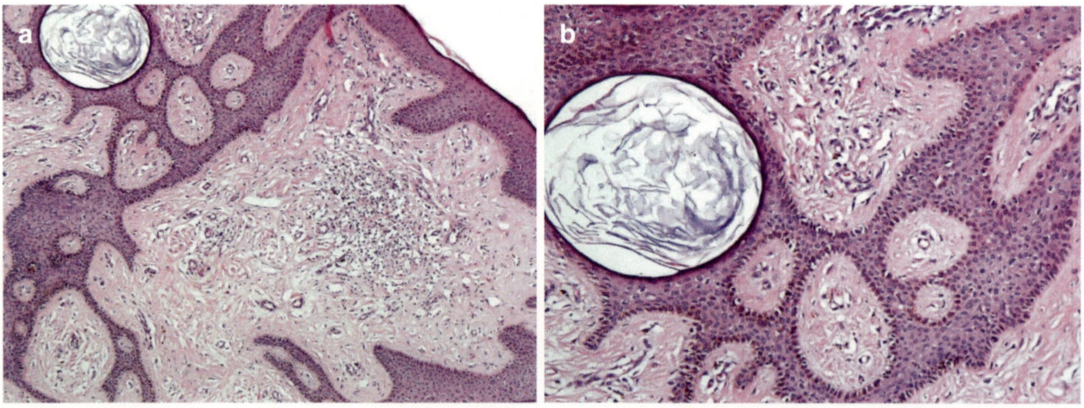


**Fig. 17.2** (**a**) HNA shows downward ramifying acanthosis, anastomosing elongation of the rete ridges, horn cyst formation, and basal hyperpigmentation (H&E, magnification ×10). (**b**) Expansion of papillary dermis with sclerotic collagen bundles and scant inflammatory cells infiltration (H&E, magnification ×20)

eration. The most important side effect of topical calcipotriol treatment is skin irritation and potential effects on calcium homeostasis [46, 47].

### 17.8.2 Ablative Modalities

Ablative modalities include cryotherapy [2, 12, 15, 21], carbon dioxide laser [2, 39], radiofrequency surgical unit [48], and shave excision [18, 22, 49]. Surgical removal of the nipple-areola complex and reconstruction with a skin graft have been used in unresponsive cases of HNA [50].

However, treatment is rarely definitive, and although HNA is a benign condition, it leads to cosmetic concerns and extreme distress in some patients and may rarely interfere with breastfeeding [51]; thus, effective treatment with an acceptable cosmetic outcome is mandatory.

**Conclusions**

Hyperkeratosis of the nipple and areola is a rare benign lesion of the nipple-areola complex presenting by verrucous thickening and pigmented plaques of the NAC. It usually presents at women of childbearing age and is correlated with hormonal changes. Men rarely are involved and disease usually seen in patients undergoing hormone therapy. Clinically, the lesions represent as verrucous thickening with brown pigmentation of the NAC. Histologically, there is thickening and downward hyperplasia of the epidermis with filiform elongation of the rete ridges associated with papillary dermis expansion by sclerotic collagen bundles and scattered inflammatory cells. Treatment includes medical and ablative modalities with variable results.

## References


1. Spyropoulou GA, Pavlidis L, Trakatelli M, Athanasiou E, Pazarli E, Sotiriadis D, Demiri E. Rare benign tumours of the nipple. J Eur Acad Dermatol Venereol. 2015;29(1):7–13.
2. Fenniche S, Badri T. Nevoid hyperkeratosis of the nipple and areola. N Engl J Med. 2010;362:1618.
3. Levy-Frankel A. Les hyperkeratoses de l'areolaet du mamelon. Paris Med. 1938;28:63–6.
4. Alpsoy E, Yilmaz E, Aykol A. Hyperkeratosis of the nipple: report of two cases. J Dermatol. 1997;24:43–5.
5. Oberste-Lehn H. Hyperkeratosenim Bereich von Mamille und Areola. Haut Geschlechtskr. 1950;8: 388–93.
6. Soden CE. Hyperkeratosis of the nipple and areola. Cutis. 1983;32:69–71. 74
7. Baykal C, Büyükbabani N, Kavak A, Alper M. Nevoid hyperkeratosis of the nipple and areola: a distinct entity. J Am Acad Dermatol. 2002;46:414–8.
8. Perez-Izquierdo J, Vilata J, Sanchez J, Gargallo E, Millan F, Aliaga A. Retinoic treatment of nipple hyperkeratosis. Arch Dermatol. 1990;126:687–8.
9. Mehanna A, Malak JA, Kibbi AG. Hyperkeratosis of thenipple and areola. Arch Dermatol. 2001;137:1327–8.
10. Chikhalkar SB, Misri R, Kharkar V. Nevoid hyperkeratosis of nipple: nevoid orhormonal? Indian J Dermatol Venereol Leprol. 2006;72(5):384–6.
11. Boussofara L, Akkari H, Saidi W, Ghariani N, Sriha B, Denguezli M, Nouira R. Bilateral idiopathic hyperkeratosis of the nipple and areola. Acta Dermatovenerol Alp Panonica Adriat. 2011;20(1):41–3.
12. Kubota Y, Koga T, Nakayama J, Kiryu H. Naevoid hyperkeratosis of the nipple and areola in a man. Br J Dermatol. 2000;142:382–4.
13. Mold DE, Jegasothy BV. Estrogen induced hyperkeratosis of the nipple. Cutis. 1980;26:95–6.
14. Marin-Bertolin S, Gonzalez-Martinez R, Marquina VP. Nevoid hyperkeratosis of the areola. Plast Reconstr Surg. 1998;102:275–6.
15. Vestey J, Bunney M. Unilateral hyperkeratosis of the nipple: the response to cryotherapy. Arch Dermatol. 1986;122:1360–1.
16. Rodallec J, Morel P, Guilaine J, Civatte J. Recurring unilateral hyperkeratosis of the areola of the nipples in a pregnant woman. Ann Dermatol Venereol 1978;105(5):527–8.
17. Aytekin S, Tarlan N, Alp S, Uzunlar AK. Naevoid hyperkeratosis of the nipple and areola. J Eur Acad Dermatol Venereol. 2003;17(2):232–3.
18. Mehregan AH, Rahbari H. Hyperkeratosis of nipple and areola. Arch Dermatol. 1977;113:1691–2.
19. Puig L, Moreno A, Noguera X, Moragas JM. Hiperqueratosis de la areola. Actas Dermo-Sifiligr. 1987;78:37–9.
20. Banuchi SR, Cohen L, Lorincz AL, Morgan J. Acanthosis nigricans following diethylstilbesterol therapy. Arch Dermatol. 1974;109:545–6.
21. Mitxelena J, Raton J, Bilbao I, Diaz-Perez J. Nevoid hyperkeratosis of the areola in men: response to cryotherapy. Dermatology. 1999;199:73–4.
22. Dupré A, Catala D, Christol D, Augustin C, Lassère J. Hyperkératose nævoïde des aréolas. Ann Dermatol Vénéréol. 1980;107:305–9.
23. Kuhlman DS, Hodge SJ, Owen LG. Hyperkeratosis of the nipple and areola. J Am Acad Dermatol. 1986;13:596–8.

24. English JC 3rd, Coots NV. A man with nevoid hyperkeratosis of the areola. Cutis. 1996;57:354–6.
25. Price NM, Fuks ZY, Hoffman TE. Hyperkeratotic and verrucous features of mycosis fungoides. Arch Dermatol. 1977;113:57–60.
26. Tyring SK, Lee PC. Hemorrhagic bullae associated with Vibrio vulnificus septicemia. Arch Dermatol. 1986;122:818–20.
27. Allegue F, Soria C, Rocamora A, Fraile G, Ledo A. Hyperkeratosisof the nipple and areola in a patient with cutaneous T-cell lymphoma. Int J Dermatol. 1990;29:519–20.
28. Ahn SK, Chung J, Lee WS, Kim SC, Lee SH. Hyperkeratosis of the nipple and areola simultaneously developing with cutaneous T-cell lymphoma. J Am Acad Dermatol. 1995;32:124–5.
29. Roustan G, Yus ES, Simon A. Nevoid hyperkeratosis of the areola with histopathological features mimicking mycosis fungoides. Eur J Dermatol. 2002;12:79–81.
30. Yalçın B, Gür G, Tabanlıoğlu-Onan D, Ekici Ö. Mycosis fungoides mimicking nevoid hyperkeratosis of the nipple and areola in an adolescent. Turk J Pediatr. 2014;56(5):565–7.
31. Rosman IS, Hepper DM, Lind AC, Anadkat MJ. Nevoid hyperkeratosi of the areola misinterpreted as mycosisfungoides. J Cutan Pathol. 2012;39:545–8.
32. PolatEkinci A, Ozturk Sari S, Buyukbabani N, Baykal C. The dilemma of coexisting nevoid hyperkeratosis of the nipple and areola in mycosis fungoides: a report of three cases. Dermatopathology (Basel). 2015;2(3):61–6.
33. Sanli H, Ekmekci P, Kusak F, Arat M, Beksaç M. Hyperkeratosis of the nipple associated with chronic graft versus host disease after allogeneic haematopoietic cell transplantation. Acta Derm Venereol. 2003;83(5):385–6.
34. Ghazeeri G, Abbas O. Syringocystadenoma papilliferum developing over hyperkeratosis of the nipple in a pregnant woman. J Am Acad Dermatol. 2014;70(4):e84–5.
35. Obayashi H, Tsuchida T, Ikeda S. Hyperkeratosis of nipple and areola. Rinsho Dermatol. 1998;40:147–50.
36. Schwartz RA. Hyperkeratosis of nipple and areola. Arch Dermatol. 1978;114:1844–5.
37. Higgins HW, Jenkins J, Horn TD, Kroumpouzos G. Pregnancy-associated hyperkeratosis of the nipple: a report of 25 cases. JAMA Dermatol. 2013;149:722–6.
38. Ghanadan A, Balighi K, Khezri S, Kamyab Hesari K. Nevoid hyperkeratosis of the nipple and/or areola: treatment with topical steroid. Indian J Dermatol. 2013;58(5):408.
39. Busse A, Peschen M, Schöpf E, Vanscheidt W. Treatment of hyperkeratosis areola mammae naeviformis with carbon dioxide laser. J Am Acad Dermatol. 1999;41:274–6.
40. Xifra M, Lagodin C, Wright D, Abburuzzeese M, Woscoff A. Nevoid keratosis of nipple. J Am Acad Dermatol. 1999;41:325–6.
41. Mayock P. Hyperkeratosis of the nipple. Arch Dermatol. 1978;114(8):1245.
42. Bayramgürler D, Bilen N, Apaydin R, Erçin C. Nevoid hyperkeratosis of the nipple and areola: treatment of two patients with topical calcipotriol. J Am Acad Dermatol. 2002;46:131–3.
43. Okan G, Baykal C. Nevoid hyperkeratosis of the nipple and areola: treatment with topical retinoic acid. J Eur Acad Dermatol Venereol. 1999;13:218–20.
44. Kartal Durmazlar SP, Eskioglu F, Bodur Z. Hyperkeratosis of the nipple and areola: 2 years of remission with low-dose acitretin and topical calcipotriol therapy. J Dermatolog Treat. 2008;19(6):337–40.
45. Bohm M, Luger TA, Metze D. Treatment of mixed-type acanthosis nigricans with topical calcipotriol. Br J Dermatol. 1998;139:932–4.
46. Lebwohl M, Ali S. Treatment of psoriasis: Part 1. Topical therapy and phototherapy. J Am Acad Dermatol. 2001;45(4):487–98.
47. Bourke JF, Mumford R, Whittaker P, Iqbal SJ, Le Van LW, Trevellyan A, Hutchinson PE. The effects of topical calcipotriol on systemic calcium homeostasis in patients with chronic plaque psoriasis. J Am Acad Dermatol. 1997;37(6):929–34.
48. Ozyazgan I, Kontas O, Ferahbas A. Treatment of nevoid hyperkeratosis of the nipple and areola using a radiofrequency surgical unit. Dermatol Surg. 2005;31:703–5.
49. Swan MC, Gwilym SE, Hollowood K, Venning V, Cassell O. Treatment of nevoid hyperkeratosis of the nipple and areola by shave excision. Ann Plast Surg. 2004;53:510–2.
50. Milanovic R, Martic K, Stanec S, Zic R, Vlajcic Z, Stanec Z. Surgical treatment of nevoid hyperkeratosis of the areola by removal of the areola and reconstruction with a skin graft. Ann Plast Surg. 2005;54:667–9.
51. Shastry V, Betkerur J, Kushalappa PA. Unilateral nevoid hyperkeratosis of the nipple:a report of two cases. Indian J Dermatol Venereol Leprol. 2006;72:303–5.

# 18 Clear Cell Acanthoma of the Areola and Nipple

Yolanda Hidalgo-García and Pablo Gonzálvo

## 18.1 Introduction

Clear cell acanthoma (CCA) is a benign epidermal lesion of epidermal keratinocytes. It was firstly described by Degos et al. [1], and it is also known as "Degos' acanthoma" or as "pale acanthoma" [2]. Firstly described as a benign epidermal tumor, at the present, it is discussed if it is a true tumor or has an inflammatory reactive origin.

## 18.2 Clinical Description

Typical CCA is a red to brown, dome-shaped, solitary papule or nodule, often covered by a thin collarette of scale. The surface is either crusted or moist, which bleeds on minor trauma. The lesions usually present on the legs in middle-aged to elderly persons, without gender predilection. It rang in size from 3 to 20 mm of diameter and has grown slowly over a period of years. Most cases are asymptomatic [2]. Although the most typical CCA is a solitary lesion, multiple lesions that can be localized or disseminated have been described [3]. It has been published clinical variants, including giant, polypoid/pedunculated, pigmented, eruptive, atypical, and cystic patterns [2].

At the present, only nine cases of CCA on the areola or the nipple have been reported in the literature [4–9]. First case was published by Kim et al. [4] in 1999, in a woman with personal history of atopy. In this location, women predilection is seen, with only a case in a man [6]. CCA presented as a chronic, erythematous, scaled, well-defined plaque, regarding chronic eczema, except in one case, presented as a polypoid lesion [7]. Some of the lesions were described as moist, exudative, bleeding, and pruritic (Fig. 18.1).

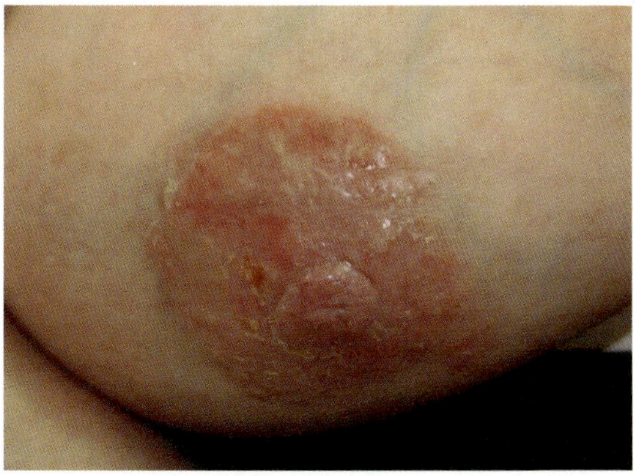

**Fig. 18.1** CCA on the right areola and nipple in a woman. Note erythema, scales, and exudative areas


Y. Hidalgo-García, M.D. (✉)
Department de Dermatología, Hospital de Cabueñes, C/ Los Prados, 395, Gijón CP 33.394, Asturias, Spain

C/ Hermanos Soria n°9, 7°G, Avilés CP 33.402, Asturias, Spain
e-mail: yhidalgog@yahoo.es

P. Gonzálvo, M.D.
Anatomopathology Department, Cabueñes Hospital, C/ Los Prados, Gijón 33.394, Asturias, Spain
e-mail: prerromanico@gmail.com



M.A. Shiffman (ed.), *Nipple-Areolar Complex Reconstruction*, https://doi.org/10.1007/978-3-319-60925-6_18

## 18.3 Histopathology

CCA has a distinctive histopathology features [1–3]. It showed well-demarcated areas of clear cell acanthosis surrounded by an epidermal collarette, organized in a psoriasiform pattern with papillomatosis and suprapapillary epidermal thinning (Fig. 18.2). The transition between normal epithelial cells and clear cells is abrupt. Common features include parakeratosis, spongiosis, and infiltration of the epidermis by neutrophils (Fig. 18.3). These clear cells are rich in glycogen and are strongly positive to periodic acid-Schiff (PAS) stain (Fig. 18.4).

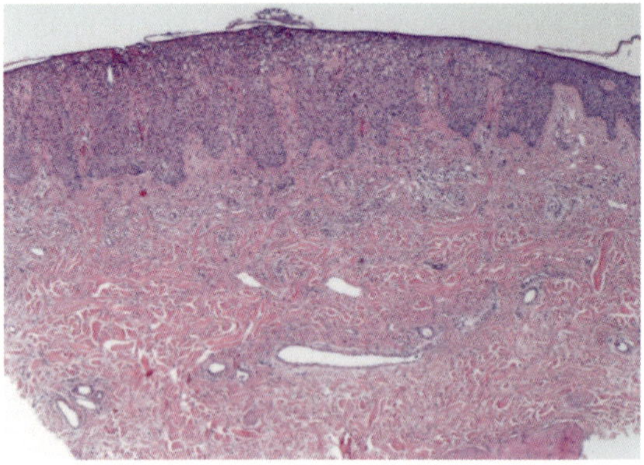

**Fig. 18.2** Clear cell acanthosis on a psoriasiform pattern in a clear cell acanthoma

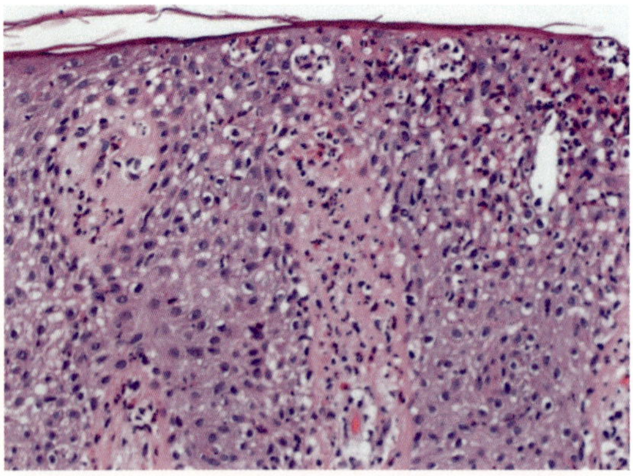

**Fig. 18.3** Agranulosis, spongiosis, parakeratosis, and intraepidermic neutrophils are typical

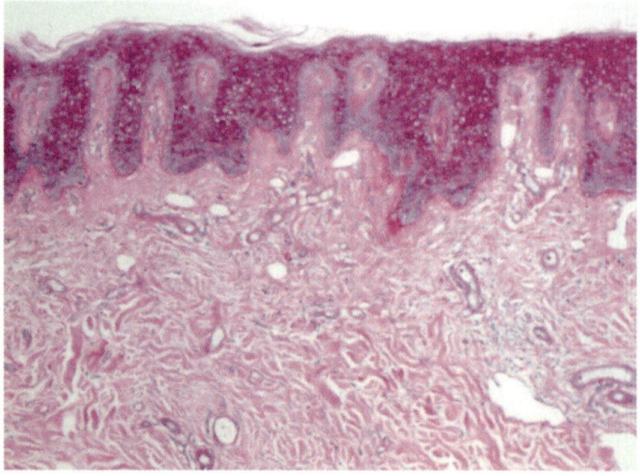

**Fig. 18.4** Periodic acid-Schiff (PAS)-positive stain in basal layers of the epidermis

## 18.4 Etiology and Histogenesis

The histogenesis and etiology of CCA remain unknown. In 1985, Fukushiro et al. [10] proposed the term "pale cell acanthosis" to define the fact that CCA is an epidermal reaction pattern rather than a neoplasm. That concept may be supported by different clinical data like eruptive forms [3], lesions on a psoriatic plaque [11], epidermal nevus [12], or a skin graft [13], as the response of some cases to topical calcipotriol [14] or corticosteroids [9].

Immunohistochemical studies also support this idea. So, Zedek et al. [15] think that CCA represents a psoriasiform reaction pattern, which stained immunohistochemically in similar pattern to normal epidermis and psoriasis. There has been also demonstrated an upregulation in expression in keratinocyte growth factor as in psoriasis [16].

Four of the CCA on the areola and nipple published had personal or familial history of atopic dermatitis, highlighting the possibility of reactive dermatosis origin [4–7].

Nonetheless, the precise nosology of this phenomenon has yet to be elucidated completely.

## 18.5 Dermoscopy Features

Dermoscopy may be useful for diagnosis of either solitary or multiple lesions, revealing a characteristic pattern consisting on widespread pinpoint-like, dotted, or glomerular vessels, linearly arranged as a string of pearls to create a network-like appearance [17]. This vascular psoriasiform pattern has been postulated as another evidence of its inflammatory origin [18].

## 18.6 Differential Diagnosis

The clinical differential diagnosis of CCA depends on the clinical presentations. Solitary forms include actinic keratosis, viral warts, pyogenic granuloma, basal cell and squamous cell carcinoma, eccrine poroma, clear cell hidradenoma, and metastatic cancer [2]. Differential diagnosis of disseminated forms includes other eruptive dermatosis as psoriasis guttata, parapsoriasis, sarcoidosis, lichen planus, or granuloma annulare [3].

Differential diagnosis of CCA of the areola or the nipple includes chronic eczema, psoriatic plaque, syringadenoma papilliferum, pemphigus vegetans, Bowen's disease, and Paget's disease [8, 9]. Two latest are the most important ones, as being malignant tumors.

The clinical differential diagnosis of a polypoid papule on the nipple includes seborrheic keratosis, histiocytoma, viral wart, nevus, and basal cell carcinoma [7].

## 18.7 Treatment

The natural course of CCA is to persist. Treatment options depend on size, location, number of lesions, and the surgical experience of the medical provider. The preferred treatment is lesion removal, although anti-inflammatory treatment should be previously done, based on reactive inflammatory dermatosis hypothesis.

Surgical treatments consist of excision, Mohs micrographic surgery, curettage, electrofulguration, cryotherapy, and carbon dioxide laser. There are very few reported cases of recurrence after excision [2].

In the few CCA of the areola and the nipple published, two cases cleared completely without recurrence with potent topical corticosteroid: 0.05% clobetasol cream [8] and betamethasone dipropionate 0.01% plus gentamicin sulfate 0.1% cream [9], avoiding surgical treatment. Other two cases were refractory to topical corticosteroids [6, 8]. Cryotherapy and surgical excision were the treatments made in the rest of the cases, including the polypoid one, with excellent results.

## References


1. Degos R, Delort J, Civatte J, Poiares Baptista A. Epidermal tumor with an unusual appearance: clear cell acanthoma. Ann Dermatol Syphiliogr (Paris). 1962;89:361–71.
2. Tempark T, Shwayder T. Clear cell acanthoma. Clin Exp Dermatol. 2012;37:831–7.
3. García-Gavín J, González-Vilas D, Montero I, Rodríguez-Pazos L, Pereiro MM, Toribio J. Disseminated eruptive clear cell acanthoma with spontaneous regression: further evidence of an inflammatory origin? Am J Dermatopathol. 2011;33: 599–602.
4. Kim DH, Kim CW, Kang SJ, Kim TY. A case of clear cell acanthoma presenting as nipple eczema. Br J Dermatol. 1999;141:950–1.
5. Um SH, Oh CW. Three cases of clear cell acanthoma on nipple and areola. Korean J Dermatol. 2003;41:85–8.
6. Nazzaro G, Cogí A, Gianotti R. A 26-year-old man with an eczematous lesion on the nipple. Arch Dermatol. 2012;148:641–6.
7. Park SY, Jung JY, Na JI, Byun HJ, Cho KH. A case of polypoid clear cell acanthoma on the nipple. Ann Dermatol. 2010;22:337–40.
8. Veiga RR, Barros RS, Santos JE, Abreu Junior JM, Bittencourt Mde J, Miranda MF. Clear cell acanthoma of the areola and nipple: clinical, histopathological, and immunohistochemical features of two Brazilian cases. An Bras Dermatol. 2013;88:84–9.
9. Hidalgo García Y, Gonzálvo P, Mallo García S, Fernández Sánchez C. Clear cell acanthoma of the areola and the nipple. Actas Dermosifiliogr. 2016;107(9):793–5.
10. Fukushiro S, Takei Y, Ackermann AB. Pale-cell acanthosis. A distinctive histologic pattern if epidermal epithelium. Am J Dermatopathol. 1985;7:515–27.
11. Finch TM, Tan CY. Clear cell acanthoma developing on a psoriatic plaque: further evidence of an inflammatory aetiology? Br J Dermatol. 2000;142:842–4.
12. Yamasaki K, Hatamochi A, Shinkai H, Manabe T. Clear cell acanthoma developing in epidermal nevus. J Dermatol. 1997;24:601–5.

13. Wang SH, Chi CC. Clear cell acanthoma occurring in a split-thickness skin-graft. Plast Reconstr Surg. 2005;116:146–9.
14. Scanni G, Pellacani G. Topical calcipotriol as a new therapeutic option for the treatment of clear cell acanthoma. An Bras Dermatol. 2014;89:803–5.
15. Zedek DC, Langel DJ, White WL. Clear-cell acanthoma versus acanthosis: a psoriasiform reaction pattern lacking trichilemmal differentiation. Am J Dermatopathol. 2007;29:378–84.
16. Kovacs D, Cota C, Cardinali G, Aspite N, Bolasco G, Amantea A, Torrisi MR, Picardo M. Expression of keratinocyte growth factor and its receptor in clear cell acanthoma. Exp Dermatol. 2006;15:762–8.
17. Zalaudek I, Kreush J, Giacomel J, Ferrara G, Catricalà C, Argenziano G. How to diagnose nonpigmented skin tumours: a review of vascular structures seen with dermoscopy: Part II. Nonmelanocytic skin tumours. J Am Acad Dermatol. 2010;63:377–86.
18. Bugatti L, Filosa G, Broganelli P, Tomasini C. Psoriasis-like dermoscopic pattern of clear cell acanthoma. J Eur Acad Dermatol Venereol. 2003;17:452–5.

# 19 Bullous Pemphigoid on the Areola of Breast

Álvaro Vargas Nevado
and Enrique Herrera Ceballos

## 19.1 Introduction

Bullous pemphigoid is a chronic autoimmune skin disorder resulting in generalized, pruritic, bullous lesions in elderly patients, although it may appear in children. Both inflammatory and immune factors are involved in its pathogenesis, and they result in the formation of vesicles and tense blisters, although the disease may appear only as an intense itching with presence of secondary excoriations from scratching. Localized bullous pemphigoid on the areola of breast is a rare form of bullous pemphigoid which is caused by the same autoantibodies that produce the generalized disease and for which we can use the same treatments. Its evolution is more favorable, and in most cases, a very aggressive treatment is not required.

## 19.2 Pathogenesis

Two kinds of factors are involved in the pathogenesis of bullous pemphigoid. The first one is characterized by the formation of antibodies directed against proteins of the hemidesmosomes, specifically against the antigens BP180 and BP 230; and the second one is determined by the action of polymorphonuclear neutrophils and eosinophils that release proteolytic enzymes and damage the dermoepidermal junction [1].

Different causes may trigger bullous pemphigoid, such as phototherapy, radiotherapy, vaccines, and viral infections, as well as in the context of acute or chronic transplant rejection. Some drugs, including spironolactone, captopril, furosemide, D-penicillamine, amoxicillin, ciprofloxacin, or potassium iodide, have also been described as causative agents.

Most cases of bullous pemphigoid on the breast are described in patients with breast carcinoma after treatment with radiotherapy. In this case, the period of time from irradiation to the beginning of the lesions is variable, so they can appear several weeks, months, or years after [2]. It is important to keep in mind that radiotherapy can also exacerbate the course of a bullous pemphigoid and the lesions may be limited to the irradiated area or appear outside this area [3–5]. The mechanism of irradiation that triggers bullous pemphigoid may be related to the radiotherapy itself. That is, radiotherapy changes antigenic properties and induces autoantibody formation through alteration of the basal membrane by unmasking the antigen. Alternatively, patients who develop bullous pemphigoid may already possess circulating anti-basement membrane antibodies, and tissue damage through radiotherapy

Á.V. Nevado, M.D. (✉) • E.H. Ceballos, M.D., Ph.D.
Department of Dermatology, Hospital Virgen de la Victoria, Campus Universitario Teatinos, 29010 Málaga, Spain
e-mail: avargasn88@gmail.com; eherrera@uma.es


M.A. Shiffman (ed.), *Nipple-Areolar Complex Reconstruction*,
https://doi.org/10.1007/978-3-319-60925-6_19

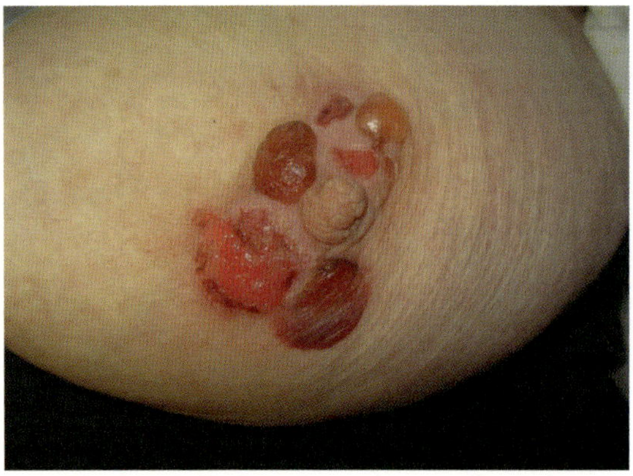

**Fig. 19.1** Tense bullae on the nipple areola complex

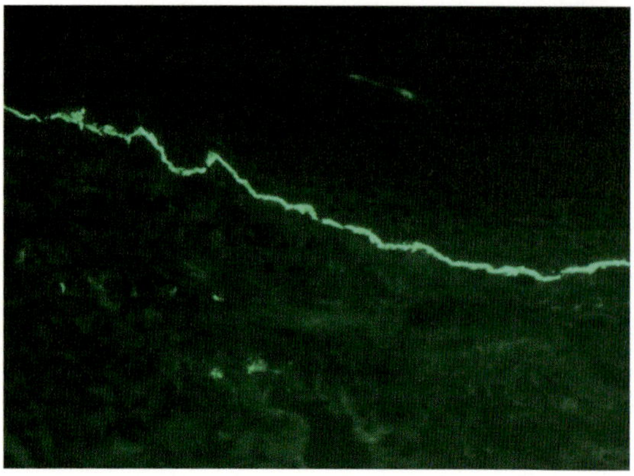

**Fig. 19.2** Direct immunofluorescence: linear deposits of IgG and C3 in the basal membrane

may enhance the deposition of antibodies, i.e., through a change in blood vessel permeability.

It can also occur after surgery, physical trauma, or burns, so these causes may trigger a Koebner phenomenon [6] in predisposed individuals. Although bullous pemphigoid is not widely considered in paraneoplastic syndromes, there is a case in which generalized bullous pemphigoid is the first manifestation of a breast carcinoma [7], so the authors suggest that this disease should be considered in the context of a cutaneous paraneoplastic syndrome and should include a careful examination for an occult breast cancer.

Finally, on other occasions, there is not any cause and the disease appears spontaneously (Fig. 19.1).

## 19.3 Clinical Features

The beginning of bullous pemphigoid is characterized by urticarial or eczematous lesions on which tense blisters and vesicles may appear. Sometimes the patient only feels intense itching so we can see excoriation. Initially vesicles may appear, but then they can turn into blisters of different sizes with a serous and hemorrhagic content. The most common site is the trunk and flexor surfaces of limbs. Nikolsky's sign is negative in most cases and mucosal involvement is rare. Patients with localized disease may evolve into a generalized bullous pemphigoid or remain with localized lesions for years, so it is necessary to make a follow-up of them.

## 19.4 Diagnosis

The diagnosis of bullous pemphigoid is based on the clinical, histological, and immunological data. When bullous pemphigoid is suspected, two biopsies must be taken, one for hematoxylin-eosin and other for immunofluorescence study. In the first one, we can see subepidermal blisters with a perivascular and inflammatory infiltrate with abundant eosinophils. In early lesions, we can find eosinophilic spongiosis [8]. The skin sample for direct immunofluorescence study should be taken from healthy perilesional or inflamed skin without blisters or vesicles. Linear deposits of IgG and C3 will be observed in the basal membrane (Fig. 19.2), although there may be deposits of other immunoglobulins as IgA and IgM of lower intensity [8, 9]. These data are observed in generalized and localized bullous pemphigoid.

Indirect immunofluorescence allows the detection of circulating anti-basement membrane zone antibodies in peripheral blood. This technique can be performed using human skin treated with a solution of 1 M sodium chloride as substrate, allowing the differentiation of bullous pemphigoid from other bullous diseases by observing deposition of antibodies in the epidermal side of the blister artificially created in the first case [8].

Finally, the ELISA technique allows to detect circulating antibodies against both antigens of bullous pemphigoid (BP230 and BP180) in a large percentage of cases. The levels of these antibodies correlate with disease activity [10].

## 19.5 Treatment

The drugs used for the treatment of bullous pemphigoid have three objectives:

1. Decrease the inflammatory activity: topical corticosteroids, sulfonamides, sulfone, tacrolimus, or antibiotics with anti-inflammatory properties such as tetracyclines.
2. Reduce the production of pathogenic antibodies: systemic corticosteroids, mycophenolate, azathioprine, methotrexate, cyclosporine, or rituximab.
3. Increase the elimination of pathogenic antibodies: high-dose intravenous immunoglobulin and plasma exchange.

Some tests should be requested in patients with bullous pemphigoid before initiation of treatments: laboratory test including blood count, biochemistry profile, and liver and kidney function; serology for HVC, HVB, and human immunodeficiency; glucose-6-phosphate dehydrogenase activity if they are to take sulfone; thiopurine S-methyltransferase activity if azathioprine is to be administered; blood pressure taking; Mantoux test [16]; and chest radiograph. It is important to keep in mind that these treatments do not cure bullous pemphigoid but rather suppress disease activity.

In the case of localized lesions, as with bullous pemphigoid on the areola of breast, they can be treated with high-potency topical corticosteroids, which may be sufficient to control the disease and would therefore be the treatment of choice [11]. Topical tacrolimus has also been useful in some cases. Blisters can be drained by piercing the base of the lesion with a sterile needle. Application of an antiseptic solution, such as chlorhexidine 0.5%, on erosive lesions reduces the risk of secondary infection. If such an infection does occur, topical antibiotics such as fusidic acid and mupirocin can be used. A course of systemic antibiotics must be started when deep cutaneous infection is suspected.

Topical or systemic corticosteroids are generally the first line of treatment in bullous pemphigoid [12]. High-potency topical corticosteroids as clobetasol propionate 0.05% are indicated in patients with mild or moderate symptoms. Very potent topical corticosteroids are also frequently used as adjuncts with systemic treatments in more severe cases.

Systemic corticosteroids are the treatment of choice in patients in whom topical treatment is insufficient. The most common agents used are prednisone and prednisolone, and the recommended dose ranges from 0.5 to 0.7 5 mg/kg/day. It is important to administer proton pump inhibitors to prevent gastroduodenal peptic ulcers and also to prescribe calcium supplements, vitamin D, and bisphosphonates from the outset to prevent steroid-induced osteoporosis. Complete remission is often achieved within 7–9 months, after which time these agents can be completely withdrawn [13]. In patients with mild or moderate disease who don't respond or respond only partially to corticosteroids, agents such as erythromycin, sulfone [14], tetracyclines, and nicotinamide [15] can be used as adjuvant treatments.

Methotrexate is one of the first-line immunosuppressive treatments for bullous pemphigoid. It can be used as corticosteroid-sparing drug in patients with moderate to severe disease, in monotherapy, or in association with topical corticosteroids in patients less severe disease [17]. It is normally used at low doses, ranging from 2.5 to 10 mg a week. The dose should not exceed 15 mg a week. It can be administered orally, subcutaneously, or intravenously. It is contraindicated in case of pregnancy, breastfeeding, cytopenia, alcoholism, severe liver or kidney failure (GFR <10 mL/min/m$^2$), or active infections.

More powerful immunosuppressive drugs such as azathioprine, mycophenolate, and cyclophosphamide are indicated for severe or refractory cases of bullous pemphigoid. Azathioprine is a drug with anti-inflammatory and immunosuppressive activities. As methotrexate, it can be used as a corticosteroid-sparing drug, being the most common one used for this purpose [18]. The therapeutic effect is achieved within 7–9 weeks of commencement of treatment. Its efficacy and secondary effects depend on the activity of thiopurine s-methyltransferase activity. The recommended doses range from 0.5 to 3 mg/kg/day. It is contraindicated in case of pregnancy and breastfeeding, allergy to azathioprine or 6-mercaptopurine, concomitant malignancy, kidney or liver failure, or history of tumor in remission.

Mycophenolate is generally used in a similar fashion to azathioprine, as corticosteroid-sparing agent, although it can be used in monotherapy with favorable results. The recommended dose is 1 g/12 h. In a recent study of patients with BP, corticosteroids combined with MPM showed similar efficacy to corticosteroids combined with azathioprine [19].

Rituximab is a humanized chimeric monoclonal antibody that selectively targets CD20 cells. The drug was initially developed to control lymphoproliferative B-cell disorders, but in recent years, used either alone or in combination with IVIG therapy, it has proven to be effective at controlling an increasing number of autoimmune diseases that do not respond to other treatments. The effects of RTX take approximately a month to appear and are maintained for 9–10 months. Its toxicity and mortality are not negligible, particularly in relation to the risk of serious opportunistic or other infections so it should only be considered in patients with severe disease who do not respond to previous treatments [20].

**Conclusions**

Bullous pemphigoid of the breast is a localized form of bullous pemphigoid. Most cases are induced by radiotherapy in patients with a history of breast carcinoma, and so far there are no reported cases in which this disease becomes generalized, so the prognosis and evolution are excellent. However, making a follow-up of these patients is recommended. In most cases, treatment with high-potency topical corticosteroids in combination with topical antibiotics may be enough.

## References

1. Mutasim DF. Autoimmune bullous dermatoses in the elderly: an update on pathophysiology, diagnosis and management. Drugs Aging. 2010;1:1–19.
2. Isohashi F, Konishi K, Umegaki N, Tanei T, Koizumi M, Yoshioka Y. A case of bullous pemphigoid exacerbated by irradiation after breast conservative radiotherapy. Jpn J Clin Oncol. 2011;41(6):811–3.
3. Mul VE, van Geest AJ, Pijls-Johannesma MC, Theys J, Verschueren TA, Jager JJ, et al. Radiation-induced bullous pemphigoid: a systematic review of an unusual radiation side effect. Radiother Oncol. 2007;82:5–9.
4. Mul VE, Verschueren TA, van Geest AJ, Baumert BG. Bullous Pemphigoid (BP) induced by radiotherapy. Radiother Oncol. 2007;82:105.
5. Anzai S, Ueo D, Fujiwara S. A case of bullous pemphigoid exacerbated by radiotherapy. Vis Dermatol. 2009;8:32–3.
6. Weiss G, Shemer A, Trau H. The Koebner phenomenon: review of the literature. J Eur Acad Dermatol Venereol. 2002;16:241–8.
7. Luliano L, Micheletta F, Natoli S. Bullous pemphigoid: an unusual and insidious presentation of breast cancer. Clin Oncol. 2003;15(8):505.
8. Vaughan Jones SA, Salas J, McGrath JA, Palmer I, Bhogal GS, Black MM. A retrospective analysis of tissue-fixed immunoreactants from skin biopsies maintained in Michel's medium. Dermatology. 1994;189(Suppl 1):131–2.
9. Yancey KB, Egan CA. Pemphigoid: clinical, histologic, immunopathologic, and therapeutic considerations. JAMA. 2000;284:350–6.
10. Iwata Y, Komura K, Kodera M, Usuda T, Yokoyama Y, Hara T, Muroi E, Ogawa F, Takenaka M, Sato S. Correlation of IgE autoantibody to BP180 with a severe form of bullous pemphigoid. Arch Dermatol. 2008;144:41–8.
11. Westerhof W. Treatment of bullous pemphigoid with topical clobetasol propionate. J Am Acad Dermatol. 1989;20:458–61.
12. Ingen-Housz-Oro S, Valeyrie-Allanore L, Ortonne N, Roujeau JC, Wolkenstein P, Chosidow O. Management of bullous pemphigoid with topical steroids in the clinical practice of a single center: outcome at 6 and 12 months. Dermatology. 2011;222:176–9.
13. Morel P, Guillaume JC. Treatment of bullous pemphigoid with prednisolone only: 0.75 mg/kg/day versus 1.25 mg/kg/day. A multicenter randomized study. Ann Dermatol Venereol. 1984;111:925–8.
14. Venning VA, Millard PR, Wojnarowska F. Dapsone as first line therapy for bullous pemphigoid. Br J Dermatol. 1989;120:83–92.
15. Fivenson D, Breneman D, Rosen G, Hersh CS, Cardone S, Mutasim D. Nicotinamide and tetracycline therapy of bullous pemphigoid. Arch Dermatol. 1994;130:753–8.
16. Kirtschig G, Khumalo NP. Management of bullous pemphigoid: recommendations for immunomodulatory treatments. Am J Clin Dermatol. 2004;5:319–26.
17. Heilborn JD, Ståhle-Bäckdahl M, Albertioni F, Vassilaki I, Peterson C, Stephansson E. Low-dose oral pulse methotrexate as monotherapy in elderly patients with bullous pemphigoid. J Am Acad Dermatol. 1999;40:741–9.

18. Burton JL, Harman RR, Peachey RD, Warin RP. Azathioprine plus prednisone in treatment of pemphigoid. Br Med J. 1978;28:1190–1.
19. Grundmann-Kollmann M, Korting HC, Behrens S, Kaskel P, Leiter U, Krähn G, Kerscher M, Peter RU. Mycophenolate mofetil: a new therapeutic option in the treatment of blistering autoimmune diseases. J Am Acad Dermatol. 1999;40(6 Pt 1):957–60.
20. Lourari S, Herve C, Doffoel-Hantz V, Meyer N, Bulai-Livideanu C, Viraben R, Maza A, Adoue D, Bedane C, Paul C. Bullous and mucous membrane pemphigoid show a mixed response to rituximab: experience in seven patients. J Eur Acad Dermatol Venereol. 2011;25:1238–40.

# 20 Paget's Disease of Nipple in Male Breast with Cancer

Uthamalingam Murali

## 20.1 Introduction

Paget's disease of the breast (also known as Paget's disease of the nipple, Paget's disease of the nipple and areola, and mammary Paget's disease) is a rare type of cancer involving the skin of the nipple and, usually, the darker circle of the skin around it, which is called the areola. It has been recognized as a distinct clinical entity for over 140 years, since its initial description by the British surgeon, Sir James Paget in 1874 [1], who noticed a relationship between the changes in the nipple and breast cancer. This chapter provides an overview of Paget's disease and describes the etiopathogenesis, clinicopathological features, differential diagnosis, and recent diagnosis and treatment modalities of Paget's diseases of the nipple in the male breast with cancer.

U. Murali, M.S., M.B.A.
Professor of Surgery, Anna Medical College Research Center, Sans Souci Road, Montagne Blanche, Mauritius
e-mail: srimuralihospital2012@gmail.com

## 20.2 Epidemiology

Worldwide breast cancers are a common cause of concern for patients as well as for doctors. Male breast cancer can account for 0.8–1% of all malignancies in men and 0.1–0.2% of male cancer deaths [2]. Paget's disease (PD) of the breast is more frequent in women than men because of the predominance of breast cancer in females. Between 1 and 4% of all female breast cancers are Paget's diseases. Thus, compared to females, Paget's disease of the male breast is clearly a rare clinical entity. However, PD represents a higher incidence in males (5%) [3]. Worldwide, the exact frequency of male PD is not clear. Evidence suggests that the highest incidence of breast cancer appears to be among the North American and British males, constituting around 1.5% of all male cancers. Jewish and African American males rank next in the highest incidence cluster [4]. So far, no racial predisposition has been reported for mammary PD.

Cancer of the male breast rarely occurs in young males. The mean age of men presenting with Paget's disease of the breast and male breast cancer is generally in the fifth or sixth decade of life, but ages range from 40 to 80 years. The average time from the onset of the first symptom to treatment is about 8–15 months, but some studies reported even up to 8 years, particularly in males [5].


M.A. Shiffman (ed.), *Nipple-Areolar Complex Reconstruction*,
https://doi.org/10.1007/978-3-319-60925-6_20

## 20.3 Etiology

Etiological factors in male breast cancer are obscure. No clinical or epidemiological factors are known to predispose patients to develop Paget's disease. Certain risk factors are recognized and may be categorized into three forms: those related to old age and radiation; those related to hormonal imbalance (estrogen and androgen) such as obesity, cirrhosis, infertility, and testicular abnormalities; and finally those related to genetic predisposition like family history, Klinefelter's syndrome (47XXY), and BRCA gene mutation [6]. Considering BRCA mutation, unlike male carriers of BRCA 1 mutation, men who inherit BRCA 2 mutation are more commonly associated (5–15%) and have an estimated risk of 6% of male breast cancer. Literature suggests that male breast cancer is also associated with Klinefelter's syndrome—a condition having reduced testosterone levels and high incidence of gynecomastia. However, gynecomastia should not be considered as a risk factor. Studies show that male breast cancer may be preceded by gynecomastia in around 20% of men [4]. Deficiency of folic acid has also been shown to be a risk factor of male breast cancer particularly in patients under methotrexate treatment [7].

**Table 20.1** Foote–Stewart original classification of invasive breast cancer

| | |
|---|---|
| I | Paget's disease of the nipple |
| II | Invasive ductal carcinoma |
| | – Adenocarcinoma—80% |
| | – Medullary—4% |
| | – Mucinous or colloid—2% |
| | – Papillary—2% |
| | – Tubular and invasive cribriform—2% |
| III | Invasive lobular carcinoma—10% |
| IV | Rare other types—adenoid cystic, squamous cell, apocrine type |

## 20.4 Pathogenesis

The pathology is similar to that of female breast cancer. Paget's disease of the nipple ranks first in the Foote–Stewart original classification of invasive breast cancer (Table 20.1). Since its description, the pathogenesis of Paget's disease of the breast is still a subject of debate. Many theories have been attributed toward the pathogenesis of Paget's disease, but only two of them have been proposed to explain properly its nature and origin. The most widely accepted theory—epidermotropic (ductal) theory—suggests that cancer cells from a tumor inside the breast migrate through the milk ducts to the nipple and areola (Fig. 20.1). It is supported by the presence of underlying intraductal or invasive carcinoma in the majority of patients as well as predominance of breast cancer markers in Paget's disease and overexpression of Her-2 protein in Paget's disease [6, 8]. This would also explain why Paget's disease of the breast and tumors inside the same breast are almost always found together. Yet another theory—intraepidermal transformation theory—proposes in situ malignant transformation of existing cells so that cancerous cells develop independently in the nipple or areola (Fig. 20.2), and this would explain the incidence of Paget's disease of the breast in few cases without tumor inside the same breast [9]. Each of the above theories is possible. However, treatment methods differ markedly depending on the theory of histogenesis which has been described at the end of this chapter.

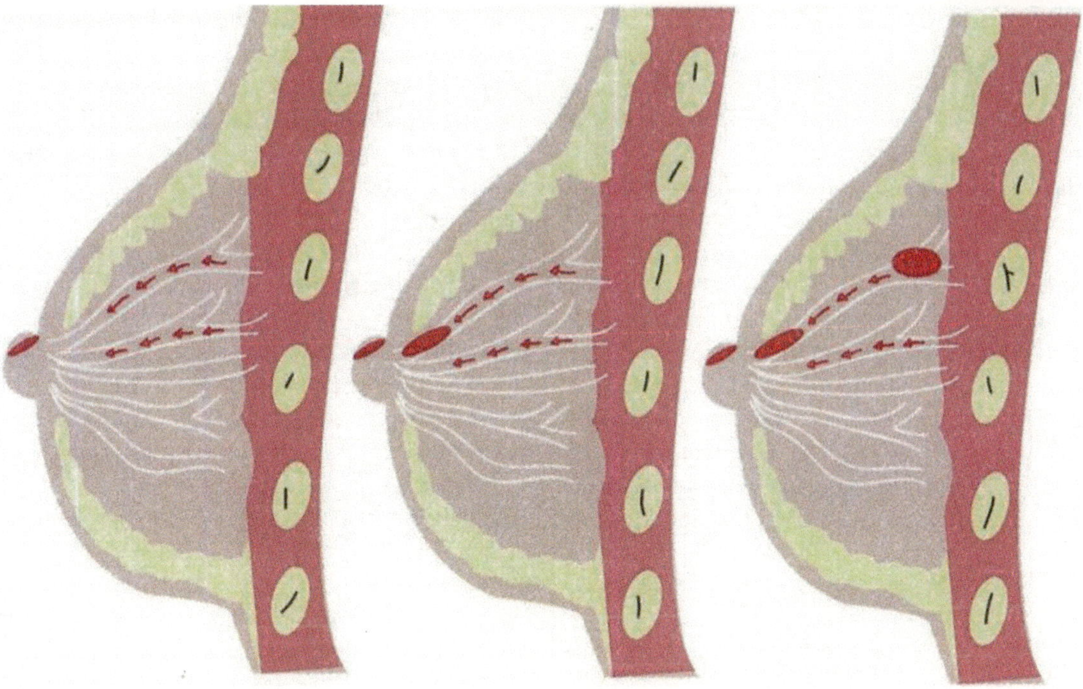

**Fig. 20.1** Epidermotropic (ductal) theory (courtesy of MuhamadIfwat Bin Zainal Abidin, second year student, Diploma in Graphic Design, Faculty of Information Science and Engineering, MSU, Malaysia)

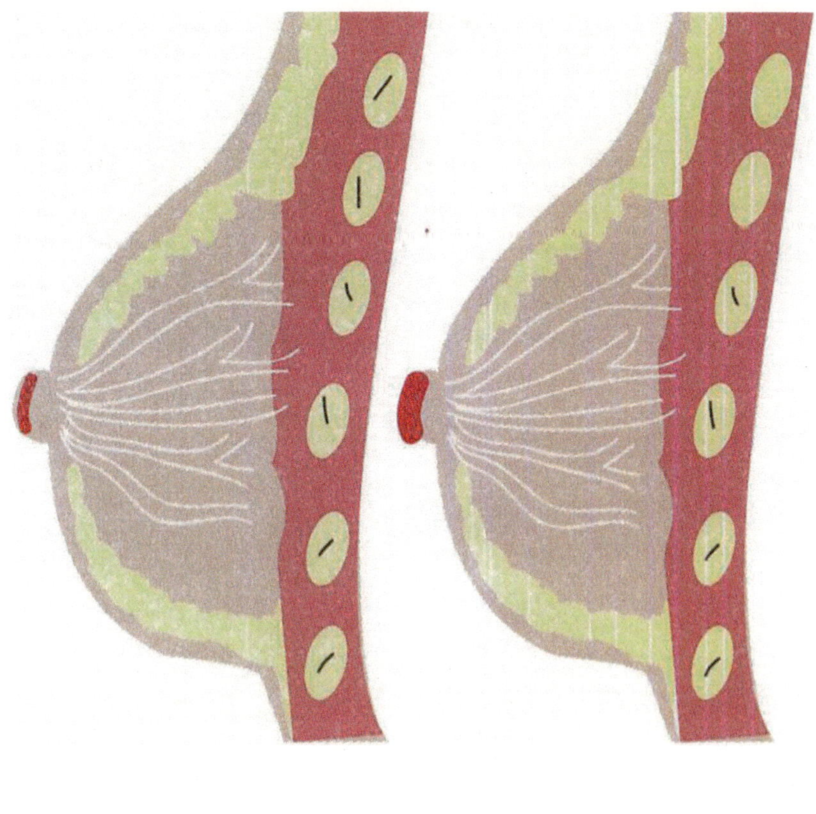

**Fig. 20.2** Intraepidermal transformation theory (courtesy of MuhamadIfwat Bin Zainal Abidin, second year student, Diploma in Graphic Design, Faculty of Information Science and Engineering, MSU, Malaysia)

## 20.5 Clinical Features

The clinical features of PD in men appear to be similar to those in women. The early presentation is, as Paget described, an erythematous, scaling or crusting, and eczema-like rash lesion involving the nipple in the initial stages and extending to the areola and surrounding skin of the breast later on (Figs. 20.3 and 20.4). This may be associated with pain or burning sensation. Itching may be a frequent complaint. These early changes may be mistaken for skin lesions such as eczema or other inflammatory lesions. Topical treatment of such eczematous lesions might mask the underlying condition causing delay in diagnosis. In more advanced stages, the lesions may progress to ulceration and cause nipple retraction or bloody discharge from the nipple [10]. This results in destruction of nipple–areolar complex. PD may be asymptomatic or cannot be clinically detected. In such cases, the pathologist would report the histological findings in the mastectomy specimen.

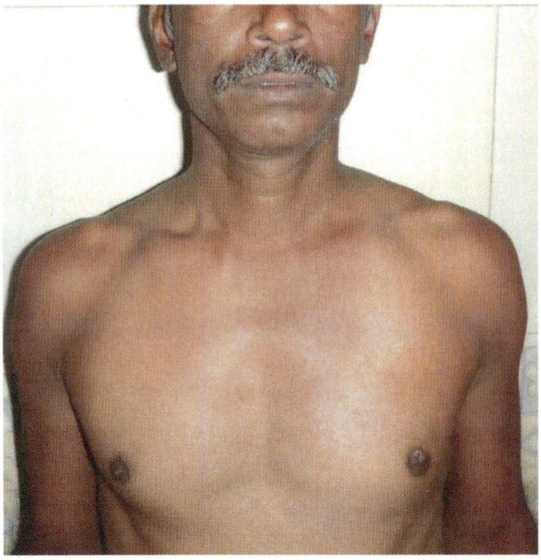

**Fig. 20.3** Male Paget's disease: scaling/crusting lesion

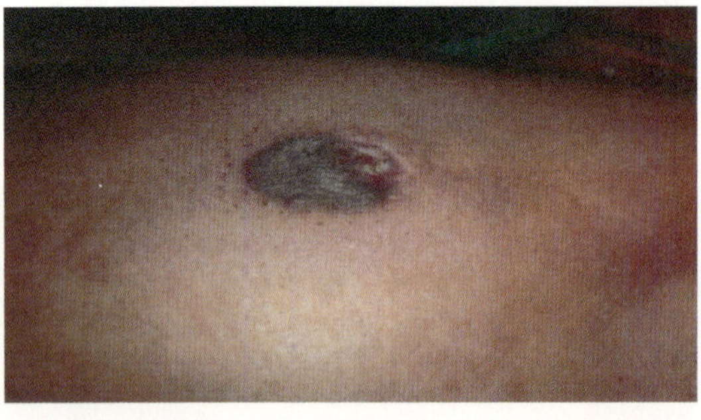

**Fig. 20.4** Male Paget's disease: lesion extending to the areola

Although mostly breast cancers are unilateral in their presentation, bilateral synchronous tumors occur in about 1% of all female breast cancers, and so far there are less than ten reported women with synchronous bilateral PD [11]. On the contrary, literatures have shown only two cases of synchronous bilateral Paget's disease of the nipple in men [3, 12]. Occasional cases of PD have been reported in the ectopic breast or accessory nipples [13, 14].

Approximately 50% of patients also present with an associated palpable mass in the breast. In these cases, underlying breast carcinoma (invasive or intraductal) is almost always associated in more than 90% of patients [3, 15]. Of note, only one case of mucinous breast carcinoma presenting as Paget's disease of the nipple in men has been so far reported [16]. On the contrary, patients without a palpable mass (40%) are more likely to have ductal carcinoma in situ (DCIS) in around 30% of cases [3, 15]. These palpable or impalpable tumors may be located close to the areola—central or at the periphery. Obviously, lymph node enlargement is found more often in cases with palpable tumor [17].

## 20.6 Differential Diagnosis

The diagnoses of male breast cancer are delayed and are often undertreated as they are mistaken for a benign dermatological condition involving the nipple. It has to be differentiated from other inflammatory lesions like eczema, psoriasis, contact dermatitis, mastitis, duct ectasia, as well as benign and malignant lesions like adenoma, papilloma, lymphomatoid papulosis, ductal carcinoma, and Bowen's disease [7, 18]. As described earlier, PD usually starts in the nipple and spreads to the areolar and skin region, while eczema and dermatitis starts in the areola and spreads to other area. In addition, in the former, there are bilateral changes with absence of nipple deformity, while in the latter, there may be presence of similar skin lesions in other areas of the body, responding to topical therapy. Long-standing lesions of PD often show prominent hyperkeratosis with epidermal hyperplasia and reactive atypia of the keratinocytes. These lesions may be misdiagnosed as Bowen's disease. Intracellular mucin, signet cells, and acini formation favor Paget's disease [19].

Recent studies suggest that any pigmented lesion of the nipple should also be included in the differential diagnosis [20, 21]. Although pigmented PD of the male breast are rare, few cases have been reported as Paget cells have similar distribution to that of junctional melanocytes [20]. Distinguishing Paget's disease from melanoma is extremely difficult when the cancer cells contain pigment melanin. Lack of acini formation along with absence of intracellular mucin helps in diagnosing melanoma. In difficult cases, immunohistochemistry is the important tool to differentiate Paget's disease from other entities. Paget cells stain positive for cytokeratin's (CK7), CAM-5.2, and Her-2 oncoprotein. But they do not express for CK 20, HMB-45, and high molecular weight keratin, which helps it to differentiate from melanomas [21].

Yet another latest in the list of differential diagnosis includes hyperplasia of mammary gland-related cells—so-called Toker cells. These Toker cells (TCs) are normal components of the nipple epidermis. Recent literatures show that Toker cells are derived from the lactiferous ductal epithelium and are referred as mammary gland precursor cells [22]. They are considered as the benign counterpart of the malignant cells of PD. It may be difficult to distinguish the Paget's cells from Toker cells, particularly in cases of Toker cell hyperplasia with cytologic atypia. In most cases, Toker cells are small- and medium-sized cells, usually dispersed singly with clear cytoplasm which may consist of a large (mucin-negative) vacuole that appears clear on routine stains. However, immunohistochemically, both these cells can be distinguished; in contrast to Paget's cells, Toker cells are usually negative for c-erbB-2, Her-2, and Ki-67 and positive to estrogen receptor (ER) [23].

## 20.7 Diagnosis

Obviously for any patient presenting with an itching or ulcerated lesion of the nipple, a tissue biopsy should be obtained to exclude the diagnosis of Paget's disease. A skin specimen containing Paget cells and a lactiferous duct secures the diagnosis and can be obtained by nipple scrape cytology or wedge biopsy. PD is characterized by the presence of Paget's cells that are large and ovoid and have abundant pale cytoplasm which contains mucin with pleomorphic and hyperchromatic nuclei [24] (Fig. 20.5). Groups of malignant Paget's cells predominantly involve the

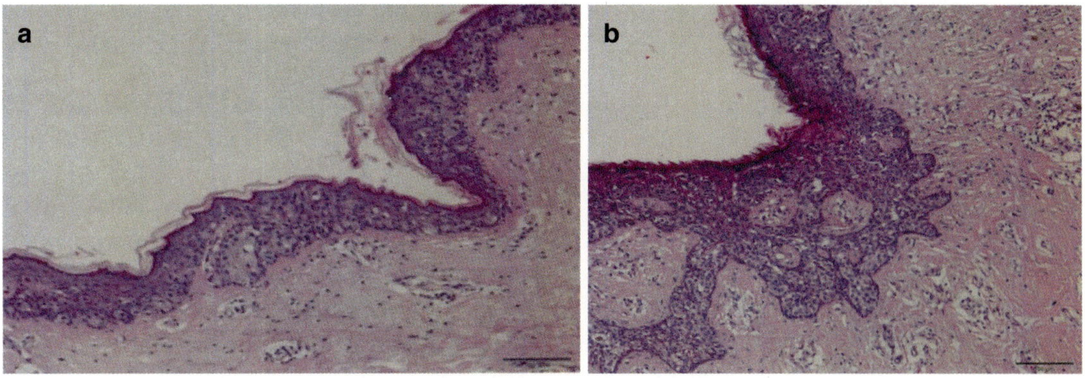


**Fig. 20.5** (**a**, **b**) Paget's cells: ovoid cells with abundant cytoplasm and hyperchromatic nuclei (courtesy of Dr. M. Akita, Department of Surgery, Hyogo Prefectural Kaibara Hospital, 5208-1 Kaibara, Kaibara-cho, Tamba, Japan)

lower layers of the epidermis. These are described as pagetoid change or pagetoid feature. In patients with nipple–areolar ulcerative skin lesions, a full-thickness biopsy of the nipple and areola or partly excision of nipple is important to make the diagnosis.

Although biopsy is considered as the standard method in diagnosis of PD, several studies have explored that immunohistochemistry allows correct diagnosis in most cases of Paget's disease of the breast in clinical practice [21–23]. Moreover, it also helps in differentiating PD from other conditions as described earlier in this chapter. Paget's cells show similar immunohistochemical staining pattern as that of malignancy growing within the breast. Paget's cells show more expression for low molecular cytokeratin (CKs) such as CK7 in most of the cases. In addition, lack of CK7 expression in Paget's cells may be associated with lack of CK7 reactivity in underlying malignancy [25]. This expression pattern will predict the association of underlying carcinoma. PD is often estrogen and progesterone receptor negative because the underlying carcinomas tend to be poorly differentiated. Usually, in most cases, there is correlation between positive staining for Her-2 oncoprotein of Paget's cells and underlying in situ or invasive breast carcinoma [26].

As PD is mostly associated with underlying in situ or invasive cancer, either fine needle aspiration or imaging methods should be performed to detect the underlying cancer [27]. It helps in the assessment and further management of the disease. Conventional imaging modality such as mammography (MMG) is limited in depicting underlying malignancy in women with Paget's disease.

MMG may show thickening of the nipple, subareolar microcalcifications, or distortion of architecture of the breast [28] (Fig. 20.6). No literatures have so far shown the role of MMG in the evaluation of male breast cancer, and hence it is not a reliable procedure for detecting PD.

On the contrary to MMG, ultrasound examination of the breast should be considered as the next imaging method in the initial evaluation. US would be useful if the patient presents with a palpable mass lesion (Fig. 20.7). In patients with

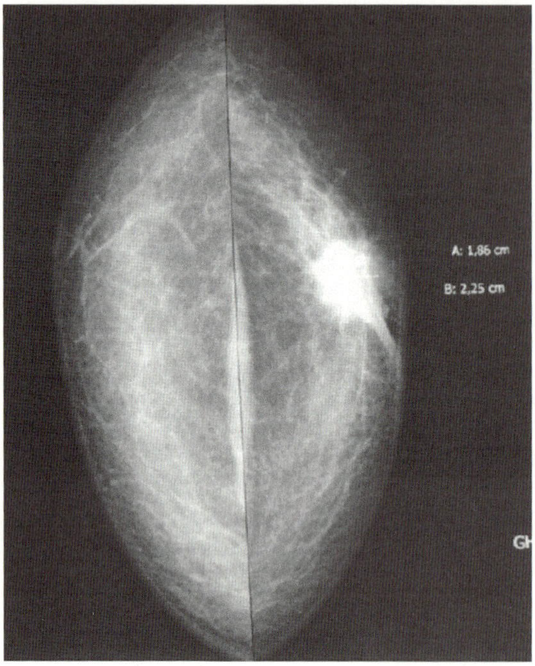


**Fig. 20.6** Mammography of the male breast—depicting breast carcinoma (courtesy of Dr. T. El Harroudi, Department of Surgery in National Institute of Oncology, Rabat, Morocco)

inconclusive mammographic or ultrasonographic findings, magnetic resonance imaging (MRI) may be used for problem solving or clarifying the lesions. Most studies suggest that breast magnetic resonance imaging plays a key role in diagnosing mammary Paget's disease (MPD) with or without lump and has a sensitivity of 95% compared to mammography and US [28]. MRI may show thickening of the nipple–areolar complex, abnormal nipple enhancement, an associated enhancing DCIS or invasive tumor, or a combination of these, even when clinically unsuspected (Fig. 20.8). In addition to MRI, the less invasive procedure such as sentinel lymph node biopsy (SLNB) has been reported to be reasonable and accurate for nodal assessment in male mammary PD without underlying invasive cancer [29]. To know the lymph node status of axilla and also to avoid second surgery, SLNB can be performed. SLNB has also shown to be effective in staging male breast cancer. Male staging of breast cancer is similar and identical to that of women. Therefore, both pathological

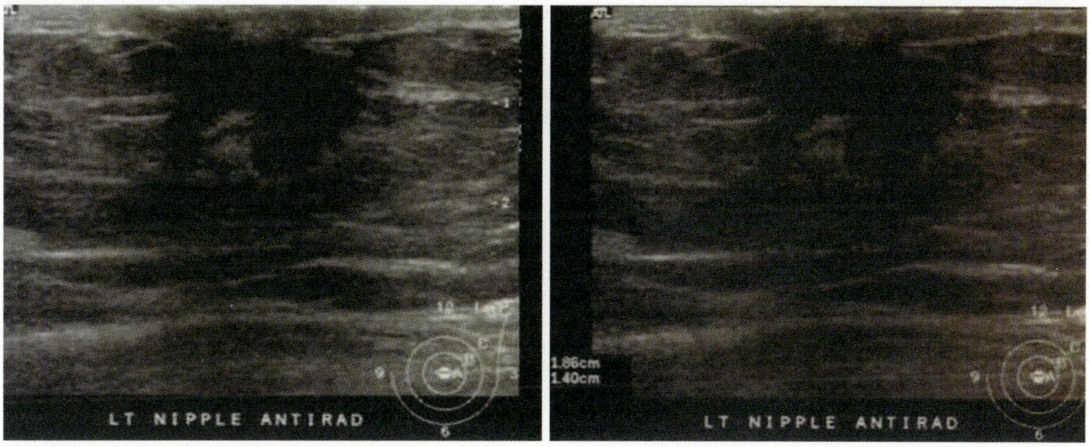


**Fig. 20.7** (*Left*, *right*) US of the male breast showing breast carcinoma (courtesy of Dr. Taco Geertsma, Radiologist, Holland)

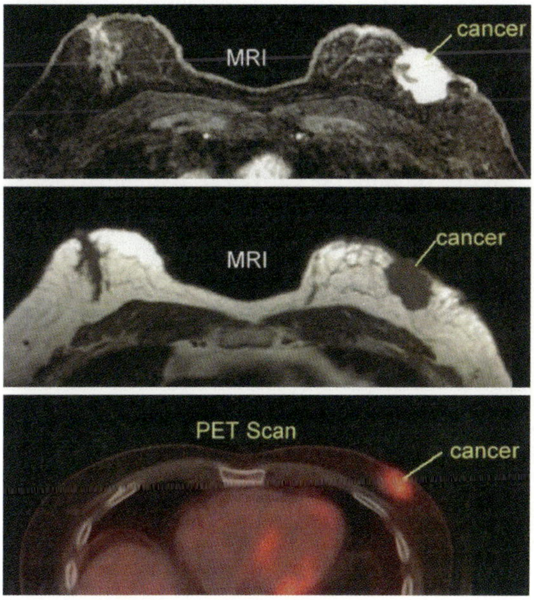


**Fig. 20.8** MRI PET scan of male breast

and imaging findings are complementary and should be correlated to confirm or exclude a diagnosis of Paget's disease.

## 20.8 Treatment

In the literature, different methods are used for the treatment. Several studies show that most patients treated with breast-conserving surgery, radiotherapy, or both had the clinical presentation of PD without a palpable mass and have concluded that these methods were not an appropriate treatment for patients with Paget's disease of the nipple due to high recurrence rates [30]. However, if breast conservative strategies such as nipple excision or central lumpectomy is planned, the patient should be carefully followed up with MMG and undergo mastectomy when relapse occurs. Of note, selected patients with Paget's disease limited to the nipple, without clinical or radiological detectable tumor, can be treated with breast radiation therapy. Recently, less invasive approaches such as photodynamic therapy (PDT) either in the form of topical or intravenous applications has shown to be effective in the treatment of mammary and extra-mammary Paget's disease [31]. PDT uses a photosensitizing agent which is activated by a light source that destroys the affected tissue and spares the healthy tissue.

Considering the surgical treatment of Paget's disease is still controversial and no randomized studies so far have compared the treatment options for mammary Paget's disease with breast cancer in men due to the relative scarcity of cases in this population. Some studies suggest treatment options like modified radical mastectomy, axillary staging, radiation therapy, or systemic chemotherapies [32]. But most studies have shown that the standard therapy for male Paget's disease even in the absence of malignancy is

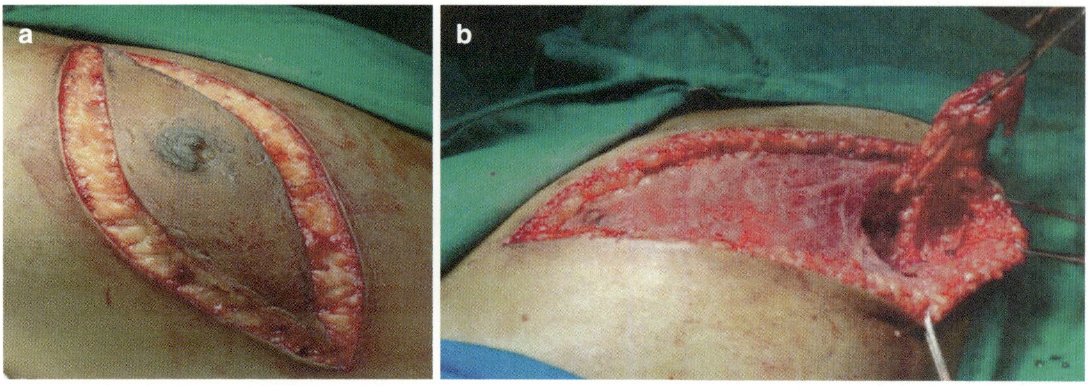

**Fig. 20.9** Modified radical mastectomy. (**a**) Skin incision. (**b**) Removal of the breast tissue

mastectomy with or without axillary lymph node dissection [5, 33] (Fig. 20.9). Finally, evidence suggests that the surgical treatment plan should be selected on the basis of careful clinical and radiological assessment as well as extent of involvement of the cancer [34].

Limited and little information are available regarding the indications for adjuvant radiotherapy and effectiveness of adjuvant chemotherapy in male patients with breast cancer. Most studies show similar recommendations and benefits in both men and women. Considering radiotherapy, local recurrence rates were less in male patients without focal skin involvement [35]. Adjuvant chemotherapy with CMF (cyclophosphamide, methotrexate, and 5-fluorouracil) lowers the risk of recurrence with good prognosis rate in male patients with stage II breast cancer. Considering the role of hormonal therapy in male breast cancer, tamoxifen is still the first and main agent in the adjuvant treatment as well as in advance disease [36]. The role of second-line drugs such as aromatase inhibitors or LHRH analogues in the treatment of male breast cancer is not defined [37].

## 20.9 Prognosis

The prognosis varies and depends on the status of invasion and the presence or absence of palpable mass. Those patients presenting with palpable mass will invariably have an associated underlying carcinoma and high rate of lymphatic spread. Most literature shows an overall survival rate of 47% in patients with positive nodes and 93% in those with negative nodes [38]. Even though the clinical and pathological description in men is similar to that of women, considering prognosis, men seems to have worst prognosis. Still this remains controversial. Estimated 5-year survival rate is around 20–30% in males compared to 30–50% in females [39]. Obviously, as mentioned earlier in the chapter, this may be due to delay in the diagnosis.

**Conclusions**

Male Paget's disease of the nipple with breast cancer, though very rare, does exist. The pathology and clinical features of male breast cancer resemble that of female breast cancer. Paget's disease of the nipple is almost always associated with an underlying invasive breast cancer. Any involvement of nipple–areolar complex should be taken seriously and there should be no hesitation in resorting to biopsy. Apart from biopsy, immunohistochemistry plays a vital role in favoring the diagnosis as well as differentiating PD from other lesions. Of the molecular markers, CK7 and Her-2 have been proposed to be specific and sensitive markers for MPD. Furthermore, breast magnetic resonance imaging is a key factor in diagnosing MPD with or without lump. The surgical treatment plan should be selected on the basis of careful clinical assessment and extent of involvement of the cancer. Postoperative adjuvant therapies should be based on the final tumor nodal status. Overall, one should be aware of both the risks of under- and overtreating patients with Paget's disease of the breast.

## References


1. Paget J. On disease of the mammary areola preceding cancer of the mammary gland. St Bartholomew Hosp Rep. 1874;10:87–9.
2. El Harroudi T, Tijami F, Otmany A, Jalil A. Paget disease of the male nipple. J Cancer Res Ther. 2010;6(1):95–6.
3. Ucar AE, Korukluoglu B, Ergul E, Aydin R, Kusdemir A. Bilateral Paget's disease of the male nipple: first report. Breast. 2008;17:317–8.
4. Hunt KK, JFR R, Bland KI. The breast. In: Brunicardi FC, Andersen DK, Billiar TR, Dunn DL, Hunter JG, Matthews JB, Pollock RE, editors. Schwartz's manual of surgery. 10th ed. Columbus, OH: McGraw-Hill Co.; 2010. p. 497–564.
5. Choudhury B, Bright-Thomas RM. Paget's disease of the male breast with underlying ductal carcinoma in situ ('DCIS'). J Surg Case Rep. 2015;4:1–2.
6. Kanitakis J. Mammary and extramammary Paget's disease. J Eur Acad Dermatol Venereol. 2007;21:581–90.
7. Fouad D. Paget's disease of the breast in a male with lymphomatoidpapulosis: a case report. J Med Case Rep. 2011;5:43.
8. Schelfhout VR, Coene ED, Delaey B, Thys S, Page DL, De Potter CR. Pathogenesis of Paget's disease: epidermal heregulin-alpha, motility factor, and the HER receptor family. J Natl Cancer Inst. 2000;92:622–8.
9. Nedelcu I, Costache DO, Costache RS, Nedelcu D, Berbecar G, Nedelcu LE. Breast Paget disease: clinical, histopathological and immunohistochemical aspects. Balkan Military Med Rev. 2006;9:71–5.
10. Sakorafas GH, Blanchard K, Sarr MG, Farley DR. Paget's disease of the breast. Cancer Treat Rev. 2001;27(1):9–18.
11. Barth D. Bilateral Paget's disease of the breast—case report of long-time misdiagnosed tumors with underlying ductal carcinomas and review of the literature. Case Rep Dermatol Med. 2014;2014:152836.
12. Nagar RC. Bilateral Paget's disease of the nipple in a male. J Indian Med Assoc. 1983;81(3–4):55–6.
13. Kao GF, Graham JH, Helwig EB. Paget's disease of the ectopic breast with an underlying intraductal carcinoma: report of a case. J Cutan Pathol. 1986;13:59–66.
14. Martin VG, Pellettiere EV, Gress D, Miller AW. Paget's disease in an adolescent arising in a supernumerary nipple. J Cutan Pathol. 1994;21:283–6.
15. Lloyd J, Flanagan AM. Mammary and extramammary Paget's disease. J Clin Pathol. 2000;53:742–9.
16. Peschos D, Tsanou E, Dallas P, Charalabopoulos K, Kanaris C, Batistatou A. Mucinous breast carcinoma presenting as Paget's disease of the nipple in a man: a case report. Diagn Pathol. 2008;3:42.
17. Yim JH, Wick MR, Philpott GW, Norton JA, Doherty GM. Underlying pathology in mammary Paget's disease. J Ann Surg Oncol. 1997;4(4):287–92.
18. Nicholson BT, Harvey JA, Cohen MA. Nipple-areolar complex: normal anatomy and benign and malignant processes. Radiographics. 2009;29(2):509–23.
19. Reed W, Oppedal BR, Eeg Larsen T. Immunohistology is valuable in distinguishing between Paget's disease, Bowen's disease and superficial spreading malignant melanoma. Histopathology. 1990;16(6):583–8.
20. Pérez A, Sánchez JL, Colón AL. Pigmented mammary Paget's disease in a man. Bol Asoc Med P R. 2003;95:36–9.
21. Mitchell S, Lachica R, Randall MB, Beech DJ. Paget's disease of the breast areola mimicking cutaneous melanoma. Breast J. 2006;12(3):233–6.
22. Di Tommaso L, Franchi G, Destro A, Broglia F, Minuti F, Rahal D, Roncalli M. Toker cells of the breast. Morphological and immunohistochemical characterization of 40 cases. Hum Pathol. 2008;39:1295–300.
23. Park S, Suh YL. Useful immunohistochemical markers for distinguishing Paget cells from Toker cells. Pathology. 2009;41:640–4.
24. Rosen PP. Paget's disease of the nipple. In: Rosen PP, editor. Rosen's breast pathology. 2nd ed. Philadelphia: Lippincott-Raven; 2001. p. 565–80.
25. Yao DX, Hoda SA, Chiu A, Ring L, Rosen PP. Intraepidermal cytokeratin 7 immunoreactive cells in the non-neoplastic nipple may represent interepithelial extension of lactiferous duct cells. Histopathology. 2002;40(3):230–6.
26. Sek P, Zawrocki A, Biernat W, Piekarski JH. HER2 molecular subtype is a dominant subtype of mammary Paget's cells. An immunohistochemical study. Histopathology. 2010;57:564–71.
27. Gunhan-Bilgen I, Oktay A. Paget's disease of the breast: clinical, mammographic, sonographic and pathologic findings in 52 cases. Eur J Radiol. 2006;60:256–63.
28. Sripathi S, Ayachit A, Kadavigere R, Kumar S, Eleti A, Sraj A. Spectrum of imaging findings in Paget's disease of the breast-a pictorial review. Insights Imaging. 2015;6(4):419–29.
29. Akita M, Kusunoki N, Nakajima T, Takase S, Maekawa Y, Kajimoto K, Ohno M. Paget's disease of the male breast: a case report. Surg Case Rep. 2015;1(1):103.
30. Chen CY, Sun LM, Anderson BO. Paget disease of the breast: changing patterns of incidence, clinical presentation, and treatment in the US. Cancer. 2006;107(7):1448–58.
31. Nardelli AA, Stafinski T, Menin D. Effectiveness of photodynamic therapy for mammary and extra-

mammary Paget's disease: a state of the science review. BMC Dermatol. 2011;11:13.
32. Bernardi M, Brown AS, Malone JC, Callen JP. Paget disease in a man. J Arch Dermatol. 2008;144(12):1660–2.
33. Dominici LS, Liao GS, Guo L, Specht M, Smith BL, Golshan M. Current surgical approach to Paget's disease. Am J Surg. 2012;204(1):18–22.
34. Uthamalingam M, Periyasamy K. Paget's disease of nipple in male breast with cancer. J Clin Diagn Res. 2016;10(2):14–6.
35. Perkins GH, Middleton LP, Garcia SM, et al. Male breast carcinoma: outcomes and predictors of local-regional failure in patients treated without radiation therapy. Breast Cancer Res Treat. 2002;76:121.
36. Bagley CS, Wesley MN, Young RC, Lippman ME. Adjuvant chemotherapy in males with cancer of the breast. Am J Clin Oncol. 1987;10:55–60.
37. Fentiman IS. Endocrine therapy for male breast cancer. J Steroids Horm Sci. 2013;4(1):112.
38. Kawase K, Dimaio DJ, Tucker SL, Buchholz TA, Ross MI, Feig BW, Kuerer HM, Meric-Bernstam F, Babiera G, Ames FC, Singletary SE, Hunt KK. Paget's disease of the breast: there is a role for breast-conserving therapy. Ann Surg Oncol. 2005;12:391–7.
39. Nakamara S, Hashimoto Y, Yokoo H. Pigmented Paget's disease of the male breast; report of a case. Dermatology. 2001;202:134–7.

# Leiomyosarcoma of the Nipple-Areola Complex

# 21

Xavier Guedes de la Puente

## 21.1 Introduction

When talking about sarcomas, we have to understand that they account for less than 1% of all malignant tumors of the breast. Primary breast leiomyosarcomas belong to an even smaller subgroup, accounting for about 5–10% of these sarcomas, making it an even rarer entity [1, 2]. In 1968 Waterworth [3] described the first convincing case of leiomyosarcoma of the breast, and since then less than 45 cases have been reported in the English literature, with only a few of these affecting the nipple-areola complex.

Leiomyosarcoma is not a rare tumor on itself. It can exist in any part of the body, but usually it affects the retroperitoneum, subcutaneous tissues, the gastrointestinal tract, and the uterus [4]. In the breast there is still controversy on the origin of this tumor. It is believed to originate from the smooth muscle cells of the vascular walls in the mammary parenchyma, and in the nipple it might originate from the smooth muscle bundles that surround the lactiferous ducts and the arrector pili muscle, with a sarcomatous change from a leiomyoma or other spindle cell tumors. The differential diagnosis will include other tumors of both mammary and cutaneous origins, such as leiomyoma, cystosarcoma phyllodes, dermatofibroma protuberans, malignant peripheral nerve sheath tumors, sarcomatoid carcinoma, spindle cell malignant melanoma, and malignant fibrous histiocytoma [2, 4].

## 21.2 Clinical Features and Diagnosis

From the cases described, we know that this tumor affects mostly postmenopausal women between the ages of 50 and 80 years old though there have been a few reports of young females and male subjects affected [5, 6]. Clinically they usually present as a painless slow-growing firm lobulated mass in the breast similar to a malignant phyllodes tumor, sometimes painful, but with no deformity, nipple discharge, nipple retraction, or skin lesions, though there is one case described with suppuration of a plaque-type lesion and in the nipple (Fig. 21.1) [2, 7]. Palpable axillary lymph nodes have been reported, but as we will discuss later, these findings will not correlate with an increase risk for lymphatic spread of the disease.

Diagnosis of this type of sarcoma can be challenging. Mammography and ultrasonography are not adequate tools for a definite diagnosis because of the difficulty in differentiating them from

X. Guedes de la Puente, M.D.
Guilleries 1, 3-2, 08500 Barcelona, Spain

Department of General Surgery,
Vic University Hospital, Barcelona, Spain
e-mail: xavierguedes@gmail.com


M.A. Shiffman (ed.), *Nipple-Areolar Complex Reconstruction*,
https://doi.org/10.1007/978-3-319-60925-6_21

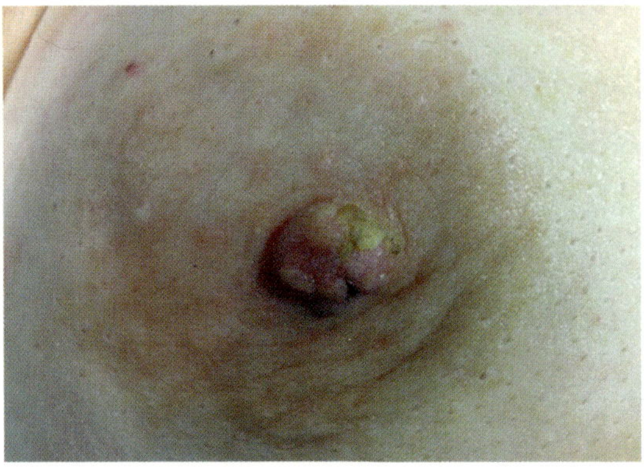

**Fig. 21.1** Nodular mass with a superficial plaque-type lesion on the left upper side of the nipple and part of the areola, being an unusual clinical presentation of leiomyosarcoma

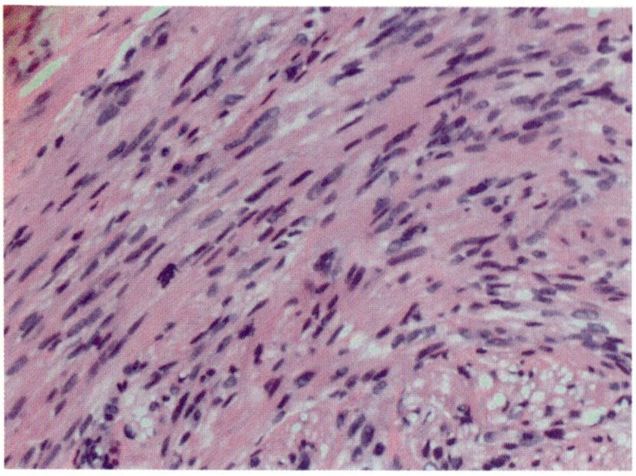

**Fig. 21.2** Smooth muscle cells with elongated nuclei and mitotic activity (visible on the left side of the sample) (HE stain)

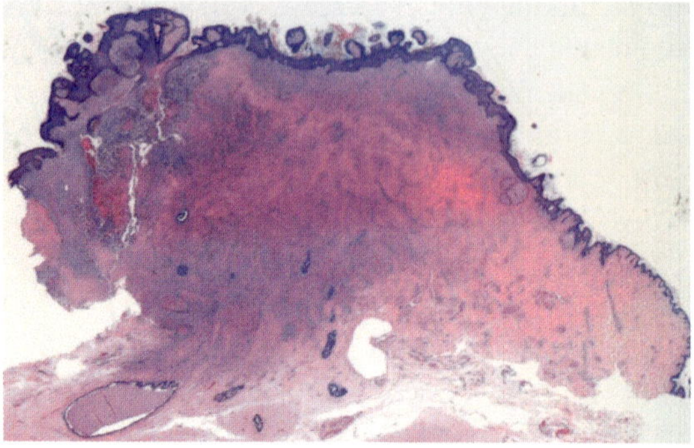

**Fig. 21.3** Leiomyosarcoma seen as a nodular lesion affecting the nipple and the left margin of the areola (HE stain)

benign lesions such as fibroadenomas, phyllodes tumors, or intracystic papillomas. Fine needle aspiration cytology (FNAC) and surgical or core needle biopsies are usually not enough for adequate diagnosis. Leiomyosarcoma is diagnosed in most cases after complete excision of the tumor with a detailed histologic examination and immunohistochemistry. This is why most cases are not diagnosed preoperatively [8, 9]. When proper diagnosis has been achieved, a chest and abdominopelvic CT scan is usually performed for neoplastic extension study.

Cytology of breast leiomyosarcomas will show large, dissociated epithelial-like cells, round or elongated, and with pleomorphic vesicular nuclei, prominent nucleoli, and usually a poorly defined cytoplasm, with numerous mitotic figures present. Hyperchromatic spindle-like shaped cells with oval and blunt-ended nuclei arranged in bundles or interdigitating fascicles are often present (Figs. 21.2 and 21.3). Mitosis is an important characteristic present in this neoplasm [10]. In previous literature, the mitosis of these tumors ranged from 2 to 21 per 10 HPF. Most authors agree that the presence of three or more mitoses per 10 HPF is what differentiates a leiomyosarcoma from a leiomyoma [11]. Necrosis can be present but is not always evident. As mentioned before, immunohistochemistry plays an important diagnostic role because the malignant spindle cells of the tumor are immunoreactive for smooth muscle actin, vimentin, caloponin, and desmin and negative for epithelial markers, neural tumor marker (PS 100), cytokeratins, hormone, and growth factor receptors [9, 11, 12]. It is important to point out that these immunohistochemical findings are not pathognomonic of this type or sarcomas, thus not diagnostic on their own. When findings are not conclusive, demonstration of myofilaments on electron microscopy can be helpful [6].

## 21.3 Treatment and Prognosis

Leiomyosarcomas of the breast including the nipple-areola complex, as with any unusual pathology with a limited amount of cases described and poor long-term follow-up, lack a clear treatment consensus.

Primary cutaneous leiomyosarcoma in other parts of the body is usually treated with wide local excision with adequate margins, usually 3–5 cm, including subcutaneous fascia and tissue, with adequate results. Wide local excision and lumpectomy have been related with higher local recurrence and metastasis, so most authors recommend simple or modified radical mastectomy as the treatment of choice. In the case of nipple-areola leiomyosarcoma, both treatments can be seen described in the literature [2, 6]. Sentinel lymph node biopsy or axillary lymph node dissection is considered unnecessary. As in other breast sarcomas, lymphatic spread and nodal metastasis occur in less than 10% of patients, and in leiomyosarcomas lymphatic spread is considered extremely uncommon [1, 13]. Adem et al. emphasize that when lymph node metastasis is present, the diagnosis of a metaplastic carcinoma should be considered even in the presence of a pure spindle cell neoplasm [1].

The need for adjuvant chemoradiotherapy is unclear. Chemotherapy has been described as a treatment option, always after adequate surgical excision, with varied results, and is considered a risk factor for developing a second malignancy after treatment. Hormone manipulation is not an option as these tumors are usually not hormone dependent [14]. The use of radiation therapy usually depends on the failure to obtain negative margins during surgical excision. The development of a secondary neoplasm after radiation therapy is well described in literature, and it has been observed that leiomyosarcoma is the more prevalent sarcoma occurring after breast cancer (data from the Surveillance, Epidemiology and End Result) with an incidence of 22.1%, followed by malignant fibrous histiocytoma (15.2%), angiosarcoma (13.7%), and liposarcoma (8.7%) [15]. Of course, increasing reports of second neoplasms after treatment of a primary breast cancer are due to the increase in survival of these patients due to multimodal treatment, and radiation-induced sarcomas have a low incidence overall. Combined or not with multimodal treatments, usually this type of sarcomas treated with adequate surgical excision presents a total remission of the disease, though leiomyosarcomas have been seen to return many years later.

Prognostic factors described for this type of neoplasm are similar to other soft tissue sarcomas. Better prognosis has been associated with smaller tumor size, extent of surgery with adequate surgical margins, and low cellular pleomorphism [1, 10].

Wong et al. [2] mentions on his review of cases that leiomyosarcoma of the nipple-areola complex has less local recurrences or metastases compared to those located on mammary parenchyma, though he admits long-term follow-up is needed. In general, prognosis of patients with leiomyosarcoma is better than in patients with other breast sarcomas [16, 17], but adequate and prolonged follow-up has to be carried out in all cases, and if adjuvant therapy has been used, the possibility of secondary neoplasms has to be taken into account.

## References

1. Adem C, Reynolds C, Ingle JN, Nascimento AG. Primary breast sarcoma: clinicopathologic series from the Mayo Clínic and review of the literature. Br J Cancer. 2004;91:23741.
2. Wong L, Huang P, Luh S, Huang C. Primary leiomyosarcoma of the nipple-areola complex: report of a case and review of literature. J Zhejiang Univ Sci B. 2008;9(2):109–13.
3. Waterworth PD, Gompertz RHK, Hennessy C. Primary leiomyosarcoma of the breast. Br J Surg. 1992;79:169–71.
4. Szekely E, Madaras L, Kulka J, Jaray B, Nagy L. Leiomyosarcoma of the female breast. Pathol Oncol Res. 2001;7:151–3.
5. Boehm D, Keller K, Schmidt M, Cotarelo C, Kern A, Lebrecht A, Koelbl H. Primary leiomyosarcoma of the male breast. World J Oncol. 2010;I(5):210–2.
6. Rane SU, Batra C, Saikia UN. Primary leiomyosarcoma of breast in an adolescent girl: a case report and review of the literature. Case Rep Pathol. 2012;2012:491984.
7. Guedes X, Medarde M, Parra T, Martinez MJ, Caralt E, Serra C. Primary leiomyosarcoma of the nipple-areola complex with an unusual clinical presentation: a case report. Int J Case Rep Images. 2014;5(1):66–70.
8. Kamio T, Nishizawa M, Aoyama K, Ohchi T, Nishikawa T, Kobayashi M, Kameoka S. Primary leiomyosarcoma of the breast treated by partial resection

of the breast including the nipple and areola: report of a case. Surg Today. 2010;40(11):1063–7.
9. Oktay Y, Fikret A. Leiomyosarcoma of the breast. J Surg Case Rep. 2011;2011(7):1.
10. Alejo-Sanchez M, Martinez MJ, Autonell J. Leiomiosarcoma de mama. Rev Esp Patol. 1999;32(1):67–70.
11. Nascimiento AG, Rosen PP, Karas M, Caron AG. Leiomyoma of the nipple. Am J Surg Pathol. 1979;3:151–4.
12. Markaki S, Sotiropoulou M, Hanioti C, Lazaris D. Leiomyosarcoma of the breast. A clinicopathologic and immunohistochemical study. Eur J Obstet Gynecol Reprod Biol. 2003;106(2):223–36.
13. Ugras S, Dilek ON, Karaayvaz M, Dilek H, Peker O, Barut I. Primary leiomyosarcoma of the breast. Jpn J Surg. 1997;27(11):1082–5.
14. Hussien M, Sivananthan S, Anderson N, Shiels A, Tracey N, Olding-Smee GW. Primary leiomyosarcoma of the breast: diagnosis, management and outcome. A report of a new case and review of literature. Breast. 2001;10(6):530–4.
15. Olcina M, Merck B, Giménez-Climent MJ, Almenar S, Sancho-Merle MF, Llopis F, Vazquez-Albadalejo C. Radiation-induced leiomyosarcoma after breast cancer treatment and TRAM flap reconstruction. Sarcoma. 2008;2008:456950.
16. El M'rabet FZ, El Kacemi H, El Mesbahi O, El Hassouni K, El Gueddari BK. Primary breast leiomyosarcoma: case report and literature review. Health. 2011;3(10):620–2.
17. Pollard SG, Marks PV, Temple LN, Thompson HH. Breast sarcoma. A clinicopathologic review of 25 cases. Cancer. 1990;66:941–4.

# 22 Leiomyoma of the Nipple

Efstratios Vakirlis

## 22.1 Introduction

Leiomyoma is a benign neoplasm of smooth muscle. Most frequently it occurs in the genitourinary and gastrointestinal tracts and less frequently in the skin. Cutaneous Leiomyomas may be further categorized in five types: (a) multiple piloleiomyomas, (b) solitary piloleiomyomas, (c) solitary angioleiomyoma, (d) genital leiomyoma, and (e) leiomyomas with additional mesenchymal elements [1]. Piloleiomyomas are believed to arise from the arrector pili muscle, and they are located on the extremities and trunk, whereas angioleiomyomas derived from tunica media of small arteries and veins and typically present on the extremities [2]. Genital leiomyomas are derived from dartos muscle of the scrotum and the labia majora or from the erectile smooth muscle of the nipple. Leiomyoma of the mammary papilla is a rare, benign, cutaneous lesion that is thought to arise from smooth muscle fibers in the subareolar tissue of the breast [3]. Diaz-Arias et al. [4] suggested that the origin of these tumors may be from (a) teratoid origin with extensive overgrowth of the myomatous elements, (b) embryologically displaced smooth muscle from nipple, (c) angiomatous smooth muscle, (d) multipotent mesenchymal cells, and (e) myoepithelial cells.

E. Vakirlis, M.D., Ph.D.
First Department of Dermatology-Venereology, Aristotle University Medical School, 3, Gr. Palama Str., Thessaloniki 54622, Greece
e-mail: svakirlis@hotmail.com

## 22.2 Background

Leiomyoma was first described by Virchow in 1854 [5], and the hereditary form, of multiple leiomyomas, was originally noted by Kloepfer et al. [6] in 1958. Leiomyoma of the nipple is of unknown epidemiology and hereditary predisposition, with only about 50 cases reported in the literature until now.

Data to determine whether a racial predilection exists are inadequate [7].

It is more frequent in women but rarely occurs also in men [8]. Approximate ratio female/male = 3:1 [9].

Sometimes cutaneous leiomyomas may be a sign of underlying systemic disease (e.g. renal malignancy) [9].

## 22.3 Clinical Presentation

The lesions are smaller than 2 cm in diameter and are usually solitary, asymptomatic for long periods, papules or nodules but in a few cases can cause pain spontaneously, or in response to stimuli such as cold, pressure, or emotional stress [9]. The pain, most probably, occurs secondary to


M.A. Shiffman (ed.), *Nipple-Areolar Complex Reconstruction*,
https://doi.org/10.1007/978-3-319-60925-6_22

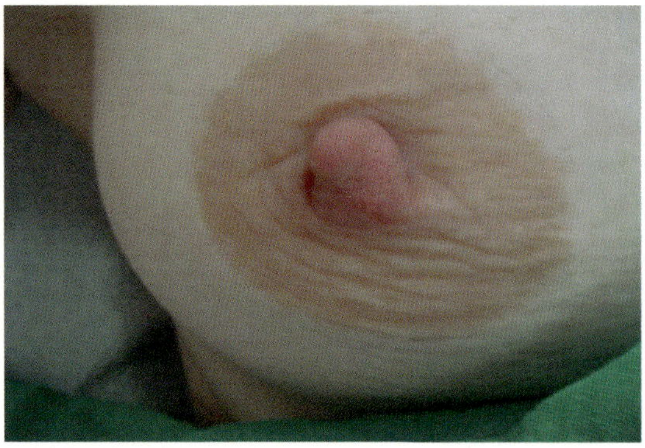

**Fig. 22.1** Nipple leiomyoma

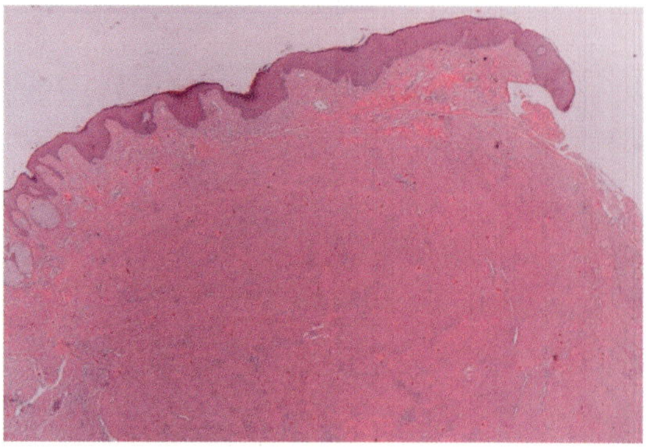

**Fig. 22.2** Skin section of the nipple with a well-circumscribed tumor in the dermis

calcium-dependent contraction of smooth muscle cells within the tumor [10], and that is why calcium channel blockers and α-adrenergic blockers are used as a palliative treatment. However, the pain may also be secondary due to pressure on nerve fibers within the tumor. Pain does not improve with time, and due to its constant presence, it affects the quality of patients' life. Nipple leiomyoma is usually unilateral, although bilateral involvement has been reported [9]. Ku et al. [11] reported multiple lesions on the areola of one nipple, while Gokdemir et al. [12] reported multiple lesions on both nipples.

Clinical examination may reveal a small, oval, red-brown or pink, firm subcutaneous papule that enlarges the nipple [12]. The nipple is becoming quite tender and indurated to palpation. Wang et al. [13] reported the only patient with nipple inversion caused by a breast leiomyoma. Breast examination reveals no abnormality, no associated regional lymphadenopathy, and no discharge from the nipple. There have been reports of leiomyomas developed in a patient receiving tamoxifen [14, 15] (a nonsteroidal antiestrogen agent), other oral contraceptives (ethinylestradiol and cyproterone acetate), and also after traumatic abrasion during breastfeeding period (Fig. 22.1) [16].

## 22.4 Imaging Studies

Ultrasonography and mammogram are indicated preoperatively, with no specific findings. Color Doppler sonogram and magnetic resonance imaging (MRI) [17] of the breast are not routinely performed, but their findings are sometimes important for differential diagnosis of the lesion.

## 22.5 Histopathology

Nipple leiomyomas are smooth muscle tumors and usually well differentiated (Fig. 22.2) [16]. Usually they occur in the reticular dermis and the adjacent mammary gland and are not encapsulated. The smooth muscle bundles of these tumors are interlaced with variable amounts of collagen. The tumor consists of interconnecting bundles of smooth muscles cells in straight or whorled arrangements. The characteristic smooth muscle nuclei are slightly elongated and blunt-ended or cigar-shaped. In cross section the eosinophilic cytoplasm of these cells appears vacuolated [18].

There is no necrosis, nuclear atypia, or mitotic activity observed, but occasional, random mitosis can be identified. The overlying epidermis may appear normal or show effacement of the rete ridge pattern, but epidermal hyperplasia (acanthosis) may be present in more than 50% of the cases [19]. In a recent article published by Lopez et al. [20], the epidermis is hyperkeratotic with increased pigmentation of the basal layer.Special stains can be used to distinguish smooth muscle from collagen, both of which are pinkish red on hematoxylin-eosin staining. Masson trichrome stain highlights smooth muscle as dark red and collagen as blue green. With aniline blue stains,

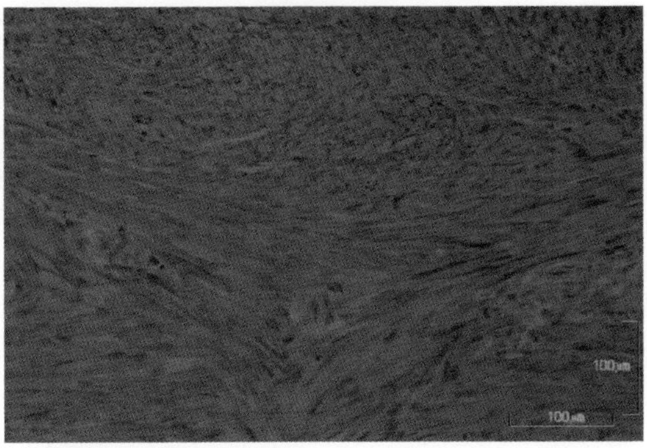

**Fig. 22.3** The neoplastic cells expressed cytoplasmic immunoreactivity for the smooth muscle actin antigen

smooth muscle becomes red and collagen blue. A van Gieson stain results in yellow smooth muscle contrasted against red collagen. With phosphotungstic acid-hematoxylin (PTAH) stain, myofibrils are purple [7]. Immunohistochemical staining for smooth muscle actin (SMA), desmin, and vimentin, but not S100 or cytokeratin, that are markers of smooth muscle cells can be performed to detect these tumor cells in nipple leiomyomas (Fig. 22.3) [16].

Chaudhary et al. [3] confirmed the relationship between subareolar smooth muscle fibers and nipple leiomyoma in females and demonstrated the consistent presence of estrogen receptor (ER) and progesterone receptor (PgR) in the normal subareolar muscle cells and their benign tumor counterpart. On the other hand, Nakamura et al. [8] described two cases of male nipple leiomyomas with negative ER and PgR.

## 22.6 Diagnosis

Diagnosis of nipple leiomyoma requires the following:

1. Patient's history.
2. Physical examination of both breasts in order to reveal any calcification, skin distortion, inflammation, discharge, or even pain during palpation.
3. Palpation for lymph nodes in axillary and supraclavicular region.
4. Imaging tests (ultrasound, color Doppler sonography, mammography, breast MRI).
5. For the establishment of the diagnosis, tissue examination is necessary. A partial or excisional biopsy of the lesion should be performed.

## 22.7 Differential Diagnosis

Multiple disease entities resemble leiomyoma of the nipple and should be differentiated [21]:

1. Angiolipoma
2. Glomus tumors
3. Paget's disease
4. Neurofibroma
5. Lymphadenosis benigna cutis
6. Myoid hamartoma
7. Breast carcinomas
8. Leiomyosarcoma of the areola
9. Erosive adenomatosis of the nipple
10. Eccrine spiradenomas
11. Mastocytoma
12. Neurilemoma
13. Nevi
14. Lipomas

## 22.8 Treatment

Surgical excision with or without skin grafting, with histologically confirmed tumor-free margins, is the treatment of choice in painful solitary leiomyomas of the nipple [16, 22]. Re-excision should be performed in the case of positive margin, with immediate reconstruction of the nipple-areola complex [23]. Despite the low incidence of the specific tumor, there are articles for cutaneous leiomyomas reporting their high rate of recurrence [11], which sometimes reaches 50% [23].

There are limited studies for the treatment of these tumors. In cases of painful lesions, calcium channel blockers, α-blockers, gabapentin, cryotherapy, nitroglycerin, hyoscine hydrobromide, lidocaine, and analgesics have been used [24]. However, surgery is sometimes contraindicated. In this case, $CO_2$ laser has been used to treat nipple leiomyomas with good results and low recurrence rate [20, 24]. The procedure is safe and rapid and enables precise selection of tissue, minimal damage to surrounding tissue, and minimal bleeding, because it promotes coagulation.

An alternative to the $CO_2$ laser is the erbium-doped yttrium aluminum garnet (Er:YAG) laser. It can vaporize the skin at a lower penetration depth than the $CO_2$ laser, but it is insufficient to promote coagulation and prevent bleeding during surgery [20].

**Conclusions**

Leiomyoma of the nipple is a rare, benign tumor that arises from smooth muscle. It usually appears as solitary tender nodule. Surgical excision with histologically confirmed tumor-free margins is the treatment of choice.

## References

1. Ragsdale B. Tumors with fatty, muscular, osseous, and cartilaginous differentiation. In: Elder DE, Elenitsas R, Jhonson BL, Murphy GF, editors. Lever's histopathology of the skin. 9th ed. Philadelphia: Wolters Kluwer-Lippincott Williams & Wilkins; 2005. p. 1061–107.
2. Malik K, Patel P, Chen J, Khachemoune A. Leiomyoma cutis: a focused review on presentation, management, and association with malignancy. Am J Clin Dermatol. 2015;16(1):35–46.
3. Chaudhary KS, Shousha S. Leiomyoma of the nipple, and normal subareolar muscle fibres, are oestrogen and progesterone receptor positive. Histopathology. 2004;44:626–8.
4. Diaz-Arias AA, Hurt MA, Loy TS, Seeger RM, Bickel JT. Leiomyoma of the breast. Hum Pathol. 1989;20:396–9.
5. Virchow R. Ueber Makroglossie und pathologische Neubildung quergestreifter Muskelfasern. Virchows Arch Pathol Anat. 1854;7:126–38.
6. Kloepfer HW, Krafchuk J, Derbes V. Hereditary multiple leiomyoma of the skin. Am J Hum Genet. 1958;10(1):48–52.
7. Horner KL. Leiomyoma. 2016. http://emedicine.medscape.com/article/1057733-overview. Accessed 25 July 16.
8. Nakamura S, Hashimoto Y, Takeda K, Nishi K, Ishida-Yamamoto A, Mizumoto T, Lizuka H. Two cases of male nipple leiomyoma: idiopathic leiomyoma and gynecomastia-associated leiomyoma. Am J Dermatopathol. 2012;34(3):287–91.
9. Deveci U, Kapakli MS, Altintoprak F, Cayırcı M, Manukyan MN, Kebudi A. Bilateral nipple leiomyoma. Case Rep Surg. 2013;2013:475215.
10. Thompson JA Jr. Therapy for painful cutaneous leiomyomas. J Am Acad Dermatol. 1985;13(5 Pt 2):865–7.
11. Ku J, Campbell C, Bennett I. Leiomyoma of the nipple. Breast J. 2006;12(4):377–80.
12. Gokdemir G, Sakiz D, Koslu A. Multiple cutaneous leiomyomas of the nipple. J Eur Acad Dermatol Venereol. 2006;20(4):468–9.
13. Wang H, Luo B, Li F. Nipple inversion caused by a breast leiomyoma. Breast J. 2012;18(4):376–7.
14. Kaufman HL, Hirsch EF. Leiomyoma of the breast. J Surg Oncol. 1996;62:62–4.
15. Son EJ, Oh KK, Kim EK, Son HJ, Jung WH, Lee HD. Leiomyoma of the breast in a 50-year-old woman receiving tamoxifen. AJR Am J Roentgenol. 1998;171(6):1684–6.
16. Pavlidis L, Vakirlis E, Spyropoulou G, Pramateftakis MG, Dionyssiou D, Demiri E. A 35-year-old woman presenting with an unusual post-traumatic leiomyoma of the nipple: a case report. J Med Case Rep. 2013;7:49–51.
17. Cho HJ, Kim SH, Kang BJ, Kim H, Song BJ, Lee AW. Leiomyoma of the nipple diagnosed by MRI. Acta Radiol Short Rep. 2012;1(9). pii: arsr.2012.120025.
18. Patterson JW. Tumors of muscle, cartilage and bone. In: Practical skin pathology: a diagnostic approach. Philadelphia: Elsevier; 2013. p. 582–3.
19. Raj S, Calonje E, Kraus M, Kavanagh G, Newman PL, Fletcher CD. Cutaneous pilar leiomyoma: clinicopathologic analysis of 53 lesions in 45 patients. Am J Dermatopathol. 1997;19(1):2–9.
20. López V, López I, Alcacer J, Ricart JM. Successful treatment of leiomyoma of the nipple with carbon dioxide laser. Actas Dermosifiliogr. 2013;104(10):928–30.
21. Khachemoune A, Rodriguez C, Lyle S, Jiang SB. Genital leiomyoma: surgical excision for both diagnosis and treatment of a unilateral leiomyoma of the male nipple. Dermatol Online J. 2005;11(1):20.
22. Malhotra P, Walia H, Singh A, Ramesh V. Leiomyoma cutis: a clinicopathological series of 37 cases. Indian J Dermatol. 2010;55(4):337–41.
23. Masamatti SS, Manjunath HR, Babu BD. Leiomyoma of nipple: a rare case report and review of literature. Int J Sci Stud. 2015;3(6):210–3.
24. Christenson LJ, Smith K, Arpey CJ. Treatment of multiple cutaneous leiomyomas with $CO_2$ laser ablation. Dermatol Surg. 2000;26:319–22.

# 23 Malignant Melanoma of the Breast

Sarah Norton, Matthew Sills,
and Gerard O'Donoghue

## 23.1 Introduction

Worldwide the incidence of cutaneous malignant melanoma has been exponentially rising [1]. Malignant melanoma accounts for 1–2% of all cancer diagnoses and 75% of skin cancer-related deaths globally [2]. Furthermore, studies have identified an increased risk in people of European origin [3, 4]. Similarly in Ireland, in a Celtic population, the incidence of malignant melanoma has been increasing yearly by 3% and 5% in females and males, respectively. More importantly, mortality rates from melanoma have also been rising with a 2.2% and a 6% yearly rise in melanoma-related deaths in women and men in Ireland, respectively [5].

Cutaneous malignant melanoma metastatic deposits account for the majority of malignant melanoma cases. However, there have been several cases of primary melanoma of the breast reported [6–9]. Similar to malignant melanoma at other sites, that which occurs on the breast is often from a pre-existing nevus. Changes in its size and shape, pigmentation, ulceration or bleeding should raise suspicion for a melanoma of the breast (Fig. 23.1).

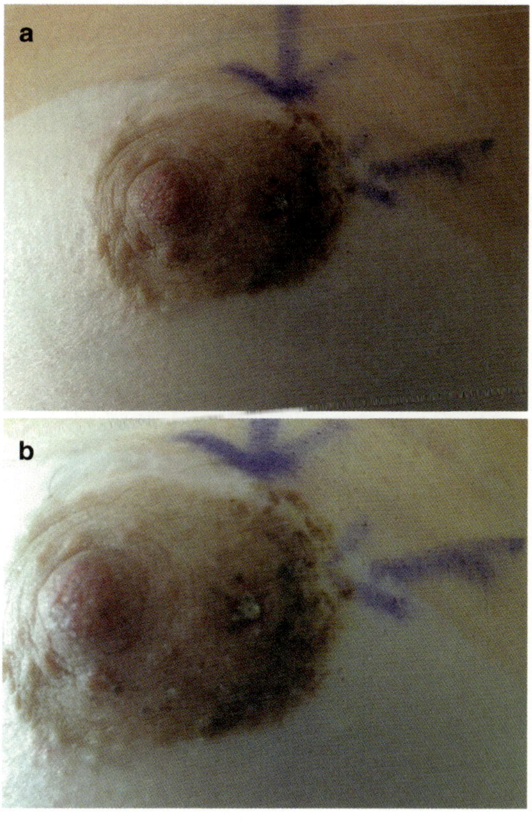


**Fig. 23.1** (**a**, **b**) Nipple-areolar complex pigmented lesion. Photos courtesy of the Department of Surgery, University Hospital Waterford

S. Norton, M.B., B.Ch., B.A.O., B.Sc., MRCSI (✉)
University Hospital Waterford, Waterford, Ireland
e-mail: sarahnorton@rcsi.ie

M. Sills • G. O'Donoghue
Department of Surgery, University Hospital
Waterford, Waterford, Ireland


M.A. Shiffman (ed.), *Nipple-Areolar Complex Reconstruction*,
https://doi.org/10.1007/978-3-319-60925-6_23

## 23.2 Diagnosing a Melanoma of the Breast

Preoperatively, an ultrasound of the breast in young patients should be performed to rule out any underlying lesions. If the patient is older, a mammogram should be performed. If the imaging is negative, an excision biopsy of the lesion should be undertaken. This allows for analysis of histology.

## 23.3 Histological Prognostic Factors

Histology allows the analysis of the subtype of melanoma, its mitotic rate, the presence of perineural or lymphovascular invasion, the involvement of the excision margins, and also whether the lesion has a vertical or horizontal growth phase pattern (Figs. 23.2 and 23.3).

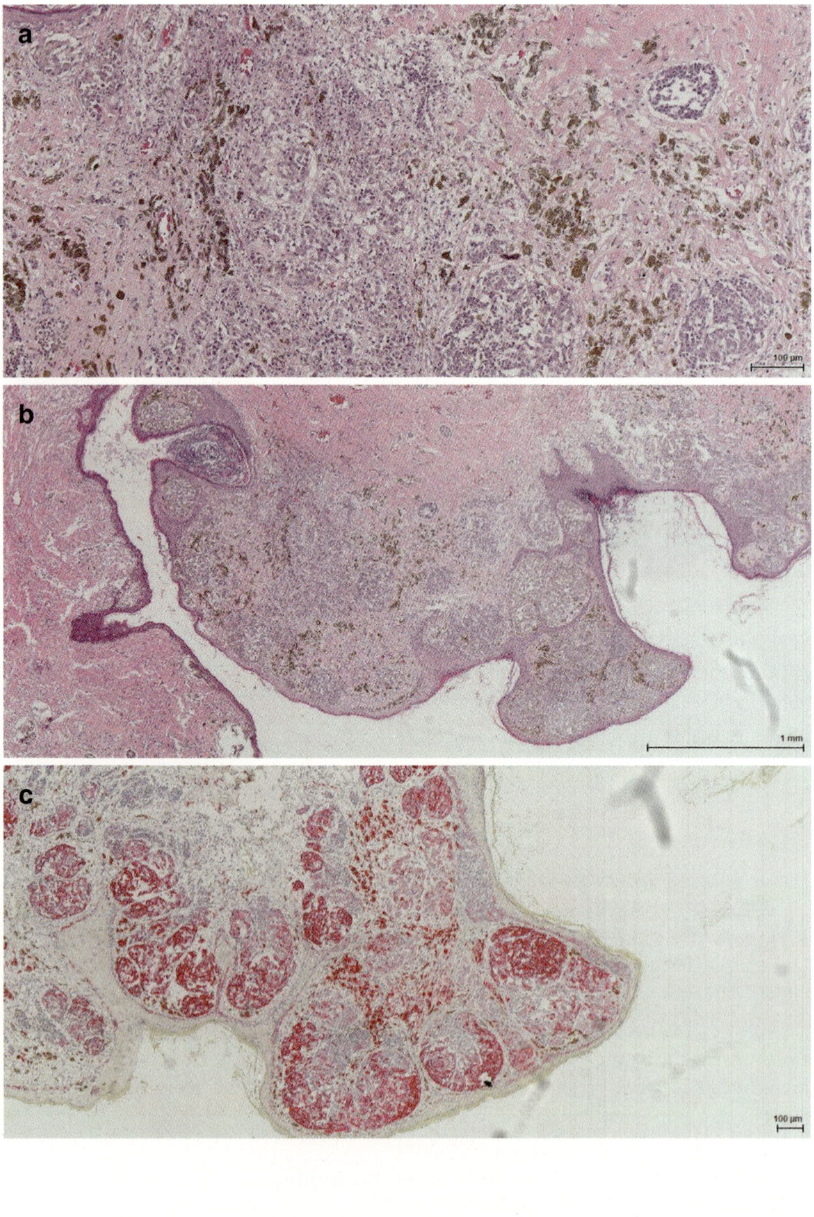


**Fig. 23.2** (**a**) High power. (**b**) Low power. (**c**) HMB 45. (**d**) Melanocytes. Photos courtesy of the Department of Surgery, University Hospital Waterford

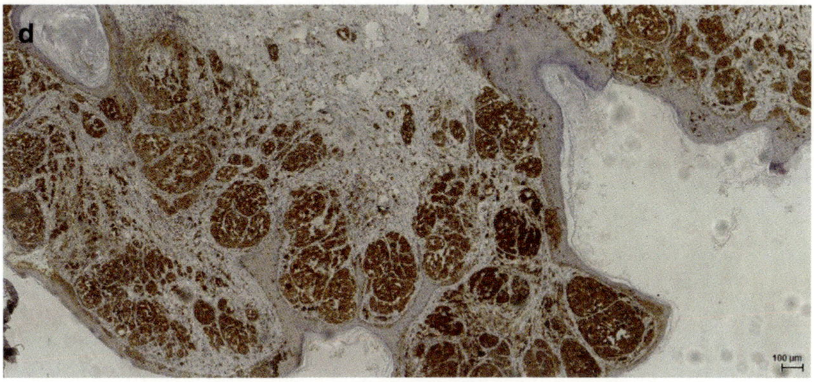


**Fig. 23.2** (continued)

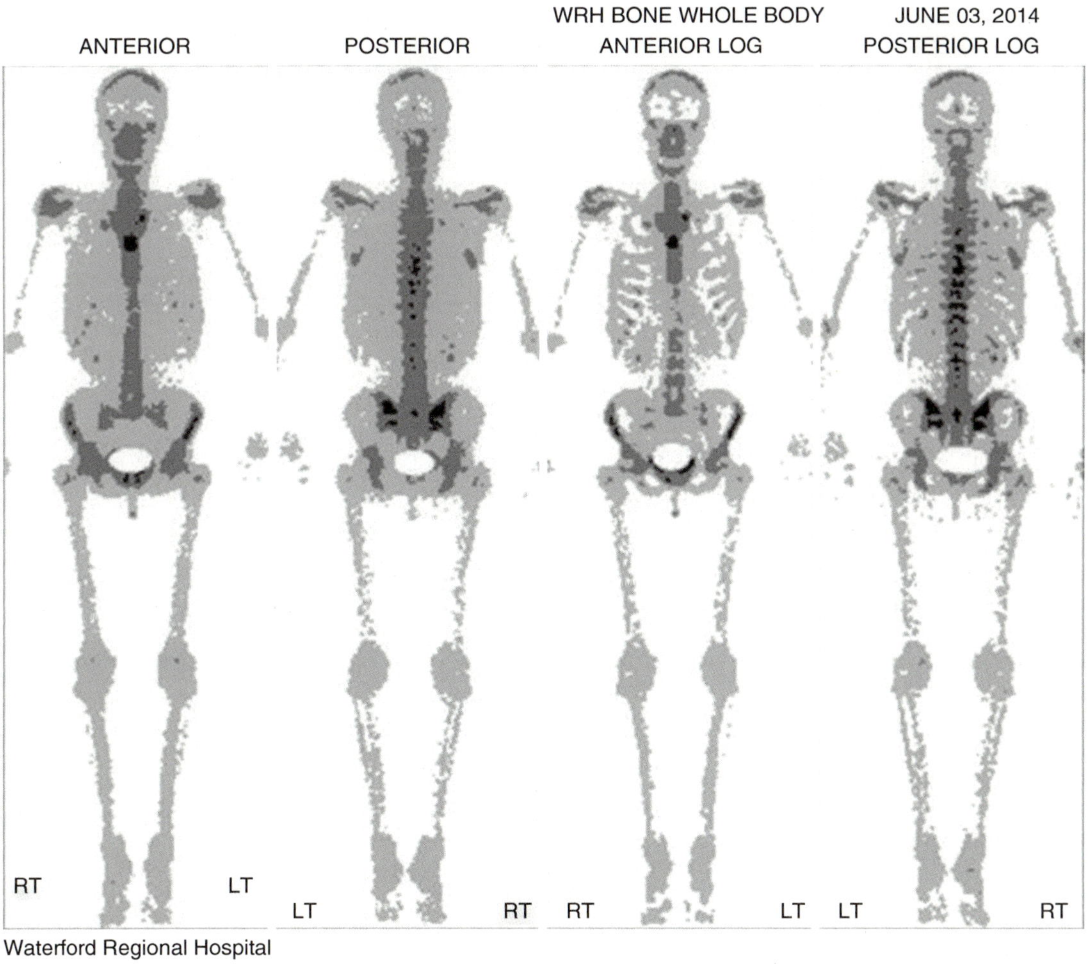


**Fig. 23.3** Nuclear medicine bone scan showing abnormal sterno-manubrial junction activity

The Breslow thickness, Clark's level and the presence of any metastatic deposits are very important prognostic indicators, as is the case for malignant melanomas at other sites on the body [10].

## 23.4 Management Following a Diagnosis

If the histology results demonstrate that the lesion is a malignant melanoma, a wide local excision of the scar should be undertaken. The aim of this is to ensure that surgical margins free of disease are obtained, and the clear margin requirement is based on Breslow thickness. This along with staging imaging should be performed, as set out by the European Society for Medical Oncology guidelines [11]. Following this diagnosis is a sentinel lymph node biopsy with lymphoscintigraphic mapping. This minimally invasive procedure is a good prognostic and survival predictor. Consultation with the medical oncology team will be required once histology is available. As highlighted in a recent paper, a patient history of tattoo ink is important to obtain. Pigmentation of nodes can occur from tattoo ink and be mistaken for a nodal metastatic deposit [6].

## 23.5 Discussion

The diagnosis of malignant melanoma is a rare one. It should be considered in a patient with a pigmented lesion that has undergone any visible change. This is important, as failure to diagnose malignant melanoma would lead to undertreatment with devastating consequences. Once the diagnosis has been confirmed by histology, a wide local excision must be undertaken with sentinel lymph node biopsy and lymphoscintigraphic mapping. A history of use of tattoo ink can result in pigmented nodes from carbon deposition with the potential for an incorrect presumptive diagnosis of malignant melanoma metastatic spread.

**Conclusions**

A consideration of a diagnosis of malignant melanoma of the breast should be made for any patient presenting with a pigmented lesion so as to ensure that it is not undertreated. On the other hand, overtreatment with nodal clearance must also be avoided by obtaining a history from the patient regarding previous tattoo ink use.

## References

1. Godar DE. Worldwide increasing incidences of cutaneous malignant melanoma. J Skin Cancer. 2011;2011:858425.
2. Lens MB, Dawes M. Global perspectives of contemporary epidemiological trend of cutaneous malignant melanoma. Br J Dermatol. 2004;150(2):179–85.
3. Merrill SJ, Subramanian M, Godar DE. Worldwide cutaneous malignant melanoma incidences analysed by sex, age, and skin type over time (1955–2007): is HPV infection of androgenic hair follicular melanocytes a risk factor for developing melanoma exclusively in people of European-ancestry? Dermatoendocrinology. 2016;8(1):e1215391.
4. Merrill SJ, Ashrafi S, Subramanian M, et al. Exponentially increasing incidences of cutaneous malignant melanoma in Europe correlate with low personal annual UV doses and suggests two major risk factors. Dermatoendocrinology. 2015;7(1):e1004018.
5. National Cancer Registry. Cancer in Ireland 1994–2012: annual report of the National Cancer Registry. Cork, Ireland: NCR; 2014.
6. Sills M, Norton S, Landers R, et al. Malignant melanoma of the breast: a case report. J Cancer Biol Res. 2016;4(1):1075.
7. Yujun HE, Jianghong MOU, Donglin LOU, Bo GAO, Yyuan WEN. Primary malignant melanoma of the breast: a case report and review of the literature. Oncol Lett. 2014;8:238–40.
8. Pressman PI. Malignant melanoma and the breast. Cancer. 1973;31:784–92.
9. Vasudevan JA, Somanathan T, Mathews A, Kattoor J. Malignant melanoma of breast: a unique case with diagnostic dilemmas. Indian J Pathol Microbiol. 2014;57:287–9.
10. Balch CM, Gershenwald JE, Soong SJ, Thompson JF, et al. Final version of 2009 AJCC melanoma staging and classification. J Clin Oncol. 2009;27(36):6199–206.
11. Drummer R, Hauschild A, Lindenblatt N, Pentheroudakis G, Keilholz U. Cutaneous melanoma: ESMO Clinical Practice Guidelines for diagnosis, treatment and follow-up. Ann Oncol. 2015;26(Suppl 5):126–32.

# Basal Cell Carcinoma of the Nipple-Areolar Complex

24

Kimberly A. Chun and Philip R. Cohen

## 24.1 Introduction

Basal cell carcinoma (BCC) accounts for approximately 80% of all nonmelanoma skin cancers; it is the most common skin malignancy [1]. The main risk factor associated with BCC development is exposure to ultraviolet radiation. However, BCCs infrequently occur in photoprotected sites such as the nipple-areolar complex (NAC). Higher rates of metastasis to regional lymph nodes of BCC of the NAC have prompted BCC in this location to be considered more aggressive [2].

Between 1893 and 2016, BCCs of the nipple and areola have been reported in 55 patients (Tables 24.1 and 24.2) [2, 4–51, 56]. To date, three cases of BCC of the NAC metastatic to the lymph nodes have been described. In comparison, from 1894 to 2011, 364 cases of metastatic BCC from all anatomic sites have only been described [3].

K.A. Chun, M.D. (✉)
Department of Dermatology, University of California San Diego, San Diego, CA, USA
e-mail: kic003@ucsd.edu

P.R. Cohen, M.D.
Department of Dermatology, University of California San Diego, San Diego, CA, USA

10991 Twinleaf Court, San Diego, CA 92131, USA
e-mail: mitehead@gmail.com

## 24.2 History

Robinson [4] described the first BCC of the NAC. He observed a rodent ulcer on the right nipple and areola of a 60-year-old man in 1893. From 1893 to 2016, an additional 34 men and 20 women were reported who had BCC of the NAC [2, 5–51, 56].

## 24.3 Epidemiology

BCCs of the NAC have been reported in 55 patients [2, 4–51, 56]. At this site, they occurred more frequently in men (35, 63.6%) than in women (20, 36.4%). The age at onset of BCC ranged from 35 to 86 years old; however, in one woman, the onset age was not mentioned [6]. In men, the median onset age was 61 years. In contrast, in women, the median onset age was 66 years.

The majority of patients with BCC of the NAC were Caucasian (28/37, 75.7%). BCCs of the NAC were also described in patients of other races: seven Asians (18.9%), one African American (2.7%), and one Hispanic (2.7%). Ethnicity or race was not described in 18 cases.


M.A. Shiffman (ed.), *Nipple-Areolar Complex Reconstruction*,
https://doi.org/10.1007/978-3-319-60925-6_24

**Table 24.1** Clinical characteristics of men with basal cell carcinoma of the nipple-areolar complex

| C | Age (Y) | Race | Loc | Morphology | Hist sub | P | Other NMSCs | Risk factors | Rx[j,k] | Outcome | Ref |
|---|---|---|---|---|---|---|---|---|---|---|---|
| 1 | 60 | NS | R N,A | Irregular ulcerated patch | NS | – | NS | NS | Simple excision and axillary LyN sampling | No recurrence. Died 18 months later of unrelated cause | Robinson [4] |
| 2 | 57 | NS | L N | NS | NS | NS | NS | NS | NS | LyN involvement. Died of disease in 8 years | Wainwright [5] |
| 3 | 43 | W | N | NS | Nod | +[a] | NS | NS | Simple mastectomy | No recurrence after 1 year | Congdon et al. [6] |
| 4 | 49 | NS | R N | Scaly and crusted lesion with ulceration and scar[b] | NS | NS | NS | NS | Wide excision | NS | Farrow [7] |
| 5 | 71 | W | R N,A | 8 cm tumor with ulceration | Nod | – | NS | NS | Simple mastectomy | LyN involved. After mastectomy, no recurrence | Wyatt [8] |
| 6 | 72 | NS | R N | Enlarged, firm R nipple[b] | Nod | – | NS | NS | Wide excision | NS | Lupton et al. [9] |
| 7 | 72 | NS | L N, A | NS | NS | NS | NS | NS | NS | NS | C2, Rahbari et al. [10] |
| 8 | 47 | NS | L A | NS | NS | NS | NS | NS | NS | NS | C22, Rahbari et al. [10] |
| 9 | 49 | W | R A | Pink, red plaque | NS | NS | NS | NS | MMS | Clear margins at surgery | Robins et al. [11] |
| 10 | 53 | W | L N | Ulcerated lesion[b] | Nod | – | NS | NS | Simple excision | Clear margins at surgery | Knudsen [12][c] |
| 11 | 51 | W | L N,A | Reddish brown, scaly, indurated plaque with pearly rolled border | S | – | None | Sun exposure | Simple excision | Clear margins at surgery | Bruce et al. [13] |
| 12 | 58 | NS | L N | Skin breakdown of L nipple[b] | M: Nod, I | – | None | None | Simple excision followed by radiotherapy | 4 years later had recurrence in axillary LyN, treated with mastectomy and LyN clearance | Shertz et al. [2] |
| 13 | 86 | NS | R N | Red, scaly, ulcerated oozing lesion[b] | F | – | BCC and SCC on face and scalp | Trauma to the chest | Simple excision[c] | NS | Nirodi et al. [14] |

| | | | | | | | | | | | |
|---|---|---|---|---|---|---|---|---|---|---|---|
| 14 | 63 | W | R N,A | Eroded plaque with crust | Nod | – | NS | None | Simple excision | No recurrence after 16 months | C1, Cain et al. [15] |
| 15 | 80 | W | R N,A | Indurated reddish brown mass with ulceration[b] | F | – | NS | NS | Wide excision | No recurrence after 8 months | C2, Cain et al. [15] |
| 16 | 68 | W | L N | 2 cm reddish brown to gray and blackish bluish nodule | Sup | +[d] | NS | NS | Simple excision | Clear margins at surgery | Titzmann et al. [16][e] |
| 17 | 57 | W | R N | 1.5 cm papule | Nod | – | BCC × 4 on face and arms | Sun exposure, although noted patient states he always wore a shirt | Simple mastectomy | No recurrence after 2 years | Benharroch et al. [17] |
| 18 | 55 | NS | N, A | NS | BCC | NS | NS | NS | MMS | NS | Weber et al. [18] |
| 19 | 57 | W | R N | Flesh colored, indurated papule | Nod | – | None | None | Wide excision | No recurrence after 5 years | C1, Betti et al. [19] |
| 20 | 39 | W | N,A | Well-limited plaque with crust | Sup | – | NS | None | Wide excision | No recurrence after 2 years | C2, Betti et al. [19] |
| 21 | 67 | W | L N,A | Ulcerated, erythematous lesion[b] | Nod | – | BCC forehead | NS | Wide excision | Clear margins at surgery | Gupta et al. [20] |
| 22 | 61 | W | L A | Pink, pearly papule | NS | NS | BCC × 2 on abdomen | Burn to chest wall from fire | MMS | Clear margins at surgery | Nouri et al. [21] |
| 23 | 78 | NS | L N, A | Erythematous nodule with crusting and swelling | Nod | – | NS | None | Simple mastectomy with LyN dissection | Clear at surgery | Kim et al. [22][f] |
| 24 | 60 | W | L N | Erythematous ulcer with scale and crust[b] | F | – | None | None | Simple mastectomy | Clear at surgery | Avci et al. [23] |
| 28 | 69 | W | L N, A | Erythematous plaque with crust | NS | NS | NS | NS | MMS | No recurrence after 6 months | Cummins et al. [24] |
| 25 | 60 | W | L N | Enlarged L nipple[b] | M: S, MN | – | BCCs | Sun | Refused excision | Lost to follow-up | Oram et al. [25] |
| 26 | 76 | W | L N | Ulcerated lesion on L nipple[b] | Nod | – | NS | NS | NS | NS | Kacerovska et al. [26] |
| 27 | 69 | W | R N | Poorly defined, pink, telangiectatic plaque with ulceration | M: Nod, S | – | None | Sun exposure | MMS | No recurrence after 2 years | Sinha et al. [27] |

(continued)

**Table 24.1** (continued)

| C | Age (Y) | Race | Loc | Morphology | Hist sub | P | Other NMSCs | Risk factors | Rx[j,k] | Outcome | Ref |
|---|---|---|---|---|---|---|---|---|---|---|---|
| 29 | 42 | W | L N, A | Poorly defined erythematous plaque | M: Nod, S | – | BCCs | BCNS, immune-suppressed | MMS | No recurrence after 3 months | Williams et al. [28] |
| 30 | 23 | NS | R N | Well-defined pink, semicircular papule with multiple pin-point pigmented macules on the nipple | NS | +[d] | NS | NS | Simple excision | No recurrence after 5 years | Brown et al. [29] |
| 31 | 78 | Asian | L N, A | Pigmented macule | Nod | +[d] | None | None | Simple excision | Disease-free at 1 year | Kalyani et al. [30] |
| 32 | 78 | Asian | R N | Pigmented mass with ulceration[b] | S[b] | +[d] | NS | Gastric cancer, chemo | Simple excision | No recurrence at 6 months | Takeno et al. [31] |
| 33 | 75 | W | R N | Erythematous ulcer on R nipple[b] | S | – | Surgical excision of nod BCC 3 years prior | NS | MMS showed lactiferous ducts were infiltrated, so simple mastectomy was performed | Clear margins after simple mastectomy | Miglino et al. [32] |
| 34 | 65 | NS | R N | Irregular, black macule | S | +[d] | NS | NS | NS | NS | Kitamura et al. [33] |
| 35[g] | 67 | W | R A | Flesh colored to Hypopigmented nodule | Nod | +[h] | BCC of L arm | None | MMS | No recurrence after 6 months | Chun et al. [56] |

*A* areola, *BCNS* basal cell nevus syndrome, *C* case, *Cm* centimeter, *CR* current report, *F* fibroepithelioma of Pinkus, *Hist sub* histologic subtype, *I* infiltrative, *L* left, *Loc* location, *LyN* lymph node, *M* mixed, *MMS* Mohs micrographic surgery, *MN* micronodular, *N* nipple, *Nod* nodular, *NS* not stated, *P* pigmented, *S* superficial, *W* white, *Y* years. Republished with permission [56]

[a]Tumor is microscopically pigmented. Clinical presentation was not stated

[b]Primary morphology not stated

[c]For this patient, the nipple was excised

[d]Tumor is both clinically and microscopically pigmented

[e]Article in German

[f]Article in Korean

[g]Clinical and pathology images in Figs. 24.1 and 24.2

[h]Tumor is microscopically pigmented, but not clinically pigmented

[i]Article in Danish

[j]Simple excision is defined as excision with narrower margins of visually normal-appearing skin

[k]Wide local excision is defined as involving a larger margin of normal-appearing skin

**Table 24.2** Clinical characteristics of women with basal cell carcinoma of the nipple-areolar complex

| C | Age (Y) | Race | Loc | Morphology | Histo | P | Other NMSCs | Risk factors | Rx | Outcome | Ref |
|---|---|---|---|---|---|---|---|---|---|---|---|
| 1 | NS | NS | N | NS | NS | NS | NS | NS | Simple mastectomy | Alive and disease-free at 2 years | Congdon et al. [6] |
| 2 | 66 | W | L N | Red, scaly nipple with induration[a] | S | – | NS | NS | Wide excision | Clear margins at surgery | Davis et al. [34] |
| 3 | 67 | W | L N,A | Erythematous, eczematous nodule | S | – | None | Smoker | Etretinate followed by simple mastectomy | Clear margins at surgery | Jones et al. [35] |
| 4 | 49 | NS | N,A | NS | NS | NS | NS | NS | No treatment | NS | Betti et al. [36] |
| 5 | 71 | W | Bilateral A | Scaly plaques. Plaque on left breast with ulceration | S | NS | BCC, melanoma | NS | Wide excision | No recurrence after 6 months | Wong et al. [37] |
| 6 | 35 | NS | L A | Red plaque with well-defined borders | S | – | None | None | Simple excision | No recurrence after 1 year | Nunez et al. [38] |
| 7 | 75 | NS | L N,A | Red, eczematous lesion[a] | M: Nod, S | – | NS | NS | Wide excision followed by radiotherapy | Clear margins at surgery | Sauven et al. [39] |
| 8 | 65 | NS | L N,A | Erythematous, indurated plaque with ulceration | M: Nod, I | – | None | Moderate sun exposure | MMS | No recurrence after 1 year | Sanchez-Carpintero et al. [40] |
| 9 | 82 | Asian | L A | Dark brown papule | Nod | +[b] | None | None | Wide Excision | Disease-free after 2 years | Yamamoto et al. [41] |
| 10 | 47 | H | L N, A | Ill-defined erythematous plaque | S | – | None | None | MMS | Clear margins at surgery | Zhu et al. [42] |
| 11 | 47 | W | L N, A | Red-brown, indurated nodule | Nod | – | None | None | Wide excision | No recurrence after 2 years | C3, Betti et al. [19] |
| 12 | 46 | Asian | R A | Well-defined, slightly crusted plaque | S | – | None | None | Initially had simple excision, but due to positive margins had a simple mastectomy and excision of an axillary sentinel LyN | Disease-free after 1 year | Huang et al. [43] |

(continued)

**Table 24.2** (continued)

| C | Age (Y) | Race | Loc | Morphology | Histo | P | Other NMSCs | Risk factors | Rx | Outcome | Ref |
|---|---|---|---|---|---|---|---|---|---|---|---|
| 13 | 49 | W | L N,A | Indurated red-brown plaque | M: S, I | – | None | Topless sunbathing | MMS with sentinel LyN biopsy | Clear margins at surgery | Rosen et al. [44] |
| 14 | 74 | NS | R N | Eczematous lesion[a] | S | – | NS | NS | Simple excision | Clear margins at surgery | Chu et al. [45] |
| 15 | 67 | Asian | R A | Black hyperkeratotic plaque | Nod | +[b] | None | None | Wide excision | Disease-free after 14 months | Jung et al. [46] |
| 16 | 48 | NS | R N, A | Hyperpigmented, erythematous plaque with ulceration | Nod | +[b] | None | None | Simple excision | Clear margins at surgery | Sharma et al. [47] |
| 17 | 72 | Asian | R N, A | Erythematous ulcer with scale and crust[a] | F | – | NS | NS | Wide excision | NS | Xu et al. [48] |
| 18 | 40 | W | R N | Ulcerated nodule | Nod | – | None | None | Simple excision | No recurrence after 18 months | Trignano et al. [49] |
| 19 | 66 | AA | L A | Lichenified, scaly, excoriated plaque | S | +[c] | NS | NS | 5-FU BID × 6 weeks | Resolved clinically but recurred after 22 months | Goddard et al. [50] |
| 20 | 82 | W | L N | Nodule | Nod | – | NS | NS | Wide excision | No recurrence after 3 years | Ozerdem et al. [51] |

*A* areola, *AA* African-American, *C* case, *F* fibroepithelioma of Pinkus, *Hist sub* histologic subtype, *I* infiltrative, *L* left, *Loc* location, *LyN* lymph node, *M* mixed, *MMS* Mohs micrographic surgery, *N* nipple, *Nod* nodular, *NS* not stated, *R* right, *S* superficial, *Y* years. Republished with permission [56]

[a]Primary morphology not stated

[b]Tumor is both clinically and microscopically pigmented

[c]Tumor is microscopically pigmented, but not clinically pigmented

[d]Simple excision is defined as excision with narrower margins of visually normal-appearing skin

[e]Wide local excision is defined as involving a larger margin of normal-appearing skin

## 24.4 Clinical Presentation

Left-sided BCCs of the nipple-areolar complex were more common (28/51, 54.9%) than the right-sided tumors (23/51, 45.1%). In 45 patients (81.8%), the nipple was affected; of these individuals, 22 patients also had tumors that affected the areola. Bilateral involvement of the areola was observed in one patient [37]. The affected side was not reported in five patients.

The clinical presentation of BCC of the NAC was variable. Tumors presented as a plaque (17/34, 50%), nodule (8/34, 23.5%), papule (6/34, 17.6%), macule (2/34, 5.9%), or patch (1/34, 2.9%) (Fig. 24.1). Eight BCCs were clinically pigmented. In addition, secondary changes were noted: erosion or ulceration (19 cases), scale (10 cases), and crust (7 cases).

There have been limited morphologic features that aid in the diagnosis of BCC of the NAC; this is likely secondary to the paucity of BCC of the NAC reported. However, a dermoscopic feature of pigmented BCC of the NAC—termed a "large black web"—was described in a recent review by Kitamura et al. [33]. Specifically, the black network structure was thicker than the typical pigment network of the areola, and the surrounding area consisted of arborizing vessels and spoke-wheel areas on dermoscopy. Indeed, the authors noted that the "large black web" was not only unique to BCC of the NAC but also appeared to avoid the hair follicles when this patient was compared with nine others diagnosed with superficial BCC of the trunk [33, 58–61].

## 24.5 Pathologic Presentation

Nodular BCC (18/42, 42.9%) was the most frequent histologic subtype (Fig. 24.2). Superficial (13/42, 30.9%), pigmented (11/42, 26.2%), mixed (7/42, 16.7%), and fibroepithelioma of Pinkus (4/42, 9.5%) were the other histologic subtypes of BCC observed. Four of the mixed subtypes were noted to have aggressive histologic features, including micronodular (1/7, 14.3%) and infiltrative (3/7, 42.9%). A histologic subtype of BCC was not provided in 13 cases.

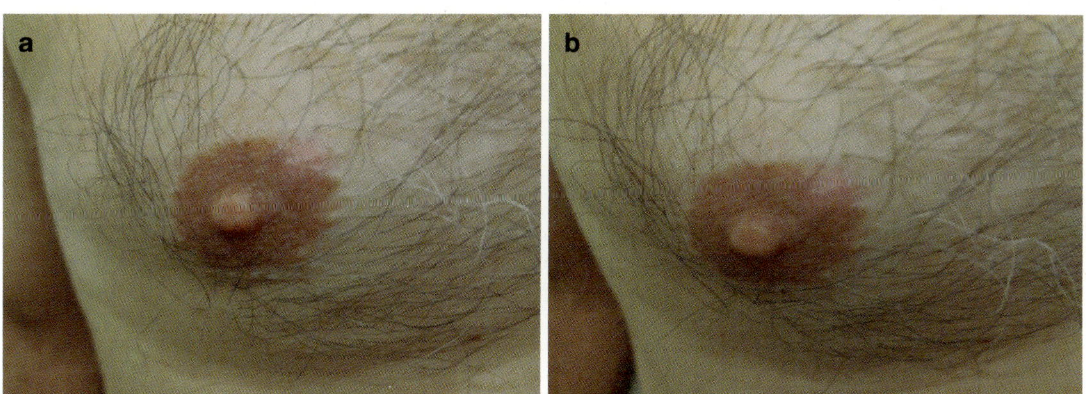


**Fig. 24.1** Clinical presentation of basal cell carcinoma of the areola. (**a**) Flesh colored to hypopigmented dermal nodule on the upper medial quadrant of the right areola in a 67-year-old Caucasian man with Fitzpatrick skin type 2. He had a prior history of basal cell carcinoma on the left arm diagnosed 3 years earlier and presented with a 6-month history of a slowly enlarging, asymptomatic lesion on the right areola and adjacent breast. He had a prior history of moderate sun exposure as a young adult. He had no exposure to ionizing radiation and had no family history of basal cell carcinoma or basal cell nevus syndrome. (**b**) The is the 7 × 7 mm flesh colored to hypopigmented dermal nodule on the upper medial quadrant of his right areola and extending into the adjacent breast. A 3 mm punch biopsy was performed. The patient in these figures is cited in Table 24.1 (Case 35). Republished with permission [56]

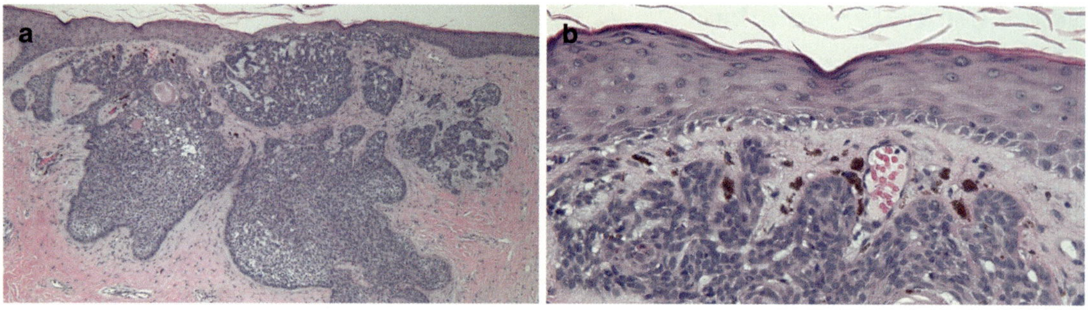


**Fig. 24.2** Pathologic presentation of the basal cell carcinoma of the areola shown in Fig. 24.1. (**a**) Low magnification views of the pigmented basal cell carcinoma shows nodular aggregates of basaloid tumor cells extending from the epidermis into the dermis. (**b**) Deposits of melanin were present not only in the tumor cells but also in dermal melanophages. The residual tumor was excised using the Mohs micrographic technique and clear margins were achieved after three stages. The final wound measured 20 × 14 mm, and a layered side-to-side closure was used to close the surgical defect. The patient in these figures is cited in Table 24.1 (Case 35). Republished with permission [56]

## 24.6 Differential Diagnosis

The clinical differential diagnoses of BCC of the NAC include adenoma of the nipple, benign nevus, Bowen's disease, erosive adenomatosis, invasive ductal carcinoma, leiomyoma, malignant melanoma, Paget disease, pigmented Paget disease, papilloma of the lactiferous duct, pigmented epidermotropic metastases, seborrheic keratosis, syringomatous adenoma, and squamous cell carcinoma [20, 25, 29, 30, 41, 43, 46].

Eight of the patients with BCC of the NAC had tumors that were clinically pigmented. Pigmented BCC of the NAC can be differentiated from melanoma by histologic examination and—if necessary—immunohistochemistry evaluation using markers such as CEA, cytokeratins, EMA, HMB-45, MART1, microphthalmia transcription factor (MiTF), and S-100 [29, 55].

## 24.7 Associated Conditions

The major risk factor for the development of BCC is ultraviolet light exposure. Other etiologies for the development of BCC include arsenic exposure, environmental exposures, genetic predisposition, ionizing radiation exposure, immunosuppression, injury (burns or trauma), light-colored skin, previous BCCs at another site, and sunburns. Indeed, the increased incidence of BCC of the NAC observed in men (35, 63.6%) versus women (20, 36.4%) [2, 4–51, 56] has been attributed to greater sun exposure of the chest in men [2, 13, 15, 20, 27, 41, 42].

The majority of patients with BCC of the NAC did not have etiologies typically associated with the development of BCC [56]. However, increased sun exposure to the chest from shirtless sunbathing was noted in two men (Table 24.1, cases 11 and 26) [13, 27] and two women (Table 24.2, cases 8 and 13) [40, 44]. In addition, a prior history of BCC was present in nine patients (9/26, 34.6%) [14, 17, 20, 21, 25, 28, 32]. Prior trauma to the chest (2/27, 7.4%) was noted in two men [14, 21]. One man had basal cell nevus syndrome (1/27, 3.7%) [28], and one man was immunosuppressed on chemotherapy for gastric cancer (1/27, 3.7%) [31].

## 24.8 Pathogenesis

The etiology of BCC remains to be determined. There is a histogenic relationship between BCCs and pilosebaceous units [52–54]. Indeed, it has been suggested that BCCs originate from the bulge region or outer root sheath of the hair follicle [23]. In addition, it has been hypothesized that BCCs may arise in proportion to the number of pilosebaceous units present [25]. The paucity of BCCs reported on the nipple and areola may be secondary to the nipple and areola being deficient in pilosebaceous units.

The patched/hedgehog signaling pathway plays a role in basal cell nevus syndrome as well as the development of sporadic BCCs. This pathway is responsible for differentiation of various tissues during embryogenesis and, afterwards, continues to regulate cell growth and differentiation. Mutations in the *PTCH* gene prevent inhibition of this pathway, allowing downstream signaling to proceed without interference. Additionally, mutations in a protein member of the receptor complex, smoothened (SMO), also lead to unregulated signaling allowing tumor growth [57].

## 24.9 Treatment

The most common treatment of BCC of the NAC is removal of the tumor (Table 24.3). Methods of surgical tumor removal most commonly included simple excision (15/50, 30%), wide excision (14/50, 28%), or Mohs micrographic surgery (11/50, 22%) with confirmation of complete tumor removal through examination of the margins. Simple mastectomies, as the initial modality of treatment, was performed in six patients (6/50, 12%). One man had a simple excision followed by radiotherapy; however, 4 years later, he developed recurrence in the axillary lymph node and thus had a simple mastectomy (2%) [2]. Another man had Mohs micrographic surgery, which showed the lactiferous ducts were infiltrated; a simple mastectomy was subsequently performed (2%) [32]. One woman had a simple excision; the tumor was present in the surgical margins and she had a partial mastectomy (2%) [43].

Two women were initially treated medically: one patient received topical 5-flourouracil (5-FU) twice daily for 6 weeks [50], and the other was treated with etretinate followed by simple mastectomy [35]. Two patients received no treatment [25, 36]. There was no mention of management for five of the men.

**Table 24.3** Initial treatment of basal cell carcinomas of the nipple-areolar complex

| Initial treatment[a] | Men[b] | Women[c] | Total[d] |
|---|---|---|---|
| Simple excision | 10[e] | 5[f] | 15 |
| Wide excision | 6 | 8[g] | 14 |
| MMS | 8[h] | 3 | 11 |
| Simple mastectomy | 5 | 1[i] | 6[j] |
| 5-Fluorouracil | 0 | 1[k] | 1 |
| Etretinate | 0 | 1[l] | 1 |
| No treatment | 1 | 1 | 2 |
| Total | 30 | 20 | 50 |

*MMS* Mohs micrographic surgery. Republished with permission [56]

[a]Initial treatment not stated in five men

[b]Number of men in which treatment was performed

[c]Number of women in which treatment was performed

[d]Total number of men and women in which treatment was performed

[e]This group includes one patient in which the nipple was excised, and excision type was not specified. Two patients had subsequent treatment including either axillary lymph node sampling or radiotherapy

[f]One woman had additional treatment: simple mastectomy and lymph node sampling

[g]One woman had additional treatment: radiotherapy

[h]Following MMS, one man had a simple mastectomy

[i]One woman was treated with etretinate and subsequently had a simple mastectomy

[j]Simple mastectomy was the initial treatment for six patients; however, nine mastectomies were eventually performed. One man was initially treated with MMS, one woman was initially treated by simple excision followed by radiotherapy, and one woman was initially treated with etretinate

[k]One woman was treated with 5-fluorouracil twice daily for 6 weeks. The BCC initially resolved, but recurred at 22 months

[l]Following etretinate therapy, one woman had a simple mastectomy

## 24.10 Prognosis

An increased metastatic potential of BCC of the NAC was reported by earlier investigators. Increased lymphatics of the NAC were hypothesized to possibly provide a direct route for tumor spread [55].

Three men with BCC of the NAC had lymph node involvement in cases 2, 5, and 12 (Table 24.1) [2, 5, 8]. This represents a minimum metastatic rate of 5.5%. One of the men died from the disease. However, this rate could potentially be higher since the outcome was not stated in ten patients, and several patients had a short duration of follow-up after surgery.

Importantly, after successful treatment of their tumor, most of the patients with BCC of the NAC had no recurrence (43/45, 95.6%). However, there was no mention of the clinical outcome for ten of the patients.

## Conclusions

From 1893 to 2016, BCC of the NAC has been described in 55 patients (Table 24.4). Men were affected more often than women. The tumor occurred more often on the left side than the right side of the body. These tumors are most commonly presented as plaques with ulceration. A nodular histology was the most frequent histologic subtype of BCC of NAC. Earlier reports suggest that there is a higher metastatic potential for BCC of the NAC than with BCCs at other anatomic sites; however, most of the patients with BCC of the NAC were successfully treated with excision of their tumor.

**Table 24.4** Summary of characteristics of basal cell carcinoma of the nipple-areolar complex

| Category | Men | Women | Total |
|---|---|---|---|
| *Epidemiology (55 patients)* | | | |
| Number | 35 | 20 | 55 |
| Age range | 23–86 years | 35–82 years | 23–86 years |
| Median | 61 years | 66 years | |
| *Clinical presentation (34 patients)* | | | |
| Plaque | 7 | 10 | 17 |
| Nodule | 4 | 4 | 8 |
| Papule | 5 | 1 | 6 |
| Macule | 2 | 0 | 2 |
| Patch | 1 | 0 | 1 |
| *Pathologic presentation (42 patients)* | | | |
| Nodular | 12 | 6 | 18 |
| Superficial | 6 | 7 | 13 |
| Mixed | 4 | 3 | 7 |
| FEP | 3 | 1 | 4 |
| *Treatment (50 patients)* | | | |
| *Surgical* | | | |
| Excision | 24 | 16 | 40 |
| Mastectomy | 5 | 1 | 6 |
| *Medical* | | | |
| 5-Fluorouracil | 0 | 1 | 1 |
| Etretinate | 0 | 1 | 1 |
| None | 1 | 1 | 2 |

*FEP* fibroepithelioma of Pinkus

## References


1. Rubin AI, Chen EH, Ratner D. Basal-cell carcinoma. N Engl J Med. 2005;353(21):2262–9.
2. Shertz WT, Balogh K. Metastasizing basal cell carcinoma of the nipple. Arch Pathol Lab Med. 1986;110(8):761–2.
3. Wysong A, Aasi SZ, Tang JY. Update on metastatic basal cell carcinoma: a summary of published cases from 1981 through 2011. JAMA Dermatol. 2013;149(5):615–6.
4. Robinson HB. Rodent ulcer of the male breast. Transact Pathol Soc London. 1893;44:147–8.
5. Wainwright JM. Carcinoma of the male breast. Arch Surg. 1927;14:836–59.
6. Congdon GH, Dockerty MB. Malignant lesions of the nipple exclusive of Paget's disease. Surg Gynecol Obstet. 1956;103(2):185–92.
7. Farrow JH. Benign and malignant lesions of the nipple. CA Cancer J Clin. 1958;8(1):16–9.
8. Wyatt AP. Basal cell carcinoma of the male breast. Proc R Soc Med. 1965;58(7):509–10.
9. Lupton GP, Goette K. Basal cell carcinoma of the nipple. Arch Dermatol. 1978;114(12):1845.
10. Rahbari H, Mehregan AH. Basal cell epitheliomas in usual and unusual sites. J Cutan Pathol. 1979;6(5):425–31.
11. Robins P, Rabinovitz HS, Rigel D. Basal-cell carcinomas on covered or unusual sites of the body. J Dermatol Surg Oncol. 1981;7(10):803–6.
12. Knudsen PJ. Basel cell carcinoma of the nipple. Ugeskr Laeger. 1982;144(12):876–7.
13. Bruce S, Tschen JA, Goldberg LH. Basal-cell carcinoma of the nipple. J Dermatol Surg Oncol. 1985;11(4):424–5.
14. Nirodi NS, Mudd DG. Basal cell carcinoma of the male nipple. J R Coll Surg Edinb. 1986;31(2):121–3.
15. Cain RJ, Sau P, Benson PM. Basal cell carcinoma of the nipple. Report of two cases. J Am Acad Dermatol. 1990;22(2 Pt 1):207–10.
16. Titzmann T, Peter RU, Thoma E, Ruzicka T. Pigmented basalioma as pseudomelanoma of the breast. Hautarzt. 1991;42(7):459–60.
17. Benharroch D, Geffen DB, Peiser J, Rosenberg L. Basal cell carcinoma of the male nipple. Case report and review of the literature. J Dermatol Surg Oncol. 1993;19(2):137–9.
18. Weber PJ, Moody BR, Foster JA. Series spiral advancement flap: an alternative to the ellipse. Dermatol Surg. 2001;27(1):64–6.
19. Betti R, Martino P, Moneghini L, Vergani R, Tolomio E, Crosti C. Basal cell carcinomas of the areola-nipple complex: case reports and review of the literature. J Dermatol. 2003;30(11):822–6.

20. Gupta C, Sheth D, Snower DP. Primary basal cell carcinoma of the nipple. Arch Pathol Lab Med. 2004;128(7):792–3.
21. Nouri K, Ballard CJ, Bouzari N, Saghari S. Basal cell carcinoma of the areola in a man. J Drugs Dermatol. 2005;4(3):352–4.
22. Kim JH, Oh JW, Shin DH, Kim SI, Park BW. Basal cell carcinoma of the nipple-areolar complex. J Korean Surg Soc. 2007;72:143–6.
23. Avci O, Pabuccuoglu U, Kocdor MA, Unlu M, Akin C, Soyal C, Canda T. Basal cell carcinoma of the nipple – an unusual location in a male patient. J Dtsch Dermatol Ges. 2008;6(2):130–2.
24. Cummins DL, Yu Y, Finn DT. Island pedicle reconstruction of partial nipple and areola defect. Dermatol Surg. 2010;36(9):1459–62.
25. Oram Y, Demirkesen C, Akkaya AD, Koyuncu E. Basal cell carcinoma of the nipple: an uncommon but ever-increasing location. Case Rep Dermatol Med. 2011;2011:818291.
26. Kacerovska D, Michal M, Kazakov DV. Basal cell carcinoma of the nipple extending into the lactiferous duct. Int J Surg Pathol. 2011;19(6):779–80.
27. Sinha A, Langtry JA. Secondary intention healing following Mohs micrographic surgery for basal cell carcinoma of the nipple and areola. Acta Derm Venereol. 2011;91(1):78–9.
28. Williams C, Hussain W. A low-risk tumour, at a high-risk site? Basal cell carcinoma of the nipple-areola complex. Br J Dermatol. 2013;168(4):901–3.
29. Brown PJ, Milch JM, Hivnor CM. Pigmented basal cell carcinoma of the nipple: a case report and review of the literature. Cutis. 2013;92(5):253–7.
30. Kalyani R, Vani BR, Srinivas MV, Veda P. Pigmented basal cell carcinoma of nipple and areola in a male breast – a case report with review of literature. Int J Biomed Sci. 2014;10(1):69–72.
31. Takeno S, Kikuchi N, Miura T, Anami K, Takahashi Y, Hashimoto T, Moroga T, Akizuki S, Kamei M, Suehiro S, Yamashita S, Kawahara K. Basal cell carcinoma of the nipple in male patients with gastric cancer recurrence: report of a case. Breast Cancer. 2014;21(1):102–7.
32. Miglino B, Tiberio R, Astolfi S, Graziola F, Boggio P, Leutner M, Valente G, Franchini R, Colombo E. Basal cell carcinoma of the nipple in a male patient: a particular case report. Breast J. 2016;22(3):339–41.
33. Kitamura S, Hata H, Yamaguchi Y, Imafuku K, Yanagi T, Shimizu H. The unique dermoscopic structure 'Large black web' in basal cell carcinoma on the areola. J Eur Acad Dermatol Venereol. 2016;30(12):e221–3.
34. Davis AB, Patchefsky AS. Basal cell carcinoma of the nipple: case report and review of the literature. Cancer. 1977;40(4):1780–1.
35. Jones R, Wayte DM, Mitchell E, Beer WE. Basal-cell carcinoma of the breast—treatment with retinoids. Clin Exp Dermatol. 1991;16(6):448–50.
36. Betti R, Urbani CE, Lodi A, Crosti C. Unusual sites of basal cell epitheliomas according to anatomical distribution and relative tumor density index. Eur J Dermatol. 1992;2:82–4.
37. Wong SW, Smith JG Jr, Thomas WO. Bilateral basal cell carcinoma of the breasts. J Am Acad Dermatol. 1993;28(5 Pt 1):777.
38. Nunez M, Marques A, de las Heras ME, Miralles ES, Ledo A. Bilateral basal cell carcinoma of the breasts in a woman. J Dermatol. 1995;22(3):226–8.
39. Sauven P, Roberts A. Basal cell carcinoma of the nipple. J R Soc Med. 1983;76(8):699–701.
40. Sanchez-Carpintero I, Redondo P, Solano T. Basal cell carcinoma affecting the areola-nipple complex. Plast Reconstr Surg. 2000;105(4):1573.
41. Yamamoto H, Ito Y, Hayashi T, Urano N, Kato T, Kimura Y, Tanigawa T, Endo W, Kurokawa E, Kikkawa N, Taniguchi H. A case of basal cell carcinoma of the nipple and areola with intraductal spread. Breast Cancer. 2001;8(3):229–33.
42. Zhu YI, Ratner D. Basal cell carcinoma of the nipple: a case report and review of the literature. Dermatol Surg. 2001;27(11):971–4.
43. Huang CW, Pan CK, Shih TF, Tsai CC, Juan CC, Ker CG. Basal cell carcinoma of the nipple-areola complex: a case report. Kaohsiung J Med Sci. 2005;21(10):480–3.
44. Rosen N, Muhn CY, Bernstein SC. A common tumor, an uncommon location: basal cell carcinoma of the nipple and areola in a 49-year-old woman. Dermatol Surg. 2005;31(4):480–3.
45. Chu PY, Teng TH, Lee CC. Primary superficial basal cell carcinoma of the nipple. Ann Saudi Med. 2007;27(4):296–7.
46. Jung HJ, Jun JH, Kim HY, Lee SJ, Kim do W, Lee WJ, Jung JH. Pigmented basal cell carcinoma of the nipple-areola complex in an elderly woman. Ann Dermatol. 2011;23(Suppl 2):S201–4.
47. Sharma A, Tambat RM, Singh A, Bhaligi DS. Basal cell carcinoma of the nipple areola complex. J Midlife Health. 2011;2(2):89–90.
48. Xu D, Tian W, Li J, Song Y. The missing nipple: a rare case of basal cell carcinoma of the nipple in a Chinese female. Breast J. 2012;18(6):606–7.
49. Trignano E, Manzo MJ, Paliogiannis P, Madonia M, Marongiu F, Lissia A, Campus GV. Basal cell carcinoma of the nipple-areola complex: report of a case and literature review. Ann Ital Chir. 2013;84(ePub).
50. Goddard L, Mollet T, Blalock T. Resident rounds: Part III. Plaque on left areola of an African-American woman. J Drugs Dermatol. 2014;13(6):767.
51. Ozerdem U, Hoda SA. Basal cell carcinoma of the nipple. Breast J. 2014;20(4):427–9.
52. Alessi E, Venegoni L, Fanoni D, Berti E. Cytokeratin profile in basal cell carcinoma. Am J Dermatopathol. 2008;30(3):249–55.
53. Pinkus H. Premalignant fibroepithelial tumors of skin. AMA Arch Derm Syphilol. 1953;67(6):598–615.
54. Wallace SA, Halpert B. Trichoma: tumor of hair anlage. Arch Pathol (Chic). 1950;50(2):199–208.
55. Ferguson MS, Nouraei SA, Davies BJ, McLean NR. Basal cell carcinoma of the nipple-areola complex. Dermatol Surg. 2009;35(11):1771–5.

56. Rogers HW, Weinstock MA, Harris AR, Hinckley MR, Feldman SR, Fleischer AB, Coldiron BM. Incidence estimate of nonmelanoma skin cancer in the United States, 2006. Arch Dermatol. 2010;146(3):283–7.
57. Requena L, Sangueza M, Sangueza OP, Kutzner H. Pigmented mammary Paget disease and pigmented epidermotropic metastases from breast carcinoma. Am J Dermatopathol. 2002;24(3):189–98.
58. Xiong YD, Ma S, Li X, Zhong X, Duan C, Chen Q. A meta-analysis of reflectance confocal microscopy for the diagnosis of malignant skin tumours. J Eur Acad Dermatol Venereol. 2016;30(8):1295–302.
59. Gonzalez S, Tannous Z. Real-time, in vivo confocal reflectance microscopy of basal cell carcinoma. J Am Acad Dermatol. 2002;47(6):869–74.
60. Menzies SW. Dermoscopy of pigmented basal cell carcinoma. Clin Dermatol. 2002;20(3):268–9.
61. di Meo N, Damiani G, Vichi S, Fadel M, Nan K, Noal C, Trevisini S, Trevisan G. Interobserver agreement on dermoscopic features of small basal cell carcinoma (<5 mm) among low-experience dermoscopists. J Dermatol. 2016; doi:10.1111/1346-8138.13426.
62. Chun KA, Cohen PR. Basal cell carcinoma of the nipple-areola complex: a comprehensive review of the world literature. Dermatol Ther (Heidelb). 2016;5(3):379–95.
63. Wicking C, McGlinn E. The role of hedgehog signalling in tumorigenesis. Cancer Lett. 2001;173(1):1–7.

# Primary Squamous Cell Carcinoma of the Nipple

# 25

Stratos S. Sofos

## 25.1 Introduction

There have been only four documented cases in the English literature with the diagnosis of primary squamous cell carcinoma (SCC) of the nipple-areola complex (NAC) [1]. Other types of skin cancers in this region are more common, such as in situ SCC or SCC secondary to radiotherapy or other forms of immunosuppression. This chapter presents a case of a primary SCC of the NAC and outlines the key steps in the management of this rare diagnosis. The patient discussed presented with an erythematous, scaly lesion on her right nipple-areola complex which strongly resembled Paget's disease; however, after histological examination, a moderately differentiated SCC was diagnosed. Due to the similar presentation to Paget's disease of the nipple, careful examination of the histology must be performed in order to ascertain a definitive diagnosis. It is highlighted that patients presenting with lesions of the NAC cannot be assumed to have either Paget's disease or SCC and biopsy should be performed before arranging further investigations or treatment, as the management pathways for the two conditions can be very different.

## 25.2 Case Presentation

The author presents the case of a 34-year-old woman who presented to the plastic surgery unit with an erythematous, scaly lesion on her right NAC (Fig. 25.1). The lesion was histologically confirmed to be an SCC and subsequently formally excised. Histology confirmed complete excision of the lesion with adequate margins with no lymphovascular or perineural invasion. The patient made a good recovery with no evidence of recurrence or metastasis at 12 months.

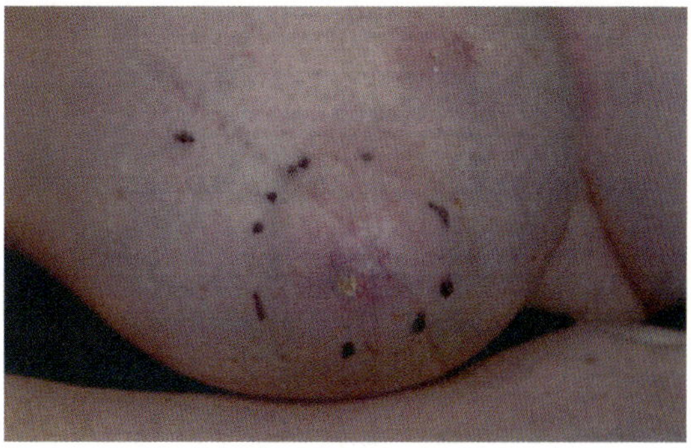

**Fig. 25.1** Scaly, erythematous lesion on the nipple-areola complex. Lesion demarcated by *dotted black lines*, depicting the excision margins

S.S. Sofos, M.B., B.Ch., M.R.C.S.
Department of Burns and Plastic Surgery, Whiston Hospital, Warrington Rd, Whiston, Prescot L35 5DR, UK
e-mail: tsofos@hotmail.com


M.A. Shiffman (ed.), *Nipple-Areolar Complex Reconstruction*, https://doi.org/10.1007/978-3-319-60925-6_25

## 25.3 Discussion

Squamous cell carcinoma is the second most common skin cancer after basal cell carcinoma. Ultraviolet exposure and immunosuppression are major risk factors for SCC of the skin, with chronic sun exposure being the strongest environmental risk factor. SCCs are generally treated by surgical excision; however nonsurgical options for the treatment of cutaneous SCC include topical chemotherapy, topical immune response modifiers, photodynamic therapy (PDT), radiotherapy, and systemic chemotherapy. Risk factors for recurrence include large diameter, anatomical site, recurrent lesions, immunosuppression, prior radiation therapy, moderate or poor differentiation, adenoid/adenos quamous/desmoplastic subtypes, depth (Clark's level IV/V or >4 mm), and perineural or vascular involvement [2]. Primary SCC of the nipple is very rare, having identified only three other cases of a primary SCC of the NAC. Other types of malignancies in this region are more common, such as in situ SCC or SCC secondary to radiotherapy or other forms of immunosuppression. Among the few reported cases, the majority have occurred in older women with rare cases seen in younger women and male patients [1]. Our patient presented with an exophytic mass of the right nipple while pregnant. As per Pendse et al., in the previously reported cases of squamous cell carcinoma of the nipple, two patients presented with an exophytic mass, and the remaining two patients', which included our case report, physical examination revealed scaling, erythema, and/or ulceration, which raised the possibility of Paget's disease [1, 3].

The most common malignancy arising in the NAC is Paget's disease, presenting initially with erythema and mild scaling and flaking of the nipple skin [4]. As early symptoms may cause only mild irritation, patients may not seek medical attention at first. At a later stage, symptoms may also include tingling, itching, increased sensitivity, burning, and pain. There may also be discharge from the nipple, which can appear flattened against the breast [4].

In most cases, Paget's disease is initially confined to the nipple, later spreading to the areola or other regions of the breast, and this helps distinguish the condition from eczema [4]. Clinically, Paget's disease of the breast can often represent one or more tumours within the same breast. If Paget's disease is suspected, then in addition to arranging for a nipple biopsy, a clinical breast examination to check for lesions or other breast masses is routinely performed. As many as 50% of people who have Paget's disease of the breast have a breast mass that can be felt in a clinical breast exam [5, 6]. Additional diagnostic tests may be performed, such as a mammogram, ultrasound, or a magnetic resonance scan to look for possible tumours. Histological diagnostic confusion can arise between Paget's disease and other neoplastic conditions affecting the skin, with the most common differential diagnoses being malignant melanoma and atypical squamous disease [7]. However, Paget's disease can be identified and differentiated by morphological appearances, the presence of intracellular mucin in many cases, and positive immunohistochemical staining for glandular cytokeratins, epithelial membrane antigen, and carcinoembryonic antigen [7].

Paget's disease associated with in situ or invasive carcinoma of the breast is often treated by excision of the NAC, but surgery is primarily based around the appropriate means of complete excision of the associated inframammary disease. As a consequence of the reported high prevalence of multifocal disease, most patients with mammary Paget's disease associated with neoplastic disease of the breast undergo mastectomy (with or without axillary sampling) rather than breast-conserving surgery such as wide local excision of tumour with excision of the NAC [7]. An invasive component to the tumour would be an indication for axillary node staging [4, 8].

The patient presented with an erythematous scaling lesion that was clinically indistinguishable from Paget's. The approach as per standard practice was to biopsy the lesion for a definitive diagnosis with subsequent wide local excision.

## Conclusions

This case report describes a rare presentation of a primary moderately differentiated SCC of the nipple. Although SCC of the nipple is a rare diagnosis, in view of its similar presentation to Paget's disease of the nipple, it must be considered, and careful examination of the histology must be performed in order to ascertain a definitive diagnosis. In addition, from the available literature, we know that primary SCC can also present as an exophytic lesion. Thus, clinicians who are presented with patients with lesions of the NAC must be suspicious of the diagnosis, and a biopsy should be performed before arranging further investigations or treatment, as the pathways for other conditions may differ.

## References

1. Pendse AA, O'Connor SM. Primary invasive squamous cell carcinoma of the nipple. Case Rep Pathol. 2015;2015:327487.
2. National comprehensive cancer network clinical practice guidelines in oncology. Basal cell and squamous cell skin cancers V.1. 2008. https://nccn.org/professionals/physician_gls/f_guidelines_nojava.asp Accessed 14 June 16.
3. Hosaka N, Uesaka K, Takaki T, Zhang Y, Takasu K, Ikehara S. Poorly differentiated squamous cell carcinoma of the nipple: unique case for marked exophytic growth, but little invasion with neuroendocrine differentiation. Med Mol Morphol. 2011;44(3):174–8.
4. Kaelin CM. Paget's disease. In: Harris JR, Lippman ME, Morrow M, Osborne CK, editors. Diseases of the breast. 3rd ed. Philadelphia: Lippincott Williams & Wilkins; 2004.
5. Harris JR, Lippman ME, Morrow M, Osborne CK, editors. Diseases of the breast. 4th ed. Philadelphia: Lippincott Williams & Wilkins; 2009.
6. Caliskan M, Gatti G, Sosnovskikh I, Rotmensz N, Botteri E, Musmeci S, Rosali dos Santos G, Viale G, Luini A. Paget's disease of the breast: the experience of the European Institute of Oncology and review of the literature. Breast Cancer Res Treat. 2008;112(3):513–21.
7. Lloyd J, Flanagan AM. Mammary and extramammary Paget's disease. J Clin Pathol. 2000;53:742–9.
8. Marcus E. The management of Paget's disease of the breast. Curr Treat Options Oncol. 2004;5:153–60.

# Part VI

# Prevention of Nipple-Areolar Complex Disorders

# Surgical Delay of the Nipple-Areolar Complex: Maximizing Nipple Viability Following Nipple-Sparing Mastectomy While Determining Clear Subareolar Margin

26

Jay Arthur Jensen

## 26.1 Introduction

Historically, nipple-sparing mastectomy has been confronted with two fundamental questions: first, "is it safe?" in the sense that it will not lead to diminished outcomes in the treatment of breast cancer, and second, "is it safe?" in the sense that it can be performed without a high incidence of complications—including nipple necrosis.

Although some consider the option of nipple-sparing mastectomy to be relatively new in the treatment of breast cancer, it was described in the modern era by Bromley Freeman in 1962 [1]. Freeman was careful to note that the observation that nipple-sparing mastectomy left a superior cosmetic outcome dated back to at least 1882. In Freeman's paper, the ideas of using an inframammary incision for the subcutaneous mastectomy and subjecting questionable mastectomy skin flaps to a surgical delay are specifically mentioned. However, Freeman addressed the use of this nipple-sparing or subcutaneous mastectomy technique for use in benign disease.

Similarly, subcutaneous mastectomies have long been performed at the Mayo Clinic [2] for patients with high-risk conditions, including a family history of breast cancer or worrisome premalignant conditions. Over a more than 30-year period from 1960 to 1993 at this center, of the 639 women with positive family histories who underwent subcutaneous mastectomies for risk reduction, only seven developed breast cancer. Of these seven, only one developed a breast cancer in a retained nipple. The Mayo Clinic series is also important because it demonstrates that nipple-sparing mastectomy is safe in the setting of BRCA-positive patients. Of the 639 patients who had previously undergone operation for risk reduction in the setting of a positive family history for breast cancer, blood samples were analyzed retrospectively on 176. Of these 176 women, 26 were found to be positive for the BRCA mutation. Therefore, this clinical experience allows us to know the outcome of nipple-sparing mastectomy in patients with the BRCA mutation: of these 26 women who were BRCA positive and followed for a mean period of 13.4 years, none developed breast cancer [3].

We must conclude that nipple-sparing mastectomy is a medically safe option for prophylactic mastectomy—indeed, more safe than patients

J.A. Jensen, M.D.
Samuel Oschin Cancer Center,
Room 5536, Cedars Sinai Medical Center, 8700
Beverly Boulevard, Los Angeles, CA 90048, USA

Division of Plastic Surgery, Geffen School of
Medicine at UCLA, Los Angeles, CA, USA
e-mail: jajensen@mednet.ucla.edu


M.A. Shiffman (ed.), *Nipple-Areolar Complex Reconstruction*,
https://doi.org/10.1007/978-3-319-60925-6_26

who do not have prophylactic mastectomy—even in the setting of patients who are genetically predisposed to breast cancer. But what about patients with invasive breast cancer: is nipple sparing a safe option?

Although nipple-sparing mastectomy in the setting of invasive operable breast cancer was first reported by Hinton and others [4] in 1984, concerns persisted about oncologic safety. Clinical reports of breast cancer recurrence [5] questioned whether the procedure was indeed safe. As recently as 2002, prominent surgeons concluded that "nipple sparing is not a reasonable option for mastectomy patients" and that "nipple-areolar complex sparing mastectomy may carry an unacceptable high risk of local relapse and should therefore not be advocated" [6, 7].

While surgeons worried about whether nipple-sparing procedures might pose unacceptably high risks for recurrence, the randomized, prospective breast conservation studies continued to add data to the more general question of the local management of breast cancer. Early reports [8] that more aggressive surgical extirpation of the breast did not add a survival advantage in early stage breast cancer were tested at multiple centers in randomized, prospective clinical trials [9, 10]. Surprisingly to many, these trials demonstrated that lumpectomy with or without radiation therapy as an initial "intention to treat" produced the same long-term survival as initial performance of modified radical mastectomy. Therefore, these studies demonstrated that initial removal of the nipple (as was done in the mastectomy group) did not confer a survival advantage over initial retention of the nipple (as was done in the lumpectomy and lumpectomy with radiation therapy groups). This extrapolation of the data from surgical oncology studies to the question of nipple-sparing mastectomy [11] allowed the conclusion that preservation of the uninvolved nipple did not compromise breast cancer survival. Multiple smaller, nonrandomized studies with shorter follow-up [12–18] are consistent with this prediction.

Understanding the scientific basis for the conclusion that nipple-sparing mastectomy does not change patient survival is important in establishing guidelines for this technique. Some authors [19] recommended arbitrary guidelines that cancers be less than 2.5 cm in diameter, be located 4 cm or more from the nipple-areolar complex, and be lymph node negative, but no survival data were cited to support such parameters. Using the guidance of the breast conservation literature and the benefit of post-nipple-sparing mastectomy radiation therapy in selected cases, the indications for nipple-sparing mastectomy can be safely expanded [20].

If nipple-sparing mastectomy is "safe" in the sense that preserving the uninvolved nipple does not compromise breast cancer survival, is it "safe" in the sense that preservation of the additional tissue will not lead to unacceptable rates of nipple necrosis?

Early studies of nipple-sparing mastectomies demonstrated significant rates of nipple necrosis: Gerber [14] reported a 10% necrosis rate, Sacchini [15] an 11% rate, and Benediktsson [16] a 7% rate. But as investigators gained experience with nipple-sparing mastectomy, nipple necrosis rates have dropped: Stolier [21] reported a series of 82 cases without any necrosis. A recent analysis performed by Gould [22] reviewed nipple necrosis rates in the literature and also reported the experience from M.D. Anderson in Houston. In this study, patients with large breasts were found to be at significantly increased risk of nipple necrosis, as were patients with hypertension or diabetes, current history of cigarette smoking, and high body mass index. Only 2% of their patients had complete nipple necrosis. Colwell et al. [23] used their large database to analyze nipple-sparing mastectomy in patients with previous breast scars and patients with previous radiation therapy [24] and demonstrated that nipple-sparing mastectomy can be safely performed in both these subgroups of patients.

Declining rates of nipple necrosis following nipple-sparing mastectomy might be explained by evolving surgical incisions which maintain nipple-areolar blood supply, thicker mastectomy skin flaps, implants held by biological or prosthetic slings so as to keep tension off from the mastectomy skin flaps, and/or better patient selection. In spite of these improvements, some patients will continue to be regarded as at higher risk for nipple-sparing mastectomy. Whether the risk factor is hypertension, diabetes, history of cigarette smoking, previous surgical scars which might restrict blood flow, high BMI, or a large (C cup or larger) breast, some patients will be at higher risk for nipple necrosis. For patients who are believed to be at higher risk for nipple necrosis or for patients who are thought to be not good candidates for nipple sparing because of the proximity of the tumor to the nipple, a nipple-areolar "delay" procedure with sub-nipple biopsy has been performed 7–21 days prior to mastectomy [25, 26]. This chapter describes our technique for nipple-areolar delay and subareolar biopsy.

## 26.2 Technique

The overriding priority of the delay procedure is to increase the probability that the nipple will survive the mastectomy procedure a week or two later. To survive the mastectomy procedure, the tissue must first survive the delay procedure. While this sounds like an obvious point, it is a point worth emphasizing. The patients usually subjected to the nipple-areolar delay/biopsy procedure are almost always the ones for whom the treating clinician has significant concerns about postmastectomy nipple necrosis: cigarette smokers, patients with scars which might limit perfusion of the nipple following mastectomy, patients with large and/or ptotic breasts, those with hypertension or microvascular disease (diabetes), and patients with high body mass index. In addition, some patients who are highly motivated for nipple sparing should undergo this procedure if they will be excluded from it on the basis of concerns about whether tumor is in the subareolar tissue.

If the patient has existing healed breast incisions, the incision for the delay procedure can be made in one of the previous incisions if the healed incision is not around the nipple. Alternatively, if the mastectomy will be performed using a different incision, the delay procedure should be done through the planned mastectomy incision. The plane of the dissection should also be considered when performing the delay procedure. As a general rule, a nipple-areolar delay/biopsy procedure should be in the same plane as the mastectomy will be performed.

The extent of the delay procedure is also open to clinical judgment: the greater the dissection, the greater the benefit of the delay procedure, but the greater the risk of losing the nipple or breast skin. Because the status of the subareolar nipple ducts is a priority, the nipple itself must always be separated from its underlying blood supply (and the underlying tissue submitted for permanent pathological evaluation), but the adjacent areola does not need to be fully undermined in cases which would seem to be particularly high risk.

The time interval between the delay procedure and the nipple-sparing mastectomy is usually set at one week. However, if the delayed tissues appear to have evidence of partial thickness loss or worrisome color changes, a longer interval is recommended (14–21 days). Shorter intervals (7 days) have the advantage of having very limited healing between the delayed tissue and the underlying breast. As time intervals lengthen, the healing process advances to the degree that sharp dissection again becomes necessary.

Prophylactic antibiotics are administered prior to the delay procedure but not continued during the postoperative course. Drains are avoided if hemostasis can be carefully maintained. Prophylaxis for deep vein thrombosis is routinely performed for both procedures. Surgeons should also realize that performing a delay procedure on the nipple-areolar complex and surrounding breast skin necessarily makes the flap a random-pattern dermal flap. As such, special precautions should be taken to avoid tension on the flap as it heals [27]. The use of a postoperative brassiere to transfer the weight of the breast to the brassiere rather than to the skin flap is strongly recommended.

## 26.3 Discussion

The history of the delay phenomenon mirrors the history of plastic surgery. Although credit for the use of the delay phenomenon to reconstruct the nose is generally given to the Italian renaissance surgeon Gaspare Taglacozzi (1545–1599), Bartolommeo Fazio (1410–1457) wrote that "Branca, the elder, and Antonius Branca, his son, Sicilians... are especially worthy to be remembered because Branca, the elder, was the inventor of an admirable and almost incredible thing. He conceived how he might repair and replace noses that had been mutilated and cut off, and developed his ideas into a marvelous art. And his son Antonius added not a little to his father's wonderful discovery. For he conceived how mutilated lips and ears might be restored, as well as noses. Moreover, whereas his father had taken the flesh for the repair from the mutilated man's face, Antonius took it from the (tissues) of his arm, so that no distortion of the face should be caused. On that arm, cut open, and into the wound itself, he bound the stump of the nose so tightly that the patient might not move his head at all, and after fifteen days, or sometimes twenty, little by little with a sharp knife he cut away the flap, which had become attached to the nose…" [28].

Although the mechanisms continue to be investigated, surgical delay of random-pattern flaps is a well-recognized method for ensuring survival of skin flaps. In their study of measured oxygen tension in delayed skin flaps, Jonsson et al. [29] concluded that "after delay, vessels were rerouted parallel to the incision and that there was considerable neovascularization… There may be, therefore, nothing particularly unique about surgical flap delay. It seems to be a useful sequence of inflammation, hemodynamic flow changes, and angiogenesis in the wound of elevation that provides a temporarily improved collateral circulation to surrounding tissue." Eriksson [30] pointed out that this was the same conclusion that Verlander [31] had come to in his 1964 thesis entitled "Vascular Changes in Tubed Pedicles."

The challenge of mastectomy to nipple survival is not a uniform question. Some surgeons leave thick mastectomy skin flaps, while others insist on maintaining traditionally thin flaps to minimize the possibility of either recurrent disease or de novo cancers. For the reason that mastectomy skin flap thickness is not a controlled variable in the nipple-sparing mastectomy necrosis literature, extrapolation of data from one surgical practice to another might not be justified. For most patients, blood flow from surrounding skin will ensure survival if 360° perfusion is maintained [21, 26]. But mastectomy skin flap survival cannot be guaranteed even in the setting of non-nipple-sparing mastectomy.

The question posed in this chapter is how the delay phenomenon can be used to maximize nipple-areolar survival following mastectomy. The first and most obvious example of using the delay phenomenon to ensure nipple, areolar, and mastectomy skin flap survival is the decision not to proceed with immediate reconstruction. In my own first cases of preserving the entire breast skin envelope, I routinely left the breast skin envelope on the chest wall following mastectomy and delayed a unipedicle "extended skin island" TRAM flap [32]. While the TRAM flap was undergoing the delay process, the skin of the mastectomy, including the nipple and areola, was also benefitting from the surgical delay. When the TRAM flap was transferred, usually at the one week mark, both components of the reconstruction, mastectomy skin and TRAM flap, had enjoyed the benefits of improved blood supply. (Final pathology was also available at the time of the flap transfer.) The practice of simply postponing the initiation of the breast reconstruction has many precedents and should be remembered in any clinical situation where the viability of the mastectomy skin and/or nipple is in serious doubt.

In the first case illustrated here, the patient had previously undergone both breast augmentation and superior peri-areolar breast biopsy (Fig. 26.1). While the breast augmentation procedure might be considered as a type of

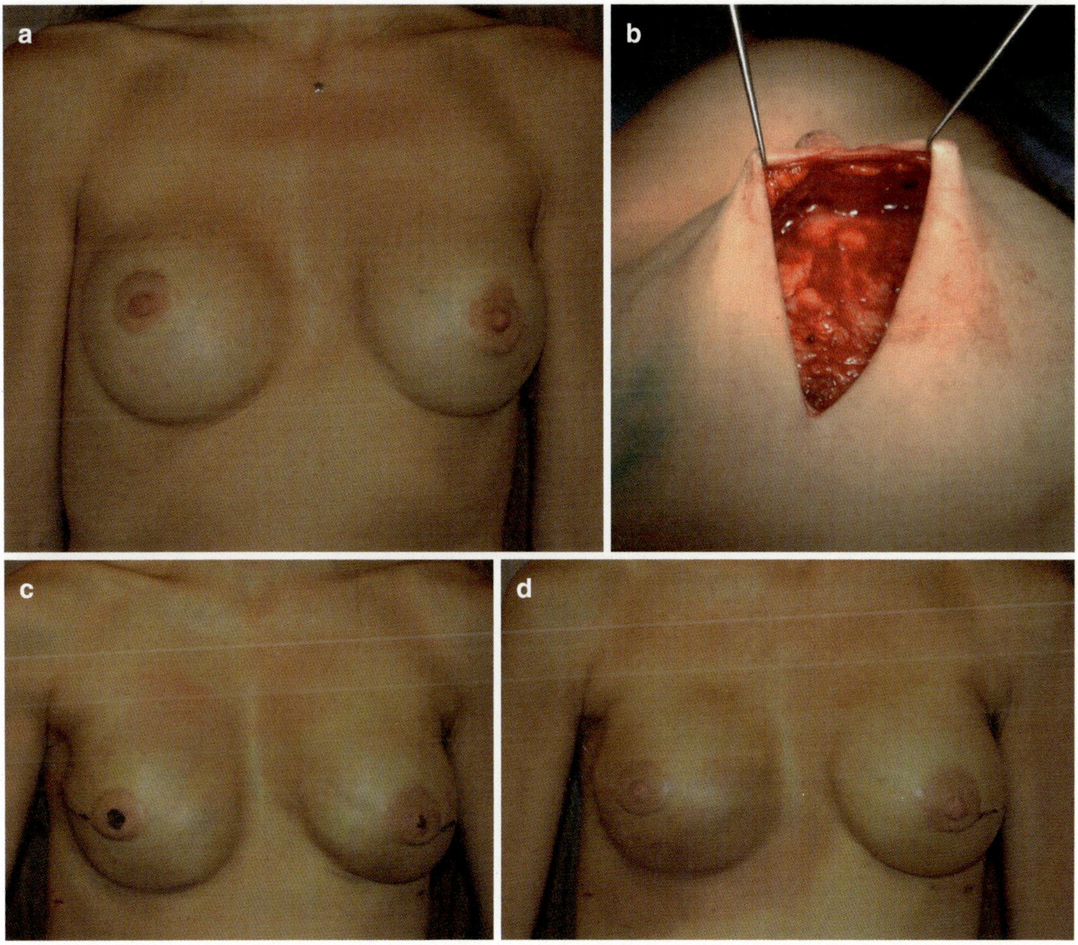


**Fig. 26.1** (**a**) The patient had previously undergone both breast augmentation and superior peri-areolar breast biopsy. (**b**) Performing the delay procedure through a lateral, radial incision preserving 360° nipple-areolar perfusion. (**c**) The patient experienced bilateral partial thickness nipple necrosis. (**d**) The improved perfusion stimulated by the delay procedure probably allowed the implant reconstruction to be successful

surgical delay procedure because it reroutes the blood supply to be parallel to the breast skin, the presence of the scars prompted the surgical team to perform the delay procedure through a lateral, radial incision preserving 360° nipple-areolar perfusion. Despite the previous rerouting prompted by the breast augmentation, this patient can be seen to have experienced bilateral partial thickness nipple necrosis. This raises the question of whether the nipples would have survived a non-delayed mastectomy procedure if they showed evidence of partial thickness loss following the delay procedure. The improved perfusion stimulated by the delay procedure probably allowed the direct to implant reconstruction to be successful.

In the second case, a patient is illustrated who would have not been considered a reasonable candidate for nipple-sparing mastectomy because she was an active cigarette smoker, had large D cup breasts, and had significant breast ptosis (Fig. 26.2). The delay procedure in her case was performed through a "hemi-batwing" pattern to allow the oncologic surgeons wide access to the breast while simultaneously lifting the nipple-areolar complex when the breast skin envelope

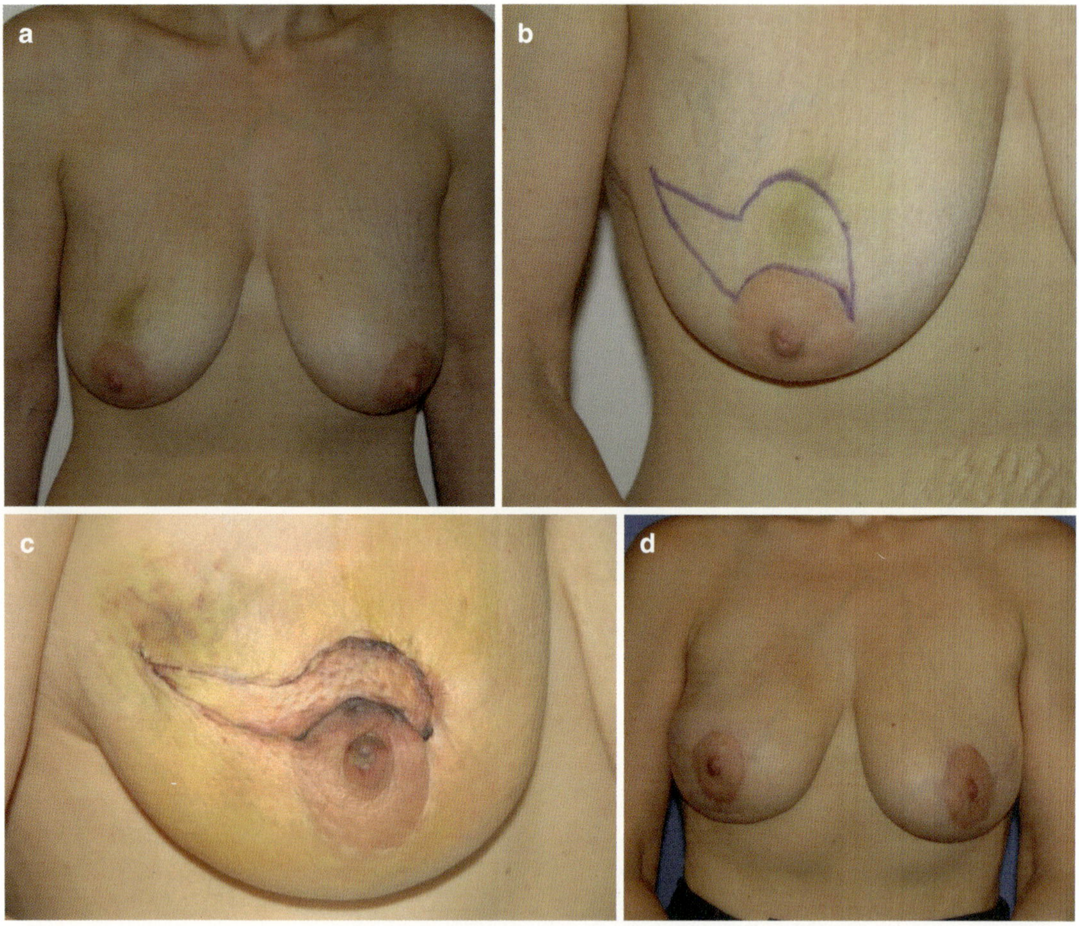

**Fig. 26.2** (**a**) This patient was an active cigarette smoker, had large D cup breasts, and had significant breast ptosis. (**b**) "Hemi-batwing" pattern to allow the oncologic surgeons wide access to the breast while simultaneously lifting the nipple-areolar complex when the breast skin envelope was reduced. (**c**) The lack of 360° perfusion of this approach probably accounts for the superficial dermal injury noted in this patient. (**d**) On the left, "hemi-batwing" reduction mammoplasty was performed and the skin envelope of the right side was filled with a muscle-sparing free TRAM flap

was reduced. The lack of 360° perfusion of this approach probably accounts for the superficial dermal injury noted in this patient but would have been significantly worse if the patient had been initially subjected to a mastectomy rather than the more limited delay procedure. On her left side, the patient underwent a "hemi-batwing" reduction mammoplasty. The skin envelope of the right side was filled with a muscle-sparing free TRAM flap.

The third illustrated case demonstrates that leaving a thick nipple-areolar skin flap (Fig. 26.3) with the intention of returning to thin out the skin flap is another way to use the delay phenomenon to ensure nipple-areolar survival. This can be done routinely in the absence of a pre-mastectomy delay procedure but can be considered a premeditated approach to delay. This approach requires careful coordination between the oncologic and plastic surgeons to be certain that a thick subareolar flap is indeed later reduced. At the later stage, the blood supply to the mastectomy skin flap has been rerouted by the wound healing changes brought on by the mastectomy procedure itself, and chances of skin loss are much reduced.

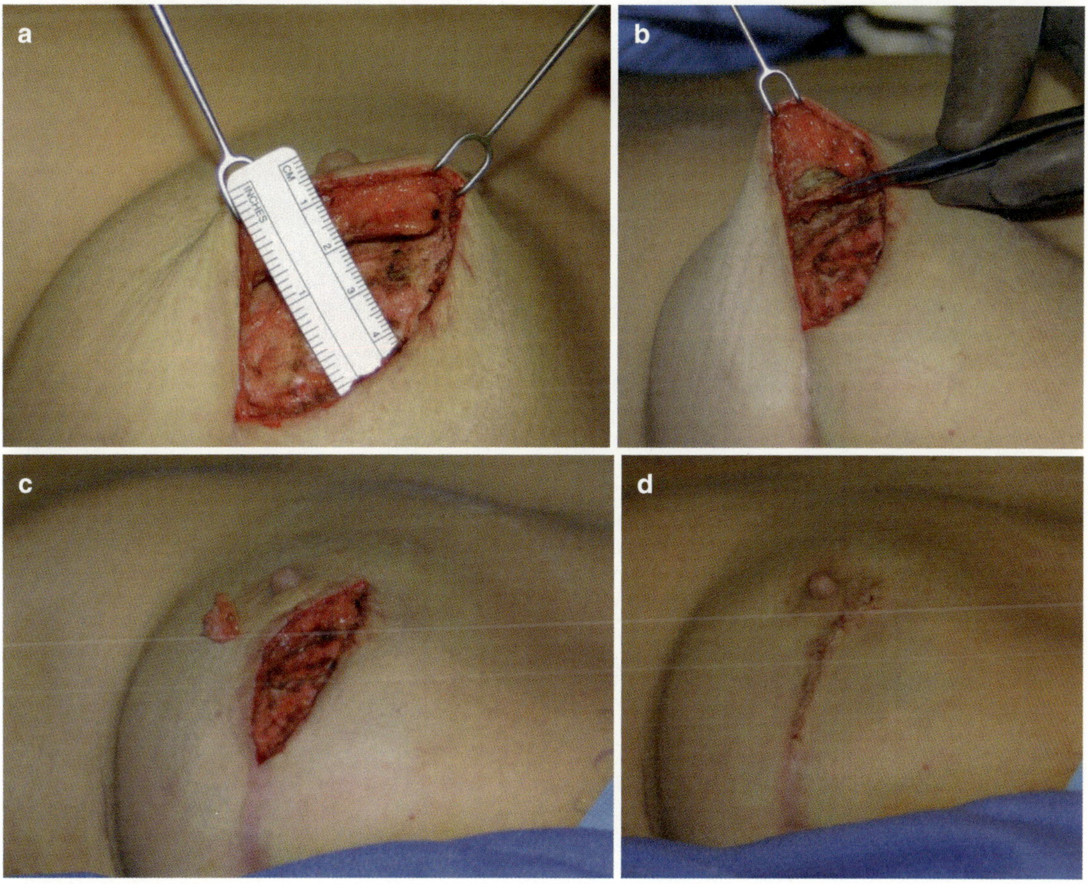

**Fig. 26.3** (**a**) Leaving a thick nipple-areolar skin flap. (**b**) Thinning out the skin flap. (**c**) Premeditated approach to delay. (**d**) Final result

## Conclusions

Nipple-sparing mastectomy has long been known to achieve superior cosmetic outcomes compared to traditional non-nipple-sparing mastectomies. Indeed, the mutilation which traditionally accompanied mastectomy might be considered the motivation behind breast conservation therapy. The relatively recent realization that nipple-sparing mastectomy is as safe or more safe as other approaches to breast conservation has stimulated wide interest and experience with this technique. Women who have been regarded as poor candidates for this procedure can be safely treated by using the principles of the delay phenomenon. A pre-mastectomy surgical delay of the nipple-areolar skin can improve the blood supply of the skin and also definitively determine the pathology of the underlying tissues. Delaying the skin envelope by postponing immediate reconstruction is also a way of using the delay phenomenon to ensure mastectomy skin survival. Leaving a thick sub-nipple-areolar skin flap (to be thinned at a later time) is also a delay technique worth consideration.

## References

1. Freeman BS. Subcutaneous mastectomy for benign breast lesions with immediate or delayed prosthetic replacement. Plast Reconstr Surg. 1962;30:676–82.
2. Hartmann LC, Schaid DJ, Woods JE, Crotty TP, Myers JL, Arnold PG, Petty PM, Sellers TA, Johnson JL, McDonnell SK, Frost MH, Jenkins RB. Efficacy

of bilateral prophylactic mastectomy in women with a family history of breast cancer. N Engl J Med. 1999;340:77–84.

3. Hartmann LC, Sellers TA, Schaid DJ, Frank TS, Soderberg CL, Sitta DL, Frost MH, Grant CS, Donohue JH, Woods JE, McDonnell SK, Vockley CW, Deffenbaugh A, Couch FJ, Jenkins RB. Efficacy of bilateral prophylactic mastectomy in BRCA1 and BRCA2 gene mutation carriers. J Natl Cancer Inst. 2001;93:1633–7.
4. Hinton CP, Doyle PJ, Blamey RW, Davies CJ, Holliday HW, Elston CW. Subcutaneous mastectomy for primary operable breast cancer. Br J Surg. 1984;71:469–72.
5. Goodnight JE Jr, Quagliana JM, Morton DL. Failure of subcutaneous mastectomy to prevent the development of breast cancer. J Surg Oncol. 1984;26:198–201.
6. Simmons RM, Brennan M, Christos P, King V, Osborne M. Analysis of nipple/areolar involvement with mastectomy: can the areola be preserved? Ann Surg Oncol. 2002;9:165–8.
7. Cense HA, Rutgers EJ, Lopes CM, Van Lanschot JJ. Nipple-sparing mastectomy in breast cancer: a viable option? Eur J Surg Oncol. 2001;27:521–6.
8. Crile G Jr, Esselstyn CB Jr, Herman RE, Hoerr SO. Partial mastectomy for carcinoma of the breast. Surg Gynecol Obstet. 1973;136:929–32.
9. Veronesi U, Cascinelli N, Mariaani L, Greco M, Saccozzi R, Luini A, Aguilar M, Marubini E. Twenty-year follow-up of a randomized study comparing breast-conserving surgery with radical mastectomy for early breast cancer. N Engl J Med. 2002;347:1227–32.
10. Fisher B, Anderson S, Bryant J, Margolese RG, Deutsch M, Fisher ER, Jeong JH, Wolmark N. Twenty-year follow-up of a randomized trial comparing total mastectomy, lumpectomy, and lumpectomy plus irradiation for the treatment of invasive breast cancer. N Engl J Med. 2002;347:1233–41.
11. Jensen JA. When can the nipple-areolar complex safely be spared during mastectomy? Plast Reconstr Surg. 2002;109:805–7.
12. Crowe JP Jr, Kim JA, Yetman R, Banbury J, Patrick RJ, Baynes D. Nipple-sparing mastectomy: technique and results in 54 procedures. Arch Surg. 2004;139:148–50.
13. Margulies AG, Hochberg J, Kepple J, Henry-Tillman RS, Westbrook K, Klimberg VS. Total skin sparing mastectomy without preservation of the nipple-areolar complex. Am J Surg. 2005;190:907–12.
14. Gerber B, Krause A, Reimer T, Müller H, Küchenmeister I, Makovitzky J, Kundt G, Friese K. Skin-sparing mastectomy with conservation of the nipple-areolar complex and autologous reconstruction is an oncologically safe procedure. Ann Surg. 2003;238:120–7.
15. Sacchini V, Pinotti JA, Barros A, Luini A, Pluchinotta A, Pinotti M, Boratto MG, Ricci MD, Ruiz CA, Nisida AC, Veronesi P, Petit J, Arnone P, Bassi F, Disa JJ, Garcia-Etienne CA, Borgen PI. Nipple-sparing mastectomy for breast cancer and risk reduction: oncologic or technical problem? J Am Coll Surg. 2006;203:704–14.
16. Benediktsson KP, Perbeck L. Survival in breast cancer after nipple-sparing subcutaneous mastectomy and immediate reconstruction with implants: a prospective trial with 13 years median follow-up in 216 patients. Eur J Surg Oncol. 2008;34:143–8.
17. Caruso F, Ferrara M, Castiglione G, Trombetta G, De Meo L, Catanuto G, Carillio G. Nipple sparing subcutaneous mastectomy: sixty-six months follow-up. Eur J Surg Oncol. 2006;32:937–40.
18. Vlajcic Z, Zic R, Stanec S, Lambasa S, Petrovecki M, Stanec Z. Nipple-areolar complex preservation: predictive factors of neoplastic nipple-areola complex invasion. Ann Plast Surg. 2005;55:240–4.
19. Spear SL, Hannan CM, Wiley SC, Cocilovo C. Nipple sparing mastectomy. Plast Reconstr Surg. 2009;123:1665–73.
20. Jensen JA. Nipple-sparing mastectomy: what is the best evidence for safety? Plast Reconstr Surg. 2009;124:2195–7.
21. Stolier AJ, Sullivan SK, Dellacroce FJ. Technical considerations in nipple-sparing mastectomy: 82 consecutive cases without necrosis. Ann Surg Oncol. 2008;15:1341–7.
22. Gould DJ, Hunt KK, Liu J, Kuerer HM, Crosby MA, Babiera G, Kronowitz SJ. Impact of surgical techniques, biomaterials, and patient variables on rate of nipple necrosis after nipple-sparing mastectomy. Plast Reconstr Surg. 2013;132:330e–8e.
23. Frederick MJ, Lin AM, Neuman R, Smith BL, Austen WG, Colwell AS. Nipple-sparing mastectomy in patients with previous breast surgery: comparative analysis of 775 immediate breast reconstructions. Plast Reconstr Surg. 2015;135:954e–62e.
24. Reish RG, Lin A, Phillips NA, Winograd J, Liao EC, Cetrulo CL, Smith BL, Austen WG, Colwell AS. Breast reconstruction outcomes after nipple-sparing mastectomy and radiation therapy. Plast Reconstr Surg. 2015;135:959–66.
25. Jensen JA, Orringer JS, Giuliano AE. Nipple sparing mastectomy in 99 patients with a mean follow-up of 5 years. Ann Surg Oncol. 2011;18:1665–70.
26. Jensen JA, Lin JH, Kapoor N, Giuliano AE. Surgical delay of the nipple-areolar complex: a powerful technique to maximize nipple viability following nipple-sparing mastectomy. Ann Surg Oncol. 2012;19:3171–6.
27. Jensen JA. Effect of tension on flap perfusion: laboratory and clinical findings. Wound Repair Regen. 2003;11:405–10.
28. Gnudi MT, Webster JP. The life and times of Gaspare Tagliacozzi, surgeon of Bologna 1545–1599. New York: Herbert Reichner; 1950. p. 110–1.

29. Jonsson K, Hunt TK, Brennan SS, Mathes SJ. Tissue oxygen measurements in delayed skin flaps: a reconsideration of the mechanisms of the delay phenomenon. Plast Reconstr Surg. 1988;82:328–35.
30. Eriksson E. Tissue oxygen measurements in delayed skin flaps: a reconsideration of the mechanisms of the delay phenomenon. Plast Reconstr Surg. 1988;82:336.
31. Velander E. Vascular changes in tubed pedicles: an animal experimental study. Acta Chir Scand Suppl. 1964;24(Suppl):322.
32. Jensen JA, Handel N, Silverstein MJ, Waisman JW, Gierson ED. Extended skin island delay of the unipedicle TRAM flap: experience in 35 patients. Plast Reconstr Surg. 1995;96:1341–5.

# Management of Nipple-Areolar Complex Complications in Nipple-Sparing Mastectomy with Prosthetic Reconstruction

27

Francesco Ciancio, Alessandro Innocenti, Domenico Parisi, and Aurelio Portincasa

## 27.1 Introduction

Nipple-sparing mastectomy (NSM) is a safe reconstructive choice in selected patients as amply demonstrated in literature [1–3]. Preserving nipple-areolar complex (NAC) provides better aesthetic outcomes than a simple mastectomy or a skin-sparing mastectomy. This technique allows good recovery of the skin envelope of the breast, including the NAC, and provides more symmetry and naturalness in the reconstructive treatment [4, 5]. Furthermore, the minor psychological impact offered by the modern techniques is a strong point in reconstructive breast surgery [6].

It is well known that one of the most frequent complications in the NSM and immediate reconstruction with implants/expander is assigned to the partial or total necrosis of the nipple-areolar complex and the skin flaps of the mastectomy [7–9]. The partial or total loss of NAC determines worse aesthetic results and requires a greater amount of time for the completion of reconstruction process; this could result in the delay of adjuvant treatment such as chemotherapy or radiotherapy [10]. A proper preoperative planning, an accurate selection of patients, and a valid management of complications after NSM would avoid a damaging loss of time for the patient's health.

## 27.2 Indications and Contraindications

The best way to reduce the possible postoperative complications is represented by proper planning of surgery. So the correct indications of NSM must be respected and all contraindicated cases must be avoided. In the literature, there are many studies concerning the correct indications in the NSM but they lack uniformity. There is a general consensus on the "absolute" contraindications such as a shorter distance of 2 cm between the neoplastic lesion and the NAC, a maximum tumor diameter of 3–4 cm, clinical suspicion of cancer involvement, or even a positive biopsy for cancer of the subareolar tissue [11, 12]. There is less consensus on the "relative" contraindications to the use of NSM and immediate reconstruction with expander/implant such as smoking, age, obesity, large breasts (weight and volume) with high degree of

F. Ciancio, M.D. (✉)
Department of Plastic and Reconstructive Surgery, University of Bari, Bari, Italy
e-mail: francescociancio01@gmail.com

A. Innocenti, M.D.
Plastic and Reconstructive Microsurgery, Careggi Universital Hospital, Florence, Italy
e-mail: innocentialessandro@alice.it

D. Parisi, M.D. • A. Portincasa, M.D.
Department of Plastic and Reconstructive Surgery, University of Foggia, Foggia 71122, Italy
e-mail: parisid@tin.it; aurelio.portincasa@unifg.it


M.A. Shiffman (ed.), *Nipple-Areolar Complex Reconstruction*,
https://doi.org/10.1007/978-3-319-60925-6_27

ptosis, previous radiation therapy, and comorbidities such as diabetes mellitus and hypertension. All of these are listed as risk factors to be considered when choosing to perform an NSM.

## 27.3 Factors that Influence the NAC Complication Rate in NSM

The reported rate of necrotic complications in NSM is highly variable in the literature because there is uniqueness in the definition of partial or total necrosis of the areola and nipple. In addition, many of these studies are characterized by poor standardization of the sample analyzed. As a general principle, partial (Fig. 27.1) or total necrosis of the NAC after NSM and immediate reconstruction with implants is around rated as <10%, and it is considered as the most frequent complication together with hematoma formation. The main identified risk factors are:

1. Type of skin incision (Fig. 27.2)
2. One-stage breast reconstruction direct with breast prosthesis or two stages with expander
3. Volume of the implants
4. Excessive inflation of breast expander
5. Dimensions of the breasts (weight and volume)
6. Smoke
7. Age
8. BMI
9. Comorbidities (diabetes and hypertension)
10. Radiotherapy
11. Experience of the surgeon

As regards on the type of skin incision, there is a widespread consensus about the superior rate of necrosis of the NAC with transareolar (81.8%) and periareolar (38.3%) incisions; in fact, these represent the approaches with greater disruption of the vascular network of the nipple-areolar complex [13]. Vertical, lateral, or radial incisions with or without extensions are safer in terms of the NAC vitality. The incisions involving the areola or nipple are those with the highest rates of necrotic complications. Interestingly, some studies have shown a higher rate of necrosis when the dissection was performed more with diathermy compared to those performed mainly with cold blade [13, 14]. In support of these data,

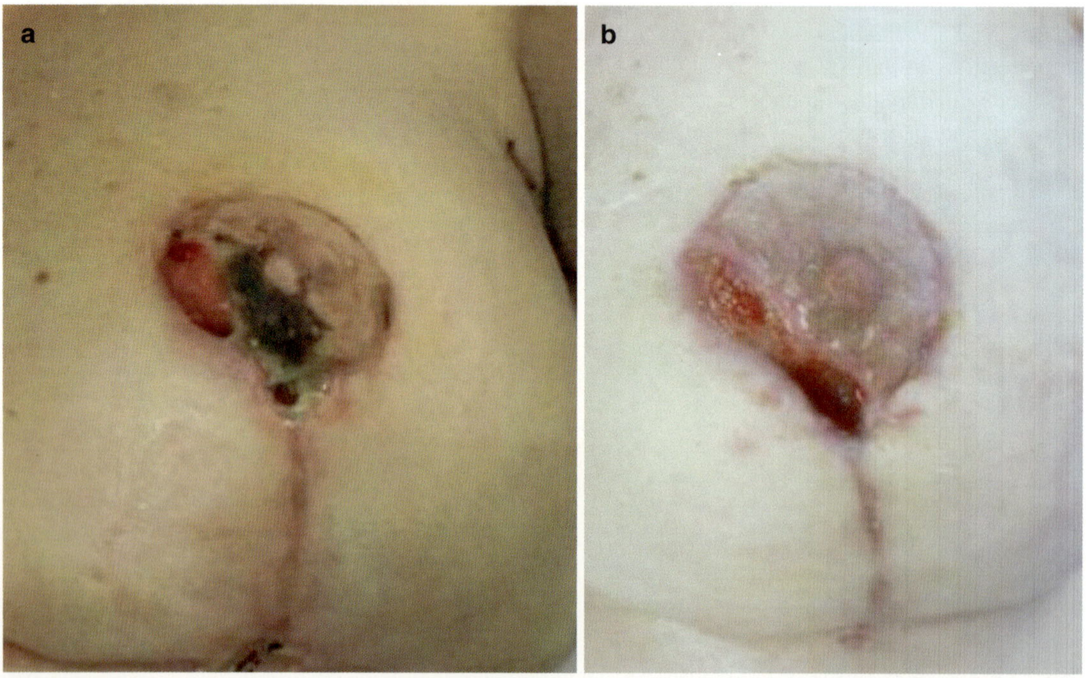

**Fig. 27.1** (**a**) Partial necrosis of the areola. (**b**) After debridement with cold blade

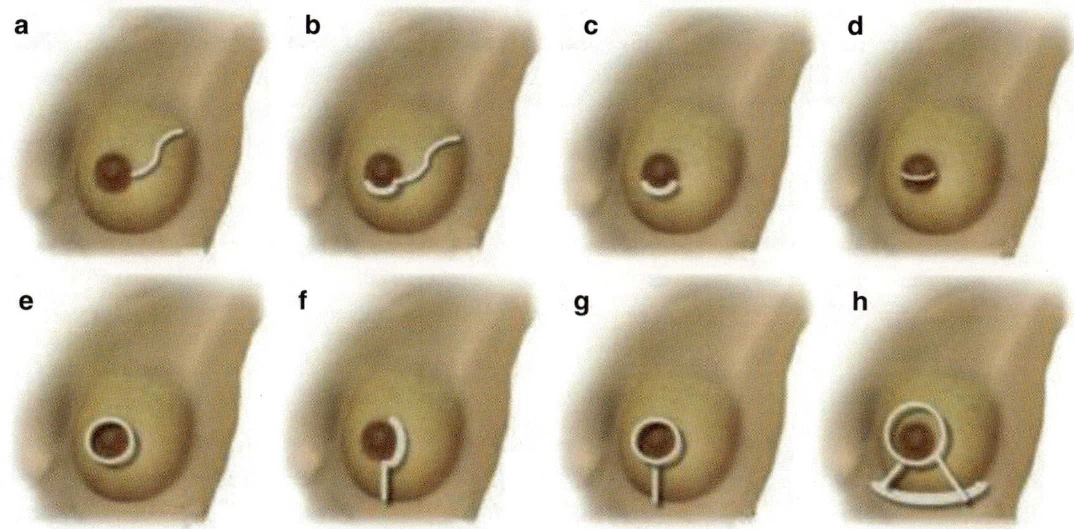


**Fig. 27.2** (**a–h**) Different types of skin incision for NSM

there are studies demonstrating the importance of the subdermal vascularization of the areola [15].

Regarding the choice of an immediate reconstruction with implants (one-stage) or in two times with expander and prosthesis (two-stage), there is no significant difference in the rate of necrotic NAC. On the other side, a higher volume of the prosthesis or an excessive intraoperative inflation of the expander appears to be more related to the NAC necrosis. A probable cause of this could be an excessive wall tension responsible for ischemia of the subdermal plexus of the NAC [3, 13].

The large breasts are characterized by a greater distance between the sternal notch and the nipple, and this determines a greater chance of vascular suffering of the NAC. Despite the fact that this consideration appears logical, in some studies, there was no significant difference in the rate of necrosis in large breasts with a high degree of ptosis undergoing NSM with implants [16], compared to medium to small breast.

In our experience, the medium or small breast patients are the ideal candidates for reconstruction with implants and savings of the nipple-areolar complex, while patients with larger breasts, skin-reducing mastectomy (SRM) should be considered as first option.

Smoking does not appear to be a statistically significant contraindication, but a general consensus exists on the greatest rate of necrotic complications of the nipple-areolar complex in smokers as well as in the case of involving microcirculation diseases such as diabetes and hypertension [13–16].

Finally, the experience of the surgeon is an element of significant difference, according to some data reported in the literature. In fact, the rate of necrotic complications after NSM is greater in series of patients performed by less expert surgeons compared to those performed by surgeons with more years of surgical activities [13–17].

## 27.4 Technique

Based on the considerations expressed in the previous paragraph, we just try to give some technical recommendations in order to minimize the rate of necrotic complications of the NAC in the NSM.

In planning the skin incision, the surgeon must consider the location of the tumor mass and the vascularization of the NAC. The transareolar incisions are to be avoided, while the periareolar incisions must not extend to more than one third of the circumference of the areola. The safest surgical approach, in our experience, is the lateral or vertical incision. The surgical dissection of the under-areolar tissue must be performed with cold knife, in order to minimize the thermal damage induced by diathermy.

A possible option is to select cases like "potentially at risk of necrosis of the NAC" and submit them to the "skin-banking technique." This method has been known for years and allows, in selected cases, to obtain good aesthetic results through two operative times [18, 19].

## 27.5 Management of Nipple-Areolar Complex Complications

The main complication of NAC is the necrosis; it may be due to a poor arterial flow or to venous congestion. For this last option, we have successfully used the continuous negative-pressure wound therapy (NPWT) at −80 mmHg in the immediate postoperative, as soon as the complication was detected for 7–10 days, resulting in a partial recovery of the NAC. The negative-pressure therapy induces an increase in perfusion of the microcirculation, reduces exudate, and reduces the bacterial load of the wound. With this step, we have saved about 80% of the NAC (Fig. 27.3) [20].

When we had areas with necrosis, the two opportunities that we could choose were either surgery or healing by secondary intention after debridement.

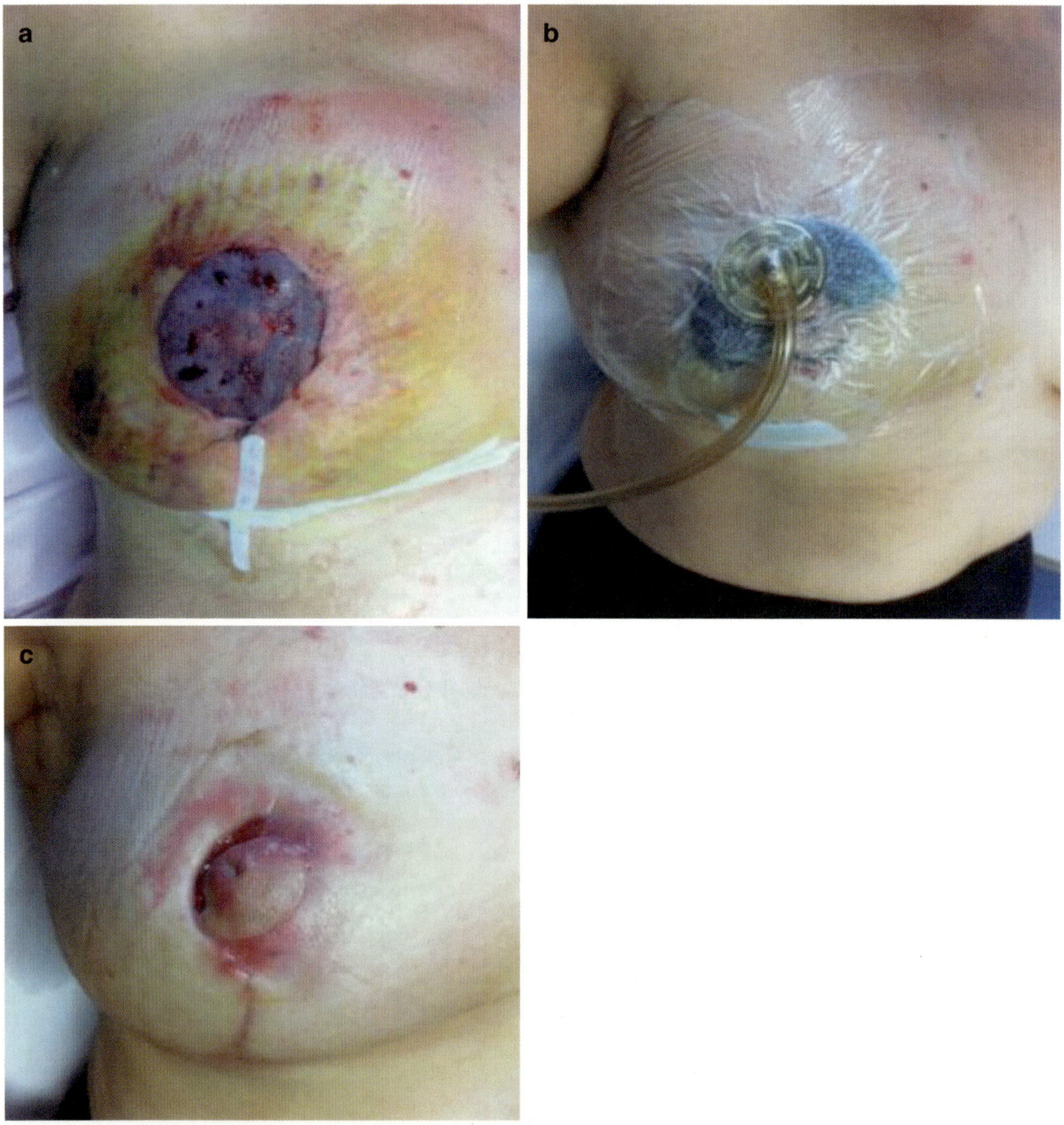


**Fig. 27.3** (**a**) Venous congestion of the NAC 24 h after surgery. (**b**) Application of negative-pressure wound therapy at −80 mmHg for 7 days. (**c**) Recovery of about 80% of the nipple-areolar complex

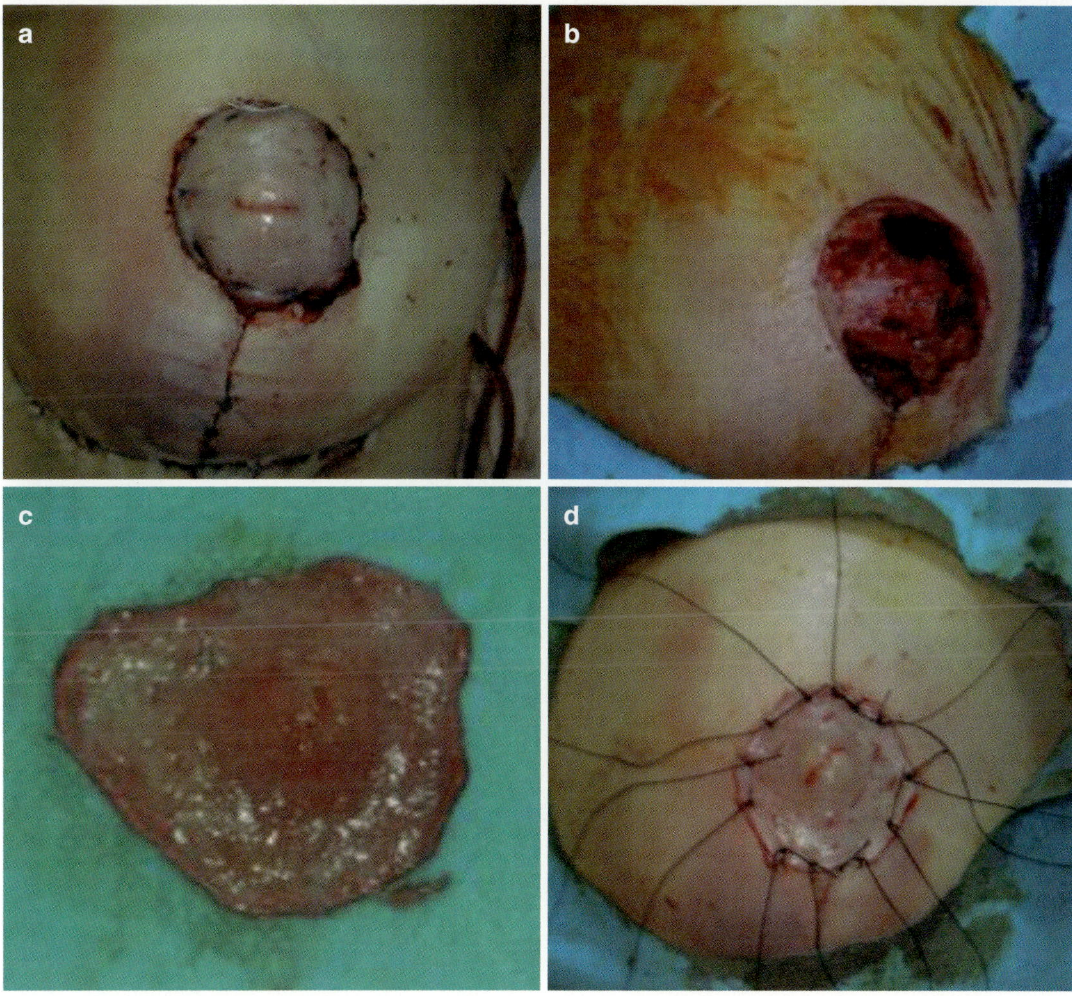


**Fig. 27.4** (**a**) Hematoma of the NAC 24 h after surgery. (**b**) Removal of nipple-areolar complex and evacuation of the hematoma. (**c**) NAC. (**d**) Graft of the NAC

Necrotic areas must be removed, and in our cases, we rarely used enzymatic debridement with collagenase, while more often, we implemented a debridement with cold blade. The choice was conditioned by the need to solve as soon as possible this complication and allow the patient the continuation of the therapeutic procedure.

In total NAC necrosis, the only choice was to remove the entire NAC, proceed to a suture by primary intention, and only later (after 2–3 months), reconstruct it with local flaps or skin grafts. In case of partial necrosis or hematoma, a debridement of necrotic areas may be indicated followed by an immediate reconstruction with local flaps and/or skin grafts taken from the contralateral areola or from donor areas like the groin (Fig. 27.4).

Healing by secondary intention requires more time, but in selected cases, we used advanced dressings as hydrofiber with excellent results (Fig. 27.5).

Epidermolysis of the nipple-areolar complex is a less frequent condition in NSM, and usually we employ dressings based on hyaluronic acid in order to stimulate the process of regeneration of the epithelium.

## 27.6 Discussion

The nipple-sparing mastectomy is an oncoplastic technique with excellent aesthetic outcomes with low psychological impact on patients and good

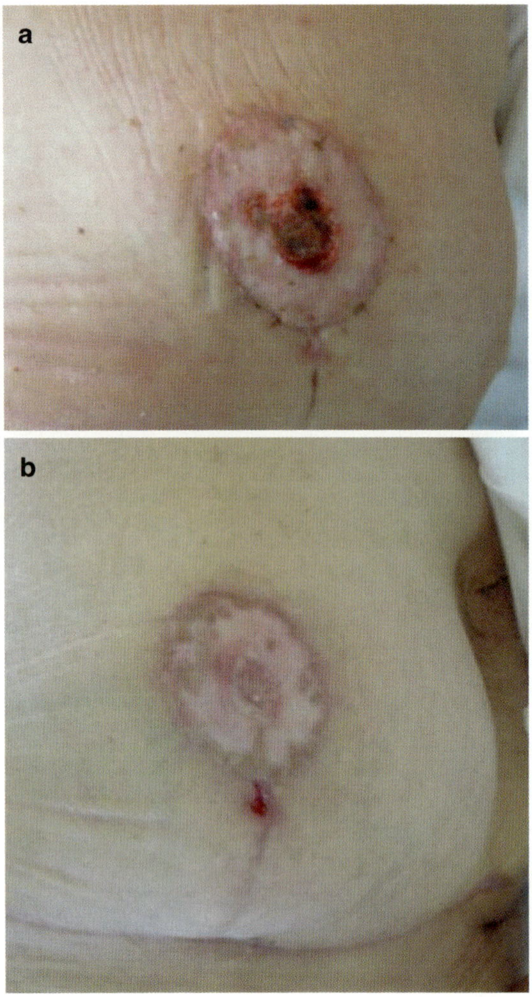

Fig. 27.5 (a) Partial necrosis of the nipple. (b) Thirty days after treatment with debridement with collagenase and hydrofiber advanced dressing

oncological radicality. There are several constitutional risk factors expressed in literature; definitely large breasts and a high degree of ptosis, smoking, and comorbidities present are items to consider when choosing a reconstructive procedure with implants or expander after nipple-sparing mastectomy.

Compliance with the indications and contraindications is the basis of the final result.

The execution of the technique must be guided by the principle of respect of tissues and even local perfusion, limiting the use of diathermy in the areas around the areola. The early recognition of complications allows us to use the appropriate and timely solutions in order to reduce the entity of the same.

**Conclusions**

The nipple-areolar-sparing mastectomy, although resulting in necrotic complications, is a valuable surgical option. The proper management of complications is an important factor for an optimal result.

## References

1. Jensen JA, Orringer JS, Giuliano AE. Nipple-sparing mastectomy in 99 patients with a mean follow-up of 5 years. Ann Surg Oncol. 2011;18:1665–70.
2. de Alcantara Filho P, Capko D, Barry JM, Morrow M, Pusic A, Sacchini VS. Nipple-sparing mastectomy for breast cancer and risk-reducing surgery: the Memorial Sloan-Kettering Cancer Center experience. Ann Surg Oncol. 2011;18:3117–22.
3. Warren PA, Foster RD, Stover AC, Itakura K, Ewing CA, Alvarado M, Hwang ES, Esserman LJ. Outcomes after total skin-sparing mastectomy and immediate reconstruction in 657 breasts. Ann Surg Oncol. 2012;19:3402–9.
4. Mallon P, Feron JG, Couturaud B, Fitoussi A, Lemasurier P, Guihard T, Cothier-Savay I, Reyal F. The role of nipple-sparing mastectomy in breast cancer: a comprehensive review of the literature. Plast Reconstr Surg. 2013;131:969–84.
5. Voltura AM, Tsangaris TN, Rosson GD, Jacobs LK, Flores JI, Singh NK, Argani P, Balch CM. Nipple-sparing mastectomy: critical assessment of 51 procedures and implications for selection criteria. Ann Surg Oncol. 2008;15:3396–401.
6. Sherman KA, Woon S, French J, Elder E. Body image and psychological distress in nipple-sparing mastectomy: the roles of self-compassion and appearance investment. Psycho-Oncology. 2017;26:337–45.
7. Bishop CC, Singh S, Nash AG. Mastectomy and breast reconstruction preserving the nipple. Ann R Coll Surg Engl. 1990;72:87–9.
8. Palmer BV, Mannur KR, Ross WB. Subcutaneous mastectomy with immediate reconstruction as treatment for early breast cancer. Br J Surg. 1992;79:1309–11.
9. Stanec Z, Zic R, Stanec S, Budi S, Hudson D, Skoll P. Skin-sparing mastectomy with nipple-areola conservation. Plast Reconstr Surg. 2003;111:496–8.
10. Eck DL, McLaughlin SA, Terkonda SP, Rawal B, Perdikis G. Effects of immediate reconstruction on adjuvant chemotherapy in breast cancer patients. Ann Plast Surg. 2015;74(Suppl 4):S201–3.

11. Garcia-Etienne CA, Borgen PI. Update on the indications for nipple-sparing mastectomy. J Support Oncol. 2006;4:225–330.
12. Alperovich M, Choi M, Karp NS, Singh B, Ayo D, Frey JD, Roses DF, Schnabel FR, Axelrod DM, Shapiro RL, Guth AA. Nipple-sparing mastectomy and sub-areolar biopsy: to freeze or not to freeze? Evaluating the role of sub-areolar intraoperative frozen section. Breast J. 2016;22(1):18–23.
13. Lee KT, Mun GH. Necrotic complications in nipple-sparing mastectomy followed by immediate breast reconstruction: systematic review with pooled analysis. Arch Reconstr Microsurg. 2014;23(2):51–64.
14. Wijayanayagam A, Kumar AS, Foster RD, Esserman L. Optimizing the total skin-sparing mastectomy. Arch Surg. 2008;143:38–45.
15. Rusby JE, Brachtel EF, Michaelson JS, Koerner FC, Smith BL. Breast duct anatomy in the human nipple: three-dimensional patterns and clinical implications. Breast Cancer Res Treat. 2007;106:171–9.
16. Chirappapha P, Petit JY, Rietjens M, De Lorenzi F, Garusi C, Martella S, Barbieri B, Gottardi A, Andrea M, Giuseppe L, Hamza A, Lohsiriwat V. Nipple sparing mastectomy: does breast morphological factor related to necrotic complications? Plast Reconstr Surg Glob Open. 2014;2(1):e99.
17. Stolier AJ, Sullivan SK, Dellacroce FJ. Technical considerations in nipple-sparing mastectomy: 82 consecutive cases without necrosis. Ann Surg Oncol. 2008;15(5):1341–7.
18. Park SW, Lee TJ, Kim EK, Eom JS. Managing necrosis of the nipple-areola complex in breast reconstruction after nipple-sparing mastectomy: immediate nipple-areola complex reconstruction with banked skin. Plast Reconstr Surg. 2014;133(1):73e–4e.
19. Kovach SJ, Georgiade GS. The "banked" TRAM: a method to insure mastectomy skin-flap survival. Ann Plast Surg. 2006;57(4):366–9.
20. Annacontini L, Ciancio F, Parisi D, Innocenti A, Portincasa A. Management of nipple-areolar complex complications in skin-sparing mastectomy with prosthetic reconstruction. A case report. Ann Ital Chir. 2016;87(ePub). pii: S2239253X16024440.

# 28 Nipple Malposition Following Nipple-Sparing Mastectomy: How Can We Prevent It?

Ioannis Flessas, Nikolaos V. Michalopoulos, Nikolaos A. Papadopulos, Constantinos G. Zografos, and George C. Zografos

## 28.1 Introduction

Nipple-sparing mastectomy is the latest evolution in mastectomy technique, providing superior cosmetic results without compromising oncological safety. A potential complication of the procedure is the malposition of the nipple in the reconstructed breast which is mainly either lateral displacement of the nipple or the so-called high-riding nipple-areolar complex (NAC). Following nipple-sparing mastectomy, immediate reconstruction is almost always applied either with a silicone breast implant or a tissue expander, under the pectoralis major muscle.

I. Flessas, M.D., Ph.D., M.Sc. (✉)
Breast Unit, General and Maternity Hospital Helena Venizelou, Helena Venizelou Square 2, Athens, Greece
e-mail: iflessas@gmail.com

N.V. Michalopoulos, Ph.D. • C.G. Zografos
G.C. Zografos, M.D., Ph.D.
1st Department of Propaedeutic Surgery, "Hippokratio" General Hospital, Medical School, University of Athens, Athens, Greece
e-mail: nmichal@med.uoa.gr; koszogra92@hotmail.com; gzografo@med.uoa.gr

N.A. Papadopulos, M.D., Ph.D.
University Hospital of Alexandroupoli, School of Medicine, Democritus University of Thrace, Alexandroupolis, Greece

University Hospital Rechts der Isar, School of Medicine, Munich Technical University, Munich, Germany
e-mail: n.papadopulos@lrz.tum.de

The high-riding nipple-areolar complex is a potential complication of cosmetic or reconstructive breast procedures. Although a number of authors have attempted to create objective measurements by which to evaluate nipple position, it is almost always obvious to the patient and physician alike when a nipple is positioned too high on the breast [1–3]. More challenging, however, is developing an operative plan to address the high-riding nipple-areolar complex based on the nature and degree of displacement.

Overelevation of the nipple-areolar complex can occur after several surgical procedures. Mastopexy and breast reduction operations are routinely designed to elevate the nipple-areolar complex, but may result in a nipple-areolar complex that appears elevated more than ideal or expected in the plan. In several revision mastopexies, breast reductions, or mastopexies followed by augmentations, there may be a tendency for the nipple-areolar complex to elevate even further. The nipple-areolar complex can also migrate superiorly and appear too high after nipple-sparing mastectomy. Unlike a skin-sparing mastectomy where the nipple-areolar complex is actively reconstructed in a staged fashion, a nipple-sparing mastectomy retains the original nipple-areolar complex position passively, and its final position is less controllable. This situation is worsened by radiation therapy, which preferentially tightens the skin above the nipple and further elevates the nipple-areolar complex. The management of the


M.A. Shiffman (ed.), *Nipple-Areolar Complex Reconstruction*,
https://doi.org/10.1007/978-3-319-60925-6_28

high-riding nipple-areolar complex is complicated in part because of the desire to avoid leaving scars that lie above the edge of the nipple-areolar complex (in the superior aspect of the breast) and the limited amount of skin available between the nipple and the clavicle. Several strategies have been described to address these issues, including elevating the inframammary fold (IMF) and the breast parenchyma, expanding the skin superior to the nipple-areolar complex, and directly repositioning the nipple by excising it and grafting it in a more appropriate location [4–7]. The high-riding nipple presents a complicated reconstructive challenge. Appreciating its cause and the available corrective surgical options may help surgeons, on the one hand, minimize the likelihood of creating nipple malpositioning and, on the other hand, help select an appropriate intervention.

## 28.2 Technique for Nipple Malpositioning Prevention

Several other solutions have been described in the literature, including techniques where the nipple is lowered through a buttonhole [8], transposed as a flap, or Z-plasty [6]. Excision and repositioning as a graft may result in the least scarring, but at the risk of nipple loss. Techniques that involve elevating the entire breast relative to the nipple have been described both by elevating the inframammary fold and with the use of implants or tissue expanders [8], but are less useful for correcting multiple vectors of displacement. Thus, given that these techniques may be complex and often provide suboptimal results [6], prevention should be preferable to cure. Following nipple-sparing mastectomy, immediate reconstruction is almost always applied either with a silicone breast implant or a tissue expander. We always try to ensure full coverage of the implant, and we place the implants underneath the pectoralis major and serratus anterior muscles. If a tissue expander is used, it is filled with saline in order to achieve the maximum possible expansion without compromising blood supply to the mastectomy flap. The patient is then turned to a sitting position to estimate the proper nipple-areolar position in the reconstructed breast in comparison with the contralateral breast [3, 4]. A mark on the proper position at the anterior surface of the pectoralis major muscle corresponding to the posterior part of the nipple-areolar complex is made. Two or three absorbable Vicryl 3-0 sutures are placed to suture the posterior border of the nipple on the marked area of the pectoralis major muscle (Fig. 28.1). Care is always taken not to puncture the submuscular implant. These sutures are placed in order to prevent migration of the nipple-areolar complex which is usually superiorly and laterally. The rest of the procedure remains unaltered.

This technique has been performed in 14 patients who underwent nipple-sparing mastectomies in our department. All patients, followed up to 12 months, had pleasant cosmetic results as nipple malposition was avoided. Therefore, we recommend this easy and quick procedure as an effective approach to optimize nipple-sparing mastectomy aesthetic outcome.

In case that the nipple malposition is not prevented, several techniques have been described in order to manage surgically the correction of this malposition. Because of the desire to avoid scars on the superior aspect of the breast and the limited availability of superior breast skin, it can be technically challenging to place the nipple-areolar complex in a lower position. Multiple surgical

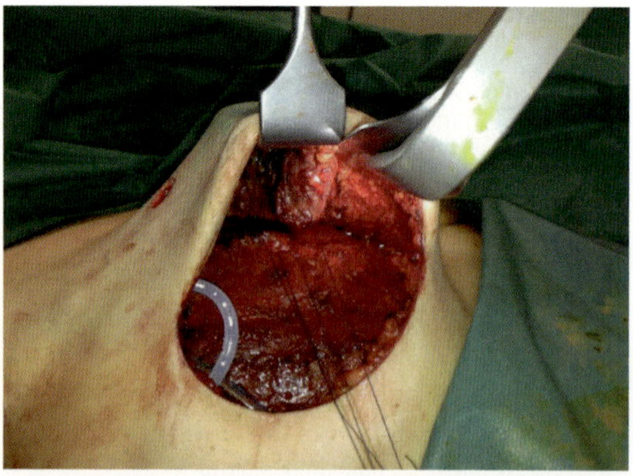

**Fig. 28.1** Suturing the posterior border of the nipple on the marked area of the pectoralis major muscle

strategies have attempted to lower it, and each has its advantages and disadvantages. Reciprocal rotation flaps have been used with success.

## 28.3 Preoperative Planning: Operative Technique of Reciprocal Flap

The surgical plan is designed with the patient upright [9]. The current nipple and areola are marked and the desired nipple location identified with a surrounding outline for the areola to ensure the two areolar outlines are adjacent. The flaps are then marked such that the blood supply of the nipple-areolar complex-carrying flap is maximized; previous scars are noted, given that all patients had previous breast surgery.

In the operating theatre, local anaesthetic is infiltrated. The flaps are sharply cut with a scalpel blade and electrocautery is kept to a minimum. If there is an underlying implant, the flap edges are taken down nearly to the level of the capsule, at which point, the edge is carefully retracted preferably with skin hooks and the flaps dissected sharply away from the capsule with a blade. The least amount of undermining that allows flap transposition is then performed. Once the flaps are raised and transposed, they are sutured in place with a few buried dermal absorbable monofilament sutures, followed by running or interrupted permanent monofilament cuticular sutures. Any standing dog's-ears are left, to avoid compromise of flap perfusion. The flaps are covered with antibiotic ointment and gauze.

## 28.4 Discussion

Z-plasty transposition to relocate the nipple-areolar complex (NAC) to a lower position following breast reconstruction is a simple and reliable technique, although it involves creation of scars. It is also important to note that a patient could have a background of radiotherapy, and the NAC relocation works well despite this. This technique was described by Mohmand and Naasan [10]. There is an important and aesthetic difference between the two techniques in the orientation of the flaps. The orientation that was described by Graeme et al. [11] provides a more aesthetic result, with minimal scarring appearing above the bra line. While Mohmand and Naasan [10] use a more rounded scar, which from their description seemed to appear above the bra line, other techniques that have been used to relocate the high-riding nipple tend to be more complex and produce a wide variety of results. Millard et al. [4] published an article in which a two-stage technique was presented: An ellipse of scarred skin is excised along the IMS, and the lower pole is tucked up behind the breast, effectively raising the whole breast while leaving the nipple in the same position. This was followed by lowering the NAC through a "buttonhole" excision of tissue at the new desired nipple position. Other authors have transposed two subcutaneous pedicled flaps in postburn malposition NAC, using the NAC as a graft and swapping this with a separate full-thickness graft at the new NAC location [12] (technique that leaves the grafted skin as scar with a potentially undesirable texture and skin colour) and trying to shorten the distance between the NAC and IMS by simply excising a transverse ellipse of skin and parenchyma, followed by a vertical wedge excision.

Conservative, meticulous dissection with flap blood supply is clearly important for a successful outcome. The outlined technique would also be suitable for other aesthetic breast cases of high-riding nipples. The patient, however, has to accept they will be gaining an additional scar as a price for correcting their nipple position.

**Conclusions**

Correction of this sometimes devastating complication can be challenging and may involve new scars [13]. Excision and repositioning as a graft may result in the least scarring, but at the risk of nipple loss. Thus, given that these techniques may be complex and often provide suboptimal results, therefore, it would be ideal if it could be prevented during the initial operation. Herein, we described a simple technique to apply immediately before skin closure which can lead to proper postoperative nipple-areolar position.

## References

1. Mallucci P, Branford OA. Concepts in aesthetic breast dimensions: analysis of the ideal breast. J Plast Reconstr Aesthet Surg. 2012;65:8–16.
2. Hauben DJ, Adler N, Silfen R, Regev D. Breast-areola-nipple proportion. Ann Plast Surg. 2003;50:510–3.
3. Hall-Findlay EJ. The three breast dimensions: analysis and effecting change. Plast Reconstr Surg. 2010;125:1632–42.
4. Millard DR Jr, Mullin WR, Lesavoy MA. Secondary correction of the too-high areola and nipple after a mammaplasty. Plast Reconstr Surg. 1976;58:568–72.
5. Elsahy NI. Correction of abnormally high nipples after reduction mammaplasty. Aesthet Plast Surg. 1990;14:21–6.
6. Colwell AS, May JW Jr, Slavin SA. Lowering the postoperative high-riding nipple. Plast Reconstr Surg. 2007;120:596–9.
7. Spear SL, Hoffman S. Relocation of the displaced nipple-areola by reciprocal skin grafts. Plast Reconstr Surg. 1998;101:1355–8.
8. Frenkiel BA, Pacifico MD, Ritz M, Southwick G. A solution to the high-riding nipple-areola complex. Aesthet Plast Surg. 2010;34:525–7.
9. Spear SL, Albino FP, Al-Attar A. Repairing the high-riding nipple with reciprocal transposition flaps. Plast Reconstr Surg. 2013;131(4):687–9.
10. Mohamand H, Naasan A. Double U-plasty for correction of geometric malposition of the nipple-areolar complex. Plast Reconstr Surg. 2002;109:2019–22.
11. Frenkiel BA, Pacifico MD, Ritz M, Southwick G. A solution to the high-riding nipple–areola complex. Aesthet Plast Surg. 2010;34:525–7.
12. Taneda H, Sakai S. Transposition technique for correction of malpositioned nipple-areola complex after reconstruction following a nipple-sparing mastectomy: a case report. Ann Plast Surg. 2001;67:579–82.
13. Flessas I, Michalopoulos NV, Zografos GC. Nipple malposition following nipple-sparing mastectomy. How can we prevent it? Breast J. 2016;22(1):131–2.

# Nipple-Areolar Complex Ischemia: Management During Aesthetic Mammoplasties

# 29

Alberto Rancati, Claudio Angrigiani, Marcelo Irigo, and Braulio Peralta

## 29.1 Introduction

Partial or total nipple necrosis after aesthetic mammoplasty surgery can be a serious complication for both the patient and surgeon. Knowledge of breast anatomy, continuous nipple-areolar complex (NAC) checking, and early identification of vascular compromise, followed by appropriate action, may help prevent total NAC loss. Intraoperative pale appearance of the NAC may be an initial sign of this complication.

Different intraoperative surgical maneuvers, other than tissue resection, can alter NAC vitality and lead to ischemia, partial/total loss, areolar sufferance, nipple projection loss, and/or hypopigmentation. This complication may arise independently of the selected technique [1–5].

NAC necrosis has been reported in 2% of the cases during breast reduction and in 1% during mastopexy; epidermolysis with blister-like formation from intra- or subdermal edema may result in 5–11% of the cases [1].

A. Rancati, M.D., Ph.D. (✉)
Department of Oncoplastic Surgery, Instituto Oncologico Henry Moore, University of Buenos Aires, Buenos Aires, Argentina
e-mail: rancati@gmail.com

C. Angrigiani, M.D.
Department of Plastic Surgery, Hospital Santojanni, Buenos Aires, Argentina
e-mail: claudioangrigiani@gmail.com

M. Irigo, M.D., Ph.D.
Department of Oculoplastic Surgery, Instituto Oncologico Henry Moore, University of Buenos Aires, Buenos Aires, Argentina
e-mail: irigomarcelo@gmail.com

B. Peralta, M.D.
Instituto Oncologico Henry Moore, University of Buenos Aires, Buenos Aires, Argentina
e-mail: brauliojperalta@gmail.com

## 29.2 Vascular Anatomy of the Breast

To understand the appearance of NAC ischemia and necrosis requires solid knowledge of breast and NAC vascular anatomy. Any surgical maneuver involving the breast parenchyma will alter not only its architecture, but its blood supply as well. Unnecessary maneuvers as detaching the parenchyma from the pectoralis fascia during mammoplasty procedures may alter not only the vascularization but also breast innervation. Regardless of the chosen pedicle, the technique, and the resected breast parenchyma, the remaining breast tissue must be mobilized without detachment from the pectoralis fascia and avoiding remaining dead spaces [6, 7].

Breast vascularization depends on:

1. Internal and external mammary systems
2. Thoracoacromial artery with perforators
3. Intercostal vessels
4. Lateral thoracic system
5. Supraclavicular branches (Fig. 29.1)


M.A. Shiffman (ed.), *Nipple-Areolar Complex Reconstruction*,
https://doi.org/10.1007/978-3-319-60925-6_29

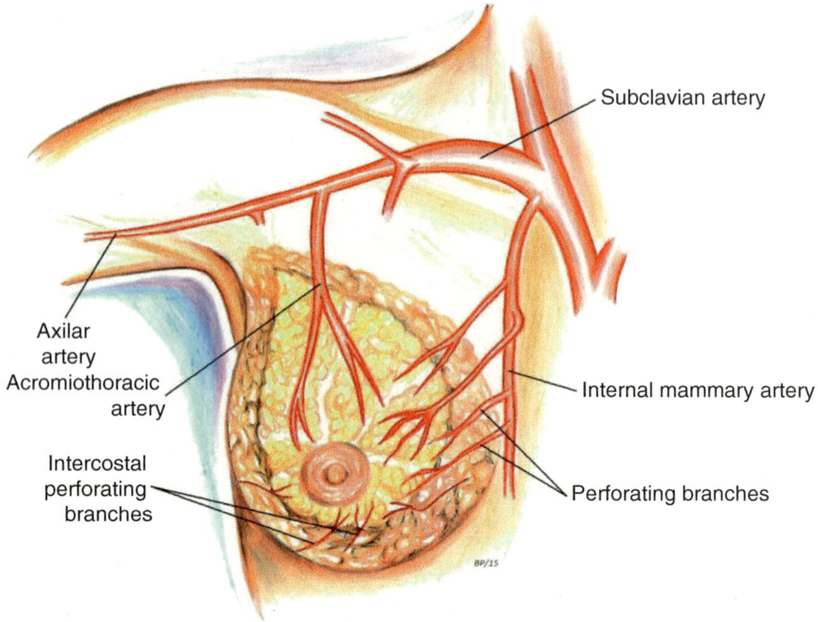


**Fig. 29.1** Breast vascular anatomy

Another key element to keep in mind previous to breast reduction revisions is the patient's history related to previous breast surgeries; pictures, if available, are ideal in these cases.

The information required goes beyond the skin scar pattern; a detailed surgical history regarding the resected tissue, the NAC pedicle, the NAC original size, the original existing relations of the NAC, (midline, inframammary fold, sternal notch), and the dates of the surgeries are considered important information to be gathered prior to surgery [1, 8–10].

Continuous nipple-areolar complex (NAC) checking and early identification of vascular compromise, followed by appropriate action, may help prevent total NAC loss.

NAC necrosis occurs commonly in the case of large reductions (resection >1000 g), where a long pedicle is created to carry the circulation of the NAC, and folding during closure can stress the circulation (Fig. 29.2) [11, 12].

1. Length of pedicle (>10 cm mobilization)
2. Large reductions (>2000 g)
3. Excessive pedicle folding, kinking, and malrotation
4. Excessive thinning of the pedicle
5. Previous periareolar scars
6. Dense gland pedicle (compression)
7. Simultaneous augmentation/mastopexy with implant hematoma compression (Fig. 29.2)
8. Reoperative reduction/mastopexy with unknown initial pedicle
9. Previous tumor resections

## 29.3 Associated Risk Factors

1. BMI >30
2. Diabetes
3. Past history of poor wound healing
4. Heavy smoking
5. Simultaneous augmentation/mastopexy
6. Previous radiotherapy
7. Previous scars around NAC
8. Post-bariatric surgery, malnutrition
9. Genetic predisposition to thrombosis
10. Malignancies, immunomodulating medication

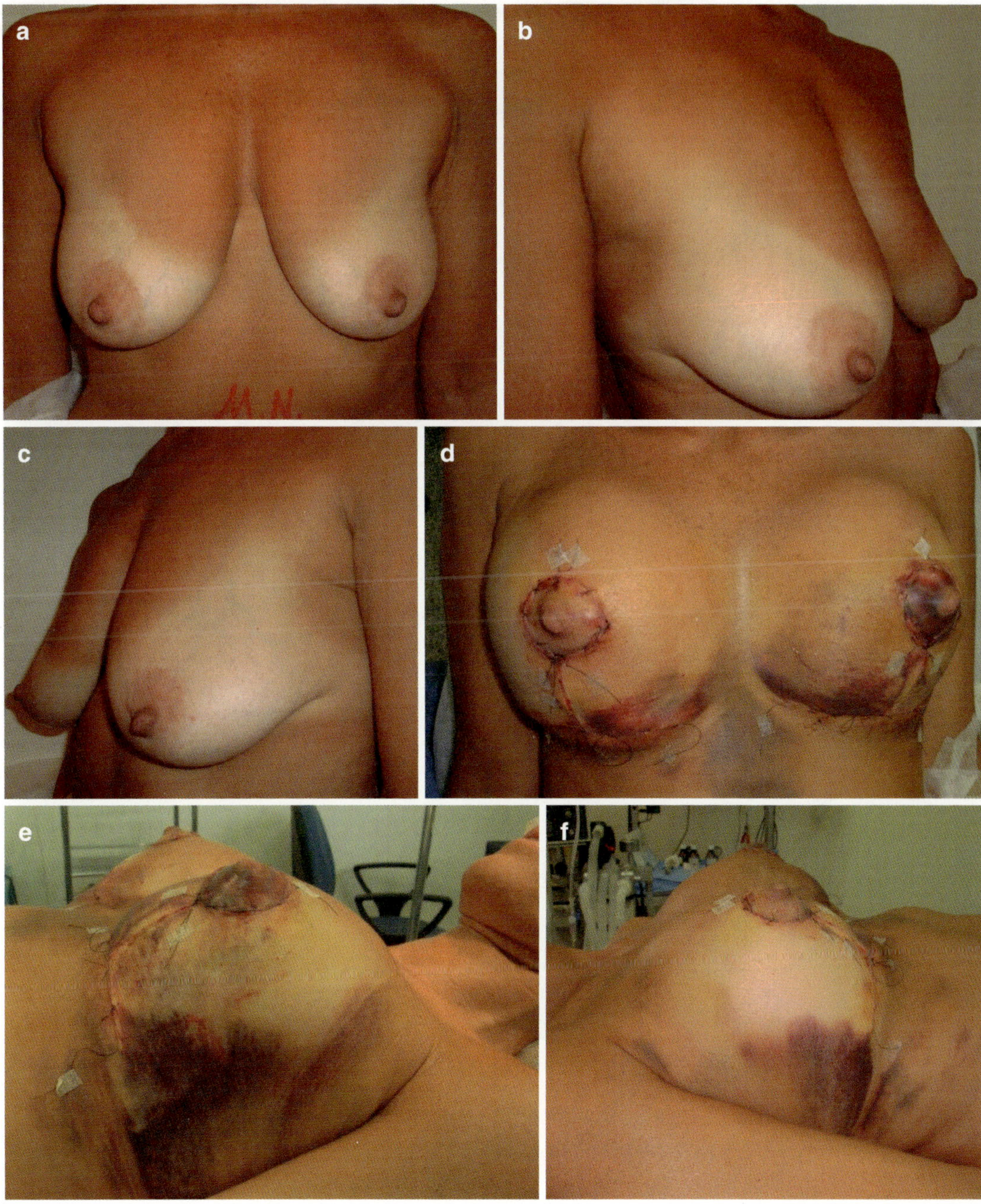


**Fig. 29.2** (**a–c**) Preoperative 50 y/o patient. (**d**, **e**) Six hours postoperative after augmentation mastopexy with 220 mL round textured implants and inverted T incision with bilateral hematoma and NAC ischemia. (**f**) Bilateral drainage and immediate closure. (**g–i**) One year postoperative

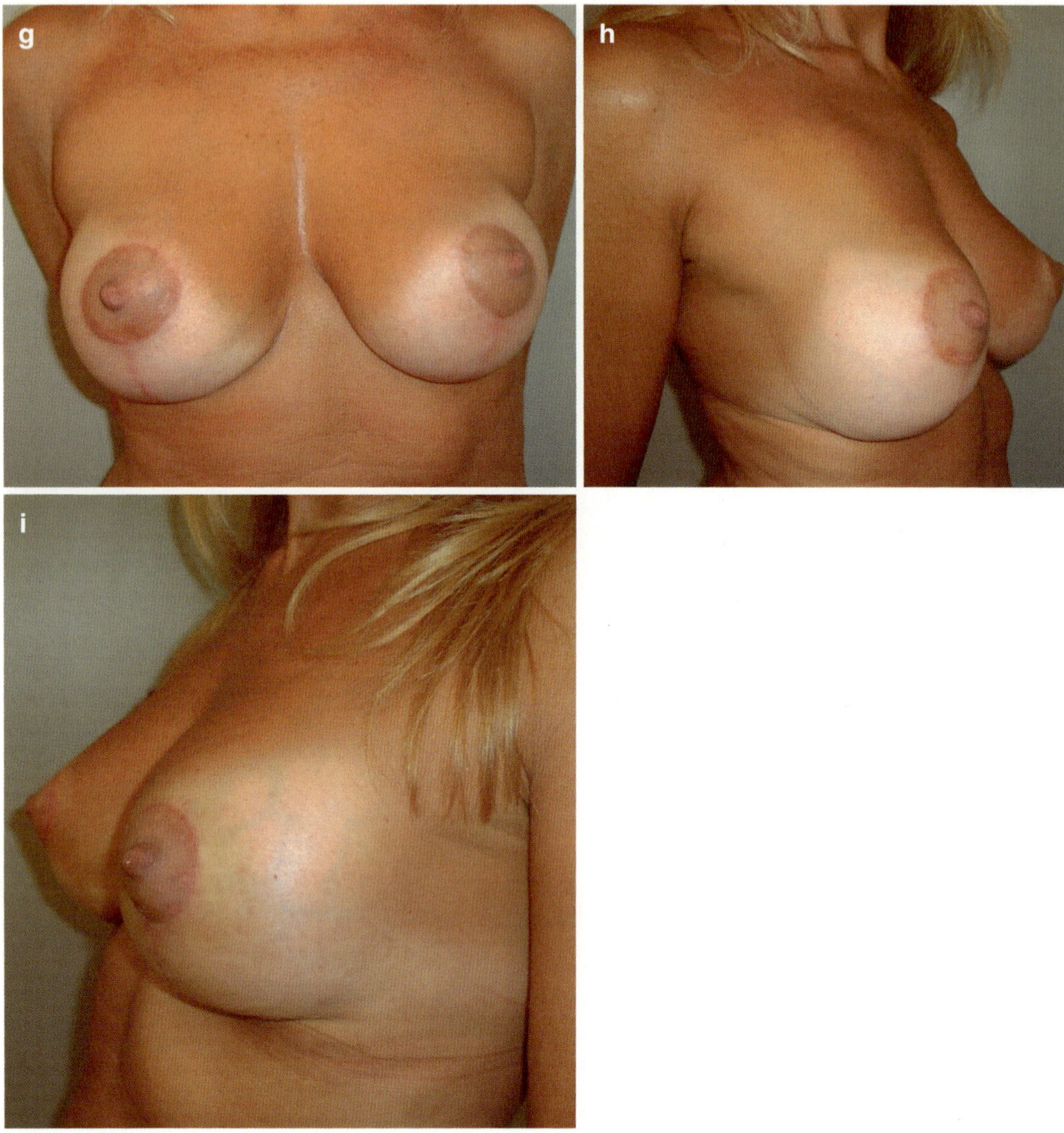


Fig. 29.2 (continued)

## 29.4 Preoperative Information

We believe that a personal history of augmented risk can be present in these cases; we therefore suggest that the following items must be checked and registered in every preoperative reduction mammoplasty patient, in order to diminish the possibilities of NAC ischemia [13–15].

1. Nutritional state, serum albumin, hemogram
2. Smoking, anemia, chemotherapy, radiation therapy, steroids
3. Recent weight loss or gain
4. Pulmonary function

## 29.5 Vitality of the NAC During Closure: An Important Factor in Mammoplasty Procedures

Vitality of the NAC can be preserved based on the previously mentioned key anatomical elements; however, despite all the care taken with regard to the selected pedicle and perfect technique, the NAC must be double-checked in order to avoid complications during closure. This time period is important for NAC vitality.

Excessive folding, compression, areolar tightening, or a bulky pedicle can stress the circulation, and if NAC is suspected, incisions must be opened and the pedicle examined. In some cases, the pedicle must be reduced in volume and the circulation reevaluated. If this improves the situation, wound reclosure must be attempted and the circulation reevaluated. If the circulation is still deficient, the pedicle might be trimmed further, and the incisions may be left open in some cases [16–18].

Changes in the NAC color may indicate its status and may be suggestive of certain rescue maneuvers [6].

1. Arterial insufficiency? White color
2. Venous congestion? Bluish color
3. Vasospasm? Try warm irrigation

## 29.6 Suspected NAC Ischemia During Surgery

See Fig. 29.3.

## 29.7 Detected NAC Ischemia After Surgery

See Fig. 29.4.

## 29.8 NAC Ischemia

A pale or bluish NAC with limited bleeding on the cut edges needs very close postoperative observation. Poor or dark blue blood flow from the deepithelialized dermis is also an indication for close monitoring [2]. In these cases, the Nitro-Bid cream can be applied to attempt vasodilatation. Patient rewarming and

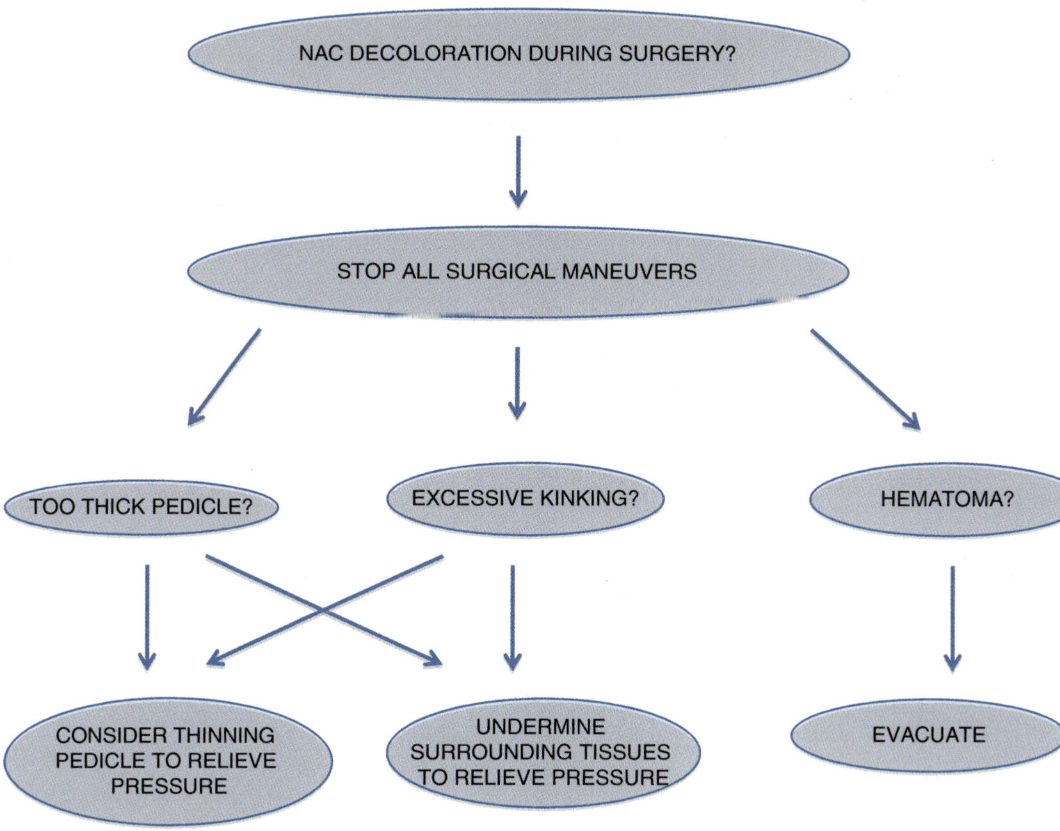


**Fig. 29.3** Suspected NAC ischemia during surgery

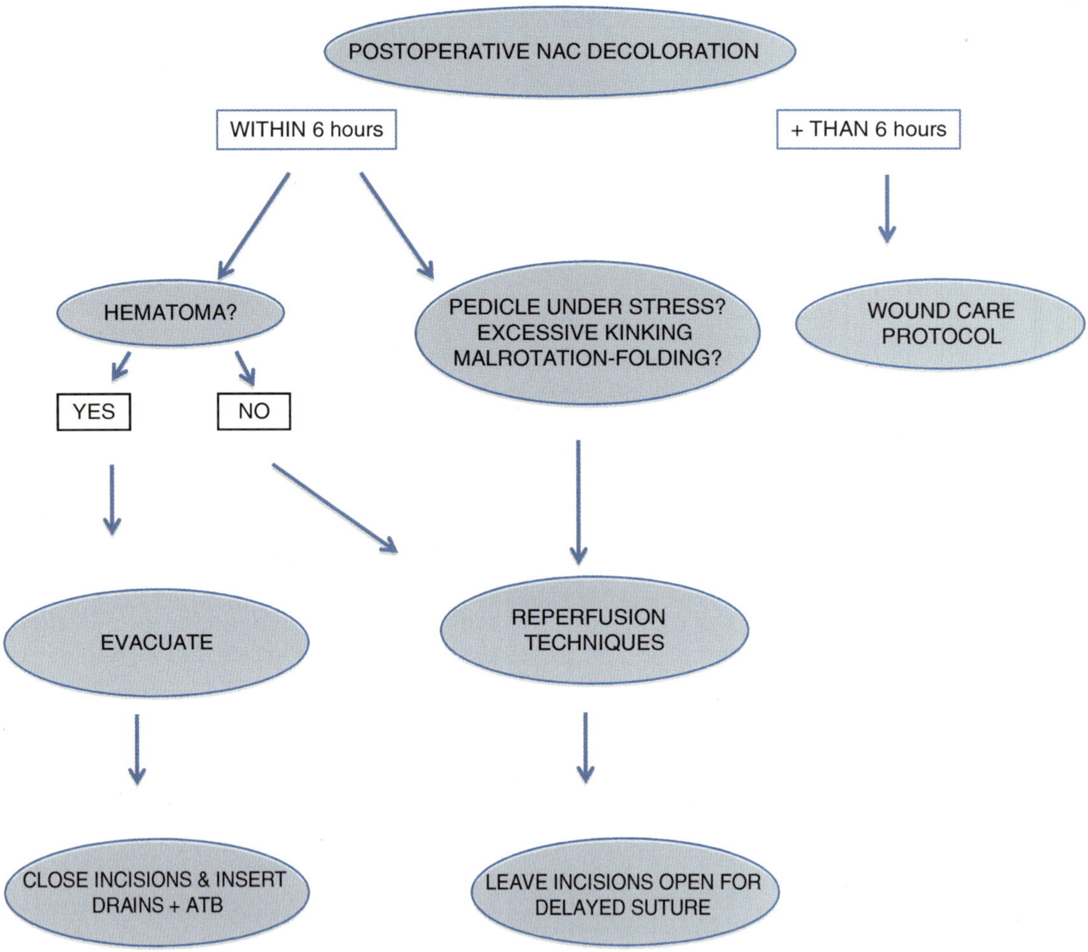


**Fig. 29.4** Detected NAC ischemia after surgery

a normal blood pressure can reverse the changes associated with poor vascularity to the NAC, and it will improve with normal capillary refill within the first hour after the end of the surgery [19–21].

In the absence of a hematoma, if the condition does not improve, the NAC should be released from its inset position, effectively relieving tension on the NAC pedicle. The NAC will generally retract 1 or 2 cm. If no immediate signs of NAC vitality are observed, the patient should be taken back to the operating room for conversion to a free NAC graft on a well-vascularized bed.

In some cases, NAC complications may not be identified in the early postoperative period to attempt salvage and are detected late to be grafted. In these cases, conservative wound care is indicated, and primary healing is the best option. NAC reconstruction is then undertaken at an appropriate time [2–4].

## 29.9 Intraoperative NAC Perfusion Evaluation

1. Clinical judgment
2. Surgical instrument pressure/capillary refill?
3. Abrading the edge of incision with gauze to check bleeding?
4. Warm irrigation to improve vasospasm?
5. Blood pressure elevation
6. Indocyanine green (ICG) dye via IV injection

## 29.10 Intraoperative NAC Reperfusion Maneuvers

1. Release sutures or tension at suture line
2. Relieve excessive kink/flexure of the pedicle
3. Evacuate hematoma, if present
4. Remove implant, if present
5. Warm water irrigation
6. Blood pressure elevation

If the problem is still not adequately solved with these maneuvers, removing the NAC from its position on the pedicle and resecting the distal portion of the pedicle and applying it as a full-thickness graft over dermis as a "free nipple graft" is recommended.

## 29.11 Free NAC Graft Indications

For extremely large (2000 g) reductions and very ptotic breasts with very long nipple to notch distances, a reliable pedicle to the NAC cannot always be preserved (Fig. 29.5). In these patients, an amputation is performed based on the Wise pattern, and the nipple is preserved and repositioned as a free graft on a deepithelialized bed. This is a safe and effective procedure for extremely large breasts and a less risky option for smokers. The nipple often undergoes desquamation in the course of healing, leading to partial pigment loss and loss of nipple projection [12, 22, 23].

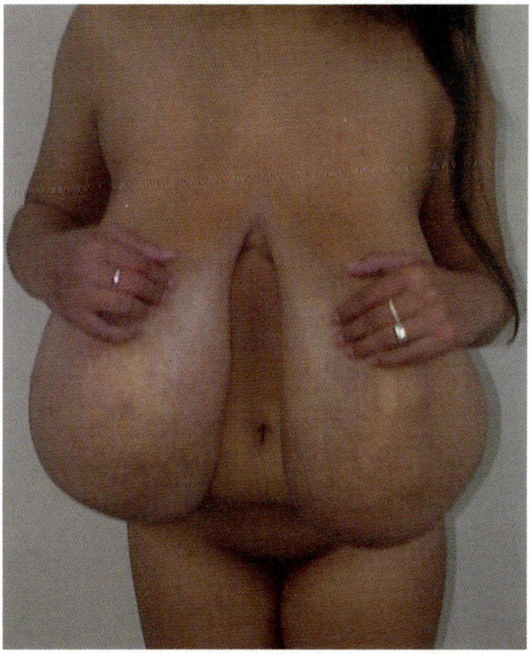

**Fig. 29.5** Gigantomastia in a 14 y/o patient with high risk of NAC necrosis

A free NAC must be grafted to healthy deepithelialized vascularized dermis. Grafting to fat or to a poorly vascularized area will not provide good results. If the nipple shows signs of ischemia in the early postoperative period (within 24 h) despite normal blood pressure and core body temperature, immediate free grafting must be undertaken.

## 29.12 When Should a NAC Free Graft Be Considered?

1. Fear of nipple necrosis
2. Excessive twisting, kinking, and pedicle compression
3. Length of pedicle (>10 cm mobilization)
4. Large reductions (>2000 g)
5. Severe ptosis, SN-N (sternal notch to nipple) 35 cm
6. Very large reductions, almost breast amputations, usually in aging women who suffer pain and discomfort
7. Patients with augmented risk factors

## 29.13 Complications of Free Nipple Grafting

1. Loss of ability to lactate
2. Loss of sensation
3. Loss of erectability
4. Possible hypopigmentation in dark-skinned patients
5. Possible non- or partial "graft take"
6. Poor cosmetic result

## 29.14 Postoperative Care (Hypothermia and Pain)

Adequate pain and postoperative body temperature control can improve cutaneous perfusion and potentially improve healing.

1. Hypothermia induces peripheral hypothermia.
2. Painful stimuli cause a diffuse adrenergic discharge leading to cutaneous vasoconstriction.

## 29.15 Wound Care for NAC Necrosis Protocol

In the case of ischemia lasting more than 24 h, consider it as an established necrosis.

In this scenario, wound care management can be mechanical, enzymatic, and surgical, with the purpose of reducing bacterial contamination and promoting rapid necrosis and reepithelialization. Non-vital tissue must be removed, and change of dressing, twice a day, is recommended [7, 24–27].

### 29.15.1 Initial Treatment

We suggest:

1. Silver iron cream dressings with ATB
2. Surgical wound debridement of nonviable surrounding tissues
3. Autolytic agents: Iruxol N or collagenase

### 29.15.2 After Debridement of All Necrotic Tissue

1. Personal contact with the patient on a weekly basis with picture documentation in the chart
2. Office follow-up every 72 h
3. Protease modulating agents, i.e., hydrogel and alginate cream (moist environment to speed healing)

## 29.16 Sequelae Treatment

NAC ischemia, in some cases, has an unfavorable outcome, and sequelae must be treated with proper patient information and consent. Depigmentation can be treated with tattooing; however, its results can vary and can be weak. Total nipple loss will require reconstruction with skin grafts, and/or local flaps, tattoos, or synthetic materials.

Bad scarring can alter NAC borders, and asymmetries produced by hypopigmentation can be observed, especially in dark-skinned patients. Tattoo scars can be a difficult task and must be repeated frequently. In some cases, scars must be resected, and nipple-areolar resuturing is needed. The interlocking suture [3] has been shown to be a good solution as it maintains uniform tension around the NAC [12, 28, 29].

### 29.16.1 Available Options

1. Intradermal tattoo (Fig. 29.6).
2. Nipple reconstruction with different pull-up flaps.
3. These can be performed as ambulatory procedures under local anesthesia and in the office setting. We usually recommend waiting at least 2 months between the nipple reconstruction and the areolar tattoo.
4. Synthetic reconstruction. For external use only (Figs. 29.7 and 29.8).

## 29.17 Can We Predict NAC Viability?

An objective assessment of the blood flow to the nipple is with the use of ICG dye via IV injection. It is a useful way to assess tissue perfusion and vitality (Spy Elite Technology), but not always available when you need it.

If there is confirmation of compromised NAC vascularity, an immediate free nipple graft should be performed.

## 29.18 ICG Intraoperative Procedure

1. 10 mg ICG IV (12.5 mg in obese patients) rapid bolus.
2. 10 mL saline rapid flush.
3. Wait 8–10 s for circulation.
4. Scan for 2–3 min.

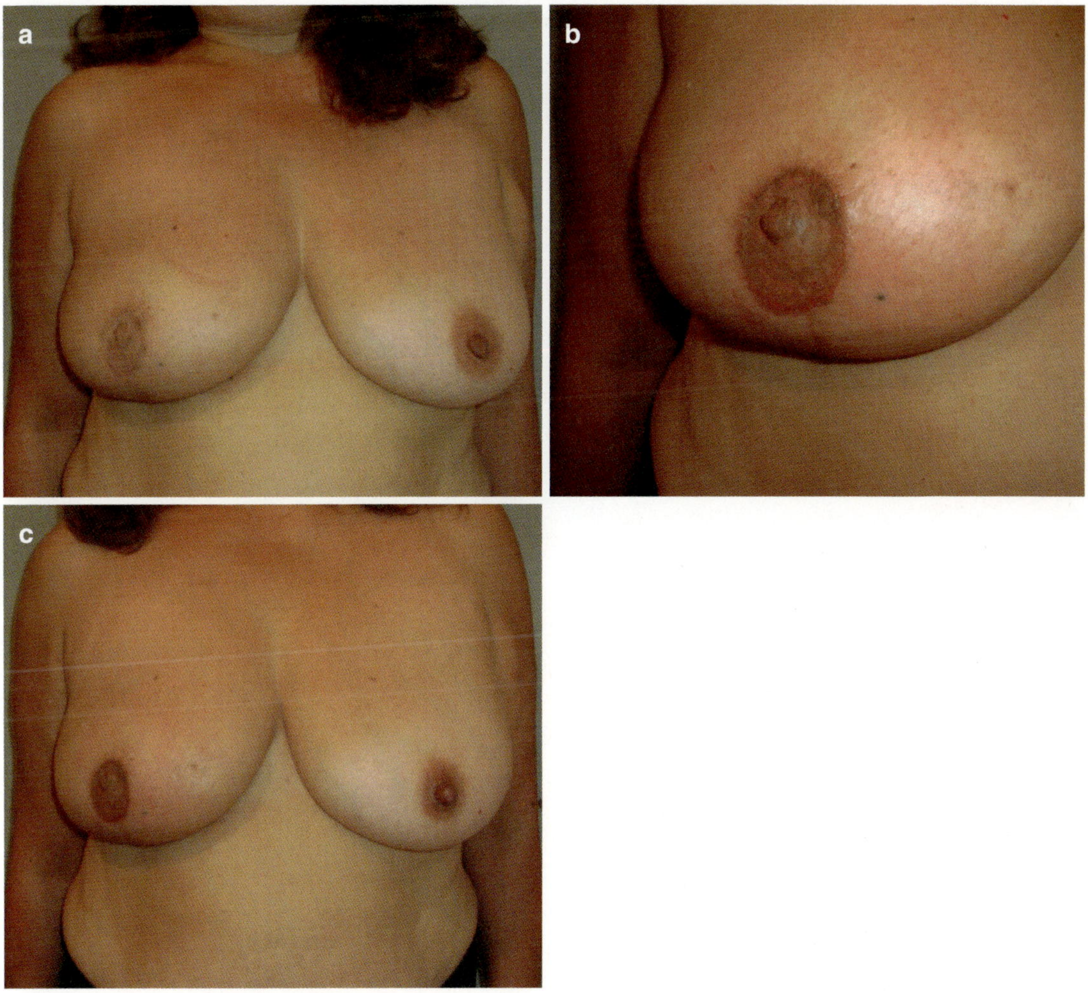


**Fig. 29.6** (**a**) Right areolar complication after mastopexy in a previously irradiated breast. (**b**, **c**) One year after NAC reconstruction and tattoo correction

5. Analyze image.
6. Repeat as desired during the procedure.

## 29.19 Importance of the Informed Consent

Informed consent must include the location of surgical scars and the possibility that these scars can widen or thicken and that they will be permanent. Temporary and permanent changes in nipple sensation, difficulty with breast-feeding or lactation, postoperative breast asymmetries, delayed wound healing, skin necrosis, partial or total nipple loss, hematoma, and seroma should be discussed. It is beneficial to share photographs demonstrating some of the possible long-term complications and less favorable outcomes. If the patient cannot accept this associated risk, this is the opportunity to reject the case.

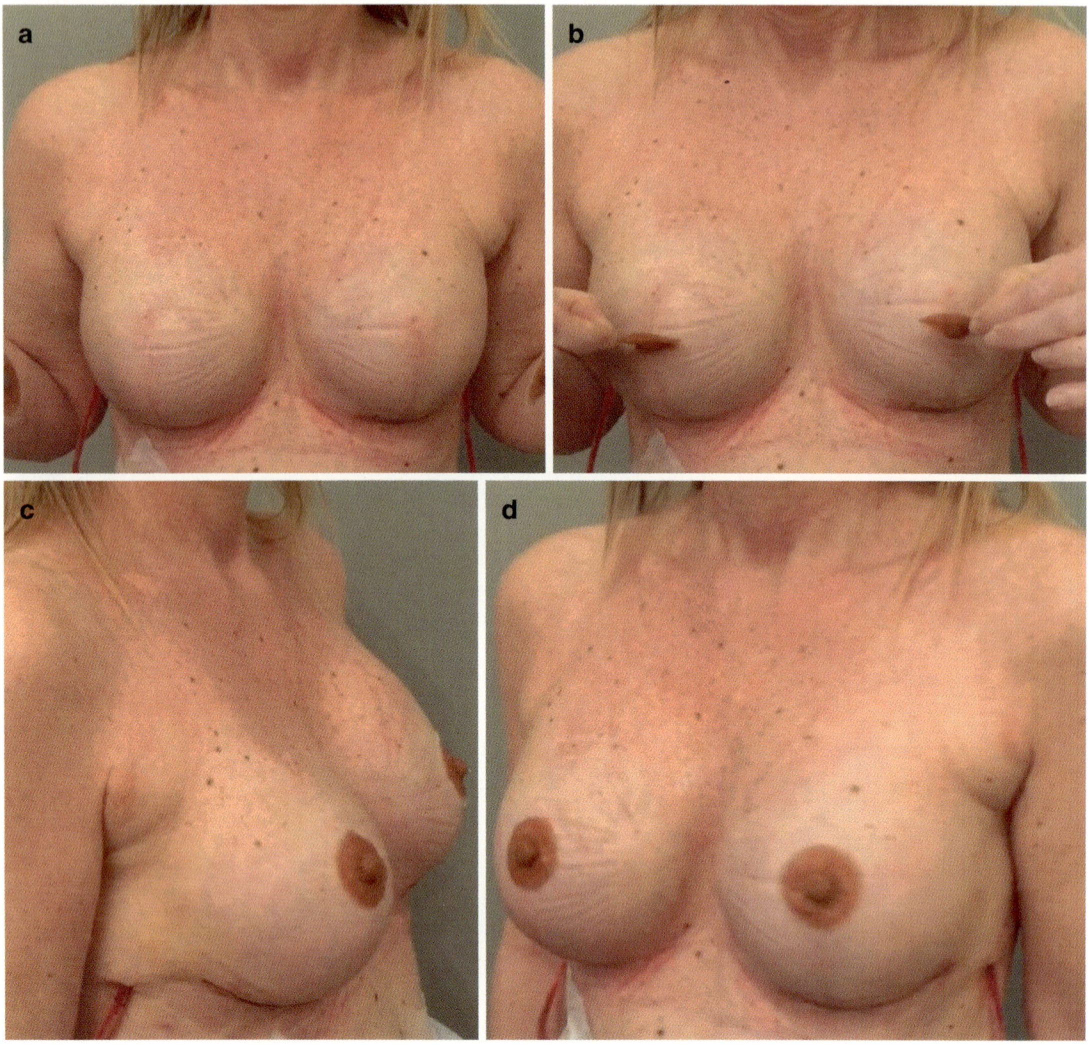


**Fig. 29.7** (**a**, **b**) 36 y/o patient with inverted T reduction mastopexy in 2004 that developed NAC necrosis. (**c**, **d**) Immediately postoperative after bilateral 255 CPG mentor implants dual plane with synthetic silicone NAC complex

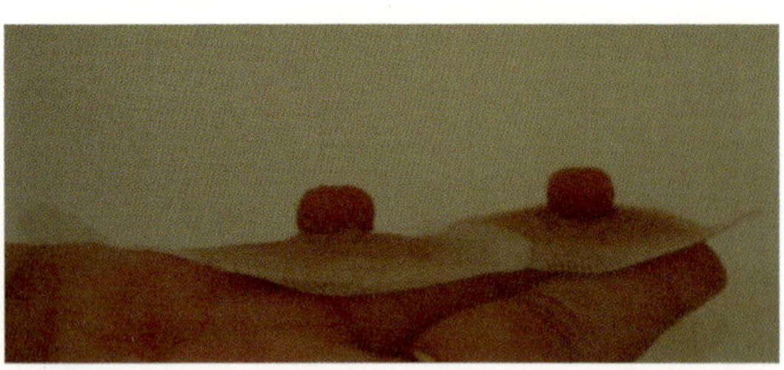

**Fig. 29.8** Synthetic silicone NAC by naturally impressive LLC

## Conclusions

Despite meticulous design, planning, marking, and execution, total prevention of NAC ischemia and necrosis is not possible. NAC loss is a potential complication in every mammoplasty procedure, and patients should be informed regarding this not a rare complication [1, 30, 31].

Assessment of the viability of a pedicled NAC after an aesthetic mammoplasty may be frustrating due to equivocal clinical signs of adequate blood supply. Our suggestion for the required action when this complication is detected differs based on the surgical period.

1. Intraoperative
2. Immediate postoperative (first 24 h)
3. Over 24 h postoperatively (Fig. 29.9)

For the first two time periods, active maneuvers have been described. For the last time period, our suggestion is to wait and resect dead tissue, treat possible infection, and allow wound healing by secondary intention.

It is the authors' opinion that conservative management of full-thickness NAC loss may provide good cosmetic results without sequelae.

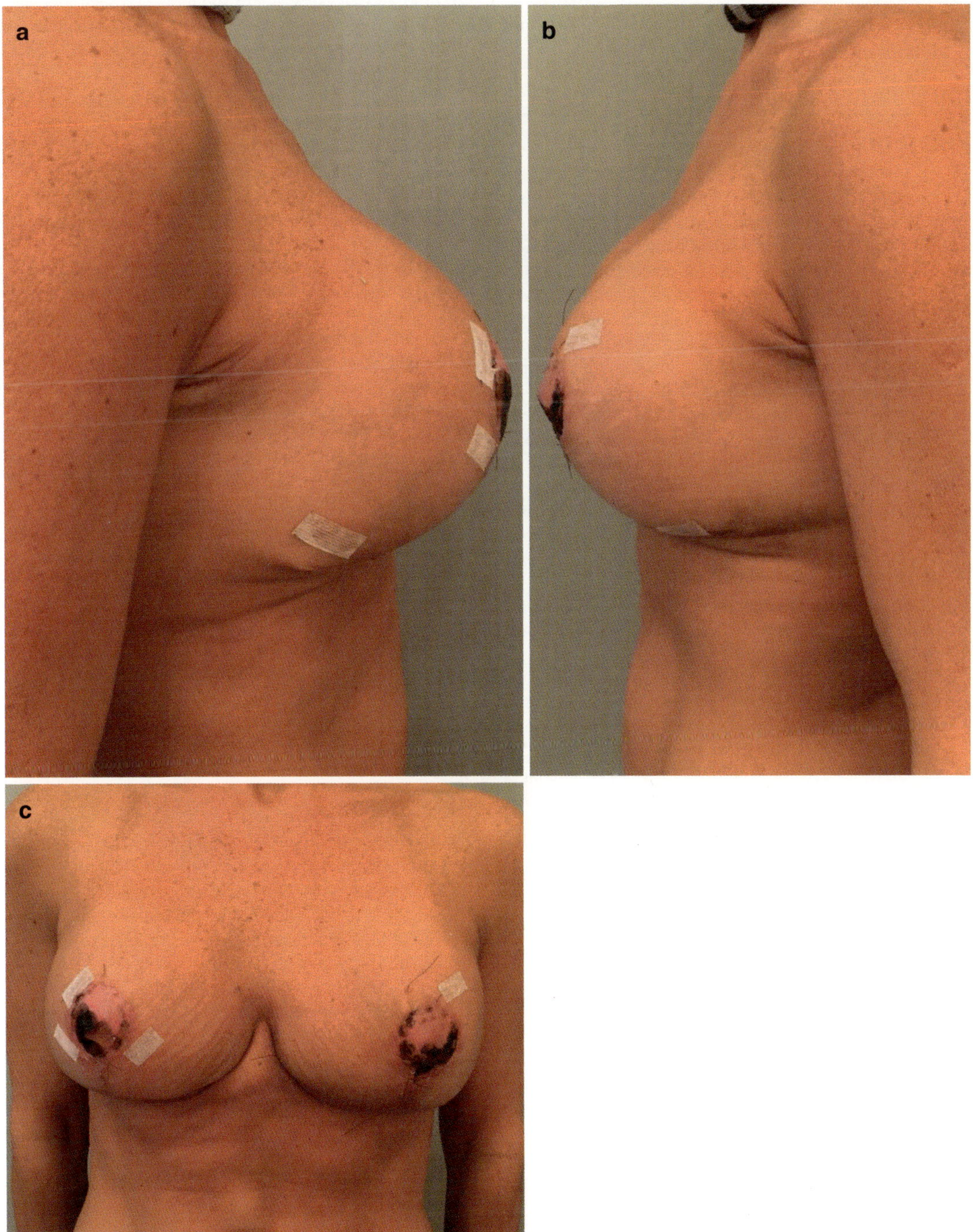

**Fig. 29.9** (**a–c**) Bilateral partial NAC necrosis 10 days postoperative after a simultaneous augmentation mastopexy with inverted T, superior pedicle in an unknown previous reduction. Conservative wound treatment

It is important to recognize NAC ischemia intraoperatively for implementation of the correct action and necrosis prevention, when possible. However, this is not always an easy task.

NAC necrosis is a real possibility in every aesthetic mammoplasty procedure and must be added to the informed consent documentation.

## References


1. Grotting JC, Neligan PC. Plastic surgery. In: Breast, vol. 5. 3rd ed. Philadelphia: Elsevier; 2012. p. 247.
2. Manahan MA, Buretta KJ, Chang D, Mithani SK, Mallalieu J, Shermak MA. An outcomes analysis of 2142 breast reduction procedures. Ann Plast Surg. 2015;74(3):289–92.
3. Stolier AJ, Levine EA. Reducing the risk of nipple necrosis: technical observations in 340 nipple-sparing mastectomies. Breast J. 2013;19:173–9.
4. Hofmann AK, Wuestner-Hofmann MC, Bassetto F, Scarpa C, Mazzoleni F. Breast reduction: modified "Lejour technique" in 500 large breasts. Plast Reconstr Surg. 2007;120:1095–104.
5. Spear SL, Rottman SJ, Seiboth LA, Hannan CM. Breast reconstruction using a staged nipple-sparing mastectomy following mastopexy or reduction. Plast Reconstr Surg. 2012;129:572–81.
6. van Deventer PV, Page BJ, Graewe FR. The safety of pedicles in breast reduction and mastopexy procedures. Aesthet Plast Surg. 2008;32:307–12.
7. Woods JE, Meland NB. Conservative management in full-thickness nipple-areolar necrosis after subcutaneous mastectomy. Plast Reconstr Surg. 1989;84:258–64.
8. Mojallal A, Comparin JP, Voulliaume D, Chichery A, Papalia I, Foyatier JL. Reduction mammaplasty using superior pedicle in macromastia. Ann Chir Plast Esthet. 2005;50(2):118–26.
9. Lugo LM, Prada M, Kohanzadeh S, Mesa JM, Long JN, de la Torre J. Surgical outcomes of gigantomastia breast reduction superomedial pedicle technique: a 12-year retrospective study. Ann Plast Surg. 2013;70(5):533–7.
10. Landau AG, Hudson DA. Choosing the superomedial pedicle for reduction mammaplasty in gigantomastia. Plast Reconstr Surg. 2008;121:735–9.
11. Hester TR Jr, Bostwick J 3rd, Miller L, Cunningham SJ. Breast reduction utilizing the maximally vascularized central breast pedicle. Plast Reconstr Surg. 1985;76:890–900.
12. Wray RC, Luce EA. Treatment of impending nipple necrosis following reduction mammaplasty. Plast Reconstr Surg. 1981;68:242–4.
13. Masia J, Larranaga J, Clavero JA, Vives L, Pons G, Pons JM. The value of the multidetector row computed tomography for the preoperative planning of deep inferior epigastric artery perforator flap: our experience in 162 cases. Ann Plast Surg. 2008;60:29–36.
14. Roth AC, Zook EG, Brown R, Zamboni WA. Nipple-areolar perfusion and reduction mammaplasty: correlation of laser Doppler readings with surgical complications. Plast Reconstr Surg. 1996;97:381–6.
15. Cunningham L. The anatomy of the arteries and veins of the breast. J Surg Oncol. 1977;9(1):71–85.
16. Findlay EH. Ischemia of the nipple, areola, and skin flaps. In: Fisher J, Handel N, editors. Problems in breast surgery: a repair manual. Boca Raton, FL: CRC Press; 2014. p. 493–5.
17. Wueringer E, Tschabitscher M. New aspects of the topographical anatomy of the mammary gland regarding its neurovascular supply along a regular ligamentous suspension. Eur J Morphol. 2002;40:181–9.
18. Hallock GG, Cusenz BJ. Salvage of the congested nipple during reduction mammoplasty. Aesthet Plast Surg. 1986;10:143–5.
19. Seamon MJ, Wobb J, Gaughan JP, Kulp H, Kamel I, Dempsey DT. The effects of intraoperative hypothermia on surgical site infection: an analysis of 524 trauma laparotomies. Ann Surg. 2012;255(4):789–95.
20. O'Dey DM, Prescher A, Pallua N. Vascular reliability of nipple-areola complex-bearing pedicles: an anatomical microdissection study. Plast Reconstr Surg. 2006;118:292–3.
21. Nahabedian MY, Mofid MM. Viability and sensation of the nipple-areolar complex after reduction mammaplasty. Ann Plast Surg. 2002;49:24–31.
22. Hammond DC, O'Connor EA, Knoll GM. The short-scar periareolar inferior pedicle reduction technique in severe mammary hypertrophy. Plast Reconstr Surg. 2015;135:34–40.
23. Lypka M, Rizvi M, Lapuerta L. The Graf/Biggs flap to increase upper pole projection in breast reductions with free nipple grafts. Aesthet Plast Surg. 2010;34:687–90.
24. Steed DL. Debridement. Am J Surg. 2004;187(5A):71S–4S.
25. Wang P, Nuveen EJ. Diagnosis and management of areolar ischemia. Am J Cosmet Surg. 2012;29(2):159–70.
26. Ramundo J, Gray M. Collagenase for enzymatic debridement: a systematic review. J Wound Ostomy Continence Nurs. 2009;36(6 Suppl):S4–11.
27. Knig M, Vanscheidt W, Augustin M, Kapp H. Enzymatic versus autolytic debridement of chronic leg ulcers: a prospective randomised trial. J Wound Care. 2005;14:320–3.
28. Colakoglu S, Khansa I, Curtis MS, Yueh JH, Ogunleye A, Haewyon C, Tobias AM, Lee BT. Impact of complications on patient satisfaction in breast reconstruction. Plast Reconstr Surg. 2011;127(4):1428–36.
29. Hallock GG. Salvage by tattooing of areolar complications following breast reduction. Plast Reconstr Surg. 1993;91:942–5.
30. Nahai FR, Nahai F. Breast reduction. Plast Reconstr Surg. 2008;121(1 Suppl):1–13.
31. Wuringer E, Mader N, Posch E, Holle J. Nerve and vessel sup plying ligamentous suspension of the mammary gland. Plast Reconstr Surg. 1998;101:1486–93.

# How to Avoid Nipple–Areola Complex Complications in High-Grade Gynecomastia Patients Treated by Mastectomy: Surgical Pearls

30

Daniele Bordoni, Giuseppe Falco, Pierfrancesco Cadenelli, Matteo Ornelli, Alberto Patriti, Ariel Tessone, Marco Serafini, and Cesare Magalotti

## 30.1 Introduction

Gynecomastia is described as an enlargement of the male breast common in both neonates and adolescent boys [1, 2] and senescence [3]. First described by Galen during the second century CE, *gyne* is derived from Greek meaning woman and *mastos* meaning breast [2]. Gynecomastia is defined as benign proliferation of male breast glandular tissue resulting from hormonal changes in the body [4] that accounts for up to 80% of all breast referrals in men [4]. Gynecomastia is observed in three key periods during life span: neonatal period, puberty, and the later years [5, 6]. The prevalence of gynecomastia is estimated to be between 60 and 90% in neonates due to the transplacental estrogens [2]. In adolescence, it is reported to be between approximately 50 and 60% [3]. However, more recent studies have identified the prevalence in males in the age group between 10 and 19 years approximately at 4% which is significantly less than previously reported [7]. In the later years, the prevalence is reported in men aged between 50 and 80 years

D. Bordoni, M.D. (✉) • M. Serafini, R.N.
C. Magalotti, M.D.
Department of Senology, Ospedale Santa Maria della Misericordia, Asur Marche Area, Vasta 1, Urbino, Italy
e-mail: dottorbordoni@gmail.com; danyburdo@hotmail.it; marco.serafini@sanita.marche.it; Cesare.magalotti@sanita.marche.it

G. Falco, M.D.
Department of Senology, Arcispedale S. Maria Nuova—IRCCS, Reggio Emilia, Italy
e-mail: giuseppe.falco81@gmail.com

P. Cadenelli, M.D.
Department of Plastic Surgery, Ospedale San Gerardo, Monza, Italy
e-mail: pierfrancesco.cadenelli@gmail.com

M. Ornelli, M.D.
Department of Plastic Surgery, Università Politecnica delle Marche, Ancona, Italy
e-mail: ornellimatteo@gmail.com

A. Patriti, M.D., PhD.
Department of General Surgery, Ospedale San Salvatore, Pesaro, Italy
e-mail: patriti@ospedalimarchenord.it

A. Tessone, M.D.
Department of Plastic Surgery, The Talpiot Medical Leadersjip Program, Sheba Medical Center, Ramat Gan, Israel
e-mail: tessonemd@icloud.com


M.A. Shiffman (ed.), *Nipple-Areolar Complex Reconstruction*,
https://doi.org/10.1007/978-3-319-60925-6_30

[5, 6]. Adolescent boys and men diagnosed with gynecomastia is an aesthetic concern with serious psychosocial implications [8].

Gynecomastia usually presents as bilateral, but patients may present with asymmetrical or unilateral findings [2]. While the etiology of gynecomastia remains unclear, an imbalance between estrogens and androgens is believed to be the primary etiology [3] with breast growth due to either physiological or pathological factors [2]. Classification of gynecomastia is based on physiologic, pathologic, pharmacologic, and idiopathic causes (Table 30.1).

Several methods of classifications for gynecomastia have been proposed by different authors over the years [9–14]. Initially, Webster [10] in 1946 classified gynecomastia as glandular, fatty glandular, and simple fatty. Simple fatty was characterized by male breast enlargement due to fat deposits and commonly known as pseudogynecomastia. Letterman and Schurter [15] proposed a classification system based on the type of surgical correction required:

- Intra-areolar incision with no excess skin
- Intra-areolar incision with mild redundancy corrected with excision of the skin through a superior periareolar scar
- Excision of the chest skin with or without shifting the nipple

Simon [11] divided gynecomastia in four grades based on skin redundancy:

- Grade 1: Minor breast enlargement without skin redundancy
- Grade 2a: Moderate breast enlargement without skin redundancy
- Grade 2b: Moderate breast enlargement with minor skin redundancy
- Grade 3: Gross breast enlargement with skin redundancy that simulates a pendulous female breast

More recently, Rohrich et al. [9] developed classification constructed on four grades without based on the utility of ultrasound-assisted liposuction in the treatment of gynecomastia:

**Table 30.1** Etiology of gynecomastia

| |
|---|
| Developmental/physiologic<br>– Neonatal<br>– Pubertal<br>– Aging |
| Drug-induced (estrogens, gonadotropins, androgens, antiandrogens, chemotherapy agents, calcium channel blockers, antihypertensive, angiotensin-converting enzyme inhibitors, antituberculous agents, central nervous system agents, digitalis, dopamine blockers, illicit drug abuse) |
| Hypogonadism (decreased androgen synthesis or increased androgen resistance)<br>– Primary<br>– Secondary<br>Acquired (trauma, infection, torsion, radiation exposure, mumps, chemotherapy)<br>Congenital<br>Hypogonadotropic, Kallmann syndrome; pituitary failure |
| Tumors (increased estrogen production)<br>• Steroid-producing (adrenal, testis)<br>• Human chorionic gonadotropin-producing (testis and others)<br>• Aromatase-producing (testis)<br>• Bronchogenic carcinoma |
| Systemic<br>• Thyrotoxicosis (altered testosterone/estrogen binding)<br>• Renal failure (acquired testicular failure)<br>• Cirrhosis (increased substrate for peripheral aromatization)<br>• Adrenal (adrenocorticotropic hormone deficiency or congenital adrenal hyperplasia) |
| Congenital disorders<br>• Klinefelter syndrome<br>• Enzyme defects of testosterone synthesis (may be late onset)<br>• Vanishing testis syndrome (anorchia)<br>• Androgen resistance syndromes<br>• True hermaphroditism and related conditions<br>• Increased peripheral tissue aromatase |
| Familial |
| Miscellaneous<br>• (HIV, chest wall trauma, psychological stress, spinal cord injury, herpes zoster infection, cystic fibrosis, alcoholism, myotonic dystrophy, malnutrition/refeeding) |
| Idiopathic |

Adapted from Glass AR. Gynecomastia. Endocrinol Metab. Clin. North Am. 1994;23:835–37 and Neuman JF. Evaluation and treatment of gynecomastia. Am. Fam. Physician 1997;55:1835–44, 1849–50, cited in Rohrich et al. [9]

- Grade I: Minimal hypertrophy (<250 g of breast tissue) without ptosis
  IA: Primarily glandular
  IB: Primarily fibrous

- Grade II: Moderate hypertrophy (250–500 g of breast tissue) without ptosis
  IIA: Primarily glandular
  IIB: Primarily fibrous
- Grade III: Severe hypertrophy (>500 g of breast tissue) with grade I ptosis
  Glandular or fibrous
- Grade IV: Severe hypertrophy with grade II or III ptosis
  Glandular or fibrous

It is important to note that with the classification by Rohrich et al. [9], a pinch test determines the fatty and glandular tissue medially, laterally, and beneath the nipple–areola complex.

In the surgical treatment of gynecomastia, contemporary surgical techniques have become increasingly less invasive [16]. There have been several surgical procedures used to treat gynecomastia including various techniques of liposuction, glandular excision [8], mastectomies, and a combination of techniques [17]. Therefore, the purpose of this chapter is to focus on avoiding nipple–areola complex (NAC) complications when a mastectomy is necessary describing a contemporary surgical technique.

## 30.2 Surgical Procedure

### 30.2.1 Preoperative Markings

The patient is marked in standing position on the day prior to the surgery. The inframmary fold (IMF) is drawn, then a straight dotted line from the subjugular notch to the umbilicus is marked. Subsequently, the anterior axillary line and a line crossing the nipple from hemi-clavicular to the IMF are marked. The distances between the notch and the NAC and between the NAC and the IMF are measured. Breast glandular or fat predominance, pinch test, degree of glandular ptosis, skin excess, and nodules must be precisely assessed. Depending on the case, the new position of the nipple is planned between 18 and 21 cm from the jugular notch. It should usually be located over the fourth intercostal space. The new areola is created maintaining a distance of 3.5–5 cm from the IMF.

### 30.2.2 Technique

With the patient in supine position and both arm abducted, the incision is performed, and then all the skin within the preoperative markings is removed. The dermis corresponding to the new NAC is incised then the skin is undermined in a mastectomy fashion (3–4 mm flap thickness) all around the NAC pedicle to free completely the gland. The gland is passed through until the pectoralis major fascial layer is reached in a slight external oblique fashion. Then, a quadrant per quadrant wide glandular excision is performed. A Monocryl 2/0 suture is placed between the posterior central NAC pedicle and the fascial layer after each quadrant glandular removal in order to avoid the kinking of the pedicle. Irrigation with saline solution is performed followed by hemostasis; then aspirative drains, when a notable bleeding is observed, are placed. PURSE-string suture with 2/0 polydioxanone (PDO) is performed to prevent centrifugal stretching of the scar followed by subcuticular and skin layers by Monocryl 3/0 and 4/0. Mild dressing of the breast is finally performed. All patients should undergo antibiotic therapy until removal of the drains. During the first two postoperative weeks, a support vest is worn to facilitate healing of areola and the chest wall flaps against the muscular fascia beneath.

### 30.2.3 Representative Cases in Technique

#### 30.2.3.1 Case 1

A 21-year-old patient with severe gynecomastia (breast type 2b) and mild breast asymmetry is shown (Fig. 30.1). Marking was performed (Fig. 30.2) at the subjugular notch and a dotted line straight to the umbilicus, the inframammary fold, the new position of the nipple (18–21 cm from the notch), the new areola, and the anterior axillary line and measurement of the distance between the notch and the NAC and between the NAC and the inframammary fold.

Incision of the new areola is defined with marker and external round incision to delimitate

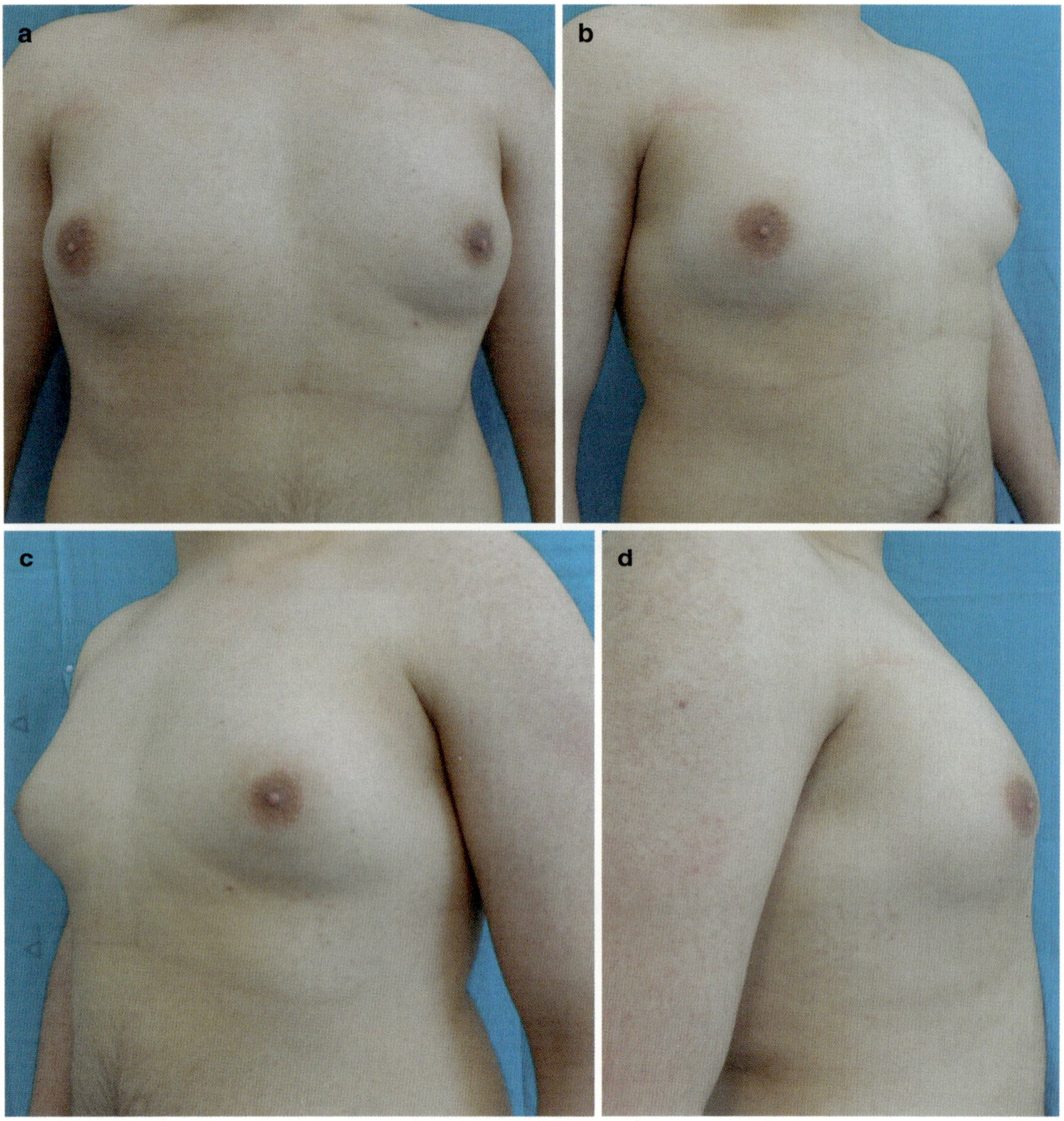

**Fig. 30.1** (**a**–**e**) Preoperative gynecomastia. Breast type 2b and asymmetry

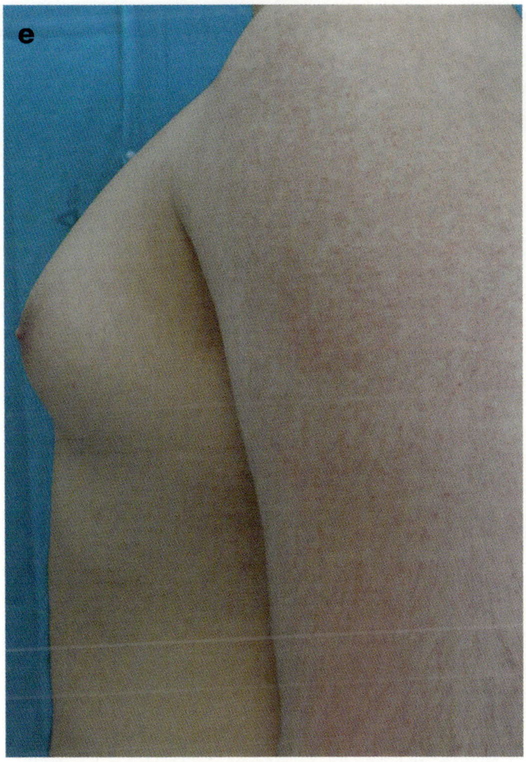


**Fig. 30.1** (continued)

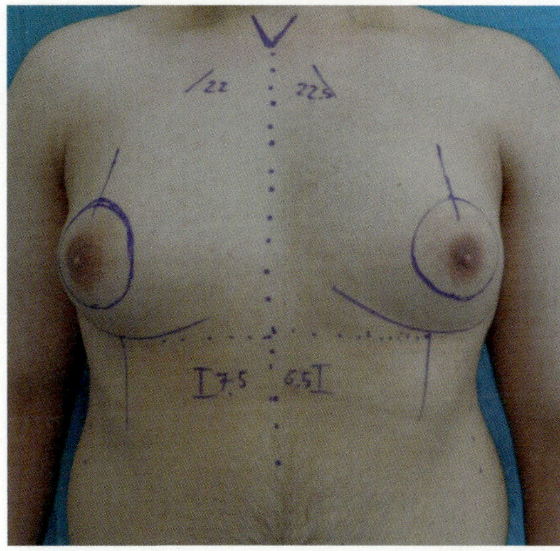

**Fig. 30.2** Marking. The subjugular notch and a *dotted line* straight to umbilicus. The inframammary fold. The new position of the nipple (18–21 cm from the notch). The new areola. The anterior axillary line. Measurement of the distance between the notch and the NAC and between the NAC and the inframammary fold

the deepithelialization area (Fig. 30.3). Deepithelialization is performed with the scalpel, the dermis surrounding the posterior central NAC pedicle is incised, the skin is undermined in a mastectomy fashion (3–4 mm flap thickness), the gland is freed up from the cutaneous envelope, and the gland is passed through until the pectoralis major fascial layer is reached in an external oblique direction. The quadrant is isolated and the Monocryl 2/0 suture is passed through the dermis of the pedicle, and the suture is passed to the pectoralis fascia. The suture is tightened and the pedicle is fixed to the pectoralis fascia. The second quadrant is isolated and the Monocryl 2/0 suture is passed through the dermis of the pedicle. The suture is passed to the pectoralis fascia, the suture is tightened, and the pedicle is fixed to the pectoralis fascia. The third quadrant is isolated and the Monocryl 2/0 suture is passed through the dermis of the pedicle, the suture is passed to the pectoralis fascia, the suture is tightened and the pedicle is fixed to the pectoralis fascia, the last quadrant is fixed to the pectoralis fascia, and the posterior central glandular pedicle is now completely fixed to the pectoralis major fascia. The round block suture is performed by PDS 2/0 and round block is tightened. The skin is closed.

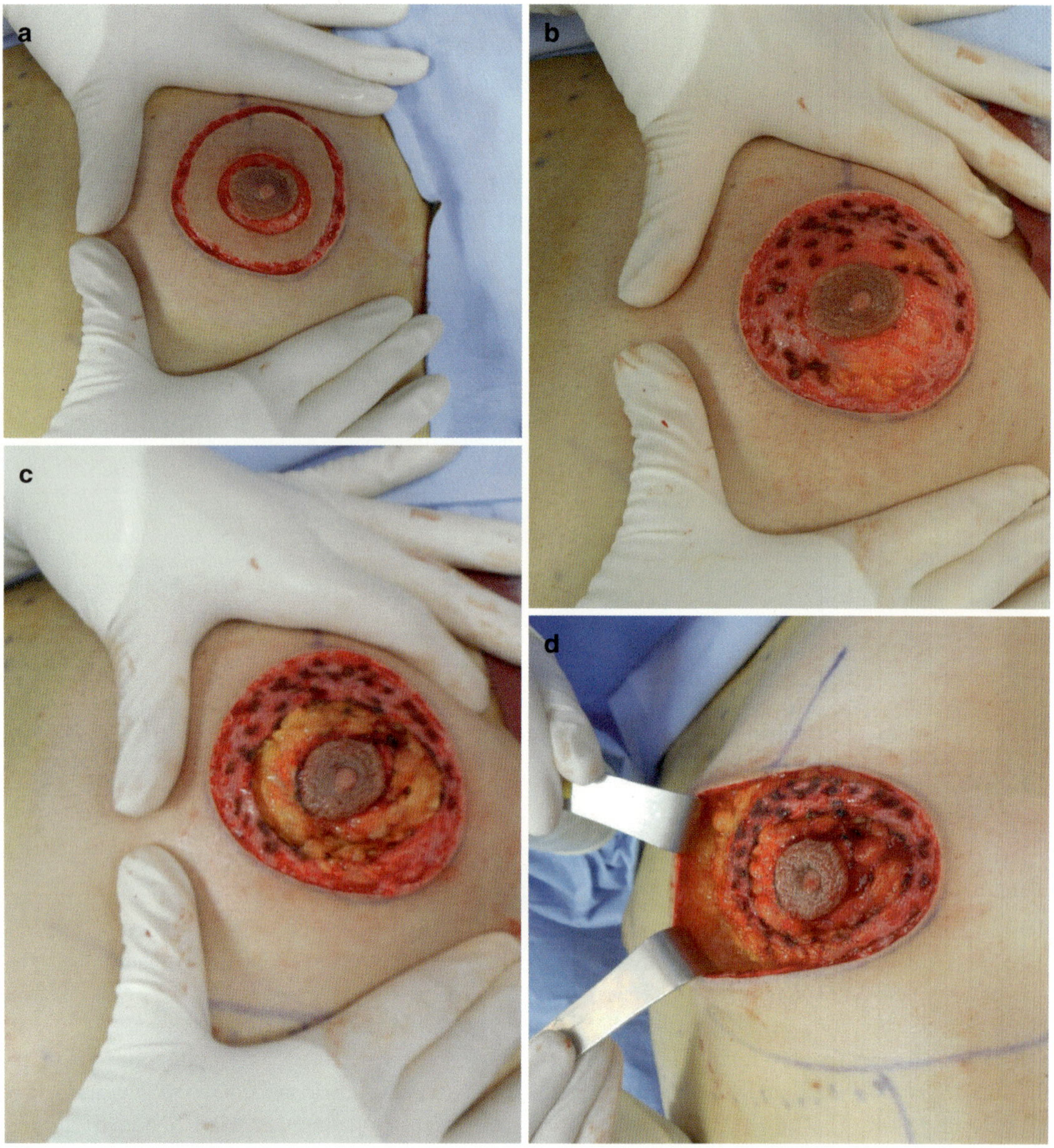


**Fig. 30.3** Deepithelialization, formation of pedicle, and reconstruction. (**a**, **b**) Deepithelialization by scalpel. (**c**) The dermis surrounding the posterior central NAC pedicle is incised. (**d**) The skin is undermined in a mastectomy fashion (3–4 mm flap thickness). (**e**) The gland is freed from the cutaneous envelope. (**f**) The gland is passed through until the pectoralis major fascial layer is reached in an external oblique direction. (**g**) The quadrant is isolated. (**h**) The Monocryl 2/0 suture is passed through the dermis of the pedicle. (**i**) The suture is passed to the pectoralis fascia. (**j**) The suture is tightened and the pedicle is fixed to the pectoralis fascia. (**k**) The second quadrant is isolated. (**l**) The Monocryl 2/0 suture is passed through the dermis of the pedicle. (**m**) The suture is passed to the pectoralis fascia. (**n**) The suture is tightened and the pedicle is fixed to the pectoralis fascia. (**o**) The third quadrant is isolated. (**p**) The Monocryl 2/0 suture is passed through the dermis of the pedicle. (**q**) The suture is passed to the pectoralis fascia. (**r**) The suture is tightened and the pedicle is fixed to the pectoralis fascia. (**s**) Excision en bloc of the breast tissue. (**t**) The last quadrant is fixed to the pectoralis fascia. (**u**) The posterior central glandular pedicle is now completely fixed to the pectoralis major fascia. (**v**) The round block suture is performed by PDS 2/0. (**w**) Breast after round block is tightened. (**x**) Final result

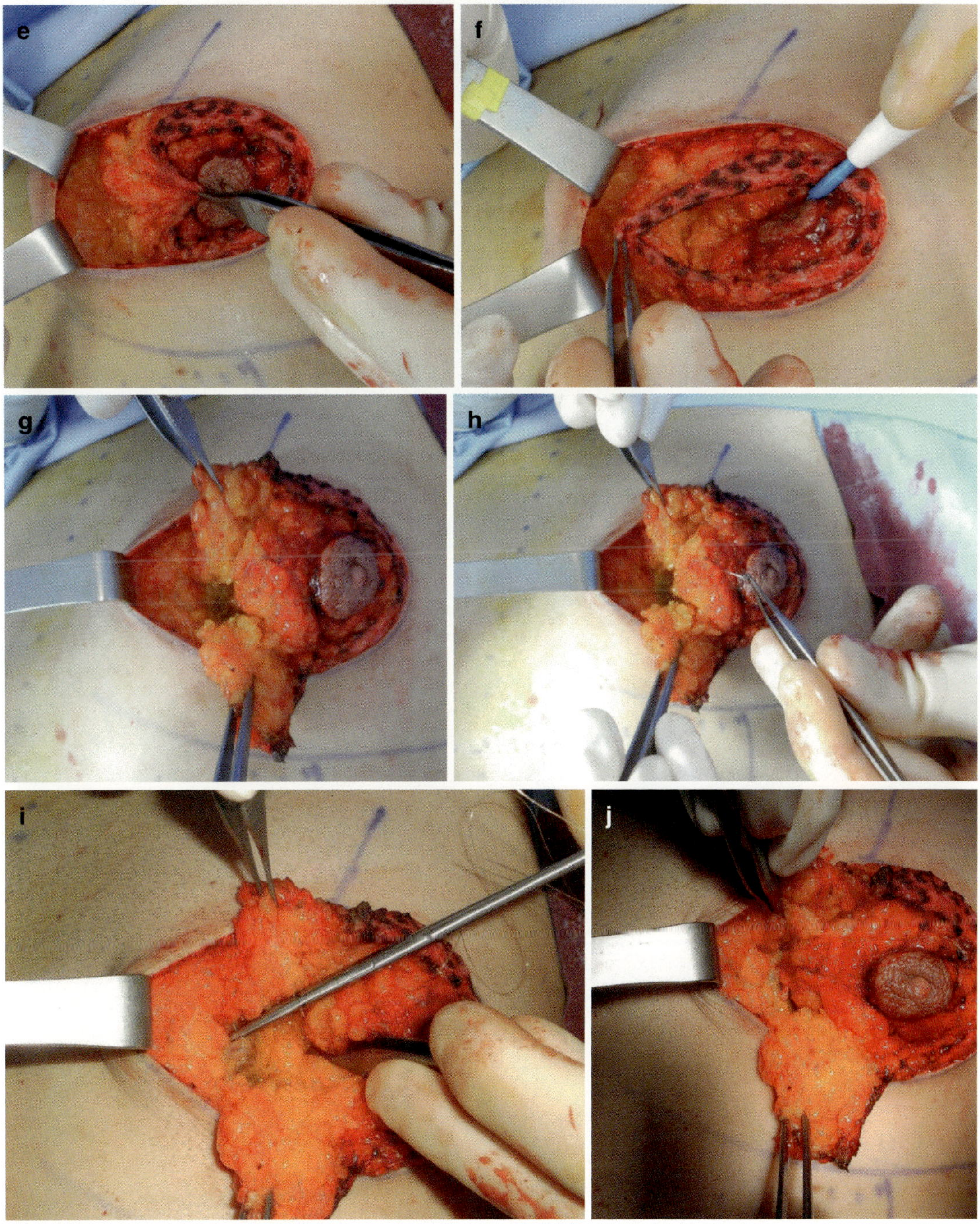


**Fig. 30.3** (continued)

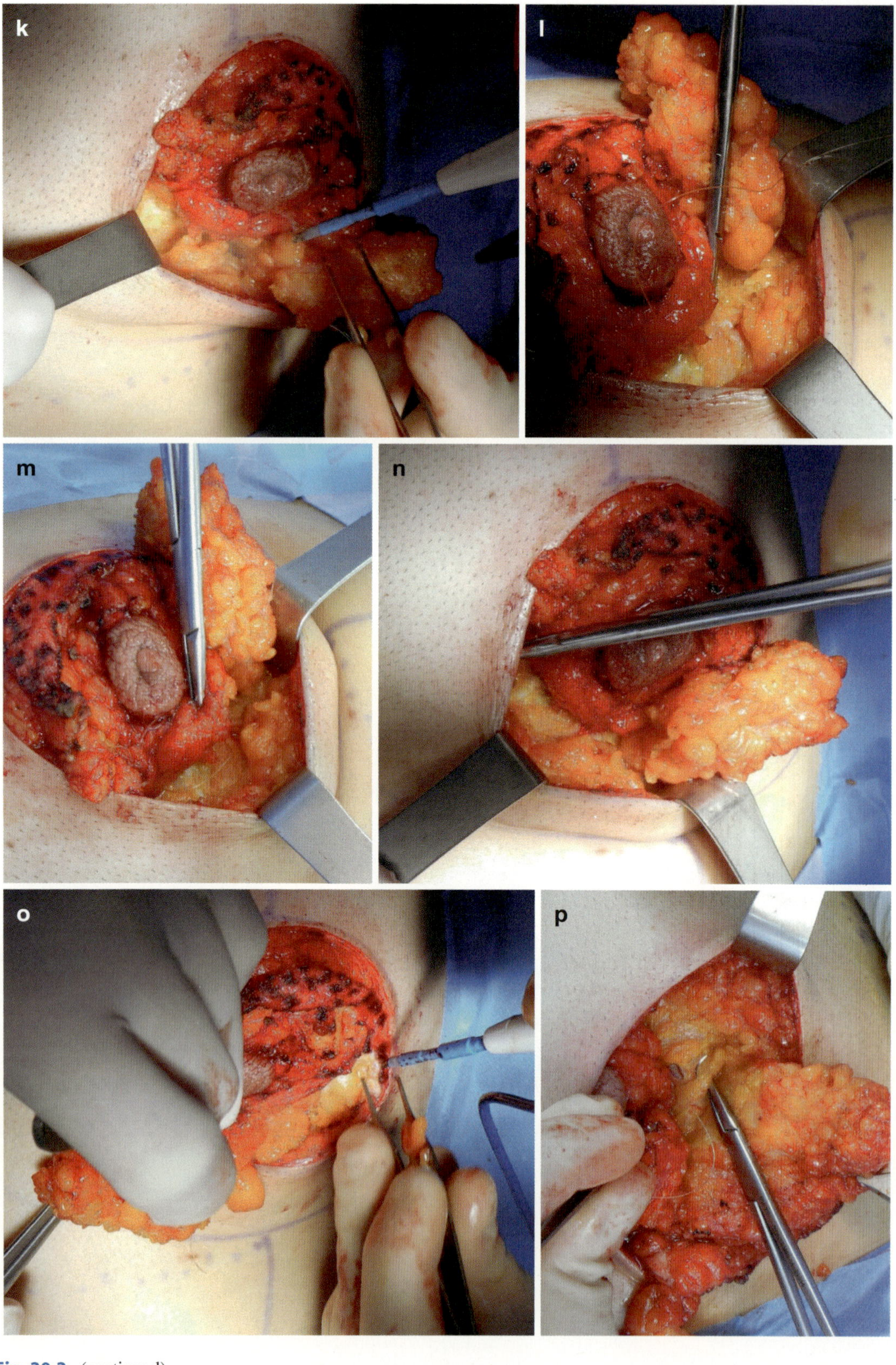


**Fig. 30.3** (continued)

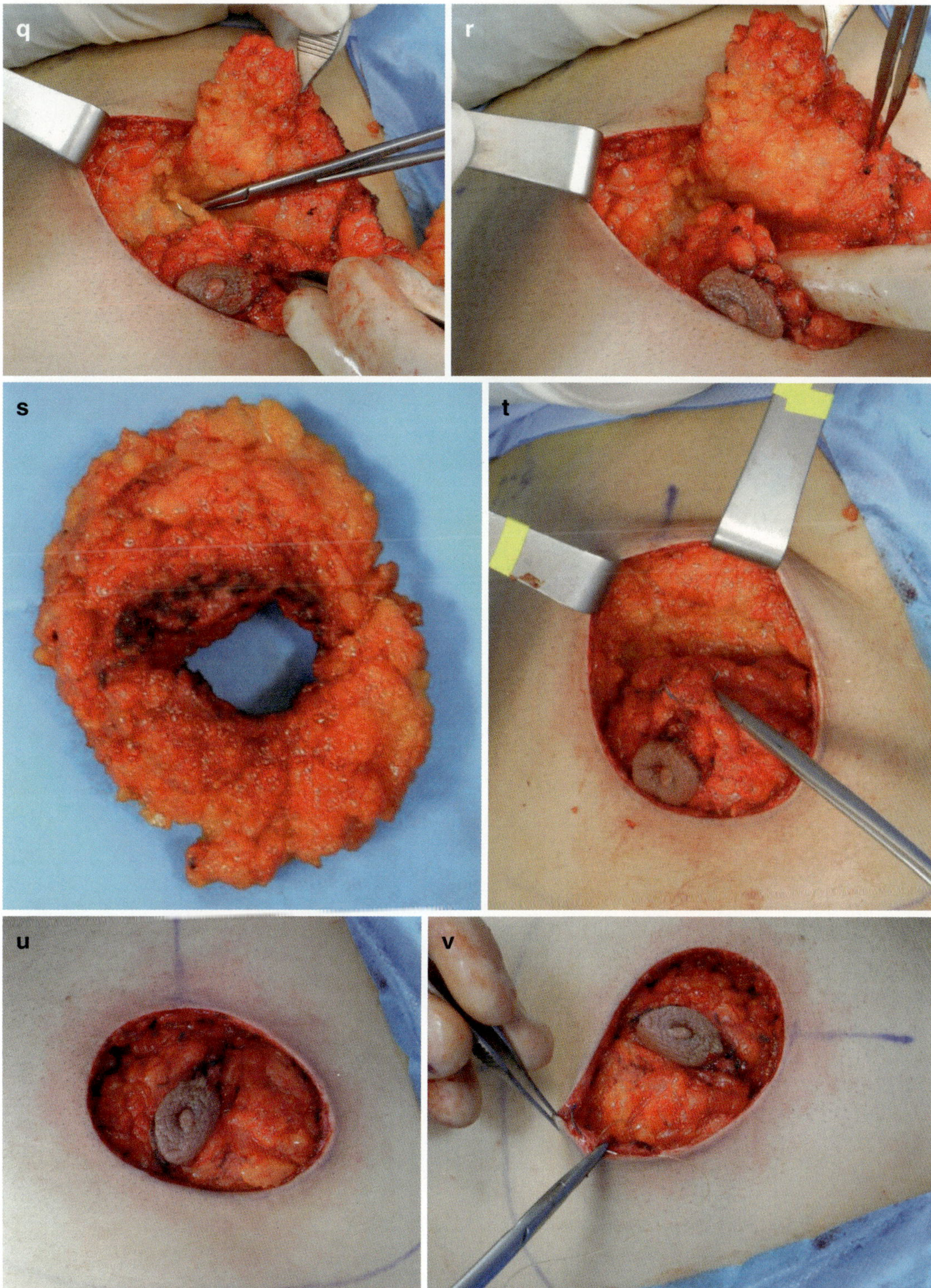


**Fig. 30.3** (continued)

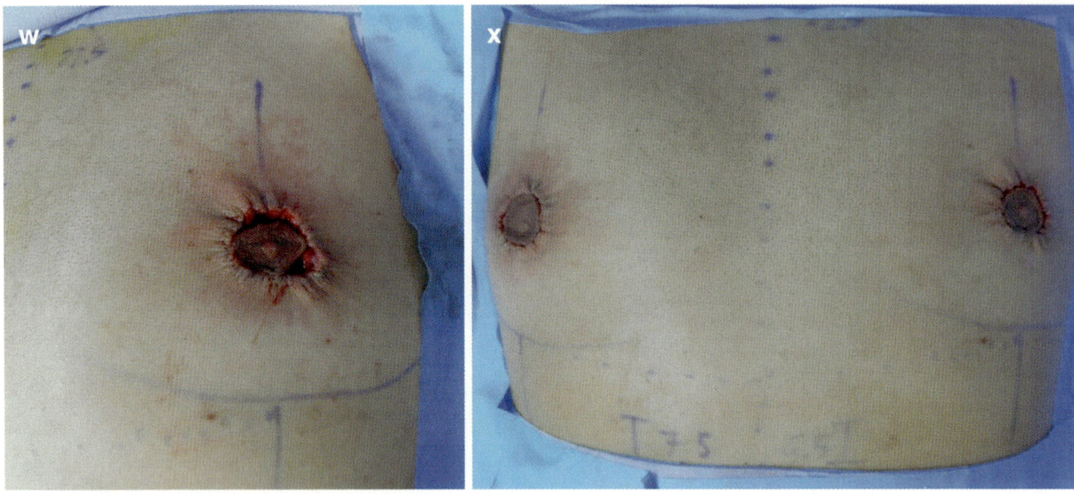


**Fig. 30.3** (continued)

The results at 4 weeks are shown in Fig. 30.4.

#### 30.2.3.2 Case 2

An 18-year-old adolescent patient with severe gynecomastia (breast type 3) is shown preoperatively (Fig. 30.5) and 6 months postoperatively (Fig. 30.6).

## 30.3 Discussion

Gynecomastia presents in male breasts as a benign proliferation of glandular tissue in three distinct periods of the life span: the neonatal, puberty, and senescence periods [3]. It is often found during autopsies in 40% of men [18]. The diagnostic evaluation begins with an adequate patient history and physical examination [18]. Nonsurgical therapeutic options for treatment of gynecomastia are based on medical therapy aimed to achieve a spontaneous regression of breast tissue regulating the hormonal imbalance. When gynecomastia lasts for a period of greater than 12 months, patients often progress to develop irreversible dense fibrosis and stromal hyalinization. In these such cases, surgical intervention becomes the treatment of choice. Rahmani et al. [18] clearly points out that the indications for surgical intervention are based on failure of medical therapy and noticeable gynecomastia to resolve spontaneously and patients presenting with moderate or large gynecomastia.

Several surgical approaches have been described and applied for the treatment of gynecomastia. Initially, low grades of gynecomastia were treated with liposuction alone, but limitations were reported when fibrous gynecomastia was present [12]. However, today its use is limited to the patients with pseudogynecomastia

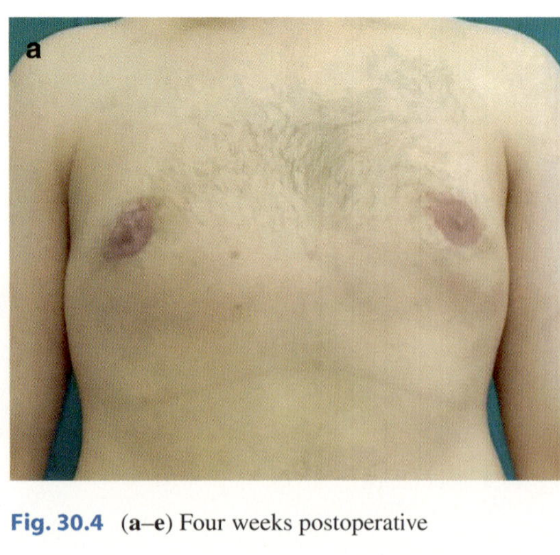


**Fig. 30.4** (**a–e**) Four weeks postoperative

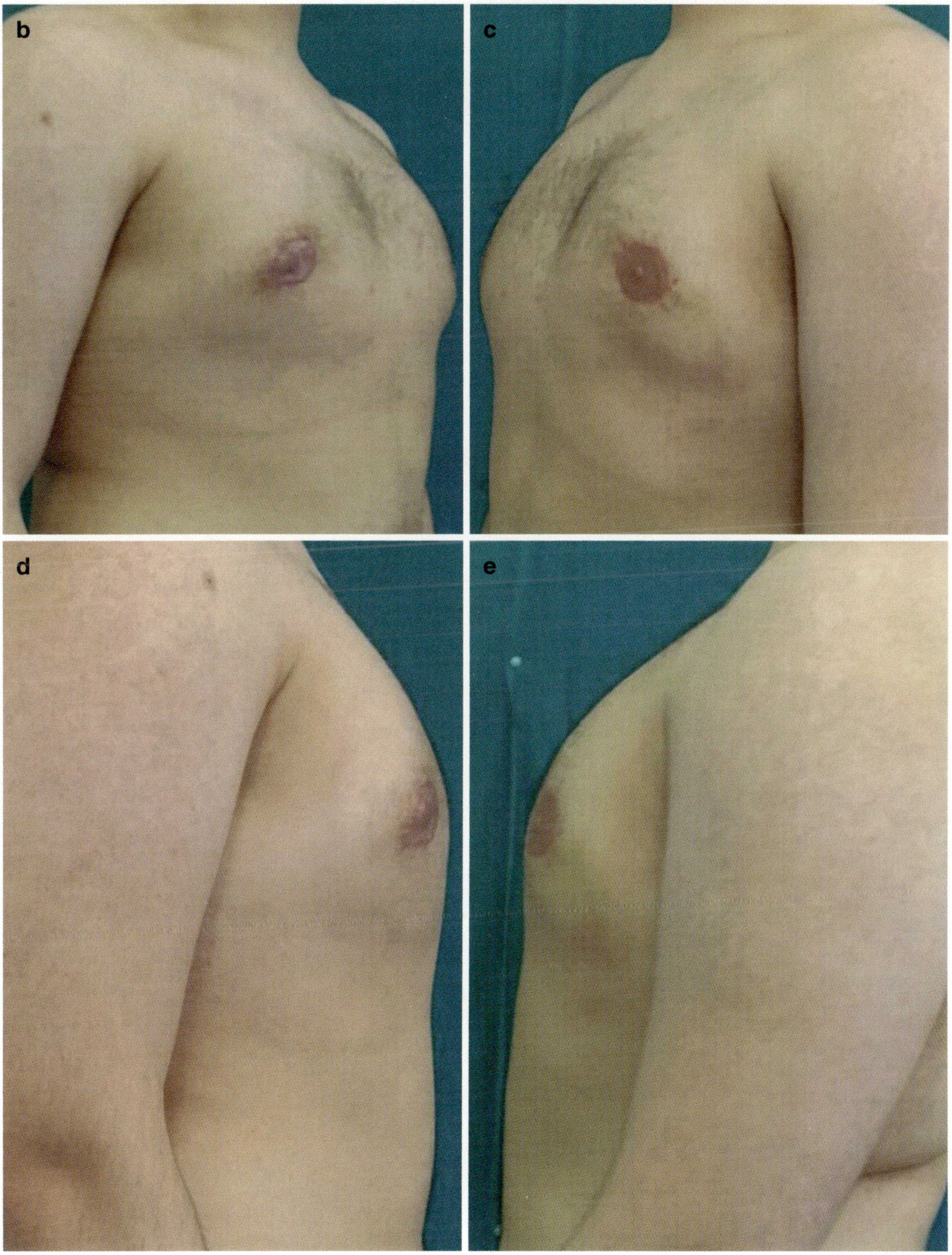


**Fig. 30.4** (continued)

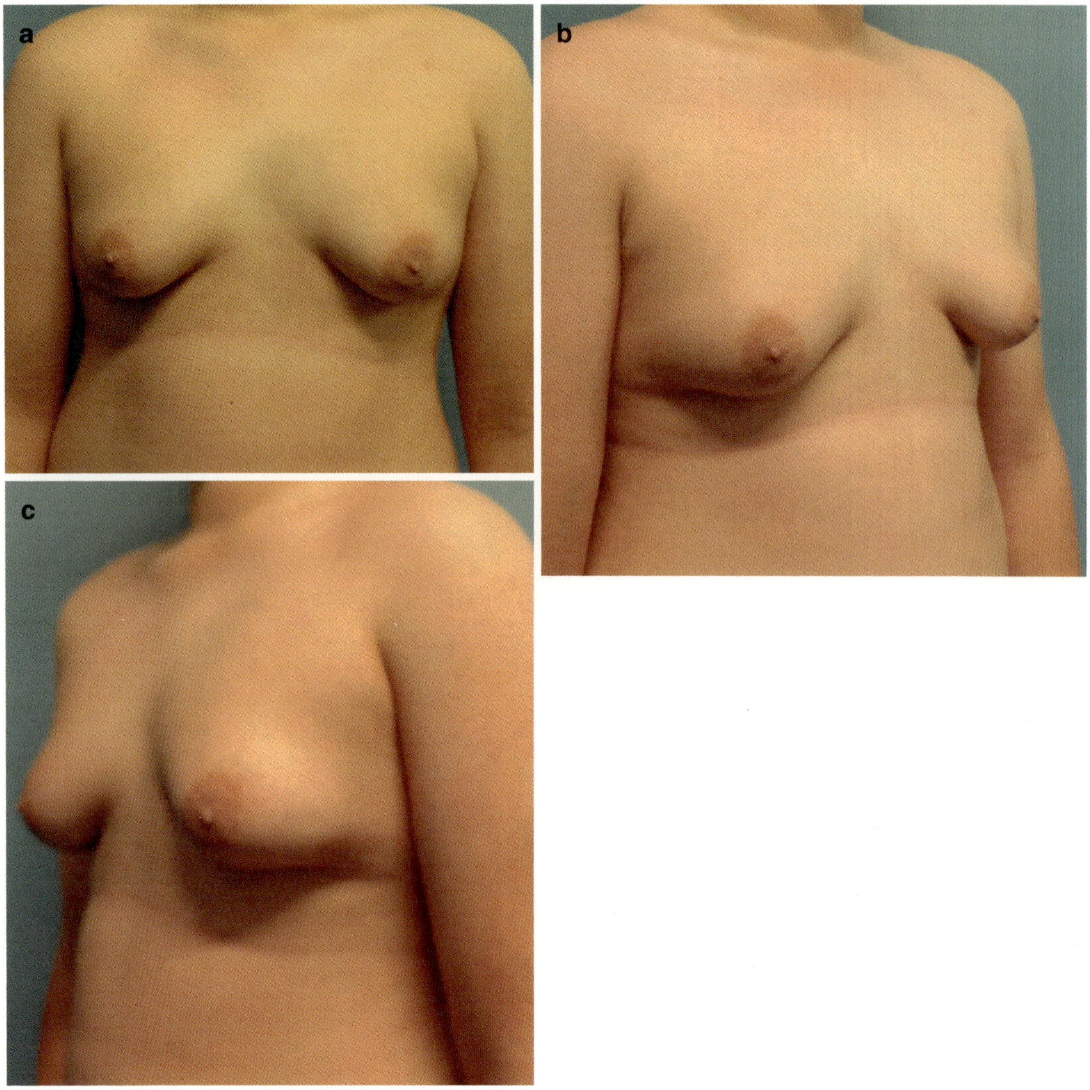

**Fig. 30.5** (**a**–**c**) Case 2 preoperative

with no sign of glandular enlargement. Low grades of fibrous gynecomastia are preferably treated with the use of ultrasound-assisted liposuction. This technique was first introduced by Zocchi [19]; it consists in the use of ultrasonic energy transmitted to the terminal ends of suction cannulas to emulsify fat while preserving adjacent nervous, vascular, and connective tissue elements. Ultrasound-assisted liposuction can effectively remove dense adipose tissues within the fibrous parenchymal framework of the male breast and cause less bruising. In a recent review of ultrasound-assisted liposuction in gynecomastia, Wong and Malata [20] state that ultrasound-assisted liposuction is an effective treatment for gynecomastia than conventional liposuction that was determined by intraoperative conversion to open surgery and the subsequent necessity for revisions. Rohrich et al. [9] refined the technique of ultrasound-assisted liposuction and defined two main advantages that demonstrated that at higher energy settings,

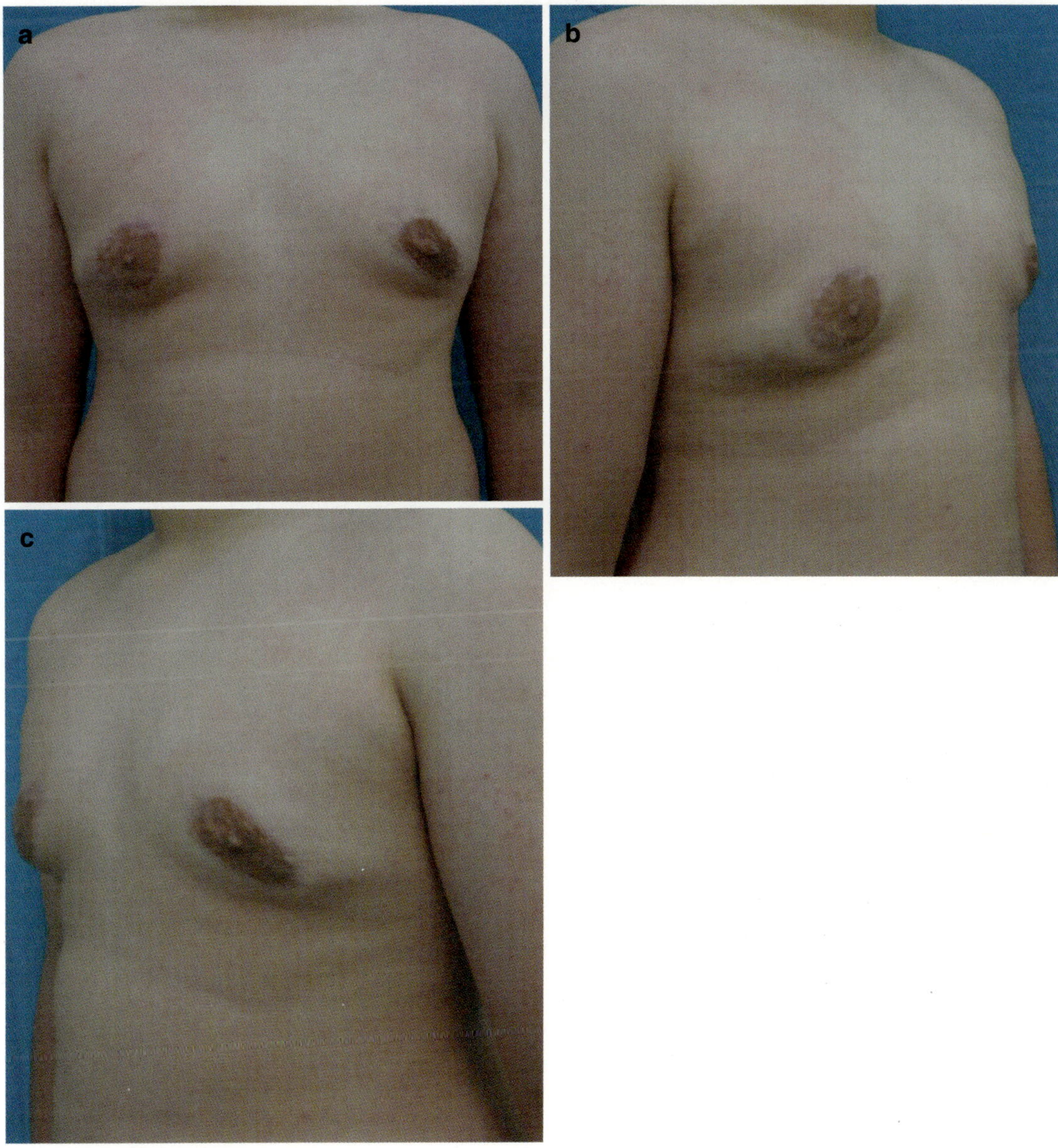

**Fig. 30.6** (**a–c**) Six months postoperative

ultrasound-assisted liposuction is effective in the removal of denser, fibrotic parenchymal tissue and also ultrasound-assisted liposuction in the subdermal plane allows skin retraction in the postoperative period. This last finding extended the indication of this technique to the intermediate grades of gynecomastia where there is mild skin redundancy.

However, when glandular-predominant gynecomastia is present, subcutaneous mastectomy is needed. Li et al. [21] prefer the semicircular-periareolar inferior incision to approach mild-to-moderate gynecomastia. Direct fat and glandular excision is performed leaving an adequate thickness of the subcutaneous tissue and a proper subareolar amount of gland. Surgeons should be aware of avoiding the potential development of a saucer-type deformity in the region under the areola and ischemia-related complications. Therefore, it is necessary to leave a thin amount of tissue under the areola to ensure a smooth surface contour and propose a limited peripheral liposuction in all directions to obtain the final contouring of the breast.

In cases of severe gynecomastia with redundant skin, the use of concentric skin excision ("Benelli type") [22] is recommended for a better aesthetic result. This procedure begins with the deepithelialization of the "doughnut"-shaped skin around the areola to reduce the redundant skin followed by the excision of the excess of glandular and fat tissue. Liposuction may be associated to ensure an aesthetic chest wall contour. At the end, a 2/0 Nylon intradermal circumareolar purse-string suture is placed. The majority of patients with high-grade gynecomastia with redundant skin can be managed with this technique.

Morselli and Morellini [23] described the "pull-through" technique combined with suction-assisted lipectomy for excision of fibroglandular breast tissue. The glandular parenchyma is removed by pulling it through two incisions previously made for liposuction. These incisions are made in the axillary pillar area and on the right side of the inframammary sulcus. The main advantage of this technique is the absence of incisions on the areola, the central aesthetic unit of the breast. Hammond et al. [24] combined the "pull-through" technique with the ultrasound-assisted liposuction from a 1 cm incision at the inferior areolar margin. Ramon et al. [25] introduced the endoscopic-assisted pull-through excision with two periareolar incisions combined with cross-chest power-assisted superficial liposuction.

An accurate preoperative physical evaluation is mandatory. The NAC should be 2–4 cm in diameter with an average of 2.8 cm, located over the fourth intercostal space at the distance of 20 cm from the sternal notch [9]. Liposuction can be performed to better manage the final contour of the breast. Cordova and Moschella [26] in 2008 proposed the goals of surgical treatment in gynecomastia. This involved flattening of the thoracic region, elimination of the inframammary fold, correct positioning of the nipple–areola complex, removal of redundant skin, symmetrization of the hemithoraxes and the areolae, and containment of scars. We completely agree with this detailed description, and we would like to focus on the main surgical problems related to the mastectomy procedure:

1. Nipple–areola complex sufferance
2. Widening of periareolar scar
3. Seroma formation

**Conclusions**

In the treatment of advanced gynecomastia, the technique we propose allows one to avoid volume deficit, shape and surface asymmetries, and scar retraction. Furthermore, the conic shape pedicle dramatically reduces the risk of nipple–areolar complex abnormalities.

## References


1. Cakan N, Kamat D. Gynecomastia: evaluation and treatment recommendations for primary care providers. Clin Pediatr. 2007;46:487–90.
2. Lemaine V, Cayci C, Simmons PS, Petty P. Gynecomastia in adolescent males. Semin Plast Surg. 2013;27:56–61.
3. Deepinder F, Braunstein GD. Gynecomastia: incidence, causes and treatment. Expert Rev Endocrinol Metab. 2014;6:723–30.
4. Al-Allak A, Govindarajulu S, Shere M, Ibrahim N, Sahu AK, Cawthorn SJ. Gynaecomastia: a decade of experience. Surgeon. 2011;9:255–8.
5. Bembo SA, Carlson HE. Gynecomastia: its features, and when and how to treat it. Cleveland Clin J Med. 2004;71:511–7.
6. Gikas P, Mokbel K. Management of gynaecomastia: an update. Int J Clin Pract. 2007;61:1209–15.
7. Kumanov P, Deepinder F, Robeva R, Tomova A, Li J, Agarwal A. Relationship of adolescent gynecomastia with varicocele and somatometric parameters: a cross-sectional study in 6200 healthy boys. J Adolesc Health. 2007;41:126–31.
8. Shirol SS. Orange peel excision of gland: a novel surgical technique for treatment of gynecomastia. Ann Plast Surg. 2016;77(6):615–9.
9. Rohrich RJ, Ha RY, Kenkel JM. Classification and management of gynecomastia: defining the role of ultrasound-assisted liposuction. Plast Reconstr Surg. 2003;111:909–25.
10. Webster JP. Mastectomy for gynecomastia through a semicircular intraareolar incision. Ann Surg. 1946;124:557–75.

11. Simon BE, Hoffman S, Kahn S. Classification of gynecomastia. Plast Reconstr Surg. 1973;51:48–52.
12. Nydick M, Bustos J, Dale JH Jr, Rawson RW. Gynecomastia in adolescent boys. JAMA. 1961;178:449–54.
13. Deutinger M, Freilinger G. Gynecomastia: attempt at a classification and surgical result. Handchir Mikrochir Plast Chir. 1986;18:239–41.
14. Rosenberg GJ. Gynecomastia: suction lipectomy as a contemporary solution. Plast Reconstr Surg. 1987;80:379–86.
15. Letterman G, Schurter M. The surgical correction of gynecomastia. Am Surg. 1969;35:322–5.
16. Brown RH, Chang DK, Siy R, Friedman J. Trends in the surgical correction of gynecomastia. Semin Plast Surg. 2015;29:122–30.
17. Schroder L, Rudlowski C, Walgenbach-Brunagel G, Leutner C, Kuhn W, Walgenbach KJ. Surgical strategies in the treatment of gynecomastia grade I–II: the combination of liposuction and subcutaneous mastectomy provides excellent patient outcome and satisfaction. Breast Care (Basel). 2015;10:184–8.
18. Rahmani S, Turton P, Shaaban A, Dall B. Overview of gynecomastia in the modern era and the Leeds Gynaecomastia Investigation algorithm. Breast J. 2011;17:246–55.
19. Zocchi M. Ultrasonic liposculpturing. Aesthet Plast Surg. 1992;16:287–98.
20. Wong KY, Malata CM. Conventional versus ultrasound-assisted liposuction in gynaecomastia surgery: a 13-year review. J Plast Reconstr Aesthet Surg. 2014;67:921–6.
21. Li CC, Fu JP, Chang SC, Chen TM, Chen SG. Surgical treatment of gynecomastia: complications and outcomes. Ann Plast Surg. 2012;69:510–5.
22. Tolba AM, Nasr M. Surgical treatment of gynaecomastia: a prospective study in 75 patients. Surg Sci. 2015;6:506–17.
23. Morselli PG, Morellini A. Breast reshaping in gynecomastia by the "pull-through technique": considerations after 15 years. Eur J Plast Surg. 2012;35:365–71.
24. Hammond DC, Arnold JF, Simon AM, Capraro PA. Combined use of ultrasonic liposuction with the pull-through technique for the treatment of gynecomastia. Plast Reconstr Surg. 2003;112:891–5.
25. Ramon Y, Fodor L, Peled IJ, Eldor L, Egozi D, Ullmann Y. Multimodality gynecomastia repair by cross-chest power-assisted superficial liposuction combined with endoscopic-assisted pull-through excision. Ann Plast Surg. 2005;55:591–4.
26. Cordova A, Moschella F. Algorithm for clinical evaluation and surgical treatment of gynaecomastia. J Plast Reconstr Aesthet Surg. 2008;61:41–9.

# Use of Magnetic Resonance Imaging to Help Avoid Skin Necrosis After Nipple-Sparing Mastectomy

# 31

Ronnie L. Shammas and Scott T. Hollenbeck

## 31.1 Introduction

### 31.1.1 Evolution of the Mastectomy

Nipple-sparing mastectomy is an increasingly popular prophylactic procedure and treatment for breast cancer [1–3]. However, the surgical management of breast cancer has evolved dramatically over the past years in order to give way to the modern-day nipple-sparing mastectomy. William Halsted is credited with the technique known as the radical mastectomy. He first performed this operation in 1882, which involved the complete removal of the breast and overlying skin, removal of the pectoralis major and minor, and removal of the axillary lymph nodes. This technique led to steep declines in mortality associated with breast cancer and thereafter became the standard of care [4]. However, due to the extreme functionally and aesthetically disfiguring nature of this procedure, less radical approaches were considered [5]. The modified radical mastectomy was introduced in 1948 and involved the removal of the entire breast and lymph nodes, with sparing of the pectoralis muscles to improve functional outcomes [6].

R.L. Shammas, B.S. • S.T. Hollenbeck, M.D. (✉)
Division of Plastic and Reconstructive Surgery, Duke University Medical Center, Durham, NC, USA
e-mail: ronnie.shammas@duke.edu; scott.hollenbeck@duke.edu


M.A. Shiffman (ed.), *Nipple-Areolar Complex Reconstruction*, https://doi.org/10.1007/978-3-319-60925-6_31

As surgical techniques advanced to further decrease patient morbidity and mortality, attention began to turn toward breast conservation therapies that involved the sparing of the nipple and native skin. In 1984, the concept of the skin-sparing mastectomy was introduced. This procedure involved the removal of the entire breast; however, <20% of the native breast skin was removed which improved cosmetic outcomes [7]. In the 1990s, as the nipple-sparing techniques began to evolve around the world, the demand for nipple-sparing mastectomies increased. While a number of approaches have been described, the most common approach utilizes the inframammary incision to accomplish complete removal of the breast with access to the axilla for oncological staging (Fig. 31.1) [8]. The successful implementation of a technique that allowed for sparing of the nipple during mastectomy procedures provided women with higher levels of satisfaction and aided patients in their ability to cope with their diagnoses [9].

### 31.1.2 Challenges of the Nipple-Sparing Mastectomy

One of the most frequent complications to be noted following a nipple-sparing mastectomy is the development of nipple-areola complex (NAC) and skin flap ischemia leading to necrosis of the spared nipple-areolar complex. Complications of this type range from 0% to 48% in the literature

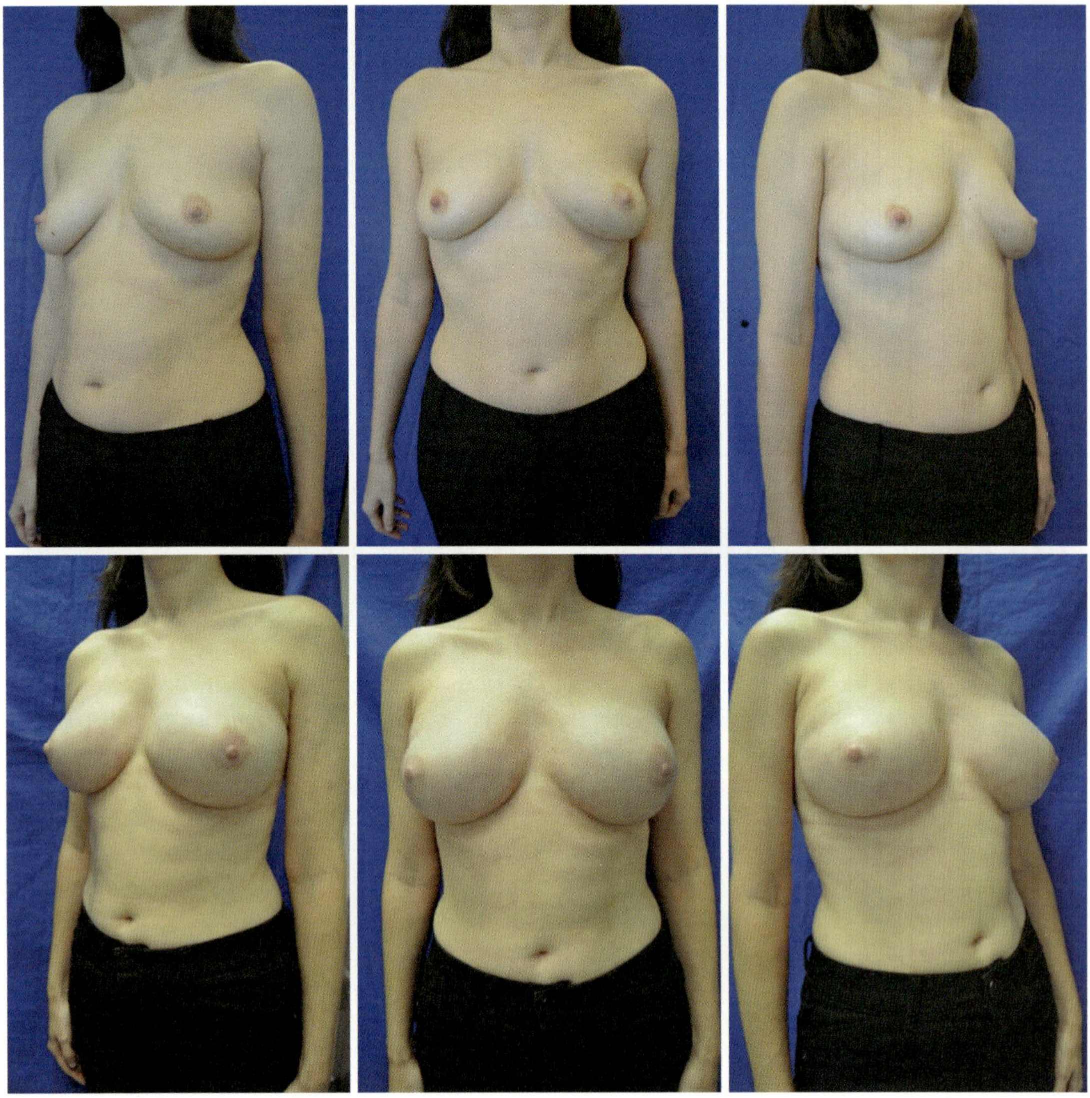

**Fig. 31.1** (*Top*) Preoperative 33-year-old female. (*Bottom*) Six months postoperative after prophylactic nipple-sparing mastectomy and 2 months after implant

[10–17]. If skin necrosis occurs, the reconstruction may be in jeopardy, and the aesthetic advantage to performing this procedure is lost.

Where the surgeon chooses to place their incision site may influence the chance of ischemic and necrotic complications and depends on many factors including the arterial distribution of the blood to the mammary gland. Inferolateral-based incisions have the advantage in that they do not cut across the skin-based blood supply to the nipple and allow for the concealment of the mastectomy scar within the inframammary fold (IMF) with sparing of the blood supply to the skin. The advantage of medial and superior incisions is that they may allow for nipple repositioning; however, these incision patterns are associated with an increased incidence of nipple necrosis due to disruption of the blood supply directly around the nipple (Fig. 31.2) [8, 18–20]. An enhanced understanding of the blood supply to the breast can help guide surgical planning and reduce the likelihood of ischemia and necrosis

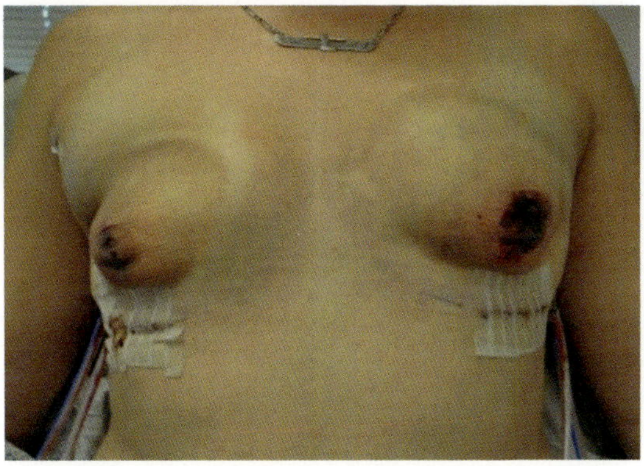

**Fig. 31.2** Postoperative left nipple and breast skin ischemia and necrosis. The patient underwent a bilateral nipple-sparing mastectomy through an inframammary fold incision. This resulted in superficial necrosis and was resolved without surgery with no further complications

following nipple-sparing mastectomy. Modern advents in imaging techniques such as MRI scanning have facilitated our understanding of the blood supply to the breast and allowed for more precise preoperative surgical planning to minimize complications of necrosis and ischemia following nipple-sparing mastectomy [21]. We have recently performed a study whereby we demonstrated the use of preoperative MRI to characterize arterial blood flow to the breast and predict nipple and breast flap ischemia and necrosis following mastectomy [21].

## 31.2 Arterial Blood Supply of the Nipple-Areolar Complex

The breast's arterial supply is primarily derived from branches of the internal mammary artery, the lateral thoracic artery, the thoracoacromial artery, and the posterior intercostal arteries. Blood is primarily supplied to the NAC by the internal thoracic artery by way of its anterior perforating branches. These anterior perforating branches are primarily responsible for the vascularization of the breast skin. However, blood supply to specific areas of the breast such as the nipple is likely to be highly variable. Furthermore, the large blood vessels that perfuse the nipple-areolar complex will likely be ligated during mastectomy, causing difficulty in predicting perfusion patterns and the viability of the nipple and breast skin following surgery.

## 31.3 Risk Factors for Developing Nipple-Areolar Complex Necrosis Following Nipple-Sparing Mastectomy

There are many risk factors that may increase the likelihood for nipple-areolar necrosis following nipple-sparing mastectomy. Patients with hypertension or diabetes mellitus have been shown to display higher rates of nipple necrosis following surgery. In addition, preoperative radiation, smoking, and higher body mass indexes have been attributed to higher rates of NAC) necrosis following surgery [12, 22, 23].

The type of incision pattern has been implicated in influencing the chance of developing nipple necrosis after nipple-sparing mastectomy, with peri-areolar incisions resulting in higher rates of nipple necrosis. This has been attributed to the peri-areolar incision disrupting the collateral blood flow to the nipple-areolar complex following mastectomy [15]. After a nipple-sparing mastectomy, the blood supply to the nipple-areolar complex is more reliant on small vessel connections that form around the areola via the medial and lateral blood supply networks. The peri-areolar incision pattern disrupts these connections, whereas lateral and inframammary incisions spare the plexus of vessels formed from the collateralization of various primary blood vessels as they advance to the nipple [13, 15].

## 31.4 Imaging Modalities Used in the Characterization of Vascular Patterns to the Nipple-Areolar Complex

We have shown that characterizing the vascular supply of the nipple by magnetic resonance imaging (MRI) can help identify vascular features that are predictive of ischemic and necrotic complications following nipple-sparing mastectomy [21].

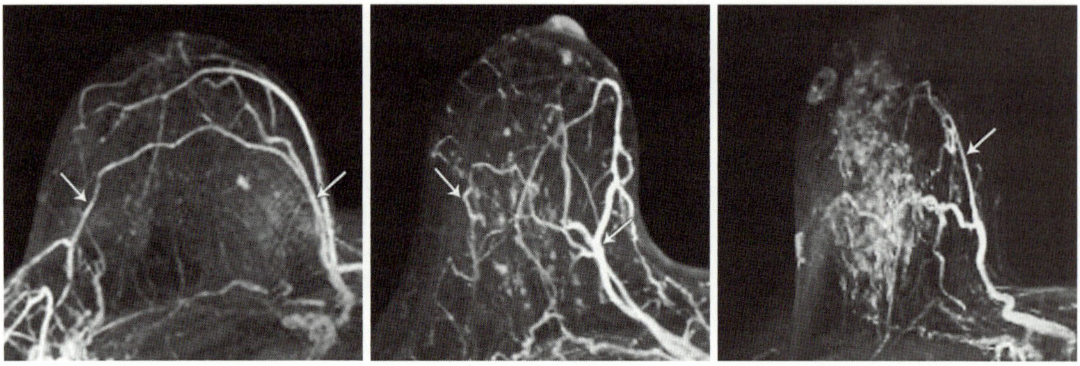

**Fig. 31.3** Axial maximum intensity projection images demonstrate different patterns of blood supply to the right breast. (*Left*) Dual blood supply with codominance of the medial and lateral vessels. (*Middle*) Dual blood supply with dominance of the medial vessel. (*Right*) Single blood supply (medial only) [21]. Reprinted with permission from the Journal of the American College of Surgeons

It is common practice to obtain a preoperative MRI in order to assess for tumor size, the degree of malignant invasion, the presence of nipple-areolar involvement, the distance between the NAC and tumor, and the amount of fibro-glandular tissue present in the NAC [24–26]. It has also been suggested that the use of preoperative MRI scans can be expanded to help predict the likelihood of NAC ischemia and necrosis following surgery by aiding in the characterization of the nipple-areola blood supply [1, 21, 27]. Our study demonstrated this concept by *using preoperative MRI scans to assess for the presence or absence of codominant dual (medial and lateral) blood supply to the nipple-areolar complex* (Fig. 31.3). We hypothesized that the presence of a dual blood supply, as seen on preoperative MRI, would increase the likelihood of preserving blood vessels and collateral flow during a mastectomy as opposed to a single blood supply [21]. We concluded that MRI characterization of breast vascularity offers clinically useful information that may be used to predict the likelihood of NAC complex necrosis and ischemia after a nipple-sparing mastectomy.

Other studies further support these conclusions by characterizing the nipple-areolar complex blood supply with preoperative MRI scans and identifying that an extensive anastomotic network exists laterally and medially around the NAC between the lateral thoracic artery and the internal mammary artery, respectively [1, 27]. As such, identification of this vascular pattern with preoperative imaging can aid surgeons in choosing their incision site to minimize the risk for postoperative complications that involve the NAC. This information may allow for a surgical approach that reduces the chance of compromising collateral flow to the NAC [1, 27]. This preoperative imaging can also be used in patient selection to help determine which patients are optimal candidates to undergo a nipple-sparing mastectomy as determined by the vascular pattern around the nipple-areolar complex.

Laser angiography is an imaging technique that has been used intraoperatively to evaluate the perfusion to the nipple-areolar complex in an attempt to minimize complications of necrosis and ischemia [28]. During intraoperative laser angiography, an injectable fluorescent dye (indocyanine green) is used to capture the inflow of blood as visualized with an infrared camera using the SPY Elite™ imaging system [28]. This technique offers the advantage of mapping blood flow patterns to the NAC in order to help guide incisions to minimize the interference with blood supply [29]. Other techniques used to evaluate perfusion intraoperatively have included tissue oximetry devices, tissue oximetry, and fluorescein; however, none of these approaches have been shown to be consistently reliable in the clinic [30]. Furthermore, it is generally felt that these techniques are more beneficial after the mastectomy has been performed to demonstrate which areas of the skin are likely to survive or develop necrosis.

**Conclusions**

Advances in surgical technique since the Halstead era have allowed surgeons to offer breast cancer patients the option of nipple-sparing mastectomies. For those eligible for this procedure, it has resulted in increased patient satisfaction and improved aesthetic outcomes. However, when offering this procedure to patients, it is important to recognize those factors which may contribute to the complication of NAC necrosis and ischemia. Imaging modalities, such as magnetic resonance imaging, offer the surgeon a noninvasive preoperative evaluation of the vascular network of the breast to enhance surgical planning and minimize the rates of postoperative skin necrosis and reconstructive failure.

## References


1. Amanti C, Vitale V, Lombardi A, Maggi S, Bersigotti L, Lazzarin G, Nuccetelli E, Romano C, Campanella L, Cristiano L, Bartoloni A, Argento G. Importance of perforating vessels in nipple-sparing mastectomy: an anatomical description. Breast Cancer (Dove Med Press). 2015;7:179–81.
2. Headon HL, Kasem A, Mokbel K. The oncological safety of nipple-sparing mastectomy: a systematic review of the literature with a pooled analysis of 12,358 procedures. Arch Plast Surg. 2016;43(4):328–38.
3. Huang NS, Wu J. Nipple-sparing mastectomy in breast cancer: from an oncologic safety perspective. Chin Med J. 2015;128(16):2256–61.
4. Halsted WS. I. The results of operations for the cure of cancer of the breast performed at the Johns Hopkins Hospital from June, 1889, to January, 1894. Ann Surg. 1894;20(5):497–555.
5. Zurrida S, Bassi F, Arnone P, Martella S, Del Castillo A, Ribeiro Martini R, Semenkiw ME, Caldarella P. The changing face of mastectomy (from mutilation to aid to breast reconstruction). Int J Surg Oncol. 2011;2011:980158.
6. Borgen P. Breast cancer in the 20(th) century: quest for the ideal therapy. Ochsner J. 2000;2(1):5–9.
7. Laronga C, Lewis JD, Smith PD. The changing face of mastectomy: an oncologic and cosmetic perspective. Cancer Control. 2012;19(4):286–94.
8. de Alcantara Filho P, Capko D, Barry JM, Morrow M, Pusic A, Sacchini VS. Nipple-sparing mastectomy for breast cancer and risk-reducing surgery: the Memorial Sloan-Kettering Cancer Center experience. Ann Surg Oncol. 2011;18(11):3117–22.
9. Didier F, Radice D, Gandini S, Bedolis R, Rotmensz N, Maldifassi A, Santillo B, Luini A, Galimberti V, Scaffidi E, Lupo F, Martella S, Petit JY. Does nipple preservation in mastectomy improve satisfaction with cosmetic results, psychological adjustment, body image and sexuality? Breast Cancer Res Treat. 2009;118(3):623–33.
10. Chattopadhyay D, Gupta S, Jash PK, Murmu MB, Gupta S. Skin sparing mastectomy with preservation of nipple areola complex and immediate breast reconstruction in patients with breast cancer: a single centre prospective study. Plast Surg Int. 2014;2014:589068.
11. Lemaine V, Hoskin TL, Farley DR, Grant CS, Boughey JC, Torstenson TA, Jacobson SR, Jakub JW, Degnim AC. Introducing the SKIN score: a validated scoring system to assess severity of mastectomy skin flap necrosis. Ann Surg Oncol. 2015;22(9): 2925–32.
12. Frey JD, Alperovich M, Chun Kim J, Saadeh PB, Hazen A, Levine JP, Ahn CY, Allen R, Choi M, Schnabel FR, Karp NS, Guth AA. Oncologic outcomes after nipple-sparing mastectomy: a single-institutional experience. Plast Reconstr Surg. 2015;136(4 Suppl):87–8.
13. Carlson GW, Chu CK, Moyer HR, Duggal C, Losken A. Predictors of nipple ischemia after nipple sparing mastectomy. Breast J. 2014;20(1):69–73.
14. Stolier AJ, Levine EA. Reducing the risk of nipple necrosis: technical observations in 340 nipple-sparing mastectomies. Breast J. 2013;19(2):173–9.
15. Rawlani V, Fiuk J, Johnson SA, Buck DW 2nd, Hirsch E, Hansen N, Khan S, Fine NA, Kim JY. The effect of incision choice on outcomes of nipple-sparing mastectomy reconstruction. Can J Plast Surg. 2011;19(4):129–33.
16. Komorowski AL, Zanini V, Regolo L, Carolei A, Wysocki WM, Costa A. Necrotic complications after nipple- and areola-sparing mastectomy. World J Surg. 2006;30(8):1410–3.
17. Wang F, Peled AW, Garwood E, Fiscalini AS, Sbitany H, Foster RD, , Alvarado M, Ewing C, Hwang ES, Esserman LJ. Total skin-sparing mastectomy and immediate breast reconstruction: an evolution of technique and assessment of outcomes. Ann Surg Oncol 2014;21(10):3223–3230.
18. Paepke S, Schmid R, Fleckner S, Paepke D, Niemeyer M, Schmalfeldt B, Jacobs VR, Kiechle M. Subcutaneous mastectomy with conservation of the nipple-areola skin: broadening the indications. Ann Surg. 2009;250(2):288–92.
19. Spear SL, Hannan CM, Willey SC, Cocilovo C. Nipple-sparing mastectomy. Plast Reconstr Surg. 2009;123(6):1665–73.
20. Wijayanayagam A, Kumar AS, Foster RD, Esserman LJ. Optimizing the total skin-sparing mastectomy. Arch Surg. 2008;143(1):38–45.
21. Bahl M, Pien IJ, Buretta KJ, Hwang ES, Greenup RA, Ghate SV, Hollenbeck ST. Can vascular patterns on preoperative magnetic resonance imaging help pre-

dict skin necrosis after nipple-sparing mastectomy? J Am Coll Surg. 2016;223(2):279–85.
22. Gould DJ, Hunt KK, Liu J, Kuerer HM, Crosby MA, Babiera G, Kronowitz SJ. Impact of surgical techniques, biomaterials, and patient variables on rate of nipple necrosis after nipple-sparing mastectomy. Plast Reconstr Surg. 2013;132(3):330e–8e.
23. Colwell AS, Tessler O, Lin AM, Liao E, Winograd J, Cetrulo CL, Tang R, Smith BL, Austen WG Jr. Breast reconstruction following nipple-sparing mastectomy: predictors of complications, reconstruction outcomes, and 5-year trends. Plast Reconstr Surg. 2014;133(3):496–506.
24. Ponzone R, Maggiorotto F, Carabalona S, Rivolin A, Pisacane A, Kubatzki F, Renditore S, Carlucci S, Sgandurra P, Marocco F, Magistris A, Regge D, Martincich L. MRI and intraoperative pathology to predict nipple-areola complex (NAC) involvement in patients undergoing NAC-sparing mastectomy. Eur J Cancer. 2015;51(14):1882–9.
25. Moon JY, Chang YW, Lee EH, Seo DY. Malignant invasion of the nipple-areolar complex of the breast: usefulness of breast MRI. AJR Am J Roentgenol. 2013;201(2):448–55.
26. Baltzer HL, Alonzo-Proulx O, Mainprize JG, Yaffe MJ, Metcalfe KA, Narod SA, Warner E, Semple JL. MRI volumetric analysis of breast fibroglandular tissue to assess risk of the spared nipple in BRCA1 and BRCA2 mutation carriers. Ann Surg Oncol. 2014;21(5):1583–8.
27. Seitz IA, Nixon AT, Friedewald SM, Rimler JC, Schechter LS. "NACsomes": a new classification system of the blood supply to the nipple areola complex (NAC) based on diagnostic breast MRI exams. J Plast Reconstr Aesthet Surg. 2015;68(6):792–9.
28. Dua MM, Bertoni DM, Nguyen D, Meyer S, Gurtner GC, Wapnir IL. Using intraoperative laser angiography to safeguard nipple perfusion in nipple-sparing mastectomies. Gland Surg. 2015;4(6):497–505.
29. Wapnir I, Dua M, Kieryn A, Paro J, Morrison D, Kahn D, Meyer S, Gurtner G. Intraoperative imaging of nipple perfusion patterns and ischemic complications in nipple-sparing mastectomies. Ann Surg Oncol. 2014;21(1):100–6.
30. Gurtner GC, Jones GE, Neligan PC, Newman MI, Phillips BT, Sacks JM, Zenn MR. Intraoperative laser angiography using the SPY system: review of the literature and recommendations for use. Ann Surg Innov Res. 2013;7(1):1.

# Part VII

# Techniques for Correction of Nipple Hypertrophy

# Correction of Nipple Hypertrophy with Nipple Circumcision Technique

32

Tolga Eryilmaz and Serhan Tuncer

## 32.1 Introduction

Nipple hypertrophy can cause significant psychosocial problems and physical discomfort to the patient. Large nipples can affect a woman's appearance. Patient may have problems with her choice of clothing especially when wearing light clothes [1, 2]. Nipple circumcision technique was first reported by Regnault [3], as a circumferential skin and superficial muscular layer excision between base and apex of the hypertrophic nipple. Lai et al. [4] modified the Regnault's technique in order to decrease the nipple height without altering the diameter. Although these techniques produce adequate nipple reduction, circumferential removal of dermal components may cause vascular flow impairment and decreased nipple sensation [1]. In order to avoid these morbidities, we are performing a modified nipple circumcision technique [5].

T. Eryilmaz, M.D. (✉)
Department of Plastic, Reconstructive and Aesthetic Surgery, Ufuk University Medical School, Dr. Ridvan Ege Hospital, Mevlana Bulvari, 86–88, Block A, 1st Floor, Balgat, Ankara, Turkey
e-mail: mdtolgaer@yahoo.com

S. Tuncer, M.D.
Department of Plastic, Reconstructive and Aesthetic Surgery, Gazi University Medical School, Gazi University Hospital, 14th Floor, Besevler, Ankara, Turkey
e-mail: serhantuncer74@yahoo.com

## 32.2 Technique

First, a circumferential incision is made approximately 5 mm above the nipple base; the second incision is made below the tip of the nipple at a level corresponding to the desired amount of reduction. The skin is deepithelialized leaving the dermal layer intact. The incision is closed with 6-0 polypropylene, vertical mattress sutures (Fig. 32.1).

Twenty-six nipple reductions were performed in 13 female patients using the modified nipple

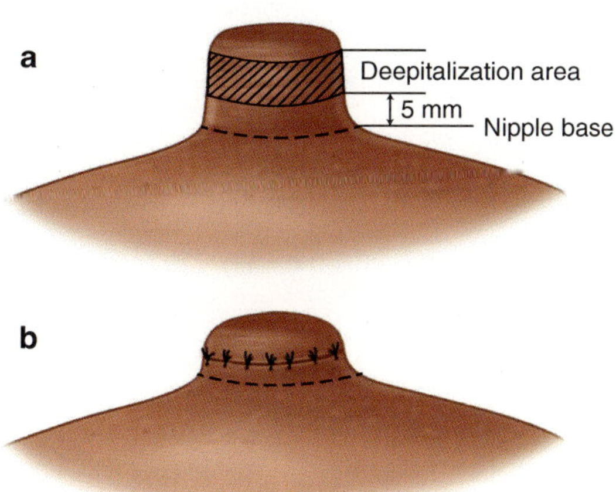


**Fig. 32.1** (**a**) First, a circumferential incision is made approximately 5 mm above the nipple base; the second incision is made below the tip of the nipple at a level corresponding to the desired amount of reduction. The skin is deepithelialized leaving the dermal layer intact. (**b**) The incision is closed with 6-0 polypropylene, vertical mattress sutures


M.A. Shiffman (ed.), *Nipple-Areolar Complex Reconstruction*,
https://doi.org/10.1007/978-3-319-60925-6_32

circumcision technique. Patient's age ranged between 24 and 41 (mean 32). Ten patients had breast hypoplasia and were requesting augmentation mammaplasty. Corrections of the nipple in seven patients were carried out simultaneously with breast augmentation using silicone implants. Three patients were operated 6 and 11 months after the breast augmentation as an outpatient procedure. The remaining three patients just complained about their nipple size, and nipple corrections were carried out as an outpatient procedure.

First, breast implants were placed and the incisions were closed, and then nipple reductions were performed in simultaneous cases. Other nipple reductions were performed under local anesthesia in the office setting. Seven patients were uniparous, two patients were multiparous, and four patients had no history of pregnancy. Patients who gave birth had a mean lactation period of 10.3 ± 5.6 (5–16) months.

Postoperative recovery in all patients was uneventful. Sutures were removed 1 week after the operation. No complications were encountered, such as ischemic problems, venous congestion, or decreased nipple sensation. The swelling and pain were minimal. There was very little discomfort in the postoperative period. The mean follow-up period was 3.2 years. The resulting scar was well concealed and almost invisible. Results were in natural appearance, and nipple sensation was preserved. Long-term aesthetic results were satisfactory, and the patients expressed a high degree of satisfaction, due to good aesthetic and functional results (Fig. 32.2).

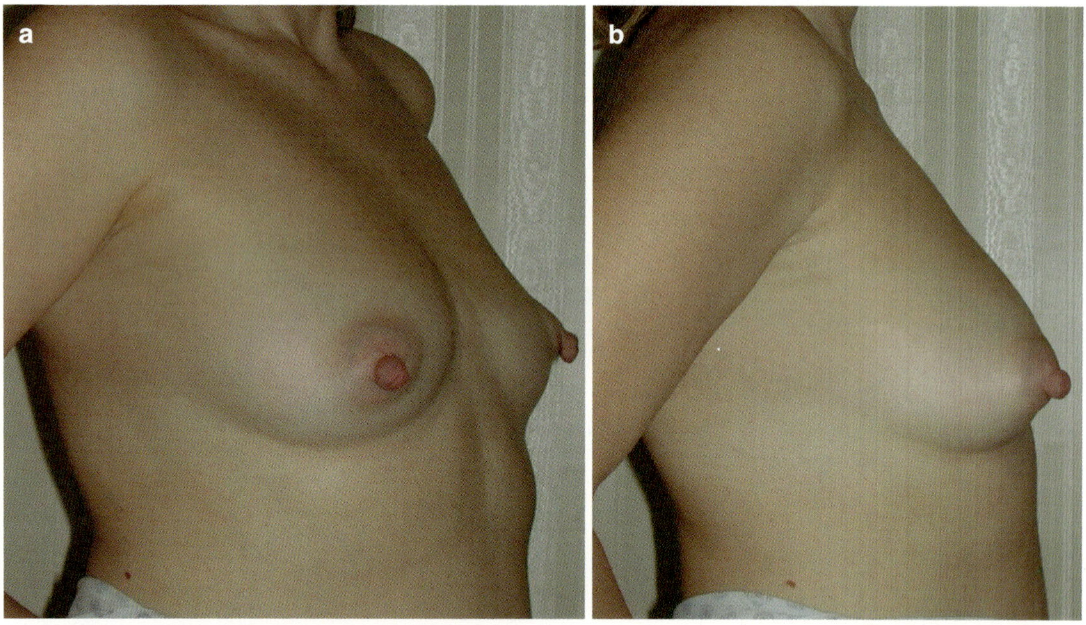


**Fig. 32.2** Breast augmentation with implant and simultaneous nipple reduction was performed to the patient. (**a**, **b**) Preoperative patient. (**c**, **d**) 1 year postoperative

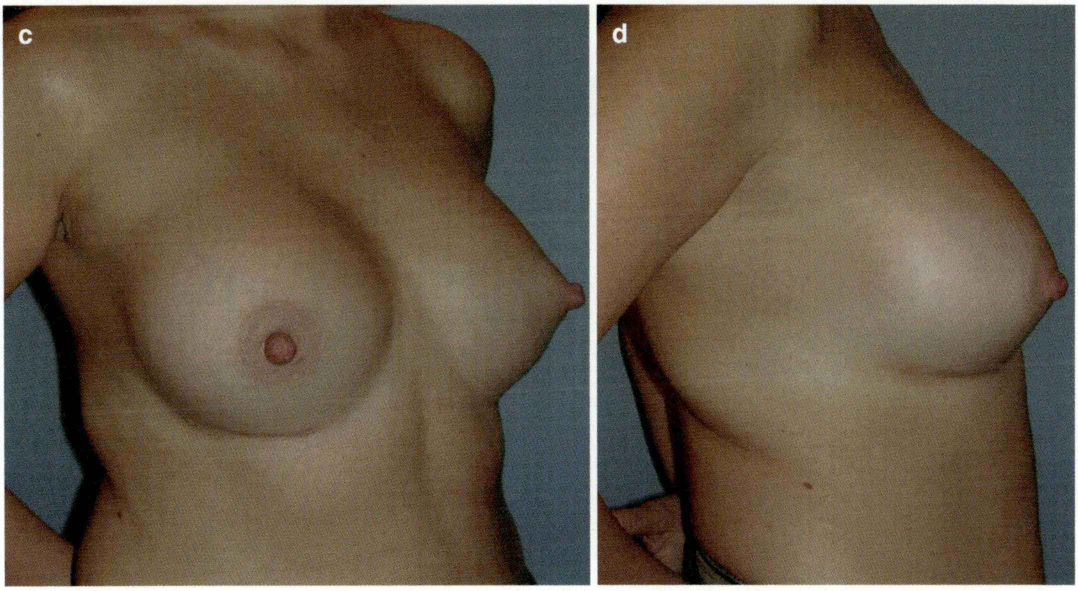


**Fig. 32.2** (continued)

## 32.3 Discussion

Nipple hypertrophy can cause significant psychosocial problems and physical discomfort to the patient. The patient may have problems with her choice of clothing especially when wearing light clothes [1, 2]. Nipple circumcision technique was first reported by Regnault [3], as a circumferential skin and superficial muscular layer excision between base and apex of the hypertrophic nipple. Lai et al. [4] modified the Regnault's technique in order to decrease the nipple height without altering the diameter. Both techniques include circumferential removal of dermal components [3, 4]. Although these techniques produce adequate nipple reduction, circumferential removal of dermal components may cause vascular flow impairment and decreased nipple sensation [1].

With the modified nipple circumcision technique, the deepithelialization avoids the removal of dermis and preserves the subdermal arterial plexus. Nipple sensation also remains unaffected, because the dermal components are preserved [5].

**Conclusions**

Modified nipple circumcision technique is safe and reliable. Nipple reduction can be done in combination with breast augmentation, breast reduction, or mastopexy. Also it can be performed as a separate procedure under local anesthesia. If there is a nipple deformity, its correction completes the breast procedure and significantly enhances outcome and patient satisfaction.

## References


1. Cheng MH, Smartt JM, Rodriguez ED, Ulusal BG. Nipple reduction using the modified top hat flap. Plast Reconstr Surg. 2006;118(7):1517–25.
2. Ferreira LM, Neto MS, Okamoto RH, Andrews J d M. Surgical correction of nipple hypertrophy. Plast Reconstr Surg. 1995;95(4):753–4.
3. Regnault P. Nipple hypertrophy. A physiologic reduction by circumcision. Clin Plast Surg. 1975;2(3):391–6.
4. Lai YL, Wu WC. Nipple reduction with a modified circumcision technique. Br J Plast Surg. 1996;49(5):307–9.
5. Tuncer S, Eryilmaz T, Atabay K. Correction of nipple hypertrophy: nipple circumcision technique revisited. J Plast Reconstr Aesthet Surg. 2010;63(9):1575–6.

# Nipple Reduction: An Adjunct to Breast Augmentation

# 33

Nabil Fanous and Amanda Fanous

## 33.1 Introduction

A review of the medical literature reveals a surprisingly limited number of publications addressing the topic of nipple hypertrophy reduction [1–9]. Nipple hyperthrophy is frequently encountered in Asian women and less commonly in Caucasian and Black females. Although the exact epidemiology remains unknown, a congenital etiology is hypothesized, as well as acquired causes linked to hormonal fluctuations during puberty, gestation, lactation, or menopause [1].

Nipple hypertrophy may be associated with significant psychosocial distress, mainly secondary to undesired esthetics. Furthermore, concealing hypertrophied nipples under light clothing or bathing suits during the summer months can prove challenging. The aim of reduction nippleplasty is to recreate the harmony between the nipple, the areola, and the breast mound by reducing the nipple projection, with or without a concomitant reduction in diameter.

In the following section, the authors will describe their personal technique, previously published in the Canadian Journal of Plastic Surgery [10]. This simple approach has the advantage of completely sparing the deep structures of the nipple, while reducing both its height and diameter in order to achieve harmonic breast proportions.

Nipple reduction can serve as an excellent adjunct to any esthetic breast surgery, especially augmentation mammoplasty. It should be part of every cosmetic surgeon's armamentarium of procedures.

## 33.2 Ideal Nipple Esthetics

There exists no formal description of detailed ideal nipple measurements. Even the exact definition of nipple hypertrophy is lacking in the medical literature. The normal nipple dimensions have been briefly reported as being around one centimeter in both diameter and projection [1]. Generally, nipples over 1–1.5 cm in either height or diameter have been considered hypertrophic.

The ideal nipple (Fig. 33.1) is cylindrical in shape, with an anterior convex surface in the form of a dome. First, it has an anterior projection (height) of around 8 mm, with an acceptable margin of 6–10 mm, depending on factors such as areola diameter and present or anticipated breast size. Second, the ideal nipple diameter, though of secondary importance, is also around 8 mm and again with a 6–10 mm margin.

N. Fanous, M.D. (✉) • A. Fanous, M.D.
The Canadian Institute of Cosmetic Surgery,
1 Westmount Square, Suite 1380, Westmount,
Montreal, Canada, H3Z 2P9


M.A. Shiffman (ed.), *Nipple-Areolar Complex Reconstruction*,
https://doi.org/10.1007/978-3-319-60925-6_33

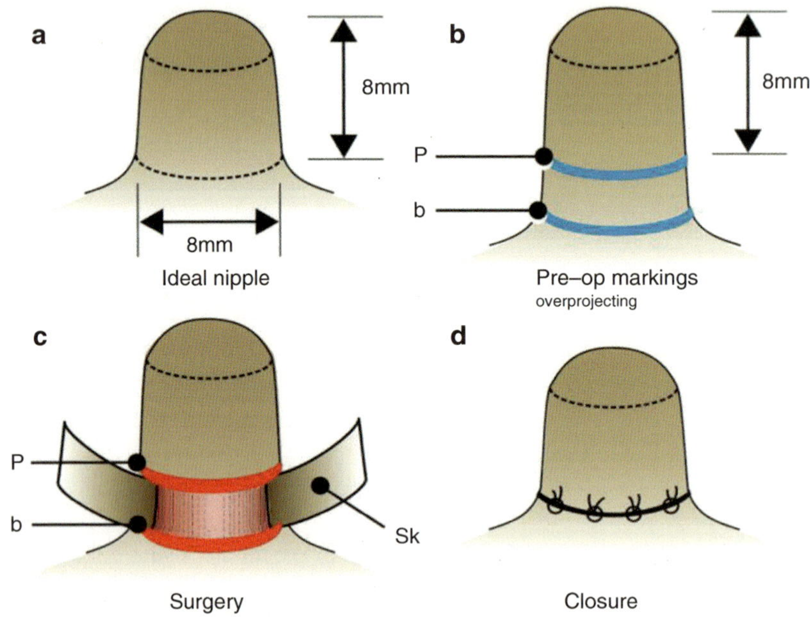


**Fig. 33.1** Ideal esthetics of the nipple: (**a**) the ideal nipple is cylindrical in shape, with an anterior convex surface in the form of a dome. It has an anterior projection (height) of around 8 mm, with an acceptable margin of 6–10 mm. The ideal nipple diameter, though of secondary importance, is also around 8 mm and again with a 6–10 mm margin. (**b**) Preoperative markings of the overprojecting nipple: firstly, the new projection of the nipple is measured 8 mm from its tip and then drawn as a circumferential line at that level (p) representing the future nipple base. Secondly, a line (b) is marked around the present base. (**c**) Surgical technique of the overprojecting nipple: a skin incision is made along the line of the future nipple base (circle p). Another incision is then made at the base of the present nipple (circle b). The skin between these two incisions is superficially dissected and excised as a thin flap (sk). (**d**) Closure: fine absorbable sutures are used to approximate the base of the new nipple to the original base. As this is done, the denuded section of the nipple is automatically buried

## 33.3 Surgical Technique

### 33.3.1 Reduction of Excessive Projection

#### 33.3.1.1 Preoperative Marking

First, the new projection of the nipple is measured 8 mm from its tip and then drawn as a circumferential line at that level (Fig. 33.1). This line represents the future nipple base. Secondly, a line is marked around the present base. Thirdly, a vertical (superior-to-inferior) line is marked across the top surface of the nipple, as well as over the areola, to serve as a guideline to the surgeon during closure.

#### 33.3.1.2 Infiltration

Using a 30 G needle and about 1–1.5 mL of 1% lidocaine with 1/100,000 epinephrine, each nipple is infiltrated at its base and across its trunk.

#### 33.3.1.3 Surgical Technique

The nipple may be stabilized with an Adson-Brown forceps, or by passing a suture through its top then holding it with a mosquito. A superficial skin incision is made along the line of the future nipple base (Fig. 33.1). Another incision is then made at the base of the present nipple. Using an Adson-Brown forceps and a No. 15 blade, the skin between these two incisions is meticulously dissected and excised as a thin flap. Occasionally, minimal electrocautery may be needed to ensure hemostasis. The closure is done by using simple interrupted 5-0 Monocryl sutures to approximate the four corners (superior, inferior, medial, lateral) of the base of the new nipple to the original base. As this is done, the denuded section of the nipple between incisions p and b (Fig. 33.1) is automatically buried and invaginated. Extra four interrupted simple 5-0 Monocryl sutures are used to complete the closure.

The detailed surgical reduction of excessive nipple projection is portrayed in a step-by-step manner in Fig. 33.2.

## 33.3.2 Reduction of Excessive Diameter

### 33.3.2.1 Preoperative Marking

Hypertrophic nipples have primarily a problem of excessive projection but may occasionally have an excessive diameter as well. In such a case, the nipple diameter needs to be simultaneously addressed. This part of the procedure is uncommon and is only required in about 10–15% of cases.

The initial preoperative markings are identical to those done for the excessive projection as described earlier (Fig. 33.1). Following this, the markings for the excessive diameter are drawn. First, the width (diameter) of the present nipple base is measured (Fig. 33.3). Then, the excess width is calculated by simply figuring out the number of millimeters exceeding 8 mm. The resultant calculated excess usually varies between 5 and 10 mm. This excess is divided by 2, producing a figure between 2 and 5 mm, which represents the width of each of the two skin rectangles to be excised later. These two rectangles of skin are marked at opposing sides, often on the inferior and superior surfaces of the new nipple. However, these two rectangles may be placed anywhere around the nipple, especially where the diameter seems to be widest.

At the top of each rectangle, two bilateral transverse incisions, measuring about 2–3 mm each, are marked just below the nipple dome.

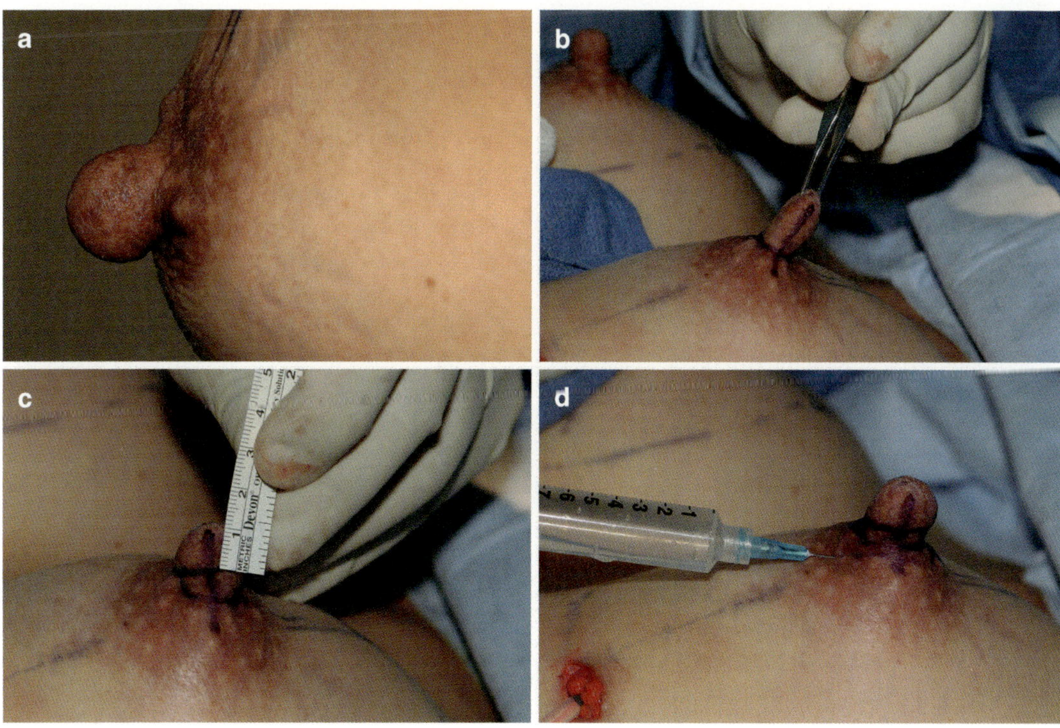


**Fig. 33.2** Surgical technique to reduce the excessive nipple projection. (**a**) A hyperttrophic nipple with excessive projection. (**b**) Preoperative marking: a circumferential line is drawn around the present base. A superior-to-inferior line is marked across the nipple and areola in order to orient the surgeon. (**c**) Preoperative marking: the new projection of the nipple is delineated at 8 mm from the top of its dome, as a circumferential line. (**d**) Infiltration of the base and core of the nipple. (**e**) Two circular incisions are done: one at the base of the original nipple and the other one at the base of the new nipple. (**f**) The extra skin between the two circular incisions is dissected and excised as a thin flap. (**g**) Interrupted fine absorbable sutures are used for closure

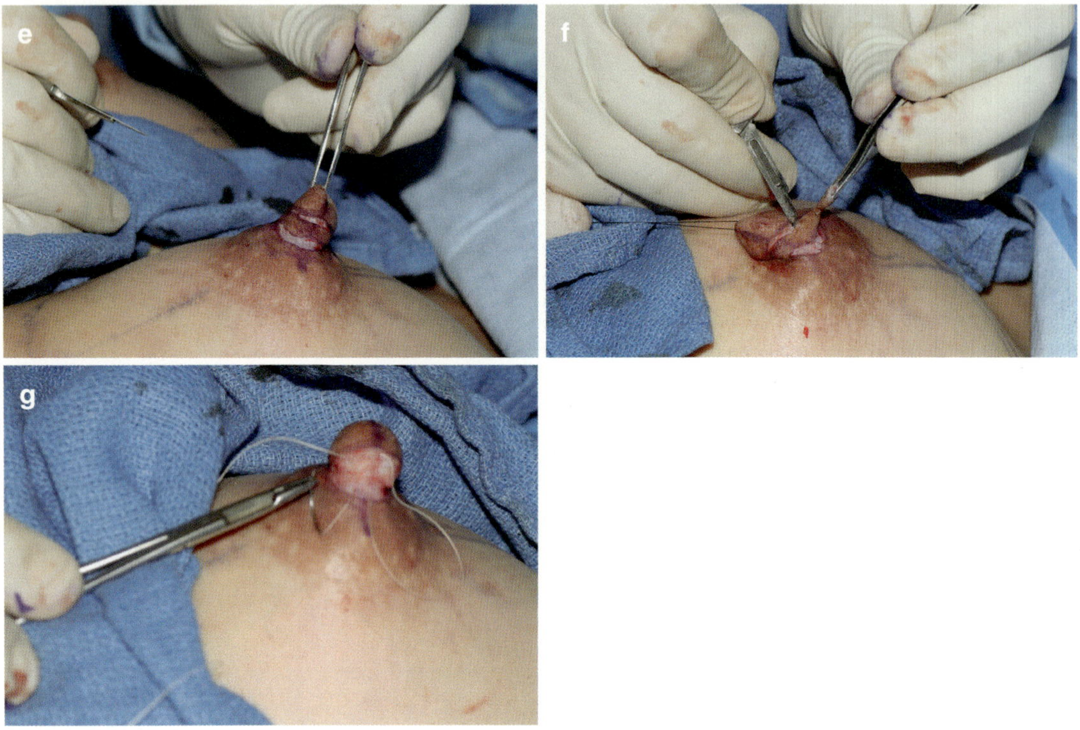


**Fig. 33.2** (continued)

This allows the movement of two advancement flaps that will close the skin defects after the excision of the triangles R and $R_2$ (Fig. 33.3).

#### 33.3.2.2 Surgical Technique

Incisions are done around the two rectangles R and $R_2$ (Fig. 33.2). Two rectangular pieces of skin are excised by superficial dissection, using an Adson-Brown forceps and a No. 15 blade. Next, two incisions are made just below the nipple dome, on both sides of the superior limit of each of the two resultant bare rectangles. Then, two advancement skin flaps are raised by a subcutaneous dissection of about 2–3 mm bilaterally and then are approximated with interrupted 5-0 Monocryl sutures.

The previous steps will result in a larger circular defect in the areola, compared to the now smaller base of the newly narrowed nipple. In order to narrow the larger diameter b, a small inferior triangle, measuring 2–4 mm at its base, is marked and excised at the circular incision b (Fig. 33.3). Minimal bilateral dissection is performed to close this triangular defect.

The step-by-step surgical approach to excessive nipple diameter reduction in the operating room is depicted in Fig. 33.4.

#### 33.3.2.3 Dressing

Two Band-Aids are used to compress the newly reduced nipple. These are placed in the form of a cross over the nipple and areola for stabilization. A dry gauze dressing is then applied.

## 33.4 Postoperative Visits

The following morning, the dressing is changed. The patient is seen at 1 week postoperatively and then every 6–12 months afterward.

## 33.5 Results

A total of 56 nipples were operated in 28 healthy females. Patients aged 24 to 42 years (average 31 years old) were included in the present series. All

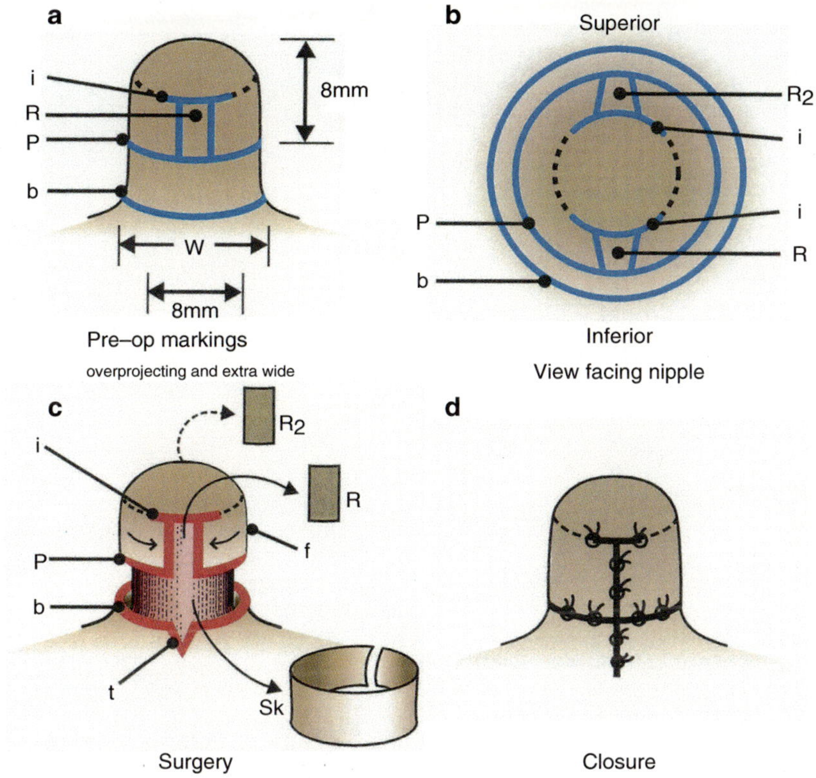


**Fig. 33.3** (**a**, **b**) Preoperative markings of an overprojecting nipple with excessive width: The width of the present nipple base is measured (*w*). Then, the excess width is calculated by simply figuring out the number of millimeters exceeding 8 mm. The resultant excess usually varies between 5 to 10 mm. This excess is divided by 2, producing a figure between 2 to 5 mm, which represents the width of each of the two skin rectangles to be excised. R and $R_2$, located on the inferior and superior surfaces of the new nipple. At the top of each rectangle, two bilateral transverse incisions, measuring about 2–3 mm each, are marked just below the nipple dome (i). This allows the movement of two advancement flaps that will close the skin defects after the excision of the triangles R and $R_2$. (**c**) Surgical technique for excessive nipple width. Incisions are done around the two rectangles "R" and "$R_2$." Two rectangular pieces of skin (R and $R_2$) are excised. Next, two incisions (i) are made on both sides of the superior limit of each of the two resultant bare rectangles. Then, two advancement skin flaps are raised by a subcutaneous dissection bilaterally (f) and are approximated with interrupted sutures. This will result in a larger circular defect in the areola (b), compared to the now smaller base of the nipple (p). In order to narrow the larger diameter b, a small inferior triangle (t), measuring 2–4 mm at its base, is marked and excised at the circular incision (b). Minimal bilateral dissection is performed to close this triangular defect. (**d**) Final closure of all incisions

patients were of Asian descent, except for three Caucasian females. The follow-up ranged from 7 months to a little over 10 years, with an average of 3 years and 2 months.

All patients had bilateral nipple hypertrophy. All scars healed surprisingly well, even in Asian patients who showed a tendency for hypertrophic scarring in the submammary incisions. There were no complaints regarding altered nipple sensation or problems with breast-feeding. This should be expected since this technique does not injure the nipple nervous network or the lactiferous ducts. In summary, there were no noted complications related to the nippleplasty.

All patients had the nipple reduction procedure combined with a breast augmentation.

Examples of the results of the nipple reduction described above are shown in Figs. 33.5, 33.6, and 33.7.

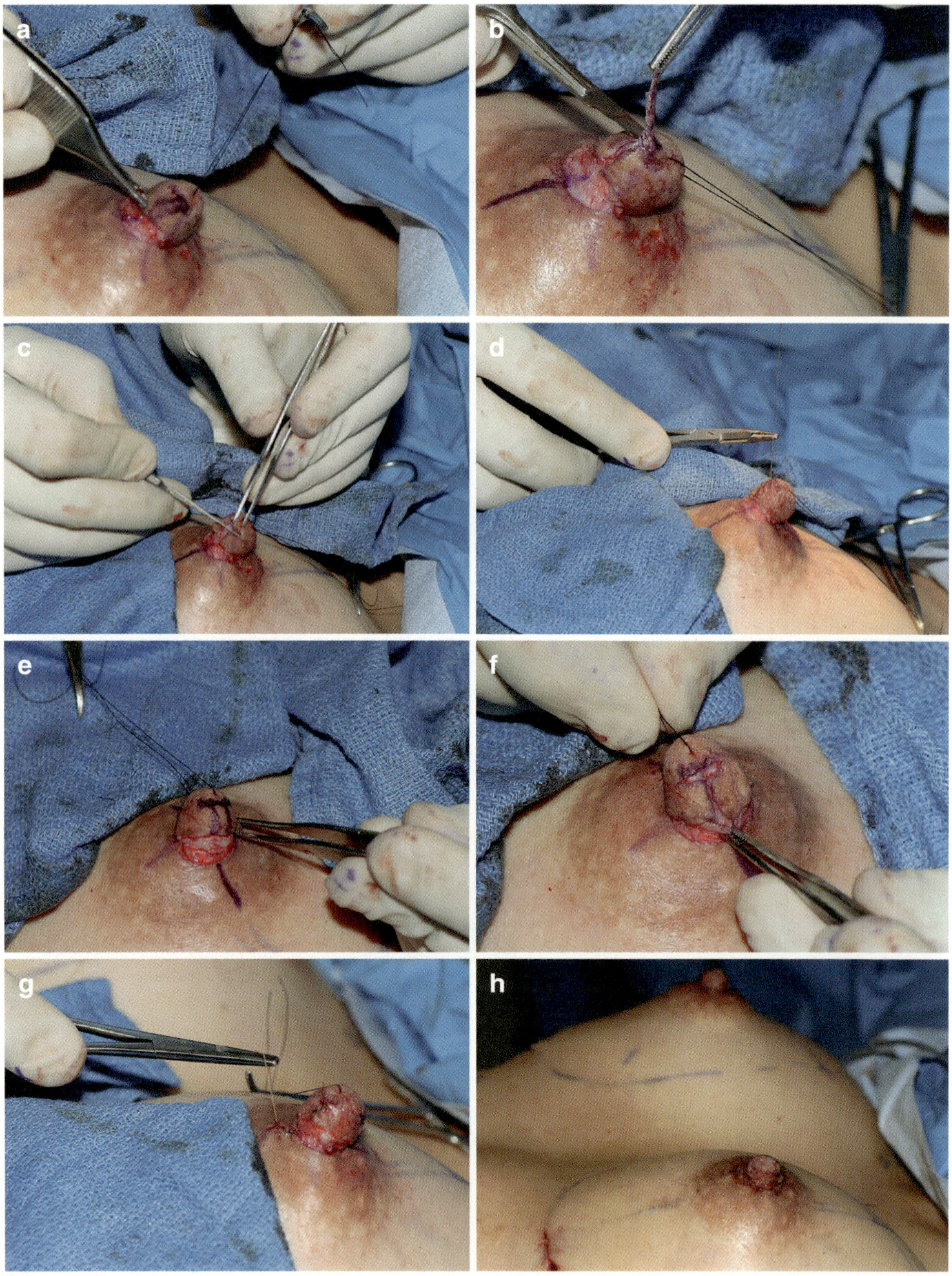


**Fig. 33.4** Surgical technique to reduce the excessive nipple diameter. (**a**) The surgical correction of the excessive nipple projection has just been done. To reduce the excessive diameter, a rectangle (measuring in width half of the total excess diameter) is drawn on the inferior surface of the new nipple. (**b**) The rectangle of skin is excised from the inferior surface of the nipple. (**c**) Two bilateral transverse incisions, on both sides of the top of the bare rectangle, are done. (**d**) Two advancement flaps are dissected, advanced, and approximated to close the rectangular defect. (**e**) The same technique is used to mark a second rectangle on the superior surface of the nipple. (**f**) Following the excision of the little skin rectangle on the superior surface of the nipple, two advancement flaps are dissected and approximated to close the defect. (**g**) In order to narrow the circular defect in the areola, a small triangle of skin is excised at the original basal incision so that it fits the new slimmer nipple. (**h**) Final bilateral result of the reduction of overprojecting and excessively wide nipples

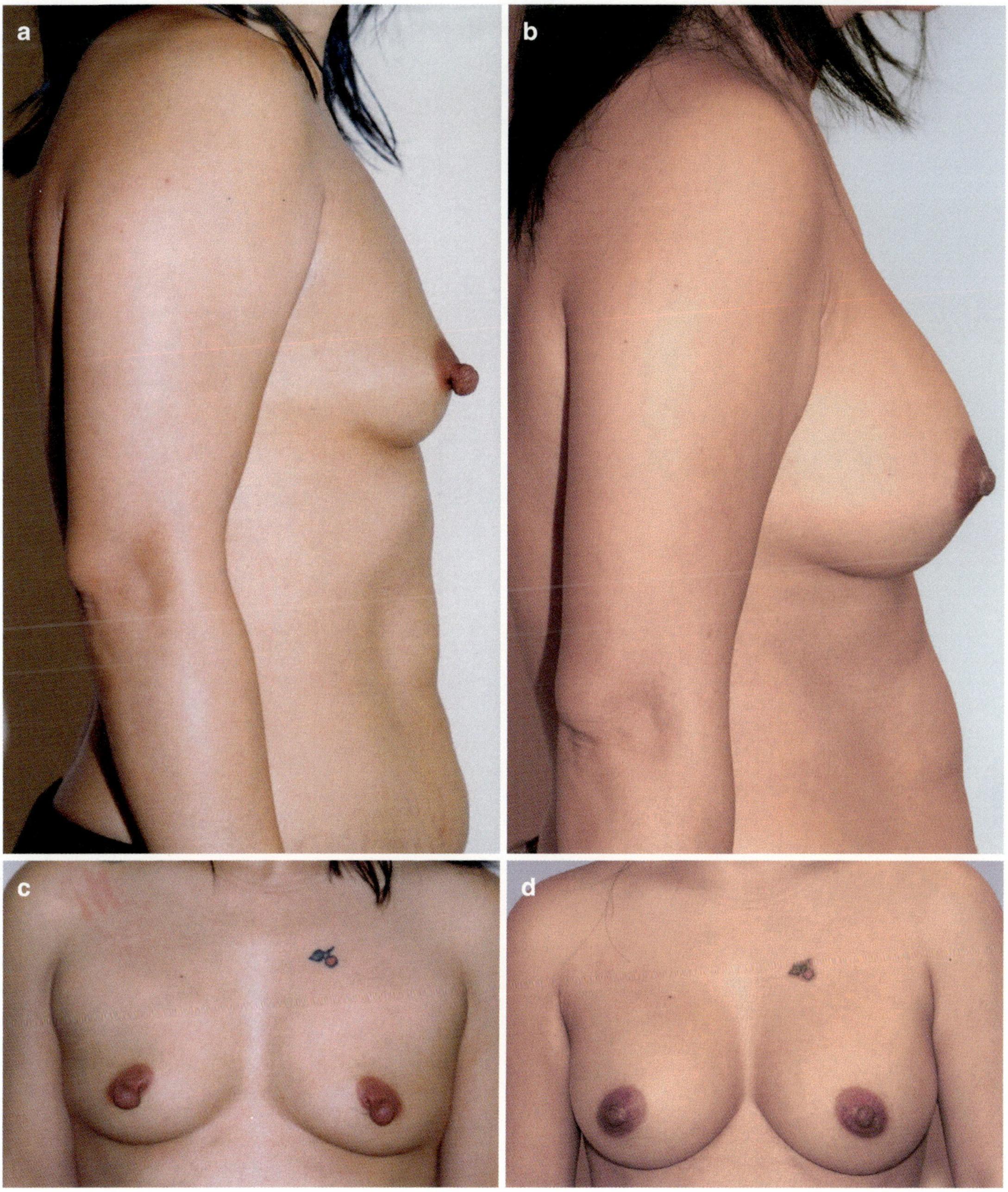


**Fig. 33.5** Example of nipple reduction case. (**a**, **c**) Preoperative 45-year-old Asian woman with severe nipple hypertrophy, including both excessive nipple projection and excessive nipple diameter. (**b**, **d**) Thirteen months postoperative after nipple reduction surgery, in combination with breast augmentation

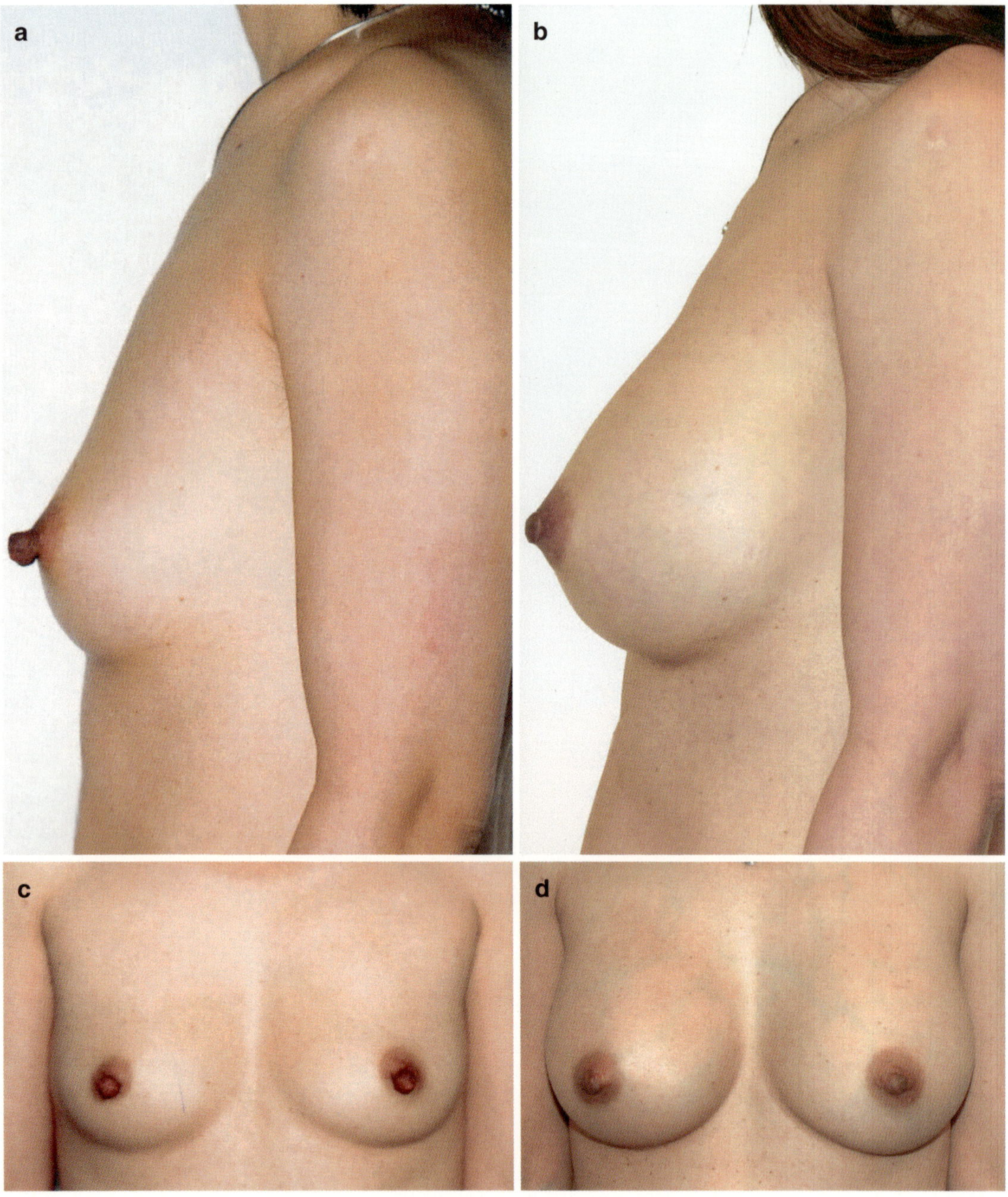


**Fig. 33.6** Example of nipple reduction case. (**a**, **c**) Preoperative 41-year-old Asian woman, suffering from excessive nipple projection. (**b**, **d**) Two and a half years postoperative after nipple reduction and breast augmentation

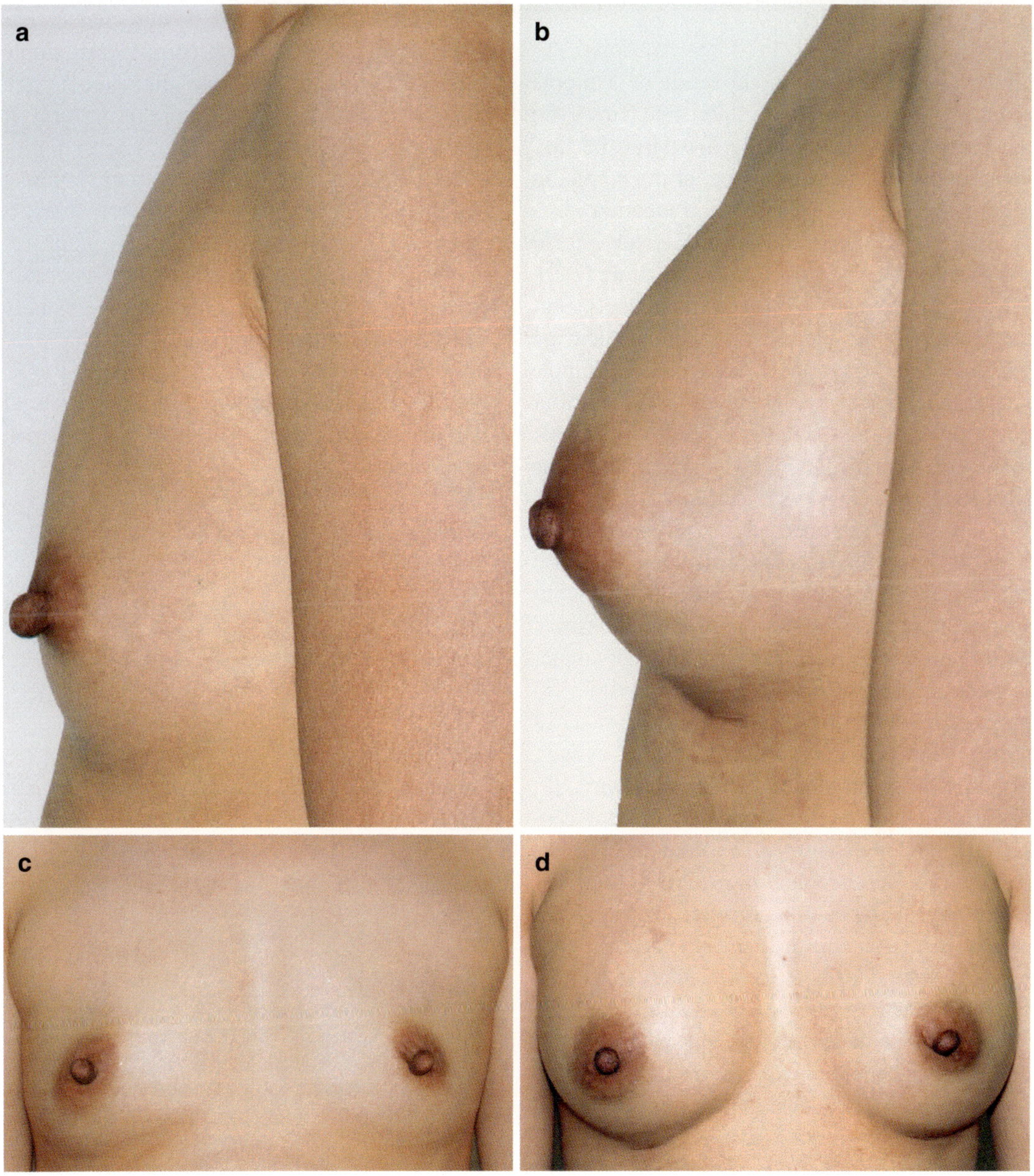


**Fig. 33.7** Example of nipple reduction case. (**a**, **c**) Preoperative 33-year-old Asian woman, suffering from excessive nipple projection. (**b**, **d**) Six months postoperative after nipple reduction and breast augmentation

## 33.6 Discussion

Understandably, the esthetic result of a nipple reduction is of paramount importance. However, the procedure should ideally not harm the nervous supply or lactiferous ducts of the nipple, in order to preserve its sensation and function.

Both conservative and nonconservative techniques have been described in the literature [1–9]. Lai's [1, 2], Regnault's [3], and Cheng's [4] techniques excise the skin high on the nipple, leaving visible scars. Vecchione [5] described a nipple amputation procedure. Marshall [6] used four quadrant flaps and a core excision for nipple reduction. Both the latter two techniques have the advantage of being easy and fast to perform. However, they both intersect the lactiferous ducts, with likely ensuing lactation difficulties. They also carry the risk of compromising the nipple nervous supply, with subsequent diminished sensation. Furthermore, they face the possibility of unpredictable scarring. Sperli's [7] and Ferreira's [8] methods to correct the height and the diameter of the nipple involve the excision of vertical wedges, resulting in a prolonged edema. Bostwick [9] described a two-variation approach including conservative and nonconservative techniques for correcting the hypertrophic nipple. His first was essentially an amputating procedure that slices the excess tissue from the top of the nipple, leaving the exposed wound to heal by secondary intention. Bostwick realized the potential adverse effects associated with this procedure and specified in his article that it should only be considered in women who have completed lactation. Bostwick's second approach was devised for patients planning future lactation. He performed a circumferential "sleeve" skin resection, and then "telescoped back" the naked part of the nipple into the areola. This technique has certain similarities with the one presented in this review. However, Bostwick did not discuss the ideal esthetics of the nipple. He suggested the new nipple projection to be no more than 2–3 mm, which is far shorter than what the authors consider ideal. Furthermore, a detailed description of the surgical technique was lacking. As well, the correction of a concomitant excessive nipple diameter was not addressed.

The technique described in this chapter has important advantages. It can correct both nipple overprojection and excessive diameter in the same surgical setting. It is simple to perform. It does not interfere with the nipple's sensation or its lactation function. As well, given the minimal dissection, the recovery period is very short. It can be safely combined with other breast procedures such as breast augmentation or mastopexy. The scar at the base of the new nipple usually heals very nicely. Its overall esthetic result is generally excellent. In a nutshell, this is a simple, practical, and safe procedure with a high rate of satisfaction and with, so far, no recorded complications.

**Acknowledgments** The authors express their thanks to "The Canadian Journal of Plastic Surgery" for granting the permission to use the figures of the original article; to Ildiko Horvath, medical artist, Montreal General Hospital, for her assistance in preparing the artwork; to Amina Flita, administrative assistant, for the typing and organizing of the manuscript; and to Minerva Khalife for her photographic contribution.

## References

1. Lai YL, Wu WC. Nipple reduction with a modified circumcision technique. Br J Plast Surg. 1996;49:307–9.
2. Lai YL, Weng CJ, Samuel Noordhoft M. Areolar reduction with inner doughnut incision. Plast Reconstr Surg. 1998;101(6):1695–9.
3. Regnault P. Nipple hypertrophy. A physiologic reduction by circumcision. Clin Plast Surg. 1975;2:391–6.
4. Cheng MH, Smartt JM, Rodriguez ED, Ulusal BG. Nipple reduction using the modified top hat flap. Plast Reconstr Surg. 2006;118(7):1517–25.
5. Vecchione TR. The reduction of the hypertrophic nipple. Aesthet Plast Surg. 1979;3:343–5.
6. Marshall KA, Wolfort FG, Cochran TC. Surgical correction of nipple hypertrophy in male gynecomastia: case report. Plast Reconstr Surg. 1977;60:277–9.
7. Sperli AE. Cosmetic reduction of the nipple with functional preservation. Br J Plast Surg. 1974;27:42–3.
8. Ferreira LM, Neto MS, Okamoto RH, Andrews J d M. Surgical correction of nipple hypertrophy. Plast Reconstr Surg. 1995;95:753–4.
9. Bostwick J III. Plastic and reconstructive breast surgery, vol. 1. St. Louis, MO: Quality Medical Publishing; 2000. p. 629–31.
10. Fanous N, Tawile C, Fanous A. Nipple reduction – an adjunct to augmentation mammaplasty. Can J Plast Surg. 2009;17(3):81–8.

# Aesthetic Surgery for Hypertrophic Nipple: A Simple Technique

# 34

Chang Yung Chia and Patricia Durgante Ritter

## 34.1 Introduction

Hypertrophic nipple is an uncommon but very distressing situation, not only for the social discomfort, as it shows under light clothing, but also for the general discomfort, pain, skin chafing, and ulceration. The author proposes a surgical technique to reduce the hypertrophic nipple, to a more suitable size and shape. It consists in splitting the nipple in three equal parts and creates three pyramidal flaps that will become the new nipple. This surgical technique works well for those nipples with diameter or height hypertrophy, as well as for those with both diameter and height hypertrophy. It is a safe procedure with good results.

C.Y. Chia, M.D. (✉)
Departamento de Microcrurgia, Hospital dos Servidores do Estado do Rio de Janeiro, Av. das Américas, 505, sala 203, Barra da Tijuca, Rio de Janeiro 22640-000, RJ, Brazil

Instituto Ivo Pitanguy, Rio de Janeiro, RJ, Brazil
e-mail: changplastica@gmail.com

P.D. Ritter, M.D.
RuaTakabumi Murata 555, casa 32, Gleba Fazenda Palhano, Londrina 86055-580, PR, Brazil
e-mail: patriciadritter@gmail.com

## 34.2 Nipple Aesthetics

There is no standard or ideal nipple size described on anatomy studies. There is, however, an aesthetic sense in different cultures and different historical periods that breast, areola, and nipple sizes should be proportional. Nipples also represent delicacy and femininity in female breast (Fig. 34.1). Considering the average women height, nipple diameter should measure between 0.8 and 1.2 cm and its height from 0.5 to 1 cm. Its attractiveness, however, is of very particular concern. The hypertrophic nipple may cause skin chafing and ulceration, general discomfort, pain, and social embarrassment as it shows under light clothing.

The nipple shape may vary from cylindrical with a marked transition from areola to nipple and a flat tip to slightly conic with a soft transition from areola to nipple and a rounded tip (Fig. 34.2).

The nipple anatomy is described below for better understanding of the surgical technique. The nipple base is the transition area from areola (horizontal level) to nipple (vertical plane)—point B (Fig. 34.3). The nipple mound is the vertical plane, which can be conical or cylindrical. The tip is the top end of the nipple. There is a lateral transition in the nipple mound, which is where the tip begins, and it may be marked, if the tip is flat, or subtle, if it is rounded. Total height is measured from the base to the top end, including the lateral wall and the tip.


M.A. Shiffman (ed.), *Nipple-Areolar Complex Reconstruction*,
https://doi.org/10.1007/978-3-319-60925-6_34

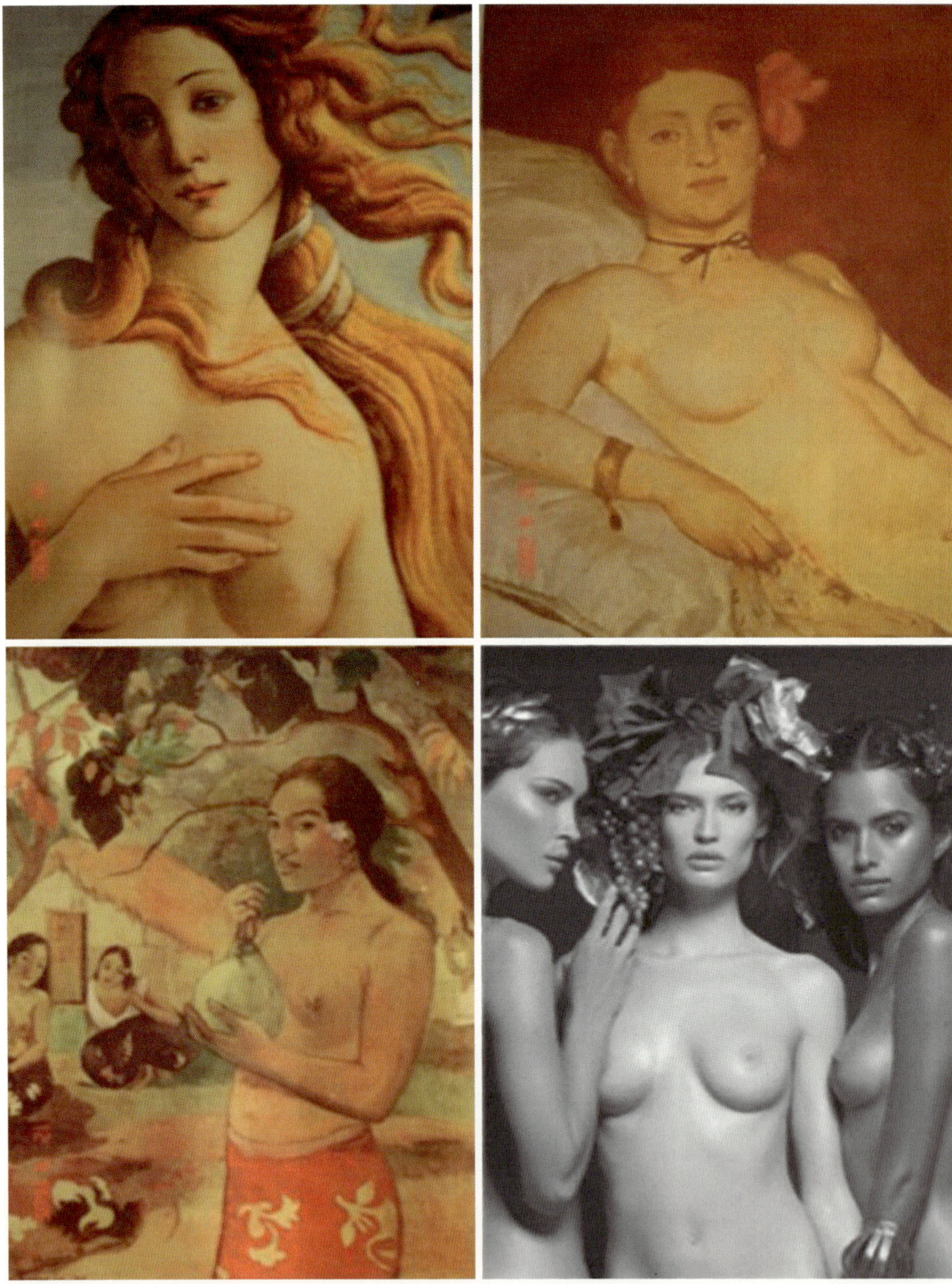

**Fig. 34.1** Beauty concept of the nipple through time in different cultures. (*Upper left*) The Birth of Venus by Sandro Botticelli—1484–1486. (*Upper right*) Olympia by Édouard Manet—1862–1863. (*Lower left*) Ea Haere Ia Oe by Paul Gauguin—1893. (*Lower right*) Karl Lagerfeld, Paris—2011

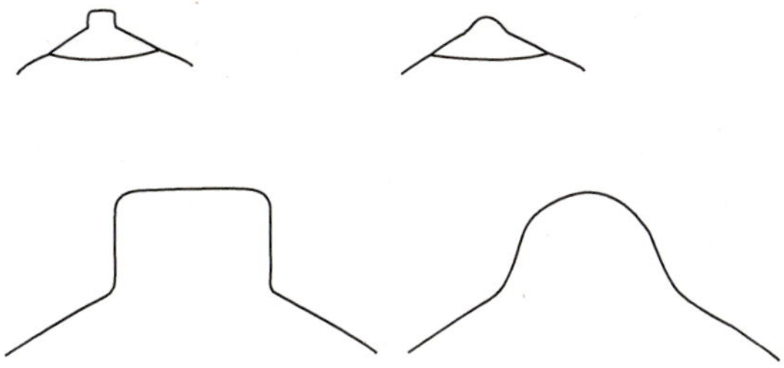

Fig. 34.2 Nipple shape variations

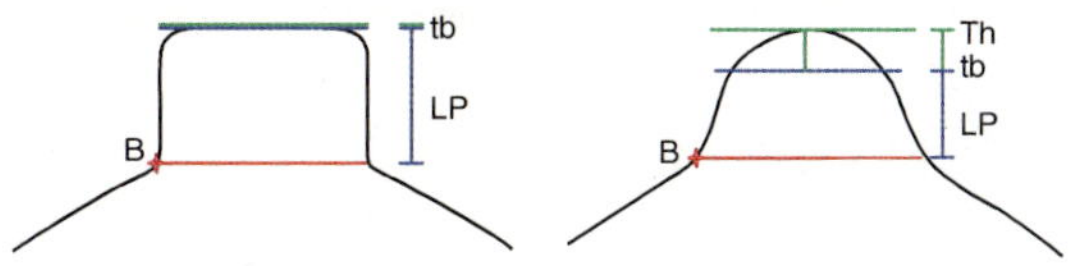


Fig. 34.3 Nipple parts. *B* = nipple base; LP = lateral projection; tb = tip base; Th = total height

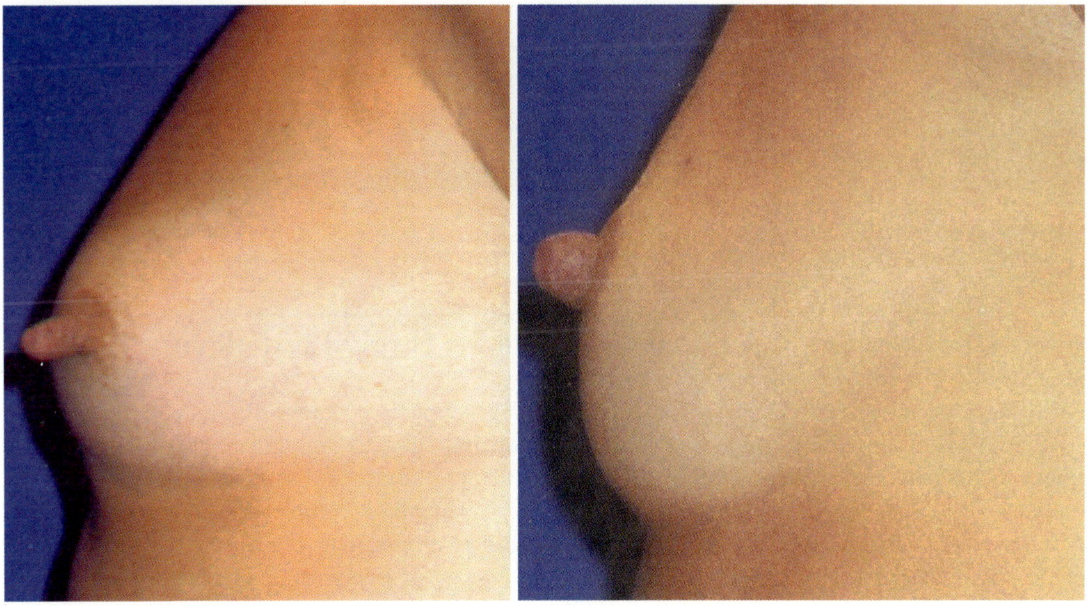

Fig. 34.4 (*Left*) Hypertrophic nipple with excessive anterior projection. (*Right*) Hypertrophic nipple including both excessive anterior projection and large diameter

## 34.3 The Unaesthetic Nipple

Nipple hypertrophy is uncommon, most often encountered in Asians. It may be genetic and may appear after onset of puberty or following pregnancy, persisting through menopause. Differences in nipple projection can be affected by age, race, weight, and hormonal changes.

The hypertrophic nipple may have an exaggerated height with a normal base diameter, an exaggerated base diameter with a normal height, or more commonly an association of both (Fig. 34.4). Other unpleasant features, such as irregularities and spherical mound with a narrow base like a pedicle may also be present (Fig. 34.5).

As no formal definition of nipple hypertrophy exits, the aim of correction is to establish satisfactory proportion of its diameter and projection.

## 34.4 Anatomy

The nipple is generally located just below the center of the breast, at the highest projection point, and is directed slightly outwards to the axilla, making breastfeeding easier.

Blood supply to the nipple comes from two intimately related plexuses, the superficial and the deep (or glandular). The small feeding vessels arise from the internal mammary (internal thoracic)

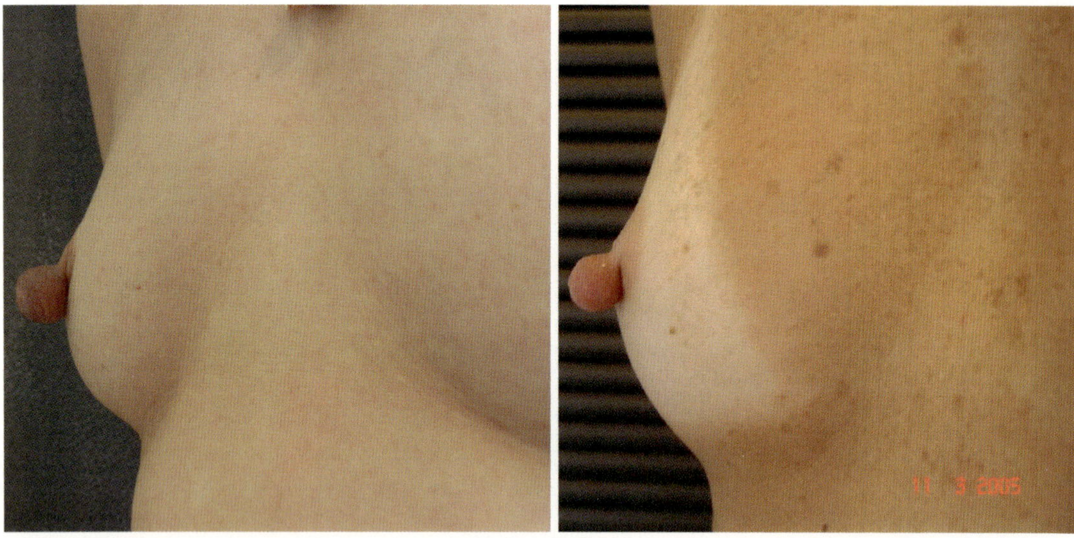


**Fig. 34.5** (*Left, right*) Unaesthetic nipple, with a hypertrophic spherical body and a narrow base like a pedicle

artery and the lateral thoracic artery. The second intercostal perforator off the internal mammary artery is the principal perforator that supplies the NAC 85% of the time. The lateral branch of the fourth intercostal nerve largely innervates the nipple.

The surface of the nipple is irregular, with a cobblestone texture and cervices that lead to the duct orifices. The epidermal skin of the nipple is continuous with the epithelium of the ducts. Piloerection of the nipple occurs with cold stimulus, arousal, or during breastfeeding due to contraction of the arrector pili muscles.

Lactiferous ducts terminals, which measure 2–4 mm of diameter, along with connective tissue and smooth muscle fibers—that are continuous with the areolar muscles disposed longitudinally and circumferentially to the nipple axis—are the nipple's main component. There continues to be discrepancies in the literature on the number of ductal orifices within the nipple between different histological techniques. According to the 3D nipple anatomy study conducted by Rusby et al., there is a central duct bundle, with a peripheral duct-free rim, which narrows to form a "waist" 2 mm beneath the level of the areola as the ducts enter the breast parenchyma.

## 34.5 Surgical Technique

The surgical technique for nipple hypertrophy consists of dividing the nipple in three flaps, excising the excess tissue, and making the flaps in an adequate volume and shape to form the desired nipple. The same principle is applied to all types of hypertrophy and irregularities. The resulting nipple shape depends on the flap design (Fig. 34.6).

In cases of height hypertrophy only, with normal diameter, the flaps are made only on the top of the nipple. First the nipple is longitudinally divided in three equal parts from tip to base (Fig. 34.7). The desired projection is determined by analyzing the lateral height (from the nipple base to tip base) and the tip height. Starting at the tip base, marks are made according to the desired new tip shape (rounded or flat). The distal excess tissue is trimmed symmetrically in a pyramidal fashion on all three sides and the flaps are brought together to make the new tip. See details ahead.

On those nipples with height and diameter hypertrophy, it is necessary to reduce its perimeter (diameter excess) and height excess (tip excess). The three flaps are marked all the way down to the base, sized and shaped as desired, for the calculated new base.

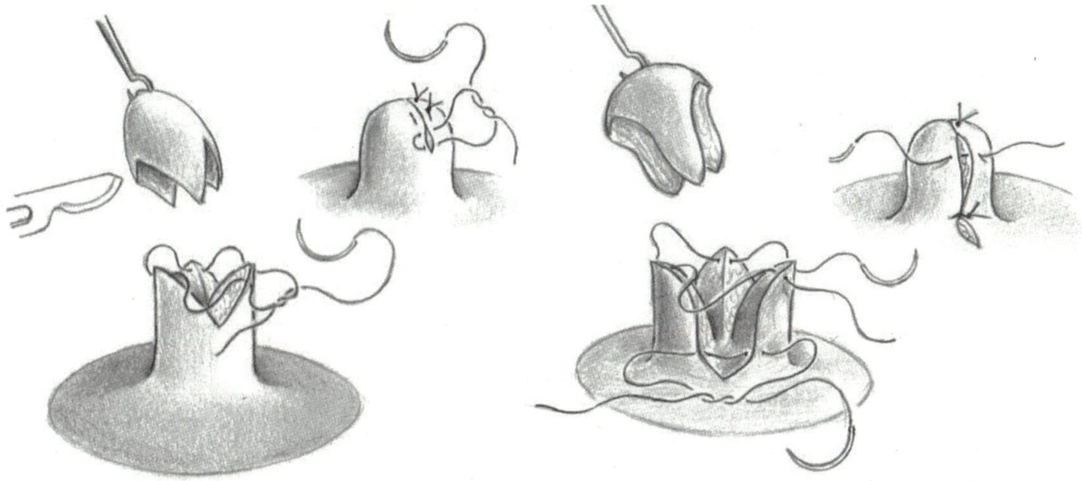

**Fig. 34.6** Surgical technique of three-flap creation. (*Left*) For height hypertrophy only. (*Right*) For height and diameter hypertrophy

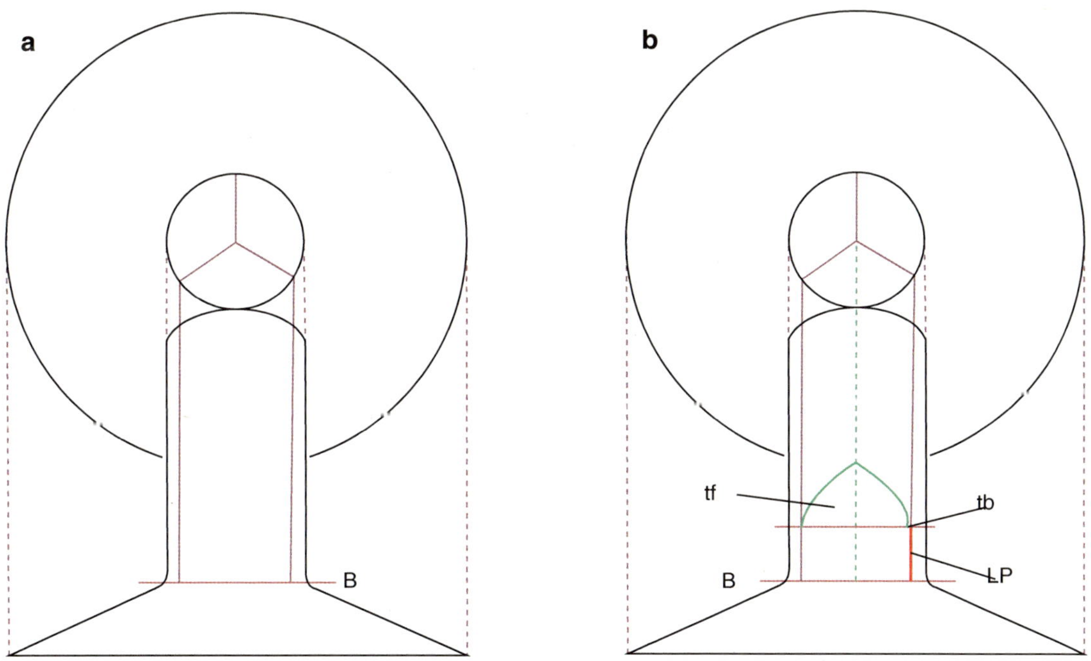


**Fig. 34.7** Nipple scheme. (**a**) Defining the base, point *B*, and division of the nipple in three longitudinal parts; (**b**) defining the lateral projection and tip base and tip flap design. *B* = nipple base; LP = lateral projection; tb = tip base; tf = nipple tip flap

The excess tissue form distal and central parts and from between the flaps is excised, taking care to make an adequate balance of volume and skin cover, thus forming three pyramidal shape flaps. The flaps are advanced to the center to unite and form the new nipple (Fig. 34.8); see scheme ahead.

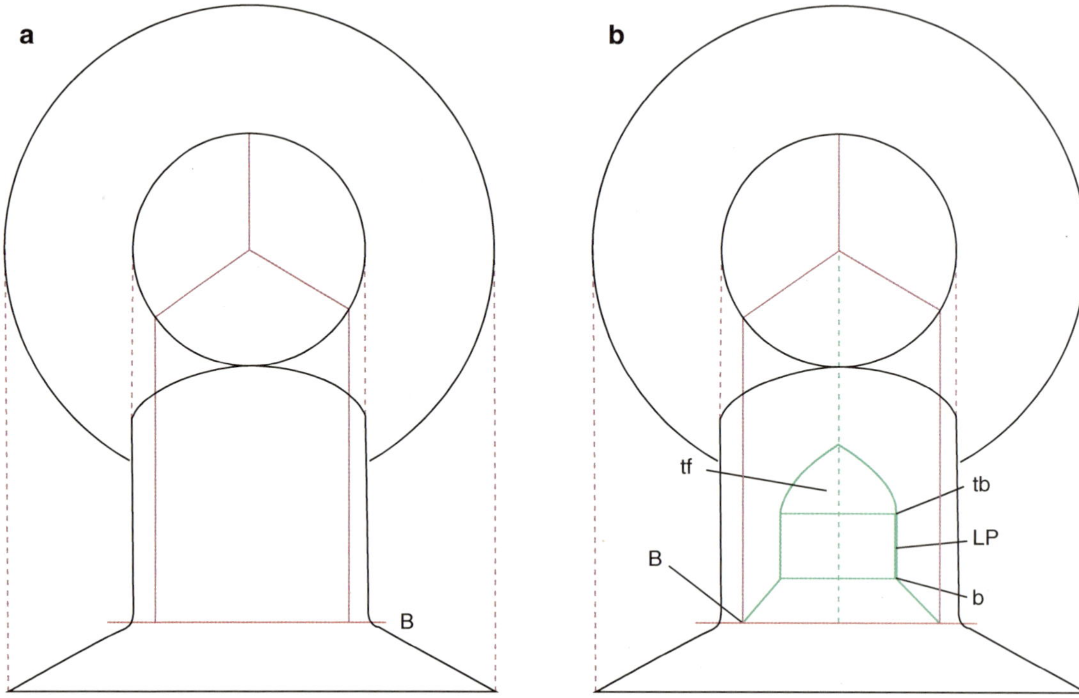


Fig. 34.8 Flap marking on a hypertrophic nipple in height and diameter. (**a**) Determining the nipple base and dividing in three longitudinal parts from nipple tip to base. (**b**) Determining the new nipple base, height and new tip flap. *B* = nipple base; *b* = new base; LP = lateral projection; tp = tip base; tf = tip flap

### 34.5.1 Flap Design

#### 34.5.1.1 Defining the Tip

The nipple tip starts at the tip base and is formed by three triangular flaps. The lateral shape of the triangles will determine the tip form: If the triangle lateral is a straight line, the transition between the lateral and the tip will be well defined and the tip will be pointy. If the triangle lateral is curved, the tip will be curved. If the triangle lateral measures the same as the base radius, the tip will be flat, and if it is longer, the tip will be projected (Figs. 34.9 and 34.10).

#### 34.5.1.2 Defining the Diameter: Flap Width

Those nipples with diameter hypertrophy need to be reduced to the desired perimeter. The perimeter is determined by the formula $P = 2r \times \pi$ ($r$ the radius and $\pi = 3.1415926535897932385$ but used simply as 3.14). The diameter is twice the radius. For example, a hypertrophic nipple that has a 2.0 cm diameter has a (2 × 3.14) 6.28 (6.3) perimeter. Dividing it in three equal parts, each one will be 2.1 cm. For a 1.0 cm diameter desired nipple, its calculated perimeter will be (1 × 3.14) 3.14 cm or 3.1 cm. Dividing it in three equal parts, each flap will be 1.03 (1.0) cm. The excess tissue to be removed is the hypertrophied perimeter less the desired perimeter, and it is resected from in between the flaps (Fig. 34.11).

Lateral flap shape and dimensions determine the diameter, projection, and nipple form. If the lateral lines are parallel, the nipple body will be cylindrical; if they are slightly convergent, from base to top, the body will be slightly conic; and if it is curved, the lateral will be rounded, and the transition from body to tip will be smooth (Fig. 34.12).

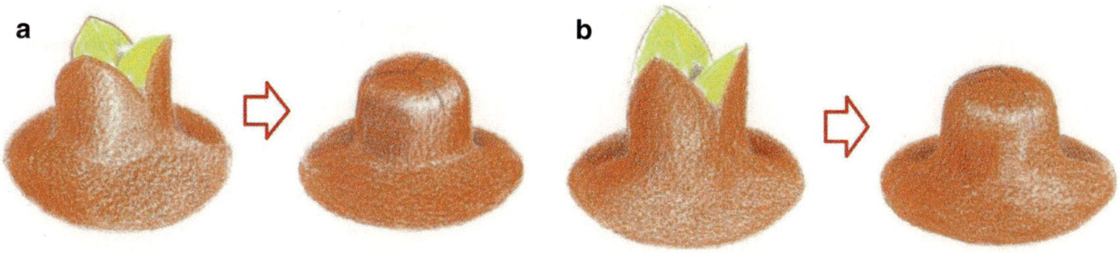


**Fig. 34.9** Tip design. (**a**) A straight line at flap lateral, measuring the same as nipple radius, results on a flat tip with well-defined tip base transition point. (**b**) A straight line at flap lateral, longer than nipple radius, results in a pointy and projected tip

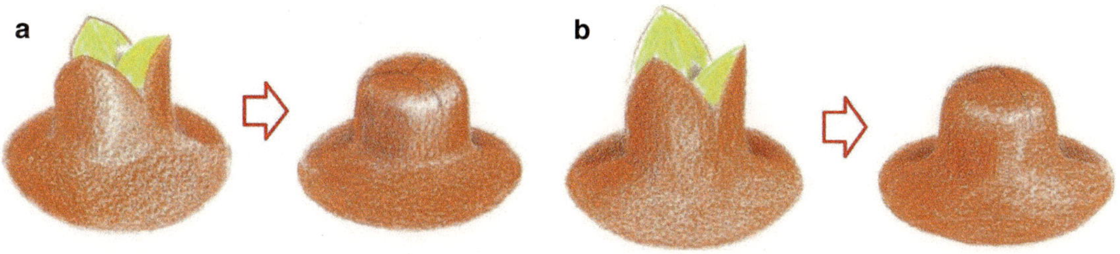


**Fig. 34.10** Tip design. (**a**) A curved line at flap lateral, measuring the same as nipple radius, results on a flat tip with a smooth transition from base to tip. (**b**) A curved line at flap lateral, longer than nipple radius, results in a rounded and projected tip

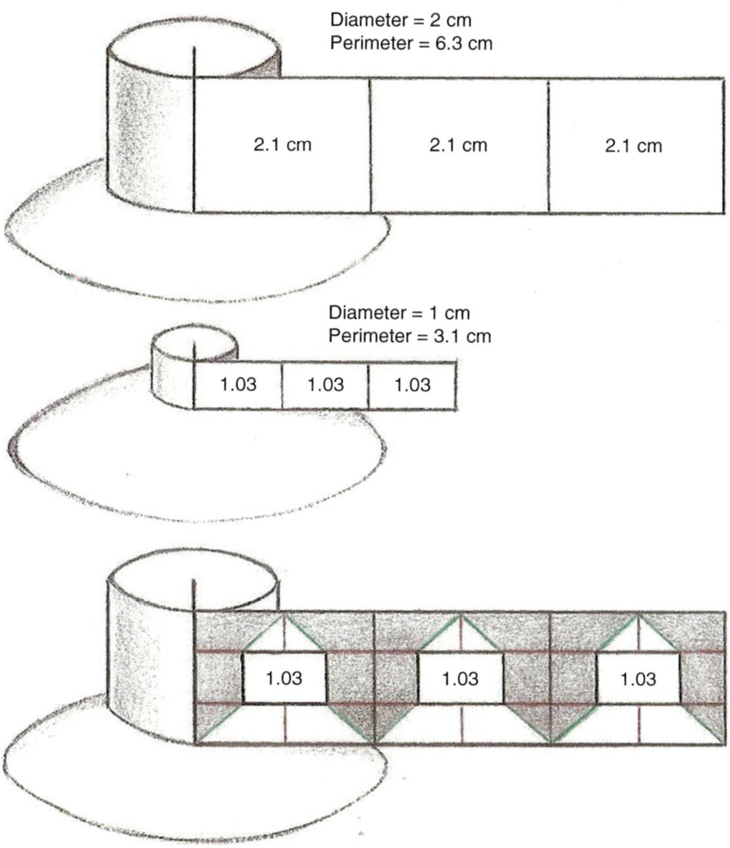


**Fig. 34.11** Lateral flap. (*Top*) 2 cm diameter nipple divided in three longitudinal parts. (*Middle*) desired nipple 1.0 cm diameter (3.14 cm perimeter) divided in three 10 cm flaps. (*Bottom*) Flap marking on hypertrophic nipple, the shadowed area represents the excessive tissue to be resected

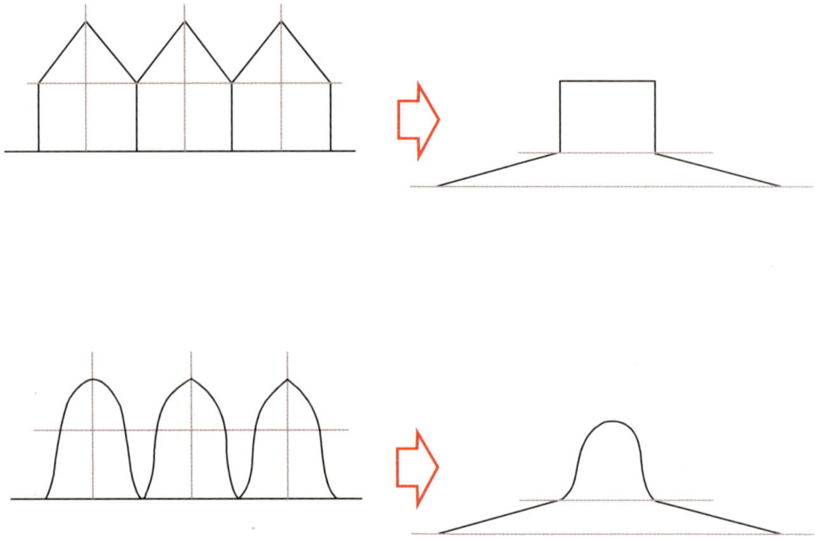

**Fig. 34.12** Flap design influences the resulting nipple shape. (*Top*) Parallel and straight lateral lines result in a cylindrical nipple. (*Bottom*) Curved lateral lines result in a conic and rounded nipple

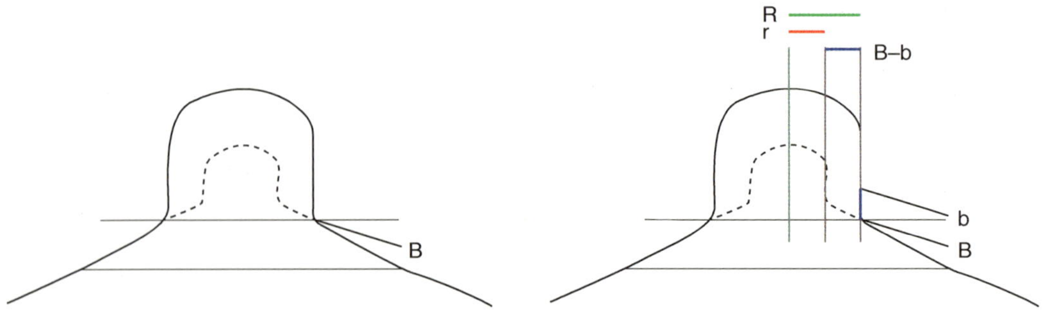


**Fig. 34.13** Determining new nipple base (*b*). (*Left*) Base of the hypertrophic nipple (*B*). *Dotted line* represents new nipple with desired size. (*Right*) The difference between the hypertrophic nipple base radius (*R*/*green line*) and new nipple base radius (*r*/*red line*) will be nearly the same distance between *B* and *b*. That means: $R - r \cong B - b$/*blue line*. New base position, point *b* will be marked at $R - r$ from point *B*

Once excess tissue is resected and flaps are made (maintaining adequate equilibrium of remaining tissue and cover skin), they are sutured in the center to form the new nipple. Note that as the flap is advanced toward the center, the base of the original nipple (vertical) will now be part of the areola (horizontal). As this is an important step of this procedure, this point should be marked carefully.

#### 34.5.1.3 Defining the Flap Base: Point *b*

The new nipple base position, of smaller diameter, is determined by the difference between the original radius (*R*) and the new radius (*r*). This difference ($R - r$) is the distance of flap advancement toward the center and nearly the same distance between the original base and the new base ($B - b$) (Fig. 34.13).

Once the new base position (*b*) is determined, lateral projection flap (LP) is marked starting at "*b*," and the tip flap (tf) is drawn, starting at the tip base (tb). The $B - b$ line that was a vertical part of the original nipple, after being advanced toward the center, becomes a horizontal part of the areola (Fig. 34.14). The bases of the new nipple are united, suturing points *b* from the two flaps aside (Fig. 34.15).

Now that the mathematic theory of the surgical technique is mastered, it is possible to adjust any

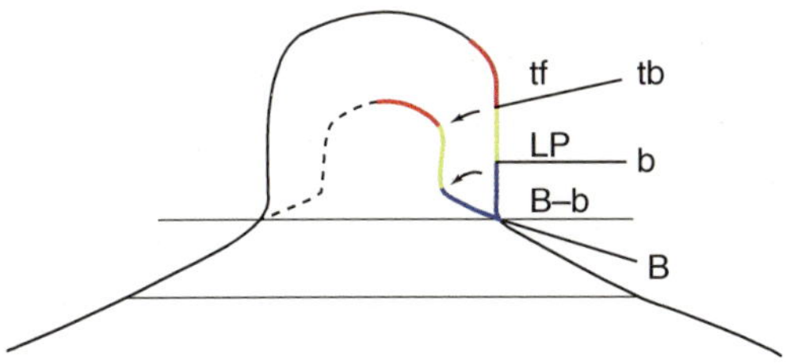


**Fig. 34.14** Starting at the new base, point *b*, the lateral projection flap is marked (LP/*yellow line*), and from the tip base (tb), the tip flap is drawn (tf/*red line*). The *B* – *b* segment that was a vertical part of the original nipple, after the flaps are advanced toward the center, becomes a horizontal segment, as part of the new areola

nipple to a desired size and shape. Usually it can be done without measurements, just as it feels right.

## 34.6 Case Illustration

The patient had small breast and areola and hypertrophic nipple. The nipple was spherical and irregular, with a narrow base. She was submitted to a breast augmentation surgery with silicone implants and nipple reduction (Fig. 34.16). The nipple was divided into three longitudinal segments, from top

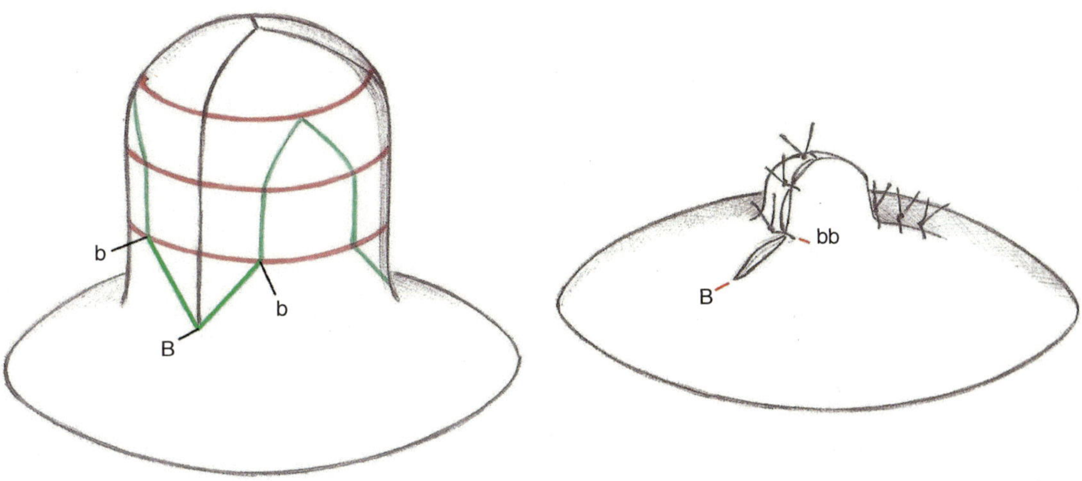


**Fig. 34.15** Points *b* from the two flaps aside are sutured, and the previously vertical segment *B* – *b* now becomes horizontal, as part of the new areola. The flaps are sutured up to the tip forming the new nipple

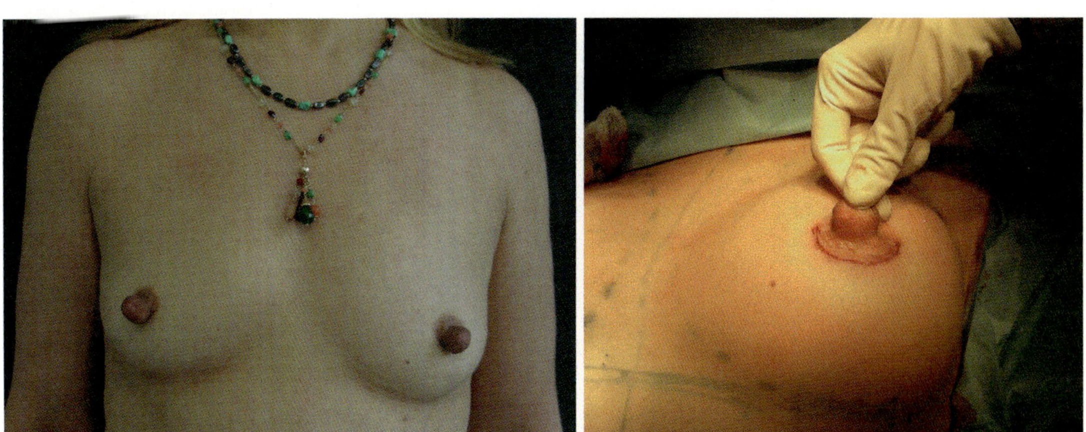

**Fig. 34.16** (*Left*) Patient with small breast and areola, and hypertrophic nipple. (*Right*) Submitted to breast augmentation surgery with silicone implants through inferior periareolar incision

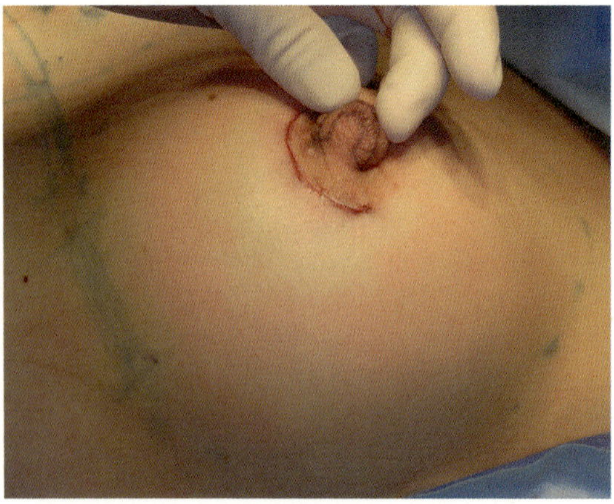

**Fig. 34.17** Marking flaps

to base (*B*). After size difference, from original to desired, was determined (*R* – *r*), the new base position was marked (*b*), and from this point, the lateral and tip flaps were drawn (Fig. 34.17). Excess tissue from the nipple core and laterals was removed, and three pyramidal flaps resulted (Fig. 34.18). After hemostasis, the suture is started at the new base as the points b from two flaps aside are met (Fig. 34.19). Next step is the suture of the apex, and the remaining sutures are placed as necessary (Fig. 34.20).

Observe in Fig. 34.21 the original base reduction. The line *B* – *b* was originally part of the nipple and now is part of the areola. Figure 34.22 shows the preoperative and postoperative difference.

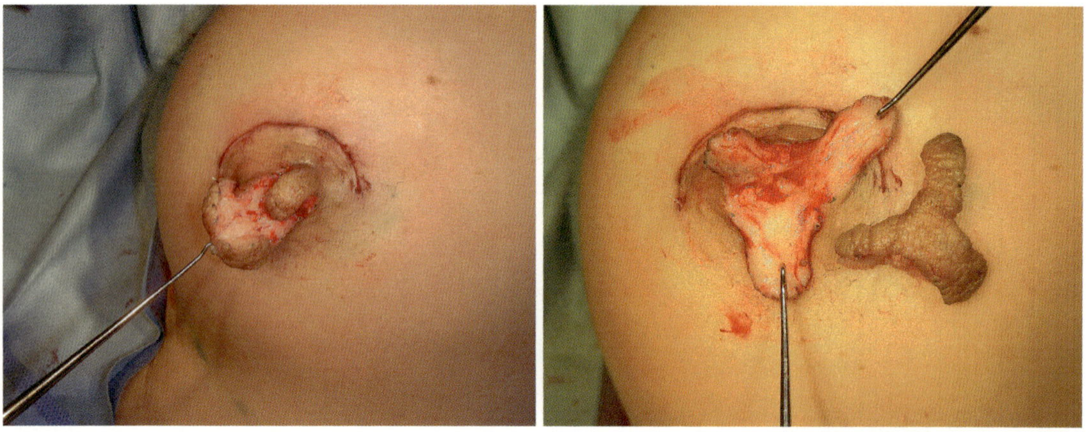

**Fig. 34.18** Flap formation. (*Left*) Excess tissue trimmed from the core and nipple laterals, (*right*) taking care to equilibrate resulting tissue and skin cover

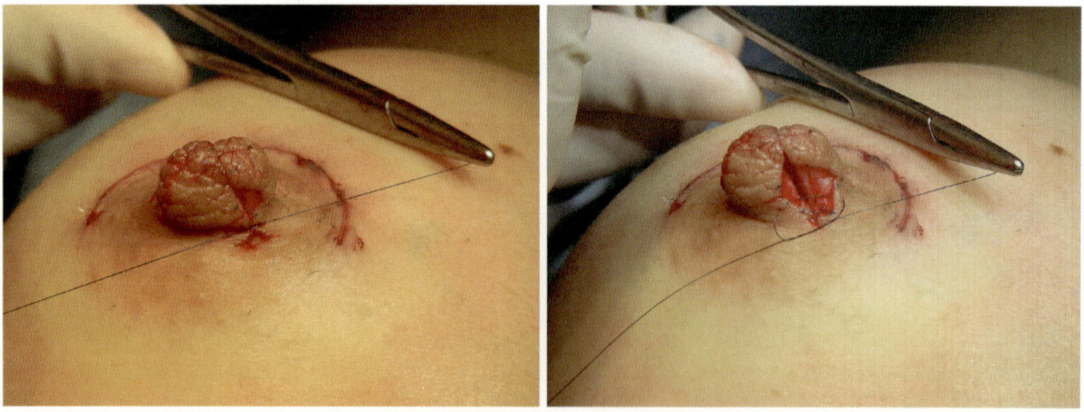

**Fig. 34.19** (*Left*, *right*) Suture of points "*b*" resulting in the new nipple base

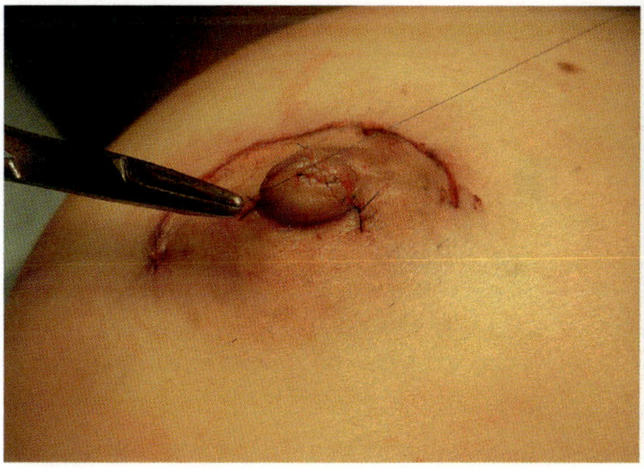

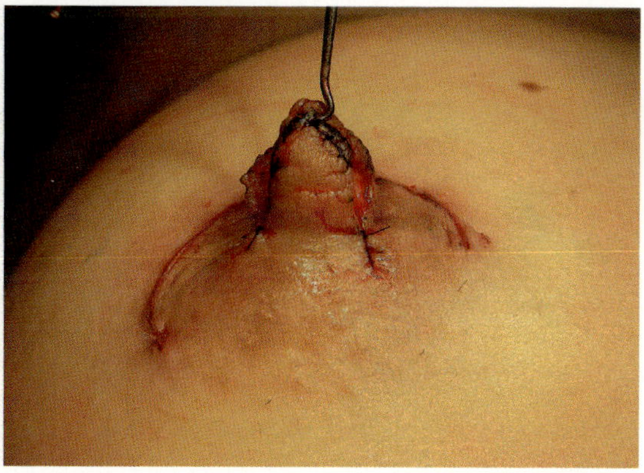

**Fig. 34.20** (*Left*) Suture of the apex. (*Right*) Suture of the lateral nipple

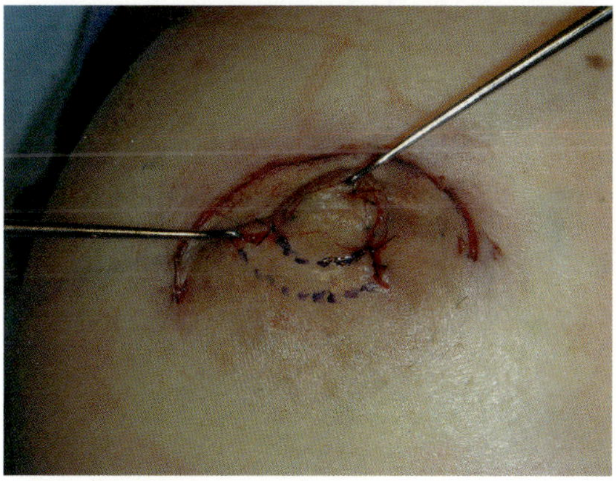

**Fig. 34.21** External dotted line is the original nipple base, and the internal is the new base

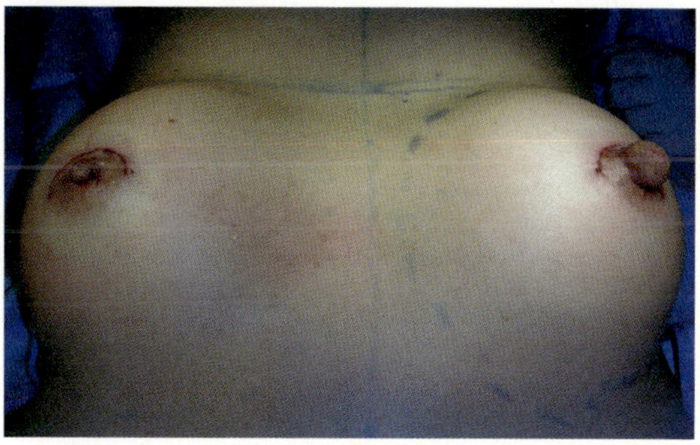

**Fig. 34.22** Difference of the nipples. (*Right breast*) Before surgery. (*Left breast*) After surgery

## 34.7 Complications

To the present, there were no ischemic or sensitive complications, probably because all incisions are longitudinal and parallel to the blood vessels and nerves. Rarely, surgical manipulation may result in small skin injuries at incision borders.

As this surgical technique removes lactiferous ducts, it might interfere with breastfeeding and it is not recommended to women who desire to breastfeed. There was one patient, however, that was able to breastfeed bilaterally after being submitted to this operation.

Subtle asymmetries in shape or volume of the nipple may occur, as in any other aesthetic surgery. Major asymmetries are easily noticed and corrected during the procedure.

There were no cases of keloid of hypertrophic scars. The nipple-areolar complex has good healing capability; however, the suture must be very precise to close borders perfectly.

## References


1. Lai YL, Wu WC. Nipple reduction with a modified circumcision technique. Br J Plast Surg. 1996;49(5):307–9.
2. Ferreira LM, Neto MS, Okamoto RH, Andrews JM. Surgical correction of nipple hypertrophy. Plast Reconstr Surg. 1995;95(4):753–4.
3. Cheffe LO. Hipertrofia de Mamilo. Tratamento com Ressecções Estrelares. Presented at Sul Bras Cirurg, Florianópolis, Brazil, Mar 1984.
4. Jaimovich CA. Mamilo Hipertrófico. Contribuição ao estudo de sua reparação cirúrgica. A técnica em "W". Rev Bras Cir. 1982;72(2):123–30.
5. Vecchione TR. The reduction of the hypertrophic nipple. Aesthet Plast Surg. 1979;3:343–5.
6. Franco T, Rebelo C, editors. Cirurgia Estética. Rio de Janeiro: Livraria Atheneu; 1977.

7. Marshall KA, Wolfort FG, Cochran TC. Surgical correction of nipple hypertrophy in male gynecomastia. Plast Reconstr Surg. 1977;60(2):277–9.
8. Singer R, Krant SM. Reconstructive problems of the nipple and areola. In: Goldwyn RM, editor. Plastic and reconstructive surgery of breast. Boston: Little Brown Co.; 1976.
9. Regnault P. Nipple hypertrophy: a physiologic reduction by circumcision. Clin Plast Surg. 1975;2(3):391–6.
10. Sperli AE. Cosmetic reduction of the nipple with the functional preservation. Br J Plast Surg. 1974;27:42–3.
11. Pitanguy I, Cansanção A. Redução do mamilo. Rev Bras Cir. 1970;61:73.
12. Cheng MH, Smartt JM, Rodriguez ED, Ulusal BG. Nipple reduction using the modified top hat flap. Plast Reconstr Surg. 2006;118:1517–25.
13. Sarhadi NS, Shaw-Dunn J, Soutar DS. Nerve supply of the breast with special reference to the nipple and areola: Sir Astley Cooper revisited. Clin Anat. 1997;10:283–8.
14. Rusby JE, Brachtel EF, Michaelson JS, Koerner FC, Smith BL. Breast duct anatomy in the human nipple: three-dimensional patterns and clinical implications. Breast Cancer Res Treat. 2007;106(2):171–9.
15. Zucca-Matthes G, Urban C, Vallejo A. Anatomy of the nipple and breast ducts. Gland Surg. 2016;5(1):32–6.
16. Stone K, Wheeler A. A review of anatomy, physiology, and benign pathology of the nipple. Ann Surg Oncol. 2015;22(10):3236–40.
17. Lee EI, Withers EH. Geometric nipple reduction technique: an approach to management of nipple hypertrophy. J Plast Reconstr Aesthet Surg. 2014;67(9):1301–3.
18. Tuncer S, Eryilmaz T, Atabay K. Correction of nipple hypertrophy: nipple circumcision technique revisited. J Plast Reconstr Aesthet Surg. 2010;63:1575–6.
19. Kerr-Valentic MA, Agarwal JP. Reduction of the hypertrophic nipple following total skin sparing mastectomy. J Plast Reconstr Aesthet Surg. 2009;62:e652–3.
20. Fanous N, Tawile C, Fanous A. Nipple reduction – an adjunct to augmentation mammaplasty. Can J Plast Surg. 2009;17(3):81–8.
21. Huang WC, Yu CM, Chang YY. Geometric incision design for reduction nippleplasty. Aesthetic Plast Surg. 2012;36:560–5.
22. Sim HB, Sun SH. Nipple reduction with the chullo-hat technique. Aesthet Surg J. 2015;35(6):NP154–60.
23. Jin US, Lee HK. Nipple reduction using circumcision and wedge excision technique. Ann Plast Surg. 2013;70(2):154–7.
24. Ren M, Wang Y, Wang B. Nipple reduction using a three-dimensional Z-shaped incision technique. J Plast Reconstr Aesthet Surg. 2013;66(6):770–5.

# 35 Reduction of the Hypertrophic Nipple Using the Crown Flap Technique

Mahlon A. Kerr and Jayant P. Agarwal

## 35.1 Introduction

Nipple hypertrophy (macrothelia) is a relatively uncommon condition that may produce both social and psychological difficulties in affected women [1]. Variation in nipple sizes and shapes are common, but aesthetically we define macrothelia as a nipple with measurements of greater than 0.8 cm in height or 1.5 cm in diameter [2]. Female patients that would like to have their nipple hypertrophy addressed are ideal candidates for combination procedures with another breast procedure. Common combinations for both authors are in breast augmentation or in breast reconstruction operations. While no ischemia has been observed in these combinations to date, the authors do not currently combine nipple reduction with any operation involving pedicled movement of the nipple-areolar complex such as a breast lift or reduction. Other authors have reported nipple reduction in combination with breast augmentation and even reduction in some cases [2, 3]. Many different techniques for addressing macrothelia exist including amputation, cylindrical, vertical, and wedge type resections [3–8]. The authors reported on the crown flap technique previously in the setting of a nipple-sparing mastectomy patient [9]. The crown flap works very well to preserve nipple blood supply and maintains excellent nipple viability.

## 35.2 Technique

The hypertrophic nipple is identified during consultation in clinic (Fig. 35.1). After sterile prep and drape, the nipple is carefully marked with the crown flap pattern (Figs. 35.2 and 35.3). The

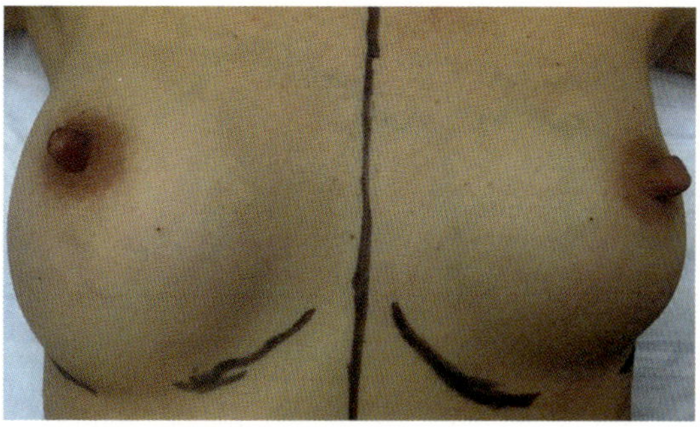

Fig. 35.1 Preoperative nipple projection

M.A. Kerr, M.D. (✉)
Plastic Surgery in Austin, Texas,
7700 Cat Hollow Drive Suite 103, Round Rock, TX 78681, USA

Department of Surgery, Texas A&M Health Sciences Center, Bryan, TX, USA
e-mail: drkerr@synergyplasticsurgery.com

J.P. Agarwal, M.D.
Department Plastic Surgery, University of Utah School of Medicine, 30 N 1900 E 3B400,
Salt Lake City, UT 84132, USA
e-mail: Jay.Agarwal@hsc.utah.edu


M.A. Shiffman (ed.), *Nipple-Areolar Complex Reconstruction*,
https://doi.org/10.1007/978-3-319-60925-6_35

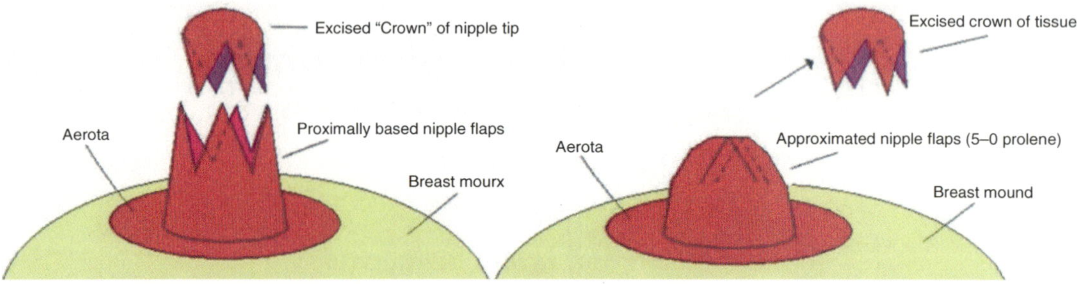


**Fig. 35.2** Crown excision technique

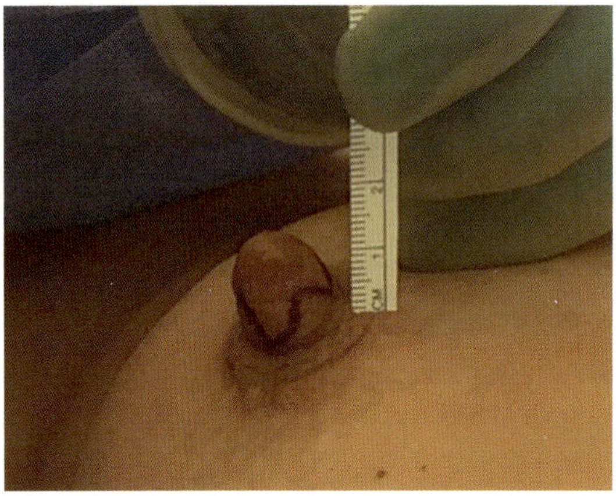

**Fig. 35.3** Crown flap marked before local injection

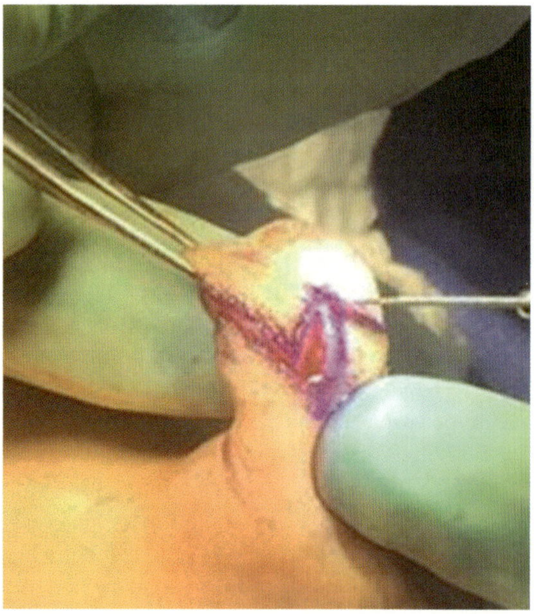

**Fig. 35.4** Intraoperative incisions

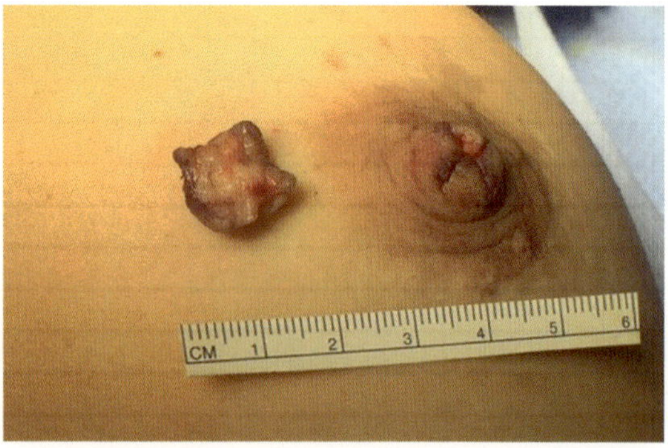

**Fig. 35.5** Nipple core excision

first author (M.A.K.) typically will mark the most proximal aspect of the crown excision approximately 1 cm above the areola, but this can be adjusted easily depending on the desired final outcome. Four separate triangle points are marked in a symmetric fashion around the base of the nipple. All proximal and distal points are marked the same distance from the areola and can be easily checked with a caliper or measuring stick. For ease of dissection and postoperative pain control, each nipple is then injected with 0.5% Marcaine with epinephrine. The crown flap is then excised full thickness and some of the central core is sharply dissected out as well. This is done with a 15-blade scalpel (Figs. 35.4 and 35.5). Bleeding, if any, is controlled, and the deeper layers are approximated with 4-0 Monocryl, and the superficial layers are approximated with 5-0 Prolene or fast gut, and attention is addressed to

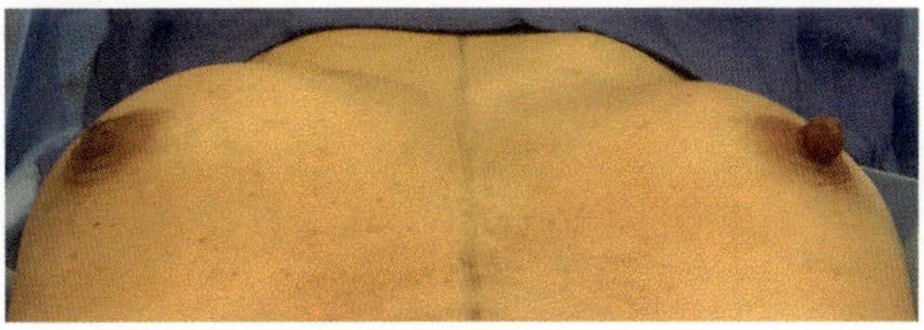

**Fig. 35.6** Post crown flap result

the opposite side in a similar fashion (Fig. 35.6). The first author (M.A.K.) will then cover with Dermabond® as it helps to support the closure. No additional bolster or dressing is required, but if done during augmentation, ABD, pads, and a 6 in. Ace wrap are typically used to support the breasts. No incisions are made at the base of the nipple.

## 35.3 Discussion

Nipple hypertrophy to the degree that requires surgical augmentation is not an everyday operation, but every plastic surgeon will certainly encounter patients who could benefit from this procedure. Cosmetic reduction of the nipple has the possibility of significant psychosocial impact on the patient and should not be overlooked or neglected. Cosmetic reduction of nipple height has been described by several authors and by these authors in conjunction with breast reconstruction after nipple-sparing mastectomy [2, 3, 9]. Our crown flap technique has been proven to have excellent healing as well as contour and shape. Scars are barely visible in a few months. The nipple reduction can be problematic in what is typically considered a necrosis prone region. Our technique avoids incisions at or near the base of the nipple which in our opinion has been helpful in reducing any ischemia problems. In addition to an appealing shape and size, our crown flap nipple reduction technique has not, in our experience, altered significantly any nipple sensation or erectile function. The effects on breastfeeding are not known, therefore caution using this method should be employed for use on patients who wish to breast feed in the future.

### Conclusions

We feel the crown technique for reduction of hypertrophic nipples is a viable option after nipple-sparing mastectomy and in the application of cosmetic surgery. We have not encountered problems with ischemia or necrosis in the postoperative setting. Nipple reduction can have a great psychosocial improvement and should not be overlooked by plastic surgeons. It can be combined with other breast operation or performed under local as a standalone procedure. The crown flap technique yields a minimal scar and excellent, shape, contour, and sensation. Breast feeding has not been assessed but we would assume that it may not be possible.

## References

1. Lai Y, Wu WC. Nipple reduction with a modified circumcision technique. Br J Plast Surg. 1996;49:307–9.
2. Basile F, Chang Y. The triple-flap nipple-reduction technique. Ann Plast Surg. 2007;59(3):260–2.
3. Regnault P. Nipple hypertrophy. Clin Plast Surg. 1975;2(3):391–6.
4. Ferreira LM, Neto MS, Okamoto RH, Andrews JM. Surgical correction of nipple hypertrophy. Plast Reconstr Surg. 1995;95(4):753.
5. van Widerden JJ. Nummular nipple hypertrophy and repair as part of an aesthetic nipple-areola unit. Aesthet Plast Surg. 1997;21:408–11.
6. Sperli AE. Cosmetic reduction of the nipple with functional preservation. Br J Plast Surg. 1974;27:42–3.
7. Marshall KA, Wolfort FG, Cochran TC. Surgical correction of nipple hypertrophy in male gynecomastia: case report. Plast Reconstr Surg. 1977;60:277–9.
8. Vecchione TR. The reduction of the hypertrophic nipple. Aesthet Plast Surg. 1979;3:343–5.
9. Kerr-Valentic MA, Agarwal JP. Reduction of the hypertrophic nipple following total skin sparing mastectomy. J Plast Reconstr Aesthet Surg. 2009;62(12):e652–3.

# Part VIII

# Techniques for Correction of Nipple Inversion

# 36 Surgical Repair of the Inverted Nipple

Adrien Aiache

## 36.1 Introduction

The nipple-areolar complex (NAC) is designed for baby breastfeeding. The color, size, and shape of the areola and the nipple vary with the subject. Men have small areolas and small nipples since it is an unnecessary anatomic unit. In women, the main problem consists of flat or inverted nipples which, in addition to the cosmetic problem, makes it difficult or impossible for breastfeeding.

Three classes of malformation have been described by Han and Hong [1]. The number one nipple classification shows a nipple which is flat at the level of the areola but can be erected by gently pushing down the areola or pulling on the nipple. Babies can usually recreate this position of the nipple and breastfeed. In number two classification, the nipple is below the surface of the areola and cannot be erected easily. In this condition the baby cannot properly breastfeed most of the time. Sometimes the baby is able to latch around the nipple and breastfeed although it is difficult. At this level of classification, special tools have been developed to help the problem. They consist of breast pumps and artificial elements that erect the nipple. In number three classification, the nipple is deeply inverted and no maneuver can get it out to erect. In these cases surgical treatment has been the only way to correct the problem.

The inverted nipple is mainly observed at puberty. Causes are varied and, in addition to genetic factors, they include trauma, breast infection, and genetic variants such as Weaver syndrome, Fryns-Aftimos syndrome or Kennerknecht-Sorgo-Oberhoffer syndrome. Anatomically, nipple inversion exhibits a retracted nipple into the breast tissue and shows that the ducts are short and sclerotic preventing elongation of the nipple and there are different degrees of this syndrome. The anatomic description of the inversion shows that the nipple end is completely inverted and is adherent to the ducts and the only way to obtain an eversion is the severance of the end of the ducts just below the skin surface and the eversion of the nipple. The condition is relatively common hovering around 10% of women; although it is a cosmetic problem for women, it becomes a functional one when they have a baby and want to breastfeed.

The surgery which is the only definitive treatment for severe nipple retraction may not allow breastfeeding. Some relatively unsuccessful techniques have been described involving vertical incision at the base of the nipple on both sides at 12 o'clock and 6:00 o'clock allowing the penetration of sharp scissors which are used to free the scar tissue from the ducts in pieces where the ducts are not completely retracted [2–18]. It can

A. Aiache, M.D.
9884 S. Santa Monica Blvd, Suite 102, Beverly Hills, CA 90212, USA
e-mail: aiachemd@gmail.com


M.A. Shiffman (ed.), *Nipple-Areolar Complex Reconstruction*,
https://doi.org/10.1007/978-3-319-60925-6_36

be relatively successful; however, its complete retraction technique is impossible.

## 36.2 Technique

The definitive surgical treatment consists of an areolar semicircular incision, inferior or superior in some cases, and is made through the skin and subcutaneous tissue down to the fat and breast tissue (Figs. 36.1, 36.2, 36.3, and 36.4). A semicircle consisting of areolar skin is elevated by sharp and brunt dissection from the breast tissue below until the re-elevation reaches the ducts.

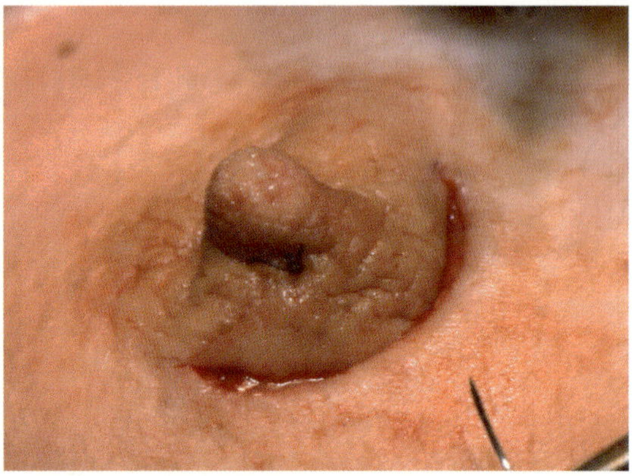

Fig. 36.2 Infra-areolar incision from one side to the other. The incision will go down toward the ducts

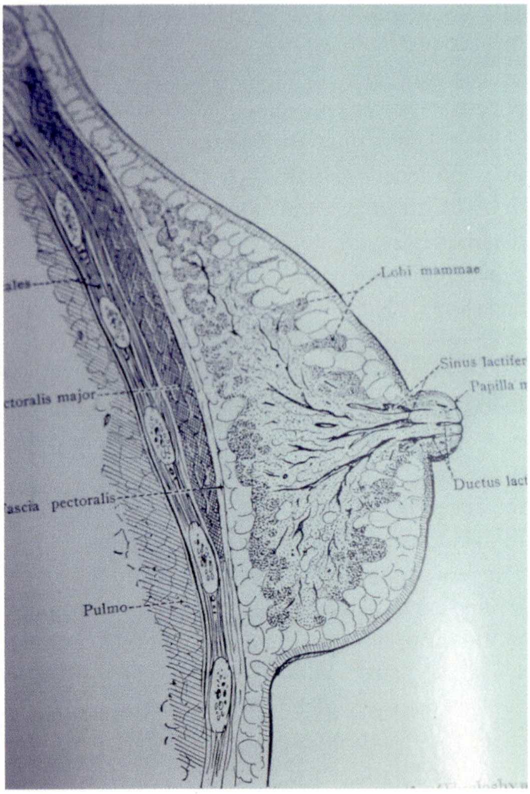


Fig. 36.1 Cross-section of the breast shows the breast tissue as well as the ducts which are going to the nipple showing the tightness of the ducts that can occur and make the operation difficult without cutting them

The ducts are then identified and they are cut off from the surrounding tissue and transected leaving a distal stump of nipple skin measuring approximately 5 mm in thickness. Then, by blunt and sharp scissor dissection, the nipple is completely disinvaginated like the finger of a grove until appropriate release and elevation is obtained and the tip of the nipple is free and visible at the end of the nipple tubular structure. Once the nipple is completely expanded and re-elevated, 4-0 Vicryl sutures (Ethicon, Johnson & Johnson, Someruille, NJ) are applied at each stage to maintain the extension and to prevent re-inversion of the tube. To preclude damaging the blood supply, strangulation of the base of the nipple is carefully avoided. The breast tissue below containing the proximal stumps of the duct is buttressed with mattress sutures to prevent the recurrence of duct shortening by their readhesion to the bases. These flaps buttressed below the nipple will provide the support for the extended nipple. Hemostasis and irrigation should be meticulous because an inverted nipple usually harbors debris and bacteria. The areola is then closed in layers and light bandages are applied (Figs. 36.5, 36.6, and 36.7). If necessary the surgeon will proceed with the implantation of a silicone prosthesis before closure of the incision.

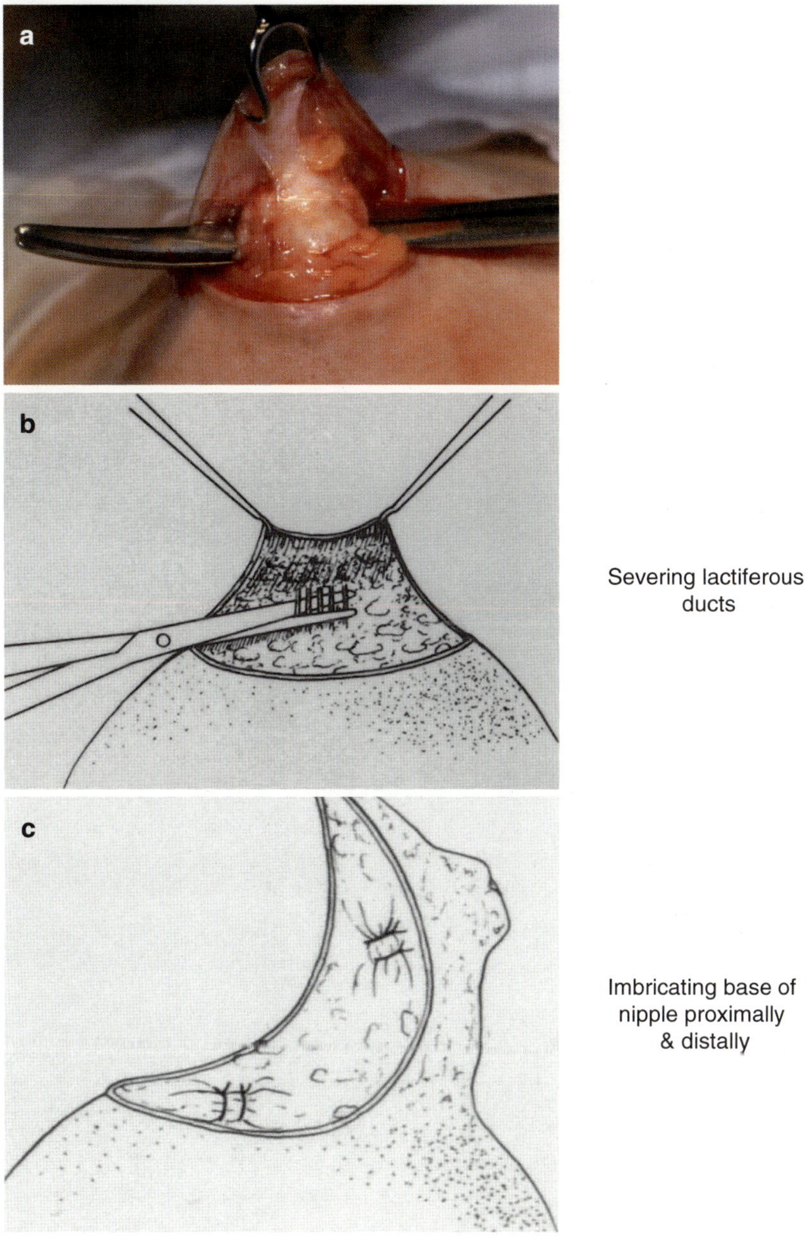


**Fig. 36.3** (**a**) The scissors are used to de-imbricate the invaginated nipple and allow its complete extension outward. (**b**) Eversion of the nipple accomplished with scissors which is de-gloving the nipple completely and turning it inside out in order to obtain a good projection. (**b**) Undermining of the lactiferous ducts which are going to be severed in a tethered nipple down to the base of the breast. (**c**) Severing the lactiferous ducts which is the only way to prevent recurrence of the condition when the ducts are completely severed from the distal attachments

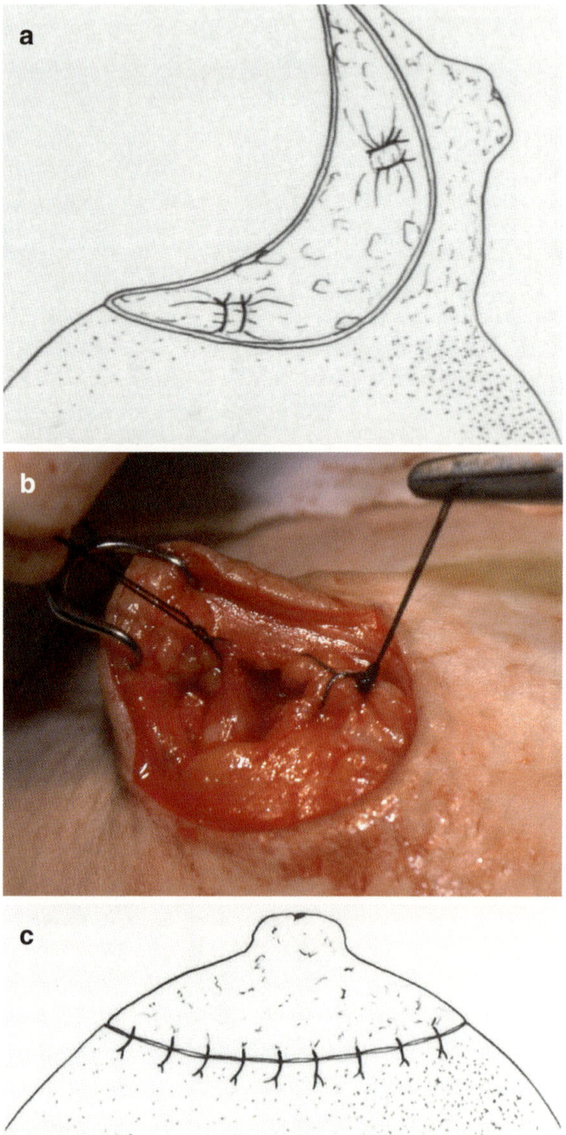


**Fig. 36.4** (**a**) Imbricating at the base of the nipple proximally and distally in order to prevent re-attachment and recurrence of the condition. (**b**) After the evagination of the nipple, a suture is applied from one side to the other avoiding complete obliteration of the vessels to prevent sloughing. This suture holds the nipple in its evaginated status. (**c**) Closure of the incision

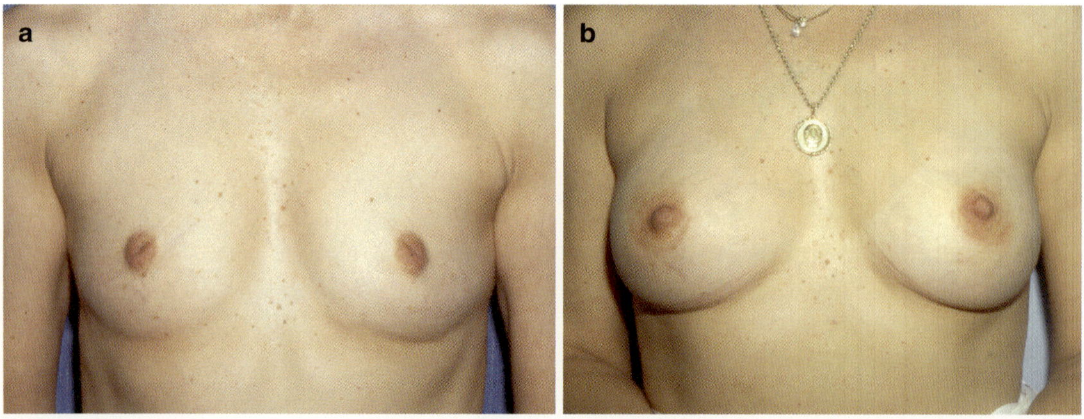


**Fig. 36.5** (**a**) Preoperative condition of inverted nipples. (**b**) Postoperative after evagination of the nipples

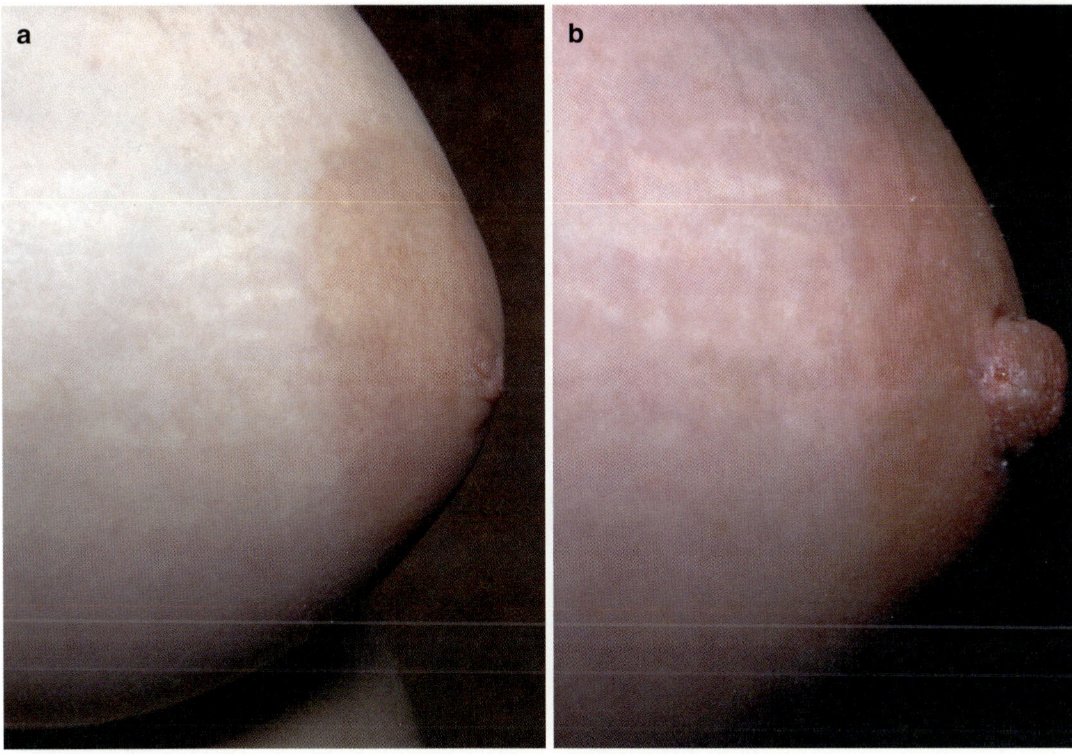

**Fig. 36.6** (**a**) Preoperative condition of an inverted nipple. (**b**) Postoperative after evagination of the nipple

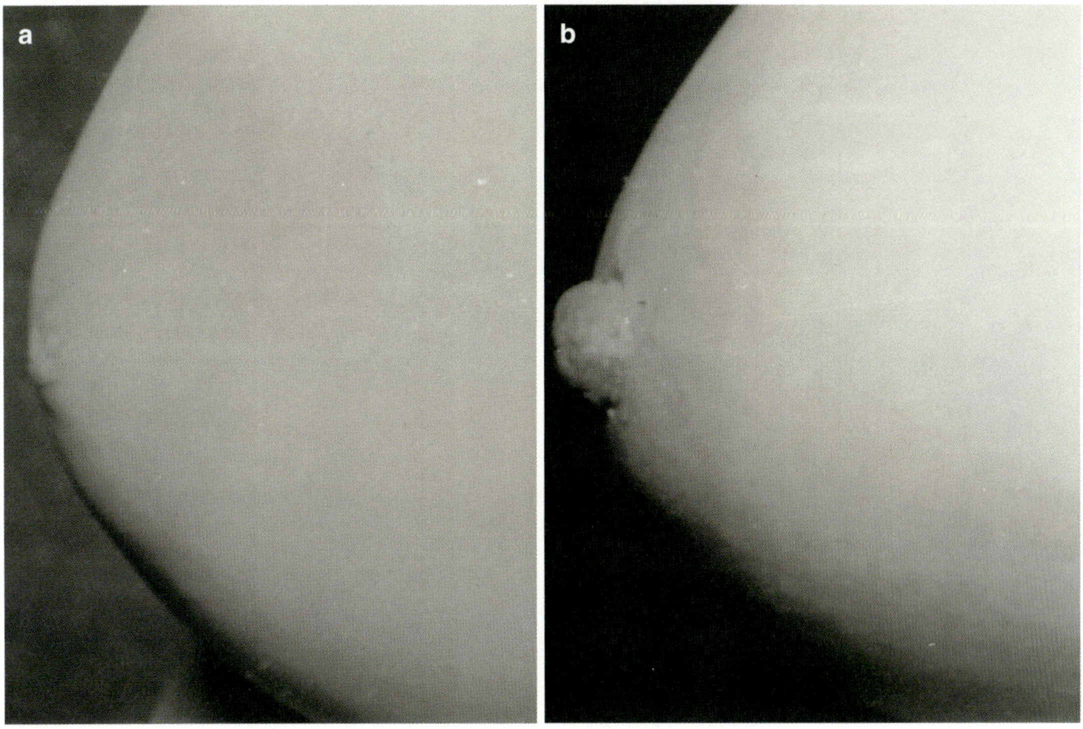

**Fig. 36.7** (**a**) Preoperative condition of an inverted nipple. (**b**) Postoperative after evagination of the nipple

## Conclusions

In most of the cases, this treatment has been shown to be a valid response to the inversion of the nipple. It is more radical than other methods and obviously prevents lactation, and patients have to decide in advance if this choice is acceptable to them.

## References


1. Han S, Hong YG. The inverted nipple: its grading and surgical correction. Plast Reconstr Surg. 1999;104(2):389–95.
2. Skoog T. An operation for inverted nipples. Br I Plast Surg. 1952;5:65–9.
3. Spina V. Inverted nipple; contribution to the surgical treatment. Plast Reconstr Surg. 1957;19:63–6.
4. Skoog T. Surgical correction of inverted nipples. J Am Med Wom Assoc. 1965;20:931–5.
5. Lamont E. Congenital inversion of the nipple in identical twins. Br J Plast Surg. 1973;26:178.
6. Schwager RG, Smith JW, Gray GF, Goulian D Jr. Inversion of the human female nipple, with a simple method of treatment. Plast Reconstr Surg. 1974;54:564–9.
7. Pitanguy I, Matta SR, Filho AF. Mamilo invertidos. Rev Bras Cirugia. 1975;64:199–207.
8. Elsahy NI. An alternative operation for inverted nipples. Plast Reconstr Surg. 1976;57:438–91.
9. Broadbent TR, Woolf RM. Benign inverted nipple: trans-nipple-areolar correction. Plast Reconstr Surg. 1976;58:673–7.
10. Hartrampf CR, Schneider WJ. A simple direct method for correction of inversion of the nipple. Plast Reconstr Surg. 1976;58:678–9.
11. D'Assumpcao E, Rosa EMS. Correction of the inverted nipple. Br J Plast Surg. 1977;30:249.
12. Gangal HT, Gangal MH. Suction methods for correcting flat nipples or inverted nipples. Plast Reconstr Surg. 1978;61:294–6.
13. Wolfort FG, Marshall KA, Cochran TC. Correction of the inverted nipple. Ann Plast Surg. 1978;1:294–7.
14. Hamilton JM. Inverted nipple. Plast Reconstr Surg. 1980;65:507–9.
15. Teirnourian B, Adham MN. Simple technique for correction of inverted nipple. Plast Reconstr Surg. 1980;65:504–6.
16. Ramakrishnan KM, Rao DK. Congenital inversion of the human nipple. Aesthet Plast Surg. 1980;4:65–72.
17. Hauben DJ, Mahler D. A simple method for the correction of the inverted nipple. Plast Reconstr Surg. 1983;71:556–9.
18. Hinderer UT, del Rio JL. Treatment of the postoperative inverted nipple with or without asymmetry of the areola. Aesthet Plast Surg. 1983;7:139–44.

# Correction of Recurrent Grade III Inverted Nipple with Antenna Dermoadipose Flap

37

Ercan Karacaoglu

## 37.1 Introduction

The nipple is the symbol of female body with the breast. It is of key importance as a visual and sexual focus of the female body with the breast. As a third focus, the nipple has a nutritive function as in breastfeeding basis. That is why body image, sexuality, and breastfeeding are adversely affected by its abnormal conditions like in the case of inverted nipple.

In order to have a normal body image and sexuality, a female should have a normal appearance in her nipple and breast. Similarly, to achieve a successful breastfeeding, an infant needs to suck the whole bulk of nipple and almost 100 to 80 percentage of the areola. That is why abnormal nipple conditions such as inverted nipple may result in problems with starting, establishing, and maintaining breastfeeding [1].

Nipple inversion may cause serious problems. These are cosmetic, functional, and psychological problems. Some of the physical signs may be irritation, inflammation, and interference with breastfeeding and lack of self-esteem [2].

Inverted nipple is defined as a non-projectile nipple [2–4] (Fig. 37.1). The nipple is located on a plane lower than the areola. The nipple is invaginated and, instead of pointing outward, is retracted into the breast parenchymal and stromal tissue. Inverted nipple is not an uncommon deformity. The frequency of inverted nipple is reported as 17.7 per 1000 women [5]. It was first described by Cooper in 1849, and Kehrer [6] first described surgical repair of the inverted nipple in 1879.

The terms inversion and retraction often are used interchangeably, but such usage is inexact. Retraction is properly applied when only a slit-shape area of the nipple is pulled inward, whereas inversion applies to cases in which the entire nipple is pulled inward occasionally, far enough to lie below the surface of the breast [7].

Inverted nipple may be seen in different shapes, forms, and structures related to the severity of fibrosis, lack of soft tissue bulk, and lactiferous ductus. In some cases, the nipple may be temporarily protruded if stimulated, but in others, the inversion remains unresponsive regardless of stimulus.

## 37.2 Anatomy, Classification, Grading, and Pathologic Basis of the Inverted Nipple

There are numerous methods to correct inverted nipple. In order to make it simplified, it would be better to start with the basic anatomic consideration of the nipple and areola. From an anatomic standpoint, it is mostly preferable to name this anatomic unit as nipple-areola complex (NAC).

E. Karacaoglu, M.D.
Department of Plastic Surgery, Bahcesehir University, Istanbul, Turkey
e-mail: drercanka@yahoo.com


M.A. Shiffman (ed.), *Nipple-Areolar Complex Reconstruction*,
https://doi.org/10.1007/978-3-319-60925-6_37

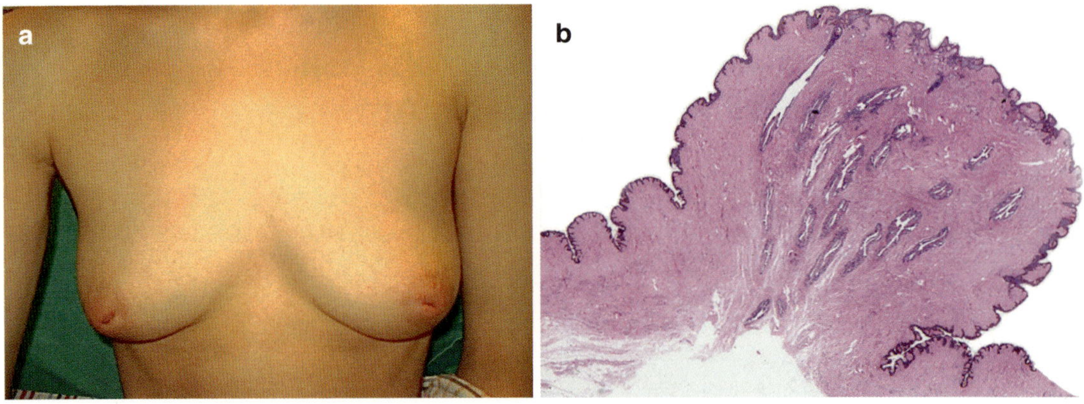


**Fig. 37.1** (**a**) A 24-year-old nulliparous woman with a history of congenital inverted nipple is seen. Inverted nipple is seen on both breasts. (**b**) The skin of the nipple is continuous with the epithelium of the ducts

## 37.3 Anatomy of the Nipple-Areola Complex (NAC)

The anatomy of nipple-areola is complex. It is therefore not surprising that the detection of disorders of the nipple-areola region may be challenging. Although the scope of this chapter is inverted nipple, a thorough understanding of anatomic variants of this complex and the imaging features specific to each is the necessary basis for a comprehensive and appropriate imaging assessment, diagnosis, and treatment. It should also be kept in mind that concurrent benign and pathologic conditions of this complex could be a fact of possibility.

Age is also a variant of nipple-areola complex anatomy. It is key to understand the maturation of breast in order to evaluate the abnormal consequences of NAC. During puberty, the breast mound increases in size. Subsequent enlargement and outward growth of the areola result in a secondary mound [8]. Finally, the areola subsides to the level of the surrounding breast tissue, leaving a single breast mound [8].

At full development, the nipple-areola complex overlies the area between the second and sixth ribs, with a location at the level of the fourth intercostal space being typical for a breast that is not ptotic. The adult breast consists of approximately 15–20 segments demarcated by mammary ducts that converge at the nipple in a radial arrangement. Like the number of segments, the number of mammary ducts may vary. The collecting ducts that drain each segment, which typically measure about 2 mm in diameter, coalesce in the subareolar region into lactiferous sinuses approximately 5–8 mm in diameter [9]. Women occasionally detect a normal lactiferous sinus as a palpable finding at self-examination. In the typical breast, there are 9–20 orifices that drain the segments at the nipple [9, 10].

The nipple-areola complex contains the Montgomery glands, large- or intermediate-stage sebaceous glands that are embryologically transitional between sweat glands and mammary glands and are capable of secreting milk [9]. The Montgomery glands open at the Morgagni tubercles, which are small (1–2-mm-diameter) raised papules on the areola. The nipple-areola complex also contains many sensory nerve endings, smooth muscle, and an abundant lymphatic system called the subareolar or Sappey's plexus. Because the skin of the nipple is continuous with the epithelium of the ducts, cancer of the ducts may spread to the nipple (Fig. 37.1) [9].

## 37.4 Classification of Inverted Nipple

Inverted nipple can be either acquired or congenital. In acquired inverted nipple, the nipple inversion is secondary to the previous breast surgery, infiltrating ductal carcinoma or mastitis, etc. In congenital inverted nipple, the inversion is not related to a known entity. Congenital inverted nipple is the most frequent type. The prevalence is reported as 2–10% [11–13].

Congenital inverted nipple is clinically classified into three subgroups: first, second, and third grade. First grade inverted nipple is the nipple that can be easily pulled out manually and maintains its projection quite well without traction. The nipple is popped out by gentle palpation around the areola. The soft tissue is intact in this form and the lactiferous ducts are normal.

Second grade inverted nipple is also popped out by palpation but not as easily as in the first grade. The nipple tends to retract. The nipple has moderate fibrosis, and the lactiferous ductus is mildly retracted but does not need to be cut to release the fibrosis. These nipples have been shown to have rich collagenous stromata with numerous bundles of smooth muscle.

Third grade inverted nipple is a severe form in which inversion and retraction are significant. Manually popping out the nipple is extremely difficult. A traction suture is needed to keep these nipples protruded. The fibrosis beneath the nipple is significant and the soft tissue is markedly insufficient. On histologic examination, the terminal lactiferous ductus and lobular units are atrophic and replaced with severe fibrosis (Fig. 37.2) [2, 3].

## 37.5 Technique

Various techniques have been reported to correct the inverted nipple [12–23]. It was also reported that no single technique is appropriate for correcting all types of nipple deformities because different grades of inverted nipple have different levels of fibrosis, soft tissue bulk, and lactiferous ductus structure [11].

The best approach for correction is supposed to be simple and reliable. In addition, a technique with low recurrence rate, with less or no scar, that requires no bulky or special dressing and that preserves lactiferous ductus function is desirable [2]. In some cases correction of the inverted nipple with simultaneous breast surgery might be required. An individualized planning still with simplicity and reliability is desirable.

Here, you will find one of the most useful techniques used to correct inverted nipple with simultaneous mastopexy. In this technique, dermoadipose flaps that are generated within the area of deepithelialization of the mastopexy are

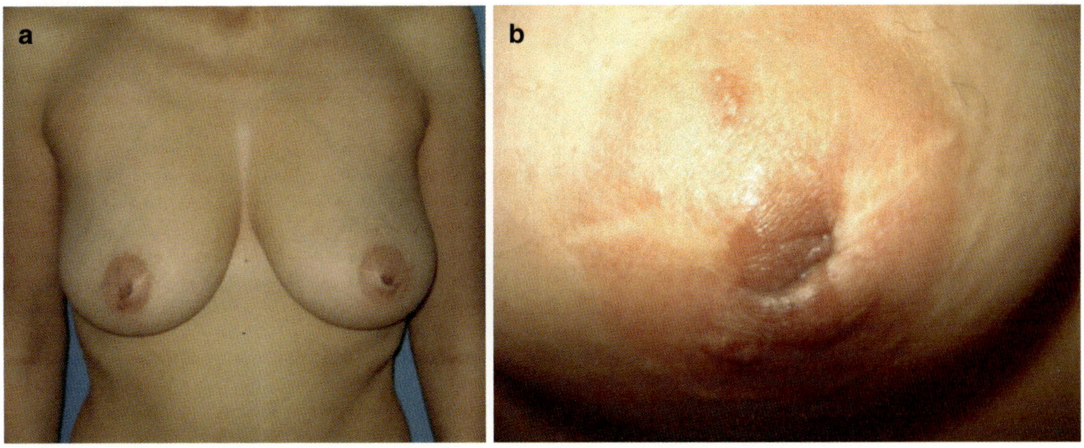


**Fig. 37.2** (**a**, **b**) A 30-year-old nulliparous woman with a history of congenital inverted nipple is seen. She had previous correction surgery for inverted nipple which resulted in failure

used. The flap is called the "antenna flap" because of its way of design.

### 37.5.1 Preoperative Marking

Preoperative planning starts with the patient standing. The preliminary marking is identical to that for circumvertical mastopexy. The midline, breast meridian with its extrapolation on the chest wall, and the inframammary fold are marked. The lateral and medial markings are made while pushing the breast laterally and medially with a slight upward rotation, in accordance with the vertical axis drawn below the breast. The new areola is then marked in a classical dome shape. Finally, the lower marking is made. This gathers the medial and lateral markings at a level 2 cm above the preexisting fold. The area below the areola is used to mark the antenna flap. Marking is done to optimally use the existing deepithelialization area (Fig. 37.3).

### 37.5.2 Surgical Technique

The operative sequence for augmentation mammoplasty is more straightforward. The marked area below the areola is deepithelialized. Antenna flaps are marked on this area (Fig. 37.3). These flaps are dissected and elevated. These flaps are left intact and the procedure goes on with augmentation mastopexy.

The breast parenchyma and adipose tissue below the nipple-areola complex are removed within the limits of the markings. A submuscular pocket is created. Once the implant is placed in the pocket, the preliminary markings around the areola

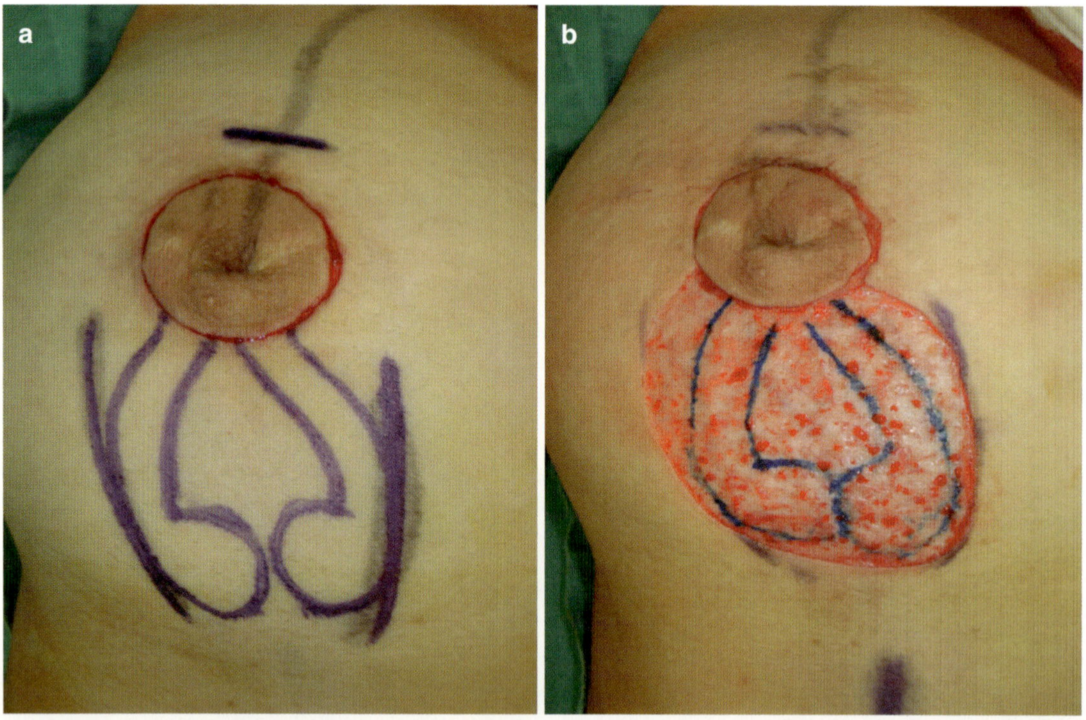


**Fig. 37.3** Technique. (**a**) The area below the areola is used to mark the antenna flap. Marking is done to optimally use the existing deepithelialization area. (**b**) The area below the areola was deepithelialized. The antenna flaps were marked on this area. (**c**) The flaps were elevated to include the dermis and 5 mm of fat tissue beneath and attached to the dermal flap using an electrocautery. (**d**) Two legs of the antenna flap are seen. (**e**) Two legs of the antenna flap are inserted into the created pocket under the nipple. A satisfactory projection of the nipple is seen at the end of the procedure. (**f**) Early postoperative

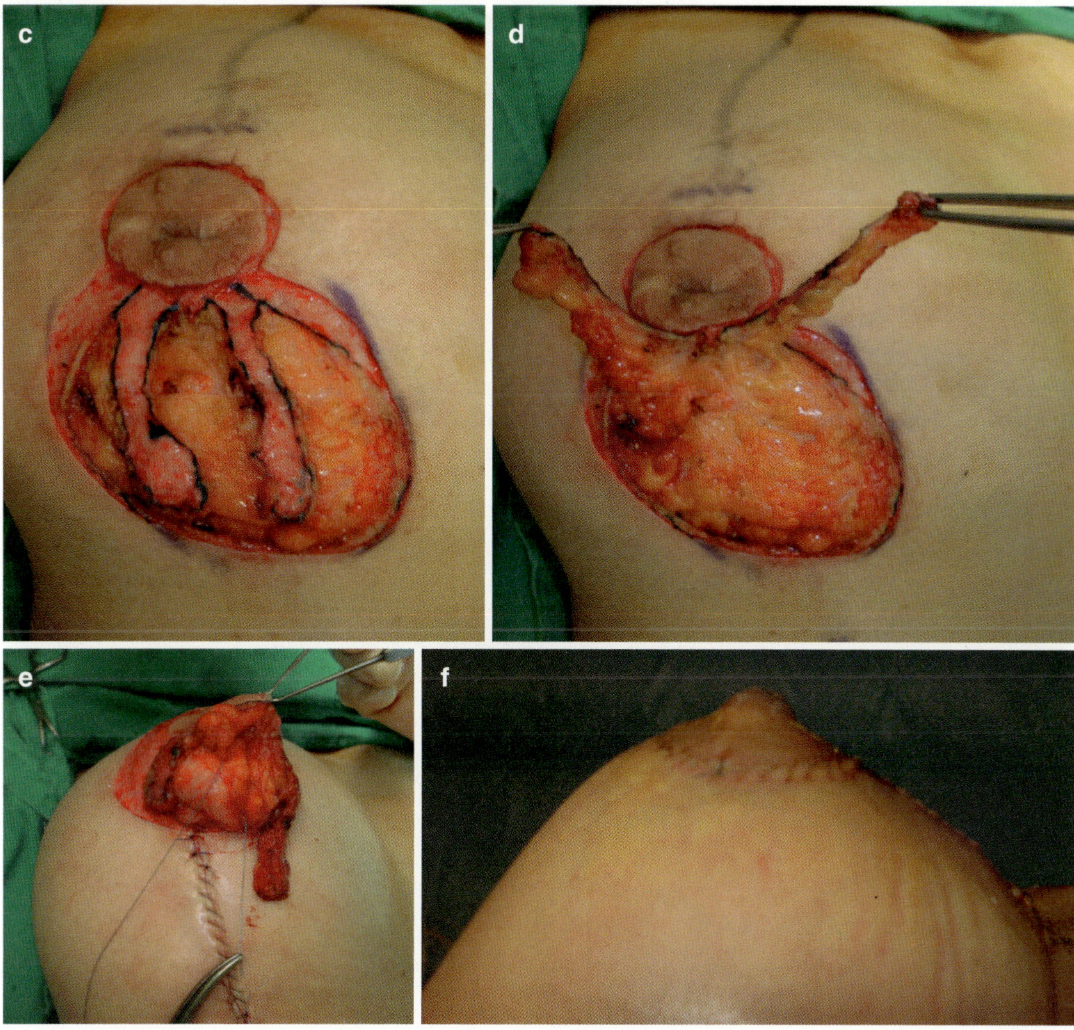


**Fig. 37.3** (continued)

and the lateral and medial markings below the areola are reevaluated. Once the implant is in place, the nipple position and planned vertical breast closure are tailor tacked with staples with the patient in a sitting position. A slight flattening of the lower pole is allowed for parenchyma and skin accommodation postoperatively. The edges of the vertical temporary closure are marked and staples removed. The amount of excess skin that could be comfortably removed in the vertical closure is thus determined. At this stage, the deepithelialization of the skin around the areola and within the medial and lateral markings is completed. Vertical incisions are closed. A pocket is created for the transposition of the antenna flaps. For that purpose a 0.5 cm vertical incision is made at the 6 o'clock position at the base of the areola. A tunnel is dissected at and through the areola and extended to the base of the nipple. The tissue beneath the nipple is dissected and the fibrosis was released. The retracting lactiferous ducts are cut mainly from the central portion of the nipple. All the fibrosis and retracting ducts are released until the nipple could maintain its eversion by itself without any traction. Two legs of the antenna flap are inserted into the created pocket (Fig. 37.3). A satisfactory projection of the nipple is seen at the end of the procedure.

Finally, the periareolar incisions are closed in layers. The periareolar portion is closed in a purse-string fashion by using nonabsorbable sutures (Fig. 37.3). After placement of Steri-Strip dressing, the newly everted nipple is maintained by a thermoplastic splint. The patient is kept in a protective splint for 2 months after surgery.

## 37.6 Discussion

In this technique, a high rate of success has been reported that no recurrence of nipple inversion reported [12]. As of patient satisfaction, the technique is promising that the shape and projection of the patient's nipple is deemed satisfactory (Fig. 37.4).

The surgical approach presented in this chapter is an option for correcting a recurrent, congenital inverted nipple. It also should be emphasized that even an alloplastic material could not have corrected the deformity in one of these cases. Two other techniques to correct

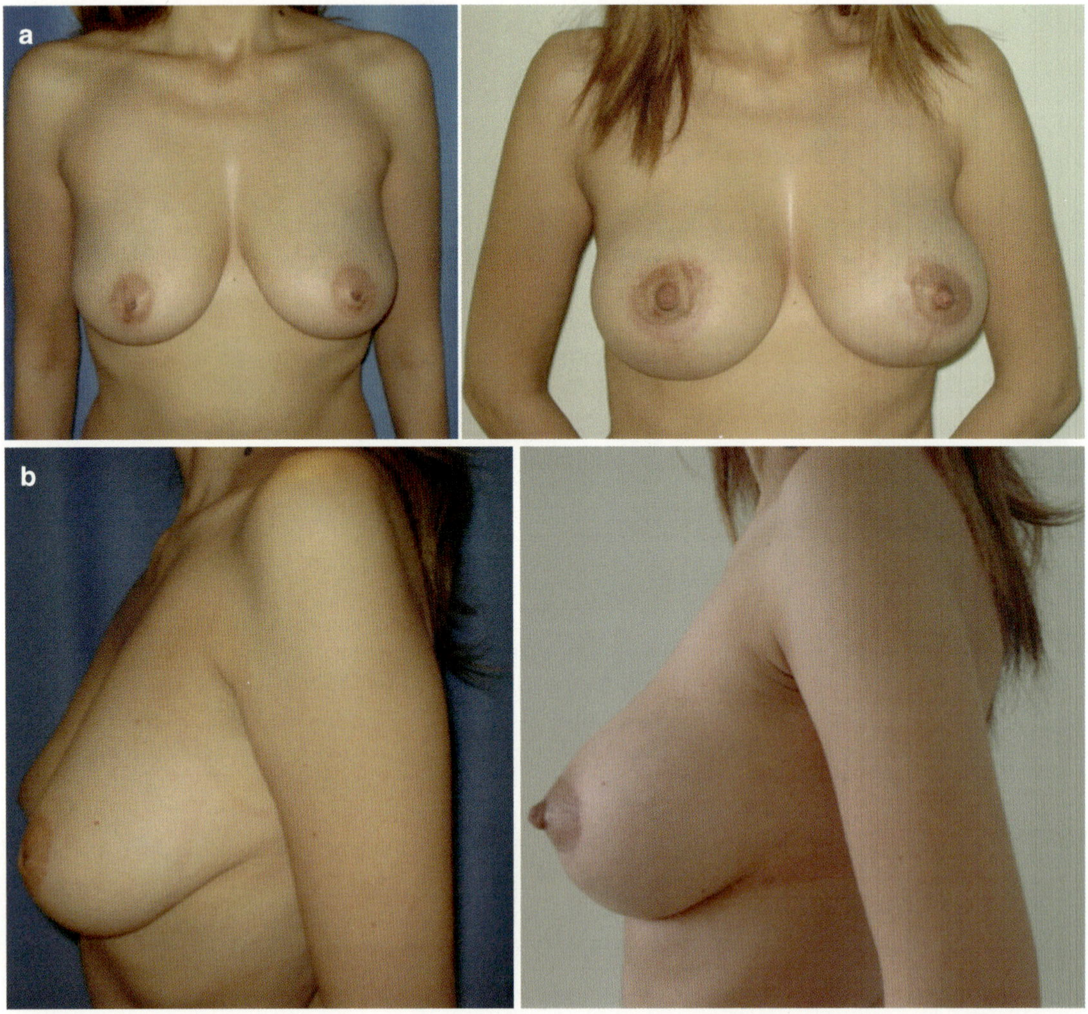


**Fig. 37.4** (**a**, **b**) Three years after surgery. (*Left*) Preoperative. (*Right*) Postoperative

inverted nipple (local flap and silicone produced for nipple projection) had already been used to correct this deformity in this particular case. But only this technique named the antenna flap ensured a satisfactory result.

This technique entails transposition of bulky dermoadipose flaps harvested from the deepithelialized area of the mastopexy into the pocket created beneath the nipple. In this technique, the dead space is filled with autologous tissue where possible complications such as extrusion that is seen with alloplastic materials is avoided. One of the advantages of this technique is the lack of scar in the areola. The disadvantage of the technique is that it is limited to those patients who are candidates for mastopexy.

The author used this technique in 20 cases since its description. All patients are reported to be happy with the results. No major complications are reported. Only in two cases suture abscesses formation is reported.

## Conclusions

As a conclusion, new vascularized tissue brought under the nipple-areola complex to correct recurrent inverted nipple yields a safe and better projection. This technique yields a satisfactory result without recurrence of inversion in 20 cases. It is strongly recommended that the technique should be considered by the surgeon for any patient contemplating correction of inverted nipple and mastopexy.

## References

1. Hytten FE. Clinical and chemical studies in human lactation: IX. Breast-feeding in hospital. Br Med J. 1954;2(2):1447–52.
2. Kim DY, Jeong EC, Eo SR, Kim KS, Lee SY, Cho BH. Correction of inverted nipple: an alternative method using two triangular areolar dermal flaps. Ann Plast Surg. 2003;51(6):636–40.
3. Han S, Yoon H. The inverted nipple: its grading and surgical correction. Plast Reconstr Surg. 1999;104(2):389–95.
4. Stevens WG, Fellows DR, Vath SD, Stoker DA. An integrated approach to the repair of inverted nipples. Aesthet Surg J. 2004;24:211–5.
5. Schwager RG, Smith JW, Gray GF, Goulian D Jr. Inversion of the human female nipple, with a simple method of treatment. Plast Reconstr Surg. 1974;54:564–9.
6. Kehrer F. Uber excision des warzenhofs bei hohlwerzen. Beitr Exp Geburtshilfe Gynaekol Gizessen. 1879;43:170.
7. Nicholson BT, Harvey JA, Cohen MA. Nipple-areolar complex: normal anatomy and benign and malignant processes. Radiographics. 2009;29(2):509–23.
8. Seltzer V. The breast: embryology, development, and anatomy. Clin Obstet Gynecol. 1994;37:879–80.
9. Kopans D. Breast anatomy and basic histology, physiology, and pathology. In: Kopans D, editor. Breast imaging. 3rd ed. Philadelphia: Lippincott Williams & Wilkins; 2007. p. 7–43.
10. Love SM, Barsky SH. Anatomy of the nipple and breast ducts revisited. Cancer. 2004;101:1947–57.
11. Lee MJ, DePolli PA, Casas LA. Aesthetic and predictable correction of the inverted nipple. Aesthet Surg J. 2003;23:353–6.
12. Alaxander JM, Campbell MJ. Prevalence of inverted and non-protractile nipples in antenatal women who intend to breastfeed. Breast. 1997;6:72–8.
13. Karacaoglu E. Correction of recurrent grade III inverted nipple with Antenna Dermoadipose Flap: case report. Aesthet Plast Surg. 2009;33:843–8.
14. Kim JT, Lim YS, Oh JG. Correction of inverted nipples with twisting and locking principles. Plast Reconstr Surg. 2006;118(7):1526–31.
15. Serra-Renom J, Fontdevila J, Monner J. Correction of the inverted nipple with an internal 5-point star suture. Ann Plast Surg. 2004;53(3):293–6.
16. Jiang HQ, Wei X, Yuan SM, Tang LM. Nipple aspirator: a self-designed instrument for inverted nipple. Plast Reconstr Surg. 2008;121(3):141e–3e.
17. Yamada N, Kakibuchi M, Kitaoshi H, Kurokawa M, Hosokawa K, Hashimoto K. A method for correcting an inverted nipple with an artificial dermis. Aesthet Plast Surg. 2004;28(4):233–8.
18. Ritz M, Silfen R, Morgan D, Southwick G. Simple technique for inverted nipple correction. Aesthet Plast Surg. 2005;29(1):24–7.
19. Huang WC. A new method for correction of inverted nipple with three periductal dermofibrous flaps. Aesthet Plast Surg. 2003;27(4):301–4.
20. Crestinu JM. The correction of inverted nipples without scars: 17 years' experience, 452 operations. Aesthet Plast Surg. 2001;25(3):246–8.
21. Pompei S, Tedesco M. A new surgical technique for the correction of the inverted nipple. Aesthet Plast Surg. 1999;23(5):371–4.
22. Jeong HS, Lee HK. Correction of inverted nipple using subcutaneous turn-over flaps to create a tent suspension-like effect. PLoS One. 2015;10(7):e0133588.
23. Gould DJ, Nadeau MH, Macias LH, Stevens WG. Inverted nipple repair revisited: a 7-year experience. Aesthet Surg J. 2015;35(2):156–64.

# Correction of Inverted Nipples with Twisting and Locking Principle

38

Jeong Tae Kim and Jagjeet Singh

## 38.1 Introduction

The causes of inverted nipples can be categorized into three major histological pathologies [1, 2] such as lack of tissue bulk at the nipple base, shortened and underdeveloped lactiferous ducts, and retractile collagen bands at the base of the nipple. Surgical repair of this type of deformity tackles these anomalies. Lack of tissue bulk at the nipple base is addressed by adding bulk and filling the dead space under the nipple with the nipple under traction. Shortened and underdeveloped lactiferous ducts would require release, which can be done either by transecting the ducts or by releasing the fibrous tissue pulling the ducts while preserving the ducts. In the case of the retractile collagen bands at the nipple base, tightness around the nipple neck should be released and the nipple base secured to prevent recurrence of the inversion [2–5]. While many ingenious methods have been introduced to correct the inverted nipple, majority of these procedures seem to suffer from recurrence of the inversion [6]. Prevention of recurrence has been commonly done by using purse-string-type techniques, but this was met with limited success [7].

It would be practical at this point in the chapter to discuss some of the earlier and more recent repair methods and highlight the similarities of these methods and the complications associated with them. Working with the three pathophysiological anomalies described above, we classify the repair methods accordingly. Among the methods that add bulk and fill up the dead space at the nipple base, there is a method reported by Broadbent and Woolf [6], who described the trans-nipple-areolar correction for inverted nipples. This method involved a right angle incision across the nipple areolar complex to release the shortened ducts, followed by elevation of the upper and lower glandular flaps that were rotated outward to fill the space under the nipple [6]. Elsahy et al. [8] described two triangular-shaped dermal flaps that were elevated opposite each other with the preservation of the ducts and vascular supply. Dermal flaps were passed beneath the nipples and anchored to each other to act as a strong sling across the base of the nipple. The main advantage of the repair was that reinversion of the nipple was prevented by the two dermal flaps which increased tissue density underneath the nipple. Teimourian and Adham [9] modified the Elsahy technique by elevating two

J.T. Kim, M.D., PhD.
Department of Plastic and Reconstructive Surgery, Hanyang University College of Medicine, Seoul, Korea
e-mail: ps360@hanmail.net; jtkim@hanyang.ac.kr; jtkim360@gmail.com

J. Singh
Department of Plastic and Reconstructive Surgery, Kuala Lumpur General Hospital, Kuala Lumpur, Malaysia
e-mail: jag.plastics@gmail.com


M.A. Shiffman (ed.), *Nipple-Areolar Complex Reconstruction*, https://doi.org/10.1007/978-3-319-60925-6_38

wider-based dermal flaps at 6 and 12 o'clock locations on the nipple-areolar complex. With the aid of nipple traction, these flaps were tunneled under the nipple with cutting of the ducts of the release of the fibrous tissue. The flaps were subsequently rotated and sutured under the nipple.

Next we outline some of the methods that were used to address the shortened underdeveloped lactiferous ducts. These methods were targeted at releasing the fibrous bands at the nipple base. In some of these techniques, it was unavoidable to sacrifice the ductal system. Pitanguy and Ceravolo [10] used a trans-nipple-areolar incision to expose the ductal system and release the fibrous tissue between the ducts. This technique resulted in no damage to the ductal tissue, and subsequently the released tissue was approximated under the nipple base to provide nipple protrusion. Crestinu [11] made a small vertical incision toward the nipple base once the nipple was elevated. The incision was described as being done in a spin top fashion, along with transection of the ductal system. This technique was later advanced to be done in a V-Y manner, along with a purse-string suture used to maintain constriction at the nipple base. Skoog et al. [4] used a 3-cm diameter circle that was marked around the nipple. Four identical triangles were marked equidistantly around the nipple and also at the area outside the circle. These triangles were spaced alternating each other and eventually were cut out. With nipple traction, the fibrous connective tissue was released and all of the triangles were closed primarily resulting in the nipple being maintained in the projected state.

Retractile collagen bands were described as another pathological factor for the cause for inverted nipples. The repair methods for addressing this issue mainly targeted at maintaining tightness around the nipple neck. Schwager et al. [12] described a periareolar incision with the undermining between the nipple and underlying breast tissue. The repair was finished off with a buried purse-string suture at the base of the nipple to maintain tightness and prevent recurrence. Hauben and Mahler [13] addressed the lack of tissue bulk at the nipple base and the retractile collagen band of the nipple by using a circumferential incision around the areolar base while the nipple was under traction. Through this incision, vertical and horizontal undermining was done and more tissue was mobilized to create a thicker nipple pedicle. Finally, a purse-string suture was used to maintain tightness around the nipple base and redundant areolar tissue was excised.

A more detailed review of more recent inverted nipple repair techniques is outlined next. Wu et al. [14] describe the correction of inverted nipple repair using two triangular areolar dermofibrous flaps. With this repair, the lack of tissue bulk at the nipple base was addressed with two triangular dermofibrous flaps. The shortened lactiferous ducts were transected to release them and an external donut dressing was used for 2 weeks to prevent recurrence from the retractile collagen band. They reported 14 nipples of nine patients with one case of recurrence. One of the disadvantages of this method is that excessive bulky dressing was needed for up to 2 weeks post procedure. Teng et al. [15] used external distraction device to achieve correction of the inverted nipple. Steel wires were used to pierce through the nipple and fixed to an external spring instrument. Distraction force was adjusted every 1–2 weeks, and the device was used for up 1–6 months to achieve overcorrection. With this method, there was no added tissue bulk at the base of the nipple. Undeveloped lactiferous ducts were released by distraction forces, and the steel wire and spring instrument prevented recurrence from taking place. They reported only one recurrence which was the result of spring device snapping. The method was simple and inexpensive with minimal disruption of local tissue; however, lengthy and persistent usage of the device proved to be a disadvantage with the technique. Burm and Kim [16] used two diamond areolar-based dermal flaps that were passed underneath the nipple. The dermal flaps were secured underneath the nipple once the periductal tissue and lactiferous ducts were released. The flaps were secured tight enough to act as suspension bridge across the nipple base. This method was combined with a donut type bolster dressing for 2–3 months. The procedures had the advantage of being easy, convenient, and accurate without having the need for using traction sutures after the operation. However, they do report one case of recurrence out of a total of 28 cases. Kolker et al. [17] presented a minimally invasive parenchymal release and percutaneous suture technique. The technique uses an 18 G needle to release the subareolar fibroductal tissue. This was followed with a 4-0 nylon suture in a purse-string manner introduced in and out through the same point every 3–5 mm around the nipple base. 31 patients with a total of 58 nipples were operated on. Seventy-eight percent of the inverted nipples required only one operative procedure. 13 recurrences were documented, and 11 of them were treated adequately with the second procedure. The remaining two needed a third procedure. There were no late recurrences documented. The method was described as simple, practical, and safe; however, a high rate of recurrence was reported. Jiang and Torina [18] used a nipple aspirator device to maintain negative pressure over the inverted nipple. The use of the device had to be for 3 months. A large series of 2000 cases were reported with no recurrence in any of their cases; however, the device needed close supervision for its effectiveness, and the patient was required to use the device all day for a period of 3 months.

From the cases that are briefly discussed here, it can be noted that the correction of inverted nipples has been described by many authors. The diversity of these methods is a clear indication of the absence of one truly reliable repair technique. Recurrence of nipple inversion still seems to be one of the major postoperative problems encountered. Several methods have been used to prevent recurrence, the most common being a purse-string suture at the nipple base or modifications of this technique. The authors will introduce the twisting and locking principle method for the correction of inverted nipples. With this method, we were able to achieve good aesthetic results and at the same time significantly lower the rate of recurrence, avoid injury to the nipple ductal system, and preserve nipple sensory innervation. This was achieved without the use of any specific postoperative dressing or devices. Herein, we describe our operative technique for the correction of inverted nipple.

## 38.2 Operative Technique

This technique involves marking three lozenge (diamond)-shaped patterns at 120° intervals around the areola (Fig. 38.1). The tip of the inner diamond is placed at the junction between the nipple tip and the areola. The two lateral aspects of the diamond are shaped at a width that would allow for primary closure of the diamond once nipple protrusion has been achieved. This results in the lateral walls of the nipple being formed by the primary closure of the inner aspect of the

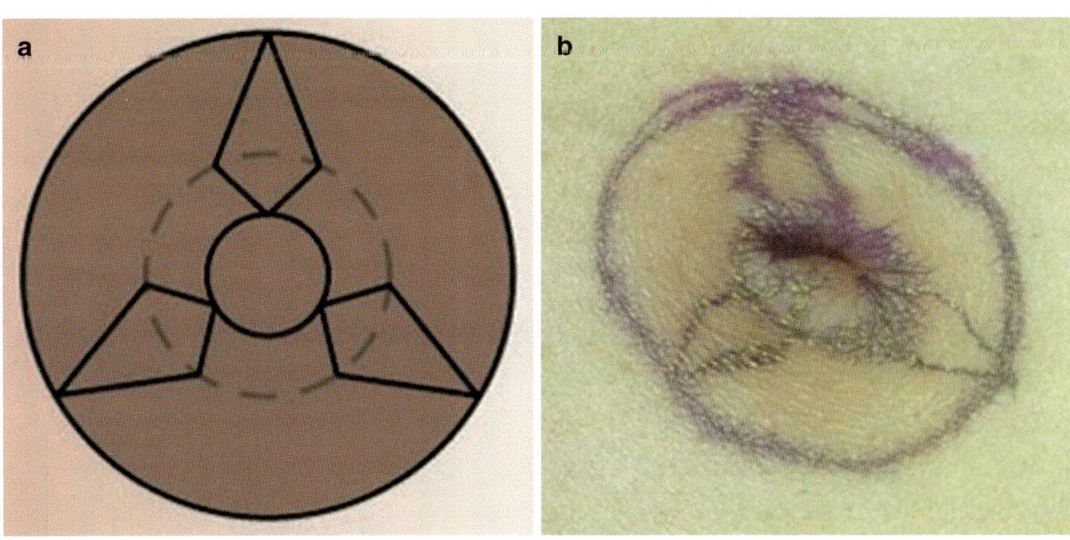


**Fig. 38.1** (**a**, **b**) The three lozenge shapes are marked out within the areolar and nipple margin

designed three diamonds (Fig. 38.2). Therefore, it is important to plan the length and the width of inner side of the diamond adequately, as it contributes to final height of the nipple projection. This factor is also the reason why the design of the diamond is usually in such way that the inner side of the diamond is shorter than the outer side. However, this ratio can be adjusted to suit the nipple prominence to areola ratio of each patient.

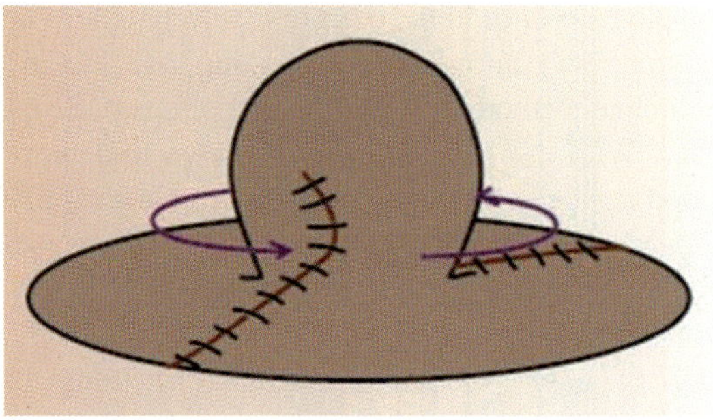

**Fig. 38.2** Placement of the suture lines once primary closure has been achieved. This leads to the lateral walls of the nipple being formed by the primary closure of the inner aspect of the three diamond design

Once the diamond shapes are satisfactorily drawn, they are carefully deepithelialized, and three triangular dermal flaps are elevated, beginning from the outer margin of the areola and working toward the nipple. It is important to note that, incisions on the areola should not extend beyond the outer margin of the areola. This is to ensure that the surgical scars are placed within the areola, and it also allows for areolar reduction procedures to be performed simultaneously (Fig. 38.3).

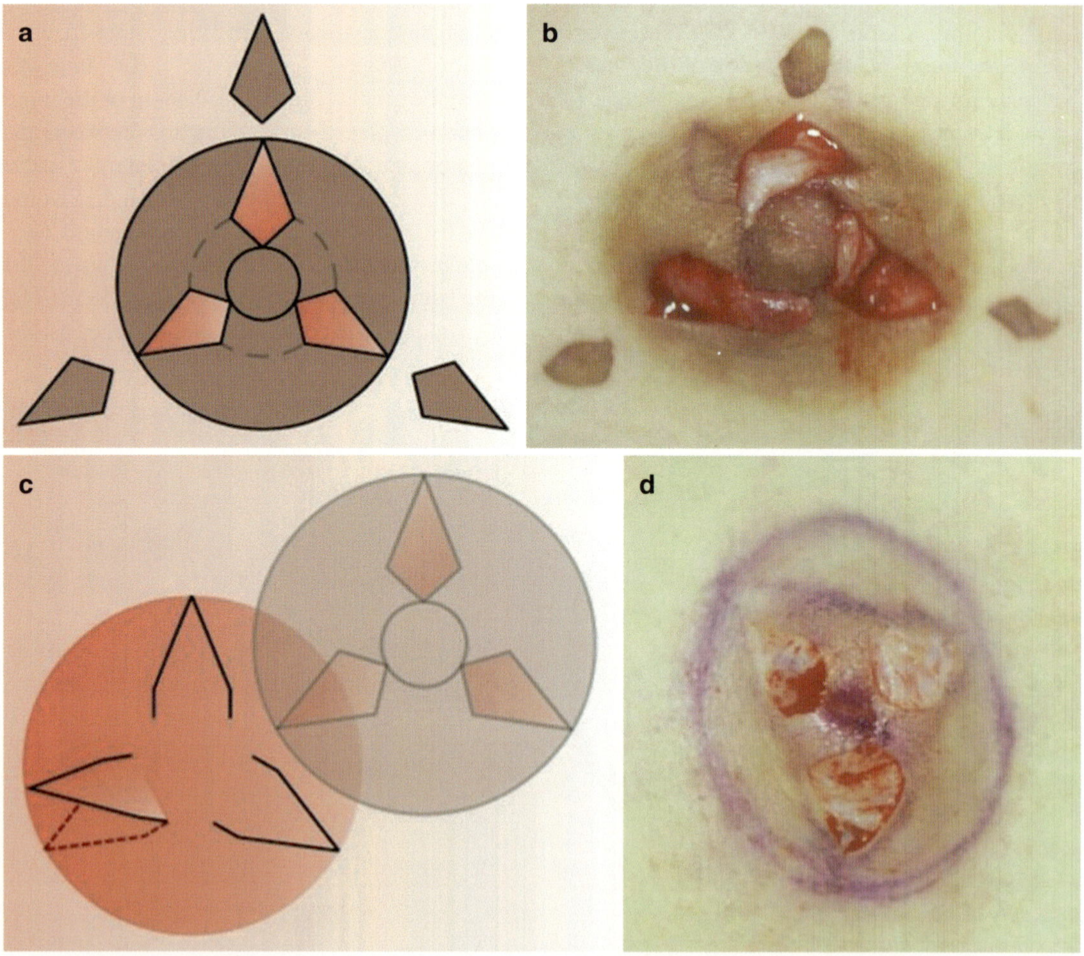


**Fig. 38.3** (**a–d**) Deepithelialization of the triangular flaps and elevation of the flaps up to the margins of the nipple

With the help of a traction suture, temporary nipple traction is provided. Next, the fibrotic bands underneath the nipple base are released using gentle blunt dissection. The aim is to make a tunnel to the next triangular dermal incision opening. This step should be done with caution as to minimize injury to the lactiferous ducts but at the same time achieve sufficient release. Gentle stretching and blunt splitting release of the fibrotic bands are performed to prevent injuries to the lactiferous ducts or the sensory nerves of the nipple (Fig. 38.4). Cutting and extensive release is avoided as this increases the risk of duct injury and sensory denervation.

Next, the elevated dermal flaps are passed through the tunnels created and sutured to the adjacent deepithelialized dermal region with 4-0 synthetic-braided absorbable sutures (Fig. 38.5).

The degree of the twisting effect is dependent on the point that is chosen on the adjacent deepithelialized triangle to anchor the dermal flaps. The twisting effect gets more profound as the anchoring point that is chosen on the neighboring deepithelialized defect becomes more distant. Temporary sutures of the dermal flaps can be placed to estimate the extent of twisting required before final fixation of the dermal flaps. The twisting of the dermal flaps at the base of the

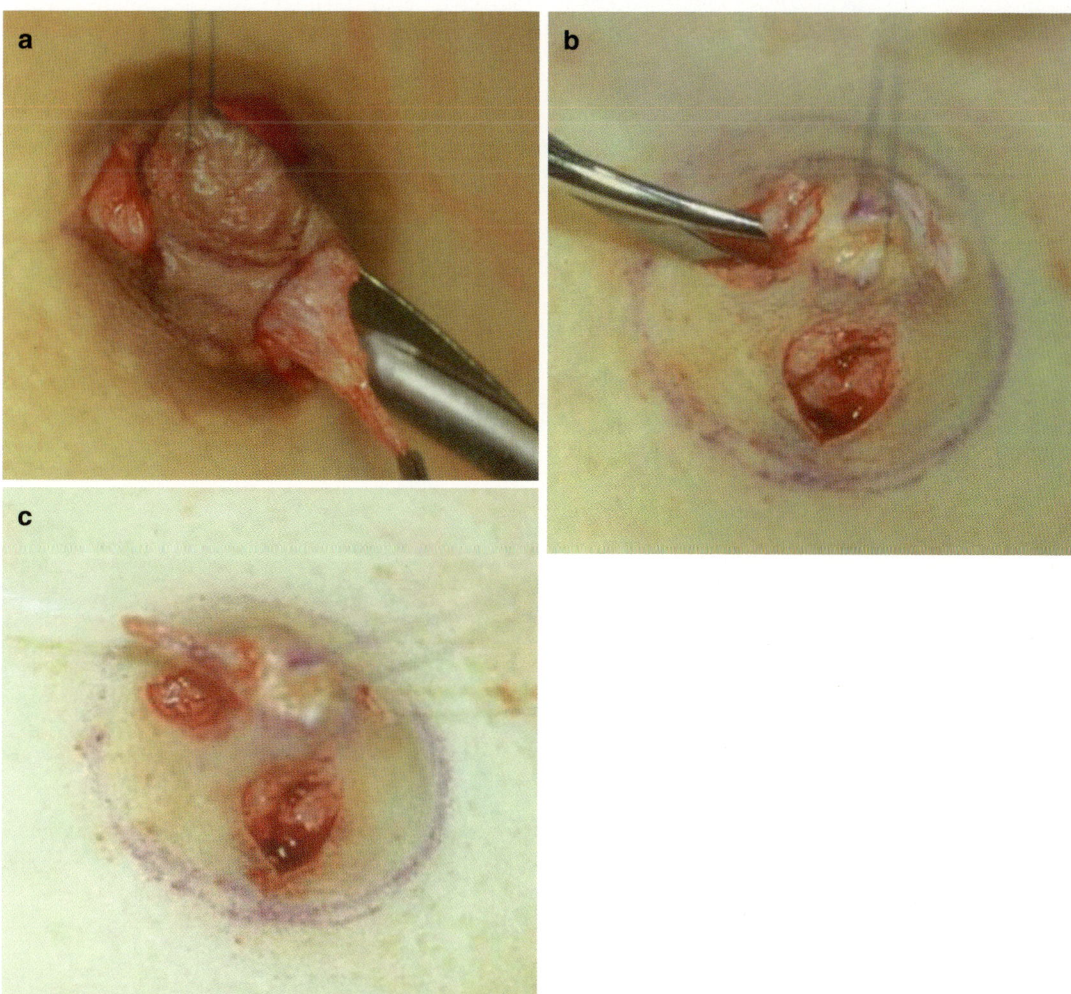


**Fig. 38.4** (**a–c**) With the help of a stay suture, temporary nipple traction is provided and the fibrotic bands underneath the nipple base are released using gentle blunt dissection

nipple creates a firm band that aids in maintaining nipple projection and helps to prevent further recurrence of nipple inversion. The shape of the projected nipple should now represent the profile of the Greek alphabet "omega" (Fig. 38.6).

The initial omega-shaped nipple might not seem ideal for some patients, but the shape changes to a round or rectangular shape with time, as we have seen in our patients. The deepithelialized defects are then closed, and primary closure can be obtained without any tension and with minimal undermining. The twisting of the dermal flaps actually has the effect of bringing the incision edges closer to each other, making closure easier and free of tension (Fig. 38.6). Dermabond® was applied over the sutures. Sutures were removed after 7–10 days, and patients were advised against using of a tight bra or compressive clothing for at least 3 weeks. No additional supportive dressings were required (Fig. 38.7).

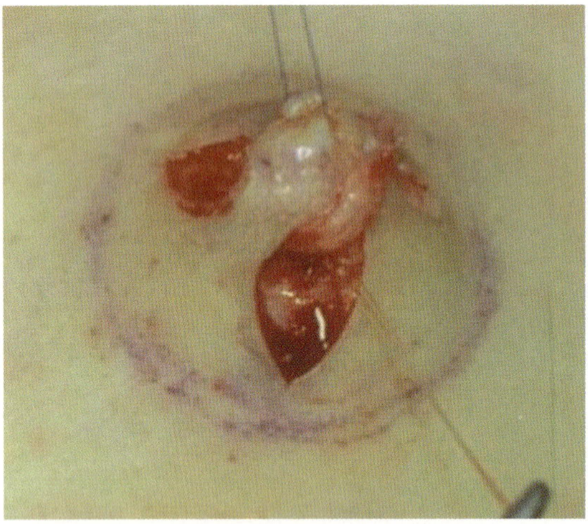

**Fig. 38.5** The elevated dermal flaps are passed through the tunnels created and sutured to the adjacent deepithelialized dermal region

## 38.3 Clinical Results

The twisting and locking principle of inverted nipple repair has shown to be an effective technique for the correction of inverted nipples (Figs. 38.8 and 38.9).

The lack of tissue bulk at the nipple base is reinforced by the three triangular dermal flaps. The shortened and fibrotic lactiferous ducts are released in three different directions and tightness at the nipple base is maintained by using the locking and twisting force provided by the three dermal flaps. The twisting and locking of the dermal flaps at the base of the nipple is adequate to maintain nipple projection without causing any strangulation of the nipple. This ensures that adequate blood supply is always maintained to the nipple and prevents the risk of necrosis.

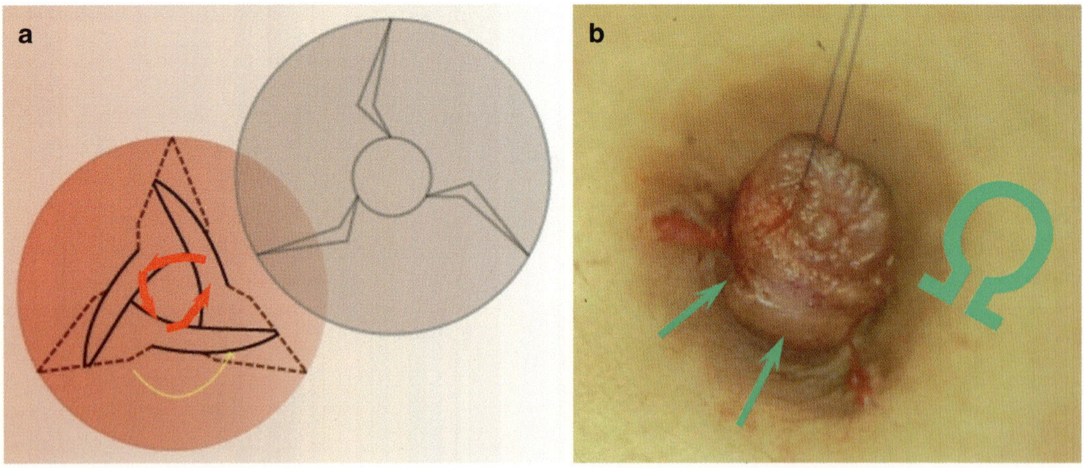


**Fig. 38.6** (**a**) Twisting of the dermal flaps at the base of the nipple creates a firm band. (**b**) Shape of the projected nipple now should represent the profile of the Greek alphabet "omega"

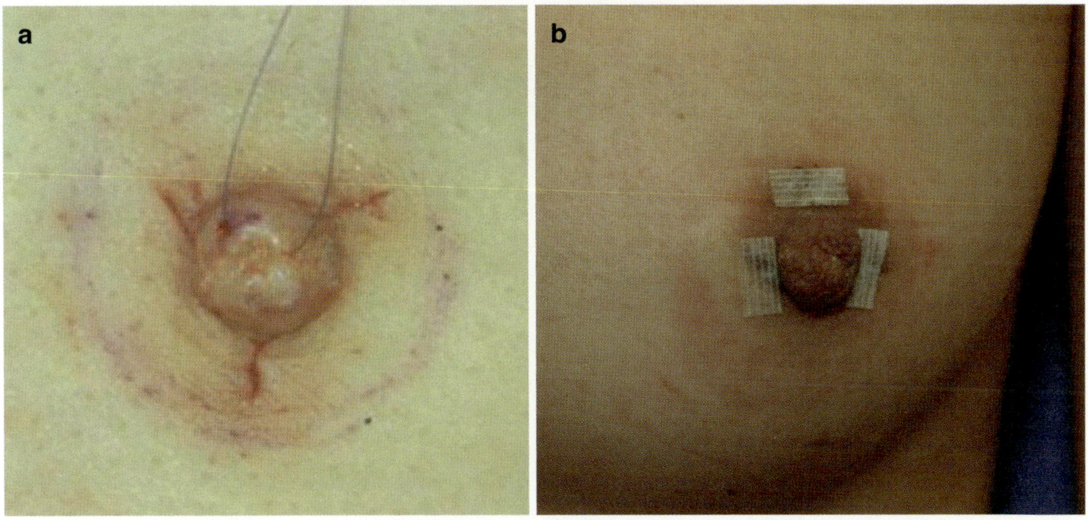

Fig. 38.7 (**a**, **b**) No additional supportive dressings were required

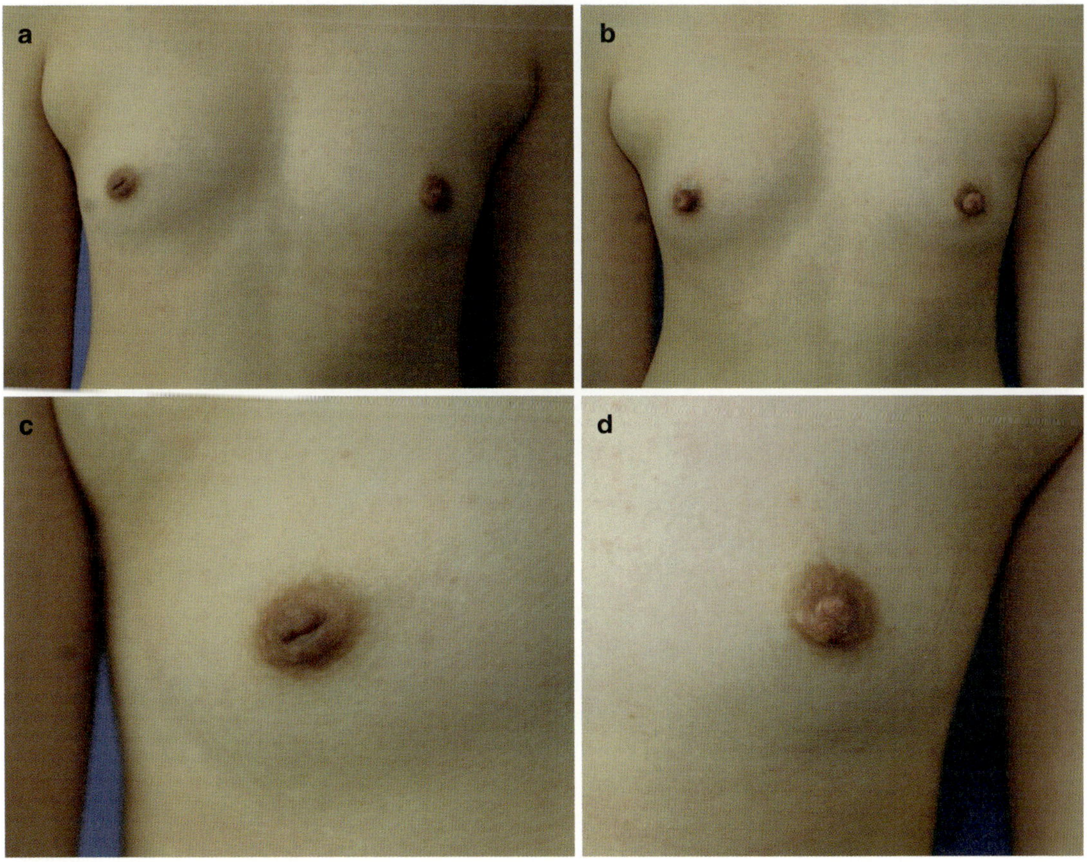

Fig. 38.8 (**a**–**h**) A patient bilateral inverted nipples with repair

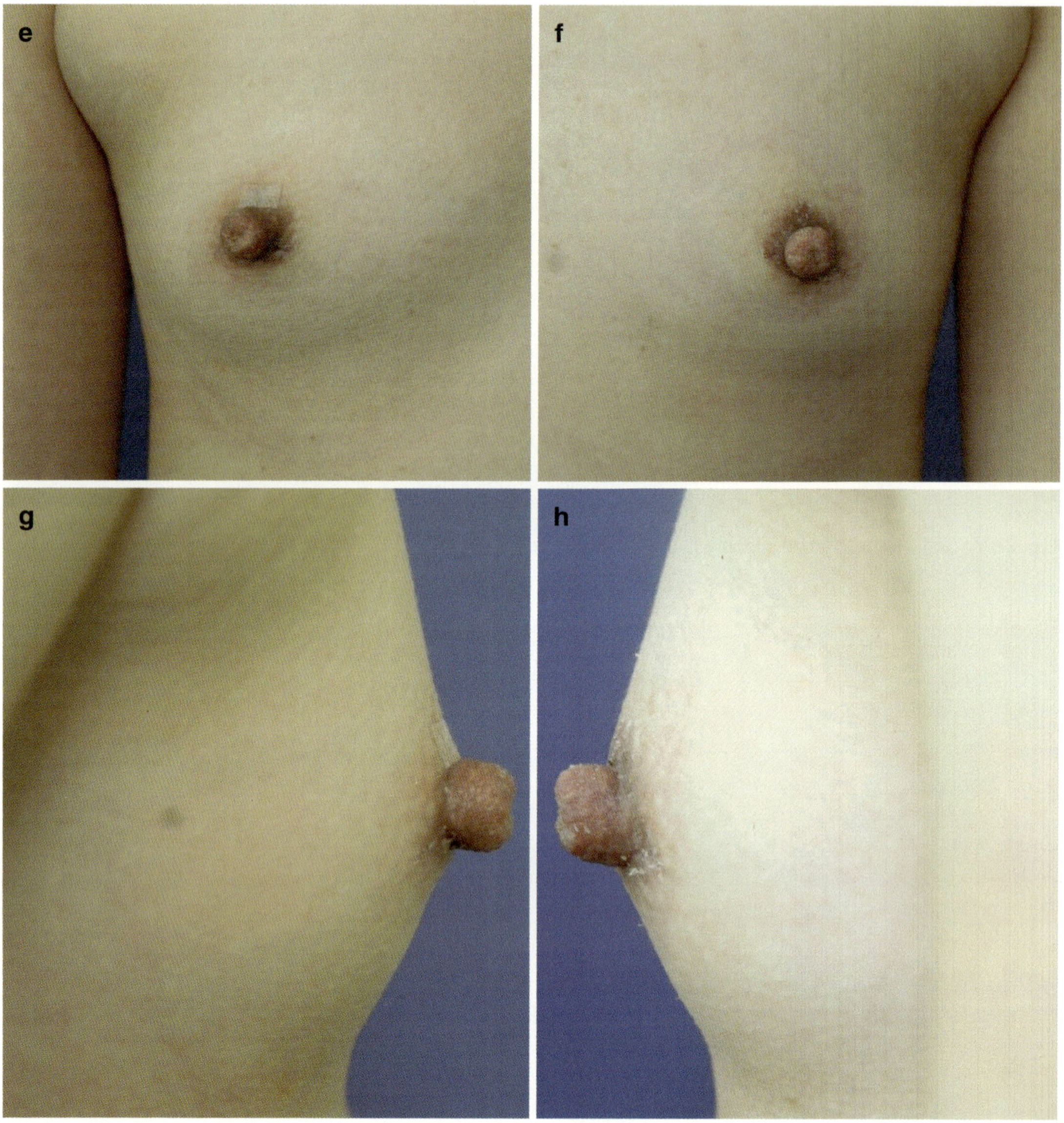


**Fig. 38.8** (continued)

Locking principle has been applied in many different types of surgeries, for example, small rectangular flaps to maintain the helical elevation in corrections for cryptotia, the M flap to keep the web space in syndactyly correction, and the C flap in Millard's method for cheiloplasty (Fig. 38.10).

No sharp dissection is required to create the tunnels for the dermal flaps and also for the release of the lactiferous ducts. This minimizes the risk of damage and transection of the lactiferous ducts, which would subsequently cause difficulty with lactation. This gentle blunt dissection also ensures that the sensation to the nipple is not damaged.

The final nipple projection and size depends on the diagonal width of lozenge, length ratio of the sides of the rhombus, pathway of tunneling, fixation level, tightening of fixation, and the tightening of the skin closure (Fig. 38.11). Nipple

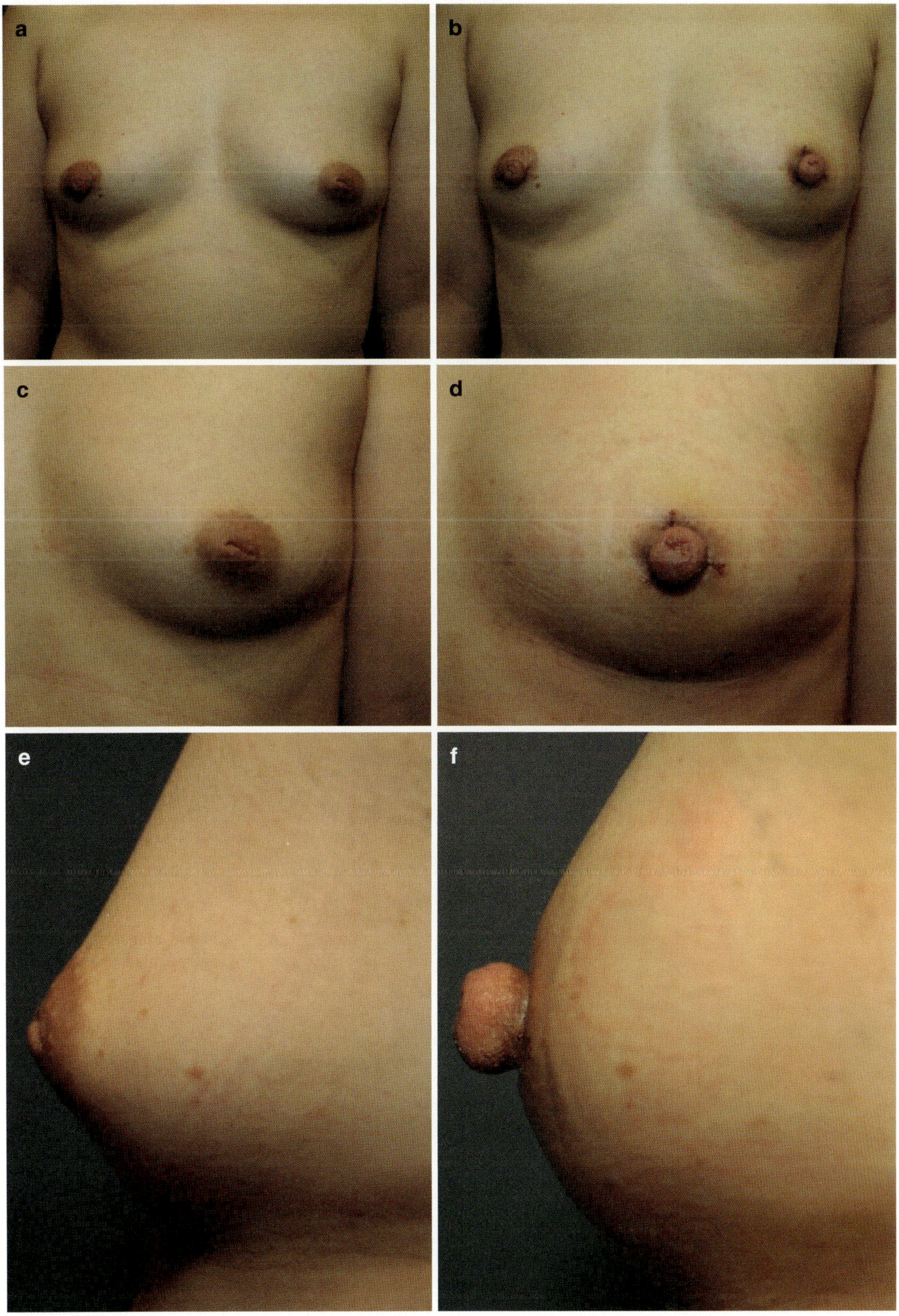


**Fig. 38.9** (**a–f**) A patient with unilateral inverted nipple with repair

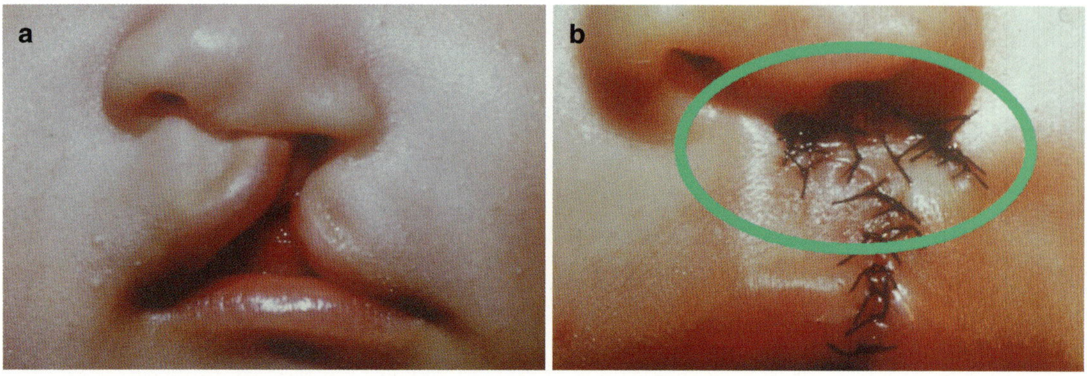


**Fig. 38.10** (**a**) Preoperative cleft lip. (**b**) The C flap in the Millard rotation advancement repair. Such a small inserting flap can occupy the space, thereby preventing the recurrence of the deformity

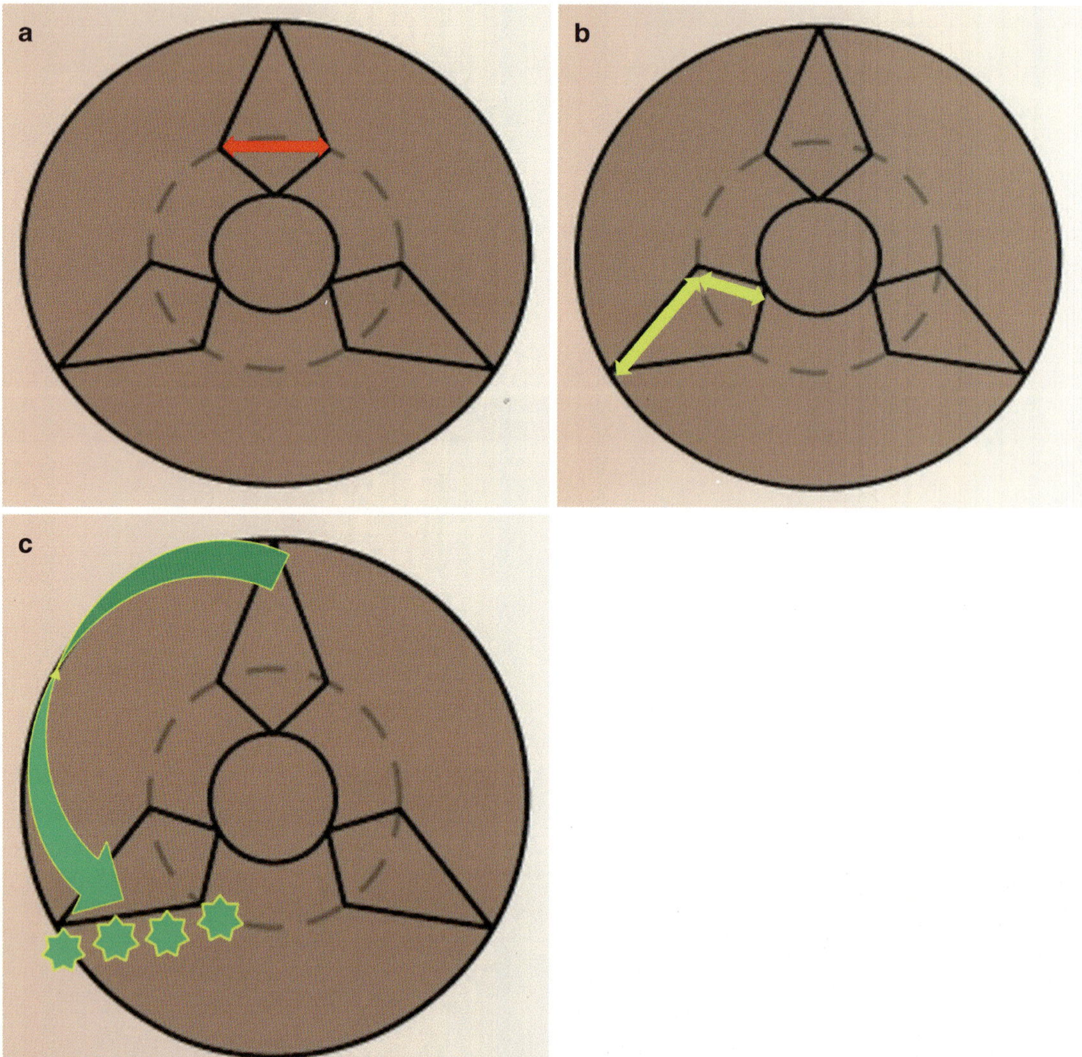


**Fig. 38.11** The final nipple projection and size depend on these several factors. (**a**) Diagonal width of the lozenge. (**b**) Length ratio of the sides of the rhombus. (**c**) Pathway of tunneling and fixation level. (**d**) Tightening of the fixation. (1) Twisting > locking. (2) Twisting < locking. (**e**) Tightening of the skin closure

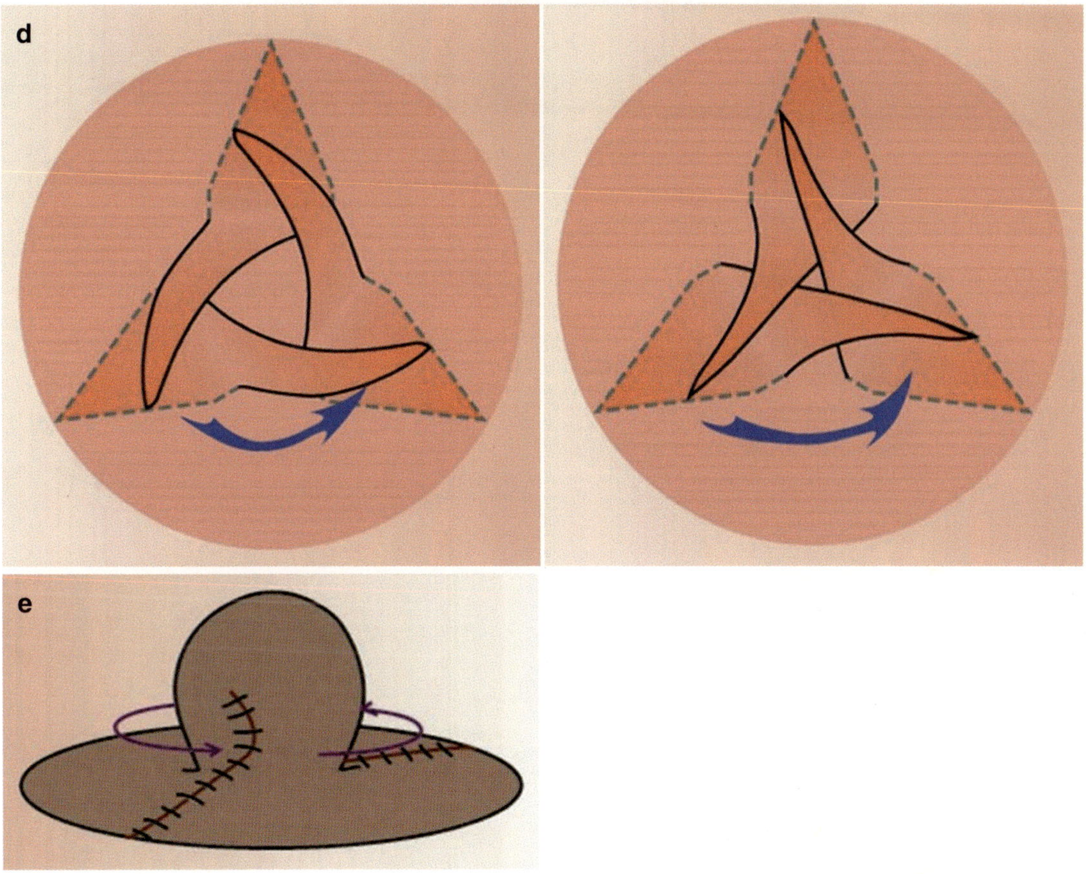


**Fig. 38.11** (continued)

shapes can be described into one of the five different types which are rectangular, round, omega, cap shaped, and slanting types (Fig. 38.12).

In a questionnaire done about the most preferred shape of the nipple, majority of women preferred the round shape followed by the rectangular. On average 25% women preferred the omega shape (Fig. 38.13). It was debated that the omega-shaped nipple appeared aged and unappealing, but in our study, it was seen that initial omega shaped changes to either the rectangular or the round variant during the follow-up period (Fig. 38.14). The procedure can also be combined with areolar reduction surgery as most women with inverted nipples also have large and pendulous breast with widened areola.

In our case series of 26 patients with a total number of 50 nipples operated on, we encountered no ischemic strangulation of any nipples. This is probably because the twisting dermal flaps maintain tension at 120° intervals and not a complete 360° band as found in the purse-string suture technique (Fig. 38.15). We encountered one patient with immediate recurrence post procedure, and this is due to the incomplete release of the contractile bands of the inverted nipples. No cases of delayed recurrence were encountered in our follow-up. No cases reported any alteration in sensation, infection, galactocele, or lactation problems.

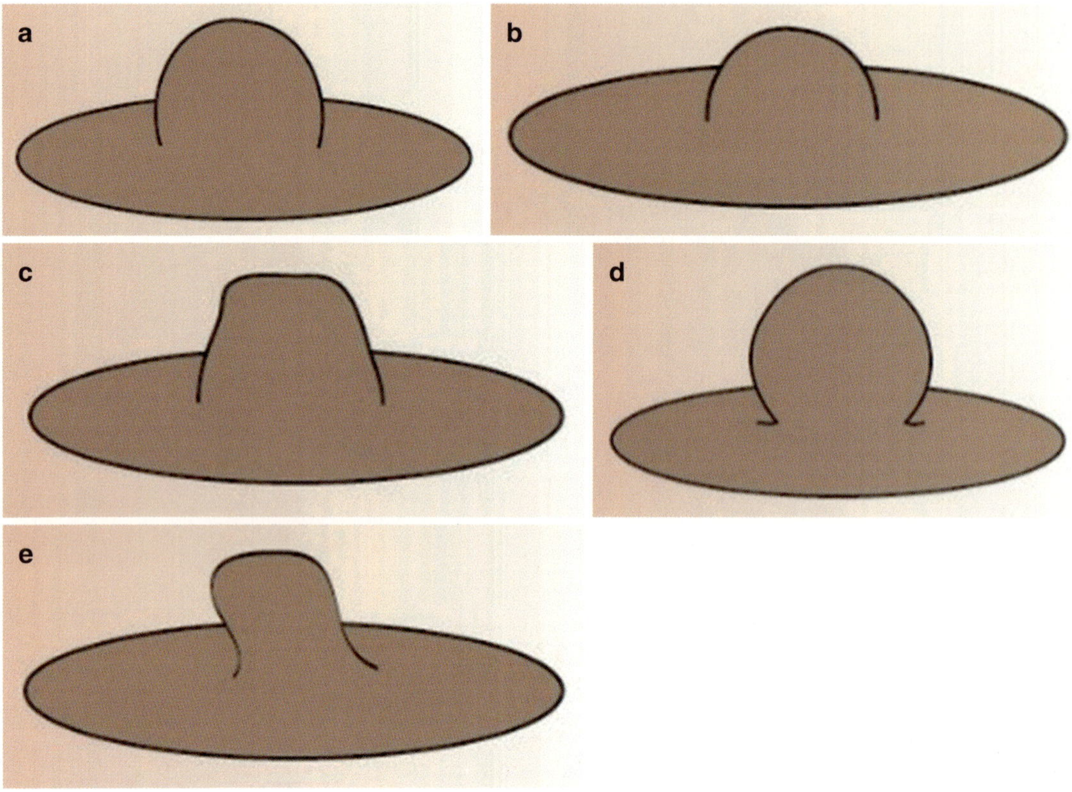


**Fig. 38.12** Nipple shapes can be described as (**a**) round, (**b**) cap shaped, (**c**) rectangular, (**d**) omega, and (**e**) slanting types

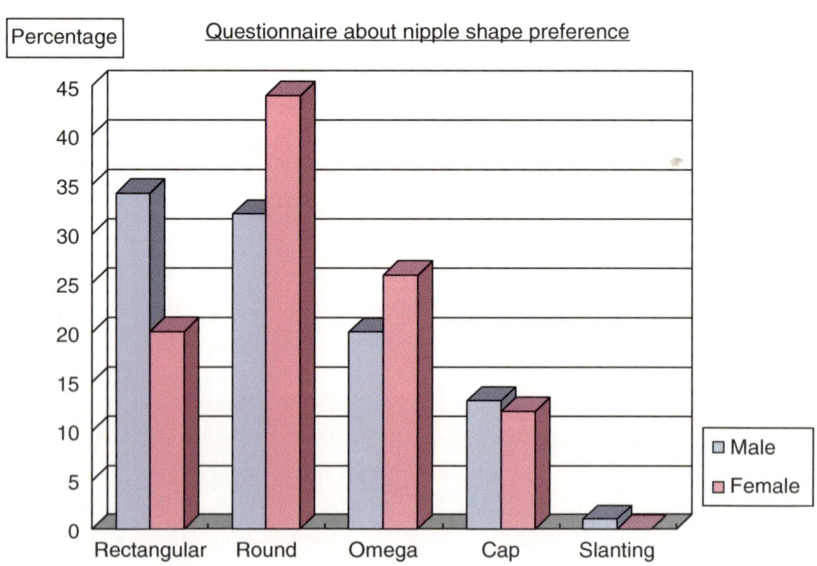


**Fig. 38.13** Questionnaire about the most preferred shape of nipple. Majority of women preferred the round shape and majority of men preferred the rectangular shape

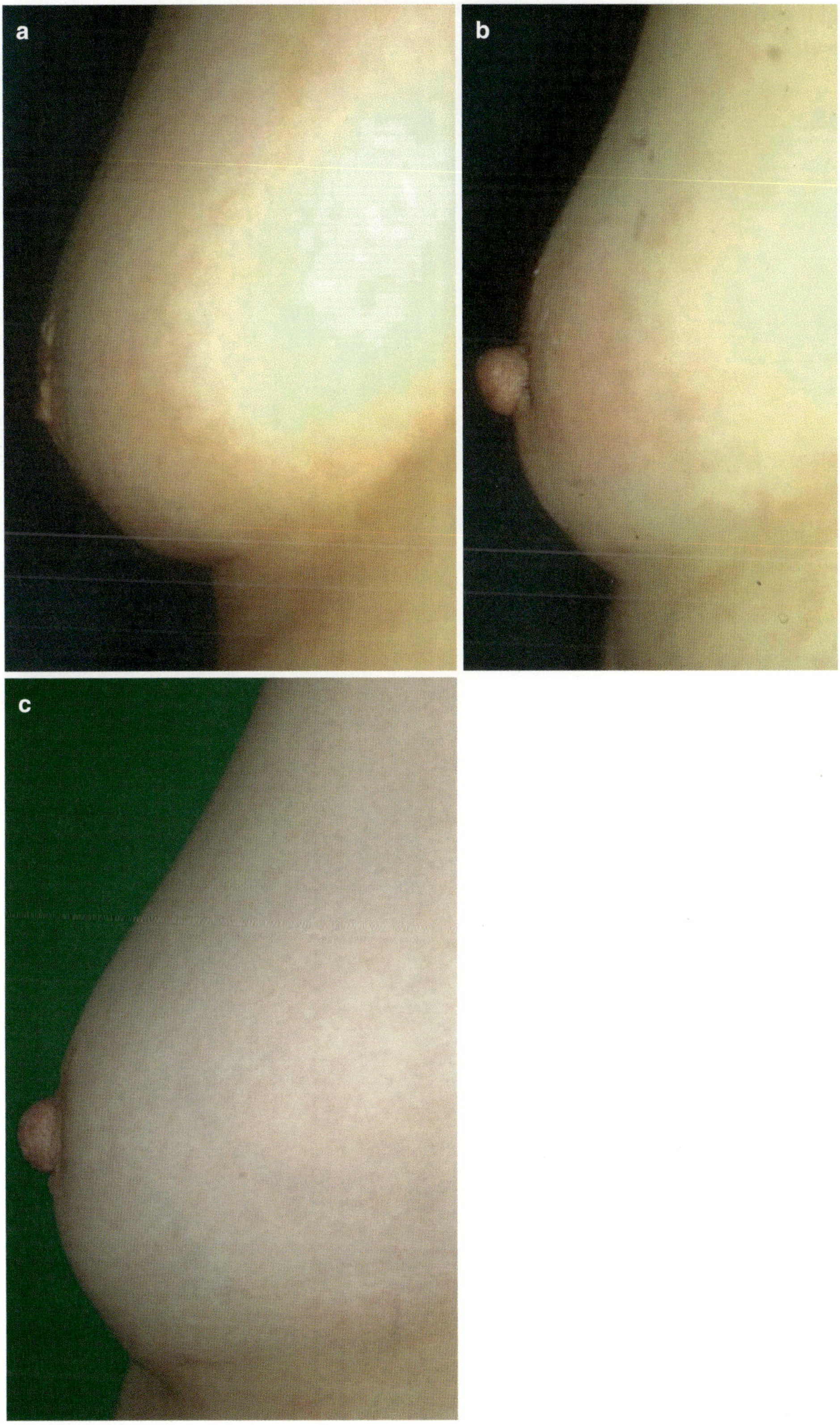


**Fig. 38.14** (**a–c**) The progression of the shape of the corrected nipple from an omega shape to that of cap shape

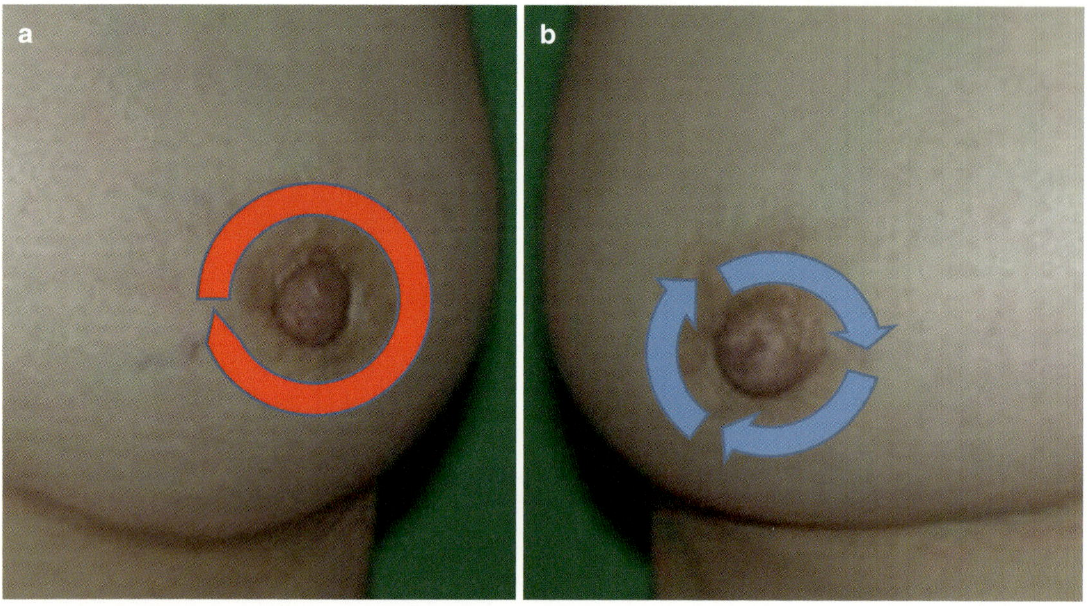


**Fig. 38.15** (**a**) Complete 360° band found in purse-string suture compared to the (**b**) 120° interval locking in the twisting locking method

**Conclusions**

The twisting and locking principle using three dermal flaps is a successful technique for the correction of inverted nipples and results in an omega-shaped and adequately projected nipple. No cases of recurrence or complications during the long-term follow-up period were seen. This simple method is highly recommended, especially considering the minimal injury inflicted on the ductal and sensory nervous systems.

## References


1. Terrill PJ, Stapleton MJ. The inverted nipple: to cut the ducts or not? Br J Plast Surg. 1991;44(5):372–7.
2. Wolfort FG, Marshall KA, Cochran TC. Correction of the inverted nipple. Ann Plast Surg. 1978;1(3):294–7.
3. Lamont E. Congenital inversion of the nipple in identical twins. Br J Plast Surg. 1973;26(2):178.
4. Skoog T. Surgical correction of inverted nipples. J Am Med Womens Assoc. 1965;20(10):931–5.
5. Teimourian B, Adham MN. Simple technique for correction of inverted nipple. Plast Reconstr Surg. 1980;65(4):504–6.
6. Broadbent TR, Woolf RM. Benign inverted nipple: trans-nipple-areolar correction. Plast Reconstr Surg. 1976;58(6):673–7.
7. Kim JT, Lim YS, Oh JG. Correction of inverted nipples with twisting and locking principles. Plast Reconstr Surg. 2006;118(7):1526–31.
8. Elsahy NI. An alternative operation for inverted nipple. Plast Reconstr Surg. 1976;57(4):438–91.
9. Teimourian B, Adham MN. Surgical correction of the tuberous breast. Ann Plast Surg. 1983;10(3):190–3.
10. Pitanguy I, Ceravolo MP. Our experience with combined procedures in aesthetic plastic surgery. Plast Reconstr Surg. 1983;71(1):56–65.
11. Crestinu JM. The inverted nipple: a blind method of correction. Plast Reconstr Surg. 1987;79(1):127–30.
12. Schwager RG, Smith JW, Gray GF, Goulian DJ. Inversion of the human female nipple, with a simple method of treatment. Plast Reconstr Surg. 1974;54(5):564–9.
13. Hauben DJ, Mahler D. A simple method for the correction of the inverted nipple. Plast Reconstr Surg. 1983;71(4):556–9.
14. Wu HL, Huang X, Zheng SS. A new procedure for correction of severe inverted nipple with two triangular areolar dermofibrous flaps. Aesthet Plast Surg. 2008;32(4):641–4.
15. Teng L, Wu GP, Sun XM, Lu JJ, Ding B, Ren M, Ji Y, Jin XL. Correction of inverted nipple: an alternative method using continuous elastic outside distraction. Ann Plast Surg. 2005;54(2):120–3.

16. Burm JS, Kim YW. Correction of inverted nipples by strong suspension with areola-based dermal flaps. Plast Reconstr Surg. 2007;120(6):1483–6.
17. Kolker AR, Torina PJ. Minimally invasive correction of inverted nipples: a safe and simple technique for reliable, sustainable projection. Ann Plast Surg. 2009;62(5):549–53.
18. Jiang HQ, Wei X, Yuan SM, Tang LM. Nipple aspirator: a self-designed instrument for inverted nipple. Plast Reconstr Surg. 2008;121(3):141e–3e.

# 39 Correction of the Inverted Nipple

Daniel J. Gould and W. Grant Stevens

## 39.1 Introduction

Nipple inversion is common, occurring in 2–10% of the female population [1]. It can be congenital or acquired, and patients report difficulty breastfeeding and interference with their sexuality when seeking treatment. Typical patients who present with an inverted nipple are self-conscious and insecure about their affected breast out of clothing. Anecdotally, it has been our experience that each of the women in our practice has complained to at least one doctor prior to seeking treatment and been told that their condition is normal and does not require intervention. Few of the patients that come to our practice are referred by another care provider, while most are self-referred through Internet search. Many seek out repair once pregnant, or after giving birth, to improve their ability to breast feed. If the inverted nipple inhibits newborn breastfeeding, it may impact parental bonding and could have lasting effects on the medical health of the child [2].

Inverted nipple is discussed with great frequency online in forums, and there are over 1,170,000 hits online for the search topic "inverted nipples affect breastfeeding." This shows the nature of the problem and the interest generated by those affected with the disorder.

Nipple inversion can be caused by failure of the lactiferous ducts to develop and grow during maturation of the breast tissue, or it can also be caused by fibrosis around the lactiferous ducts due to inflammation (mastitis, cancer, previous breast surgery) [3]. Early in the development of the fetus, the breast buds form along the milk line around the sixth week. Mammary glands develop as epithelial down growths into the mesenchymal tissue. Later, during the eighth to ninth month of development, a pit forms at the entry to the ducts. As the mesenchymal tissue and fat proliferates below the pit, this causes it to elevate above the nascent skin and forms the projection of the nipple. Failure of the growth of the mesenchyme or of lengthening of the lactiferous ducts can cause congenital inverted nipples [4].

Inverted nipples may be classified into three different categories. On review of the different classification systems, including anatomical, histological, and functional grades, we found

D.J. Gould, M.D., Ph.D. (✉)
Department of Plastic and Reconstructive Surgery, University of Southern California, 1500 San Pablo Street, Los Angeles, CA 90030, USA
e-mail: Daniel.Gould@med.usc.edu

W. Grant Stevens, M.D.
Department of Plastic and Reconstructive Surgery, University of Southern California, 1500 San Pablo Street, Los Angeles, CA 90030, USA

Marina Plastic Surgery Associates, 4644 Lincoln Boulevard, Suite 552 Marina Del Rey, Los Angeles, CA 90292, USA
e-mail: DrStevens@hotmail.com


M.A. Shiffman (ed.), *Nipple-Areolar Complex Reconstruction*,
https://doi.org/10.1007/978-3-319-60925-6_39

**Table 39.1** Inverted nipple grading system [23]

| Nipple grade | Physically retractable | Projection | Milk ducts | Breastfeeding | Fibrosis | Histology | Lactiferous ducts |
|---|---|---|---|---|---|---|---|
| 1 | Easily pulled out | Maintains projection occasionally pops up w/out manipulation | Not compromised | Possible | Minimal or none | Soft tissue deficiency present | Normal/no retraction |
| 2 | Can be pulled out | Inverted | Compromised | Very difficult if possible | Moderate | Rich collagenous stroma smooth muscle bundles | Mildly retracted/do not need to be cut for fibrosis release |
| 3 | Severely retracted/ inverted requires surgery to be protracted | Inverted | Constricted | Impossible | Remarkable fibrosis sometimes suffer from rashes infection/ poor nipple hygiene | Insufficient soft tissue, atrophic terminal duct lobular units, and severe fibrosis | Short and severely retracted |

Several different classification systems and findings are shown. Notice the key physical exam findings as well as the correlated histological findings

several different ways to delineate the different grades of inversion. We sought to form a unified grading system, which combines all of the different descriptors of the different grades of nipples. Here, in Table 39.1 we combine all the known classification systems and common findings for easy reference. Nipple inversion may be stratified based on the amount of eversion possible and the projection that can be maintained with traction. The surgical treatment of the inverted nipple relies on several basic principles, including maintenance of as many of the functional lactiferous ducts as possible, meticulous dissection of the fibrous attachments surrounding the duct system, mattress suture placement at the nipple base to oppose the underlying tissue and close the dead space maintaining eversion, running suture at the base of the nipple in selected cases, and the use of a stent to maintain the nipple in a projected state as it heals [3].

Several articles have described different techniques [5–8] for the correction of the inverted nipple. In this chapter we review the technique previously published in the Aesthetic Surgery Journal by Stevens et al. in 2004 [6], and we explore the demographics of our patients and complications specifically for recurrence.

## 39.2 Surgical Technique

Nipple eversion is primarily achieved using gentle traction with a single skin hook (Fig. 39.1). Then, the nipple base is freed up through an inferior incision at the nipple base. Fibrous bands which constrict the base of the nipple are freed up through blunt dissection using a vertical spreading technique parallel to the ducts. This helps to restore nipple projection. Ductal structures should be easily visualized and preserved during dissection. The ducts are easily visually identified—they are tubular nonvascular structures, which are larger with different consistency than nerves. They do not appear similar to scar tissue. Only when necessary, selective ductal division may be performed to achieve complete eversion with normal projection. This technique releases tension by incrementally dividing the peripheral lactiferous ducts under direct vision. Two external 4-0 Vicryl horizontal mattress sutures are then placed, one from 12 o'clock to the 6 o'clock positions and one from the 3 o' clock to the 9 o'clock positions. It is important to make the entry and exit points of the suture as close together as possible to avoid vascular embarrassment. These

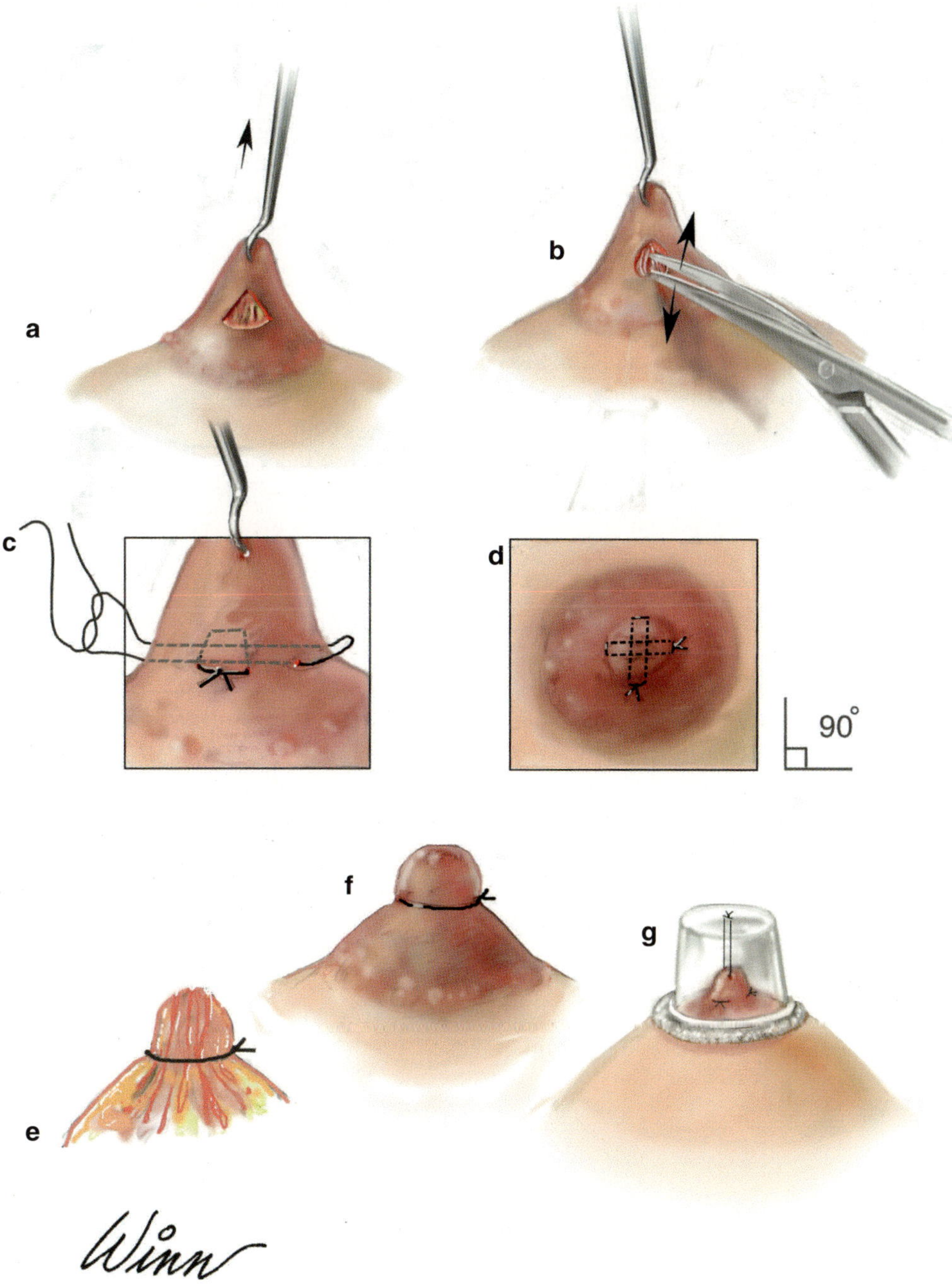


**Fig. 39.1** Technique for the repair of the inverted nipple. (**a**) This process involves a dissection down to the lactiferous ducts, (**b**) followed by vertical spreading to prevent unnecessary division of ducts. (**c**, **d**) Then the bolster sutures are passed at 90° opposition to draw the nipple skin together around the ducts. (**e**, **f**) An external purse string can be passed, and the most important step is (**g**) applying a nipple stent by placing a nylon suture through a medicine cup and through the nipple to apply upward traction as the nipple heals

sutures serve to draw together opposing nipple-areolar dermal flaps, providing stability and reducing dead space. It is important to obliterate the dead space but to avoid compromising vascular flow and to avoid constricting the lactiferous ducts. Theoretically the orientation of the sutures should minimize restriction of the ducts, because the sutures are longitudinally oriented, parallel to duct structures. But in practice, the surgeon has to be careful to apply the correct tension and to ensure exact placement of the sutures to avoid circumscribing the ducts, and to avoid tamponading the ducts through pressure from the nipple complex. An external 4-0 chromic purse-string suture may then be run at the junction of the nipple-areola border (Fig. 39.1). The perpendicular sutures are placed very close together to limit vascular disruption. The cerclage suture is placed in the dermis not affecting the parenchymal/ductal blood supply to the nipple. We have not had any cases of vascular embarrassment, although the nipple is checked before the patient is discharged (30 min after procedure) and on postoperative day 1. Last, a 4-0 nylon traction suture is placed through the point of highest projection of the nipple and affixed to a stent consisting of a medicine cup and gauze padding. This traction helps to exert an anteriorly directed force that maintains the nipple in an overcorrected position and it serves as a stent. Traction is maintained for 2–5 days, and this time period is selected based on ease of retraction—if the nipple retracts easily, traction is 2 days (grades 1 and 2), and if it is densely fibrotic, the stent is maintained for 5 days (grade 3). If there is any sign of vascular compromise, the stent is removed. In follow-up evaluations we assess maintenance of nipple eversion and subjective patient satisfaction. If the nipple is corrected but the patient desires more projection, fillers may help augment the projection, but there is no data on how they may affect the lactiferous ducts, and this not a standard on label use of the product. Since there is a significant recurrence rate, it is a standard protocol within this practice to frequently schedule follow-up appointments, to provide appropriate patient counseling and to offer secondary surgery for recurrent nipple inversion. When there is a recurrence of the inverted nipple, we repeat the same procedure; with the hope the repeated release of the nipple will free the underlying stromal attachments.

## 39.3 Results

Figures 39.2, 39.3, and 39.4 are typical of the inverted nipple repair. Note the improved nipple projection, without manual extraction. The nipples are proud and react to stimulation and temperature. Several patients undergoing this repair anecdotally experienced improved body image and improved breastfeeding behaviors, though this data was not expressly documented in each case.

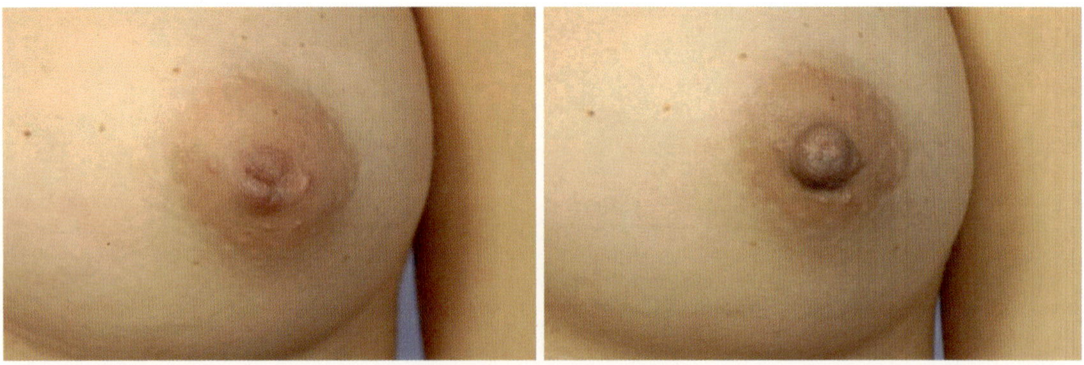

**Fig. 39.2** Long-term follow-up. (*Left*) Preoperatively this 23-year-old female was reported as a 34 B, who came in for bilateral repair. (*Right*) Fourteen months postoperative

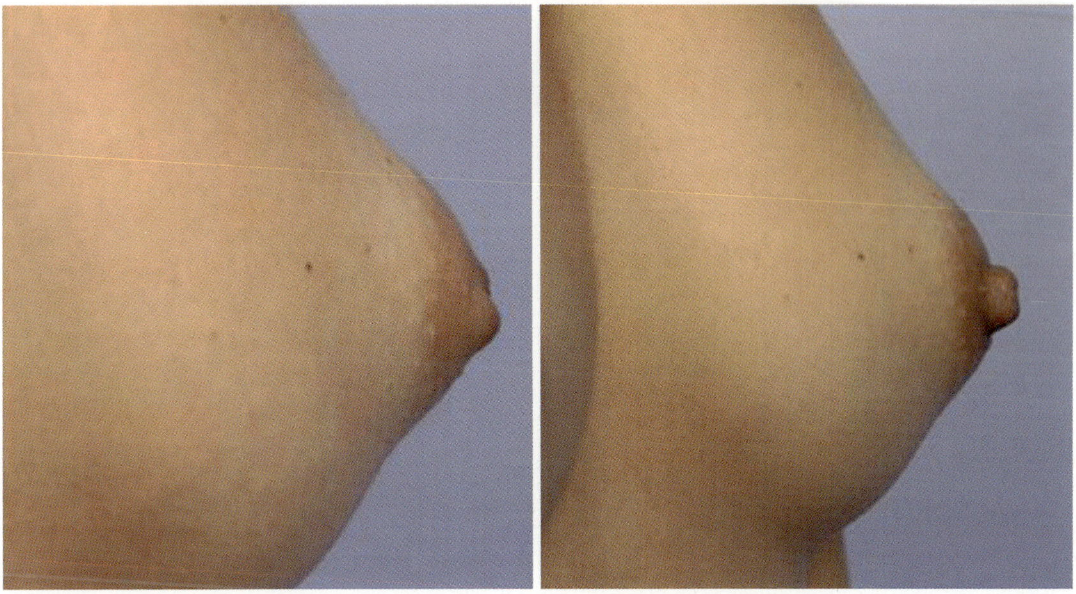

**Fig. 39.2** (continued)

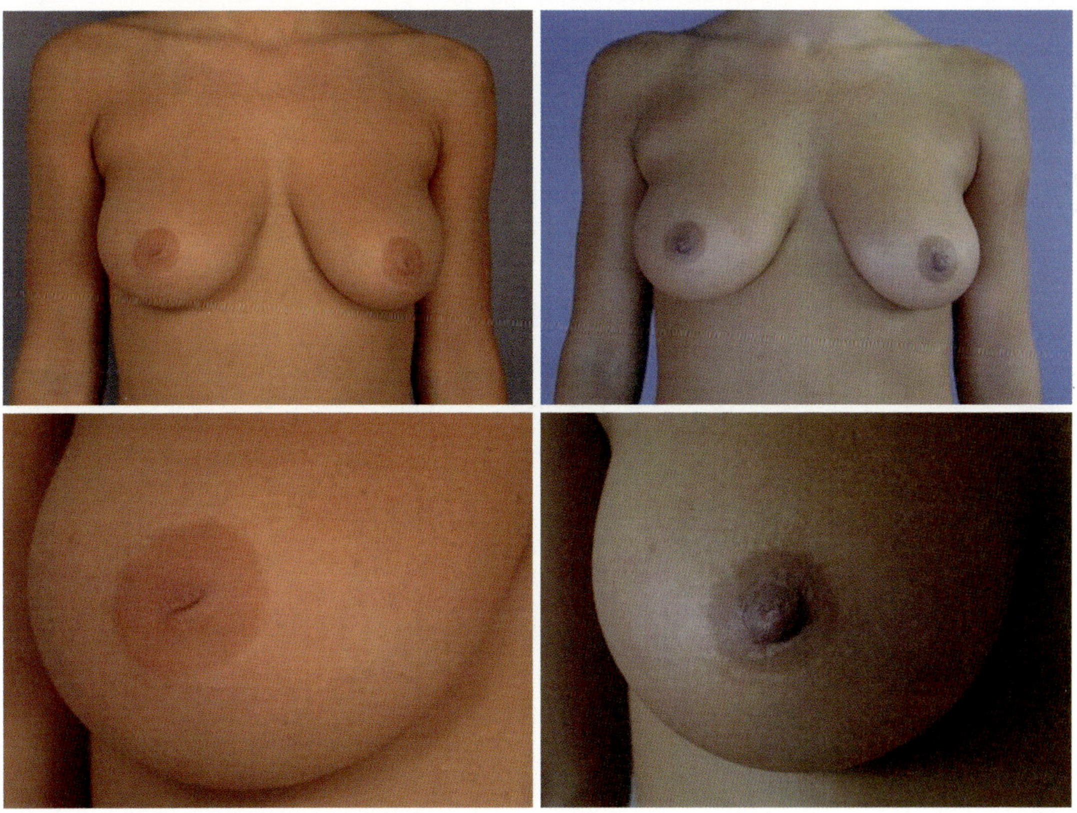

**Fig. 39.3** Long-term follow-up. (*Left*) Preoperative 23-year-old female was reported as a 34 C who came in for bilateral repair. (*Right*) Fifteen months after inverted nipple repair

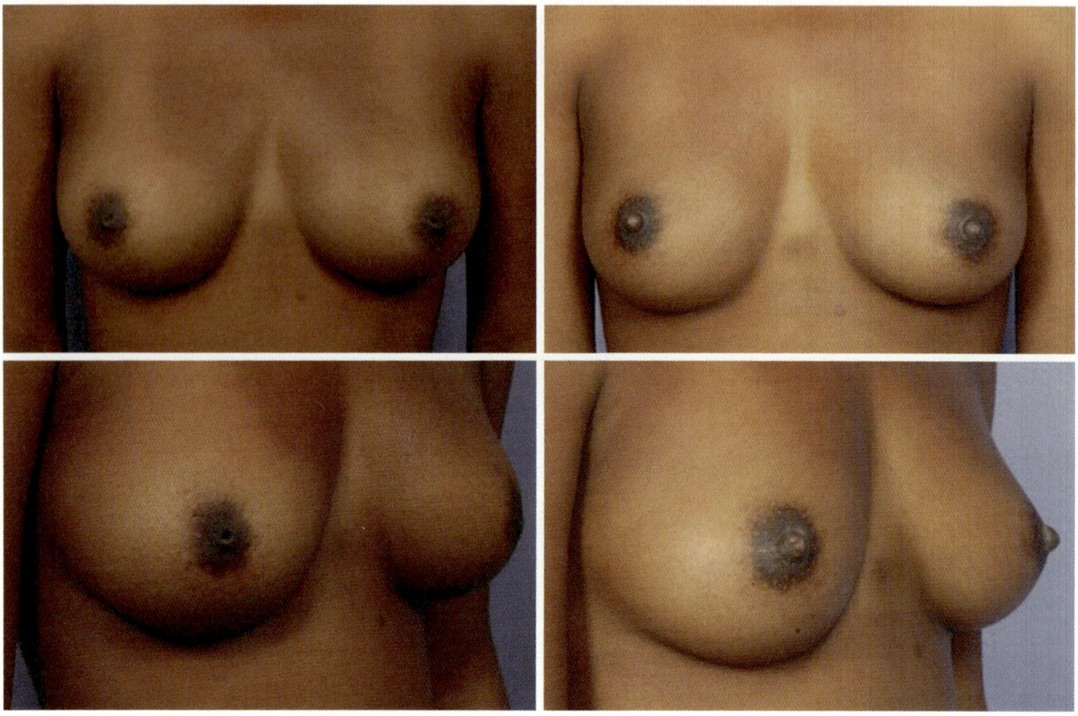

**Fig. 39.4** Inverted nipple repair in an African-American woman. (*Left*) Preoperative 23-year-old female with a 34 C bra size who presented due to deformity of the nipples which she said affected her relationship with her current boyfriend. At 6 weeks postoperative, there was improved projection without significant scarring. (*Right*) Fourteen months postoperative

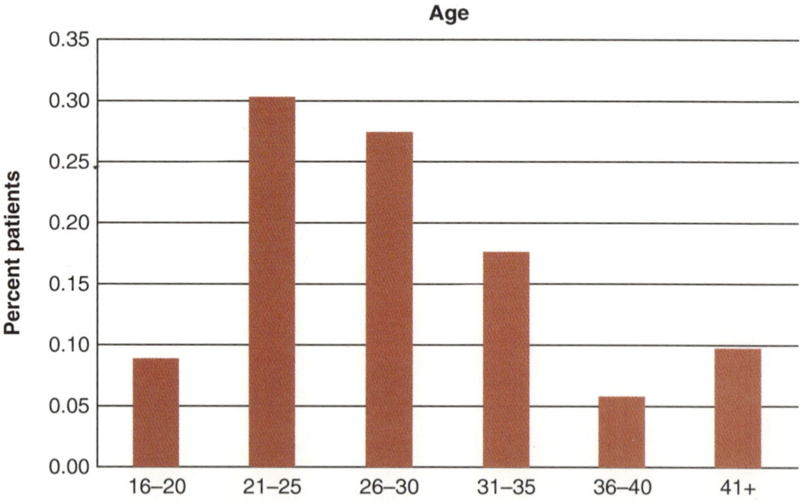


**Fig. 39.5** Age histogram. The ages of the women who chose to undergo this surgery with most being between 20 and 30 years old

The age of the patients seen for inverted nipple repair is fairly young, with most being in their twenties (Fig. 39.5). Several very young females sought this procedure out and care was made to be sure they had achieved appropriate complete breast development prior to offering surgery. These young women were often self-referred through the Internet though a small number were referred by their primary care doctors.

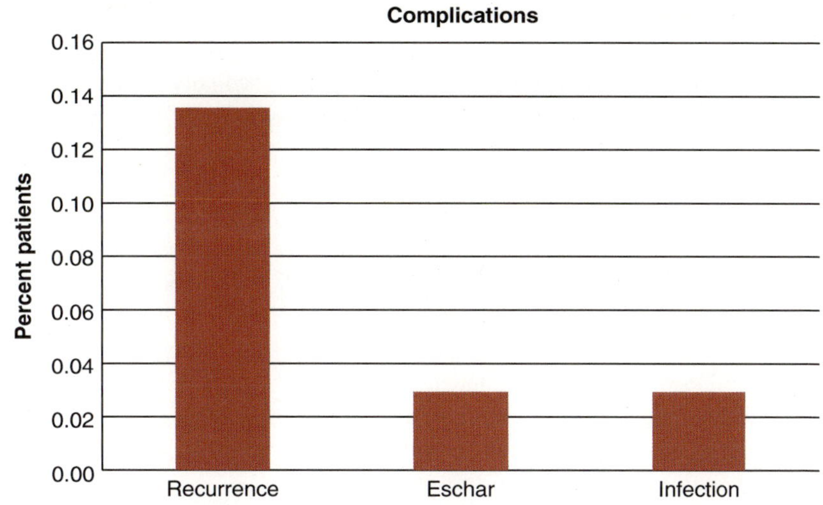


**Fig. 39.6** Rate of complications per patient, not per nipple procedure. Most complications involved recurrence with a small number of cases of infection or eschar. When normalized per procedure, the rate of recurrence is 7% and the rate of complication either eschar or redness and possible infection is 3%

## 39.4 Complications

The total rate of complications, including recurrence, partial nipple epidermolysis, eschar, or breast cellulitis when corrected per nipple surgery is approximately 10% (Fig. 39.6). The vast majority of the complication rate is attributed to recurrence. In our recent study, four women received injections of filler to augment nipple projection, and each time they were injected with calcium hydroxylapatite microspheres in a water-based gel carrier.

## 39.5 Discussion

A review of the literature was conducted to revisit some of the past reported techniques for inverted nipple repair in an effort to compare and contrast reported rates of complications and outcomes. Many methods were found which have been used to correct the inverted nipple, some being more invasive then others [9–22].

In our review in 2015 [23] we found several good retrospective studies with relevance [9–22], though only three studies had high numbers of patients [12, 13, 21] and one of these studies had no data on recurrence rates or complications [13]. One study had a high number of operations (452 nipples) but only described one recurrence and no complications, without data on postoperative long-term follow-up [21]. Several other studies involved between 11 and 17 patients and described no recurrence [9–11], with one study describing only one out of 16 patients [10]. In the most comprehensive study of these, they described 53 patients with a 1-year follow-up, no recurrences, and a 5% complication rate [12]. The caveat to this study is that they required all of their patients to wear nipple retractors for at least 6 months. This requires extreme patient compliance and diligence on behalf of the surgeon and may only be practical in a controlled setting.

In comparison our recent study shows a complication rate of about 3% per patient, and 7% recurrence rate per patient (happening in at least one nipple). The higher rate of recurrence may be due to differences in nipple retractor length of use, but also may be due to differences in demographics of patients with different BMI and ethnicity, and thus intrinsic differences in rates of contracture and fibrosis.

Some of the limitations of this study include that it was done in a retrospective manner, without prospective cohorts. There was no opportunity to prospectively track changes in self-image and patient satisfaction. Also there were no standardized reporting forms for the tracking of patient outcomes and no set follow-up dates. Importantly, there were some women who sought correction for aesthetic reasons, and it is unknown if they later became pregnant and were able to breast feed. This information would be valuable to our understanding of how this procedure affects breastfeeding and the lactiferous ducts. An important limitation is in our ability to asses lactiferous duct patency and disruption. In this procedure, the ducts are directly visualized which should reduce disruption. Also many patients have gone on to breastfeed, which has been discussed in follow-up visits although not formally recorded. Most of the literature discussing techniques so far has included very small sample sizes and is therefore inaccurate in terms of reporting recurrence rates or complication. The few studies that approach this study in size have better recurrence rates but require long-term external wires (6 months) [12] or complete disruption of the ducts [13].

### Conclusions

In this chapter we examine inverted nipple repair. Inverted nipple is a fairly common condition, but it is uncommonly repaired surgically. In our experience, this procedure is safe and effective. This condition can greatly affect the psyche of those with the deformity. Repair benefits not only the patient and their body image, but also their ability to bond with newborns and to effectively breastfeed in some cases. Here we show that inverted nipples can be repaired with relative efficacy, with a recurrence rate of approximately 13% of patients, or 7% of nipples. That being said in our practice, the potential for failure is always and should always be discussed in depth with the patient to ensure informed consent and to plan for repeated surgery if needed.

Interestingly, very few referrals for this corrective and reconstructive procedure came from primary care physicians or OB-GYN physicians, despite the fact that almost all of the patients reported having mentioned their concerns to these practitioners. Most of the patients at our practice had researched inverted nipple repair online and had located the practice based on our 2004 publication and online forums. Future studies documenting the psychosocial and breastfeeding benefits of this procedure in an objective manner would likely help bridge the referral gap.

**Conflict of Interest Statement** This research received no specific grant from any funding agency in the public, commercial, or not-for-profit sectors. The individual authors have no conflicts of interest to declare as they relate to this study and the findings.

## References

1. Park HS, Yoon CH, Kim HJ. The prevalence of congenital inverted nipple. Aesthet Plast Surg. 1999;23(2):144–6.
2. Leung AK, Sauve RS. Breast is best for babies. J Natl Med Assoc. 2005;97(7):1010–9.
3. Schwager RG, Smith JW, Gray GF, Goulian D Jr. Inversion of the human female nipple, with a simple method of treatment. Plast Reconstr Surg. 1974;54(5):564–9.
4. Koyama S, Wu HJ, Easwaran T, Thopady S, Foley J. The nipple: a simple intersection of mammary gland and integument, but focal point of organ function. J Mammary Gland Biol Neoplasia. 2013;18(2):121–31.
5. Persichetti P, Poccia I, Pallara T, Delle Femmine PF, Marangi GF. A new simple technique to correct nipple inversion using 2 V-Y advancement flaps. Ann Plast Surg. 2011;67(4):343–5.
6. Stevens WG, Fellows DR, Vath SD, Stoker DA. An integrated approach to the repair of inverted nipples. Aesthet Surg J. 2004;24(3):211–5.
7. Kolker AR, Torina PJ. Minimally invasive correction of inverted nipples: a safe and simple technique for reliable, sustainable projection. Ann Plast Surg. 2009;62(5):549–53.
8. Chen SH, Gedebou T, Chen PH. The endoscope as an adjunct to correction of nipple inversion deformity. Plast Reconstr Surg. 2007;119(4):1178–82.
9. Lee MJ, Depoli PA, Casas LA. Aesthetic and predictable correction of the inverted nipple. Aesthet Surg J. 2003;23(5):353–6.
10. Durgun M, Ozakpinar HR, Selcuk CT, Sarici M, Ceran C, Seven E. Inverted nipple correction with dermal flaps and traction. Aesthet Plast Surg. 2014;38(3):533–9.
11. Lee HB, Roh TS, Chung YK, Kim SW, Kim JB, Shin KS. Correction of inverted nipple using strut reinforcement with deepithelialized triangular flaps. Plast Reconstr Surg. 1998;102(4):1253–8.
12. Long X, Zhao R. Nipple retractor to correct inverted nipples. Breast Care (Basel). 2011;6(6):463–5.

13. Min KH, Park SS, Heo CY, Min KW. Scar-free technique for inverted-nipple correction. Aesthet Plast Surg. 2010;34(1):116–9.
14. Alexander J, Campbell M. Prevalence of inverted and non-protractile nipples in antenatal women who intend to breast-feed. Breast. 1997;6(2):72–8.
15. Kim JT, Lim YS, Oh JG. Correction of inverted nipples with twisting and locking principles. Plast Reconstr Surg. 2006;118(7):1526–31.
16. Serra-Renom J, Fontdevila J, Monner J. Correction of the inverted nipple with an internal 5 point star suture. Ann Plast Surg. 2004;53(3):293–6.
17. Jiang HQ, Wei X, Yuan SM, Tang LM. Nipple aspirator: a self-designed instrument for inverted nipple. Plast Reconstr Surg. 2008;121(3):141e–3e.
18. Yamada N, Kakibuchi M, Kitayoshi H, Kurokawa M, Hosokawa K, Hashimoto K. A method for correcting an inverted nipple with an artificial dermis. Aesthet Plast Surg. 2004;28(4):233–8.
19. Ritz M, Silfen R, Morgan D, Southwick G. Simple technique for inverted nipple correction. Aesthet Plast Surg. 2005;29(1):24–7.
20. Huang WC. A new method for correction of inverted nipple with three periductal dermofibrous flaps. Aesthet Plast Surg. 2003;27(4):301–4.
21. Crestinu JM. The correction of inverted nipples without scars: 17 years' experience, 452 operations. Aesthet Plast Surg. 2000;24(1):52–7.
22. Pompei S, Tedesco M. A new surgical technique for the correction of the inverted nipple. Aesthet Plast Surg. 1999;23(5):371–4.
23. Gould DJ, Nadeau MH, Macias LH, Stevens WG. Inverted nipple repair revisited: a 7-year experience. Aesthet Surg J. 2015;35(2):156–64.

# Convenient Nipple Splint Using Aquaplast Thermoplastic (Optimold) After Surgical Correction of the Inverted Nipple

# 40

Seong Cheol Yu

## 40.1 Introduction

There are various surgical techniques to correct an inverted nipple, but no one is free from its recurrence. It is well known that postoperative suspension of the pulled up nipple is helpful to avoid relapse [1–3]. But inconvenience of attaching the suspension device for several days is another problem. A comfortable nipple suspension device using a heat-malleable material of Aquaplast Thermoplastic (Optimold) was newly designed and introduced here.

## 40.2 Technique

A 1 mm thickness sheet of Optimold is tailored into a piece of about 15 × 50 mm with a pair of scissors. It is soaked in a hot water bath of 80–90 °C. In about 10 seconds, it turns very malleable and is taken out. Then it is flipped on a towel several times to drain residual water and manually molded into "Ω" shape which has a dome and two base plates. The dome should be slightly larger and higher than the corrected nipple. In a few minutes, it becomes hard and cool to room temperature. After completion of pulling up procedures for the retracted nipple, regardless of operation technique, it was applied on the nipple-areolar complex as a kind of a nipple splint. Its dome was placed right on the projected nipple and its base plates on areola (Fig. 45.1). Two pieces of 3-0 nylon thread are prepared as traction sutures which pierce the top of the nipple. One end of each thread is arranged upward from it and the other end downward to be tied on the roof of the splint. The raised nipple is suspended from the dome of the nipple splint in proper tension. It is usually maintained for about 7 days (Figs. 40.1 and 40.2) [4].

Every patient is routinely educated to check the condition of the operated nipple 3–4 times per day for herself at home and return to clinic if she finds any significant changes in color, ecchymosis, edema, turgor, pain, bleeding, etc.

## 40.3 Discussion

Though a lot of surgical techniques for correcting inverted nipples have been reported, occasional recurrence is inevitable. To prevent or reduce this tricky situation, postoperative nipple support by suspension of the corrected nipple is known to be useful in terms of protecting pressure on the nipple and stabilizing eversion state.

S.C. Yu, M.D., Ph.D.
Department of Plastic and Reconstructive Surgery, Gangneung Asan Hospital, University of Ulsan, College of Medicine, 415 Bangdong-ri, Sacheon-myeon, Gangneung-si, Gangwon-do 210-711, Republic of Korea
e-mail: sugarglass@hanmail.net


M.A. Shiffman (ed.), *Nipple-Areolar Complex Reconstruction*,
https://doi.org/10.1007/978-3-319-60925-6_40

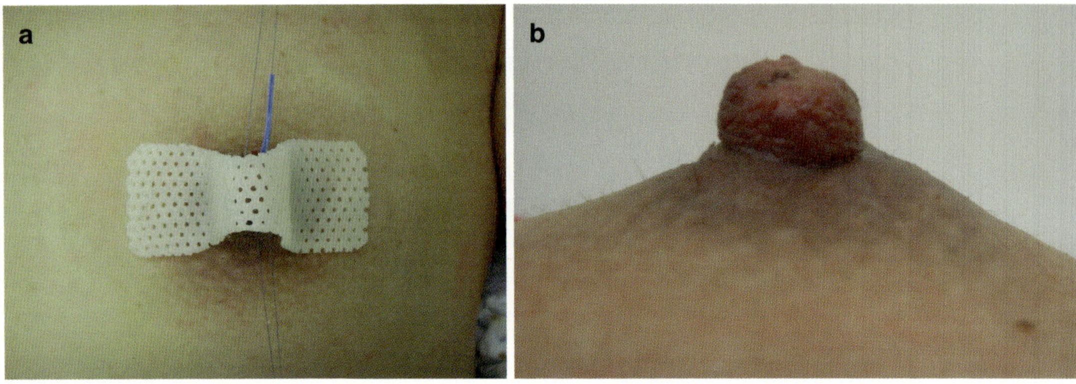


**Fig. 40.1** (**a**, **b**) Application of "Ω" shape nipple splint as suspension device using a heat-malleable material of Aquaplast Thermoplastic (Optimold). The everted nipple was suspended by two traction sutures with 3-0 nylon on top of the splint for 7 days

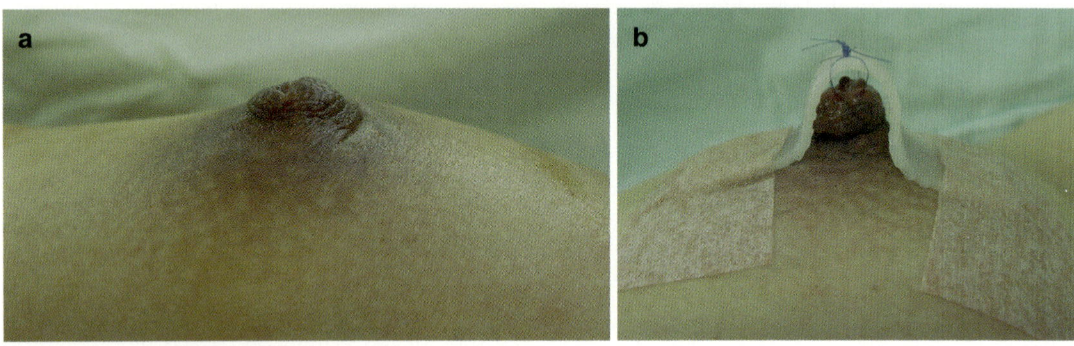


**Fig. 40.2** Correction of the inverted nipple. (**a**) Preoperative patient was a 36-year-old female with retracted nipple on her left breast. (**b**) One month after operation

Several suspension devices are reported [1–3]. But attaching and maintaining those devices cause additional discomforts to patients. As mentioned in other articles, Kurihara's [3] thick paper model is complicated to make and easily breakable; Han's [2] Sombrero (Mexican hat) splint is also difficult to make to proper shape and size. Lee's [1] plastic container (biopsy bottle) is a little bulky and uncomfortable to wear.

This "Ω" shape nipple suspension device is a kind of nipple splint using a heat-malleable material of Aquaplast Thermoplastic (Optimold). On account of its plasticity in hot water, this splint is quick and simple to make. It is also easily made to be tightly adaptive. Other advantages of lightness, compact size, durability, and slim fit wearing give patients much comfort in routine activities for several days. Postoperative impairment of nipple circulation is unusual; nevertheless, it may occur in simple procedures. As is well known, checking out the operated nipple, especially its circulation, is important to avoid rarely probable but serious situation such as nipple necrosis. So, easy monitoring is necessary for patients and surgeons, but most suspension devices have common drawback of difficult monitoring. With open sides of the splint, it enables patients and surgeons to conveniently monitor the blood circulation of the operated nipple without disturbing the dressing (Fig. 40.1). This can be a significant merit for patients who are far away or have difficulty visiting the clinic again due to personal reasons. Because of easy self-monitoring, frequent checking out and early detection of compromised nipple are possible. It is a prerequisite for early action to salvage the nipple in danger [4].

## Conclusions

Regardless of correction techniques, nothing is free from the recurrence of the inverted nipple. Postoperative suspension of the projected nipple is helpful to avoid tricky relapse but causes considerable discomfort to patients and surgeons. This "Ω" shape nipple splint using a heat-malleable sheet of Aquaplast Thermoplastic (Optimold) is a comfortable nipple suspension device which is simple, small, and light. It is simple and quick to make. It also gives effective, stable suspension of the everted nipple and easy self-monitoring.

## References

1. Lee TJ, Kim WR. Nipple Suspension Using biopsy bottle after surgical correction for inverted nipple. J Korean Soc Aesthet Plast Reconstr Surg. 2004;10(2):115–7.
2. Han SH, Hong YG. The inverted nipple: its grading and surgical correction. Plast Reconstr Surg. 1999;104(2):389–95.
3. Kurihara K, Maexawa N, Yanagawa H, Imai T. Surgical correction of the inverted nipple with a tendon graft: Hammock procedure. Plast Reconstr Surg. 1990;86(5):999–1003.
4. Kim JK, SC Y. Convenient nipple suspension method using Aquaplast Thermoplastic (Optimold) Splint after surgical correction of inverted nipple. J Korean Soc Aesthet Plast Reconstr Surg. 2007;13(1):89–91.

# Chandler's Modified Technique for Simple Correction of Inverted Nipple Deformities

41

Diego Schavelzon, Miguel Mussi Becker, Guido Ariel Blugerman, and Guillermo Blugerman

## 41.1 Introduction

The nipple plays an important role in the aesthetic appearance of the breast. An inverted nipple is a common deformity characterized by the relative shortness of the lactiferous ducts, which tether the nipple and prevent it from projecting [1]. This deformity can be either congenital or acquired [2]. It has been widely described and graded, and many procedures have been performed to restore the normal anatomic configuration. Historically, it was first described by Sir Ashley Cooper on his book *On the Anatomy of the Breast* published at England in 1840 [3], and the first corrective operation was reported by Kehrer in 1888 [4]. By 1990, Chandler [5] described a surgical technique for the permanent repair of inverted nipples under local anesthesia.

Patients who have invaginated nipples are unable to breastfeed, and it causes cosmetic, functional, psychological, sexual, and even hygiene problems. Although several methods for the correction of an inverted nipple brought satisfactory outcomes, an under-correction, prominent scars, failure to breastfeed, and sensory disturbances have been noted. A pleasing appearance without scars can contribute to the patients overall satisfaction with the results.

D. Schavelzon, M.D. • M.M. Becker
G.A. Blugerman • G. Blugerman, M.D. (✉)
B&S Centro de Excelencia en Cirugía Plástica,
Laprida 1579, Buenos Aires, Argentina
e-mail: schavelzon@clinicabys.com;
schavelzon@centrosbys.com;
blugerman@centrosbys.com

## 41.2 Anatomy

### 41.2.1 Embryologic Development

The development of the nipple-areolar complex begins in the 12th–16th week of gestation. This event is quickly followed by the development of special apocrine glands into the Montgomery glands. In the first stage of glandular development, between 8 and 12 mammary ducts form. These ducts are associated with sebaceous glands near the epidermis. Differentiation of the breast parenchyma and development and pigmentation of the nipple-areolar complex begin around the 32nd week and continue to the 40th week [6].

### 41.2.2 Nipple-Areolar Complex

The nipple-areolar complex contains the Montgomery glands, large intermediate-stage sebaceous glands that are embryologically transitional between sweat glands and mammary glands and are capable of secreting milk. The nipple-areolar complex also contains many sensory nerve endings, smooth muscle, and an abundant lymphatic system called the subareolar or Sappey plexus.


M.A. Shiffman (ed.), *Nipple-Areolar Complex Reconstruction*,
https://doi.org/10.1007/978-3-319-60925-6_41

The adult breast consists of approximately 15–20 segments demarcated by mammary ducts that converge at the nipple in a radial arrangement. Like the number of segments, the number of mammary ducts may vary. Because the skin of the nipple is continuous with the epithelium of the ducts, cancer of the ducts may spread to the nipple [7].

### 41.2.3 Nipple Retraction or Inversion

The terms *retraction* and *inversion* often are used interchangeably, but such usage is inexact. *Retraction* is properly applied when only a slit-like area is pulled inward (Fig. 41.1), whereas *inversion* applies to cases in which the entire nipple is pulled inward—occasionally, far enough to lie below the surface of the breast (Fig. 41.2) [8]. Both retraction and inversion may be either congenital or acquired and either unilateral or bilateral. Bilateral and slowly progressive or long-standing nipple retraction is likely benign and may be a normal variant. A woman with an acquired unilateral nipple inversion may have an underlying malignancy or inflammatory condition and should undergo evaluation with mammography and possibly US or magnetic resonance (MR) imaging. The differential diagnosis in a case of acquired nipple retraction or inversion includes inflammatory conditions such as duct ectasia (common), periductal mastitis, and tuberculosis, as well as malignancy. Central, symmetric, slit-like retraction usually indicates a benign process, whereas inversion of the whole nipple with distortion of the areola is typically a result of malignancy [8].

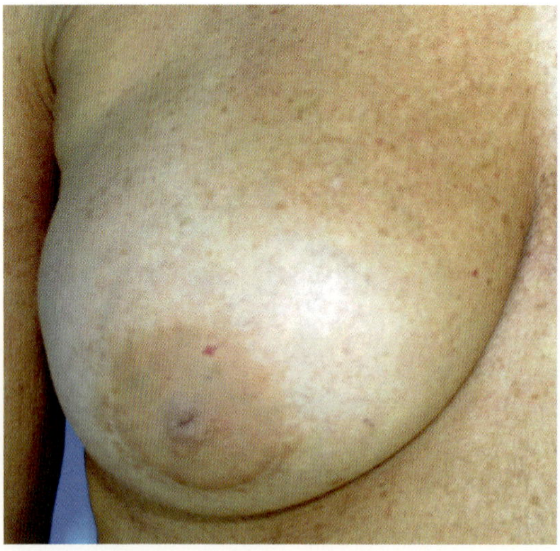

**Fig. 41.1** Retracted nipple

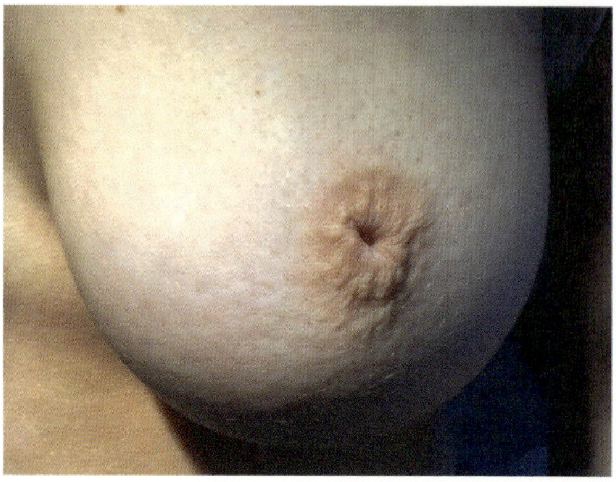

**Fig. 41.2** Inverted nipple

## 41.3 Classification and Grading

The Han and Hong [9] system grading was made by preoperative evaluation of severity of nipple retraction and was confirmed by the surgical findings. It has been widely adopted because of its direct implication on surgical correction.

Grade I: The nipple is easily pulled out manually and maintains its projection quite well. Grade I nipples are believed to have minimal fibrosis; thus, manual traction and a single, buried purse-string suture are enough for the correction.

Grade II: The nipples can be pulled out but cannot maintain projection and tend to go back again. The majority of inverted nipples belong to grade II.

Grade III: To which the least number of inverted nipple cases belong, the nipple can hardly be pulled out manually. Severe fibrosis made it impossible to reach optimal release of the fibrotic band with the preservation of the ducts.

## 41.4 Technique

We propose a Chandler's modified technique, which involves the actual release of the fibrous tissue between the ducts with a direct approach made through a trans-nipple stab, to correct grades I, II, and III inverted nipples. First, the nipple is pulled up anteriorly by its apex with a simple curve needle. Then, it is everted and maintained in gentle traction (Fig. 41.3). Following this, a small incision is made at the nipple-areola junction with a 14-G flexible FEP polymer intravenous (IV) catheter (Fig. 41.4) at 12 o'clock, and the lactiferous ducts are dissected free from surrounding fibrous tissue and released by sharp dissection (Fig. 41.5); this gives the nipple the needed projection. Without pulling out, the same catheter is passed through the nipple base at 6 o'clock (Fig. 41.6), then the shaft of the catheter is removed, and the FEP polymer cannula is left through the nipple acting as a supporter (Fig. 41.7).

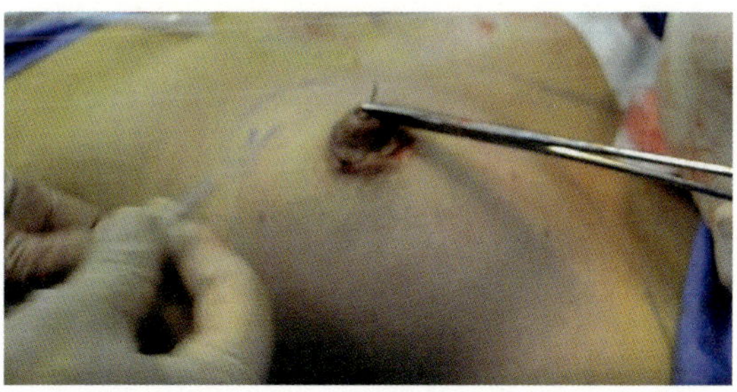

**Fig. 41.3** The nipple is pulled up with a needle

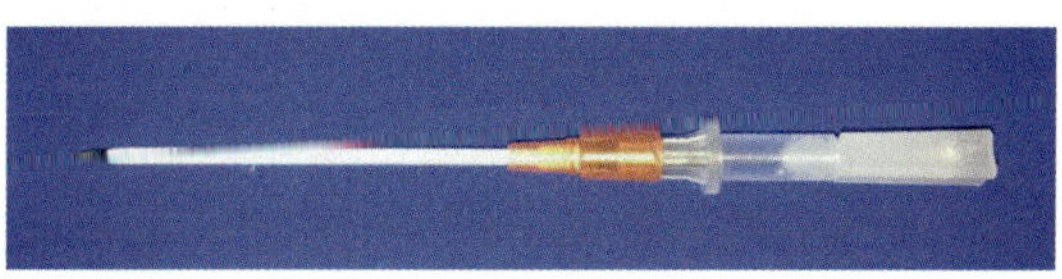

**Fig. 41.4** 14-G flexible FEP polymer IV catheter

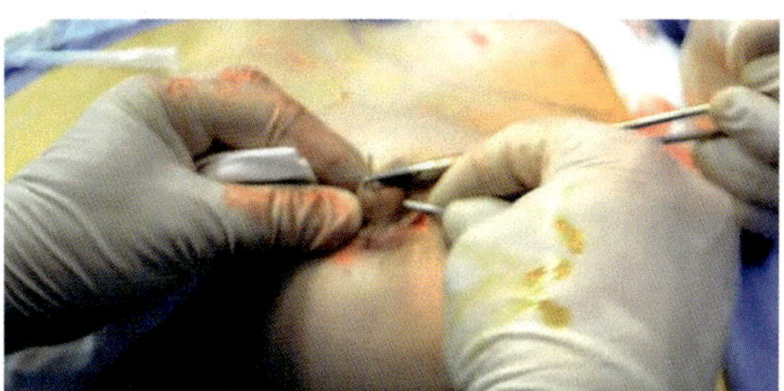

**Fig. 41.5** Dissection of surrounding fibrous tissue

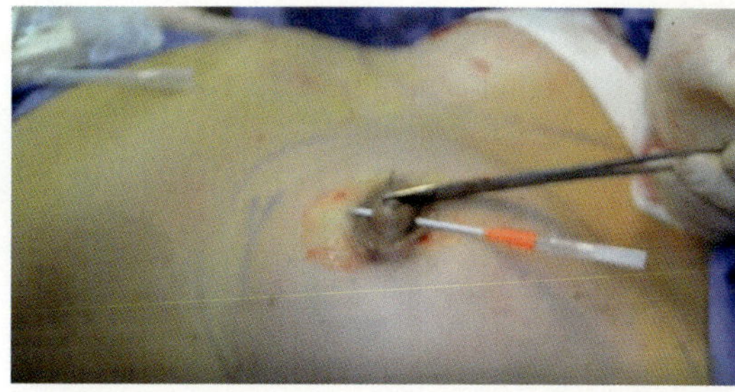

**Fig. 41.6** Catheter is passed through the nipple

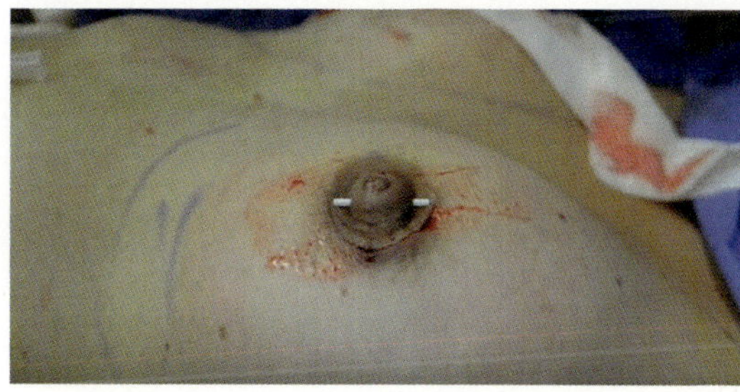

**Fig. 41.7** Catheter's FEP polymer cannula as supporter

This supporting frame must be kept in place for at least 10 days during which the fibrous scar tissue will be developed under the released nipple.

## 41.5 Discussion

This technique offers many advantages such as:

1. No scars on the surface of the areola.
2. Adequate blood and nerve supply.
3. No risk of nipple necrosis.
4. It preserves the sensitive function.
5. The procedure can be performed under local anesthesia.
6. It is reproducible, reliable, and easy to perform.

Definitive results can be appreciated 12 days after the procedure (Fig. 41.8). We believe that more incisions and dissections carry a higher risk of complications.

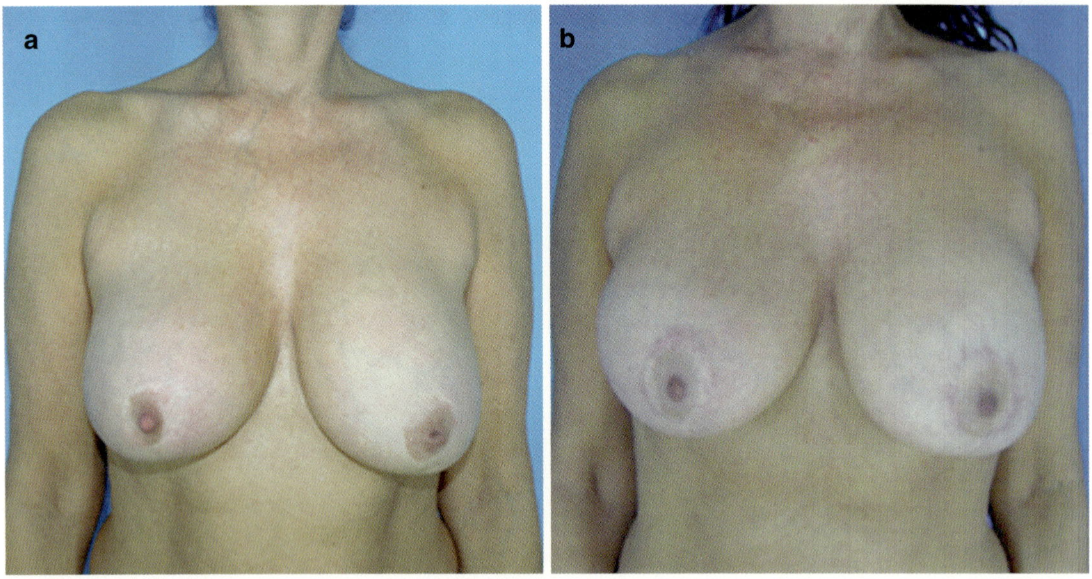


**Fig. 41.8** (**a**) Preoperative patient with left inverted nipple. (**b**) After procedure

## References


1. Park HS. The prevalence of congenital inverted nipple. Aesthet Plast Surg. 1999;23:144–6.
2. Schwager RG, Smith JW, Gray GF, Goulian D. Inversion of the human female nipple, with a simple method of treatment. Plast Reconstr Surg. 1974;54:564–9.
3. Cooper A. On the anatomy of the breast, vol. 2. London: Longman's; 1840. p. 1–89.
4. Sanghoo H, Yoon H. The inverted nipple: its grading and surgical correction. Plast Reconstr Surg. 1999;104(2):389–95.
5. Chandler PJ Jr, Hill SD. A direct surgical approach to correct the inverted nipple. Plast Reconstr Surg. 1990;86:352–4.
6. Osborne MP. Breast development and anatomy. In: Harris J, Hellman S, Henderson I, Kinne D, editors. Breast diseases. 2nd ed. Philadelphia, PA: Lippincott; 1991. p. 1–13.
7. Kopans D. Breast anatomy and basic histology, physiology, and pathology. In: Kopans D, editor. Breast imaging. 3rd ed. Philadelphia, PA: Lippincott Williams & Wilkins; 2007. p. 7–43.
8. Dixon J, Bundred N. Management of disorders of the ductal system and infections. In: Harris J, Lippman M, Morrow M, Osborne C, editors. Diseases of the breast. 3rd ed. Philadelphia, PA: Lippincott Williams & Wilkins; 2004. p. 47–56.
9. Han S, Hong YG. The inverted nipple: its grading and surgical correction. Plast Reconstr Surg. 1999;104:389–95.

# Part IX

# Nipple-Areolar Complex Reconstruction

# Reconstruction of the Nipple-Areola Complex

**42**

Johanna N. Riesel and Yoon S. Chun

## 42.1 Introduction

Breast cancer is the second most common cancer in women in the United States. Approximately 12% of women in the United States will develop invasive breast cancer in their lifetime. According to the American Cancer Society, almost 250,000 new cases of breast cancer will be diagnosed in 2016, and there are currently 2.8 million breast cancer survivors [1]. Of these, many will go on to pursue breast reconstruction. Since the passage of the Women's Health and Cancer Rights Act in 1998, there has been a 200% increase in breast reconstruction with implants [2]. Following mastectomy, as many as 38% of patients will elect to pursue immediate breast reconstruction [3]. Notably, as breast surgery techniques improve, there has been an increase in nipple-sparing mastectomies that, when performed successfully, obviate the need for nipple and areola reconstruction [4]. However, for many women with breast ptosis or with specific oncologic characteristics, the nipple-sparing mastectomy is not an option, and reconstructing the nipple-areola complex (NAC) can be an important final step in their breast reconstruction.

The significance of the NAC to patients, artists, and anatomists cannot be understated. Nipple-areolar reconstruction, though fully elective, often gives the breast reconstruction patient a sense of completeness, and patients who undergo nipple-areolar reconstruction report higher rates of satisfaction with their breast reconstruction and overall psychosocial well-being [5, 6].

## 42.2 Anatomy

The NAC is a unique structure seldom replicated between breasts of one individual let alone among those in the general population. There is great variability in native NAC position, size, color, projection, and texture. In general, a raised mound in the center of a pigmented area on the breast represents the nipple. Another generalization allows us to estimate that in the average B–C cup breast, the areola has a diameter of 4.2–5 cm, with the nipple diameter and projection equal to one-third to one-fourth of the areola diameter. Nipple projection is the result of the coalescence of mammary ducts and either direct or neural stimuli.

J.N. Riesel, M.D. (✉)
Department of Plastic and Reconstructive Surgery, Harvard Combined Plastic Surgery Residency Program, 75 Francis Street, Boston, MA 02115, USA
e-mail: Jriesel@partners.org

Y.S. Chun, M.D.
Department of Plastic Surgery, Brigham and Women's Hospital, Harvard Medical School, 1153 Centre Street, Suite 21, Boston, MA 02130, USA
e-mail: ychun@bwh.harvard.edu


M.A. Shiffman (ed.), *Nipple-Areolar Complex Reconstruction*,
https://doi.org/10.1007/978-3-319-60925-6_42

Not all properties of the native NAC can be recreated with reconstruction. For example, its contractile and neural properties are not currently replicable. However, the appearance of the NAC can often be mimicked with a variety of reconstructive options, irrespective of whether the breast mound was reconstructed with autologous tissue or with alloplastic materials. Autologous reconstructions generally allow for more soft tissue bulk for the Nipple Areolar Reconstruction (NAR) and do not run the risk of potential implant exposure and/or loss (see complications below), but both can generally be used. As with any reconstructive surgery, (NAR) designs must take into account prior biopsy and mastectomy scars so as not to compromise the viability of skin flaps used in NAR.

## 42.3 Technique

### 42.3.1 Surgical Options

In the non-irradiated patient or in patients with flap-based reconstruction, NAR is usually performed 3 months after the breast reconstruction as an outpatient procedure under local anesthesia. Alternatively, it can be performed in the operating room under general anesthesia if the patient desires or if it is combined with other refining procedures such as fat grafting to the reconstructed breasts. Surgical options for NAR include but are not limited to:

1. CV flap
2. Star flap [7]
3. Skate flap [8]
4. Bell flap [9]
5. Double-opposing tab flap [10]
6. Top-hat flap, twin flap [11]
7. Nipple-sharing procedure
8. S flap [12]
9. Rolled dermal fat flap [13]

The use of acellular dermal matrixes or injectable fillers has also been reported to create nipple projection [14–16].

After the nipple mound has been surgically created and allowed to completely heal (anywhere from 2 to 5 months), it is often tattooed either by the reconstructive team or by a professional tattooist to match the color and texture of the native NAC (if present on the contralateral side) or the patient's preference in the case of bilateral reconstructions.

### 42.3.2 Preoperative Planning

Achieving symmetry between breasts is important in yielding an aesthetically pleasing outcome. When a native NAC is present, this can be used as a template for reconstruction. Projection and ptosis of the native breast as compared to the reconstructed breast must be taken into consideration when deciding on placement of the NAC. If the native NAC is particularly large, one may discuss the possibility of a NAC reduction procedure with the patient.

In the scenario of a bilateral NAR, the NAR should be designed along the breast meridian, approximately 11 cm from the sternal midline, and at the most projecting point of the breast mound. This is generally 21–23 cm from the sternal notch and 5–7 cm from the inframammary fold. However, these measurements are mere guidelines, and the ultimate placement of the NAR should be the result of collaboration between the reconstructive surgeon and the patient.

### 42.3.3 Intraoperative Details

There are multiple approaches to creating the nipple both with available, local, and distant tissue. In general, the principles are similar: astute attention must be paid to preserving the blood supply to the nipple flaps; when available, subcutaneous adipose tissue should be incorporated into the flap for greater bulk; initial nipple size and projection should be made 2–3 times larger, if possible, than the native nipple to account for inevitable contraction with scar remodeling; donor defects can often be closed primarily or with small skin grafts. We will discuss several reconstructive options here. Descriptions of the remaining procedures can be found in their respective references.

When performing unilateral reconstruction, the surgeon has the advantage of a natural template on the contralateral side. The size and placement of the reconstructed nipple and areola should be determined by the contralateral native areola, provided the patient does not have plans to modify the natural NAC's position or size. The reconstructed NAC should also be in an aesthetically pleasing position (confirm placement with sternal notch-nipple and inframammary fold-nipple measurements) and positioned with the blood supply to the NAR away from mastectomy scars. If the surgeon is embarking on a bilateral NAR, position and size should be determined both by anatomic landmarks (sternal notch-nipple distance, position on breast mound, distance from inframammary fold) and with the patient's input to ensure a satisfactory result.

#### 42.3.3.1 Star Flap

The star flap procedure is a local tissue rearrangement that creates nipple projection using three "arms" of a star. Mark the areola such that it matches the contralateral areola diameter. Within this circle, draw the three limbs of a star, with the base of the star at the margin of a circle in the center of the areola and the diameter equal to approximately one-fifth of the areola diameter. The flaps should be approximately 2 cm in length and 1 cm at their widest dimension. Raise the three arms of the star in the subcutaneous tissue plane, including more subcutaneous fat as the base is approached. Once elevated, the lateral arms are wrapped toward the midline, resting on top of each other, forming a cylindrical mound. The central limb then rests on top of this mound, creating a roof on top of the cylinder. The flaps are secured to each other and the surrounding skin with permanent or absorbable suture based on the surgeon preference. This flap is commonly performed on flap-based breast reconstructions where there is more available local tissue.

#### 42.3.3.2 CV Flap (Fig. 42.1)

The CV flap is similar to the star flap as a method of NAR reconstruction using a local tissue rearrangement. Again, the areola is marked to match the contralateral areola. In the center of that circle mark is a 5 cm horizontal line that will account for the two lateral limbs (2 cm each) and the central base (1 cm). In between the two lateral limbs, draw a c-shaped curve that connects the two limbs. Lift the lateral limbs toward the midline in the subcutaneous tissue plane. Include some subcutaneous fat if it is available to optimize vascularity and soft tissue volume. Some prefer to deepithelialize the most distal part of the C-flap to provide a "shelf" on which the flap can sit. After about 0.5 cm of deepithelialization, deepen the dissection to the subcutaneous tissue plane such that it meets with the dissection plane of the lateral limbs. The lateral limbs are wrapped toward each other, creating a cylindrical structure. The C-flap creates the roof on the cylinder. The advantage of the CV flap over the star flap includes the use of less local tissue and the elimination of the vertical, third scar.

#### 42.3.3.3 Skate Flap (Fig. 42.2)

Mark the position and size of the new areola based on the contralateral areola. The axis of the skate flap is oriented to fall on the underside of the reconstructed nipple and is marked twice as long as the contralateral nipple height to compensate for eventual contraction of the flap. The base of the flap is drawn three times the diameter of the contralateral nipple. Beginning laterally, the lateral wings of the flap are dissected in the deep dermal layer until the lateral perimeter of the body of the skate flap. At this point, subcutaneous fat is elevated with the body of the flap to give greater bulk to the structure. The lateral wings are wrapped around the body and secured with finely absorbable suture. Donor sites can sometimes be closed primarily. However, if there is undue tension on the closure, a skin graft can be used to close the defect. Some prefer to take a skin graft along nearby scar lines on the breast; others have advocated to take a skin graft from the posterior thigh or upper buttock to offer a

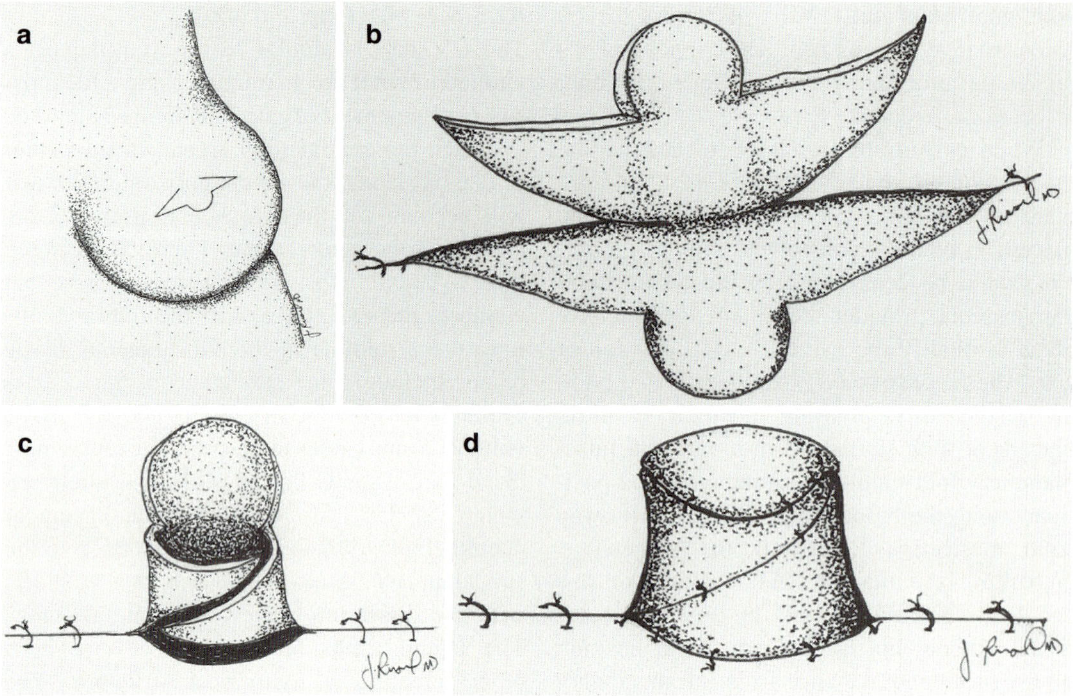


Fig. 42.1 (**a**) The CV flap is composed of two lateral, v-shaped flaps, measuring 2 cm in length, separated by a 1 cm gap where the central, c-shaped flap is designed. (**b**) The lateral and central flaps are raised in the subcutaneous plane, taking with them some underlying adipose tissue, if available, as the dissection moves centrally. (**c**) The lateral limbs are wrapped toward each other. The donor sites are closed primarily. (**d**) The lateral limbs are secured to themselves and the surrounding tissue with either absorbable or permanent suture. The central, C-flap forms the "roof" of the nipple and is also secured with suture of the surgeon's choosing

darker color appearance that might avert the need for tattoo of the areola later on.

#### 42.3.3.4 Nipple Sharing

The nipple-sharing procedure is a controversial topic in unilateral reconstruction as dogma implores the reconstructive surgeon to "not ruin the good side." In proceeding with a nipple-sharing procedure, the surgeon is at risk of decreasing or eliminating both projection and sensation to the only erogenous structure remaining on the patient's chest. However, a study by Haslik et al. [17] found that of 26 patients who underwent a nipple-sharing procedure, the majority (88%) were either very satisfied or somewhat satisfied with nipple sensitivity in the donor nipple and with appearance, projection, color, and shape of their nipples.

Nipple-sharing procedures may be a good option when the unaffected NAC is displeasingly large and projecting and/or the reconstructed side does not have adequate tissue to use for local flap rearrangement. In the nipple-sharing procedure, the most anterior portion of the native nipple or a wedge resection of the native nipple is used as a composite graft for the reconstructed NAC. The areola can be tattooed either pre- or postoperatively.

### 42.3.4 Postoperative Care

Most surgeons favor covering the newly reconstructed NAC with a protective dressing or splint. This can be fashioned in a variety of ways, the limits of which are confined to the surgeon's imagination. Common dressings include covering the reconstruction in antibiotic ointment or a petroleum jelly dressing, with a hole cut in the center. A tower of stacked, 2 × 2 gauze with a central hole for the new nipple or a "nest" of gauze can be placed on top to protect the nipple. One can

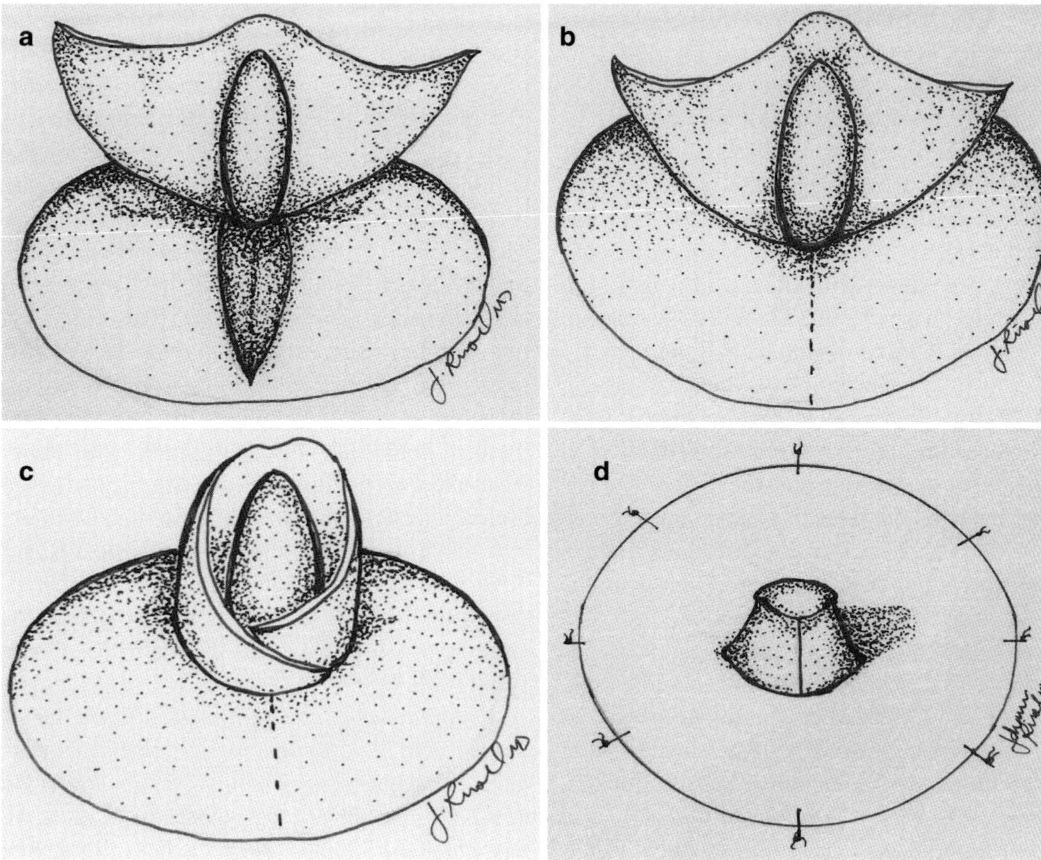

**Fig. 42.2** (**a**) The skate flap employs a column of adipose tissue in the creation of the body of the nipple for enhanced projection. (**b**) The adipose tissue donor site is closed primarily. This may constrict a portion of the circular deepithelialized area intended for the skin graft that will create the appearance of an areola. If this occurs, simply re-deepithelialize the constricted margins to create a more circular wound bed. (**c**) The full thickness "wings" of the skate flap wrap around the central body of the nipple. (**d**) A skin graft is placed around the newly constructed nipple mound. A graft from the buttocks or upper thigh may offer a darker pigment that can avert the need for tattooing in some cases. Another alternative is to close the circular deepithelialized area primarily and avoid a skin graft and the subsequent donor site completely

also protect the reconstructed nipple with a prefabricated nipple guard or one made from a medicine cup or syringe. This dressing should be changed often and maintained for 2 weeks.

## 42.4 Contraindications

Few contraindications exist for NAR, with the exception of poor skin quality in the potential location of the NAR as may be the case following postmastectomy radiation especially in implant-based breast reconstruction. In these cases, proceeding with a local tissue rearrangement to build the nipple mound could result in implant loss secondary to exposure due to skin breakdown or due to infection as a result of intraoperative capsule violation. In these cases, most surgeons will delay NAR to allow the skin to heal further. However, a frank conversation must be had with the patient, so they are aware that NAR may never be an option for them if the risk of breast mound reconstruction failure due to implant loss outweighs the benefits of nipple reconstruction.

## 42.5 Complications

Complications of NAR include wound infection, wound breakdown or necrosis, loss of nipple projection, and implant exposure and loss. Higher rates of complications are seen in patients with a history of radiation and/or implant-based reconstructions [18]. If pursuing nipple-areolar reconstruction in a patient with chest wall radiation, it is imperative to ensure all acute radiation-induced skin changes have resolved and that mastectomy skin flaps are appropriately thick. Synthetic materials used for enhanced nipple projection are associated with higher complications than when allogeneic or autologous grafts are used. The latter two have similar rates of postoperative nipple projection [19]. If wound complications such as dehiscence or flap distal tip necrosis occur in the setting of autologous reconstruction, they can generally be managed with local wound care, as nearly all will heal via secondary intention. However, if such complications occur in an implant-based reconstruction, a heightened sense of vigilance must be employed as the implant, generally below a fairly thin layer of tissue, is at increased risk of exposure and subsequent loss.

## 42.6 Nonsurgical Options

Nonsurgical options include nipple prostheses and nipple-areola tattoo. The use of nipple prostheses is less common as women frequently opt for a more permanent solution. However, such prostheses can be an appealing temporizing measure for the patient who is uncertain whether she wants to pursue nipple-areolar reconstruction or for the patient who has healed from breast reconstruction and is awaiting reconstruction.

The nipple-areola tattoo can be performed by the reconstructive surgeon and team or, more recently, by a professional tattooist. The advent of "three-dimensional (3-D) tattoos" offers a realistic-appearing NAC for both women who have undergone surgical reconstruction and those who have not [20]. However, patients must understand that the tattoo alone is an optical illusion: it does not provide nipple projection. For some patients who do not like the continuous projection of the nipple, this may be preferred. The tattooist is able to create this appearance of projection by employing artistic shadowing within the tattoo. The tattooist can also create realistic-appearing nuances including Montgomery glands and other details to either match an unaffected NAC on the contralateral side or a patient's premastectomy NAC in the setting of bilateral reconstruction (Fig. 42.3). Most tattoos by professional tattooists do not require revisions for color fading, unlike tattoos using medical-grade ink that may fade with time. Regardless of ink used, tattoos can be, and often are, repeated to enhance faded colors. Women who have undergone breast reconstruction and NAR with tattoo shave found significant satisfaction with tattoos, and the majority would opt for another tattoo if they had to make the choice again [21].

Unfortunately, such professional-grade three-dimensional NAC tattoos are expensive, and insurance companies may be reluctant to cover the costs. This is an ever-evolving issue, but since the passage of the Women's Health and Cancer Rights Act, patients have found some success in insurance coverage of these procedures. Furthermore, access to three-dimensional tattoos may be limited due to scarce number of professional tattooists who are able to perform three-dimensional NAC tattoos. Accordingly, there is a need for greater collaboration between medical professionals, health insurance companies, and professional tattooists to provide the most complete reconstructive options for mastectomy patients.

## 42.7 Discussion

When considering NAR after non-nipple-sparing mastectomy and reconstruction, it is important to construct an NAC of the appropriate size, shape, color, and location, or it will compromise the entire aesthetic outcome of the reconstructed breast. Long-term outcomes are variable and largely influenced by individual patient charac-

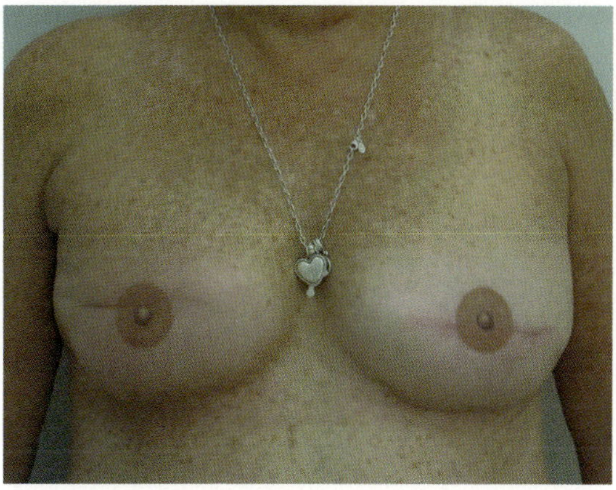

**Fig. 42.3** Bilateral three-dimensional nipple tattoo following bilateral skin-sparing mastectomy and reconstruction with implants

teristics including tissue thickness and quality, history of radiation, and trauma. Patients should be counseled that most NAC reconstruction will contract and flatten over time and tattoos will frequently fade over time. Options should be provided in the event of nipple flattening or color fading such as revision of the NAC with local flaps, fillers, repeat tattoo, and 3-D tattoos.

Traditionally, the greater clinical import has been placed on reconstruction of the breast mound, and NAC has been considered more of an elective, secondary procedure. However, it is important to recognize the added psychosocial benefits that patients might experience from NAC reconstruction [5, 6], even though it may prolong the patient's overall timeline of reconstruction. Many reconstructive surgeons advocate for allowing the reconstructed breast to "settle" before NAC reconstruction such that placement of the reconstructed nipple can be as precise as possible. Patients may also wait to pursue NAC reconstruction to give themselves a respite from multiple surgical procedures. As a result, some patients fatigue from recurrent procedures and never pursue NAC reconstruction, potentially forgoing the added psychosocial benefits of reconstruction. As such, some have advocated for NAC reconstruction at the time of autologous-free tissue flaps to minimize the total number of procedures [22]. This may be a viable option, but the final decision will fall to the discretion of both the reconstructive surgeon and the patient.

## Conclusions

NAR is an important element of breast reconstruction and can provide significant benefit to patients following non-nipple-sparing mastectomy. The procedure is well tolerated, requires minimal postoperative care, and can result in higher patient satisfaction with an improved sense of completion and well-being. There are multiple options for NAR, and they should be presented to all appropriate candidates.

## References


1. American Cancer Society. What are the key statistics about breast cancer? http://www.cancer.org/cancer/breastcancer/detailedguide/breast-cancer-keystatistics. Accessed 20 June 2016.
2. Albornoz CR, Bach PB, Mehrara BJ, Disa JJ, Pusic AL, McCarthy CM, Cordeiro PG, Matros E. A paradigm shift in US breast reconstruction: increasing implant rates. Plast Reconstr Surg. 2013;131(1):15–23.
3. Alboronoz CR, Matros E, Lee CN, Hudis CA, Pusic AL, Elkin E, Bach PB, Cordeiro PG, Morrow M. Bilateral mastectomy versus breast-conserving surgery for early stage breast cancer: the role of breast reconstruction. Plast Reconstr Surg. 2015;135(6):1518–26.
4. Gerber B, Krause A, Reimer T, Muller H, Kuchenmeister I, Makovitzky J, Kundt G, Friese K. Skin-sparing mastectomy with conservation of the nipple-areola complex and autologous reconstruction is an oncologically safe procedure. Ann Surg. 2003;238(1):120–7.
5. Wellisch DK, Schain WS, Noone RB, Little JW 3rd. The psychosocial contribution of nipple addition in breast reconstruction. Plast Reconstr Surg. 1987;80(5):699–704.
6. Momoh AO, Colakoglu S, de Blacam C, Yueh JH, Lin SJ, Tobias AM, Lee BT. The impact of nipple reconstruction on patient satisfaction in breast reconstruction. Ann Plast Surg. 2012;69(4):389–93.
7. Few JW, Marcus JR, Casas LA. Long-term predictable nipple projection following reconstruction. Plast Reconstr Surg. 1999;104(5):1321–4.
8. Bogue DP, Mungara AK, Thomposon M, Cederna PS. Modified technique for nipple-areolar reconstruction: a case series. Plast Reconstr Surg. 2003;112(5):1274–8.

9. Eng JS. Bell flap nipple reconstruction – a new wrinkle. Ann Plast Surg. 1996;36(5):485–8.
10. Kroll SS, Reece GP, Miller MJ. Comparison of nipple projection with the modified double-opposing tab and star flaps. Plast Reconstr Surg. 1997;99(6):1602–5.
11. Ramakrishnan VV, Mohan D, Villafane O. Twin flap technique for nipple reconstruction. Ann Plast Surg. 1997;39(3):241–4.
12. Lossing C, Brongo S, Holmstrom H. Nipple reconstruction with a modified S-flap technique. Scand J Plast Reconstr Surg Hand Surg. 1998;32(3):275–9.
13. Tanabe HY, Tai Y, Kiyokawa K. Nipple-areola reconstruction with a dermal-fat flap and rolled auricular cartilage. Plast Reconstr Surg. 1997;100(2):431–8.
14. Garramone CE, Lam B. Use of AlloDerm in primary nipple reconstruction to improve long-term nipple projection. Plast Reconstr Surg. 2007;119(6):1663–8.
15. Nahabedian MY. Secondary nipple reconstruction using local flaps and AlloDerm. Plast Reconstr Surg. 2005;115(7):2056–61.
16. Evans KK, Rasko Y, Lenert J. The use of calcium hydroxylapatite for nipple projection after failed nipple-areolar reconstruction: early results. Ann Plast Surg. 2005;55(1):25–9.
17. Haslik W, Nedomansky J, Hacker S, Nickl S, Shroegendorfer KF. Objective and subjective evaluation of donor-site morbidity after nipple sharing for nipple areola reconstruction. J Plast Reconstr Aesthet Surg. 2015;68(2):168–74.
18. Satteson ES, Reynolds MF, Bond AM, Pestana IA. An analysis of complication risk factors in 641 nipple reconstructions. Breast J. 2016;22(4):379–83.
19. Winocour S, Saksena A, Oh C, Wu PS, Laungani A, Baltxer H, Saint-Cyr M. A systematic review of comparison of autologous, allogenic, and synthetic augmentation grafts in nipple reconstruction. Plast Reconstr Surg. 2015;137(1):14e–23e.
20. Halvorson EG, Cormican M, West ME, Myers V. Three-dimensional nipple-areola tattooing: a new technique with superior results. Plast Reconstr Surg. 2014;133(5):1073–5.
21. Spear SL, Arias J. Long-term experience with nipple-areola tattooing. Ann Plast Surg. 1995;35:232–6.
22. Williams EH, Rosenberg LZ, Kolm P, de la Torre JI, Fix RJ. Immediate nipple reconstruction on a free TRAM flap breast reconstruction. Plast Reconstr Surg. 2007;120:1115–24.

# Nipple-Areola Complex Reconstruction

# 43

Andrea Sisti, Juri Tassinari, Roberto Cuomo, Cesare Brandi, Giuseppe Nisi, Luca Grimaldi, and Carlo D'Aniello

## 43.1 Introduction

Reconstruction of the nipple-areola complex (NAC) completes the final aesthetic step of breast reconstruction and restores the body image of breast cancer patients who have undergone mastectomy [1–3]. The absence of the nipple has important consequences on a woman's psyche. Patients that have suffered the loss of this anatomical structure continue to experience psychological discomfort for a long time; conversely, the reconstruction of this complex can alleviate this discomfort [4, 5].

An ideal reconstruction should provide a good symmetry as regards color, texture, and projection compared to the contralateral nipple. The nipple can be reconstructed using a local flap, a local flap with synthetic/allogeneic/autologous graft inside, a skin graft, or a subdermal pocket.

The areola is reconstructed by a split skin graft from hyperpigmented areas or from the contralateral areola or by tattooing.

NAC prosthesis or of the three-dimensional tattoo allows the reconstruction of the nipple and areola simultaneously, with only one method [6–13].

## 43.2 Nipple Reconstruction Using Local Flap

The local flap is the most frequently used technique for nipple reconstruction. It is generally performed 3 months after the breast mound creation, as an outpatient procedure, under local anesthesia. This method includes the preparation of a local skin flap in the area where you want to re-create the nipple.

To date, more than 60 local flap surgical techniques have been described to reconstruct the nipple (Figs. 43.1 and 43.2) [2]. The first description of the nipple reconstruction using a local skin flap dates back to 1946 and belongs to Berson (Fig. 43.2) [39]. The epithelium is undermined from the periphery to 1 cm from the center, exposing the dermal surface of the skin. On the loose epithelium (which is shrunken and stretched), three identical triangular sections are

A. Sisti, M.D. (✉) • J. Tassinari, M.D. • R. Cuomo, M.D.
C. Brandi, M.D. • G. Nisi, M.D. • L. Grimaldi, M.D.
C. D'Aniello, M.D.
Plastic and Reconstructive Surgery Unit, Department of Medicine, Surgery and Neuroscience, S. Maria alle Scotte Hospital, University of Siena, Siena, Italy
e-mail: asisti6@gmail.com; juritassinari@gmail.com; robertocuomo@outlook.com; cesarebrandi@virgilio.it; pipponisi@gmail.com; lucagrimaldi.mail@gmail.com; daniello@unisi.it



M.A. Shiffman (ed.), *Nipple-Areolar Complex Reconstruction*,
https://doi.org/10.1007/978-3-319-60925-6_43

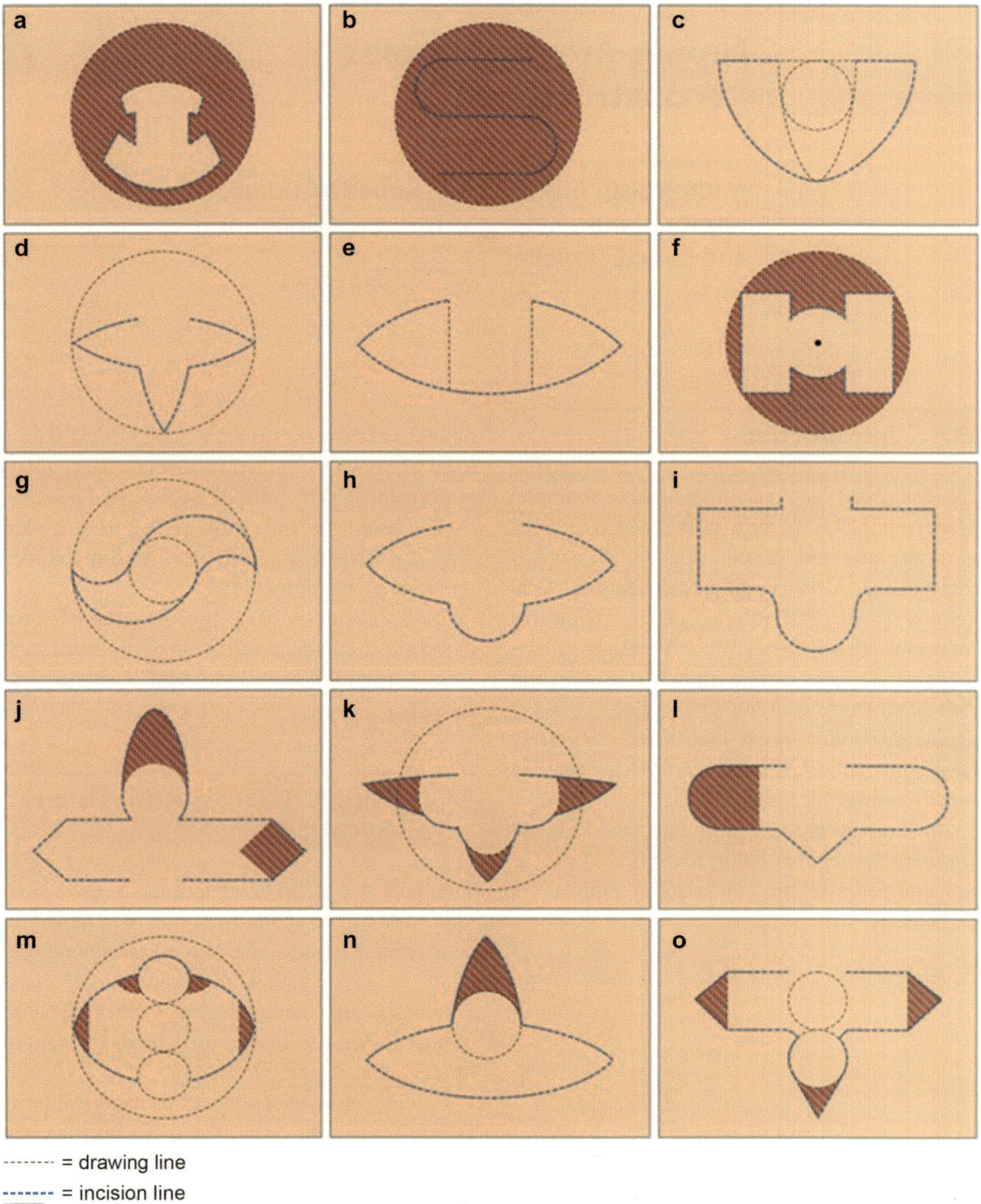


**Fig. 43.1** Preoperative marking of 15 local flaps for the nipple reconstruction (adapted from Sisti [2]). (**a**) T-flap, as described by Chang in 1984 [14]. (**b**) S-flap, as described by Cronin in 1988 [15]. (**c**) Skate flap, as described by Little [16] in 1988. (**d**) Star flap, as described by Anton in 1991 [17]. (**e**) Wrap flap, as described by Anton in 1991 [17]. (**f**) H-flap, as described by Hallock in 1993 [18]. (**g**) Propeller flap, as described by Teimourian in 1994 [19]. (**h**) First description of C-V flap [20]. (**i**) Local flap as described by Thomas in 1996 [21]. (**l**) Arrow flap, as described by Rubino in 2003 [22]. (**m**) Fleur-de-lis flap technique, as described by Germanò in 2006 [23]. (**n**) Cigar roll flap, as described by Jamnadas-Khoda in 2011 [24]. (**o**) Angel flap, as described by Wong in 2013 [25]. (**p**) V-V flap, as described by Witt in 2013 [54]. (**q**) Rolled triangular dermal- fat flap, as described by Temiz [55] in 2015

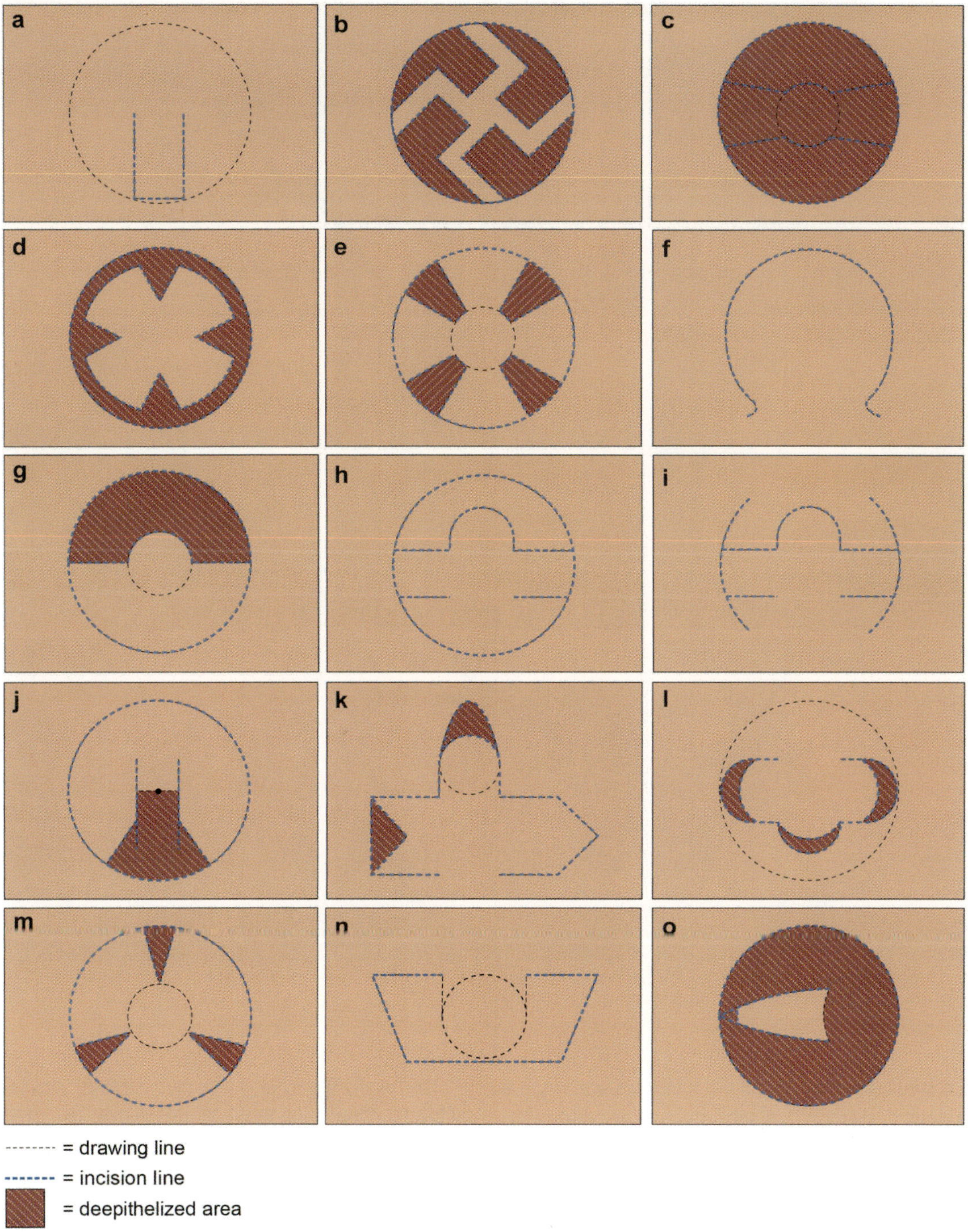


**Fig. 43.2** Preoperative marking of 15 local flaps for the nipple reconstruction (adapted from Sisti [2]). (**a**) Rectangular flap, as described by Dini in 2006 [26]. (**b**) Pinwheel flap, as described by Cohen [27] in 1986. (**c**) Double dermal-fat flap, as described by Muruci [28] in 1978. (**d**) Di Pirro technique flap, as described by Di Pirro [29] in 1970. (**e**) Quadrapod flap, as described by Little [30] in 1983. (**f**) Omega flap, as described by Hartrampf [31] in 1984. (**g**) Silversmith technique, as described by Silversmith [32] in 1983. (**h**) Hammond flap, as described by Hammond [33] and Shestak [34] in 2007. (**i**) Modified Hammond flap, described by Yang [35] in 2014. (**l**) Bell flap, as described by Eng [36] in 1996. (**m**) Modified arrow flap, as described by Farace [37] in 2010. (**n**) Modified C-V flap, as described by Brackley [38] in 2009. (**o**) Berson technique, as described by Berson [39] in 1946. (**p**) Double flag flap, as described by Grosdidier [40] in 2014. (**q**) Inchworm flap, as described by Puckett [41] in 1992

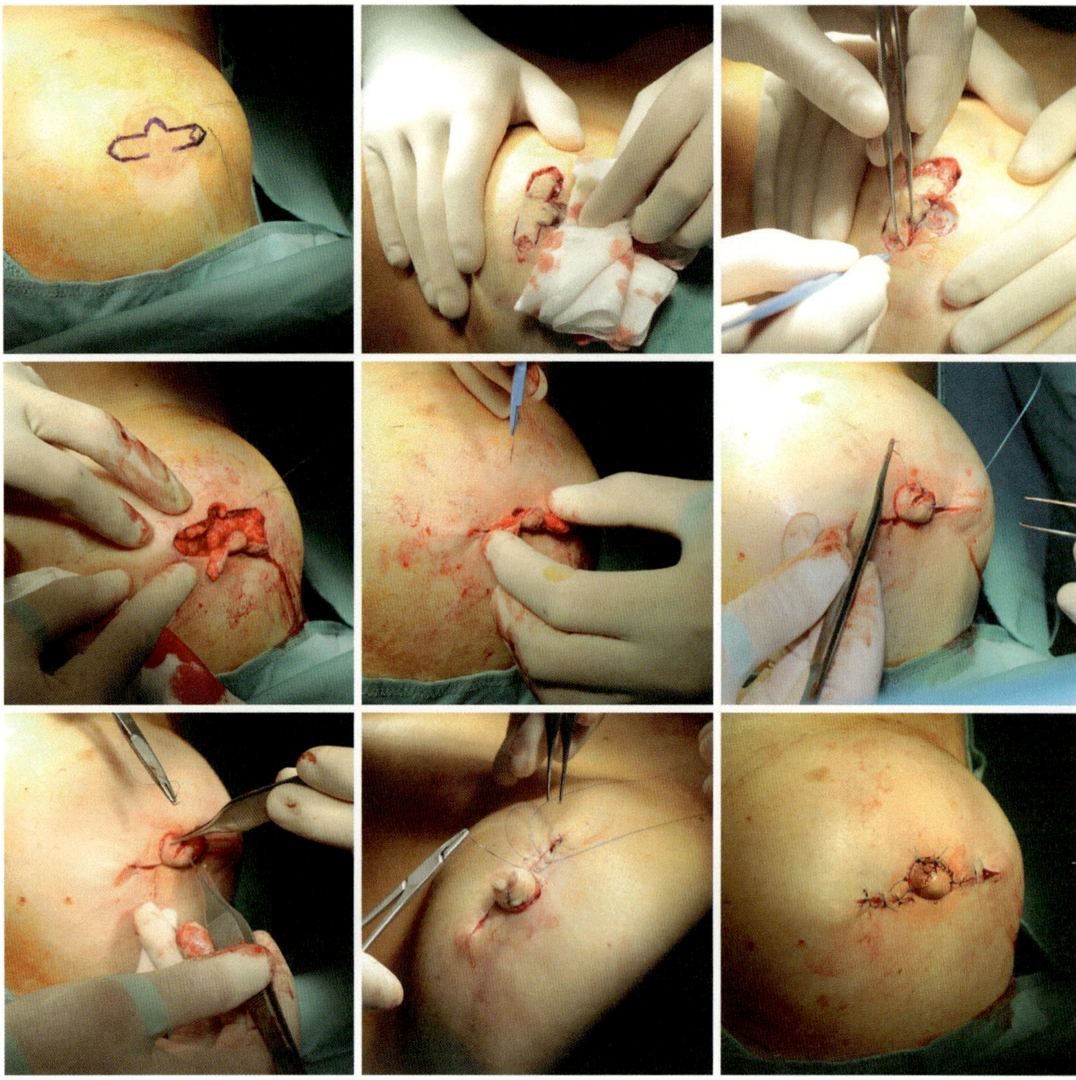

**Fig. 43.3** Surgical steps of a modified arrow flap technique [47]

excised; the margins of the triangles are sutured together; skin graft is subsequently used to cover the areola and the upper face of the flap.

Cronin, in 1988 [42], described the "S-flap" (Fig. 43.1). The first step of this technique consists in the total deepithelialization of the round area where the future nipple-areola complex will rise. Subsequently, an S-shaped incision is performed and two facing flaps are raised. These are sutured together and then entirely covered by a skin graft. S-flap was modified by Lossing (1998) [43] and Narra (2008) [44].

The "skate flap" (Fig. 43.1), the "star flap," and the "wrap flap" were the first effective and, at the same time, easy to perform techniques, described in literature [16, 17]. Several modifications to the original star flap were proposed over the years [23, 45, 46].

Jones and Bostwick, in 1994, [20] provided the first description of C-V flap (Fig. 43.1). It is a simple and easily reliable technique, which does not include any deepithelialization. Afterward, several minor modifications to this technique have been proposed (Figs. 43.2, 43.3, 43.4, and 43.5) [38, 48–55].

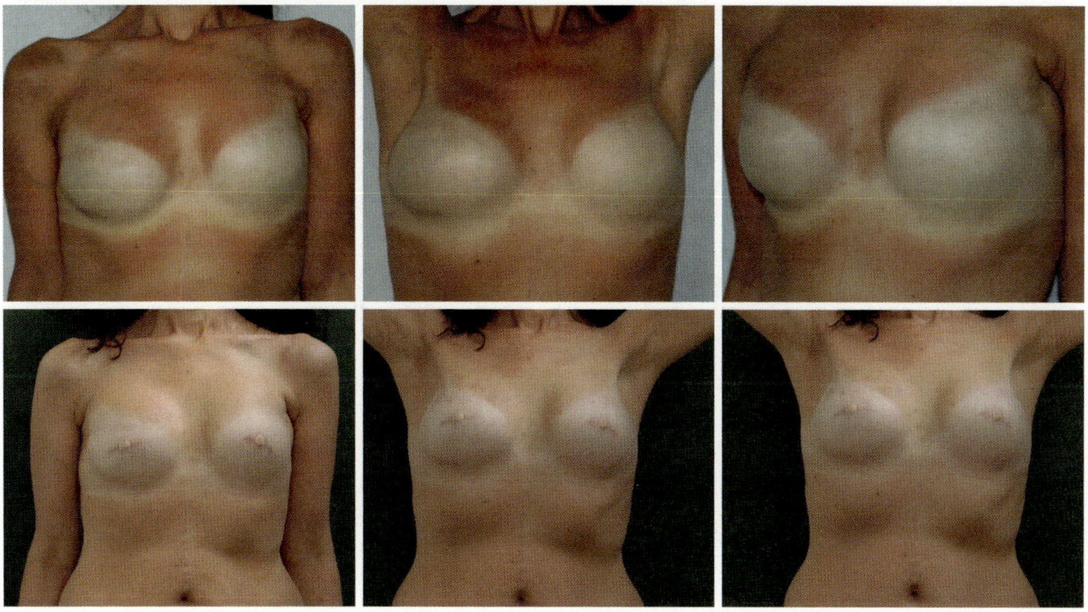

**Fig. 43.4** (*Top*) Preoperative. (*Bottom*) 6 months after nipple reconstruction with modified arrow flap technique [47]

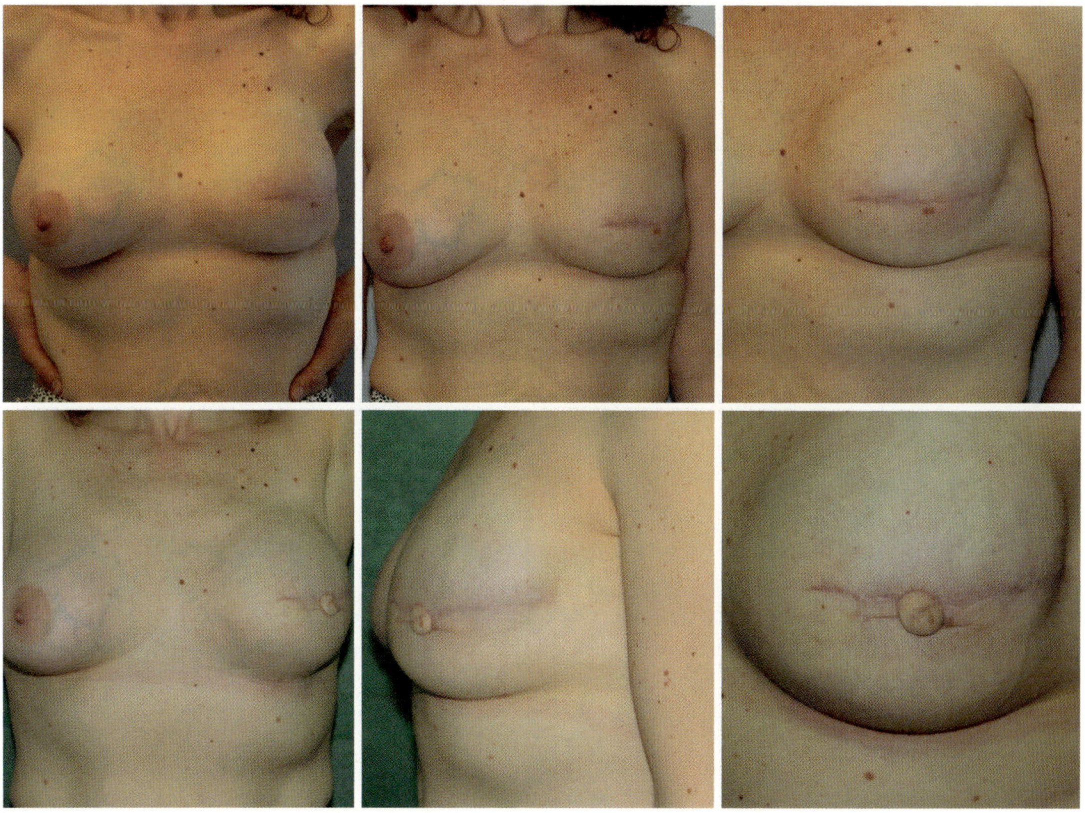

**Fig. 43.5** (*Top*) Preoperative. (*Bottom*) 6 months after nipple reconstruction with modified arrow flap technique [47]

In 2003, Rubino [22] and Guerra [56] (in two independent papers) described the "arrow flap" (Fig. 43.1), a modification of the previously described "Thomas flap" [21]. It involves the deepithelialization of two areas, leading to the formation of a flap in the shape of an arrow. In subsequent years, this type of local flap was subjected to minor changes [37, 47, 57, 58].

Hammond [33] and Shestak [34], in 2007, proposed a double-opposing peri-areolar flap, modifying the skate flap with a purse-string design; today it is commonly called the Hammond flap (Fig. 43.2). It was modified in 2014 by Yang [35], as minimal incision version, obtaining excellent results and by Saleh [59], as double-breasted dermal flap.

Wong, in 2013, [25] described the angel flap (Fig. 43.1). The preoperative design is very interesting and includes four small areas of deepithelialization and a main body of the flap that is similar to two angel's wings.

Other described local flap techniques are the top hat technique [60–64], the V-Y flap [65, 66], the double-opposing TAB [67, 68], dome technique with double pedicle [69], bipedicled dermal flap [70], inferiorly pedicled dermal flap [71], the omega flap [31], cigar roll flap [24, 72], the quadrapod flap [30], Barton's technique [73], the spiral flap [74], the badge flap [75], the H-flap [18], the e-flap [76], the T-flap [14, 77], and the two-step purse-string suture technique [78]. Preoperative drawings of other local flap techniques are represented in (Figs. 43.1 and 43.2).

In general, due to contraction, overcorrection of 25–50% of the desired result is advisory when adopting local flaps, in order to prevent loss of projection [2].

In 2016, Kim [79] described a technique that uses local flaps to improve the lost projection of reconstructed nipples. Deepithelialized triangular flaps were made on all four sides of the nipple and buried in the opposite corners in order to augment the volume of the nipple. Anchoring sutures were used to attach each triangular flap on the side opposite their point of origin, and the resulting defects were closed directly.

Postoperative complications include nipple necrosis, tip loss, wound infection, and wound breakdown. Complication rate after nipple reconstruction using local flap is between 7% and 8% [2, 80, 81].

## 43.3 Nipple Reconstruction Using Local Flap with Synthetic/ Allogeneic/Autologous Graft

This technique includes the addition of a synthetic/allogeneic/autologous graft inside the flap, in order to augment the projection of the nipple and ensure the long-term maintenance of the projection [1]. A variety of materials are available for projection augmentation, including autologous (hallux pulp graft, auricular cartilage, composite tissue, contralateral breast tissue, labia minora, costal cartilage, fat graft, rolled dermal graft), allogeneic (acellular dermal matrix, bone graft, costal cartilage, ECM collagen-rolled cylinder), and synthetic (polyurethane, silicone rods, polytetrafluoroethylene, calcium hydroxylapatite gel) materials [3].

The use of these augmentation grafts in nipple reconstruction showed a minor loss of nipple projection but may expose to a relative increased number of postoperative flap necrosis [2].

Winocour, in 2016, [3] performed a systematic review to study the efficacy, projection, and complication rates of different materials used in nipple reconstruction. The results of this review revealed heterogeneity in the type of material used within each category and inconsistent methodology used in outcome assessment in nipple reconstruction. Overall, the quality of evidence is low. Synthetic materials have higher complication rates, and allogeneic grafts have nipple projection comparable to that of autologous grafts. Further investigation with high-level evidence is necessary to determine the optimal material for nipple reconstruction.

## 43.4 NAC Reconstruction Using Skin Graft

This technique involves the reconstruction of the NAC with a skin graft. The suitable areas are those that have a texture and a pigmentation similar to the nipple such as the small lips of the vagina, the contralateral nipple (nipple sharing), the axilla, the perineal region, or the inguinal region.

The first description of skin graft for reconstruction of missing nipple dates to 1949 [82]. In this case report, the skin from the labium minor was used to reconstruct the nipple. The graft was harvested from labium minor, and it was next spread out over the recipient area of the breast, cut to proper shape, and attached around the periphery with fine silk. The central portion of the graft was left a little loose and sutured to give the appearance of a nipple.

Millard, in 1971, described the use of contralateral nipple graft, and this remained a popular method for nipple reconstruction in patients with excess contralateral nipple projection [83, 84].

Combination of these grafts can be performed for the reconstruction of nipple and areola [85]. Nowadays, the local flap is the most frequently used for the reconstruction of the nipple, whereas the graft is eventually used for the reconstruction of the areola.

Areola can also be grafted before the reconstruction of the nipple with local flap, as described by Dini (Fig. 43.2) [26]. In this case, the local flap is performed in a second time, on the previously grafted areola

In a recent review, complications in areola reconstruction were 10.1% after graft while only 1.6% after areola tattoo [2]. Fading of the areola's pigmentation with time is a common issue.

## 43.5 NAC Reconstruction with Tattoo

The tattoo of the NAC is performed after the reconstruction of the nipple with local flap. Making the tattoo before surgery is an interesting shrewdness; it allows to avoid the difficulties of tattooing the already projected nipple in a second time [86]. Tattooing of the nipple-areola complex has become standard procedure in reconstruction following a mastectomy. It is a simple, quick, and safe procedure.

The NAC is designed, using natural pigments and by relating the color and size, to the contralateral nipple. A professional tattoo artist usually performs it, 3–4 months after breast reconstruction. Intradermal tattooing may also constitute alone a definitive reconstructive method for the reconstruction of the nipple-areola complex, without the flap local.

In 2014, Halvorson [8] described the reconstruction of the NAC through a three-dimensional tattoo. The illusion of three dimensionality, although the drawing is in two dimensions, is obtained by the combination of light and dark.

NAC tattoos are prone to significant fading, leading patients to seek revisions [87]. Color asymmetry is another significant issue after this procedure. An objective assessment of tattooing using a computer software program can be a useful tool in reviewing the outcome [88].

Moreover, dermabrasion could be performed before starting the tattoo. Dermabrasion allows better penetration of the pigments inside the dermis and thus offers two advantages: a more durable result over time and reduced operation time by reducing the number of passing of the machine tattoo [42].

## 43.6 NAC Reconstruction Using Prosthesis

The principle of this technique is to perform an exact reproduction of the NAC [6, 9–13]. The procedure appears to be minimally invasive and rapid. It is a quick and inexpensive alternative to surgical nipple reconstruction. This method offers substantial cost benefits in comparison to surgical reconstruction, which involves both theater and inpatient time.

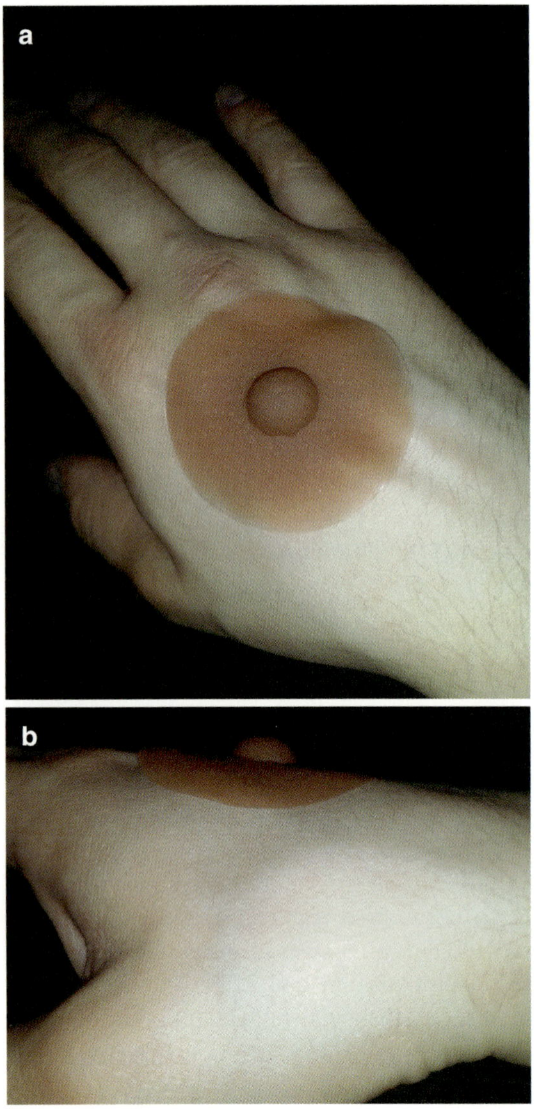


**Fig. 43.6** (**a**, **b**) External prosthesis

The prosthesis can be external (Fig. 43.6a and b) or internal. The role of an internal nipple prosthesis, although perhaps of some value as a salvage procedure, appears to offer few advantages over other accepted methods of reconstruction that do not use any foreign body [7].

## 43.7 Reconstruction of the Nipple with a Subdermal Pocket

In 2009, Colwell and Breuing [89] described the introduction of an acellular dermal matrix cylinder into a subdermal pocket to simulate a normal nipple. This construct offers the look and feel of the autologous nipple-areola complex without jeopardizing the underlying implant. The nipple reconstruction with acellular dermal matrix (without the use of autologous dermal flap) is reserved for select patients with thin skin following breast implant reconstruction.

## References


1. Nimboriboonporn A, Chuthapisith S. Nipple-areola complex reconstruction. Gland Surg. 2014;3(1):35–42.
2. Sisti A, Grimaldi L, Tassinari J, Cuomo R, Fortezza L, Bocchiotti MA, Roviello F, D'Aniello C, Nisi G. Nipple-areola complex reconstruction techniques: a literature review. Eur J Surg Oncol. 2016;42(4):441–65.
3. Winocour S, Saksena A, Oh C, Wu PS, Laungani A, Baltzer H, Saint-Cyr M. A systematic review of comparison of autologous, allogeneic, and synthetic augmentation grafts in nipple reconstruction. Plast Reconstr Surg. 2016;137(1):14e–23e.
4. Levison J. Breast reconstruction; a patient's view. Plast Reconstr Surg. 1984;73(4):703.
5. Wellisch DK, Schain WS, Noone RB, Little JW 3rd. The psychological contribution of nipple addition in breast reconstruction. Plast Reconstr Surg. 1987;80(5):699–704.
6. Clarkson DJ, Smith PM, Thorpe RJ, Daly JC. The use of custom-made external nipple-areolar prostheses following breast cancer reconstruction. J Plast Reconstr Aesthet Surg. 2011;64(4):e103–5.
7. Hallock GG. Polyurethane nipple prosthesis. Ann Plast Surg. 1990;24(1):80–5.
8. Halvorson EG, Cormican M, West ME, Myers V. Three-dimensional nipple-areola tattooing: a new technique with superior results. Plast Reconstr Surg. 2014;133(5):1073–5.
9. Janes S. Custom-made nipple prosthesis: a long-term satisfaction survey. J Cancer Res Ther. 2005;1(2):111–3.
10. Roberts AC, Coleman DJ, Sharpe DT. Custom-made nipple-areola prostheses in breast reconstruction. Br J Plast Surg. 1988;41(6):586–7.
11. Sainsbury R, Walker VA, Smith PM. An improved nipple prosthesis. Ann R Coll Surg Engl. 1991;73(2):67–9.
12. Ullmann Y, Peled IJ, Laufer D, Blumenfeld I. Nipple-areola reconstruction with a custom-made silicone ectoprosthesis. Ann Plast Surg. 1992;28(5):485–7.
13. Ward CM. The uses of external nipple-areola prostheses following reconstruction of a breast mound after mastectomy. Br J Plast Surg. 1985;38(1):51–4.
14. Chang WH. Nipple reconstruction with a T flap. Plast Reconstr Surg. 1984;73(1):140–3.
15. Cronin ED, Humphreys DH, Ruiz-Razura A. Nipple reconstruction: the S flap. Plast Reconstr Surg. 1988;81(5):783–7.

16. Little J, Spear S. The finishing touches in nipple-areola reconstruction. Perspect Plast Surg. 1987;2(1):1–17.
17. Anton LE, Hartrampf CR. Nipple reconstruction with local flaps: star and wrap flaps. Perspect Plast Surg. 1991;5:67–78.
18. Hallock GG, Altobelli JA. Cylindrical nipple reconstruction using an H flap. Ann Plast Surg. 1993;30(1):23–6.
19. Teimourian B, Duda G. The propeller flap: a one-stage procedure for nipple-areola reconstruction. Aesthet Plast Surg. 1994;18(1):81–4.
20. Jones G, Bostwick J 3rd. Nipple-areolar reconstruction. Oper Tech Plast Reconstr Surg. 1994;1:35–8.
21. Thomas SV, Gellis MB, Pool R. Nipple reconstruction with a new local tissue flap. Plast Reconstr Surg. 1996;97(5):1053–6.
22. Rubino C, Dessy LA, Posadinu A. A modified technique for nipple reconstruction: the 'arrow flap'. Br J Plast Surg. 2003;56(3):247–51.
23. Germano D, De Biasio F, Piedimonte A, Parodi PC. Nipple reconstruction using the fleur-de-lis flap technique. Aesthet Plast Surg. 2006;30(4):399–402.
24. Jamnadas-Khoda B, Thomas R, Heppell S. The 'cigar roll' flap for nipple areola complex reconstruction: a novel technique. J Plast Reconstr Aesthet Surg. 2011;64(8):e218–20.
25. Wong WW, Hiersche MA, Martin MC. The angel flap for nipple reconstruction. Can J Plast Surg. 2013;21(1):e1–4.
26. Dini GM, Ferreira LM. The graft said, "when I grow up, I want to be a flap": nipple reconstruction with the graft flap. Plast Reconstr Surg. 2006;117(1):333–4.
27. Cohen IK, Ward JA, Chandrasekhar B. The pinwheel flap nipple and barrier areola graft reconstruction. Plast Reconstr Surg. 1986;77(6):995–9.
28. Muruci A, Dantas JJ, Noguerira LR. Reconstruction of the nipple-areola complex. Plast Reconstr Surg. 1978;61(4):558–60.
29. DiPirro ME. Reconstruction of the nipple and areola after a burn. Case report. Plast Reconstr Surg. 1970;46(3):299–300.
30. Little JW 3rd, Munasifi T, McCulloch DT. One-stage reconstruction of a projecting nipple: the quadrapod flap. Plast Reconstr Surg. 1983;71(1):126–33.
31. Hartrampf CR Jr, Culbertson JH. A dermal-fat flap for nipple reconstruction. Plast Reconstr Surg. 1984;73(6):982–6.
32. Silversmith PE. Nipple reconstruction by quadrapod flaps. Plast Reconstr Surg. 1983;72(3):422.
33. Hammond DC, Khuthaila D, Kim J. The skate flap purse-string technique for nipple-areola complex reconstruction. Plast Reconstr Surg. 2007;120(2):399–406.
34. Shestak KC, Nguyen TD. The double opposing periareola flap: a novel concept for nipple-areola reconstruction. Plast Reconstr Surg. 2007;119(2):473–80.
35. Yang JD, Ryu JY, Ryu DW, Kwon OH, Bae SG, Lee JW, et al. Our experiences in nipple reconstruction using the Hammond flap. Arch Plast Surg. 2014;41(5):550–5.
36. Eng JS. Bell flap nipple reconstruction—a new wrinkle. Ann Plast Surg. 1996;36(5):485–8.
37. Farace F, Bulla A, Puddu A, Rubino C. The arrow flap for nipple reconstruction: long term results. J Plast Reconstr Aesthet Surg. 2010;63(10):e756–7.
38. Brackley PT, Iqbal A. Enhancing your C-V flap nipple reconstruction. J Plast Reconstr Aesthet Surg. 2009;62(1):128–30.
39. Berson MI. Construction of pseudoareola. Surgery. 1946;20(6):808.
40. Grosdidier A, Lebeau J, Ochala C, Payan R, Bettega G. "Double flag" flap nipple reconstruction. Clinical evaluation on 70 cases. Ann Chir Plast Esthet. 2014;59(2):123–9.
41. Puckett CL, Concannon MJ, Croll GH, Welsh CF. Nipple reconstruction using the "inchworm" flap. Aesthet Plast Surg. 1992;16(2):117–22.
42. Riot S, Devinck F, Aljudaibi N, Duquennoy-Martinot V, Guerreschi P. Tattooing of the nipple-areola complex in breast reconstruction: technical note. Ann Chir Plast Esthet. 2016;61(2):141–4.
43. Lossing C, Brongo S, Holmstrom H. Nipple reconstruction with a modified S-flap technique. Scand J Plast Reconstr Surg Hand Surg. 1998;32(3):275–9.
44. Narra K, Diaz LM, Papay FA. A new approach to nipple reconstruction: the modified S-flap. Plast Reconstr Surg. 2008;122(2):89e–90e.
45. Eskenazi L. A one-stage nipple reconstruction with the "modified star" flap and immediate tattoo: a review of 100 cases. Plast Reconstr Surg. 1993;92(4):671–80.
46. Sierakowski A, Niranjan N. Star flap with a dermal platform for nipple reconstruction. J Plast Reconstr Aesthet Surg. 2011;64(2):e55–6.
47. Cuomo R, Sisti A, Grimaldi L, D'Aniello C. Modified Arrow Flap Technique for Nipple Reconstruction. Breast J. 2016;22(6):710–11.
48. El-Ali K, Dalal M, Kat CC. Modified C-V flap for nipple reconstruction: our results in 50 patients. J Plast Reconstr Aesthet Surg. 2009;62(8):991–6.
49. Katerinaki E, Sircar T, Sterne GD. The C-V flap for nipple reconstruction after previous skin-sparing mastectomy and immediate breast reconstruction: refinements of donor-site closure. Aesthet Plast Surg. 2011;35(4):624–7.
50. Kim JY, Gust MJ, Connor CM, Davila A, Hansen NM, Nguyen KT. The weave technique for nipple reconstruction. J Plast Surg Hand Surg. 2013;47(2):135–8.
51. Macdonald CR, Nakhdjevani A, Shah A. The "Swiss-Roll" flap: a modified C-V flap for nipple reconstruction. Breast. 2011;20(5):475–7.
52. Mori H, Hata Y. Modified C-V flap in nipple reconstruction. J Plast Reconstr Aesthet Surg. 2008;61(9):1109–10.
53. Otterburn DM, Sikora KE, Losken A. An outcome evaluation following postmastectomy nipple reconstruction using the C-V flap technique. Ann Plast Surg. 2010;64(5):574–8.
54. Witt P, Dujon DG. The V-V flap—a simple modification of the C-V flap for nipple reconstruction. J Plast Reconstr Aesthet Surg. 2013;66(7):1009–10.
55. Temiz G, Yesiloglu N, Sirinoglu H, Sarici M. A new modification of c-v flap technique in nipple reconstruction: rolled triangular dermal-fat flaps. Aesthet Plast Surg. 2015;39(1):173–5.

56. Guerra AB, Khoobehi K, Metzinger SE, Allen RJ. New technique for nipple areola reconstruction: arrow flap and rib cartilage graft for long-lasting nipple projection. Ann Plast Surg. 2003;50(1):31–7.
57. Lebeau J, Lopes TR, Gallodoro A, Raphael B. Nipple reconstruction: technical aspects and evolution in 14 patients. Plast Reconstr Surg. 2006;117(3):751–6.
58. Schoeller T, Schubert HM, Pulzl P, Wechselberger G. Nipple reconstruction using a modified arrow flap technique. Breast. 2006;15(6):762–8.
59. Saleh DB, Mohammed PD. The double-breasted dermal flap in nipple reconstruction. J Reconstr Microsurg. 2013;29(6):421–2.
60. Cheng MH, Ho-Asjoe M, Wei FC, Chuang DC. Nipple reconstruction in Asian females using banked cartilage graft and modified top hat flap. Br J Plast Surg. 2003;56(7):692–4.
61. Cheng MH, Rodriguez ED, Smartt JM, Cardenas-Mejia A. Nipple reconstruction using the modified top hat flap with banked costal cartilage graft: long-term follow-up in 58 patients. Ann Plast Surg. 2007;59(6):621–8.
62. De Biasio F, Nadalig B, Salemi S, Parodi PC. Re: Nipple reconstruction: the top hat technique. Ann Plast Surg. 2006;56(2):224.
63. Gamboa-Bobadilla GM. Nipple reconstruction: the top hat technique. Ann Plast Surg. 2005;54(3):243–6.
64. Hamori CA, LaRossa D. The top hat flap: for one stage reconstruction of a prominent nipple. Aesthet Plast Surg. 1998;22(2):142–4.
65. Lesavoy M, Liu TS. The diamond double-opposing V-Y flap: a reliable, simple, and versatile technique for nipple reconstruction. Plast Reconstr Surg. 2010;125(6):1643–8.
66. Riccio CA, Zeiderman MR, Chowdhry S, Wilhelmi BJ. Review of nipple reconstruction techniques and introduction of v to y technique in a bilateral wise pattern mastectomy or reduction mammaplasty. Eplasty. 2015;15:e11.
67. Kroll SS. Nipple reconstruction with the double-opposing tab flap. Plast Reconstr Surg. 1999;104(2):511–4.
68. Kroll SS, Hamilton S. Nipple reconstruction with the double-opposing-tab flap. Plast Reconstr Surg. 1989;84(3):520–5.
69. Tatlidede S, Yesilada AK, Egemen O, Bas L. A new technique in nipple reconstruction: dome technique with double pedicle. Ann Plast Surg. 2008;60(2):141–3.
70. Turgut G, Sacak B, Gorgulu T, Yesilada AK, Bas L. Nipple reconstruction with bipedicled dermal flap: a new and easy technique. Aesthet Plast Surg. 2009;33(5):770–3.
71. Rem K, Al Hindi A, Sorin T, Ozil C, Revol M, Mazouz Dorval S. Nipple reconstruction after implant-based breast reconstruction in radiated patients: a new safe dermal flap. J Plast Reconstr Aesthet Surg. 2016;69(5):617–22.
72. Lee S, Jung Y, Bae Y. Immediate nipple reconstruction as oncoplastic breast surgery: the cigar roll flap with inner dermal core technique. Aesthet Plast Surg. 2015;39(5):706–12.
73. Barton FE Jr. Latissimus dermal-epidermal nipple reconstruction. Plast Reconstr Surg. 1982;70(2):234–7.
74. Di Benedetto G, Sperti V, Pierangeli M, Bertani A. A simple and reliable method of nipple reconstruction using a spiral flap made of residual scar tissue. Plast Reconstr Surg. 2004;114(1):158–61.
75. Chen SG, Chiu TF, Su WF, Chou TD, Chen TM, Wang HJ. Nipple-areola complex reconstruction using badge flap and intradermal tattooing. Br J Surg. 2005;92(4):435–7.
76. Karabagli Y, Kose AA, Mangir S, Cetin C. e-Flap nipple reconstruction in amputation mammaplasty. Aesthet Plast Surg. 2012;36(5):1140–3.
77. Kon M. Latissimus dorsi three-flap nipple reconstruction. Aesthet Plast Surg. 1984;8(4):243–5.
78. Van Laeken N, Genoway K. Nipple reconstruction using a two-step purse-string suture technique. Can J Plast Surg. 2011;19(2):56–9.
79. Kim JH, Ahn HC. A revision restoring projection after nipple reconstruction by burying four triangular dermal flaps. Arch Plast Surg. 2016;43(4):339–43.
80. Satteson ES, Reynolds MF, Bond AM, Pestana IA. An analysis of complication risk factors in 641 nipple reconstructions. Breast J. 2016;22(4):379–83.
81. Zhong T, Antony A, Cordeiro P. Surgical outcomes and nipple projection using the modified skate flap for nipple-areolar reconstruction in a series of 422 implant reconstructions. Ann Plast Surg. 2009;62(5):591–5.
82. Adams WM. Labial transplant for correction of loss of the nipple. Plast Reconstr Surg (1946). 1949;4(3):295–8.
83. Millard DR Jr. Nipple and areola reconstruction by split-skin graft from the normal side. Plast Reconstr Surg. 1972;50(4):350–3.
84. Nagura-Inomata N, Iwahira Y, Hayashi N, Komiya T, Takahashi O. The optimal reconstruction size of nipple-areola complex following breast implant in breast cancer patients. Spring. 2016;5:579.
85. Mendelson BC. Results of nipple areola reconstruction. Aust N Z J Surg. 1983;53(1):63–6.
86. White CP, Gdalevitch P, Strazar R, Murrill W, Guay NA. Surgical tips: areolar tattoo prior to nipple reconstruction. J Plast Reconstr Aesthet Surg. 2011;64(12):1724–6.
87. Levites HA, Fourman MS, Phillips BT, Fromm IM, Khan SU, Dagum AB, et al. Modeling fade patterns of nipple areola complex tattoos following breast reconstruction. Ann Plast Surg. 2014;73(Suppl 2):S153–6.
88. El-Ali K, Dalal M, Kat CC. Tattooing of the nipple-areola complex: review of outcome in 40 patients. J Plast Reconstr Aesthet Surg. 2006;59(10):1052–7.
89. Colwell AS, Breuing KH. Primary nipple reconstruction with AlloDerm: is a dermal flap always necessary? Plast Reconstr Surg. 2009;124(5):260e–2e.

# V-Y Nipple Reconstruction

# 44

Matthew R. Zeiderman and Bradon J. Wilhelmi

## 44.1 Introduction

Nipple-areola complex reconstruction (NAR) is the final procedure in breast reconstruction after mastectomy. Studies have demonstrated that timely completion of nipple and areola construction leads to improved psychological well-being in addition to patient and partner satisfaction and represents the defining feature of the female breast [1, 2]. Many technical descriptions regarding nipple reconstruction exist, but there is little evidence-based consensus establishing which techniques are superior. Therefore, no definitive indications dictate when a certain technique should be employed. Nipple reconstructions are often complicated by scars or previous nipple reconstruction. This makes the procedure more challenging as it frequently relies on randomly based flaps. The V-Y advancement flap for nipple reconstruction was first described by Riccio et al. in 2015 [3] and serves as a straightforward option for nipple reconstruction. It is an ideal choice for the breast compromised by vertical mastectomy scar at ideal site of nipple reconstruction, Wise-pattern reduction mammoplasty, or secondary nipple reconstruction.

The V-Y flap is a modified advancement flap with a local pedicle which allows for structure elongation and is commonly used for the closure of small to medium cutaneous defects of the face [4]. The V-Y NAR is ideal for any case where other well-known methods would be technically challenging or likely produce a poor result secondary to compromised blood flow through pre-existing scar.

M.R. Zeiderman, M.D.
Division of Plastic and Reconstructive Surgery, University of California, Davis, 2221 Stockton Blvd, Room 2125, Sacramento, CA 95817, USA
e-mail: mrzeiderman@ucdavis.edu

B.J. Wilhelmi, M.D. (✉)
Division of Plastic and Reconstructive Surgery, University of Louisville School of Medicine, Louisville, KY, USA

Leonard J. Weiner Professor and Chief, Department of Plastic Surgery, University of Louisville, Louisville, KY, USA

Hiram C. Polk Jr. Department of Surgery, University of Louisville, Louisville, KY, USA
e-mail: Bradon.wilhelmi@louisville.edu

## 44.2 Technique

Flap design is the same as a traditional V-Y flap. The position of the new nipple is outlined and the base of the flap is set as the margin of the new nipple (Fig. 44.1). The apex of the V is designed for the two arms of the V to be 2 cm in length. This provides 2/3 cm nipple projection. The arms may be designed 3 cm in length if 1 cm projection is desired. Incisions are made through the skin to subcutaneous fat. The flap is elevated by dissection in the deep subcutaneous plane,


M.A. Shiffman (ed.), *Nipple-Areolar Complex Reconstruction*,
https://doi.org/10.1007/978-3-319-60925-6_44

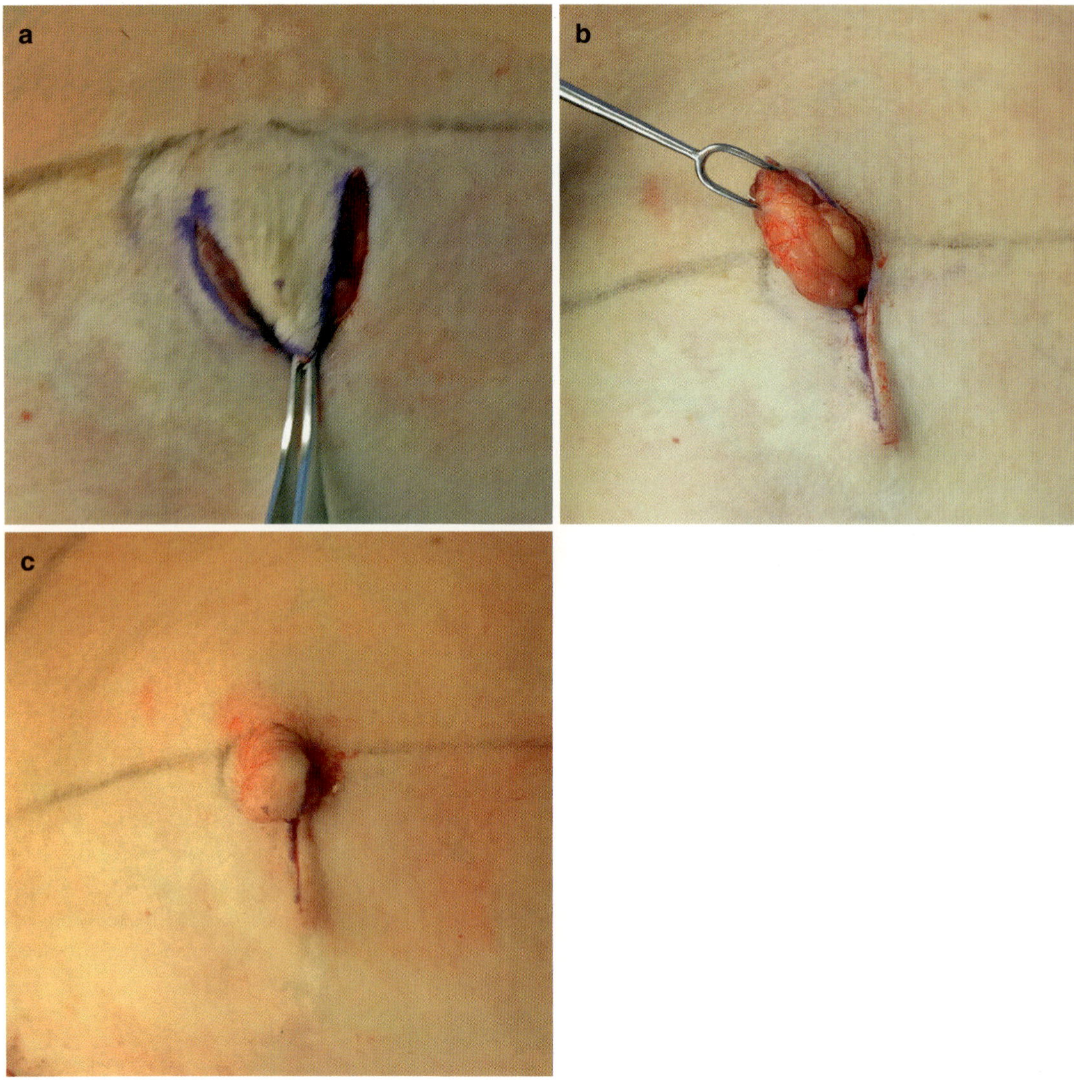


**Fig. 44.1** (**a**) Flap design. (**b**) Demonstration of flap dissection. (**c**) Flap inset and final appearance

just above the muscle or implant capsule. The secondary defect at the apex of the flap is subsequently closed in linear fashion with deep and superficial sutures (Image 2). The apex of the flap is folded upon itself and the edges are approximated (Fig. 44.1). All tissue should be closed as much as possible while remaining tension free.

The superior base of the flap allows incorporation of previous scars into one of the borders of the flap (Fig. 44.2). Consequently, the scar at the donor site is concealed on the inferior surface of the nipple, yielding a more aesthetically pleasing result for the patient.

V-Y NAR has distinct advantages stemming from linear site closure. The procedure forms only one new scar. Linear closure of the small donor site prevents distortion and flattening of the breast tissue. Primary closure of the donor site obviates the need for a full-thickness skin graft. This avoids complications of graft ischemia and creation of a new donor site. The native skin of the breast is left intact. Areolar tattooing is subsequently easier to perform and more likely

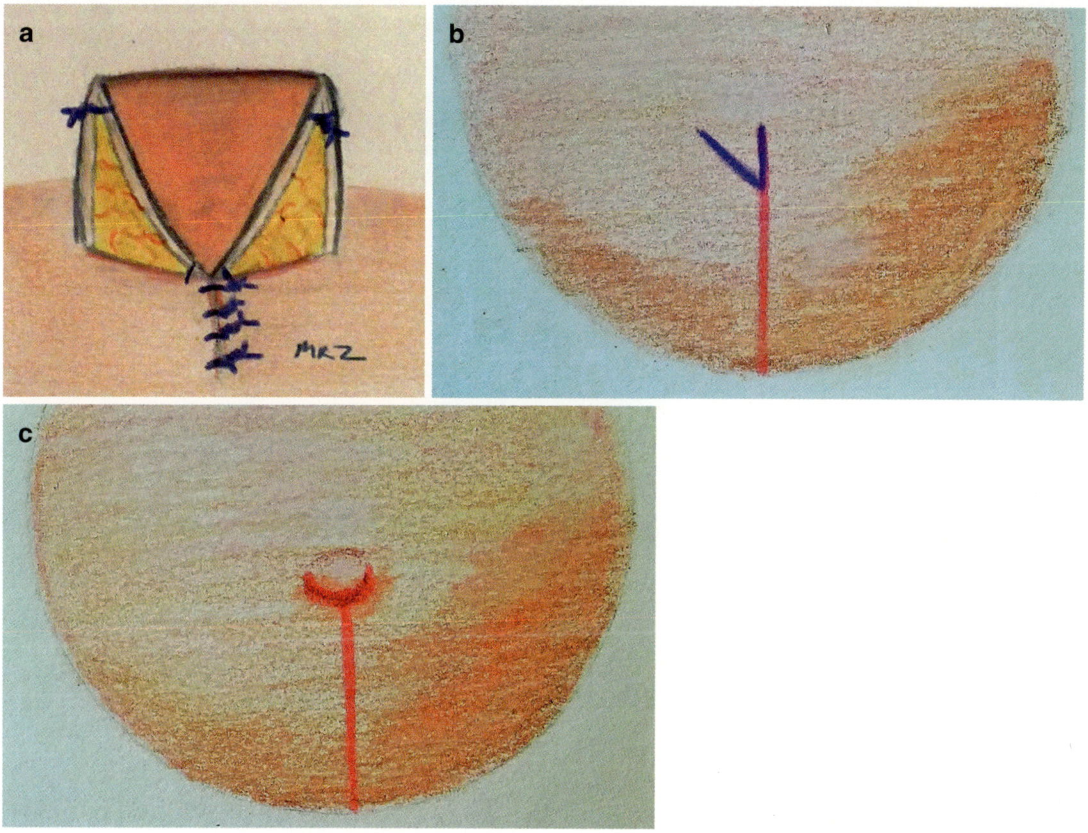


**Fig. 44.2** (**a**) Demonstration of beginning of flap inset and fold-over. (**b**, **c**) Incorporation of scar

to maintain long-term pigmentation, whereas donor grafts frequently taken from the inner thigh less reliably maintain tattoo pigmentation due to the fragility of the graft tissue.

Possible integration of mastectomy scar into the reconstructed nipple better maintains long-term nipple projection due to decreased fat resorption from scar tissue. As a subdermal pedicle flap, the V-Y is not subject to the same retraction forces as centrally based flaps, which helps to maintain long-term projection. Preservation of the subdermal pedicle and subcutaneous fat decreases fat resorption and necrosis because the native vascular architecture is not disrupted. By including the subdermal fat in the newly reconstructed nipple, the use of cartilage or synthetic fillers can be avoided. This is desirable, as cartilage filler results in a firm, unnatural feeling nipple and carries risk of extrusion, which requires subsequent revision or removal. Furthermore, cartilage graft can cause wound dehiscence, implant exposure, and infection, all of which may necessitate implant removal.

## Conclusions

The V-Y flap is a simple option for NAR with minimal operative morbidity and scar burden. The method produces acceptable aesthetic results for patients with unfavorable anatomy for other NAR techniques or who are seeking revision of previous nipple reconstruction.

## References

1. Momeni A, Becker A, Torio-Padron N, Iblher N, Stark GB, Bannasch H. Nipple reconstruction: evidence-based trials in the plastic surgical literature. Aesthet Plast Surg. 2008;32(1):18–20.
2. Few JW, Marcus JR, Casas LA, Aitken ME, Redding J. Long-term predictable nipple projection following reconstruction. Plast Reconstr Surg. 1999;104(5):1321–4.
3. Riccio CA, Zeiderman MR, Chowdhry S, Wilhelmi BJ. Review of nipple reconstruction techniques and introduction of v to y technique in a bilateral wise pattern mastectomy or reduction mammaplasty. Eplasty. 2015;15:e11.
4. Braun M Jr, Cook J. The island pedicle flap. Dermatol Surg. 2005;31(8 Pt 2):995–1005.

# Three-Dimensional Nipple-Areola Tattooing

45

Joseph A. Ricci and Eric G. Halvorson

## 45.1 Introduction

Breast reconstruction represents one of the most common procedures performed annually by reconstructive surgeons [1, 2]. While breast reconstruction can be accomplished with a variety of techniques including implants and/or autologous tissue, many patients desire reconstruction of the nipple-areola complex (NAC). To a degree, the need for nipple reconstruction has somewhat decreased as the popularity of nipple-sparing mastectomy has increased [1, 2]. Although optional, many women consider NAC reconstruction an essential element of breast reconstruction following mastectomy. Furthermore, construction of a nipple and subsequent areola tattooing completes an emotional and complex process of feeling whole again for many women.

There are several different strategies for NAC reconstruction and a wide range of reported techniques [3]. Typically, nipple reconstruction is performed with various local flaps, and the literature is filled with numerous variations of local flap designs for nipple reconstruction. Areola reconstruction has been achieved with skin grafting, labial grafts, dermabrasion, tattooing, or a combination of the above. Unfortunately, nipple projection can be difficult to maintain, especially in patients with thin or irradiated soft tissue [3–7], and the color of the areola can be unpredictable.

Despite the benefits of nipple reconstruction, it is important to recognize that some patients choose or are best served by tattoo-only NAC reconstruction. To date there has been a minimal amount published on this technique, and outcome evaluations are needed [8]. Some patients may not like the fact that reconstructed nipples maintain projection at all times. Others forego surgical approaches because they do not want another surgical procedure. Lastly, in patients who have undergone radiotherapy or those with extremely thin mastectomy flaps, tattooing alone may be the safest option, considering the increased risk of complications with thin, tight, or atrophic skin. Tattooing alone likely decreases the risk of infection and potential subsequent implant exposure in these patients.

In one series of patients with long-term follow-up, Spear and Arias [9] reported that 84% were satisfied with their tattoo and 86% would opt for tattooing again. Recently, three-dimensional (3D) tattoo techniques have allowed for superior esthetic results over traditional techniques for tattoo-only NAC reconstruction, and it is likely that patient satisfaction is even higher. In this article, we describe 3D NAC tattoo and demonstrate outcomes for the reader to evaluate.

J.A. Ricci, M.D. • E.G. Halvorson, M.D. (✉)
Department of Plastic Surgery, Brigham and Women's Hospital, Harvard Medical School, 75 Francis Street, Boston, MA 02115, USA
e-mail: jaricci@partners.org; ehalvorson@partners.org


M.A. Shiffman (ed.), *Nipple-Areolar Complex Reconstruction*,
https://doi.org/10.1007/978-3-319-60925-6_45

## 45.2 Technique

Most NAC tattoos are performed in the clinic by a mid-level practitioner without supervision. Traditionally, these tattoos use lighter ink for the areola and a central circle of darker ink for the nipple (Fig. 45.1). Although these traditional tattooing techniques produce satisfactory results, newer methods, inspired by the work of professional tattoo artist Vinnie Myers [10], have become popular with improved results.

The 3D technique is essentially the inverse of traditional NAC tattoo. Ideally, like traditional tattooing, it is best performed more than 3 months following breast reconstruction, after the postoperative swelling has receded completely, and a stable result has been achieved. In addition, immature scars do not accept dye well. The areola is created according to the patient's preferred diameter and color. The final areolar diameter and location on the breast should be marked with the patient standing before the procedure, taking the patient's preference into account (Fig. 45.2).

For 3D tattoos, instead of using a darker inner circle to create the appearance of a nipple, a lighter inner circle is created with a dark border.

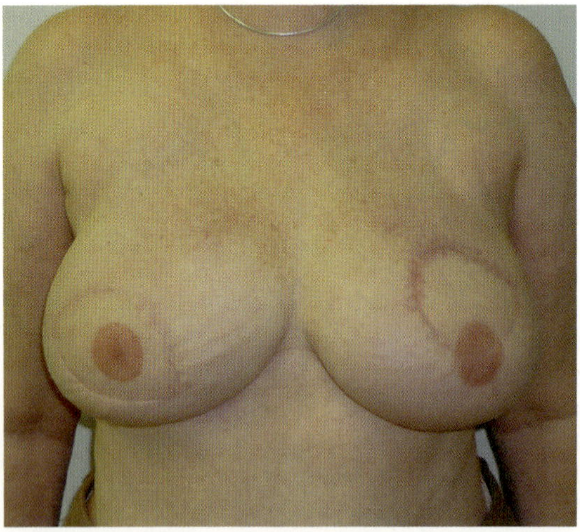

**Fig. 45.1** Nipple-areola complex reconstruction using standard tattoo-only technique. The nipple is tattooed darker than the areola and lacks the illusion of projection

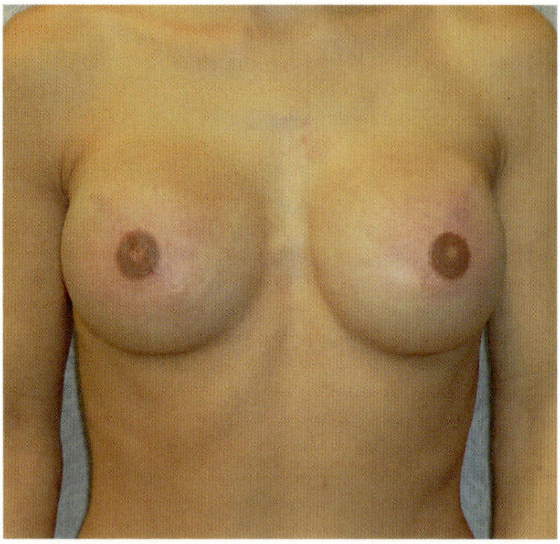

**Fig. 45.2** Three-dimensional nipple-areola complex reconstruction by a clinic nurse using standard clinic medical equipment. Note the nipple is tattooed lighter than the areola

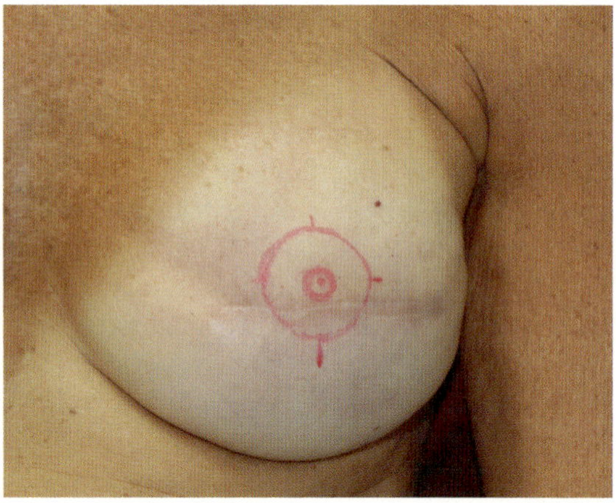

**Fig. 45.3** Pre-procedure markings for three-dimensional nipple-areola complex tattooing by a professional tattoo artist (Photograph courtesy of Vinnie Myers)

This border is then thickened inferiorly to create a shadow effect. A satisfactory result can be achieved with standard medical tattooing equipment (Figs. 45.3 and 45.4); however, a professional tattoo artist with specialized equipment and ink can produce an outstanding result, including tattooing of Montgomery glands (Figs. 45.5 and 45.6).

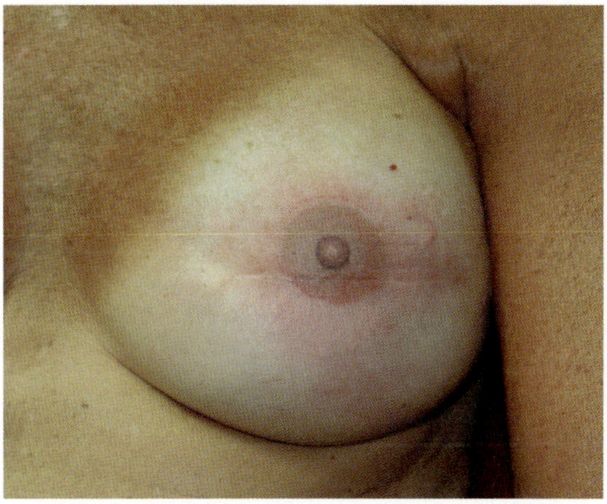

**Fig. 45.4** Second step in professional three-dimensional nipple reconstruction after the addition of a dark rim that is thicker inferiorly, giving a shadow effect and the appearance of more projection (Photograph courtesy of Vinnie Myers)

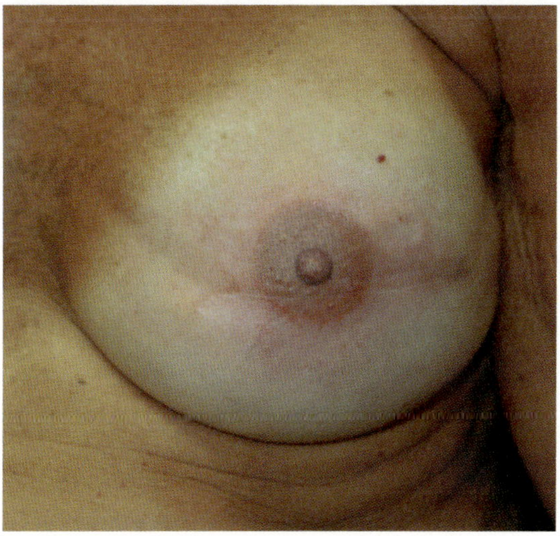

**Fig. 45.5** Three-dimensional tattoo-only nipple-areola complex reconstruction performed by professional tattoo artist. Note the inclusion of Montgomery glands (Photograph courtesy of Vinnie Myers)

## 45.3 Discussion

The plastic surgery community takes pride in its artistic sensibility. With respect to NAC tattoo, however, our simple assumptions have resulted in an artistic blunder. Professional artists have long

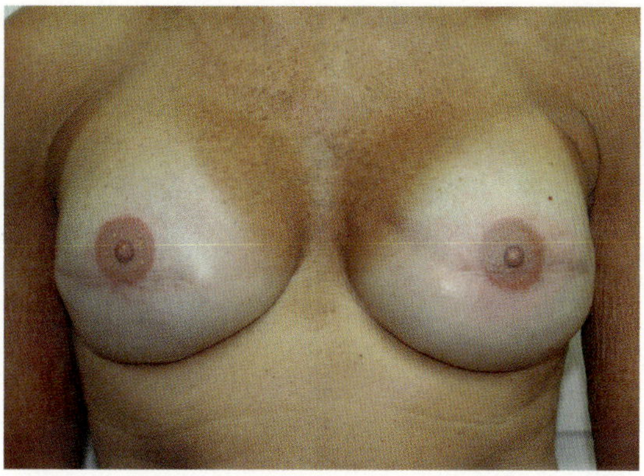

**Fig. 45.6** Bilateral three-dimensional tattoo-only nipple-areola complex reconstruction performed by a professional tattoo artist (Photograph courtesy of Vinnie Myers)

recognized that the juxtaposition of light and dark colors can simulate shadows, creating an artificial sense of depth on an otherwise two-dimensional object. Objects in light stand out, whereas those in shadow appear recessed. This was well recognized by Burget and Menickin [11] on their classic article on nasal subunits. Any prominence such as the nose, ear, or in this case, the nipple, will achieve three-dimensionality when light and shadow are used appropriately in two dimensions. This artistic principle serves as the basis for the 3D NAC tattoo technique presented.

Traditional medical tattooing procedures ignore the basic fundamentals of professional tattooing with respect to machine speed, needle type, and color mixing. Practitioners often use preset speeds in excess of 180 cycles per second which is twice the frequency of traditional tattooing. These extra needle punctures are especially problematic when medical practitioners work on patients with thin or compromised skin. The heightened frequency and increased numbers of needle punctures can result in increased healing time, scarring, and poor pigment retention. Poor pigment retention also results from the use of medical-grade pigments which are not as vibrant or long lasting as the ink typically used by professional artists. With medical tattoos, it is not uncommon for patients to require two sessions for adequate pigmentation, in addition to occasional touch-ups.

Pigments used in medical facilities are typically vegetable oil-based dyes or metal salt pigments mixed very thin and available in a small range of colors, limiting the choices available (which can make it difficult to match the coloration of a native contralateral NAC). It is widely known that medical tattoos fade with time, sometimes becoming invisible after several years. By using traditional tattoo pigments and a color wheel, excellent color match can be achieved by professional artists with significantly improved pigment retention. Unfortunately, there is a significant disconnect between the cosmetic and traditional tattoo industries, a discussion of which is beyond the scope of this chapter. It is our belief that improved results for our patients will be realized when these two industries share best practices and establish education programs.

Although referring patients to professional tattoo artists for 3D NAC reconstruction may take some business away from a surgeon's practice, it is our obligation to offer patients the best results possible. Still, some patients and surgeons alike are wary of tattoo parlors and prefer to have their NAC tattoo performed in a medical facility. It is our hope that tattoo artists and health care providers will collaborate to bring the technology and skills required into the medical arena. Some tattoo artists are willing to work in a medical facility on a periodic basis. At the Brigham and Women's Hospital, we have partnered with the Vinnie Myers Team to have them come to our clinic on a quarterly basis. This has been a very popular addition to our armamentarium of reconstructive options for our breast reconstruction patients. Additionally, some artists are willing to demonstrate their techniques to mid-level providers who care for patients in the medical setting on a routine basis. Although it is unlikely that they will achieve similar results with medical equipment and dyes, it should still improve their results.

Searching the Internet for local tattoo shops and speaking with them by phone is a good way to establish contact with interested tattoo artists. Several websites, such as Pink Ink Project (www.pinkinkproject.com), have a list of tattoo artists who are willing to perform nipple-areola tattooing for patients [12]. The cost of 3D NAC tattoo varies by location and tattoo artist. In our experience, the typical cost for a unilateral tattoo (45 min) is approximately $400, while the cost for a bilateral tattoo (60 min) is approximately $600 [8]. Additionally, the cost for 3D NAC tattooing may also vary based on whether the hospital, patient, or tattoo artist seeks insurance reimbursement. In our experience with these procedures, most insurance companies reimburse patients between $300 and $400 on average [8]. Most professional tattoo artists will not accept insurance in their private tattoo parlors and instead will charge the patient directly for the work, leaving the patient to obtain reimbursement from their insurance provider secondarily.

With a professional 3D tattoo, it is unusual for a patient to require more than one session for a durable result. The 3D technique can also be used after formal nipple reconstruction as well and is particularly helpful to address asymmetries following surgical NAC reconstruction. By adjusting the darker ring of color around the nipple, the tattoo artist can account for asymmetries in nipple projection without the need for further surgical intervention. Furthermore, when projection is almost or completely lost, this technique can give the illusion of projection again without surgical revision. The 3D NAC tattoo technique has also changed how we perform surgical nipple reconstruction with areola tattooing. Whereas we used to tattoo the nipple construct darker than the areola (effectively decreasing the illusion of projection), we now forego tattooing of the nipple construct and only tattoo the surrounding areola.

More recently, 3D NAC tattoo has been used as an adjunct to nipple-sparing mastectomy (NSM). Following NSM, there can be complete or partial loss of the NAC as well as asymmetries in pigmentation, diameter, and nipple projection. Three-dimensional NAC tattooing, especially when performed by a professional tattoo artist, can dramatically improve such asymmetries and optimize the esthetic outcomes of NSM.

**Conclusions**

The technique of 3D NAC tattooing presented above is a significant advance in obtaining improved esthetic results for women undergoing breast reconstruction. Given the long-standing disconnect in knowledge sharing between medical practitioners and professional tattoo artists, we have only begun to explore the possible applications of medical tattoos in plastic surgery. The application of 3D techniques or "realism" in tattoo artistry has the potential to expand the role of medical tattooing and may allow us to enhance the esthetic results of not only breast reconstruction but other areas like head and neck reconstruction (e.g., eyebrow, lip vermillion tattoo) and extremity reconstruction (e.g., nail bed tattoo) as well.

## References

1. Chun YS, Verma K, Rosen H, Lipsitz S, Morris D, Kenney P, Eriksson E. Implant-based breast reconstruction using acellular dermal matrix and the risk of postoperative complications. Plast Reconstr Surg. 2010;125:429–36.
2. Breuing KH, Warren SM. Immediate bilateral breast reconstruction with implants and inferolateral AlloDerm slings. Ann Plast Surg. 2005;55:232–9.
3. Winocour S, Saksena A, Oh C, Wu PS, Laungani A, Baltzer H, Saint-Cyr M. A systematic review of comparison of autologous, allogeneic, and synthetic augmentation grafts in nipple reconstruction. Plast Reconstr Surg. 2016;137:14e–23e.
4. Zhong T, Antony A, Cordeiro P. Surgical outcomes and nipple projection using the modified skate flap for nipple-areolar reconstruction in a series of 422 implant reconstructions. Ann Plast Surg. 2009;62:591–5.
5. Richter DF, Reichenberger MA, Faymonville C. Comparison of the nipple projection after reconstruction with three different methods. Handchir Mikrochir Plast Chir. 2004;36:374–8.
6. Boccola MA, Savage J, Rozen WM, Ashton MW, Milner C, Rahdon R, Whitaker IS. Surgical correction and reconstruction of the nipple-areola complex: current review of techniques. J Reconstr Microsurg. 2010;26:589–600.
7. Jabor MA, Shayani P, Collins DR Jr, Karas T, Cohen BE. Nipple-areola reconstruction: satisfaction and clinical determinants. Plast Reconstr Surg. 2002;110:457–63.
8. Halvorson EG, Cormican M, West ME, Myers V. Three-dimensional nipple-areola tattooing: a new technique with superior results. Plast Reconstr Surg. 2014;133:1073–5.
9. Spear SL, Arias J. Long-term experience with nipple-areola tattooing. Ann Plast Surg. 1995;35:232–6.
10. Myers V. Vinnie Myers Tattoos. Available at: www.vinniemyers.com. Accessed 15 June 2016.
11. Burget GC, Menick FJ. The subunit principle in nasal reconstruction. Plast Reconstr Surg. 1985;76:239–47.
12. Project PI. 3D nipple areolar tattooing. www.pinkink-project.com. Accessed 12 June 2016.

# 46 Total Single-Stage Autologous Breast Reconstruction with Free Nipple Grafts: A Modified Goldilocks Procedure

Jean-Claude D. Schwartz

## 46.1 Introduction

The "Goldilocks mastectomy" was originally described in 2012 by Richardson and Ma [1] as an alternative postmastectomy reconstructive technique that was useful in patients with comorbidities who were not good candidates for traditional reconstructive approaches. The original description involved a skin-sparing mastectomy with deepithelialization of the mastectomy flaps to create an autologous breast mound and closure using a standard Wise pattern. Some patients chose this option who did not want a breast amputation but were not fully committed to the multiple surgeries typically required to complete a reconstruction. The author noted its limited applicability in patients with small, non-ptotic breasts and deemed this the "Goldilocks mastectomy" as it was neither amputation of the breast nor a full reconstruction. In women with significant macromastia and ptosis, this technique could be used to complete a full reconstruction in a single stage [2]. Free nipple grafts were added at the same setting to make this a more definitive reconstruction. This chapter describes the technique for creating an autologous breast mound in a single stage from the residual mastectomy flaps with subsequent free nipple grafting or nipple-areolar complex (NAC) reconstruction. Strategies are described for completely autologous reconstructions using this technique followed by subsequent skin tailoring and lipofilling in patients who are too small for a single-stage approach [3]. This approach has also been combined with subsequent implant-based surgery (unpublished results) and discuss the benefits of initially proceeding with Goldilocks mastectomy. This is a versatile reconstructive technique with low risk for immediate complications that allows the patient significant flexibility to pursue future additional volume supplementation on her own time schedule. In some patients, this technique completes their reconstruction in a single stage. The Goldilocks mastectomy is useful in patients requiring radiotherapy (unpublished results).

## 46.2 Technique

The ideal candidates for a single-stage autologous reconstruction have large, ptotic breasts with an average or above-average body mass index (BMI) (Fig. 46.1). The author excludes smokers from consideration and requires cessation for 4 weeks before surgery and until complete healing postoperatively. There are no stringent exclusions requiring the upper limits on BMI and have had very good results with patients with BMIs

J.-C. D. Schwartz, M.D., Ph.D.
Georgia Breast Surgery, PC, 631 Professional Drive, #240, Lawrenceville, GA 30046, USA
e-mail: gabreastsurgery@gmail.com


M.A. Shiffman (ed.), *Nipple-Areolar Complex Reconstruction*,
https://doi.org/10.1007/978-3-319-60925-6_46

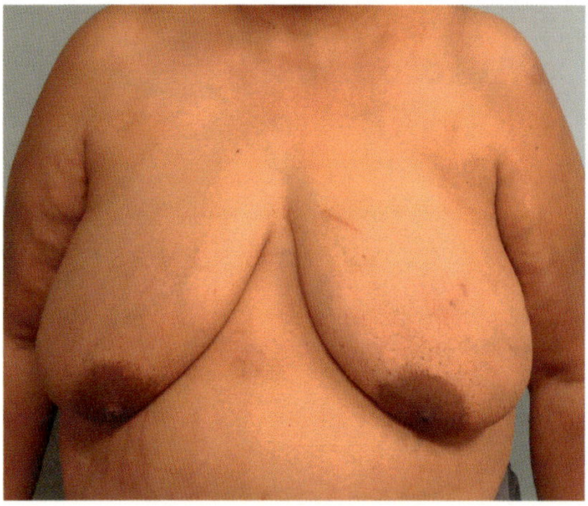

**Fig. 46.1** Ideal candidate for a single stage Goldilocks postmastectomy reconstruction with free nipple grafts. She is 66 with multifocal right breast DCIS and requires a mastectomy. She is obese and diabetic. She is a poor candidate for any other type of breast reconstruction

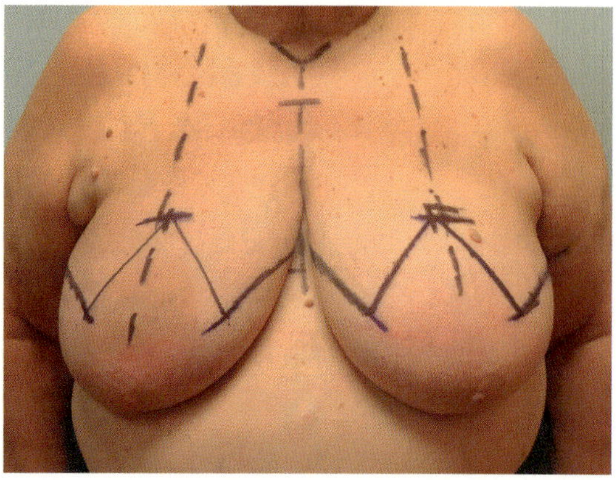

**Fig. 46.2** Wise markings as we would design for a standard reduction mammoplasty. The skin markings are slightly more aggressive as we do not have to close over a large pedicle. This has to be compromised with the fact that the blood flow to these flaps is less robust as all the breast tissue will be completely removed

between 40 and 50 whom are typically excluded from consideration for other reconstructive techniques. Patients with diabetes are at higher risk for wound healing complications but are not excluded. This technique has been performed on a single patient with recurrent breast cancer and a previous history of radiotherapy after breast conservation without complication (her nipples were not grafted as it was felt the recipient dermal bed would be compromised).

The patient is marked in the standing position as is a standard Wise reduction mammoplasty (Figs. 46.2 and 46.3). The author is more aggressive with the skin resection to allow us to maximize the amount of tissue to be deepithelialized and involuted and used to create a breast mound. This is possible because a skin closure is not performed over a pedicle as would be done in a standard reduction mammoplasty. The apex of the Wise pattern is typically 10 cm from the midline at the desired level of the most superior point of the NAC. Medial and lateral limbs measuring 11 cm (7 cm for the vertical limb and 4 cm for the NAC) are drawn with 10–14 cm between the distal ends of the limbs depending on the size of the breasts and laxity of the skin. Standard extensions to the inframammary fold (IMF) are drawn with an attempt to maximize the amount of lateral breast skin incorporated into the pattern as this skin will be used to help create the final breast mound. The meridian at the IMF is set at 10 cm with shorter or longer distances acceptable depending on chest wall dimensions.

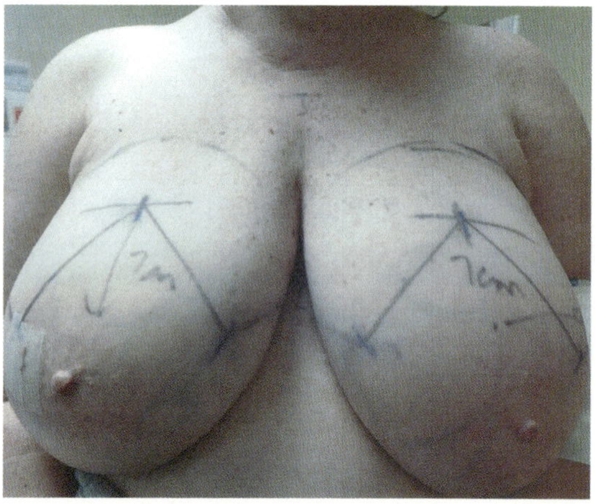

**Fig. 46.3** Preoperative Wise mammoplasty markings on an ideal single-stage Goldilocks reconstruction candidate. Note the 7 cm marking above the IMF where the most superior point of our autologous breast mound will be secured to the pectoralis. This concentrates the reconstruction at the IMF in the meridian and ensures adequate nipple projection. Additional height and projection is provided by the overlying skin flaps upon closure

The surgery is optimally performed by two surgeons with training in breast reconstruction at least one of whom should also be capable of performing the cancer resection. The cancer side is started and then the NAC is immediately resized and resected and placed in a saline-soaked laparotomy pad for later grafting. The back of the NAC is sampled and this is sent for frozen section. Full thickness incisions are made through the lateral and medial extensions from the vertical limbs to the inframammary fold. The vertical limbs are not incised as it was found that the involuted dermis and fat between the vertical limbs add important additional projection to the breast mound upon closure. The medial and lateral incisions are combined to create a single incision through the breast which typically lies above the NAC. A standard mastectomy using oncological principles is started. All breast tissue is excised leaving behind just fat and skin. If it is felt that the cancer is close to the overlying skin, this skin is sacrificed. An intraoperative gross and/or frozen section is often performed, and the author makes use of intraoperative ultrasound to give confidence that the margins will be clear. If the overlying skin is not sacrificed, it marked with clips in case it is necessary to return for inadequate margins. This requires good coordination between radiology, pathology, and surgery and surgeons with good awareness of the location of the tumor and its proximity to the overlying soft tissue. The sentinel node is then evaluated with frozen section without the need for an additional incision. A positive frozen section typically mandates an axillary dissection although definitive plans for postmastectomy radiotherapy may make this a less stringent requirement.

At this point, gowns, gloves, and instruments are changed. One surgeon then proceeds to the prophylactic mastectomy side (the overwhelming majority of patients choose to have bilateral mastectomy), and the other surgeon works on deepithelializing the skin within the Wise pattern on the cancer side. This deepithelialization is a meticulous process with an attempt to conserve as much dermis as possible to maximize both the final volume and blood flow to the underlying conserved fat (Figs. 46.4, 46.5, 46.6, and 46.7).

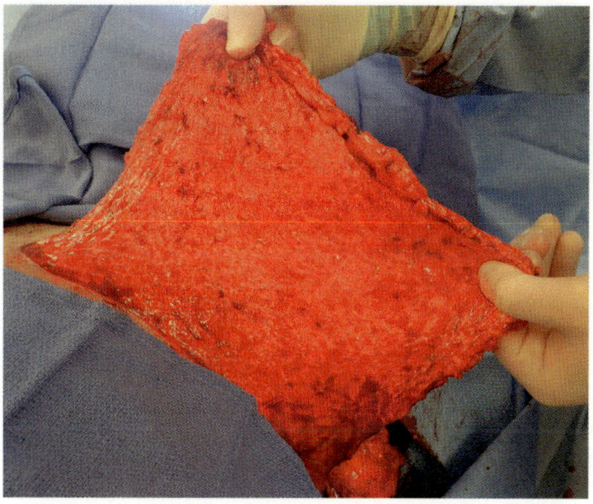

**Fig. 46.4** Inferior dermal flap meticulously dissected to preserve dermis and blood flow to the underlying subcutaneous tissue

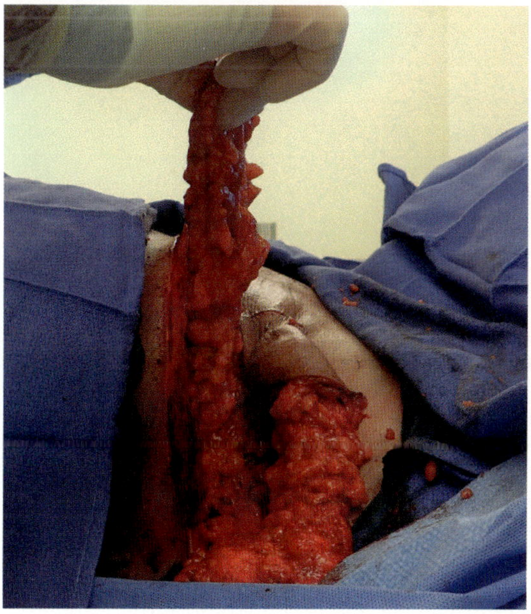

**Fig. 46.5** Mediolateral view of the dermal flap with underlying fatty tissue to demonstrate complete extirpation of the glandular breast tissue

This minimizes postoperative fat necrosis. The prophylactic nipple is similarly resized, resected, and saved for later grafting. The prophylactic mastectomy is performed in an identical fashion to the therapeutic side although there is often a subconscious more aggressive resection on the cancer side which typically leaves behind less

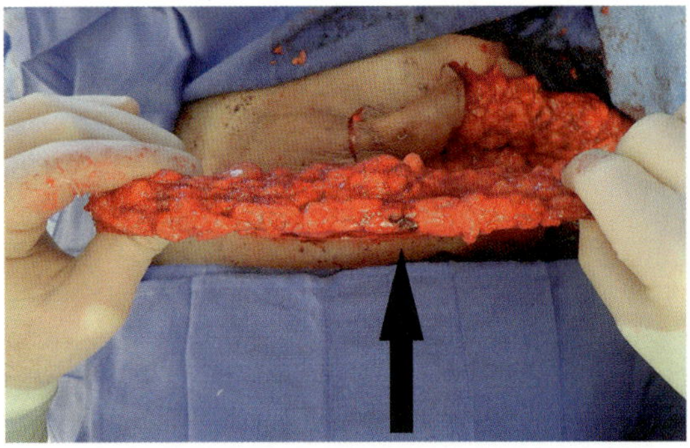

**Fig. 46.6** View of the dermal flap from above demonstrating no residual breast tissue. *Black arrow points* to the IMF

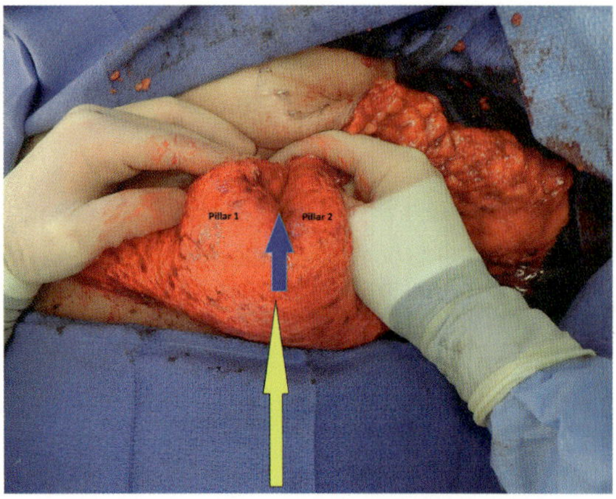


**Fig. 46.8** The dermal flap has been folded to create a breast mound. It is first folded in half, on a transverse axis, perpendicular to the vertical axis drawn by the *yellow arrow*. It is then folded in half again, around a vertical axis creating the structure shown. The two pillars of tissue shown are sewn to each other starting posteriorly near the IMF with interrupted 2-0 absorbable suture. I usually use four interrupted sutures until I reach the apex seen above (the *blue arrow* demonstrates the apical suture keeping these two pillars together). I use additional suture to secure the reconstructed mound to the chest wall approximately 7 cm superior to the IMF

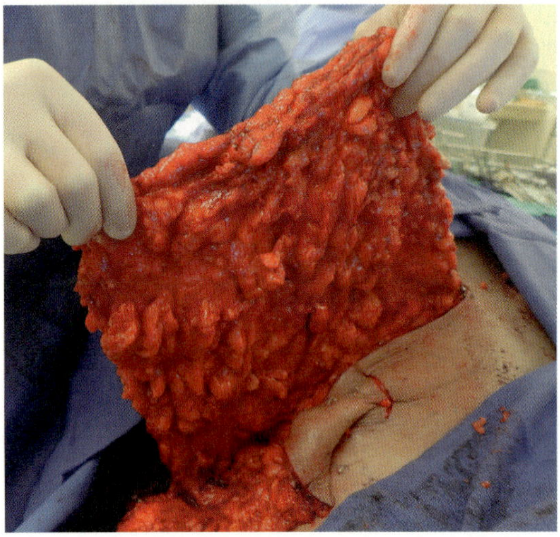

**Fig. 46.7** Underlying subcutaneous tissue of the dermal flap. Note the significant fatty tissue that will provide the volume to the reconstructed breast mound

soft tissue. After the prophylactic mastectomy is performed and the deepithelialization of the cancer side is complete, one surgeon works on creating a breast mound on the cancer side (Figs. 46.8, 46.9, and 46.10), while the other surgeon deepithelializes the prophylactic side and prepares the nipples for grafting.

The inferior dermal flap and associated subcutaneous tissue comprise the majority of tissue that will help create the breast mound (Figs. 46.4–46.7). Additional volume and projection will be obtained from bringing the vertical limbs down to the meridian in the IMF upon closure and involuting the intervening dermis and fat. In order to maximize the amount of volume available for reconstructing a breast mound centered on the meridian, it is useful to divide the dermis in the inframammary fold laterally, leaving two thirds connected medially (Fig. 46.9). This allows the shift of tissue from its lateral location to a more medial position where it is more useful. In patients with diabetes or history of tobacco abuse, one should be less aggressive with this division. The dermal flap is folded on itself on a transverse axis which creates a double thickness flap. This folded flap is then folded again on itself on a vertical axis (the vertical axis should in essence be equivalent to the meridian). At this point, a longer-lasting 2-0 absorbable suture is used to stabilize the reconstructed breast mound by suturing the dermal flaps to each other at the base near the IMF (Fig. 46.8). The interrupted suturing is continued superiorly to the apex of the reconstructed mound. This reconstructed mound is sutured to the pectoralis major muscle. A point is chosen 6–7 cm above the IMF as the most superior point

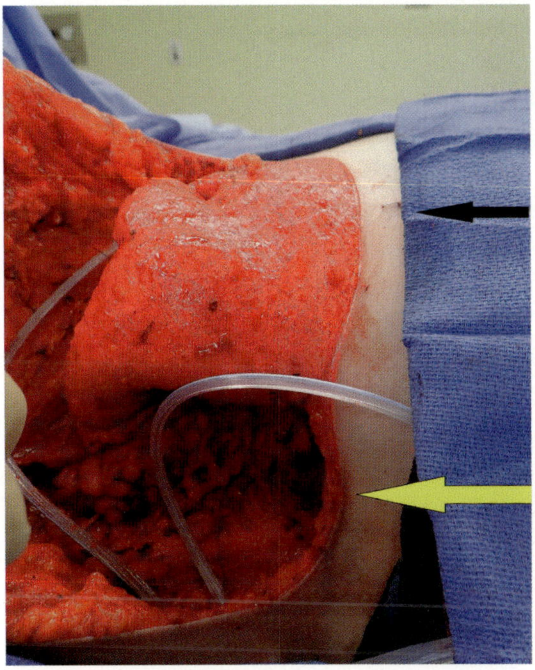

**Fig. 46.9** After the main mound is created and secured with suture, the excess lateral tissue is recruited to supplement the reconstruction. This lateral tissue is derived from dividing the lateral one third of the IMF (*yellow arrow*). This allows the mobilization of the lateral flap and transposing it medially and slightly above and behind the main mound providing additional projection and height. The author always works to keep the mound oriented centrally on the meridian (*black arrow*). Drains are shown in place. Aggressive preoperative skin markings allow us to maximally recruit additional lateral soft tissue to supplement the reconstruction

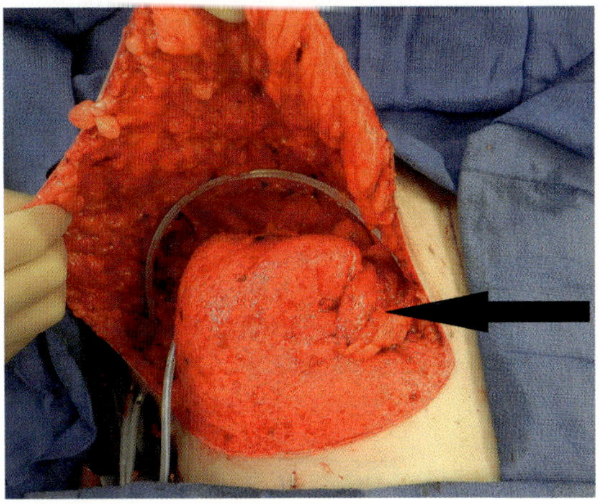

**Fig. 46.10** The lateral flap tissue is transposed medially, above and slightly posterior to the reconstructed breast mound. The tip is sutured down in a parasternal location (*black arrow*) and represents tissue that was initially at the most lateral point of the divided IMF

on the pectoralis where the mound is sutured in place (Fig. 46.3). This concentrates the bulk of the tissue inferiorly near the IMF where the author wants it to create lower pole fullness which will give a good breast shape and projection behind the nipple. Finally, the lateral excess tissue is recruited and swings it as far medially as possible over the reconstructed breast mound and sutured down to the pectoralis major muscle in a parasternal location (Fig. 46.10) which gives additional projection and height. A drain is placed behind the reconstructed mound and another one above it. One surgeon then closes as one would close a standard reduction mammoplasty. The other surgeon goes to the other side to reconstruct the contralateral breast in a similar fashion. Asymmetries between the two breasts are often noted at this point, and they can be corrected by resecting additional tissue or planning on returning at a second stage for fat grafting and/or implant placement. The patient is requested preoperatively their willingness to undergo a second-stage procedure for improved symmetry.

Finally, at the apex of the vertical limbs, a disc of the skin is deepithelialized and then the NACs are grafted in place. It is pie-crusted and sutured in place with interrupted 4-0 absorbable suture and a running 4-0 chromic suture. Sponges, wrapped in petrolatum gauze, are then placed over the NACs which are held in place with 3-0 nylon sutures (Fig. 46.11). These remain

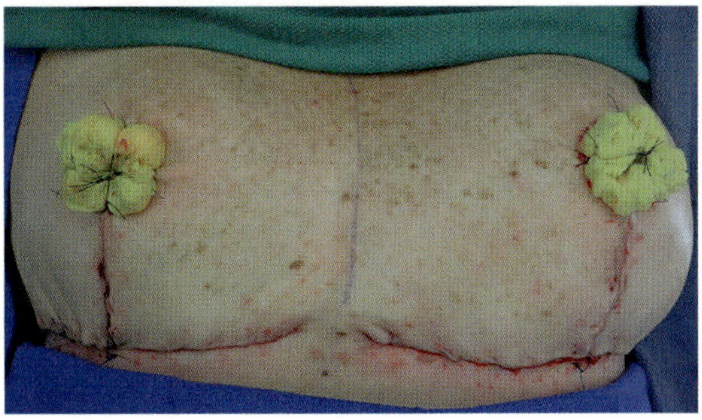

**Fig. 46.11** Finally, the overlying Wise pattern flaps are brought over the reconstructed breast mound and closed to complete the reconstruction supplying the last bit of volume. The wider the pattern is drawn at the outset, the more involuted tissue is available between the vertical limbs to give the breast mound the most possible additional projection. Finally, the nipples are grafted into position using standard techniques and the bolsters are secured for 7 days

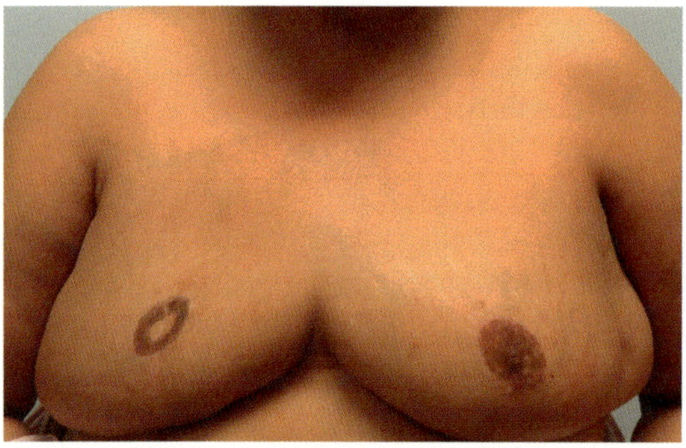

**Fig. 46.12** Reconstructed right NAC from the excess left NAC available as the right NAC was in close proximity to cancer and needed to be sacrificed. The center of the right NAC is actually a disc of skin from right mastectomy skin flap left in place surrounded by grafted, donated left areolar skin

in place for 7 days. In the case where a nipple frozen section is positive for carcinoma, excess areolar skin is taken from the contralateral side to reconstruct the areola and leave a disc of skin in place to serve as the nipple (Fig. 46.12). The breasts are dressed with bacitracin, petrolatum gauze, abdominal pads, and an elastic bandage. The entire procedure (resection and reconstruction) takes approximately 2½–4 h depending on the size of the breasts.

Patients are typically admitted overnight and discharged the following day. Drains are typically removed within a week. Persistent drainage has not been seen since the extensive dermal surface that is buried is quite reactive and is quickly adherent to the tissues. The bolsters are removed within a week and there is typically an 80–100% take of the NAC grafts. Wounds are dressed daily with bacitracin and gauze for a few weeks. Wound healing complications are commonly seen in the obese, diabetics, and patients of more advanced age. In the event of close or positive margins, the reconstruction is taken down and the area marked with clips or suture is resected. This invariably compromises the quality of the reconstruction and is best avoided with initial aggressive resection of the skin overlying the cancer and the use of intraoperative pathology and radiology. The overwhelming majority of patients are healed within 4 weeks and are prepared to proceed with adjuvant chemotherapy and or radiotherapy (Fig. 46.13).

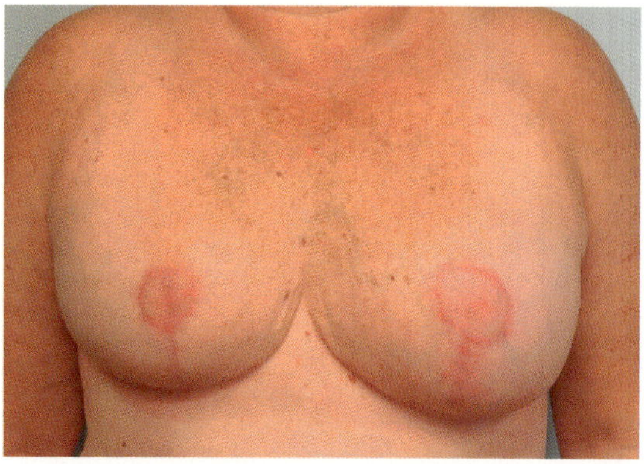

**Fig. 46.13** Four months after reconstructive surgery depicted in Figs. 46.4–46.11. Note the asymmetry between the right and left breasts which will be corrected with an implant and lipofilling on the right. The patient had agreed preoperatively to a second-stage surgery if necessary. It was decided to keep the larger, more ideal left breast with plans for future volume supplementation on the right. Other women demand a single-stage procedure which mandates reducing the size of the larger breast regardless of its ideal shape

## 46.3 Discussion

The technique described above is most suited for patients with macromastia, ptosis, and some excess adipose tissue. For these patients, bilateral mastectomy, lymph node evaluation, and single-stage autologous reconstruction with free nipple grafts may be performed in less than 4 h. For some patients with a high BMI or excessive ptosis and macromastia, this may be the preferred reconstructive option as these patients have notoriously poor results with other reconstructive approaches. This technique does not require a donor site and does not have the complications associated with using a prosthetic. This technique has been extended with success to patients with BMIs over 40 who typically would not be considered good candidates for reconstruction (Figs. 46.14 and 46.15) [4]. In addition, patients who require post-mastectomy radiotherapy do well, and the reconstruction performs similar to patients who have undergone breast conservation followed by whole breast radiotherapy (unpublished results).

After a standard mastectomy, the vast majority of recurrences are detected by palpation in the skin flaps. With the technique described here,

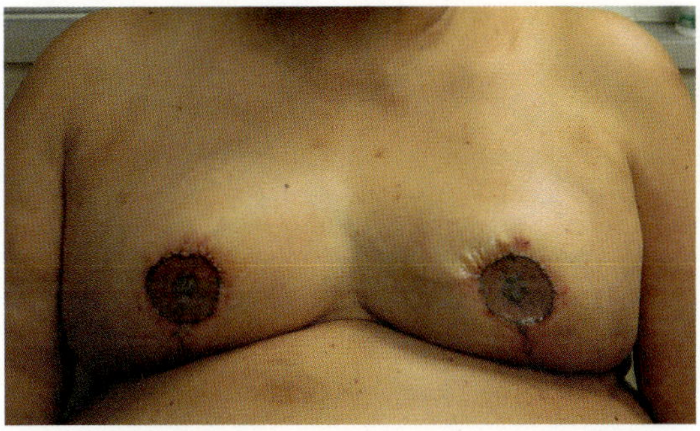

**Fig. 46.14** Two weeks postoperative for patient in Fig. 46.1 (BMI 44) after single-stage autologous reconstruction with free nipple grafts.

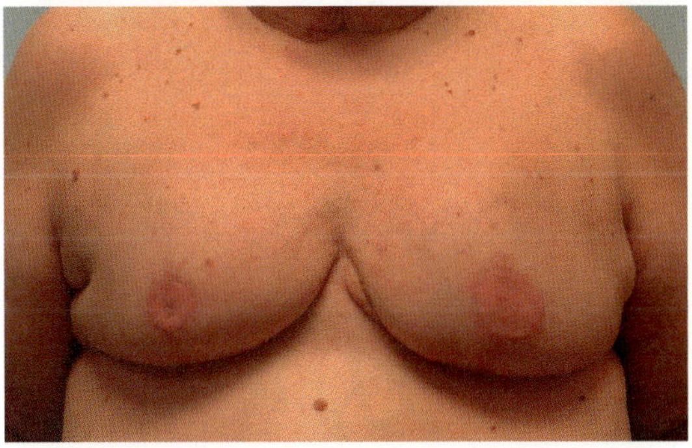

**Fig. 46.15** Four months postoperative for patient in Fig. 46.2 (BMI 46) after single-stage autologous reconstruction with free nipple grafts

the deepithelialized flaps are layered and buried potentially making detection of a recurrence more difficult. This is not the first description of burying a deepithelialized mastectomy flap after cancer surgery. The "Bostwick autoderm" involved a deepithelialized inferior mastectomy flap that was used to cover a prosthetic and sewn to the inferior edge of the pectoralis muscle [5]. There have been multiple other descriptions of similar techniques [4, 6, 7]. While there has never been a discussion regarding imaging surveillance in these patients, the Goldilocks patients may benefit from mammographic surveillance as the dermal flaps are buried and folded on each other in a more complex fashion which may mask detection to a greater degree than previously described techniques.

The majority of patients encountered will not have enough residual mastectomy flap tissue to complete their reconstruction in a single stage and will require a second stage (or more) to complete their reconstruction. For patients who demand a completely autologous reconstruction, a second-stage procedure that involves further deepithelialization and involution of the skin flaps (if there is laxity in the flaps) followed by immediate fat grafting is performed (Fig. 46.16) [3]. For a minimum of 3 months after the initial procedure, a second stage can be performed.

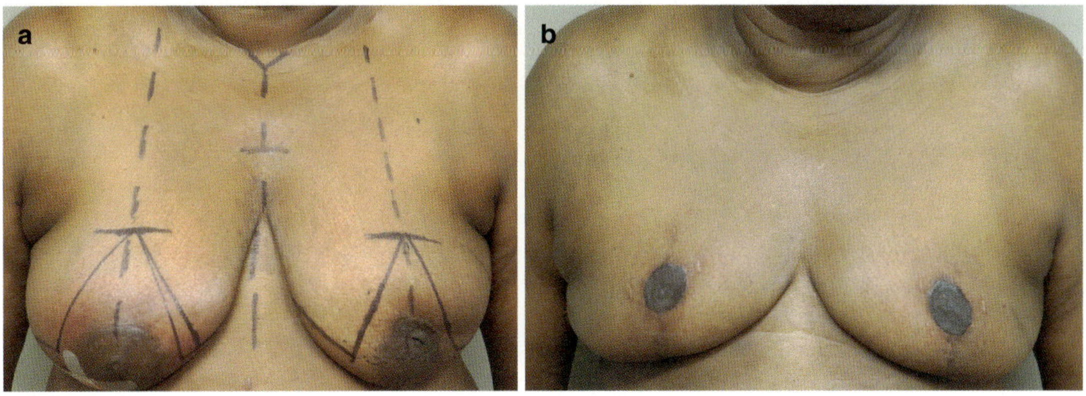


**Fig. 46.16** (**a**) 67-year-old female with multicentric right breast cancer desiring mastectomy and autologous reconstruction. She is bruised after her biopsy. Wise markings before single-stage mastectomy and immediate autologous reconstruction with free nipple grafts. (**b**) Four months after single-stage autologous reconstruction with free nipple grafts. She has a satisfactory result but requests additional autologous volume supplementation. (**c**) Intraoperative photograph demonstrating triangle of deepithelialized mastectomy flaps to help cone the breast and add additional volume. After involution of these flaps and closure, both reconstructed breasts undergo lipofilling. (**d**) One week postoperative after surgery

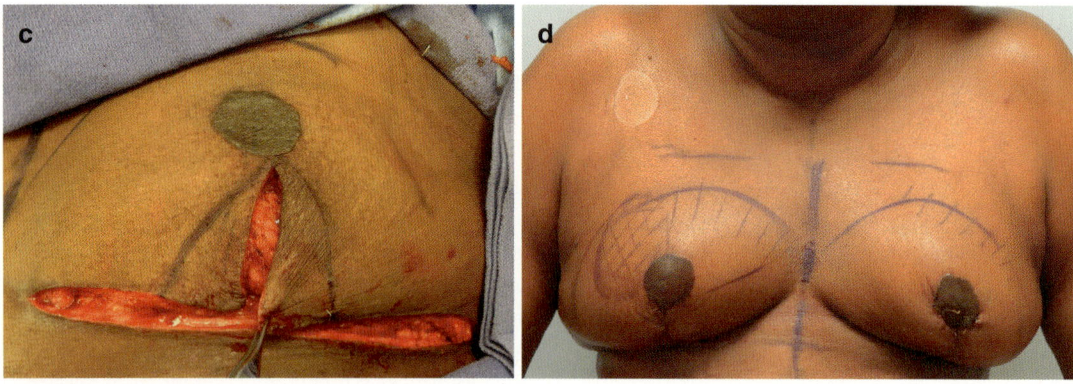


**Fig. 46.17** (continued)

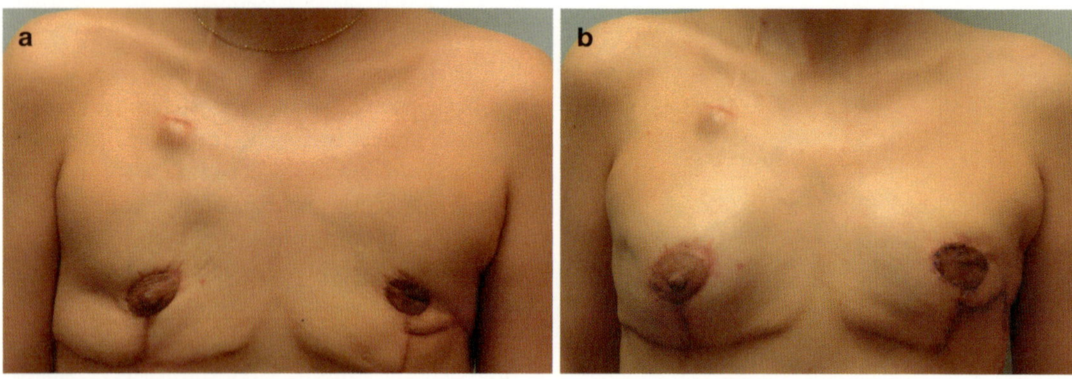


**Fig. 46.17** (**a**) 52-year-old female with multicentric left breast cancer not amenable to breast conservation. Despite being a poor candidate for this approach because of her low BMI (she did have significant ptosis), she wanted to avoid an implant-based reconstruction. On the right, there was not enough tissue to shape a mound, and therefore the inferior deepithelialized mastectomy flap was allowed to lie flat to support the NAC which was preserved on a pedicle. The left nipple needed to be disconnected and grafted because of the proximity to the cancer. Some of the inferolateral left mastectomy skin needed to be sacrificed as well because of oncological considerations. (**b**) This patient finally accepted an implant as she did not have significant excess fatty tissue for lipofilling. She did not want to commit to flap surgery. After she completed chemotherapy, she underwent placement of 11 cm short height, variable projection tissue expanders filled to 120 mL on table (150 mL capacity). There is a dramatic improvement in the shape of the reconstruction after implant placement

In some patients who realize that their target breast volumes cannot be achieved in a reasonable amount of fat grafting sessions (secondary to lack of excess adipose tissue or desire for much larger breasts), tissue expanders are placed in a second-stage procedure (Fig. 46.17). In this procedure, the pectoralis is completely released at the inframammary fold and medially to the 3 o'clock (right breast) or 9 o'clock (left breast) positions, and the expander has dual plane coverage of muscle above and deepithelialized mastectomy flap below with complete autologous cover and is expanded aggressively on table. Definitive implants could be placed at this stage, and the author would attempt this in the appropriate candidate taking into consideration their size goals and existing soft tissue envelope. In the event a second-stage implant procedure is required or planned from the outset, one might question the utility of the initial Goldilocks procedure versus placement of immediate tissue expanders after mastectomy. The Goldilocks offers the surgeon the ability to immediately address the excess skin in the first stage and utilize this for coverage of the implant in the second stage. The second-stage procedure, which is in essence a delayed implant-based reconstruction, is safer with regard to prosthetic infection, extrusion, and capsular contracture as documented by multiple previous studies [8, 9]. This strategy also allows the surgeon to obtain the final pathology and determine the need for radiotherapy which might have deleterious effect on an immediate implant-based reconstruction. These ptotic patients with higher BMIs also tend to be at higher risk for infectious complications after implant-based reconstruction in the immediate setting [4]. Implant malposition is more likely in the immediate setting as the seroma after mastectomy delays incorporation of the textured expander to a greater extent than seen in a delayed reconstruction (unpublished observations). This strategy also allows the patient the flexibility of proceeding with a second stage as this can be performed as early as 3 months after the first stage or years later (as opposed to an expander which should be exchanged within 6 months). In a way, these second-stage implant patients can be approached as those presenting for an elective subpectoral breast augmentation. Salvage of the nipple as a graft is superior to a future NAC reconstruction. The safety of delayed expander or implant placement may also be superior in the setting of radiotherapy as the underlying preserved deepithelialized flaps offer enhanced soft tissue coverage and protection of the implant.

### Conclusions

Patients with significant skin excess, ptosis, macromastia, and above-average BMIs are poor candidates for traditional reconstructions. They are, however, ideal candidates for the single-stage reconstruction described here. In smaller patients that cannot be reconstructed in a single stage who demand a completely autologous approach, one or two additional outpatient skin tailoring and/or lipofilling procedures can usually complete their reconstruction. In patients who are smaller and accept an implant, placement of the prosthetic in a delayed procedure provides us with enhanced safety, more reliable positioning and better soft tissue coverage of the implant compared to the standard implant-based reconstructions and obviates the need for the use of an acellular dermal matrix. These "hybrid-Goldilocks" procedures may have a more natural feel and look as they can be thought of as intermediate between an elective subpectoral breast augmentation and a traditional implant-based reconstruction. These strategies require careful study and long-term follow-up to determine their role in the postmastectomy reconstructive process.

**Acknowledgments** I thank my colleague Dr. Piotr Skowronski for his generosity of time and intellectual input that allowed for the development of many of these techniques. I thank my mentors across the world, Dr. Cicero Urban (Curitiba, Brazil), Gustavo Zucca-Matthes (Barretos, Brazil), John Harman (Auckland, New Zealand), Krishna Clough and Claude Nos (Paris, France), Mario Rietjens (Milan, Italy), and Mark Gittos (London, UK) who patiently mentored and taught me the basics of oncoplastic breast surgery.

## References

1. Richardson H, Ma G. The goldilocks mastectomy. Int J Surg. 2012;10(9):522–6.
2. Schwartz JC, Skowronski P. Total single-stage autologous breast reconstruction with free nipple grafts. Plast Reconstr Surg Glob Open. 2016;3(12):e587.
3. Schwartz JC, Skowronski P. Extending the indications for autologous breast reconstruction using a two stage modified goldilocks procedure: a case report. Breast J. 2017;23(3):344–7.
4. De Vita R, Pozzi M, Zoccali G, Costantini M, Gullo P, Buccheri FM, Varanese A. Skin-reducing mastectomy and immediate breast reconstruction in patients with macromastia. J Exp Clin Cancer Res. 2015;14(34):120–31.
5. Bostwick J. Prophylactic (risk reducing) mastectomy and reconstruction. In: Bostwick J, editor. Plastic and reconstructive breast surgery, vol. II. St. Louis: Quality Med Publishing; 1990. p. 1369–73.
6. Ladizinsky DA, Sandholm PH, Jewett ST, Shazad F, Andrews K. Breast reconstruction with the Bostwick Autoderm technique. Plast Reconstr Surg. 2013;132(2):261–70.
7. Torstenson T, Boughey JC, Saint-Cyr M. Inferior dermal flap in immediate breast reconstruction. Ann Surg Oncol. 2013;20:3349.
8. Quinn TT, Miller GS, Rostek M, Cabalag MS, Rozen WM, Hunter-Smith DJ. Prosthetic breast reconstruction: indications and update. Gland Surg. 2016;5(2):174–86.
9. Voineskos SH, Frank SG, Cordeiro PG. Breast reconstruction following conservative mastectomies: predictors of complications and outcomes. Gland Surg. 2015;4(6):484–96.

# 47 Nipple-Areolar Complex Reconstruction with Acellular Dermal Matrix

Steven P. Davison and Kelly A. Scriven

## 47.1 Introduction

Acellular dermal matrix (ADM) was first introduced in 1994 and has numerous uses in tissue reconstruction. It is derived from cadaveric human skin, which through processing is decellularized so that an extracellular matrix remains. The remaining acellular matrix can ultimately be repopulated by the recipient patient's own cells and revascularized. Several types of ADM are available commercially, most notably AlloDerm™, and have been used in oral surgery, neurosurgery, abdominal surgery, and plastic and reconstructive surgery.

The use of ADM in breast reconstruction in particular has been well established for several years. Numerous authors including Spear et al. [1] and Salzberg [2] have shown ADM to improve cosmetic outcomes in breast reconstruction with tissue expanders and implants. In these cases, ADM can be used as a pectoralis extender to provide soft tissue after implant placement that ultimately revascularizes. More recently, the combination of pre-pectoral prosthetic devices and ADM has been used to avoid animation deformity.

In this chapter, we will discuss the use of ADM specifically in nipple reconstruction, which has been complicated by modern advances in breast surgery. In the era of genetic screening, prophylactic mastectomies in younger patients pose a unique challenge to the reconstructive surgeon given young patients' lack of skin laxity and skin graft donor sites. Additionally, matching a nipple-sparing mastectomy on one breast to a skin-sparing mastectomy on the other poses another significant challenge.

The reconstruction of the nipple-areolar complex is the key final step in breast reconstruction. After reconstruction of the nipple with one of various local flap techniques, the surgeon is left with a paucity of skin for areolar reconstruction. This is particularly problematic in the case of tissue expander or implant reconstruction, which leaves significantly less available skin than autogenous flap reconstruction. Primary skin closure of the nipple-areolar complex often leaves a flattened breast contour that is not cosmetically favorable. Additionally, obtaining a full-thickness skin graft from another site necessitates an additional incision with donor site morbidity, which is particularly problematic in the young patient with no previous scars

S.P. Davison, D.D.S., M.D. (✉)
DaVinci Plastic Surgery, 3301 New Mexico Ave., NW, Suite 236, Washington, DC 20016, USA
e-mail: davisonplastic@yahoo.com

K.A. Scriven, M.D.
Department of Otolaryngology-Head and Neck Surgery, MedStar Georgetown University Hospital, 3800 Reservoir Rd NW, Washington, DC 20007, USA
e-mail: Kelly.a.scriven@gmail.com


M.A. Shiffman (ed.), *Nipple-Areolar Complex Reconstruction*,
https://doi.org/10.1007/978-3-319-60925-6_47

or skin laxity. This chapter discusses the use of acellular dermal matrix as an onlay graft for reconstruction of the nipple-areolar complex, negating the secondary defect. The thinner the AlloDerm™ graft, the faster and more complete the reepithelialization. The 4 × 7 cm thin sheet designed for tympanic membrane reconstruction is ideal, with the 12 × 4 sheet a reasonable substitute.

## 47.2 Technique

In using ADM as an onlay graft, the first step is to mark a proposed areolar complex on the reconstructed breast. This is based on the contralateral areola if present or, if absent, is set at about 40–45 mm (Fig. 47.1). A standard nipple reconstruction technique such as a skate flap is then executed, leaving a denuded pattern on the breast. A contiguous circle the size of the proposed areola is marked out. More often than not, the nipple flap is raised superiorly and the areolar circle is adjusted accordingly. The proposed area is then deepithelialized, taking care to leave an adequate dermal base (Fig. 47.2). Next, the ADM is prepared and cut to the appropriate size. Note that acellular dermal matrix does not have primary contraction and therefore can be sized exactly to meet the defect in question.

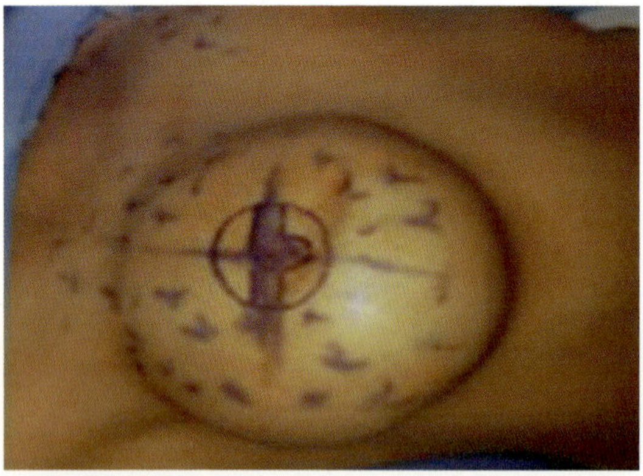

**Fig. 47.1** Perioperative markings, in which a standard nipple reconstruction of choice is outlined. This breast with thin tissue coverage and paucity of excess envelope would be distorted by primary closure of the defect

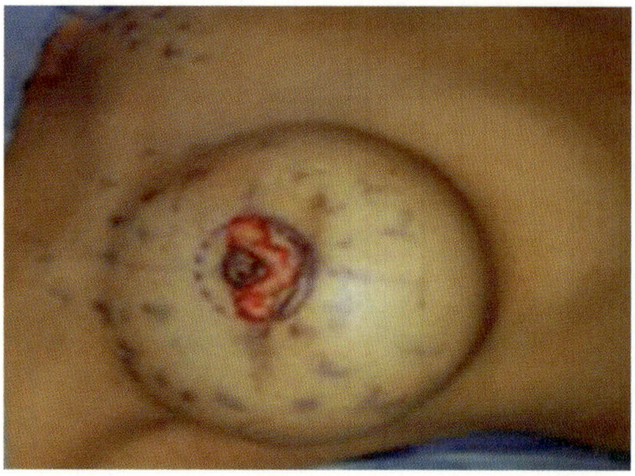

**Fig. 47.2** The concentric areolar area is deepithelialized with minimal defect depth and a circular ADM pattern cut. The center is perforated and ADM dermis side down applied

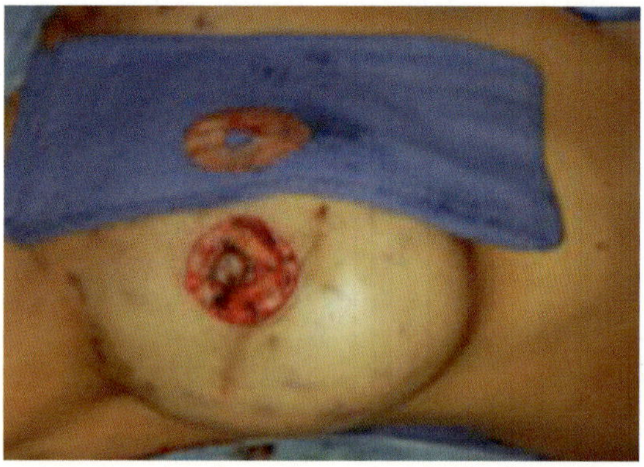

**Fig. 47.3** The sewn in ADM graft, which is tacked centrally and circumferentially closed with a running absorbable suture. A standard bolster dressing of surgeon choice is applied for 5–6 days

The ADM is then prepared for projection of the nipple flap by creating a cruciate opening in its center. Once the nipple flap is brought out the opening, ADM can be used to cover the deepithelialized area. The circular part of the ADM is then sutured in place to complete the reconstruction of the nipple-areolar complex (Figs. 47.3 and 47.4). A bolster for the nipple flap is then applied and sewn in place for 5 days. After the bolster is removed, the area must be kept moist with ointment until reepithelialization is complete, which typically is about 8 weeks postoperatively [3].

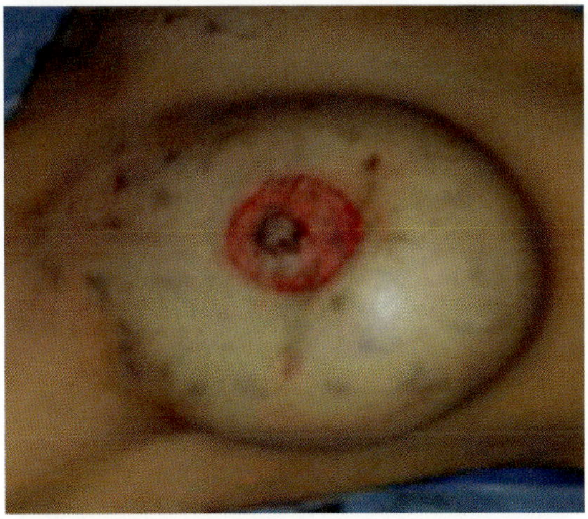

**Fig. 47.4** The subsequent excision of nipple-areolar complex after a nipple-sparing mastectomy is a graftable reconstruction. Primary closure with a delayed envelope is not possible

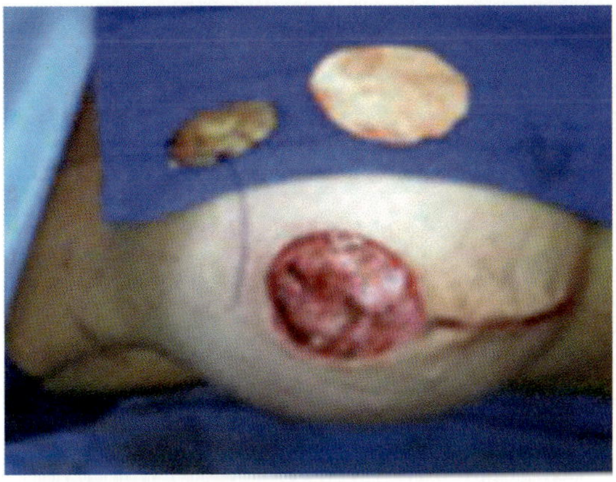

**Fig. 47.5** Here is a revascularized neo-areola after six weeks of reepithelialization. Note there is no contracture of the soft tissue envelope

The technique is modified slightly for reconstruction of a secondary defect created by delayed nipple excision. A delayed nipple removal from a nipple-sparing mastectomy dictated by the subareolar pathology leaves a circular defect on the peak of the reconstructed breast mound. The edge of the areolar excision is marked with blue marking pen, and a slightly moist ADM is used as a template. The ADM circular disk is cut to fit the defect and sewn into place, dermal side down. A bolster is then sewn in place for 5–6 days (Figs. 47.5, 47.6, and 47.7).

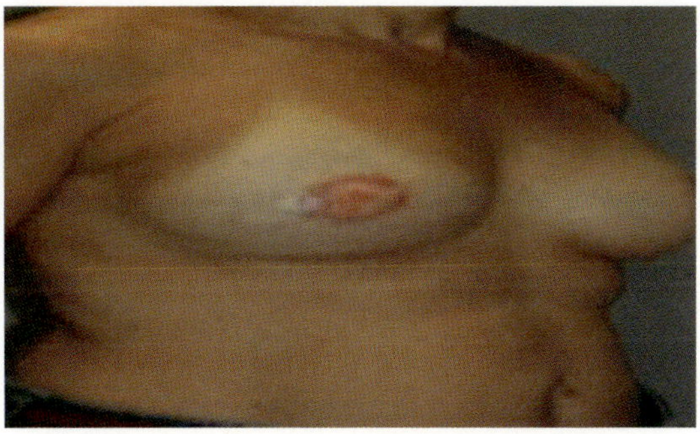

**Fig. 47.6** Before and after ADM areolar grafting after tattoo color augmentation

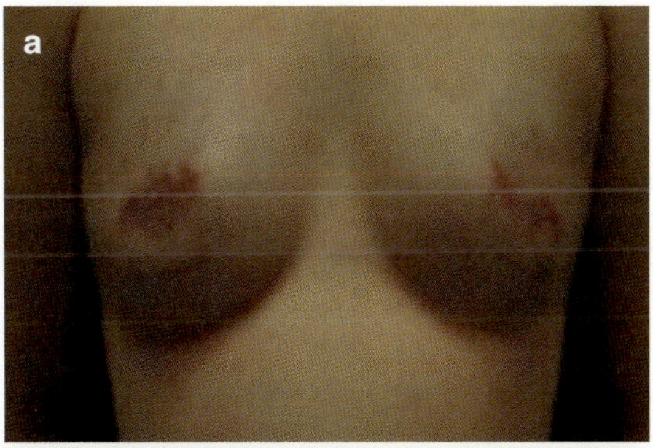

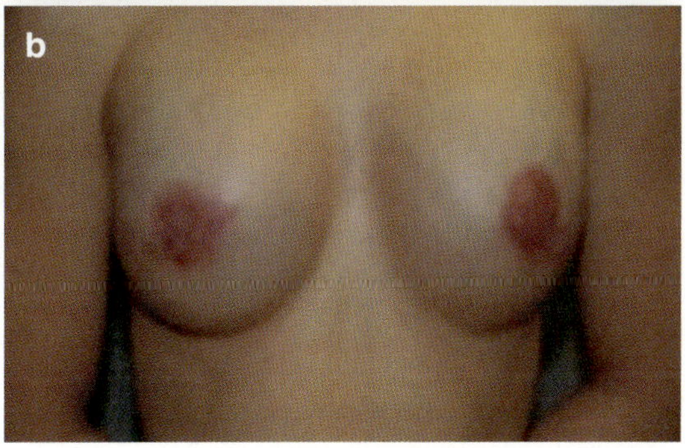

**Fig. 47.7** (**a**) Preoperative. (**b**) After ADM areolar grafting and tattoo color augmentation

## 47.3 Discussion

Acellular dermal matrix has been used for years in breast reconstruction, and its use is expanding. This author described a novel technique as outlined above for the use of ADM in reconstruction of the nipple-areolar complex. This method has both advantages and disadvantages compared to the use of a skin graft for the same purpose. Patients with existing scars from abdominal flaps, caesarian sections, or hysterectomies can undergo a full-thickness skin graft with minimal donor site morbidity. However, thin women with no prior surgical scars may be left with a cosmetically unfavorable outcome from the harvest of a full-thickness skin graft. In areolar reconstruction, the average areolar size of 4 cm often necessitates a scar up to 12 cm at the donor site of a full-thickness skin graft. In women with no prior scars, the use of ADM completely avoids this. It should also be noted that the harvest of a skin graft also contributes significantly to postoperative pain. These factors should be weighed against the cost of ADM, with AlloDerm costing approximately 30 dollars per square centimeter.

In a study published by this author, 19 patients underwent reconstruction of the nipple-areolar complex with AlloDerm. All 24 areolas studied revascularized, and the graft had 100% take in 23 of 24. Two patients were able to use the AlloDerm graft to create areolar coverage in a staged operation, and 19 of the areolar complexes were subsequently tattooed for color. Additionally, all patients who completed a postoperative satisfaction survey expressed that they would choose to undergo the same procedure again [3]. Subsequent to this study, the neo-areolar complex made from AlloDerm has been used to create a skate flap in two patients who underwent staged removal of the nipple-areolar complex, emphasizing its robust revascularization.

Other studies have used ADM in various ways for nipple reconstruction. Nahabedian [4] previously described the use of AlloDerm for nipple reconstruction in which the piece of ADM is folded on itself to create vertical projection of the nipple. In this method, the AlloDerm is incorporated into the base of the nipple between opposing local skin flaps. Other authors have noted a disadvantage of decreased nipple projection when using ADM for nipple reconstruction as compared to standard techniques [5]. In the study discussed above, however, patients noted satisfaction with the cosmetic outcome of their nipple reconstruction with no major complaints of nipple deprojection.

The reconstruction of the nipple-areolar complex is a critical step in breast reconstruction and, when done well, has an immense positive impact on cosmetic outcomes. This author advocates the use of an acellular dermal matrix onlay graft as a substitute for a skin graft in reconstruction of the nipple-areolar complex. This method has demonstrated favorable results with no donor site morbidity.

## References

1. Spear SL, Parikh PM, Reisin E, Menon NG. Acellular dermis-assisted breast reconstruction. Aesthetic Plast Surg. 2008;32(3):418–25.
2. Salzberg CA. Non-expansive immediate breast reconstruction using acellular dermal matrix graft (AlloDerm). Annals Plast Surg. 2006;57:1–5.
3. Rao SS, Seaman BJ, Davison SP. The acellular dermal matrix onlay graft for areolar reconstruction. Ann Plastic Surg. 2012;72(5):508–12.
4. Nahabedian MY. Nipple reconstruction. Clin Plast Surg. 2007;34:131–7.
5. Nimboriboonporn A, Chusapisith S. Nipple-areola complex reconstruction. Gland Surg. 2014; 3(1):35–42.

# 48 Nipple-Areola Complex Reconstruction with Dermal-Fat Flaps: Technical Improvement from Rolled Auricular Cartilage to Artificial Bone

Hiroko Yanaga and Katsu Yanaga

## 48.1 Introduction

Nipple reconstruction methods can roughly be classified into methods of reconstruction with composite grafts [1–3] and those with local flaps [4–15]. Obviously the goal is to create a nipple that most resembles the healthy nipple in shape, color tone, and texture [1–3]. Therefore, when the healthy nipple is large, a composite graft is the first choice. However, a composite graft is not applicable in (1) cases where the healthy nipple is small and cannot serve as a donor, (2) cases of bilateral breast cancer, (3) cases where future breast feeding is desired, and (4) cases where the patient does not desire the healthy side to be damaged.

Various types of nipple reconstructions using local flaps have been tried up until now [4–15]. However, a problem with this method is that the nipple projection cannot be maintained for a long period of time after the operation. This is because with local flaps, mainly soft tissue is used and the support is often lost when the scar softens after the operation.

The authors inserted cartilage or artificial bone in between two dermal-fat flaps as a means to maintain the support of the nipple. An advantage is that it is formed at the section between the two dermal-fat flaps, so retraction does not occur as with a subcutaneous pedicle flap. Using this method blood circulation at the formed base in between the two flaps is stable, so necrosis of the flaps does not occur, and there is low risk of exposure of the cartilage or artificial bone. A distinguishing feature of this method is that cartilage or artificial bone is used as the support tissue that serves as the core of the nipple [16–18].

However, as a problem, there is the demerit of imposing donor sacrifice by collecting cartilage from another site for nipple reconstruction and requiring additional operating time for the collection. In order to solve this problem, artificial bone (composition is hydroxyapatite (HAP) + tricalcium phosphate (TAP) complex; trade name, Ceratite (Kobayashi Medical Device, Osaka)) was used in place of auricular cartilage. More than 400 cases of the NAC reconstruction method using dermal-fat flaps and Ceratite have been performed up until now. Results reported have indicated no case of total flap necrosis and the operative procedure has been safe and stable.

Also with NAC reconstruction using the conventional dermal flap method, the nipple is initially reconstructed with a flap and tattooing is performed secondarily to add color to the flap [2, 3, 19–23]. Although tattooing enables the color tone to match the healthy side closely, a demerit is that, due to tattooing of precordial skin, the

H. Yanaga, M.D. (✉) • K. Yanaga, M.D.
Yanaga Clinic and Tissue Culture Laboratory, 1-2-12 Tenjin, Chuo-ku, Fukuoka 810-0001, Japan
e-mail: force@yanaga-cl.com


M.A. Shiffman (ed.), *Nipple-Areolar Complex Reconstruction*,
https://doi.org/10.1007/978-3-319-60925-6_48

reconstructed nipple texture and luster are different from that of the opposite healthy side. Also, the medical dye disappears in 4–5 years and the tattooing must be repeated again.

The authors use a method of full-thickness skin grafting (FTFG) from a proximal portion of the inner thigh [17, 18, 24] for adaptation to the texture and color tone of the NAC. This method enables NAC reconstruction in one step. The NAC reconstruction operation technique using dermal-fat flaps and artificial bone with FTSG is described in detail in this chapter.

## 48.2 Technique

### 48.2.1 Evaluation of the Positions and Sizes of the Nipple and the Areola

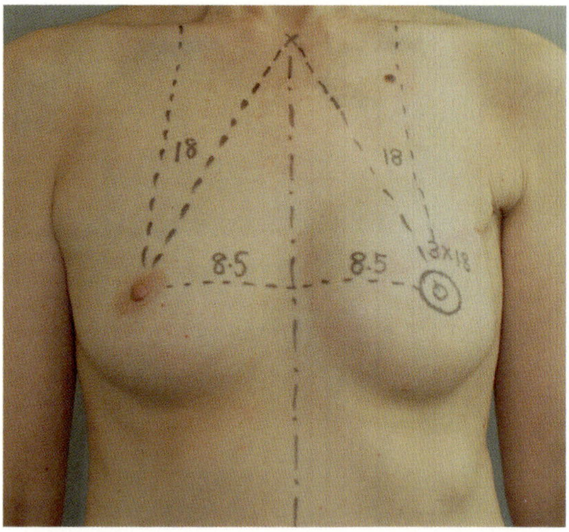


**Fig. 48.1** Case of a 55-year-old: *Left side*; 6 months after breast reconstruction operation by tissue expander/implant following mastectomy with conservation of pectoral muscle (modified mastectomy, Auchincloss method). In this case, the healthy nipple and areola are both small and the NAC must thus be reconstructed anew. Design prior to operation: A key point is to mark the distance from the sternal notch to the nipple and the distance from the nipple to the midline to be equidistant. The triangle is measured accurately. The distance from the clavicular midpoint to the nipple is also measured and checked to determine if it is equidistant or not

Prior to operation, the distance from the affected nipple midline to the opposite side nipple in the upright position is measured accurately. Next, upon measuring the long axis and lateral axis sizes of the healthy areola and carefully observing the shape of the areola, the shape is drawn symmetrically at the affected side with a felt-tip pen. Also, with an oval areola, the long-axis direction is directed somewhat obliquely and therefore the mark should be made carefully in consideration of this point as well (Fig. 48.1). The position of the nipple is also marked. Although the nipple is positioned at the center of the areola in many cases, care must be taken because it may be biased in some cases (Fig. 48.2).

### 48.2.2 Operative Procedure

In the operation, immediately after sterilization, a 24 G needle is loaded with gentian violet dye, and tattooing is performed on the NAC drawn with gentian violet before the operation. Next, deepithelialization of the NAC area is performed and graft wound bed preparation is performed. The tattooing is performed because whereas the marks disappear in the process of deepithelialization, the marked positions can be left accurately with the tattoo. The deepithelialization is performed to about a depth at which petechial hemorrhaging occurs. When the areolar edge is designed in a zigzag form to prevent contracture of the areolar edge and bring out the effects of degradation of pigmentation at the periphery, a natural areolar shape can be obtained. The designs of the nipple and the two dermal-fat flaps are drawn using the position of the nipple tattooed in advance as a guide (Fig. 48.3).

In order to preserve the subcutaneous vascular network, the two dermal-fat flaps are elevated at the thickness of the dermis with the fat attached.

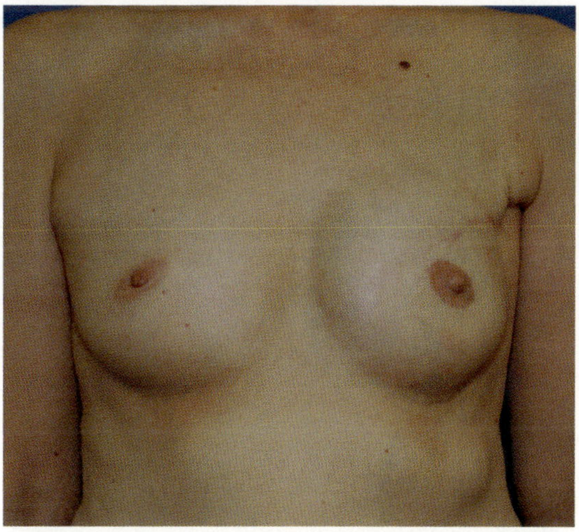

**Fig. 48.2** Same patient, one year after reconstruction by shaping with dermal-fat flaps and Ceratite. Satisfactory bilateral balance was achieved in terms of the size, shape, position, color tone, and texture of the opposite NAC

If the fat is thin, the pectoralis muscular fascia is elevated together. If the fat is thick, elevation is performed at the intermediate fat layer. The already shaped artificial bone (Ceratite) is placed at the dermal portion at the center of the two dermal-fat flaps. The artificial bone is wrapped in the two elevated dermal-fat flaps, and the dermal-fat flaps are sutured with 5-0 PDS so as not to form any dead space. Next, FTSG, collected from a proximal portion of the inner thigh, is grafted onto the graft wound bed and tie-over dressing is applied (Fig. 48.3). When cartilage is used, the cartilage is wrapped and enclosed at the center of the two dermal-fat flaps, and the procedure is thereafter the same [18, 19].

### 48.2.3 Postoperative Care

The tie-over dressing is removed one week after the operation. By this time, the FTSG will have taken and blood circulation is maintained satisfactorily. Suture removal at the areolar portion is performed after two weeks, and suture removal in the nipple portion is performed at the third week. For 2 weeks after removal of the tie-over dressing, a comparatively thick gauze with a hole in the center is applied to the nipple to protect the nipple from deformation. Also, after the FTSG portion has stabilized to the degree of being capable of withstanding external force, the nipple is protected for 3 months with a donut-shaped sponge (a circularly cut Reston sponge with a hole in the center). Thereafter, the donut-shaped sponge is put on only during the day and only when wearing a tight undergarment, a bra, or when performing exercise.

The long term results are shown in (Figs. 48.4, 48.5, 48.6 and 48.7).

## 48.3 Complications

### 48.3.1 Necrosis of Dermal-Fat Flaps

So far, total necrosis of the dermal-fat flaps has not been observed. However, partial necrosis has occurred in some cases when the circulation was poor. Skin necrosis of the areolar portion might occur partially in some cases, but this does not present a problem because epithelialization occurs quickly.

### 48.3.2 Exposure of Auricular Cartilage or Artificial Bone

Although exposure of auricular cartilage hardly occurs, exposure of artificial bone has been observed in 5% of the cases [18]. This has mostly occurred after several years in cases where the flaps were thin. In case of exposure, the remaining dermal flaps can be elevated to reconstruct the nipple again. Because the present method uses two dermal-fat flaps, the dermal-fat flaps at portions that have not been elevated can be used (Fig. 48.8).

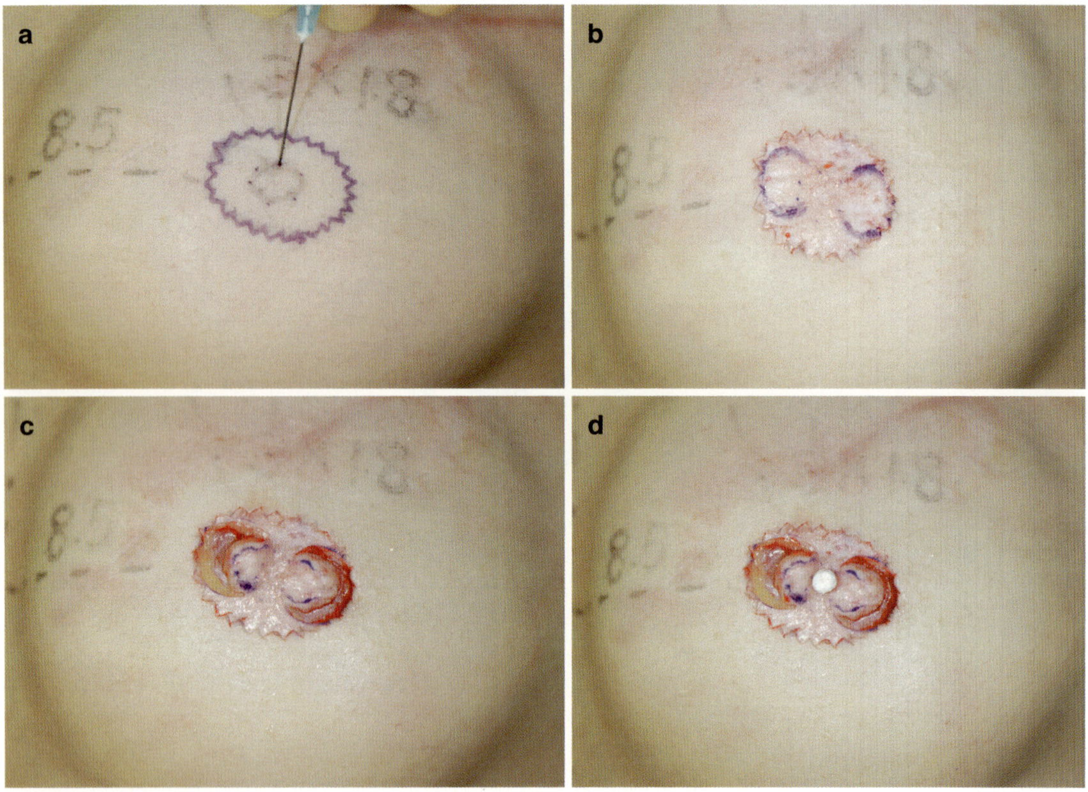

**Fig. 48.3** Operative procedure. (**a**) The areolar edge to be reconstructed, which was marked in advance before the operation, is designed in a zigzag form. This is performed to prevent contracture of the areolar edge and bring out the effects of degradation of pigmentation at the periphery. By designing the areolar edge in a zigzag form, a natural areolar shape can be obtained. A 24 G needle is loaded with gentian violet dye and tattooing is performed at the position of the drawn NAC. Tattooing is performed because whereas the marks disappear in the process of deepithelialization, the marked positions can be left accurately with the tattoo. (**b**) Deepithelialization of the NAC portion is performed and graft wound bed preparation is performed. The deepithelialization is performed to about a depth at which petechial hemorrhaging occurs. Deepithelialization of the to-be-reconstructed NAC site has been performed, and the two flaps have been designed with gentian violet. (**c**) Elevation of the two dermal-fat flaps. Elevation is performed with the fat and the pectoralis major muscle fascia attached to the dermal flaps. (**d**) Artificial bone (Ceratite) that has been shaped is placed on the central portion between the dermal flaps. (**e**) The projection of the artificial bone (Ceratite) can be discerned. (**f**) The Ceratite is wrapped in the two dermal-fat flaps and suturing with 5-0 PDS absorbable sutures is performed. Suturing is performed roughly so as not to obstruct blood flow at the dermal-fat flaps. (**g**) The projection of the dermal-fat flaps can be discerned well. (**h**) Full-thickness skin graft (FTSG), collected from a proximal portion of the inner thigh, placed on its side. (**i**) Fine holes are made in the FTSG using an 18 G needle. This is performed not only for drainage but also to simulate Montgomery glands. (**j**) A hole is opened in the center of the fusiform FTSG. The nipple portion is passed through the hole and the FTSG is grafted onto the areolar portion. The two excess triangular portions at the respective ends of the FTSG are grafted onto the nipple. The nipple and the FTSG were sutured with 5-0 nylon. (**k**) Tie-over dressing is performed to fix the grafted FTSG securely to the areolar portion. (**l**) In the fixing process, cotton and gauze, which have been cut out in a donut form, are used to prevent compression of the nipple portion. (**m**) One week after the operation. Taking of the graft is satisfactory. (**n**) Two weeks after the operation. Suture removal is performed at this point. (**o**) Three weeks after the operation. (**p**) The affected side 6 months after the operation. The color tone and form of the NAC are satisfactory. (**q**) A cubical Ceratite and a Ceratite shaped to have the form of a core of a nipple are shown at the right. A carving knife and the Ceratite are shown side by side at the upper.

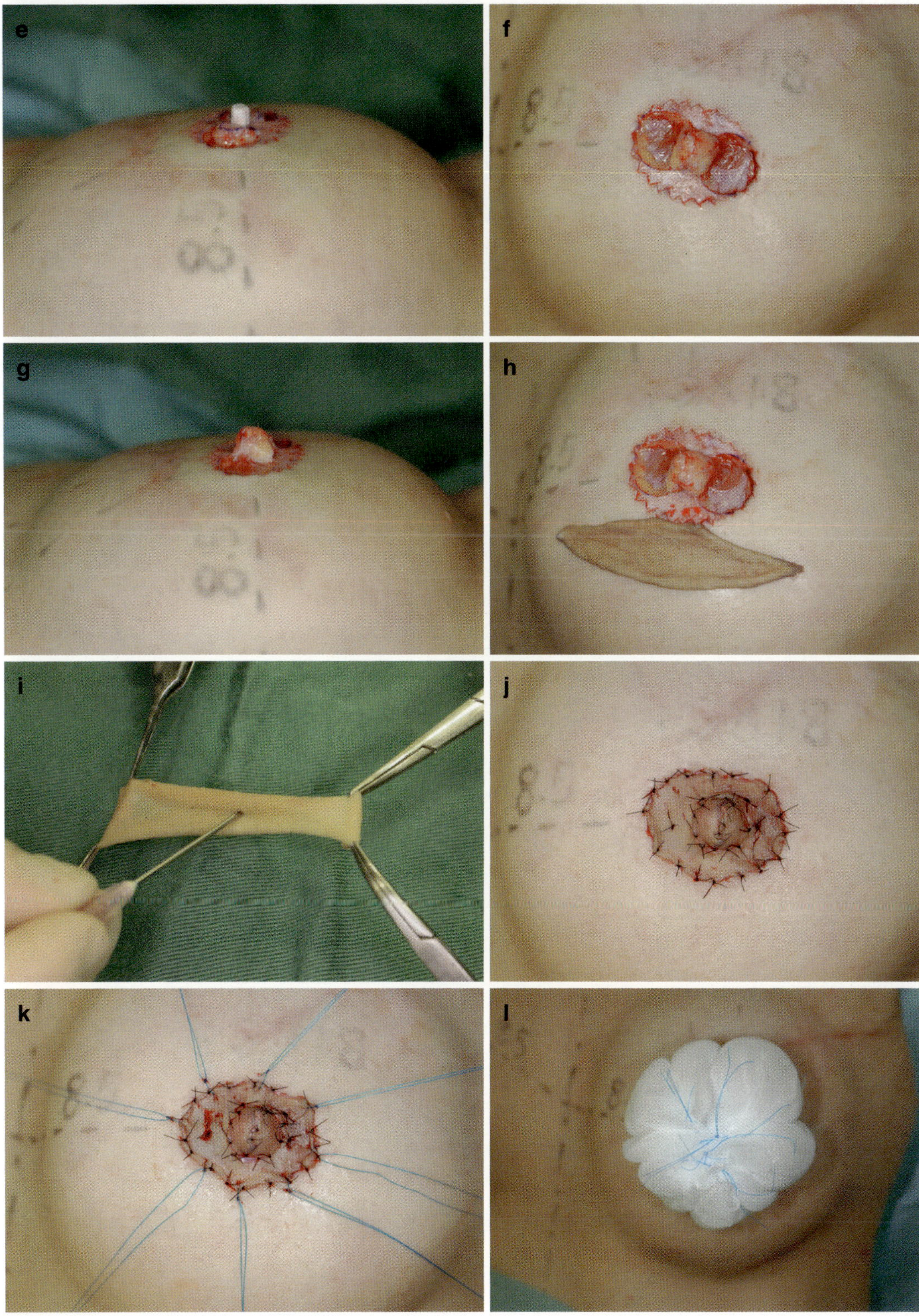


**Fig. 48.3** (continued)

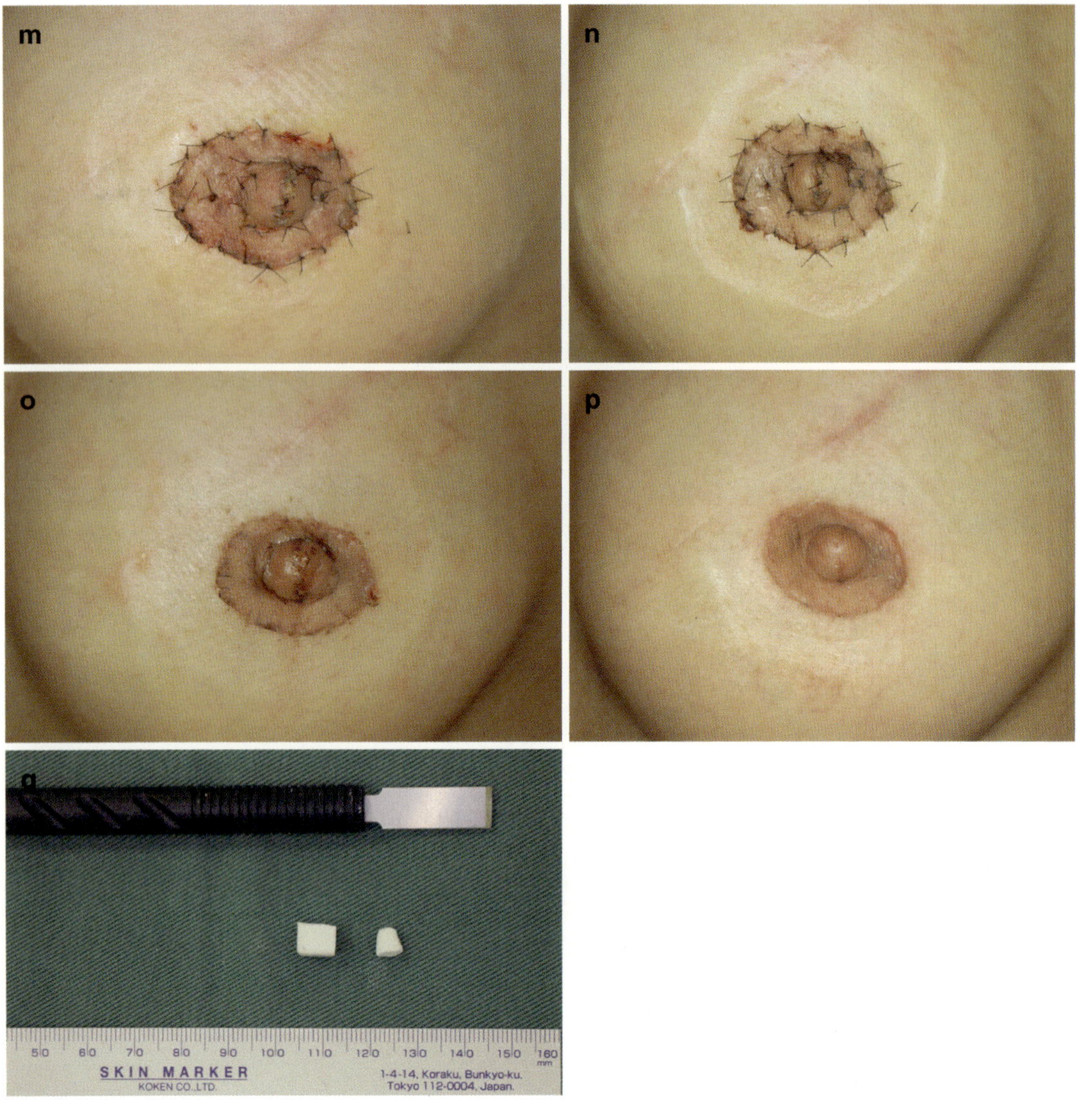


**Fig. 48.3** (continued)

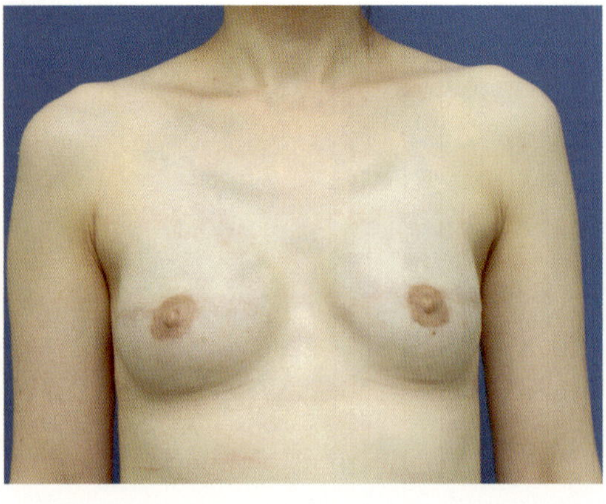

**Fig. 48.4** Bilateral NACs shaped with dermal-fat flaps and Ceratite, 3 years after reconstruction. The shape, color tone, and texture of the NACs are expressed symmetrically. The outlines look natural because the peripheries have zigzag forms

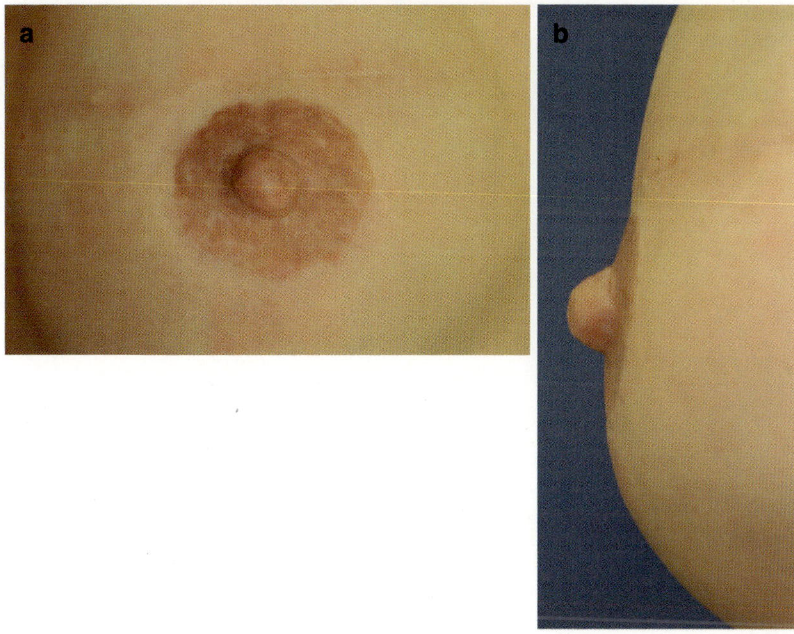


**Fig. 48.5** Right NAC, shaped with dermal-fat flaps and Ceratite, 4 years after reconstruction. (**a**) The shape, color tone, and texture of the NAC are expressed well. The outline looks natural because the periphery has a zigzag form. Montgomery glands are also simulated well. (**b**) The reconstructed NAC—a sufficient projection is obtained

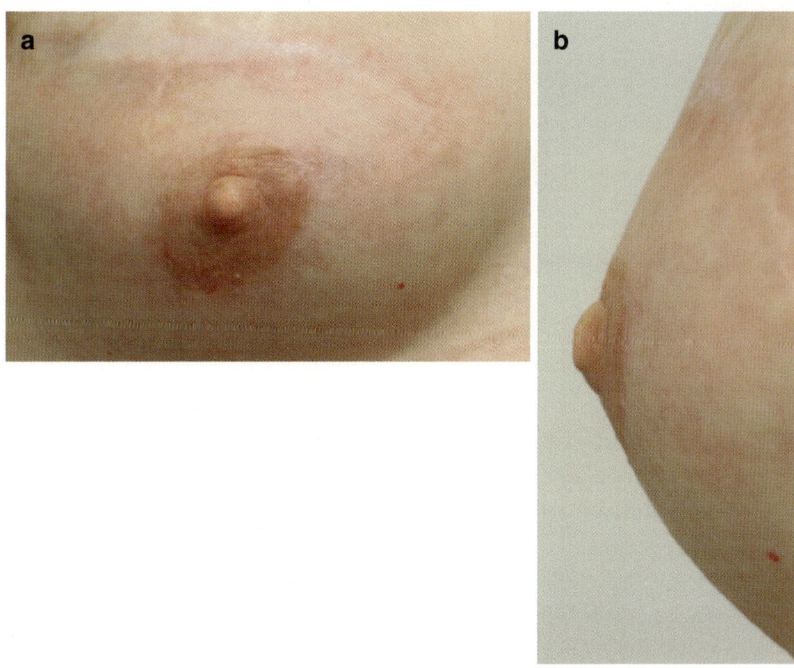


**Fig. 48.6** Right NAC, shaped with dermal-fat flaps and Ceratite, 6 years after reconstruction. (**a**) The shape, color tone, and texture of the NACs are expressed well. The outlines look natural because the peripheries have zigzag forms. (**b**) The bilateral reconstructed NACs—sufficient projections were obtained

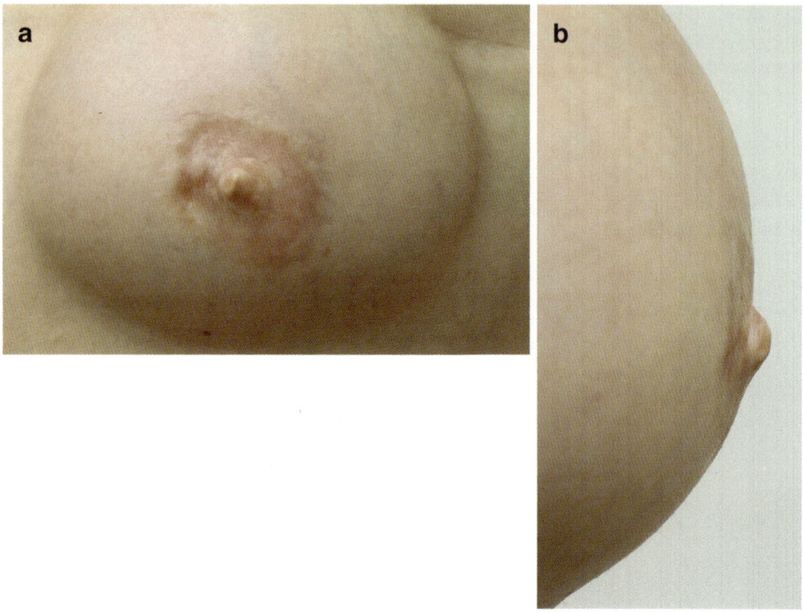


**Fig. 48.7** Left NAC, shaped with dermal-fat flaps and Ceratite, 13 years after reconstruction. (**a**) Although the shape and texture of the NAC are expressed well, the color tone has become somewhat lighter, and the color does not disappear. (**b**) The reconstructed NAC—a sufficient projection has been maintained

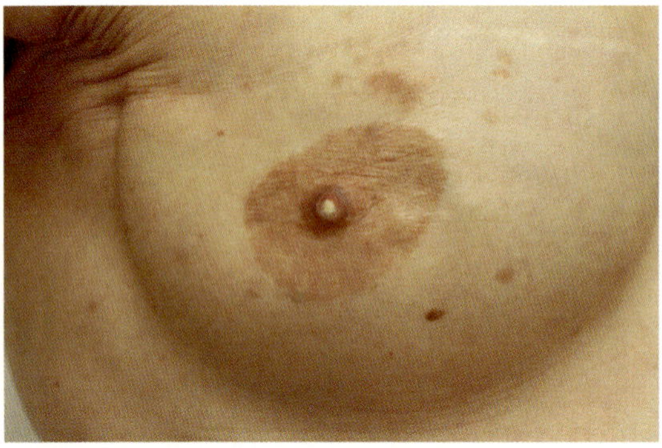

**Fig. 48.8** Ceratite became exposed in the 10th year after NAC reconstruction. Note, there is no absorption of Ceratite

### 48.3.3 Possibility of Absorption of Auricular Cartilage or Artificial Bone

With both cartilage and artificial bone, there is a possibility of absorption in the long term. However, the support is maintained in comparison to NAC reconstruction using only flaps.

### 48.3.4 Skin Necrosis

Although skin necrosis of the nipple and the areolar portion occurs partially in some cases, this does not present a problem because epithelialization occurs quickly.

## 48.4 Discussion

Up to date, various NAC reconstruction methods have been tried up until now. However, in most methods, reconstruction is performed using mainly soft tissue. Therefore, in many cases, the nipple projection cannot be maintained longer than 6 months. We thus considered the use of hard tissue instead of soft tissue to maintain the nipple projection. Cartilage tissue is suitable as the hard tissue for nipple reconstruction, and auricular cartilage was first selected from the point of low donor sacrifice. We thus rolled auricular cartilage into a roll shape as a means to provide projection and considered a method of wrapping the cartilage in two dermal-fat flaps [17]. We then changed the operation method to one where the auricular cartilage, rolled into the roll shape, is supported with a bridge of the dermal base and wrapped in two dermal-fat flaps. In cases of reconstruction by this method, the results of maintenance of the nipple projection for a long period of time and the unlikelihood of occurrence of nipple retraction deformation were obtained. Also, after the operation, complications, such as partial necrosis of the flaps and graft, exposure of the cartilage, etc., were not observed so we can conclude that the method is safe. When using this method, blood circulation is maintained well, and because nipple volume is obtained, it can be adapted to both cases of breast reconstruction using a myocutaneous flap [18] and cases of breast reconstruction using a tissue expander/implant. As a problem in terms of procedure, it takes a long time to collect the auricular cartilage. However, scarring at the collection portion is hardly noticeable, and it is thus believed that auricular cartilage is useful for nipple reconstruction. Costal cartilage can also be used instead of auricular cartilage [25]. By collecting costal cartilage and banking it in the abdominal region, when autologous tissue breast reconstruction is performed, the cartilage can be used when performing NAC reconstruction later.

Presently, with the newly improved method, artificial bone (Ceratite) is supported at the center of the dermal base, and therefore satisfactory form and the support are maintained without subcutaneous subsidence. The method was also found to be safe in terms of blood circulation. Out of 100 cases examined, total flap necrosis did not occur in any case, and partial flap necrosis occurred in 5% of the cases. Exposure of Ceratite was also observed in 5% of the cases [18]. It was possible to handle the Ceratite exposure cases by taking out the Ceratite and reinserting it upon carving with Luer forceps to reduce the projection. The dermal-fat flaps at the portions that were not elevated were used to reconstruct the nipple again. Hence, the best method for avoiding complications is to use Ceratite of a size that would not apply tension to the dermal-fat flaps. The proportion of the nipple projection with respect to the projection of the healthy nipple as 100% was 80.5% after 3 years [18]. Further, to examine how the artificial bone Ceratite changes within the soft tissue after grafting, mammography photography was performed several years after the operation. Neither deformation nor absorption of the Ceratite was observed by mammography 6 years after the operation (Fig. 48.9). Satisfactory results were obtained in regard to the recommended form and nipple projection reconstructed by the present method.

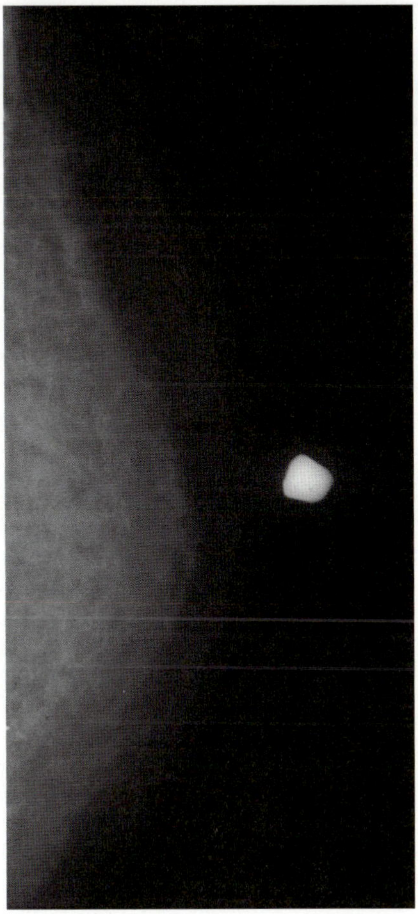

**Fig. 48.9** Mammography 6 years after the operation. Neither deformation nor absorption of Ceratite was observed

The artificial bone is wrapped in the dermal-fat flaps, and the underlying tissue is supported by the dermal base so that even if an external force is applied, bounding occurs, subsidence is unlikely to occur, and the nipple returns to its previous position [18]. The NAC differs in terms of texture match from the skin of the precordium, and therefore full-thickness skin from the proximal portion of the inner thigh was grafted to approximately match the healthy NAC in terms of texture and color. It was possible to perform color match adjustment according to each case by observing the color of the skin of the proximal portion of the inner thigh and collecting from the thigh side in cases where the NAC was light colored and collecting from a vulva side portion in dark color cases. The skin is thin and somewhat dark in color tone at the proximal portion of the inner thigh. Also, the hue of the areola can be controlled by controlling the dermal thickness of the skin. Although a problem is that the color tone becomes somewhat lighter after a few years, the color does not disappear as with a tattoo.

## Conclusions

NAC reconstruction using dermal-fat flaps and rolled auricular cartilage is an excellent method because the auricular cartilage maintains the support of the nipple. However, by using artificial bone (Ceratite) as the material for maintaining the support of the nipple, donor sacrifice is not necessary and the support is further stabilized. It can thus be concluded that the treatment method was improved. Here the author also presented long-term follow-up cases, sufficient projection of the NAC was maintained over the follow up period.

## References


1. Millard DR Jr. Nipple and areolar reconstruction by split-skin graft from the normal side. Plast Reconstr Surg. 1972;50:350–3.
2. Bostwick J III. Plastic and reconstruction breast surgery. 2nd ed. St. Louis: Quality Medical Publishing; 2000.
3. Spear SL. Surgery of the breast, vol. 2. 2nd ed. Philadelphia: Lippincott Williams & Wilkins; 2006.
4. Little JW 3rd, Munasifi T, McCulloch DT. One-stage reconstruction of a projecting nipple: the quadrapod flap. Plast Reconstr Surg. 1983;71:126–33.
5. Hartrampf CR Jr, Culbertson JH. A dermal-fat flap for nipple reconstruction. Plast Reconstr Surg. 1984;73:982–6.
6. Chang WH. Nipple reconstruction with a T flap. Plast Reconstr Surg. 1984;73:140–3.
7. Cohen IK, Ward JA, Chandresekhar B. The pinwheel flap nipple and barrier areola graft reconstruction. Plast Reconstr Surg. 1986;77:995–9.
8. Little JW 3rd, Spear SL. The finishing touches in nipple-areolar reconstruction. Perspect Plast Surg. 1988;2:1.
9. Weiss J, Herman O, Rosenberg L, et al. The S nipple-areola reconstruction. Plast Reconstr Surg. 1989;83:904–6.
10. Kroll SS, Hamilton S. Nipple reconstruction with the double-opposing-tab flap. Plast Reconstr Surg. 1989;84:520–5.
11. Anton MR, Eskenazi LB, Hartrampf CR Jr. Nipple reconstruction with local flaps: star and wrap flaps. Perspect Plast Surg. 1991;5:67–78.
12. Thomas SV, Gellis MB, Pool R. Nipple reconstruction with a new local tissue flap. Plast Reconstr Surg. 1996;97:1053–6.
13. Losken A, Mackay GJ, Bostwick J 3rd. Nipple reconstruction using the C-V flap technique: a long-term evaluation. Plast Reconstr Surg. 2001;108:361–9.
14. Hammond DC, Khuthaila D, Kim J. The skate flap purse-string technique for nipple-areola complex reconstruction. Plast Reconstr Surg. 2007;120:399–406.
15. Shestak KC, Gabriel A, Landecker A, et al. Assessment of long-term nipple projection: a comparison of three techniques. Plast Reconstr Surg. 2002;110:780–6.
16. Brent B, Bostwick J. Nipple-areola reconstruction with auricular tissues. Plast Reconstr Surg. 1977;60:353–61.
17. Tanable HY, Tai Y, Kiyokawa K, Yamauchi T. Nipple-areola reconstruction with a dermal-fat flap and rolled auricular cartilage. Plast Reconstr Surg. 1997;100:431–8.
18. Yanaga H. Nipple-areola reconstruction with a dermal-fat flap: technical improvement from rolled auricular cartilage to artificial bone. Plast Reconstr Surg. 2003;112:1863–9.
19. Becker H. The use of intradermal tattoo to enhance the final result of nipple-areola reconstruction. Plast Reconstr Surg. 1986;77:673–6.
20. Hugo NE, Sultan MR, Hardy SP. Nipple-areola reconstruction with intradermal tattoo and double-opposing pennant flaps. Ann Plast Surg. 1993;30:510–3.
21. Eskenazi L. A one-stage nipple reconstruction with the "modified star" flap and immediate tattoo: a review of 100 cases. Plast Reconstr Surg. 1993;92:671–80.
22. Spear SL, Convit R, Little JW 3rd. Intradermal tattoo as an adjunct to nipple-areola reconstruction. Plast Reconstr Surg. 1989;83:907–11.
23. Wong RK, Banducci DR, Feldman S, et al. Pre-reconstruction tattooing eliminates the need for skin grafting in nipple areolar reconstruction. Plast Reconstr Surg. 1993;92:547–9.
24. Broadbent TR, Woolf RM, Metz PS. Restoring the mammary areola by a skin graft from the upper inner thigh. Br J Plast Surg. 1977;30:220–2.
25. Guerra AB, Khoobehi K, Metzinger SE, et al. New technique for nipple areola reconstruction: arrow flap and rib cartilage graft for long-lasting nipple projection. Ann Plast Surg. 2003;50:31–7.


## Note

1. In reference 17, the author name H. Tanable (Hiroko Tanable) has been changed to H. Yanaga (Hiroko Yanaga) in 1999.

# 49 Regrafting of Nipple-Areola Complex During Pectoralis Major Myocutaneous Flap Reconstruction

Basavaraj R. Patil and Adarsh Kudva

## 49.1 Introduction

Pectoralis myocutaneous flap for reconstruction of head and neck defects [1] is still considered as one of the popular reconstructive options in developing countries in the era of free flaps.

In the use of large skin paddle for reconstruction of large defects, it is necessary to involve the nipple-areola complex, which results in unacceptable cosmetic deformity on the chest wall of the donor site.

To overcome this cosmetic deformity, it is essential to transfer the nipple-areola complex to donor site on the chest wall, to provide esthetically pleasing appearance to the patient. The position of the nipple in young adults of both the sexes is approximately 20–23 cm from the suprasternal notch in the midclavicular line and 20–23 cm apart in the horizontal plane. The areola is a disk of the skin, which encircles the base of nipple, varying in color from pink to dark brown depending on the parity and race [2].

We describe a simple and effective technical note to regraft the nipple complex to achieve symmetry of the chest wall.

## 49.2 Technique

Skin paddle is marked; nipple-areola complex is incised using sharp dissection in subdermal plane and preserved in saline (Fig. 49.1). Flap is harvested and chest incision is closed primarily by undermining the adjacent area on the chest wall. The position of the nipple graft is marked using the opposite side nipple as a reference, along with the abovementioned landmarks.

The split thickness skin is removed in a circular fashion over the chest, the nipple-areola complex is sutured, and bolster dressing is placed over it (Fig. 49.2).

Healing resembles that of split skin graft, and nipple-areola complex is taken up well on donor site with esthetically pleasing results.

B.R. Patil
Department of Surgical Oncology, Karnataka Cancer Therapy and Research Institute,
Navanagar, Hubli, India

A. Kudva, M.D.S., M.O.M.S., R.C.S (✉)
Department of Oral and Maxillofacial Surgery, Manipal College of Dental Sciences, Manipal University, Madhav Nagar, Manipal, Karnataka 576104, India
e-mail: dradarshkudva@gmail.com


M.A. Shiffman (ed.), *Nipple-Areolar Complex Reconstruction*,
https://doi.org/10.1007/978-3-319-60925-6_49

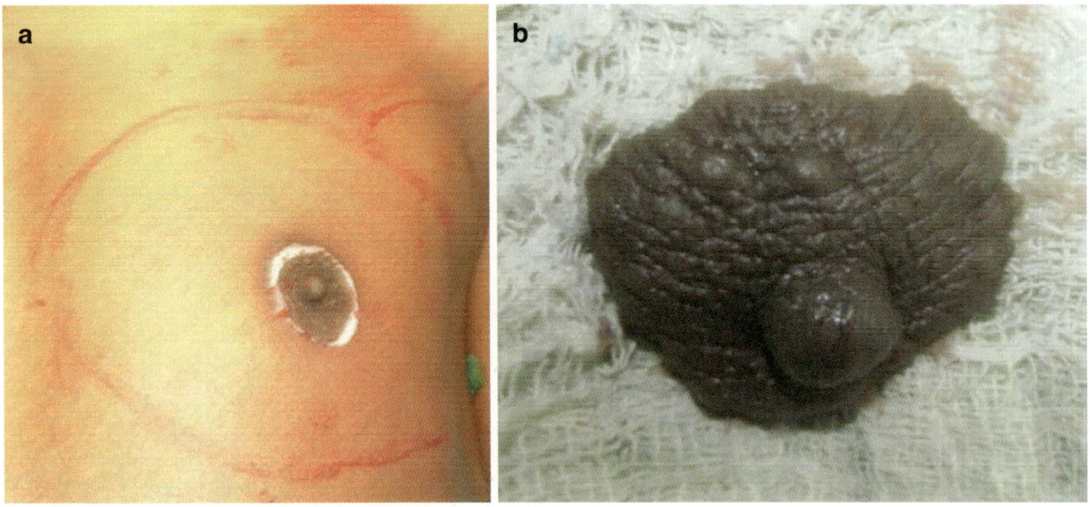


**Fig. 49.1** (**a**) Incision around areola. (**b**) Split thickness removal of nipple-areola complex

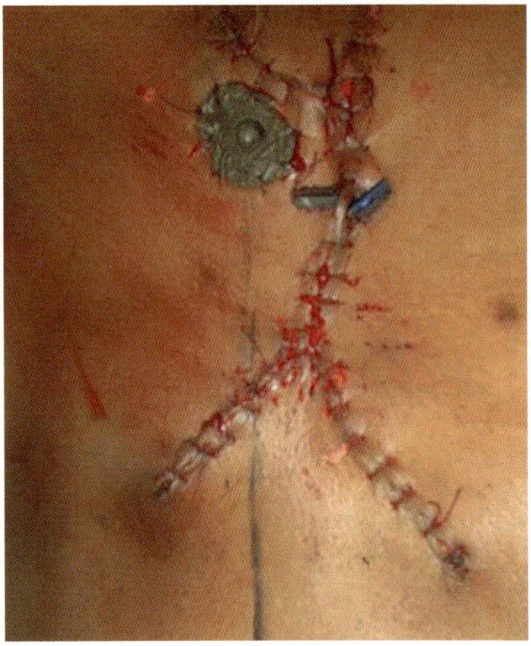

**Fig. 49.2** Resutured nipple-areola complex to the chest wall

## References

1. Ariyan S. The pectoralis major myocutaneous flap. Aversatile flap for reconstruction in head and neck. Plast Reconstr Surg. 1976;63:73–81.
2. Gray H, Standring S, Ellis H, Berkovitz BKB. Gray's anatomy: the anatomical basis of clinical practice. Edinburgh: Elsevier Churchill Livingstone; 2005.

# 50 Free Nipple Grafting: An Alternative for Patients Ineligible for Nipple-Sparing Mastectomy

Heather Curtis and Paul Smith

## 50.1 Introduction

Nipple reconstruction plays an important role in completion of breast reconstruction; however, a natural appearance of the reconstructed nipple is difficult to obtain with local flap reconstruction. In fact, patients often note more complaints of dissatisfaction surrounding the nipple-areolar complex (NAC) reconstruction than the breast mound reconstruction [1]. A simple solution to this problem is preservation of the native nipple via nipple-sparing mastectomy or free nipple grafting which provides the most natural appearance and is therefore the ideal form of reconstruction. While there were initially concerns of transplantation of cancer with this procedure, it has been proven that when certain criteria are met, there is no increased risk of local recurrence above the general population.

## 50.2 Anatomy

When considering the benefits of nipple preservation during mastectomy, it is important to first understand the unique anatomical characteristics of the nipple and why it is such a difficult structure to reconstruct. An anatomical review paper by Zucca-Matthes et al. [2] describes the nipple-areolar complex as being composed of two components: the papillary nipple and the surrounding areolar complex. The nipple itself is composed of smooth muscle and milk ducts. The areolar complex is the surrounding pigmented tissue which is composed of small sebaceous glands called tubercles of Morgagni. The tubercles of Morgagni form soft, slightly raised areas all along the nipple. It is the opinion of the author that these provide an appearance which is difficult to replicate with local flaps and can result in noticeable asymmetries, particularly in a unilateral reconstruction (Fig. 50.1).

## 50.3 History

Free nipple grafting was first described in the context of amputation mammoplasty as early as the 1920s for patients with symptomatic gigantomastia, although popularity did not gain until the 1940s [3]. These early amputations were performed essentially as a mastectomy, and required nipple transplantation to the chest wall in the

H. Curtis, M.D. (✉)
2319 W. Bristol Ave. #205, Tampa, FL 33606, USA
e-mail: hcurtis1@health.usf.edu

P. Smith, M.D.
Department of Plastic Surgery,
University of South Florida, Tampa, FL, USA
e-mail: paul.smith@moffitt.org


M.A. Shiffman (ed.), *Nipple-Areolar Complex Reconstruction*,
https://doi.org/10.1007/978-3-319-60925-6_50

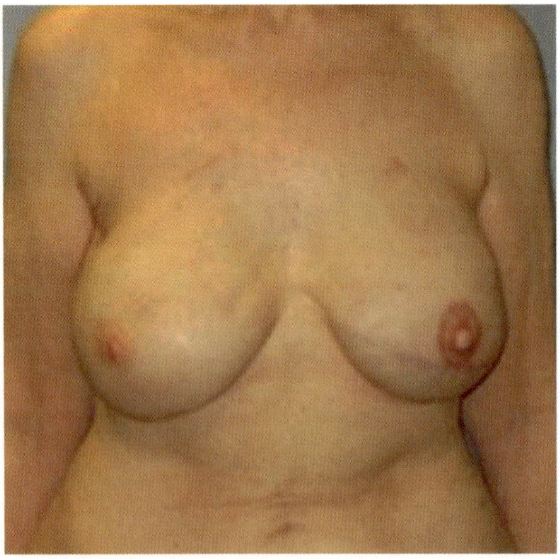

**Fig. 50.1** Patient had bilateral nipple-sparing mastectomy with subsequent loss of NAC requiring nipple reconstruction via skate flap. Note the perceptible differences in the reconstructed nipple compared to the native nipple including the absence of tubercles of Morgagni

form of a full-thickness skin graft as the use of pedicles had not yet been identified with respect to mammoplasty. The final result was that of a non-projecting breast mound which was not aesthetically ideal.

Technical refinements subsequently followed to allow better breast shape and contour in reduction mammoplasty as compared with breast amputation alone. The technique was performed similar to what is now referred to as a "Wise" pattern reduction using the keyhole pattern of closure; however, the inferior pole of the breast was resected, thus obliterating the blood supply to the nipple and requiring the nipple to be harvested and replaced on the most projecting portion of the new breast mound as a free nipple graft [4]. In addition, in patients with nipple projection greater than 5 cm, amputation and direct closure of the tip were considered to improve graft take. Another modification ensured that the vertical limb of the reduction was intentionally closed with a dog ear at the apex (new nipple position) which improved long-term nipple projection[4]. Good results were obtained; however, there was at least partial hypopigmentation in all patients, most notably in those with Fitzpatrick type IV skin [5].

In the 1960s–1970s, breast reconstruction following mastectomy became increasingly more popular. The subcutaneous mastectomy with immediate or delayed prosthetic reconstruction was introduced in 1967 by Freeman and was felt to be advantageous due to the preservation of the nipple-areolar complex with the procedure and thus retention of female form [6]. This procedure largely fell out of favor due to high complication rates including seroma, nipple, and skin necrosis, asymmetries, and cancer recurrence [7]. This led to a new technique where the nipple was often transplanted to the groin and preserved until the time of final reconstruction to minimize some of the complications associated with immediate reconstruction. This technique also became undesirable to many surgeons later in the decade due to several case reports which were published demonstrating development of infiltrating carcinoma at the transplantation site in the groin requiring wide local excision and inguinal lymph node dissection [8, 9].

These cases all occurred in patients either with positive subareolar tissue or large tumor size, which prompted authors to develop guidelines to improve oncologic safety of the procedure. These criteria are gross signs of nipple involvement (ulceration, crusting, retraction, or inversion of the nipple; fixation to the tumor; or discharge from the nipple), signs of poor prognosis (fungating or inflammatory lesions, peau d'orange), location within 2 cm of the areola, size larger than 2 cm, bilateral tumors, subareolar involvement, multicentricity, or nodal involvement [8]. Despite these recommendations, most surgeons stopped using free nipple grafting in an oncologic setting for many years.

In the early 2000s, nipple preservation during mastectomy was revisited as an option for reconstruction after a review of the literature involving nipple-sparing mastectomy by Kissin and Kark [10]. The data revealed that the current literature all showed comparable recurrence rates between traditional modified radical mastectomy and nipple-preserving techniques when the above criteria were met. The authors' argument against nipple-preserving procedures is that breast conserving therapy could be used instead. Despite this, a new found fervor for nipple-sparing mastectomy was launched as surgeons realized that patients may opt for mastectomy rather than breast conserving therapy due to the psychological effects of possible recurrence [11]. It is now a relatively common procedure and becoming more accepted as an oncologically sound procedure, although it still remains controversial.

Recurrence was not the only risk associated with nipple-sparing mastectomy. There is also a significant risk of nipple necrosis particularly in women with large or ptotic breasts [12]. This risk can be decreased or alleviated with the use of free nipple grafting.

## 50.4 Indications

Free nipple grafting may be indicated for patients who meet oncologic criteria for a nipple-sparing mastectomy, but who are precluded by body habitus [13, 14]. Criteria for keeping the nipple either as a nipple-sparing mastectomy or a free nipple graft are somewhat variable but include invasive tumor size <4 cm, DCIS <2 cm, and tumor location >2 cm from the nipple. Relative exclusion criteria for nipple-sparing mastectomy from a patient perspective include large breast weight (cited as greater than 700 grams), grade II–III ptosis, radiation, and periareolar scars[15]. In these selected individuals, they may still receive the benefits that go along with nipple-sparing mastectomy in respect to fewer operations and more natural appearance of the nipple by undergoing free nipple grafting at the time of the mastectomy (Fig. 50.2).

This technique is most commonly used in patients undergoing autologous reconstruction after mastectomy as the final nipple position is difficult to predict in tissue expander to implant reconstruction due to settling of the implants in the pocket. The exception is when performing immediate implant-based reconstruction as a one-staged procedure. This was described by King et al. as an addition to a technique combining wWise pattern reduction markings with an inferior dermal flap which can be used similar to AlloDerm to allow complete coverage of the implant [15–18]. This technique is reserved for patients with predicted breast weight >500 g and ptotic breasts [15].

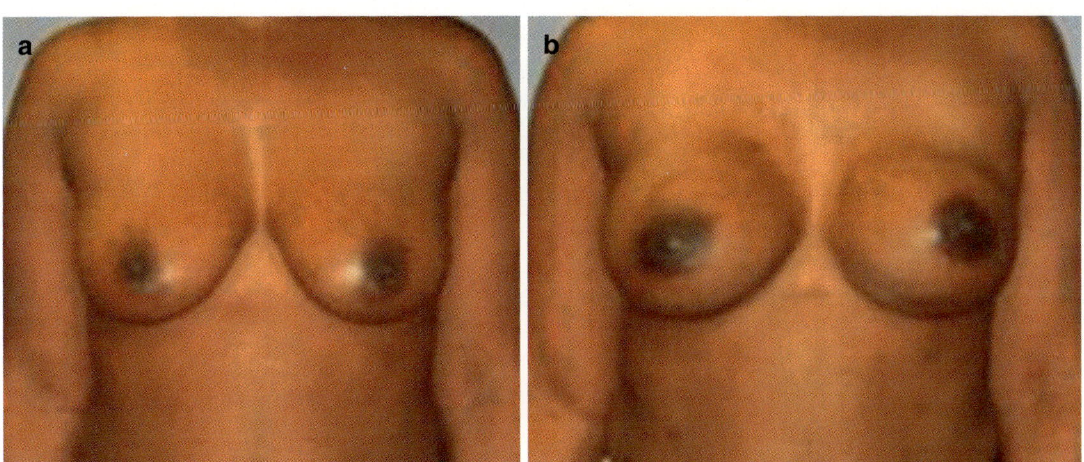


**Fig. 50.2** (**a**) Preoperative patient undergoing prophylactic mastectomies secondary to strong family history of breast cancer. (**b**) Postoperative patient after reconstruction with buried latissimus dorsi flap reconstruction and free nipple grafting bilaterally showing no hypopigmentation and excellent nipple projection. Note there is some widening of the areolar complex and minor asymmetries in nipple position

## 50.5 Technique

Patients who otherwise meet criteria for nipple-sparing mastectomy but demonstrated prior periareolar incisions, breast weight greater than 700 g, and with grade II or III ptosis or with prior radiation are considered candidates for free nipple grafting at the time of their breast reconstruction. Skin-sparing mastectomies are performed by the breast team. Once this is completed, the nipples are harvested as a full-thickness skin graft with a 10 blade scalpel (Fig. 50.3). Tissue is harvested from the base of the nipple and sent to pathology for frozen section. If pathology returns as clear, the nipple is then defatted leaving only a thin layer of dermis. Recipient site on the newly reconstructed breasts is then marked with a 38 or 42 cookie cutter (depending on patient's preoperative areolar size) and deepithelialized to create a vascular bed for the nipple graft. The nipple graft is then secured to the wound bed using 4-0 chromic sutures at the cardinal and ordinal points. The grafts are then secured with a bolster composed of Xeroform and wet cotton balls which are sutured into place with a 3-0 nylon which is used to tack the graft between the chromic sutures for additional adherence.

## 50.6 Oncologic Safety

It has been reported in the literature that rates of involvement of the nipple-areolar complex by tumor can range anywhere from 5 to 58% [15, 19–24]. These rates, however, do not take into account that involvement of the nipple has been shown to be dependent on many factors including distance of tumor from nipple, type of tumor, and size of tumor [8, 19, 20]. Given this and the prior history of transplantation of cancer to the groin where nipples were banked prior to transplantation in earlier years, there was a need to demonstrate the oncologic safety of free nipple grafting in breast reconstruction. A retrospective study was performed by Wirth et al. [15] to evaluate the rates of nipple-areolar complex tumor involvement at a single institution. Retroareolar tissue was sent for pathologic inspection if the tumor was at least 1 cm from the nipple. This was performed whether or not the nipple was intended to be replanted. The findings demonstrated that there was a 9.1% rate of involvement of the subareolar tissue which is comparable to other studies. Along with this, there was a 75% false-negative rate of initially frozen pathology resulting in subsequent removal of the transplanted nipple. Despite these findings, there was no evidence of recurrence originating from the transplanted nipple and no increase in local recurrence rates compared to standard mastectomy suggesting that free nipple grafting can be a reconstructive alternative in individuals who meet inclusion criteria. Further studies evaluating skin-sparing mastectomy specimens for nipple involvement demonstrated correlating results to the previous study suggesting that nipple-areolar complex involvement is rare in patients with small, peripheral tumors and negative axillary lymph nodes [23–25].

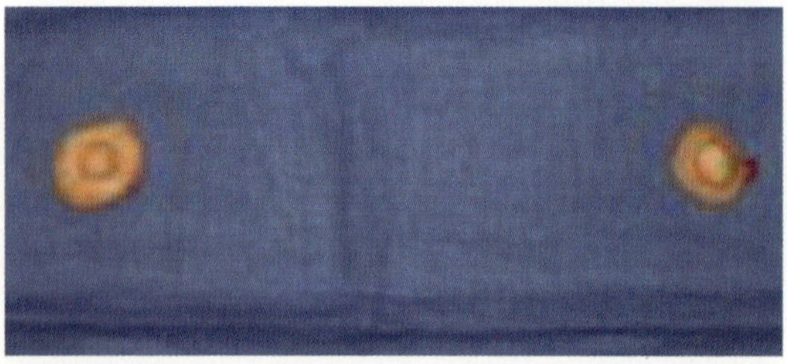

Fig. 50.3 Free nipple grafts harvested

## 50.7 Complications

The most frequent complication associated with free nipple grafting is loss of nipple sensation. There is complete absence of sensation immediately after the procedure; however, most patients do eventually recover at least partial sensation. The most troublesome complication, however, is loss of nipple projection which occurs in close to 50% of patients. Techniques have been attempted to reduce the amount of projection loss including avoidance of compression on the newly transplanted nipple, transplanting the nipple and areola as separate grafts, and reducing already large nipples to reduce the metabolic demand; however, outcomes remain similar

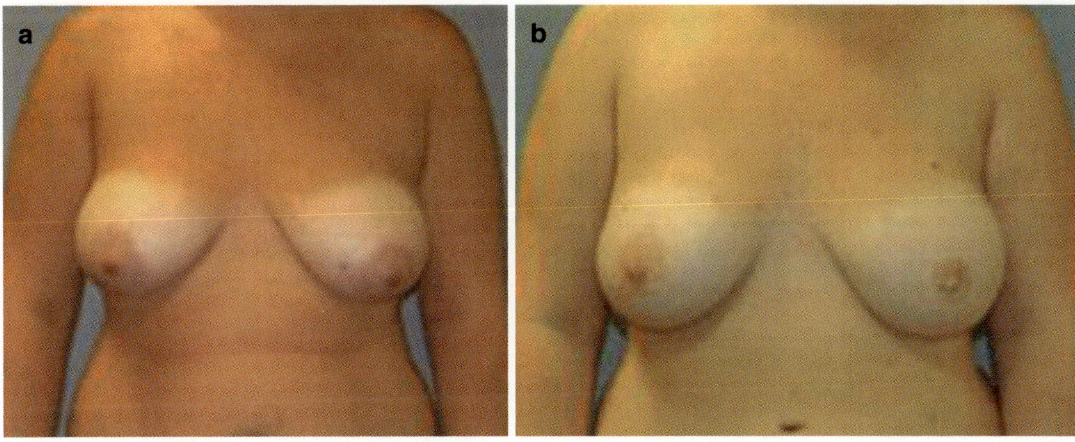


**Fig. 50.4** (**a**) Preoperative patient had bilateral prophylactic mastectomies due to BRCA positivity. (**b**) Postoperative after bilateral breast reconstruction with TRAM flaps and free nipple grafting. Note the patchy hypopigmentation of the grafted nipples

over time. Other complications include hypopigmentation (20%) and partial or complete graft loss (18%) (Fig. 50.4) [12]. These can be managed with tattooing or attempts at traditional local flap methods of nipple reconstruction if bothersome to the patient [15].

## Conclusions

Free nipple grafting should be considered as an option in patients undergoing breast reconstruction whom would otherwise be a candidate for nipple-sparing mastectomy but are precluded by body habitus. In appropriate candidates, it is oncologically equivalent to standard skin-sparing mastectomy as far as tumor recurrence and offers a more natural result compared to most described nipple reconstruction techniques.

## References

1. Jabor MA, Shayani P, Collins DR Jr, Karas T, Cohen BE. Nipple areola reconstruction: satisfaction and clinical determinants. Plast Reconstr Surg. 2002;110:457–63.
2. Zucca-Matthes G, Urban C, Vallejo A. Anatomy of the nipple and breast ducts. Gland Surg. 2016;5(1):32–6.
3. Thorek M. Possibilities in the reconstruction of the human form. N Y Med J. 1922;116:572.
4. Oneal R, Goldstein J, Rohrich R, Izenberg P, Pollock R. Reduction mammoplasty with free-nipple transplantation: indications and technical refinements. Ann Plast Surg. 1991;26:2.
5. Casas LA, Byun MY, Depoli PA. Maximizing breast projection after free-nipple-graft reduction mammaplasty. Plast Reconstr Surg. 2001;107(4):955–60.
6. Freeman BS. Subcutaneous mastectomy for benign breast lesions with immediate or delayed prosthetic replacement. Plast Reconstr Surg Transplant Bull. 1962;30:676–82.
7. Freeman BS. Complications of subcutaneous mastectomy with prosthetic replacement, immediate or delayed. South Med J. 1967;60(12):1277–80.
8. Allison AB, Howorth MB Jr. Carcinoma in a nipple preserved by heterotopic auto-implantation. N Engl J Med. 1978;298:1132.
9. Cucin R, Gaston J. Case report: Implantation of breast cancer in a transplanted nipple: A plea for preoperative screening. CA Cancer J Clin. 1981;31(5):281–3.
10. Kissin MW, Kark AE. Nipple preservation during mastectomy. Br J Surg. 1987;74(1):58–61.
11. Chung AP, Sacchini V. Nipple-sparing mastectomy: where are we now? Surg Oncol. 2008;17(4):261–6.
12. Cense HA, Rutgers EJ, Lopes Cardozo M, Van Lanschot JJ. Nipple-sparing mastectomy in breast cancer: a viable option? Eur J Surg Oncol. 2001;27(6):521–6.
13. Komorowski AL, Zanini V, Regolo L, Carolei A, Wysocki WM, Costa A. Necrotic complications after nipple- and areola-sparing mastectomy. World J Surg. 2006;30:1410–3.
14. Chidester JR, Ray AO, Lum SS, Miles DC. Revisiting the free nipple graft: an opportunity for nipple sparing mastectomy in women with breast ptosis. Ann Surg Oncol. 2013;20(10):3350.
15. Wirth R, Banic A, Erni D. Aesthetic outcome and oncological safety of nipple areola complex replantation after mastectomy and immediate breast reconstruction.

Department of Plastic and Hand Surgery, Inselspital, University of Bern, Bern, Switzerland, received 12 Apr 2009; accepted 18 Aug 2009.
16. Doren EL, Van Eldik Kuykendall L, Lopez JJ, Laronga C, Smith PD. Free nipple grafting: an alternative for patients ineligible for nipple-sparing mastectomy? Ann Plast Surg. 2014;72:S112–5.
17. King CC, Harvey JR, Bhaskar P. One-stage breast reconstruction using the inferior dermal flap, implant, and free nipple graft. Aesthet Plast Surg. 2014;38:358–64.
18. Ross GL. One stage breast reconstruction following prophylactic mastectomy for ptotic breasts: the inferior dermal flap and implant. J Plast Reconstr Aesthet Surg 2012;65(9):1204–8.
19. Bostwick J. Prophylactic (risk-reducing) mastectomy and reconstruction. In: Bostwick J, editor. Plastic and reconstructive breast surgery, vol. II. St. Louis: Quality Medical Publishing; 1990. p. 1369–73.
20. Smith J, Payne WS, Carney JA. Involvement of the nipple and areola in carcinoma of the breast. Surg Gynecol Obstet. 1976;143:546–8.
21. Parry RG, Cochran TC, Wolfort FG. When is there nipple involvement on carcinoma of the breast? Plast Reconstr Surg. 1977;59:535–7.
22. Lagios MD, Gates EA, Westdahl PR, Richards V, Alpert BS. A guide to the frequency of nipple involvement in breast cancer. A study of 149 consecutive mastectomies using a serial subgross and correlated radiographic technique. Am J Surg. 1979;138:135–41.
23. Laronga C, Kemp B, Johnston D, Robb GL, Singletary SE. The incidence of occult nippleeareola complex involvement in breast cancer patients receiving skin-sparing mastectomy. Ann Surg Oncol. 1999;6:609–13.
24. Vlajcic Z, Zic R, Stanec S, Lambasa S, Petrovecki M, Stanec Z. Nipple-areola complex preservation: predictive factors of neoplastic nipple-areola complex invasion. Ann Plast Surg. 2005;55:240–4.
25. Gerber B, Krause A, Reimer T, Muller H, Kuchenmeister I, Makovitzky J, et al. Skin-sparing mastectomy with conservation of the nippleeareola complex and autologous reconstruction is an oncologically safe procedure. Ann Surg. 2003;238:120–7.

# 51 Maximizing Nipple Graft Survival After Performing Free Nipple-Areolar Complex Reduction Mammaplasty

Aris Sterodimas

## 51.1 Introduction

Gigantomastia, characterized by massive breast enlargement during adolescence or pregnancy, is thought to be caused by an abnormal and excessive end organ response to a normal hormonal milieu. It requires a surgical reduction of more than 1500 g of breast tissue per breast and poses a unique problem to the reconstructive surgeon. Various procedures have been described for reduction mammoplasty with specific skin incisions, patterns of breast parenchymal resection and blood supply to the nipple-areolar complex [1]. There are different types of techniques that have been used to achieve aesthetically acceptable results with the basis and the knowledge of the blood supply and innervation to the breasts in order to avoid distortion and ischaemia of the nipple-areolar complex (NAC) and alteration of nipple sensation apart from the good aesthetic outcome and maintaining ability for breastfeeding function. Among all the techniques using different pedicle such as superior, inferior, medial, lateral central/posterior or combinations of pedicles that are suitable for different types of patient according to degree of hypertrophy, ptosis and particular surgeon's preference or expertise. To date, only small case reports and series are available which specifically address the surgical management of this specific group. In cases of massive hypertrophy, the free nipple graft technique is still being performed by some surgeons out of fear of losing the nipple-areolar complex (NAC) [2–5]. In patients that the free NAC technique is chosen, there are cases that partial epidermolysis or complete loss of the areola has been reported [6]. A 32-year-old patient presented to our unit after massive reduction (2200 mL of breast tissue on each side) with signs of NAC necrosis after performing free NAC graft in a different institution (Fig. 51.1). In 2008 the author published a modified technique of NAC free graft in the selected cases of gigantomastia that the surgeon decides to perform the reduction mammoplasty combined

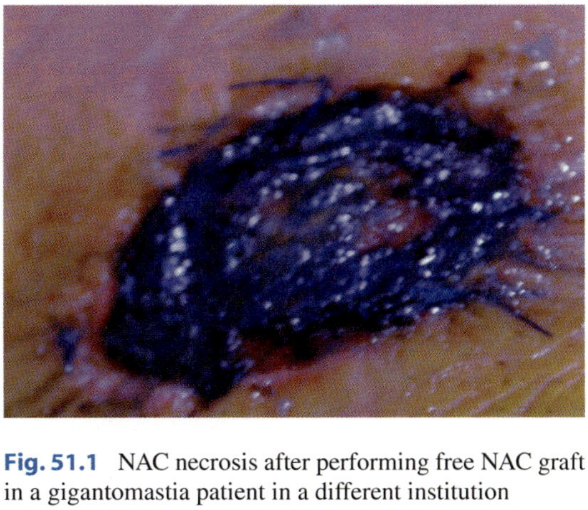

**Fig. 51.1** NAC necrosis after performing free NAC graft in a gigantomastia patient in a different institution

A. Sterodimas, M.D., M.Sc.
Department of Plastic Surgery, IASO General Hospital, 264 Mesogeion Avenue, Athens, Greece
e-mail: aris@sterodimas.com


M.A. Shiffman (ed.), *Nipple-Areolar Complex Reconstruction*,
https://doi.org/10.1007/978-3-319-60925-6_51

with a free transplantation of the NAC [7]. This modified technique of free NAC graft has shown better revascularization of the NAC graft, avoiding epidermolysis and total necrosis of NAC.

## 51.2 Technique

Rebuilding the central mound of the breast and repositioning it on the chest wall is a necessity in these patients. Using internal sutures to shape the breast mound has become an essential component to the surgical technique in these patients. The principal benefits of shaping sutures are to facilitate central projection and to prevent the bulk of the long pedicle from displacing laterally. To this end, sutures are placed in a manner to tack the breast parenchyma medially and may occasionally be placed to secure the pedicle itself medially to the chest wall to achieve maximal central projection and to keep the breast mound central to the axis of the breast. Closure of the nipple-areolar complex is accomplished by choosing the appropriate position and size. Nipple diameter is selected at 38–42 cm depending on ultimate breast size and patient preference. This circle is then deepithelialized, and the dermis is then incised radially from the 9 to 3 o'clock position and from the 6 to 12 o'clock position. A circular dermo-dermic round block using a 2-0 Mononylon™ (Ethicon Ltd., USA) is then performed as shown in Fig. 51.2. This was based on the principle of the periareolar 'round block' described by Benelli [8, 9]. The NAC graft is then placed as a free, thick, split-thickness skin graft. The graft is sutured with 5-0 Mononylon™ (Ethicon Ltd., USA). The bolus tie-over 'pressure' dressing is used. On the seventh post-operative day, removal of the tie-over dressing is done. This technique guarantees the maintenance of the nipple mount in the nipple-areolar complex (Fig. 51.3).

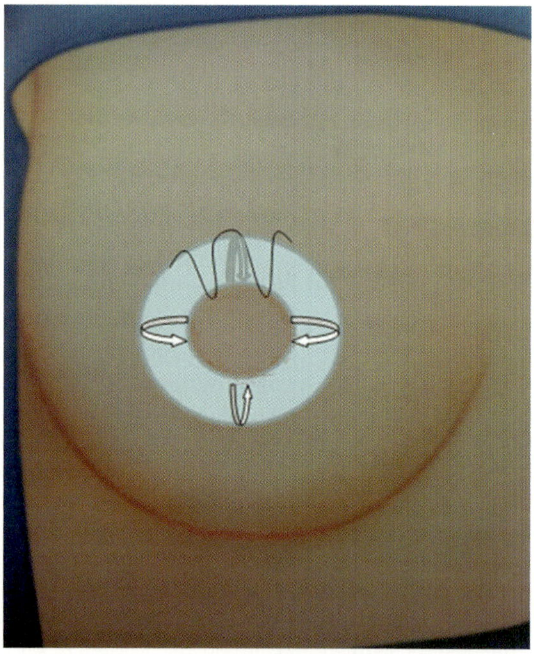

**Fig. 51.2** A circular dermo-dermic round block using a 2-0 Mononylon™ is performed before the NAC graft

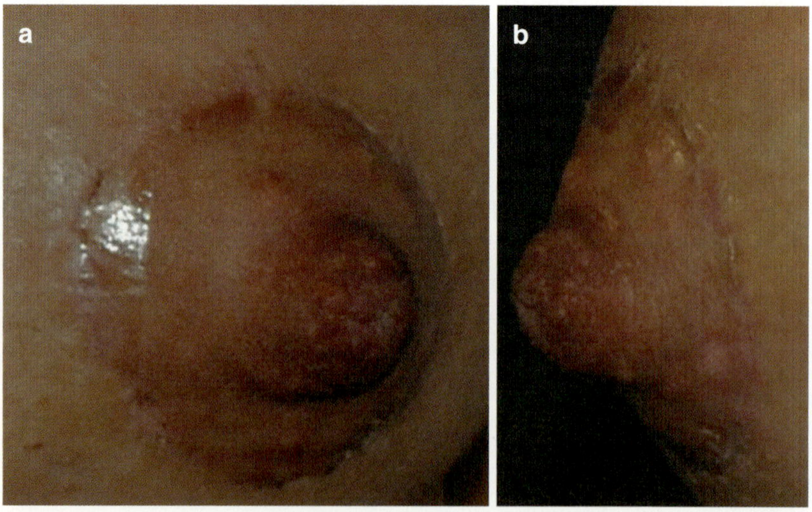

**Fig. 51.3** (**a**, **b**) Post-operative view of the nipple-areolar complex after modified NAC graft technique

## 51.3 Discussion

Various procedures have been described for reduction mammoplasty with specific skin incisions, patterns of breast parenchymal resection and retained blood supply to the remaining breast tissue and areolar complex; however, not all of these techniques can be applied successfully in the setting of gigantomastia [10, 11]. There are numerous techniques currently available for breast reduction in gigantomastia cases. Techniques relying on nipple-areolar complex transposition, rather than grafting, have been described with inferior, superomedial and medial pedicles [2, 12]. The technique chosen usually depends on the personal experience and expertise of the surgeon, as well as the requirements of the individual patient. Breast reduction by the inferior pedicle technique is one of the most commonly performed operations for macromastia and has been shown to be consistently reliable. A major advantage of this technique is that it usually preserves the main nerve to the nipple and areola, the deep branch of the lateral cutaneous branch of the fourth intercostal nerve. Many surgeons recommend this operation for all patients and all breast types. It necessitates, however, extensive undermining of skin flaps and relies on a vascularized dermo-parenchymal pedicle. In patients in whom the skin flaps and nipple survival are at risk, the inferior pedicle technique may be relatively contraindicated [13] The superomedial pedicle (SMP) reduction mammoplasty technique has been demonstrated as a safe and effective method of reduction in cases of mild to moderate hypertrophy [14, 15]. Central (posterior) reduction

satile pedicle due to its good blood supply and innervation for maintaining of nipple sensation with unremarkably long-term complication and proven in preservation of breastfeeding function. It is one of the options to correct breast hypertrophy in gigantomastia cases [16]. Operative techniques have been adapted to the management of gigantomastia to reduce the rates of surgical complications, including minor complications such as asymmetry, hematoma, seroma, focal superficial skin necrosis and nipple-areolar complex hypopigmentation, and major complications such as reoperation and nipple-areolar complex necrosis [17].

Reduction mammoplasty has been shown to improve or eliminate pain, restores physical activity and quality of life and has one of the highest patient satisfaction rates of any procedure performed by plastic surgeons [18]. For selected patients, however, breast reduction with free nipple-areolar grafting may be the procedure of choice. The traditional indication for this procedure is the patient with massive breast hypertrophy or gigantomastia. Other indications are poor-risk elderly patients, patients with severe systemic disease, patients with operative scars in the region of potential pedicles or skin flaps and patients in whom resection of tissue is indicated in the region of the inferior pedicle [19, 20]. The disadvantages of free nipple grafts include loss of sensation, poor nipple projection, uneven pigmentation due to partial epidermolysis, loss of lactation and total necrosis [21]. The most common part of epidermolysis is the central part of the nipple, which is an expected sequela of free nipple graft procedures [22]. As a result, there is loss of the nipple mount and hypopigmentation.

This modified technique of free NAC graft described by Sterodimas contributes in the prevention of partial and/or complete epidermolysis and as a consequence preserves the nipple mount in the breast (Fig. 51.3). The deepithelialized dermal bed is telescoped outward by the 'round block', pushing against the graft and thus promoting a better contact with the free nipple-areolar graft. This tissue contact contributes in the better revascularization of the NAC graft. In Fig. 51.4 a 45-year-old female patient who underwent reduction mammoplasty combined with modified NAC free graft is shown preoperatively and 4 months post-operatively. The 'round block' also assists in decreasing the tension upon the NAC graft, preventing the epidermolysis of the central part of the areola and eviting possible necrosis. In Fig. 51.5 a 65-year-old female patient who underwent reduction mammoplasty combined with modified NAC free graft is shown preoperatively and 12 months post-operatively.

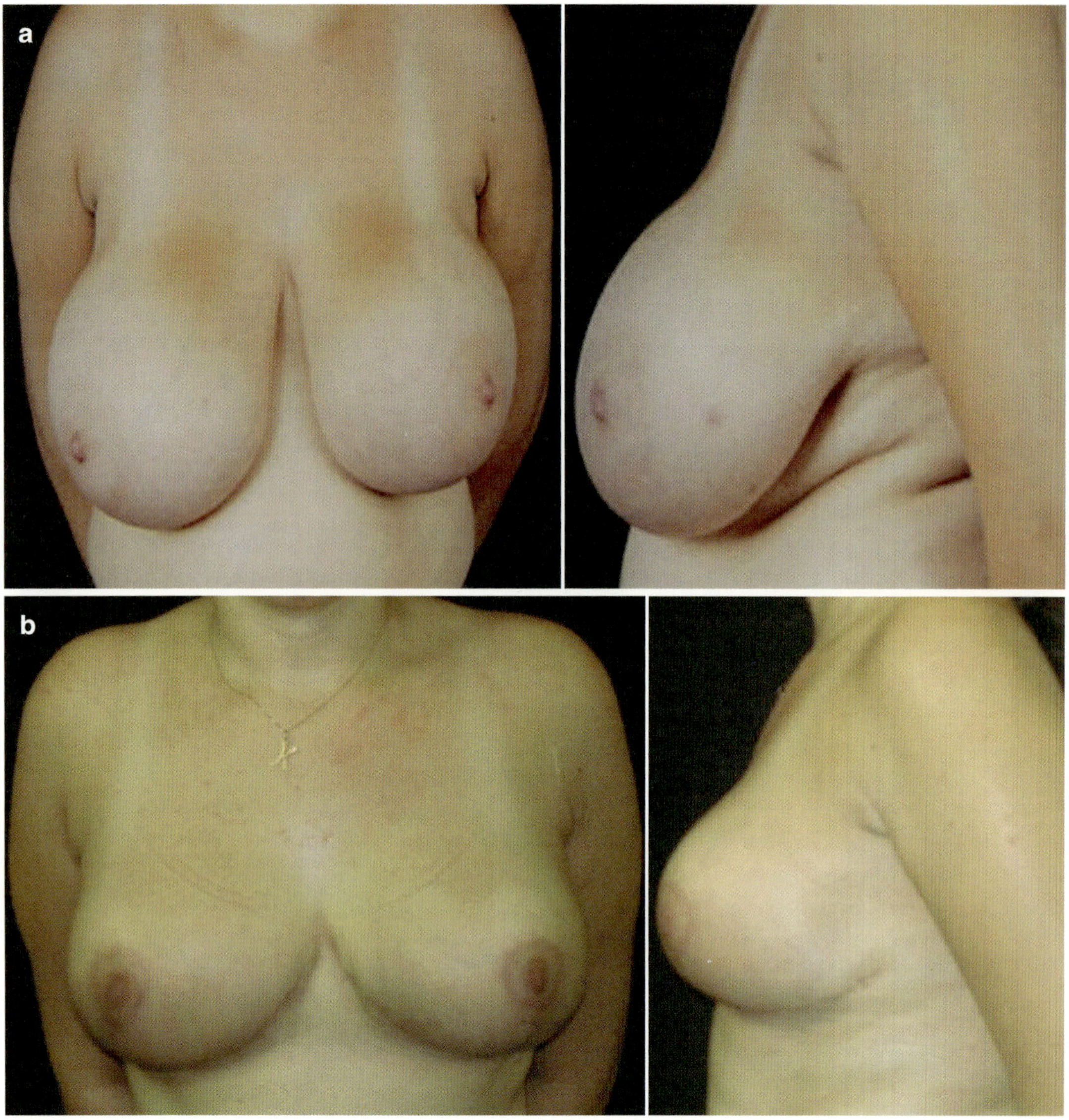

**Fig. 51.4** (**a**) Preoperative 45-year-old female patient. (**b**) Four months after reduction mammoplasty combined with modified NAC free graft

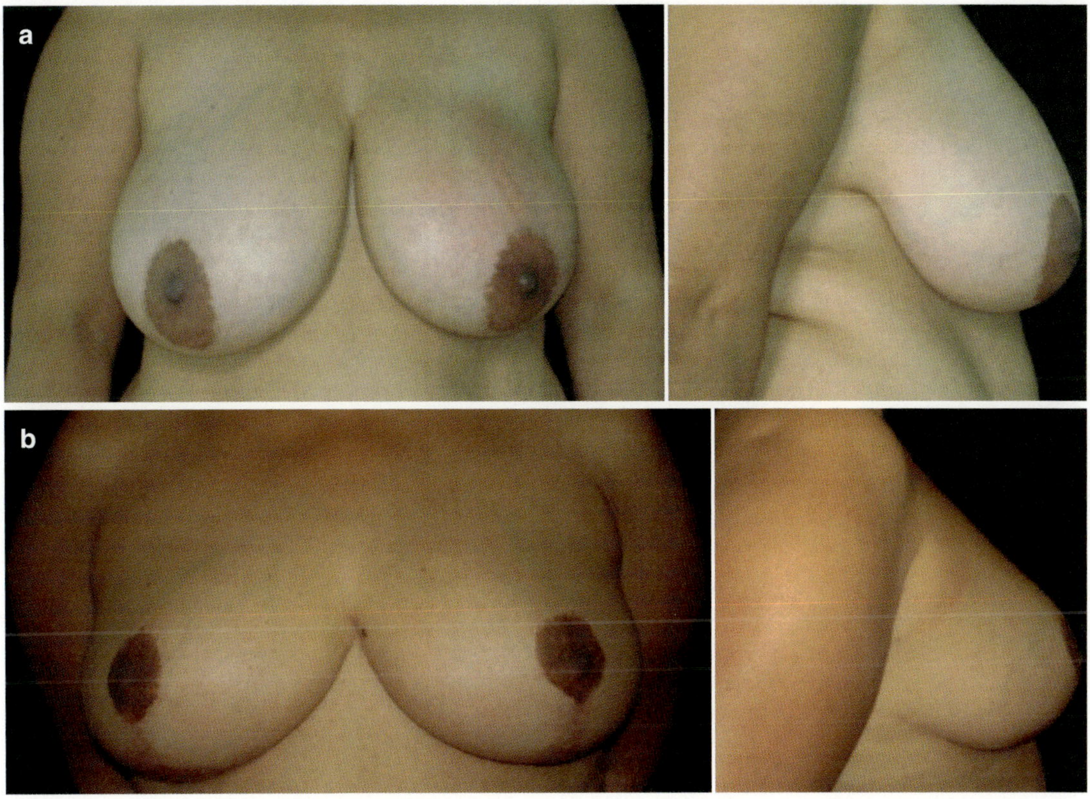


**Fig. 51.5** (**a**) Preoperative 65-year-old female patient. (**b**) Twelve months following reduction mammoplasty combined with modified NAC free graft

## Conclusions

The author strongly recommends using the modified free NAC graft in the selected cases of gigantomastia where the surgeon chooses to use free NAC graft and believes that the 'round block' can possibly be an additional measure in order to maximize the survival of the NAC graft in the reduction mammoplasty cases.

## References

1. Sterodimas A, Vargas A, Radwanski HN, Pitanguy I. The use of buflomedil in reduction mammaplasty for a previously irradiated breast: a case report. Aesthet Plast Surg. 2008;32(2):383–5.
2. Dafydd H, Roehl KR, Phillips LG, Dancey A, Peart F, Shokrollahi K. Redefining gigantomastia. J Plast Reconstr Aesthet Surg. 2011;64:160–3.
3. Casas LA, Byun MY, Depoli PA. Maximizing breast projection after free-nipple-graft reduction mammaplasty. Plast Reconstr Surg. 2001;107(4):955–60.
4. Koger KE, Sunde D, Press BH, et al. Reduction mammaplasty for gigantomastia using inferiorly based pedicle and free nipple transplantation. Ann Plast Surg. 1994;33:561–4.
5. Basaran K, Saydam FA, Ersin I, Yazar M, Aygit AC. The free-nipple breast-reduction technique performed with transfer of the nipple-areola complex over the superior or superomedial pedicles. Aesthet Plast Surg. 2014;38(4):718–26.
6. Rietjens M, De Lorenzi F, Andrea M, Chirappapha P, Martella S, Barbieri B, Gottardi A, Giuseppe L, Hamza A, Petit JY, Lohsiriwat V. Free nipple graft technique to correct nipple and areola malposition after breast procedures. Plast Reconstr Surg Glob Open. 2013;1(8):e69.

7. Sterodimas A, Pineda EF, Meirelles V, Pitanguy I. Maximizing nipple graft survival after performing free nipple-areolar complex reduction mammaplasty. J Plast Reconstr Aesthet Surg. 2008;61(8):971–2.
8. Benelli L. A new periareolar mammaplasty: the "round block" technique. Aesthet Plast Surg. 1990;14(2):93–100.
9. Sterodimas A, Nicaretta B, Boriani F. Modified round block mastopexy versus traditional round block mastopexy. Eur Rev Med Pharmacol Sci. 2015;19(3):350–6.
10. Manahan MA, Buretta KJ, Chang D, Mithani SK, Mallalieu J, Shermak MA. An outcomes analysis of 2142 breast reduction procedures. Ann Plast Surg. 2015;74(3):289–92.
11. Dancey A, Khan M, Dawson J, Peart F. Gigantomastia—a classification and review of the literature. J Plast Reconstr Aesthet Surg. 2008;61(5):493–502.
12. Wettstein R, Christofides E, Pittet B, Psaras G, Harder Y. Superior pedicle breast reduction for hypertrophy with massive ptosis. J Plast Reconstr Aesthet Surg. 2011;64(4):500–7.
13. Kling RE, Tobler WD Jr, Gusenoff JA, Rubin JP. Avoiding complications in gigantomastia. Clin Plast Surg. 2016;43(2):429–39.
14. Lugo LM, Prada M, Kohanzadeh S, Mesa JM, Long JN, de la Torre J. Surgical outcomes of gigantomastia breast reduction superomedial pedicle technique: a 12-year retrospective study. Ann Plast Surg. 2013;70(5):533–7.
15. Amini P, Stasch T, Theodorou P, Altintas AA, Phan V, Spilker G. Vertical reduction mammaplasty combined with a superomedial pedicle in gigantomastia. Ann Plast Surg. 2010;64(3):279–85.
16. See MH. Central pedicle reduction mammoplasty: a reliable technique. Gland Surg. 2014;3(1):51–4.
17. Fischer JP, Cleveland EC, Shang EK, Nelson JA, Serletti JM. Complications following reduction mammaplasty: a review of 3538 cases from the 2005-2010 NSQIP data sets. Aesthet Surg J. 2014;34(1):66–73.
18. Kececi Y, Sir E, Gungor M. Patient-reported quality-of-life outcomes of breast reduction evaluated with generic questionnaires and the breast reduction assessed severity scale. Aesthet Surg J. 2015;35(1):48–54.
19. Kalliainen LK, ASPS Health Policy Committee. ASPS clinical practice guideline summary on reduction mammaplasty. Plast Reconstr Surg. 2012;130(4):785–9.
20. Fırat C, Gurlek A, Erbatur S, Aytekin AH. An autoprosthesis technique for better breast projection in free nipple graft reduction mammaplasty. Aesthet Plast Surg. 2012;36(6):1340–6.
21. Lacerna M, Spears J, Mitra A, Medina C, McCampbell E, Kiran R, Mitra A. Avoiding free nipple grafts during reduction mammaplasty in patients with gigantomastia. Ann Plast Surg. 2005;55(1):21–4.
22. Spear SL, Pelletiere CV, Wolfe AJ, Tsangaris TN, Pennanen MF. Experience with reduction mammaplasty combined with breast conservation therapy in the treatment of breast cancer. Plast Reconstr Surg. 2003;111(3):1102–9.

# 52 The Free Nipple Breast Reduction Technique Performed with Transfer of the Nipple-Areola Complex over the Superior or Superomedial Pedicles

Karaca Basaran and Idris Ersin

## 52.1 Introduction

Patients with gigantomastia refer to plastic surgeons due to problems with self-esteem caused by the negative body image, limitation in exercise and daily activities, and other physical complaints [1]. Numerous techniques for breast reduction have been developed until today, all with certain advantages and disadvantages [2–7]. Although there are many alternatives for patients with moderate breast hypertrophy, surgical options for patients with massive breast hypertrophy or severe ptosis are more limited. In this latter group of patients, the free nipple reduction technique described by Thorek in 1922 is still used frequently [8] despite disadvantages such as hypopigmentation, graft loss, lactation disorders, reduced sensitivity, and projection loss [9–11].

In the method described, the NAC is transferred over the full-thickness superomedial or superior pedicles which we believe provides more satisfactory results with respect to projection. In this technique, it's possible to minimize the projection loss resulting from the conventional free nipple technique.

## 52.2 Technique

### 52.2.1 Patient Markings

The markings were made according to the classical Wise pattern (Figs. 52.1 and 52.2). With the patient standing, the sternal midline, inframammary fold, suprasternal notch, and breast meridian were marked. The new nipple position was determined as the point where the IMF intersected with the breast meridian. The amount of excision was determined by moving the breast medially and laterally. The length of the vertical limb beginning from the lower edge of the areola was 6.5 cm (9 cm from the nipple). The length of the superior or superomedial pedicle was determined according to the estimated amount of resection. The maximum pedicle length was determined as 10 cm to prevent compression in the vertical plane. The superomedial pedicle allowed a longer pedicle length due to the rotational advantage; mean length was 11 cm (range: 8–14 cm). In the superior pedicle, the base of the pedicle was planned as wide as the areolar opening, whereas it had an average width 8 cm in the superomedial pedicle. When deemed necessary, 8 × 8 cm rectangular

K. Basaran, M.D. (✉)
Department of Plastic and Reconstructive Surgery, Bagcilar Research and Training Hospital, Merkez Mahallesi Mimar Sinan Caddesi, 6. Sokak Bagcilar, Istanbul, Turkey
e-mail: basarankaraca@gmail.com

I. Ersin, M.D.
Department of Plastic and Reconstructive Surgery, Urla Public Hospital, Torasan Mahallesi Özbek Yolu Caddesi No:15, Urla, İzmir, Turkey
e-mail: idrisersin@yahoo.com


M.A. Shiffman (ed.), *Nipple-Areolar Complex Reconstruction*,
https://doi.org/10.1007/978-3-319-60925-6_52

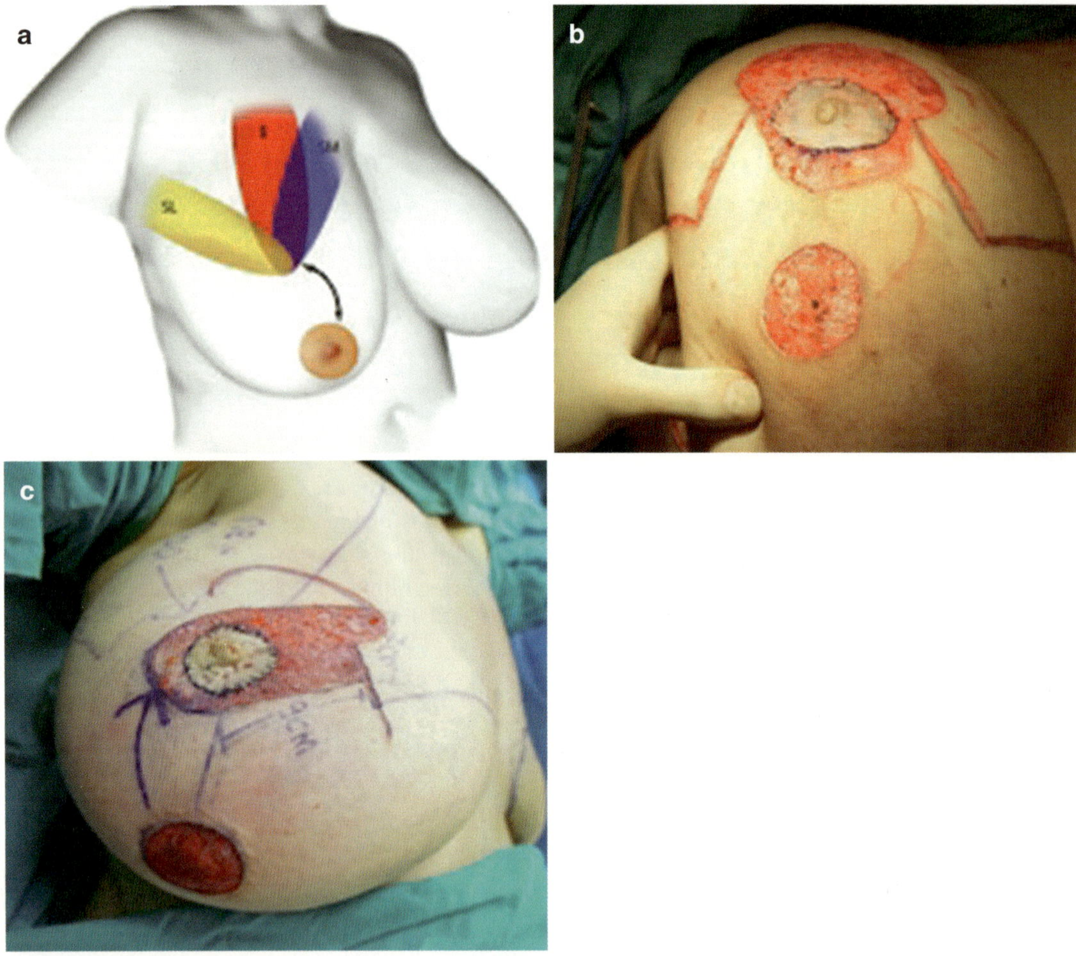


**Fig. 52.1** (**a**) Major pedicle options for NAC transfer. *S* Superior, *SM* Superomedial, *SL* Superolateral. (**b**) Superior pedicle prepared for NAC transfer, (**c**) Superomedial pedicles prepared for NAC transfer

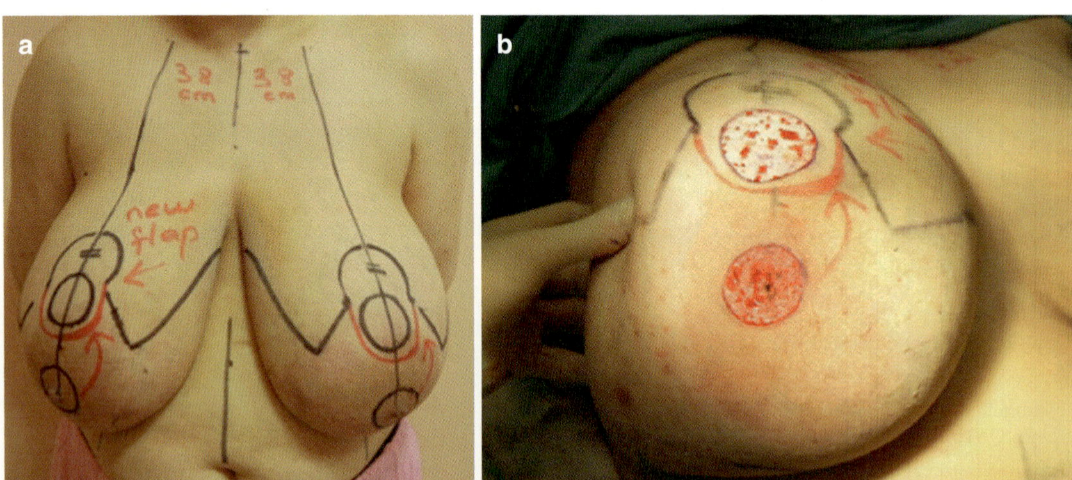


**Fig. 52.2** (**a**) Preoperative markings. (**b**) NAC is taken as a full-thickness skin graft (FTSG). (**c**) 3 × 2 cm dermal rectangular flaps are prepared centrally to increase the nipple projection. (**d**) Adaptation of the NAC to its new place on the superior pedicle

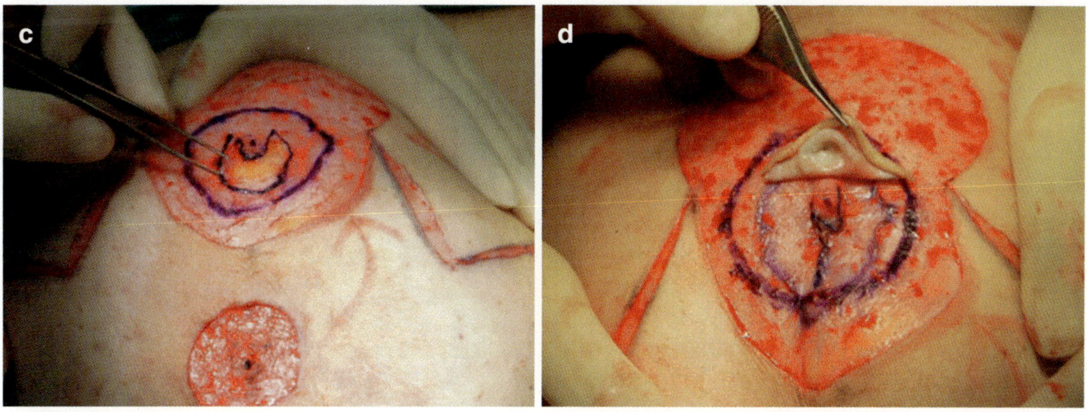

Fig. 52.2 (continued)

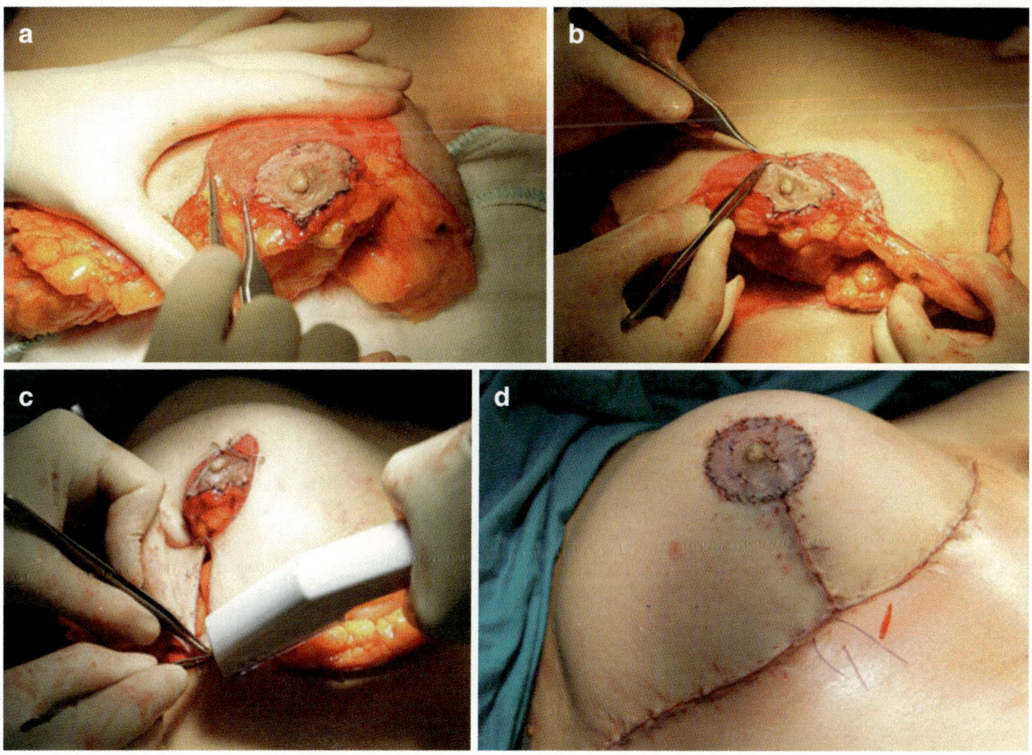

Fig. 52.3 (**a**) The glandular resections performed with leaving a full-thickness superior pedicle. (**b**) Adaptation of the NAC to its new place. (**c**) Skin flap closure. (**d**) Final result with considerable breast projection

flaps were planned to further increase the inferior projection.

## 52.2.2 Surgical Technique

Standard Wise pattern breast reduction skin incisions were made. First, the NAC was taken as a full-thickness skin graft (FTSG), (Fig. 52.2). Then superior or superomedial flaps were prepared and deepithelialized. The new determined site of the areola was marked on these pedicles using a marker. In order to increase the nipple projection, 3 × 2 cm dermal rectangular flaps were prepared in the middle of the new NAC area. The NAC prepared as a FTSG was placed directly over this pedicle. Therefore the subsequent stages of the operation were converted into a superior or superomedial pedicled reduction mammaplasty technique. The inferior, medial, and lateral glandular tissues around the pedicle were resected as a single piece (Fig. 52.3). Depending on the pedicle, the NAC was placed into its new location with rotational (superomedial pedicle) or direct vertical (superior pedicle). During shaping, care was taken to avoid excessive thinning of the full-thickness dermoglandular pedicles or shearing them from the thoracic wall. In order to decrease the tension in the NAC and to provide stabilization, the full-thickness pedicles were sutured to the pectoral fascia at the level of the second intercostal space using 2/0 PDS sutures. In conditions where there were severe skin laxity and inadequate projection, 8 × 8 cm inferior rectangular flaps were prepared as described above. These deepithelialized flaps were pulled upward and stabilized to the pectoral fascia at six points using 2/0 PDS. After hemostasis, glandular and skin sutures were placed, and vacuum drains were inserted. The NAC applied as a FTSG was covered using a tie-over dressing with mild compression.

### 52.2.3 Postoperative Care

The tie-over dressing on the nipple graft is removed at the postoperative seventh to tenth day. Antibacterial impregnated gauze dressing is applied on the NAC area daily. Drains are

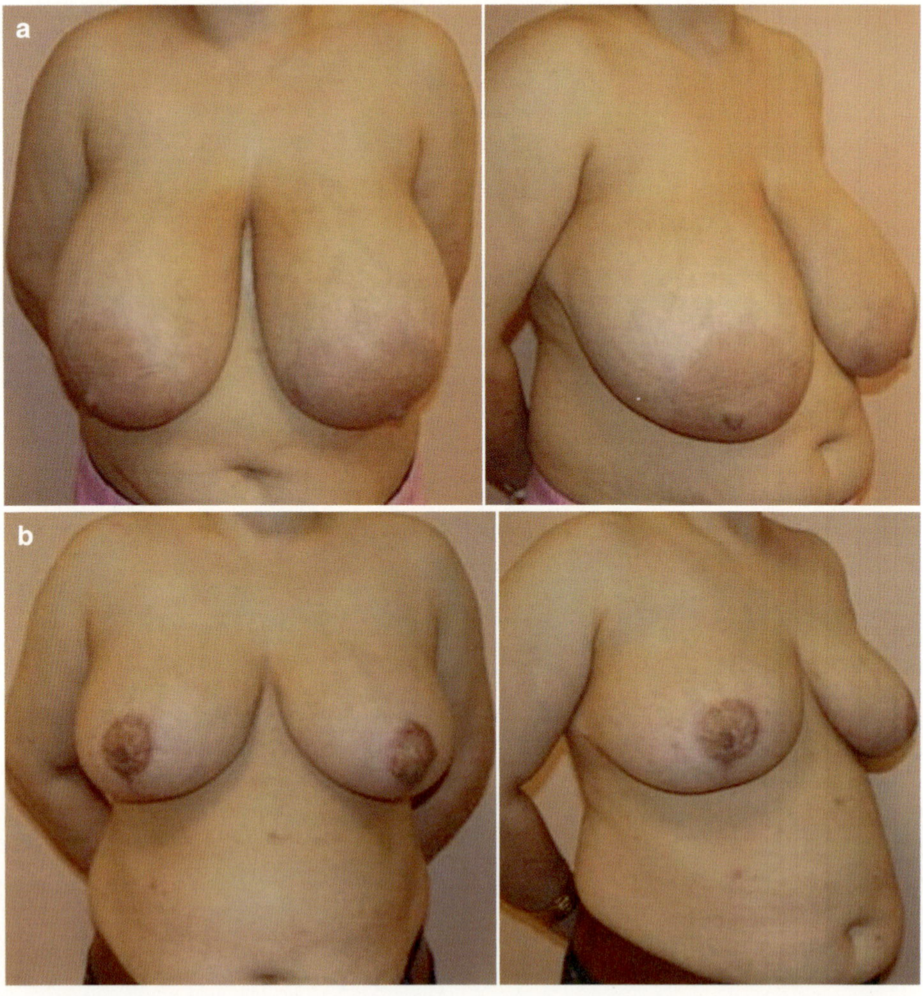


**Fig. 52.4** (**a**) Preoperative. (**b**) Thirteen months postoperative after reduction performed with the transfer of the NAC on the superomedial pedicle

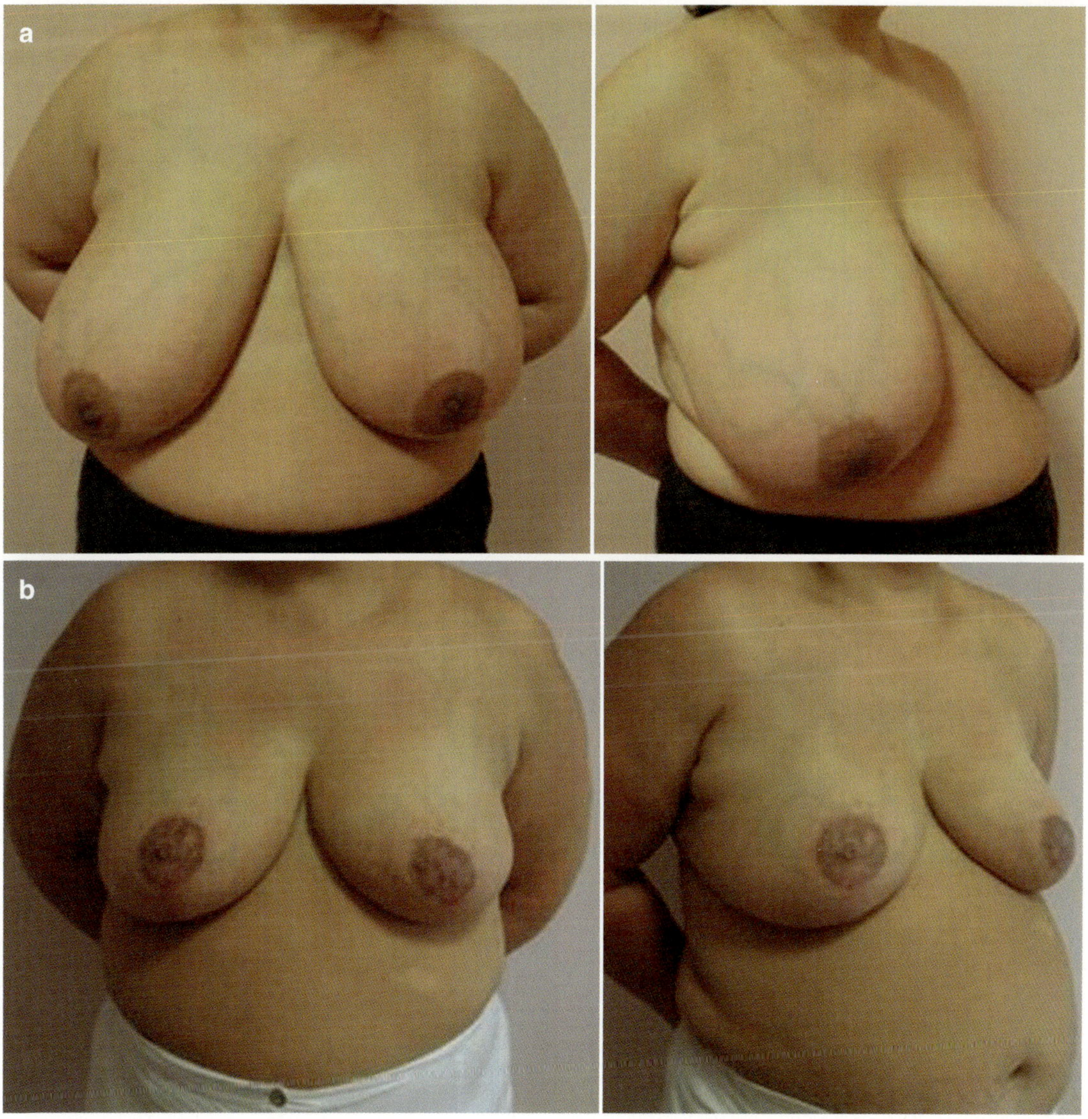

**Fig. 52.5** (**a**) Preoperative. (**b**) Fifteen months postoperative after reduction performed with the transfer of the NAC on the superior pedicle

removed at the discretion of the physician based on the amount. A surgical bra is instructed to be worn for a month. Patient results are demonstrated in Figs. 52.4, 52.5, and 52.6.

## 52.3 Discussion

There are numerous options described previously for breast reduction: the inferior, lateral, superolateral, superior, superomedial, central, and bipedicled ones are among the most commonly used [2–7, 12]. Most of these techniques provide satisfactory results in mild or moderate levels of macromastia. The main problem occurs in patients who require large amounts of resection.

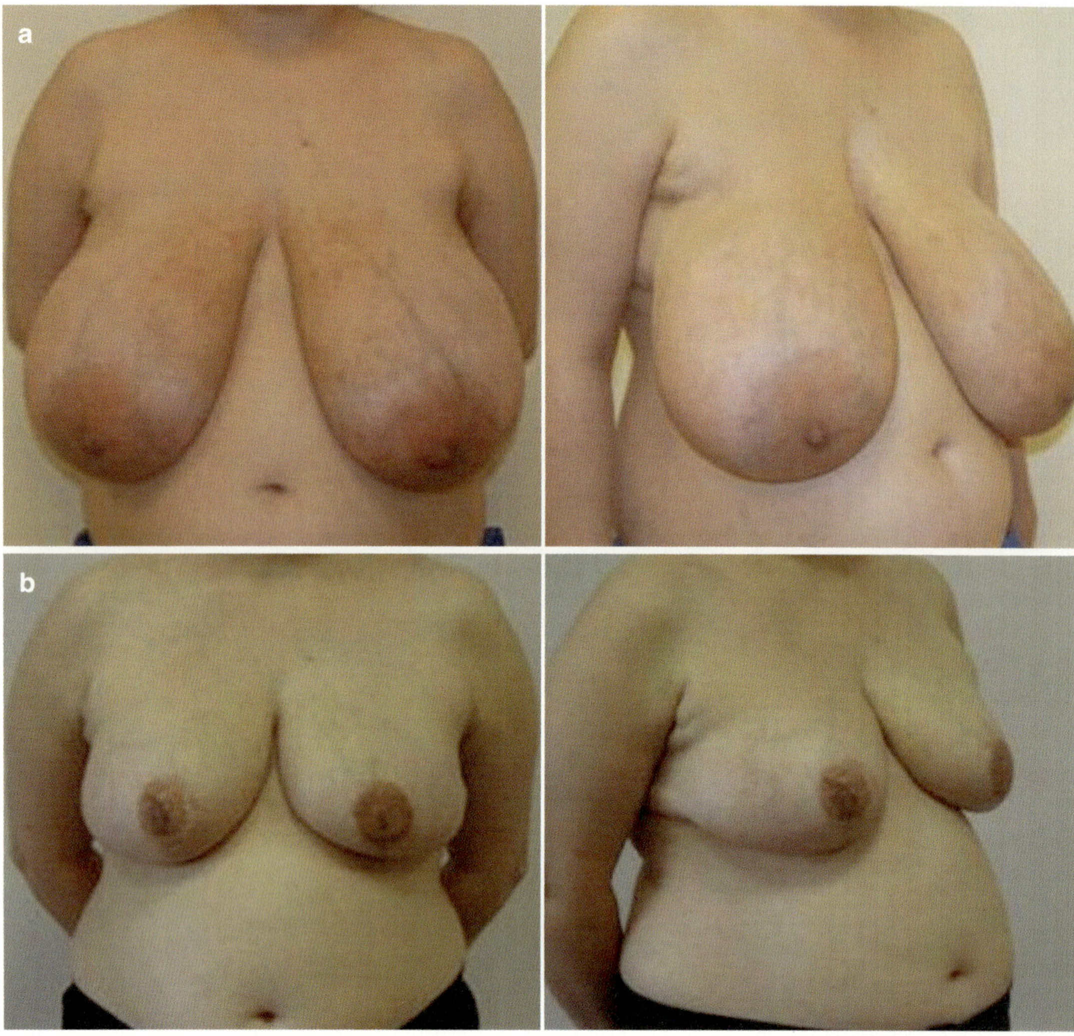

**Fig. 52.6** (**a**) Preoperative. (**b**) Fourteen months postoperative after reduction performed with the transfer of the NAC on the superior pedicle

In patients with severe hypertrophy, most of the pedicled techniques risk the NAC circulation due to pedicle length and greater amounts of resection.

In cases with severe gigantomastia, breast amputation and free nipple graft application is a useful and a reliable method; however, it has disadvantages including hypopigmentation, graft loss, failure to lactate, decreased sensation, and decreased breast projection [9–11]. Therefore some authors have tried to avoid the free nipple method and modified the pedicled reduction methods to achieve more reliable and aesthetically more pleasing methods [10, 13–16]. Nahabedian et al. [13] modified the medial pedicle reduction mammaplasty method. He stated that the pedicle length and the associated limitation in the rotational arch limited the use of the superomedial pedicle in large breasts and tried to solve the problem by narrowing the pedicle base and detaching the superior connections of the pedicle. Gerzenshtein et al. [15] emphasized the contribution of the perforators to the NAC circulation in inferior pedicle breast reduction, and they safely used the inferior pedicle in severely hypertrophic breasts by maximal preservation of the connections to the chest wall. In 2010, Wettstein et al. [14] published a series of 10 patients with average SN-N distance 44 cm, and who underwent a mean resection amount of 1450 grams. They showed that by thinning the pedicle, the superior pedicle breast reduction technique could be used in patients with massive hypertrophy and ptosis in a way that could provide superior fullness and projection. Basaran et al. [16] tried to solve this problem by introducing a patient-based approach in another study. The technique relies on determining the major pedicle by using a color Doppler USG and designing a pedicle that includes these vessels. This method has enabled a safer reduction in patients with severe macromastia.

Although various modifications of the pedicled breast reduction methods have been attempted, free nipple breast reduction method is unfortunately inevitable in some patients. The free nipple technique may be preferred especially in patients who have comorbidities such as diabetes mellitus, hypertension, vascular disease, and metabolic syndrome or in patients who are considered to be candidates for delayed wound healing and complications due to risk factors like obesity and smoking [17, 18]. The classical free nipple reduction mammaplasty often results in a widely based breast without projection, and recently various dermoglandular pedicles have been used for providing augmentation of the central breast mound [9, 11, 19–22]. These flaps are mostly inferior- or superior-based flaps; they have been dissected free from the pectoral fascia up to a certain extent in order to be shaped and transferred to where needed. For example, in 2007, Gorgu et al. [19] described the inferior dermaglandular pedicled modification for free nipple reduction mammaplasty. They folded the inferior dermaglandular pedicle which was planned 0.5 cm above the original inframammary sulcus and sutured it to the pectoralis major fascia. Romano et al. [23] placed the superiorly based dermal pedicles under the lateral and medial skin flaps and reported that they did not observe projection loss or flattening. Misirlioglu and Akoz [21] backfolded the superior dermaglandular pedicle, aiming to increase the central projection. Karsidag et al. [22] described a modification of the free nipple technique where a superior dermaglandular flap was used with the vertical technique. They preserved the superior dermaglandular pedicle and sutured it to the fascia. In 1997, Abramson [24] used two dermaglandular pedicles, superior and inferior, to increase the projection. Guven et al. [9] modified the same technique by backfolding the superior flap and obtained successful results in 24 patients.

In our technique, we used a different approach to increase the projection where we could not avert a free nipple procedure in patients with severe gigantomastia. The NAC was transposed to the full-thickness superomedial or superior dermaglandular pedicles during the first stage, in contrast to other studies. After this stage, the surgical procedure resembled a pedicled breast reduction. The pedicle that carried the NAC graft could thus be reduced and thinned in a way customized for each patient. On the other hand, in all of the methods described above, after shaping and suturing of the flaps that increase the projection, the NAC is sutured directly to its final position as a standard. Although our technique shows similarities to the other techniques using the superior flaps, the thickness of the flap constructed in all of them has a thickness that ranges between 1 and 4 cm [9–11]. This is because the authors have seen this necessary for handling the flap [11, 22]. In contrast, the pedicles we prepared are pedicles that have not detached from their connections with the pectoral fascia. This has provided a significant amount of central breast tissue, thereby achieving a conical shape. The effect of this modification is not limited to only providing an effective projection. The pedicle that has been constructed feeds from both the superficial subcutaneous tissues (the second and third intercostal branches of the internal mammary artery and the lateral thoracic artery) and the deep pectoral perforators [16]. In clinical practice, this condition provides the best viability for the NAC that is placed as a full-thickness graft.

We believe that the technique we used has some advantages. The biggest advantages are its effectiveness in providing breast projection equivalent to pedicled breast reduction techniques and allowing the surgeons to use the method that they are accustomed to and that they believe yields good results. Although superior and superomedial pedicle techniques are more popular today, some surgeons may prefer to use a different pedicle that they are more comfortable to work with. In addition, the internal mammary artery that provides significant perfusion to the breast was included in these two pedicles, which has been influential in our decision.

When choosing between two pedicles, the superomedial pedicle may be advantageous in achieving a larger breast due to its rotational advantage. The superior pedicle has folding limitation in a single plane and vertical axis. Therefore it should be remembered that a more limited flap may be constructed with the superior pedicle. Also, although this technique was applied to the Wise pattern incisions where the skin excisions are determined during patient markings, it should be remembered that the technique can be adapted to vertical pattern reductions. In that respect, this technique can be used by adapting to superolateral, central, or even inferior pedicle reduction techniques (Fig. 52.1).

Although we consider that we have obtained aesthetically successful results, the disadvantages of the free nipple technique, including loss of sensation and lactation and depigmentation risk, are valid also for our technique. Dog-ear deformity and minimal wound dehiscences especially in T-region were noted to be the most common complications with this technique.

### Conclusions

The technique we described differs from the previous free nipple reduction mammaplasty modifications in many aspects. In the abovementioned previous techniques, the designed dermoglandular flaps were used independently of the nipple-areola complex. In contrast, in this technique, the pedicles are used as a carrier and individually tailored for each patient. Therefore, various single or multiple pedicle designs can be utilized according to the preference of the surgeon and patient characteristics.

## References

1. Roehl K, Craig ES, Gómez V, Phillips LG. Breast reduction: safe in the morbidly obese? Plast Reconstr Surg. 2008;122(2):370–8.
2. Robbins TH. A reduction mammaplasty with the areola-nipple based on an inferior dermal pedicle. Plast Reconstr Surg. 1977;59(1):64–7.
3. Skoog T. A technique of breast reduction; transposition of the nipple on a cutaneous vascular pedicle. Acta Chir Scand. 1963;126:453–65.
4. Cárdenas-Camarena L. Reduction mammoplasty with superolateral dermoglandular pedicle: details of 15 years of experience. Ann Plast Surg. 2009;63(3):255–61.
5. Lejour M. Vertical mammaplasty and liposuction of the breast. Plast Reconstr Surg. 1994;94:100–14.
6. Balch CR. The central mound technique for reduction mammaplasty. Plast Reconstr Surg. 1981;67(3):305–11.
7. McKissock PK. Reduction mammaplasty by the vertical bipedicle flap technique. Rationale and results. Clin Plast Surg. 1976;3(2):309–20.
8. Thorek M. Possibilities in the reconstruction of the human form. N Y Med J. 1922;116:572.
9. Güven E, Aydin H, Başaran K, Aydin U, Kuvat SV. Reduction mammaplasty using bipedicled dermoglandular flaps and free-nipple transplantation. Aesthet Plast Surg. 2010;34(6):738–44.
10. Lacerna M, Spears J, Mitra A, Medina C, McCampbell E, Kiran R, Mitra A. Avoiding free nipple grafts during reduction mammaplasty in patients with gigantomastia. Ann Plast Surg. 2005;55(1):21–4.
11. Ozerdem OR, Anlatici R, Maral T, Demiralay A. Modified free nipple graft reduction mammaplasty to increase breast projection with superior and inferior dermoglandular flaps. Ann Plast Surg. 2002;49(5):506–10.
12. Hall-Findlay EJ. A simplified vertical reduction mammaplasty: shortening the learning curve. Plast Reconstr Surg. 1999;104(3):748–59.
13. Nahabedian MY, McGibbon BM, Manson PN. Medial pedicle reduction mammaplasty for severe mammary hypertrophy. Plast Reconstr Surg. 2000;105(3):896–904.
14. Wettstein R, Christofides E, Pittet B, Psaras G, Harder Y. Superior pedicle breast reduction for hypertrophy with massive ptosis. J Plast Reconstr Aesthet Surg. 2011;64(4):500–7.
15. Gerzenshtein J, Oswald T, McCluskey P, Caplan J, Angel MF. Avoiding free nipple grafting with the inferior pedicle technique. Ann Plast Surg. 2005;55(3):245–9.
16. Başaran K, Ucar A, Guven E, Arinci A, Yazar M, Kuvat SV. Ultrasonographically determined pedicled breast reduction in severe gigantomastia. Plast Reconstr Surg. 2011;128(4):252e–9e.
17. Chen CL, Shore AD, Johns R, Clark JM, Manahan M, Makary MA. The impact of obesity on breast

surgery complications. Plast Reconstr Surg. 2011;128(5):395e–402e.
18. Aydin H, Bilgin-Karabulut A, Tümerdem B. Free nipple reduction mammaplasty with a horizontal scar in high-risk patients. Aesthet Plast Surg. 2002;26(6):457–60.
19. Gorgu M, Ayhan M, Aytug Z, Aksungur E, Demirdover C. Maximizing breast projection with combined free nipple graft reduction mammaplasty and back-folded dermaglandular inferior pedicle. Breast J. 2007;13(3):226–32.
20. Koger KE, Sunde D, Press BH, Hovey LM. Reduction mammaplasty for gigantomastia using inferiorly based pedicle and free nipple transplantation. Ann Plast Surg. 1994;33(5):561–4.
21. Misirlioglu A, Akoz T. Familial severe gigantomastia and reduction with the free nipple graft vertical mammoplasty technique: report of two cases. Aesthet Plast Surg. 2005;29(3):205–9.
22. Karsidag S, Akcal A, Karsidag T, Yesiloglu N, Yesilada AK, Ugurlu K. Reduction mammaplasty using the free-nipple-graft vertical technique for severe breast hypertrophy: improved outcomes with the superior dermaglandular flap. Aesthet Plast Surg. 2011;35(2):254–61.
23. Romano JJ, Francel TJ, Hoopes JE. Free nipple graft reduction mammoplasty. Ann Plast Surg. 1992;28(3):271–6.
24. Abramson DL. Increasing projection in patients undergoing free nipple graft reduction mammoplasty. Aesthet Plast Surg. 1999;23(4):282–4.

# One-Stage Breast Reconstruction Using the Inferior Dermal Flap, Implant, and Free Nipple Graft

53

Ian C.C. King and James R. Harvey

## 53.1 Introduction

There are many evolving reconstructive options following treatment for breast cancer. These are broadly implant based or centered on autologous tissue techniques. Such techniques include tissue expanders or implant-based prostheses alone; pedicled flaps, typically the latissimus dorsi or transverse rectus abdominis myocutaneous (TRAM) flaps; or free flap reconstructions such as free deep inferior epigastric perforator (DIEP) or transverse upper gracilis (TUG) flaps. Options are dependent on patient preference and physical factors, such as disease location or extent, previous scarring, and tissue available. Free and pedicled flap reconstructions are widely accepted as being the aesthetically most satisfactory options, particularly when combined with nipple reconstruction and tattooing. However, such flaps require considerable surgical and nursing skills and resources with lengthy operations, physical and psychological stress to patients undergoing the procedures and resultant donor site morbidity, and the potential for further ancillary procedures being required.

Breast cancer incidence increases with age, as do comorbidities. An increase in the incidence of screen-detected cancers in an aging population means that many women are either unfit for autologous reconstruction or simply do not wish to affect their current level of performance or lifestyle with a prolonged recovery following a significant operation. Immediate implant-based breast reconstruction following skin-sparing mastectomy is an appealing option for women who wish to have the most straightforward and minimally invasive procedure available and avoid the donor site morbidity resultant from autologous tissue transfer. Implants are usually covered superiorly using a raised pectoralis major pocket, with lower pole coverage provided by either acellular dermal matrices [1], serratus anterior [2], or using an inferior dermal flap [3, 4].

Single-stage reconstruction, as described initially by Bostwick [3], can be achieved through the creation of a pocket of deepithelialized inferiorly based dermal tissue which is attached to the pectoralis muscle to enclose a permanent implant. The fully vascularized pocket for an implant provided by an inferior dermal flap which maintains its own blood supply is advantageous over acellular dermal matrices, which lack this important feature.

I.C.C. King, M.A. (Oxon), M.B.B.S., M.R.C.S.Ed. (✉)
Department of Plastic Surgery,
St George's Hospital, London, UK
e-mail: ianccking@doctors.org.uk

J.R. Harvey, M.B.B.S., Ph.D.
University of Manchester, Manchester Academic Health Science Centre, Manchester, UK

Nightingale Centre, University Hospital of South of Manchester, Southmoor Road, Manchester, UK
e-mail: James.Harvey@uhsm.nhs.uk


M.A. Shiffman (ed.), *Nipple-Areolar Complex Reconstruction*,
https://doi.org/10.1007/978-3-319-60925-6_53

The subcutaneous fat attached to the inferior dermal flap provides a thick layer of tissue to cover the implant, giving a more natural feel to the breast. The breast is shaped by this supportive suspension of the soft tissue envelope [3, 5, 6].

We describe a method of breast reconstruction for patients with ptotic breasts which we have found to offer a reliable, aesthetically pleasing, and safe breast following mastectomy [7, 8]. This single-stage procedure utilizes elements from commonly performed dermal flap augmentations [9, 10] with additional immediate resiting of the nipple as a free graft to complete the aesthetic of the reconstructed breast. Similar approaches without the use of free nipple grafts have been described for prophylactic mastectomies [11] and cancer mastectomies [3, 4, 12, 13]. We offered this procedure to all women with a larger ptotic breast who had expressed a preference for an immediate implant-based reconstruction and had a low risk of cancer involvement of the nipple [14].

## 53.2 Technique

The key to dermal sling reconstruction is that the patient has significant ptosis of at least second degree. The nipple must lie at least 2 cm below the inframammary fold (IMF). This is important to ensure that the dermal sling coverage is sufficient to cover the lower pole of the breast to the level of pectoralis major. Patients with grade 3 ptosis and a large breast (over 600 mL) will almost certainly have enough dermal sling to cover the lower pole. Patients with smaller breasts and moderate ptosis can present a challenge as they are too ptotic for an acellular dermal matrix but may not have enough dermal sling to cover the whole lower pole.

We certainly find it advantageous to mark the patient in the preoperative clinic setting. We specifically mark the lower border of pectoralis major, the site of the new nipple height. From here we can measure the length of the Wise pattern limbs and can calculate the height of the dermal sling coverage. If this is sufficient to span the distance from the IMF to pectoralis major, then this operative option is feasible.

Oncologically, we prefer evidence of no tumor involvement with the nipple. Free grafting of the nipple was only performed if the invasive tumor was less than 4 cm in size, if there was less than 2 cm of ductal carcinoma in situ (DCIS) and the tumor was more than 2 cm from the nipple-areola complex.

Preoperative Wise pattern markings are drawn [15], allowing for a 7.5 cm vertical incision [16]. The vertical lines are marked as close to the areola as possible, and these converge as near to the superior edge of the areola as the tissue allows (Fig. 53.1). The nipple is harvested as a full-thickness graft prior to the mastectomy and placed aside in a wet gauze. The Wise pattern markings are then incised and the skin below the markings is deepithelialized inferiorly to the level of the IMF. This deepithelialized area will form the inferior dermal flap. A standard mastectomy following fascial planes is subsequently performed at the superior junction of deepithelialized and epithelialized skin, using the length of the incision to optimize access.

Once the breast has been dissected from the pectoral fascia, pectoralis major is raised superiorly. The most lateral border of the deepithelialized dermal flap of the skin is sutured to the lateral

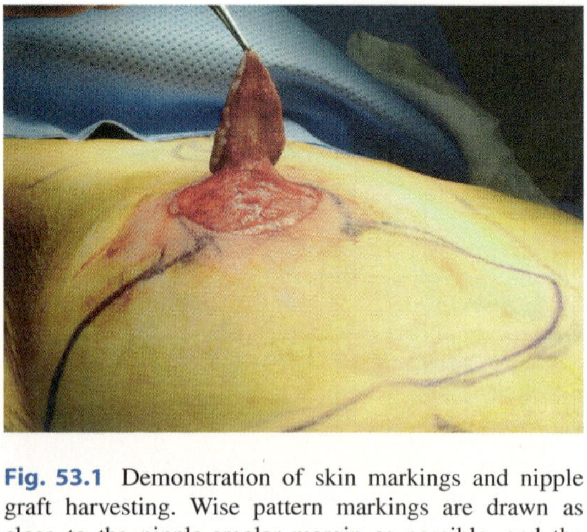

**Fig. 53.1** Demonstration of skin markings and nipple graft harvesting. Wise pattern markings are drawn as close to the nipple-areolar margin as possible, and the nipple is harvested as a full-thickness graft prior to deepithelialization

edge of the pectoralis major to close the lateral free space. The remaining deepithelialized flap is attached to the free edge of the pectoralis major, creating an inferior dermal flap (Fig. 53.2) which will surround the implant. An implant sizer is used prior to insertion of the textured silicone implant. The use of the inferior dermal flap elevates the ptotic breast enough to enable the skin to close in a standard Wise pattern to the IMF (Fig. 53.3).

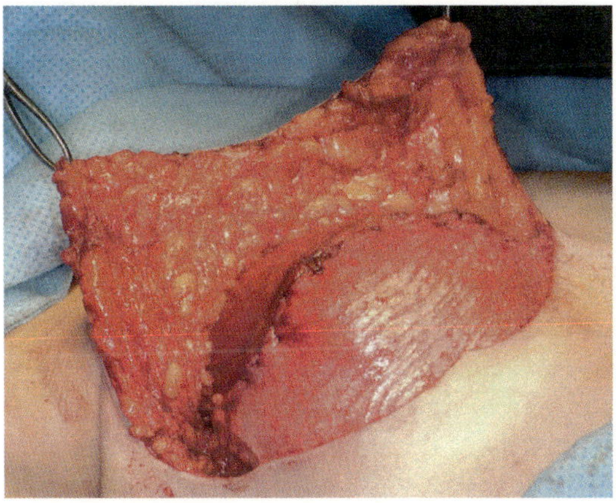

**Fig. 53.2** Implant in pocket below pectoralis major and inferior dermal flap. The deepithelialized inferior dermal sling is sutured end to end to pectoralis major, which has been divided from its inferior and medial attachments, to create a fully vascularized pocket into which a permanent implant has been placed

Two 12Ch suction drains are placed, one superficial to the dermal flap and one deep to the flap. Our preference is for the procedure to be performed as a single-stage procedure using a permanent implant. A two-stage procedure is usually unnecessary in the presence of adequate skin redundancy and lack of skin tension as in a standard breast reduction. Where potential for closure under tension is encountered, a tissue expander with integrated port is a useful alternative to a permanent implant.

The full-thickness nipple graft is thinned posteriorly until the nipple appears to be almost translucent and approximately 1 mm thick. Retroareolar biopsies are taken which are sent for histology to assess the remaining tissue attached to the nipple. The nipple site is centered on the breast's apex. The nipple donor site is centered 7.5 cm superior to the IMF at the apex of the vertical incision. This donor site is deepithelialized after partial skin closure (Fig. 53.4) and the nipple sutured with interrupted 5/0 Vicryl Rapide. A tie-over dressing comprised of Jelonet and gauze is used to secure graft with four radial 3/0 polypropylene sutures. Dressings are left in place for 10 days. The standardized follow-up regimen includes wound review with discussion of pathology results at 2 weeks (Fig. 53.5), followed by

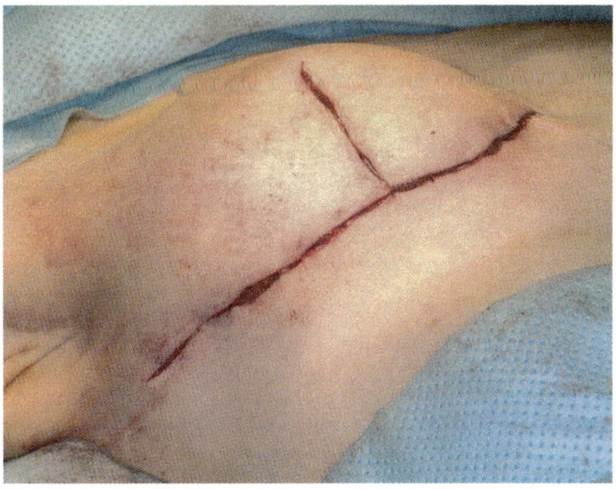

**Fig. 53.3** Closure of Wise pattern. Standard closure of Wise pattern incision including closure of all skin with subcuticular sutures prior to determination of the site for nipple placement

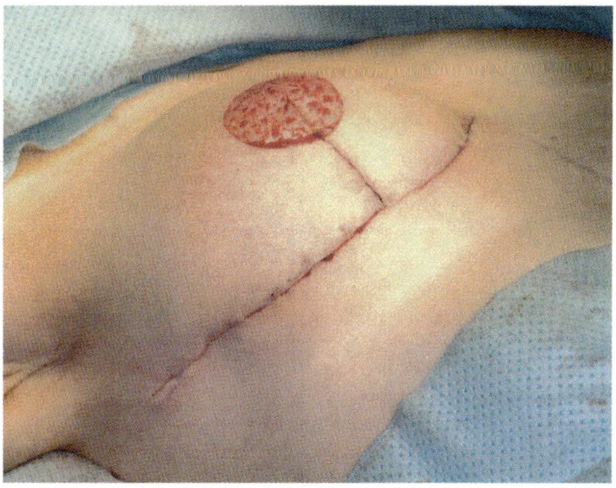

**Fig. 53.4** Deepithelialization of new nipple site. The new nipple site is deepithelialized at apex of implant; usually the center of the nipple is sited approximately 7.5 cm superior to the IMF

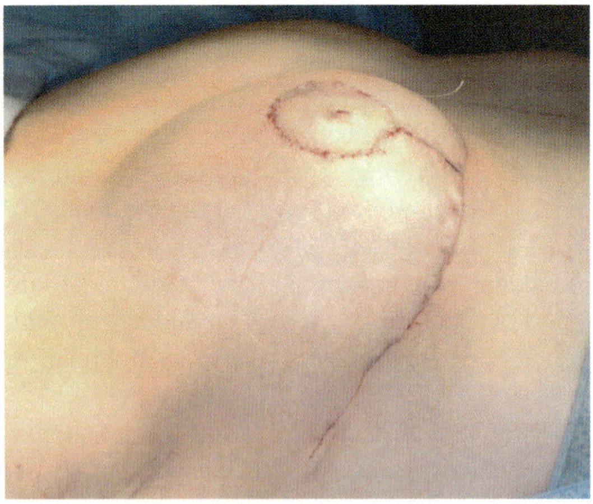

**Fig. 53.5** Final appearance of breast reconstruction with nipple graft in place

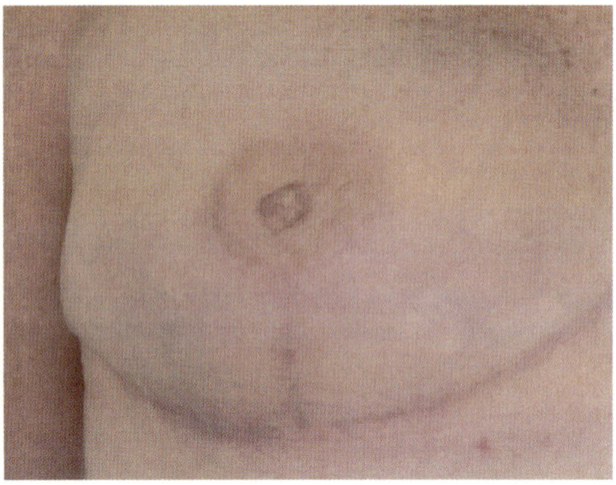

**Fig. 53.6** Four months postoperative after breast reconstruction

further wound checks if required, and thereafter 6 monthly reviews for 2 years and annual review with mammography for a total of 5 years after cancer treatment (Fig. 53.6).

## 53.3 Discussion

The reconstruction of large ptotic breasts using implant-based techniques has traditionally been a challenge. The use of inferior dermal flaps enables the creation of an aesthetic breast shape using a local tissue sling which has its own viable blood supply. For those women with a ptotic breast wishing to avoid the donor site and general morbidity and recovery associated with autologous reconstruction, the dermal flap is considered a safe option [17]. This technique of breast reconstruction involves removal of the tumor with an aesthetically acceptable, straightforward, and potentially safe outcome. Our recently published case series has demonstrated a relatively short operative time for the reconstruction with very few complications and excellent feedback from patients [7]. Excellent outcomes have been reported by Kijima et al. [18] combining this technique with a partial mastectomy and breast reconstruction.

An immediate cosmetic result is achieved for patients by using an immediate free nipple graft. In our experience the nipple graft gives a far superior cosmetic outcome in comparison with that produced by postoperative areolar tattooing. This free graft is a perfect pigment match for the contralateral nipple and avoids the need for painful tattooing or for a second procedure. It is essential to thin the nipple to translucency prior to suturing to the donor site in order to maximize nutrient uptake to promote graft viability. In our experience to date, owing to the excellent cosmetic result, no patients opting for free nipple grafts have requested further nipple reconstruction to recreate the nipple prominence [7].

Since Thorek's [19] initial description of free nipple grafting in combination with reduction mammoplasties for the treatment of massive breast hypertrophy, free nipple grafting has been widely reported elsewhere [20]. Criticisms of free nipple grafts focus on grafted nipples being flatter and having poor projection [21] though many modifications have been proposed to address this aesthetic concern [22, 23]. Contralateral composite nipple grafts may be used for reconstruction, but these are associated with contralateral donor morbidity and deformity [24] which can be avoided by using the ipsilateral nipple as the graft's donor site.

A potential problem with the use of free nipple grafts in breasts with disease is the chance of residual malignancy in the graft itself. We reduce this risk by not offering this option to patients with DCIS greater than 2 cm in size, those with tumors larger than 4 cm, or those with disease near the nipple-areolar complex. Removal of almost all ductal tissue through thinning prior to placement of the graft means that the risk of locally recurrent disease is expectantly lower than that associated with a nipple-sparing procedure [14]. Should the retroareolar biopsies demonstrate pathologically cancerous cells, excision of the nipple graft can be undertaken under local anesthetic, and a full-thickness graft could be transferred from another donor site. We ensured that all our patients were fully informed of this risk and are carefully monitored for any evidence of malignancy.

The preservation of nipples offers an aesthetic advantage to a reconstructed breast. Preservation can take the form of a pedicle or of a free graft when combined with a dermal sling. We favor the use of a free nipple graft over a pedicled flap due to the risk reduction offered by a thinned free nipple graft. Nipple-sparing mastectomy using a pedicled flap has been demonstrated to be equivalent to a skin-sparing mastectomy with respect to the oncological outcome in carefully selected patients [25]. The free nipple graft offers good cosmesis and conveys further oncological safety and reduced risk as the nipple is thinned down to skin alone, reducing the amount of residual breast tissue compared with that left in a pedicled nipple. Preserving nipples with pedicles is a good option that is offered to some women by surgeons, especially in the prophylactic setting.

Complications with this procedure are minimal [7]. We reported three patients encountering a minor breakdown of the T-junction where the mastectomy flap skin was draped over the vascularized dermal flap and closed in the standard Wise pattern. These were managed conservatively with dressings as the vascularized dermal flap both prevented exposure of the implant and acted as a scaffold for epithelialization.

Most importantly, performing the procedure in one step, including the contralateral reduction, enables women to achieve their final cosmetic result without the need for multiple follow-up appointments or operations. Women also do not need to have a significant period spent with an unfinished breast while awaiting contralateral procedures or nipple reconstructions/tattooing. Patients are extremely satisfied with waking up with a finished looking breast, and it also has quality of life benefits such that they can get back to normal social and functional aspects of their life sooner as they are not putting their lives on hold waiting for the next operation.

## Conclusions

This novel approach to breast reconstruction uses a combination of techniques that address both shape and global aesthetic of the reconstructed breast. Our experience has shown this modification to be a valuable reconstructive option for patients reporting a preference for a one-step procedure. This option is only appropriate for a minority of patients, in particular those who are suitable for immediate reconstruction, who have a large ptotic breast, and who have a low likelihood of disease involving the nipple. The combination of the two safe techniques, employing a dermal sling and a free nipple graft further, conveys a cosmetic benefit. The safety of dermal slings and free nipple grafts has been described widely in the literature [4, 5, 9, 11, 18, 20, 23]. The conversion of a ptotic breast to a younger non-ptotic breast shape does mandate that a majority of women might be anticipated to opt for a balancing contralateral breast reduction or mastopexy which we will perform concurrently. This combination of techniques appears to be a safe method of implant based breast reconstruction that gives an excellent cosmetic result in a single procedure and negates the need for subsequent procedures on that breast.

## References

1. Breuing KH, Warren SM. Immediate bilateral breast reconstruction with implants and inferolateral AlloDerm slings. Ann Plast Surg. 2005;55(30):232–9.
2. Saint-Cyr M, Dauwe P, Wong C, Thakar H, Nagarkar P, Rohrich RJ. Use of the serratus anterior fascia flap for expander coverage in breast reconstruction. Plast Reconstr Surg. 2010;125(4):1057–64.
3. Bostwick J. Prophylactic (risk-reducing) mastectomy and reconstruction. In: Bostwick J, editor. Plastic and reconstructive breast surgery, vol. II. St Louis: Quality Medical Publishing; 1990. p. 1369–73.

4. Goyal A, Wu JM, Chandran VP, Reed MW. Outcome after autologous dermal sling-assisted immediate breast reconstruction. Br J Surg. 2011;98(9):1267–72.
5. Echo A, Guerra G, Yuksel E. The dermal suspension sling: shaping the inferior pedicle during breast reconstruction. Aesthet Plast Surg. 2011;35(4):608–16.
6. Spear SL, Sher SR, Al-Attar A. Focus on technique: supporting the soft-tissue envelope in breast reconstruction. Plast Reconstr Surg. 2012;130(5 Suppl 2):89S–94S.
7. King ICC, Harvey J, Bhaskar P. One stage breast reconstruction using the inferior dermal flap, implant and free nipple graft. Aesthet Plast Surg. 2014;38(2):358–64.
8. King ICC, Harvey J. One stage breast reconstruction using the inferior dermal flap, implant and free nipple graft. In: Shiffman MA, editor. Breast reconstruction: art, science and new clinical techniques. Berlin: Springer; 2015. p. 467–73.
9. Aydin H, Bilgin-Karabulut A, Tumerdem B. Free nipple reduction mammoplasty with a horizontal scar in high-risk patients. Aesthet Plast Surg. 2002;26(6):457–60.
10. Munhoz AM, Montag E, Arrunda EG, Aldrighi C, Gemperli R, Aldrighi JM, Ferreira MC. Superior-medial dermoglandular pedicle reduction mammoplasty for immediate conservative breast surgery reconstruction: technical aspects and outcome. Ann Plast Surg. 2006;57(5):502–8.
11. Ross GL. One stage breast reconstruction following prophylactic mastectomy for ptotic breasts: the inferior dermal flap and implant. J Plast Reconstr Aesthet Surg. 2012;65(9):1204–8.
12. Rosato RE, Fink PJ, Horton CE, Payne RL Jr. Immediate postmastectomy reconstruction. J Surg Oncol. 1976;8(4):277–80.
13. Ladizinsky DA, Sandholm PH, Jewett ST, Shahzad F, Andrews K. Breast reconstruction with the Bostwick autoderm technique. Plast Reconstr Surg. 2013;132(2):261–70.
14. Spear SL, Willey SC, Feldman ED, Cocilovo C, Sidawy M, Al-Attar A, Hannan C, Seiboth L, Nahabedian MY. Nipple-sparing mastectomy for prophylactic and therapeutic indications. Plast Reconstr Surg. 2011;128(5):1005–14.
15. Wise RJ. A preliminary report on a method of planning the mammoplasty. Plast Reconstr Surg. 1956;17:367–75.
16. Regnault P. Breast ptosis: definition and treatment. Clin Plast Surg. 1976;34(2):193–203.
17. National Mastectomy and Breast Reconstruction Audit 2011. 22 Mar 2011. http://www.ic.nhs.uk/mbr. Accessed 31 Aug 2012.
18. Kijima Y, Yoshinaka H, Hirata M, Mizoguchi T, Ishigami S, Arima H, Nakajo A, Ueno S, Natsugoe S. Oncoplastic surgery combining partial mastectomy with breast reconstruction using a free nipple-areola graft for ductal carcinoma in situ in a ptotic breast: report of a case. Surg Today. 2011;41(3):390–5.
19. Thorek M. Possibilities in the reconstruction of the human form 1922. Aesthet Plast Surg. 1989;13(1):55–8.
20. Koger KE, Sunde D, Press BH, Hovey LM. Reduction mammoplasty for gigantomastia using inferiorly based pedicle and free nipple transplantation. Ann Plast Surg. 1994;33(5):561–4.
21. Casas LA, Byun MY, Depoli PA, Gradinger GP. Maximizing breast projection after free-nipple-graft reduction mammoplasty. Plast Reconstr Surg. 2001;107:955–60.
22. Bektas G, Cinpolat A, Bicici P, Unal K, Coskunfirat OK. A new application to free-nipple-graft reduction mammoplasty for breast and nipple projection. Eplasty. 2012;12:e37.
23. Guven E, Aydin H, Basaran K, Aydin U, Kuvat SV. Reduction mammoplasty using bipedicled dermoglandular flaps and free-nipple transplantation. Aesthet Plast Surg. 2010;34(6):738–44.
24. Lee TJ, Noh HJ, Kim EK, Eom JS. Reducing donor site morbidity when reconstructing the nipple using a composite nipple graft. Arch Plast Surg. 2012;39(4):384–9.
25. Rusby JE, Smith BL, Gui GP. Nipple-sparing mastectomy. Br J Surg. 2010;97(3):305–16.

# Nipple Reconstruction Using a Two-Step Purse Suture Technique

# 54

Krista Genoway and Nancy Van Laeken

## 54.1 Introduction

The nipple-areolar complex is often described as the defining feature of the female breast [1]. Traditionally reconstructed as a final stage in breast reconstruction, NAC reconstruction is often performed under local anesthesia on an outpatient basis [2]. Though a minor procedure, the appearance of the NAC has a significant impact on the overall symmetry, shape, and esthetics of the breast.

Since the first documented NAC reconstruction in 1949, many techniques have been described [3]. Techniques have utilized local flaps, autologous grafts, and non-autologous material in the search of attaining symmetry in nipple position, shape, size, pigmentation, and texture [2, 4–17]. An update by Farhadi et al. [2] identified that the majority of surgeons utilize various forms of local pedicled flap with or without the adjunct of skin grafting and tattooing. The described technique employs a two-step surgical procedure to independently create the nipple-areola complex. This chapter will highlight the indications, contraindications, surgical technique, and possible modifications.

K. Genoway, M.D. (✉)
Division of Plastic Surgery, Department of Surgery, University of British Columbia, Vancouver, BC, Canada
e-mail: kgenoway@gmail.com

N. Van Laeken, M.D. (✉)
Division of Plastic Surgery, Department of Surgery, University of British Columbia, Vancouver, BC, Canada

Department of Surgery, Providence Health Care, Vancouver, BC, Canada
e-mail: nvanlaeken@providencehealth.bc.ca

## 54.2 Surgical Indications

1. Stable breast and soft tissue envelope
2. Realistic patient expectations

## 54.3 Surgical Contraindications

1. Medically unfit patient with contraindications to regional or general anesthesia
2. Wound-healing complications
3. An oncologically unstable patient requiring additional surgical or radiation therapy
4. Poor soft tissue envelope in the setting of radiation

## 54.4 Surgical Technique

After discussion with the patient and evaluation of the breast the nipple position is chosen. This ideally is situated on the most projecting position of the breast and at the mid humeral level. Patients are marked preoperatively in the upright position. During the creation of the NAC, small adjustments to the breast mounds can occur to help improve symmetry.


M.A. Shiffman (ed.), *Nipple-Areolar Complex Reconstruction*,
https://doi.org/10.1007/978-3-319-60925-6_54

One of the key features to generating an aesthetic nipple is creating a distinction between the nipple-areolar complex and nipple. It is felt that there needs to be areola elevation as well as nipple elevation. One of the features of the two-step technique is the creation of a distinct NAC independent of the underlying breast and nipple. The technique has been designed to create this three-dimensional complex with a gradation in elevation between the areola and the nipple itself.

A full-thickness skin graft is used for the areola reconstruction. There are several options for skin graft harvest site. The chosen site is often dictated by the patient's prior surgical incisions. Utilizing the lateral aspect of the mastectomy scar can prove beneficial if a scar revision on breast mound shaping is required. In the setting of autologous reconstruction, the lateral aspect of the abdominal incision can be selected (Fig. 54.1).

A full thickness skin graft is harvested in the diameter in the desired areola. The size can be designed to match the patient's contralateral breast or template based on standard NAC breast templates. The donor site is then closed primarily, and the graft is defatted and stored in saline.

Attention is then directed to creating the areola on the breast mound. The outer incision of the areola is marked corresponding in size to the previously harvested full-thickness skin graft (Fig. 54.2). The disc for the areola is deepithelialized similar to the deepithelialization that one would do for an inferior pedicle breast reduction (Fig. 54.3). The central core of the elevated skin graft is left attached to a central disc. The diameter of this retained complex is chosen to match the diameter of the non-operated breast. If the nipple reconstruction is bilateral, a diameter ranging between 5 and 10 mm is created. The attached central core of the skin acts to provide blood flow to the elevated nipple complex.

The elevated areola skin can be trimmed in accordance with the size of nipple or degree of elevation desired. A purse-string suture around the remaining outer disc facilitates elevation (Fig. 54.4). A 4-0 Mersilene or similar suture is used. The degree of nipple elevation can be fine-tuned by securing and tightening the purse-string suture. The purse-string suture is left in place for 6 weeks.

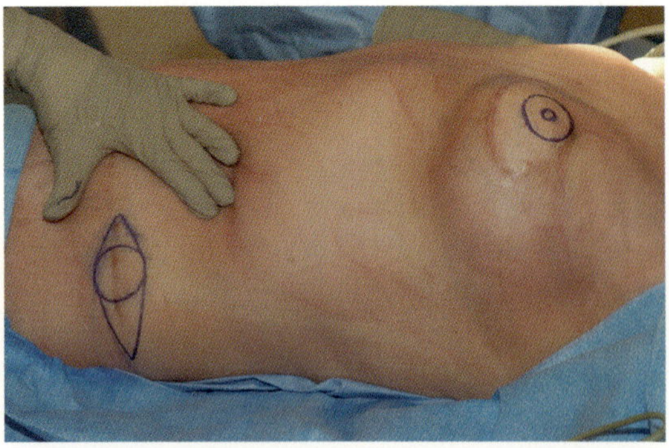

**Fig. 54.1** Of autologous reconstruction, the lateral aspect of the abdominal incision can be selected

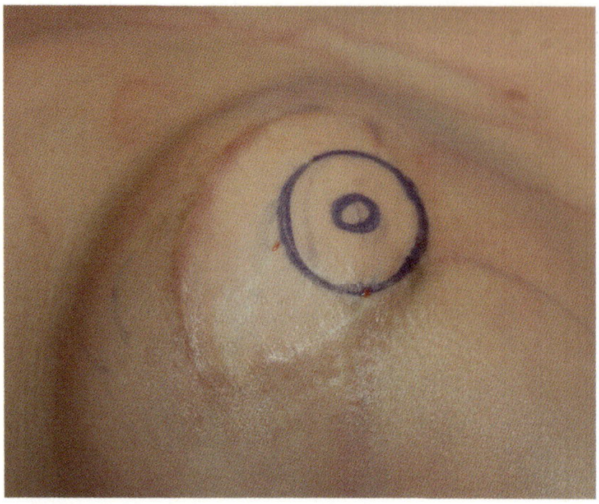

**Fig. 54.2** The outer incision of the areola is marked corresponding in size to the previously harvested full-thickness skin graft

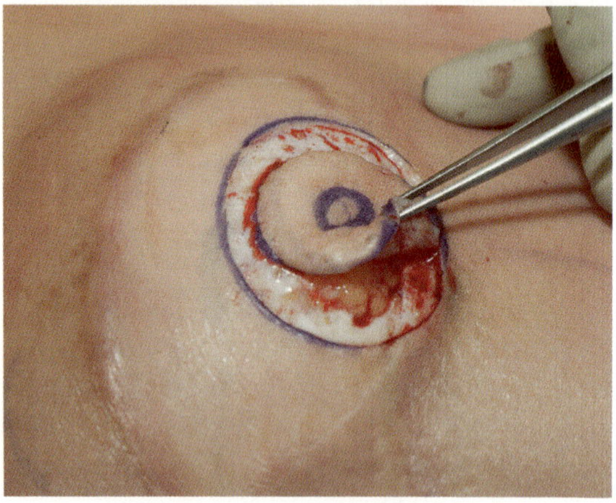

**Fig. 54.3** The disc for the areola is deepithelialized

The remaining deepithelialized areola undergoes grafting with the harvested full-thickness skin graft (Fig. 54.5). A central hole is made in the middle of the skin graft, and the newly created nipple is pulled through creating a three-dimensional nipple complex (Fig. 54.6). A tie-over dressing is secured over the graft to encourage graft take (Fig. 54.7). An opening is left in the tie-over dressing centrally, and the nipple is passed through. This maneuver helps to prevent flattening of the projected nipple. Tattooing is completed approximately 6 months after the nipple reconstruction (Fig. 54.8).

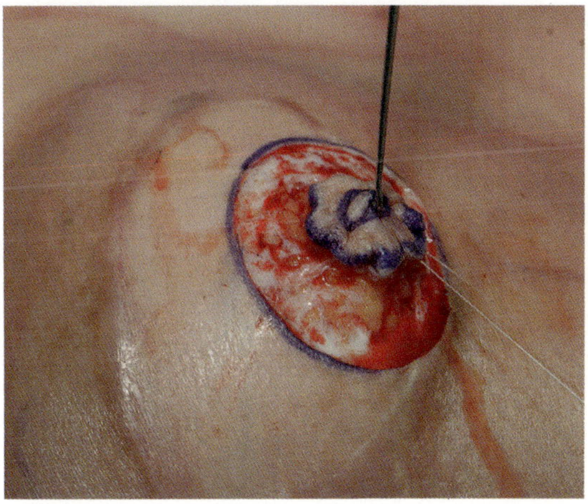

**Fig. 54.4** A purse-string suture around the remaining outer disc

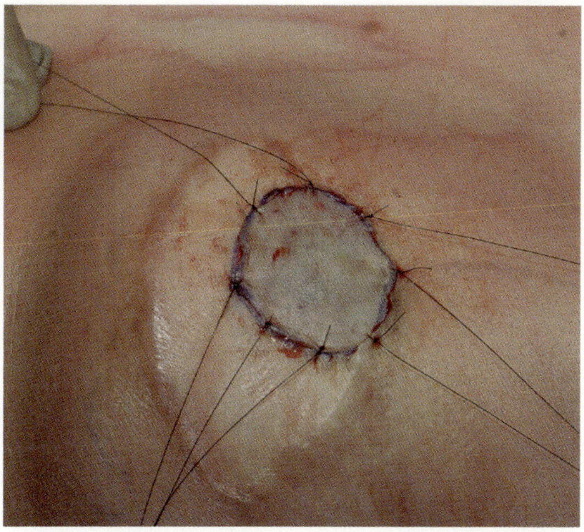

**Fig. 54.5** The deepithelialized area of the areola undergoes grafting with the harvested full-thickness skin graft

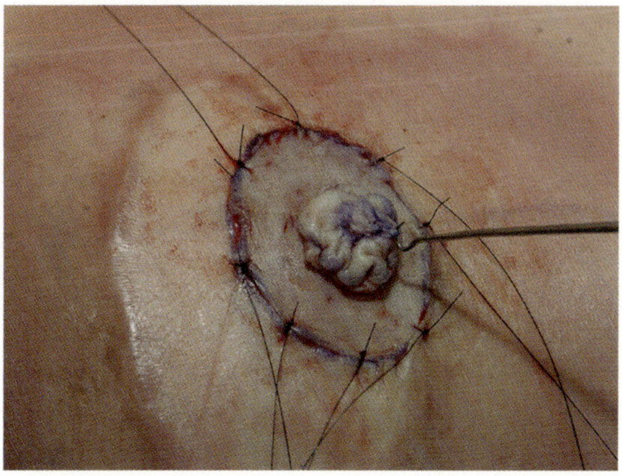

**Fig. 54.6** The newly created nipple is pulled through the middle of the skin graft

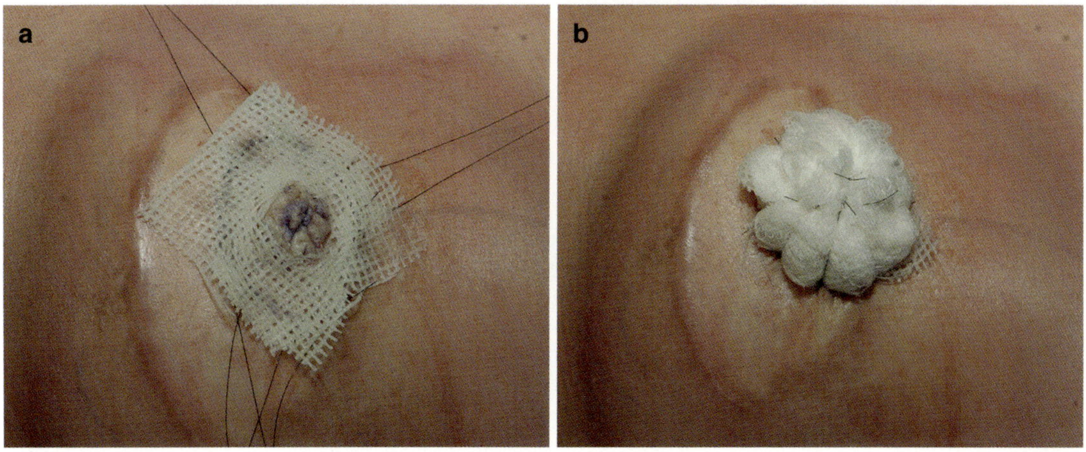

**Fig. 54.7** (**a**, **b**) A tie-over dressing is secured over the graft

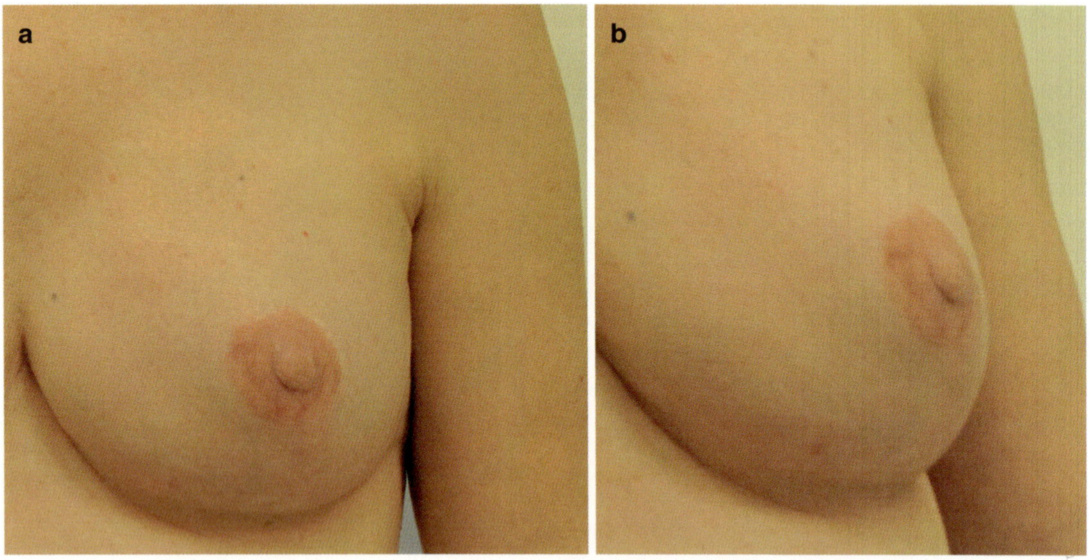


Fig. 54.8 (a, b) Tattooing is completed approximately 6 months after the nipple reconstruction

## 54.5 Key Technique Features

Creation of an aesthetic, well-placed nipple with lasting projection remains a challenge for the reconstructive surgeon [12]. Criticism and complications of nipple reconstructive techniques included NAC distortion secondary to contractile forces on local tissue during healing and NAC atrophy secondary to loss of adipose tissue and NAC tissue necrosis secondary to a poor vascular supply [12–14]. Together, these postoperative changes contribute to loss of nipple projection and poor aesthetic outcomes. Techniques of nipple "overbuilding" are often advocated to compensate for loss of nipple projection overtime. The literature has estimated loss of nipple projection to be between 25 and 50% [4, 12]. The described technique aims to avoid the pitfall of other techniques by not relying on rearrangement of local flaps prone to distortion and flattening over time. By creating the nipple-areola complex independent of one another, long-term projection is achieved. The degree of projection can be varied depending on the extent of dermis that is undermined prior to suture placement.

A crucial component in maintaining long-term projection is the lack of devascularization of the central core of the nipple. In other surgical techniques, a local flap is elevated and rotated with the vascular supply being distant for the central core. Here the vascular supply to the nipple remains unaltered as the central aspect has not been undermined or dissected. This healthy vascular supply minimizes the chance of tissue atrophy and necrosis which are major factors contributing to the loss of nipple projection [15, 16]. Similarly, creating the nipple-areola complex independent of one another further reduces local contraction forces on the nipple.

## 54.6 Technique Pitfalls

Graft take with this surgical technique is usually excellent; however, one must take extreme care when operating on thin and irradiated patients. In such cases, deepithelialization must be performed superficially to allow for the maintenance of a well-vascularized tissue bed. The site of graft harvest must also be carefully chosen in irradiated patients. Full-thickness graft harvest away from the radiation field is preferred.

In the setting of the under-projected nipple, delayed fat grafting under the nipple or the use of acellular dermal matrix provides promising results.

## Conclusions

The two-step purse suture nipple areola complex reconstructive technique provides aesthetic long-lasting results. It is straightforward to perform and reliable in producing a three-dimensional nipple complex projection. Over a 20-year period, the surgical results prove satisfactory to both surgeon and patient.

## References

1. Few JW, Marcus JR, Casas LA, Aitken ME, Redding J. Long-term predictable nipple projection following reconstruction. Plast Reconstr Surg. 1999;104:1321–4.
2. Farhadi J, Maksvytyte GK, Schaefer DJ, Pierrer G, Scheufler O. Reconstruction of the nipple-areola complex: an update. J Plast Reconstr Aesthet Surg. 2006;59:40–53.
3. Adams WM. Labial transplant for correction of loss of the nipple. Plast Reconstr Surg. 1949;4:295–8.
4. Guerra AB, Khoobehi K, Metzinger SE, Allen RJ. New technique for nipple areola reconstruction: arrow flap and rib cartilage graft for long-lasting nipple projection. Ann Plast Surg. 2003;50:31–7.
5. Weiss J, Herman O, Rosenberg L, Shafir R. The S nipple-areola reconstruction. Plast Reconstr Surg. 1989;83:904–6.
6. Cronin TD, Upton J, McDonough JM. Reconstruction of the breast after mastectomy. Plast Reconstr Surg. 1977;59:1–14.
7. Little JW III, Munasifi T, McCulloch DT. One-stage reconstruction of a projecting nipple: the quadrapod flap. Plast Reconstr Surg. 1983;71:126–33.
8. Hallock GG, Altobelli JA. Cylindrical nipple reconstruction using an H flap. Ann Plast Surg. 1993;30:23–6.
9. Thomas SV, Gellis MB, Pool R. Nipple reconstruction with a new local tissue flap. Plast Reconstr Surg. 1996;97:1053–6.
10. Cohen IK, Ward JA, Chandrasekhar B. The pinwheel flap nipple and barrier areola graft reconstruction. Plast Reconstr Surg. 1986;77:995–9.
11. Kroll SS, Hamilton S. Nipple reconstruction with the double-opposing-tab flap. Plast Reconstr Surg. 1989;84:520–5.
12. Turgut G, Sacak B, Gorgulu T, Yesilada AK, Bas L. Nipple reconstruction with bipedicled dermal flap: a new and easy technique. Aesthet Plast Surg. 2009;33:770–3.
13. Rubino C, Dessy LA, Posadinu A. A modified technique for nipple reconstruction: the 'arrow flap'. Br J Plast Surg. 2003;56:247–51.
14. Dolmans GH, Van de Kar AL, Van Rappard JH, Hoogbergen MM. Nipple reconstruction: the "Hammond" flap. Plast Reconstr Surg. 2008;121:353–4.
15. Weinfeld AB, Somia N, Codner MA. Purse-string nipple areolar reconstruction. Ann Plast Surg. 2008;61:364–7.
16. Tatlidede S, Yesilada AK, Egemen O, Bas L. A new technique in nipple reconstruction dome technique with double pedicle. Ann Plast Surg. 2008;60:141–3.
17. Van Laeken N, Genoway K. Nipple reconstruction using a two-step purse suture technique. Can J Plast Surg. 2011;19(2):56–9.

# Immediate Nipple Reconstruction Using the Everted Umbilicus

# 55

Christian A. El Amm

## 55.1 Introduction

Women considering unilateral immediate or delayed reconstruction may be candidates for abdominally sourced flaps (TRAM, free TRAM, and DIEP) with immediate nipple reconstruction using the everted umbilicus [1, 2]. The umbilical stalk and surrounding skin is included in the harvested flap. Periumbilical perforators provide blood supply to the ipsilateral half of the umbilical stalk, and the contralateral half is supplied by a preserved subdermal plexus. A neo-umbilicus is recreated on the abdominal wall in an esthetically pleasing location.

The single-stage reconstruction described below produces a naturally ptotic mound, a nipple with generous and long-term projection, and a patch of glabrous skin around the nipple that emulates the texture of the areola. This technique may be attractive to women who, for cultural or personal reasons, prefer to avoid scars on the contralateral breast required for symmetry procedures and in most cases avoid the use of silicone implants. Single-stage procedures, although technically challenging, may represent a more efficient use of resources compared to the typical multistage protracted process of expander-implant reconstruction with secondary nipple-areola reconstruction.

Long-term nipple projection is still unpredictable for most locally based flap techniques. The everted umbilicus is most promising on that basis, being a naturally created inverted funnel of skin, repurposed in a symmetrical everted configuration. The native nipple is of opposite shape to the umbilicus but essentially identical geometry.

Relative contraindication to the use of the everted navel includes a history of umbilical hernia repair or other umbilical surgery. These result in a high incidence of partial necrosis of the reconstructed nipple. Small umbilical incisions without undermining or dissection such as insertion of laparoscopy ports have not adversely affected the outcome of the reconstruction. Patients with a very large pannus, pannus lymphedema, and extensive striae represent a hazard for abdominal-based reconstructions in general, and similar warnings extend to the use of the everted umbilicus. Extensive striae are associated with disruption of the subdermal anastomotic plexus and present a particular challenge to deepithelialization techniques required for reconstruction after skin-sparing mastectomies.

Disadvantages of the technique include a more superiorly located transverse abdominal scar and a 2-week course of wound care for reconstruction of a neo-umbilicus.

C.A. El Amm, M.D.
Department of Plastic, Reconstructive Surgery, and Craniofacial Surgery, University of Oklahoma, 825 NE 10th St Suite 1G, Oklahoma City, OK 73104, USA
e-mail: Christian-elamm@ouhsc.edu


M.A. Shiffman (ed.), *Nipple-Areolar Complex Reconstruction*,
https://doi.org/10.1007/978-3-319-60925-6_55

Complications overall are relatively minor and include partial necrosis of the reconstructed nipple (14%) and unsatisfactory neo-umbilicus reconstruction (6%).

Operative planning and close communication with the ablative surgeon are critical for proper execution. The contralateral breast is used as a template, and it is assumed that no intervention to modify the shape of the contralateral breast is expected. Planning may be conceived in three steps:

1. Mapping the defect: Precise marking of the planned excisional defect, in coordination with the ablative surgeon where immediate reconstruction is planned. Mapping the skin defect on the vertical and transverse breast meridians, centering on the nipple.
2. Creation of a template of the resection on the contralateral breast. Transposition of the template to the abdominal flap centered on the umbilicus.
   (a) Asymmetrical breasts and delayed reconstruction
   (b) Symmetrical breasts
   (c) Skin-sparing mastectomy
   (d) Ptosis Grades 1–2
   (e) Ptosis Grade 3
3. Sizing and inset: This is accomplished intraoperatively.

## 55.2 Mapping the Defect

Vertical and transverse meridians are marked on both breasts, extending from mid-clavicle to mid-IMF including the nipple and from midline to lateral edge of breast (anterior axillary line) crossing the vertical meridian at the nipple. The cardinal points are thus defined as mid-sternum, mid-IMF, median projection of nipple, and lateral projection of nipple (Fig. 55.1).

For cases when immediate reconstruction is planned, the ablative surgeon marks the planned incision line and the resulting skin defect, including likely required margins. The intersection of the planned incision with the breast meridians is marked, and the distance of these points to the four cardinal points defined above is measured (Fig. 55.2).

When delayed reconstruction is performed, the intersection of the existing mastectomy scar

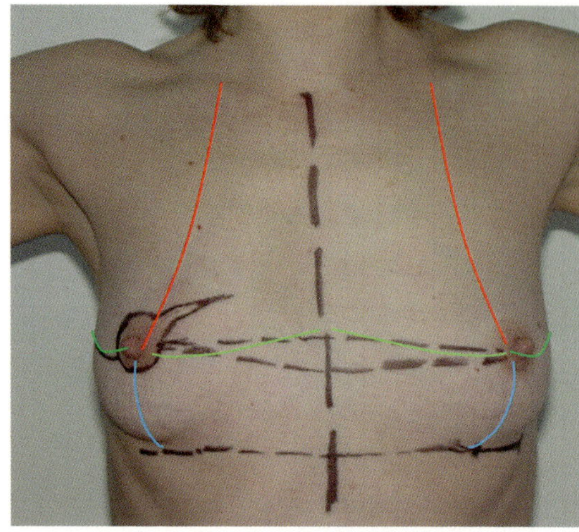

**Fig. 55.1** Identification and conceptualization of the vertical (*Red* and *Blue lines*) and horizontal meridians (*Green* and *Yellow lines*). The four cardinal points are mid-clavicle, lowest point of the inframammary fold (IMF), point on sternal midline level with the nipple, and lateral point on anterior axillary line level with the nipple

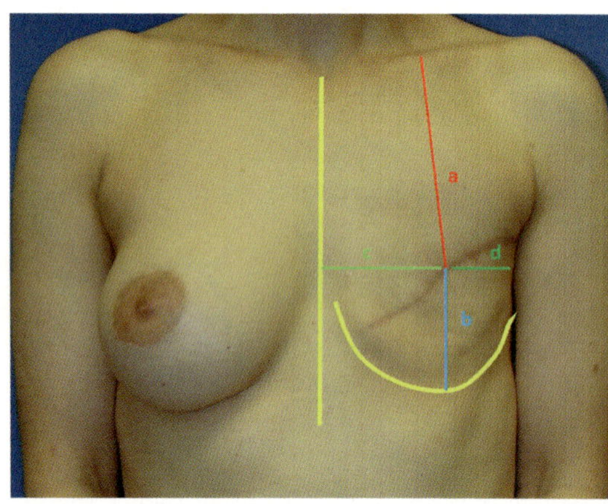


**Fig. 55.2** Operative planning for immediate reconstruction: The ablative surgeon marks the planned location of the skin excision. The meridians are marked on the patient as described in Fig. 55.1. The distance from the planned incision to the four cardinal points is measured. In this patient, the distance to the superior cardinal point is 13 cm, the distance to the medial cardinal point is 7 cm, etc. (*a*) Mid-clavicle to nipple. (*b*) Nipple to IMF. (*c*) Nipple to midline. (*d*) Nipple to anterior axillary line

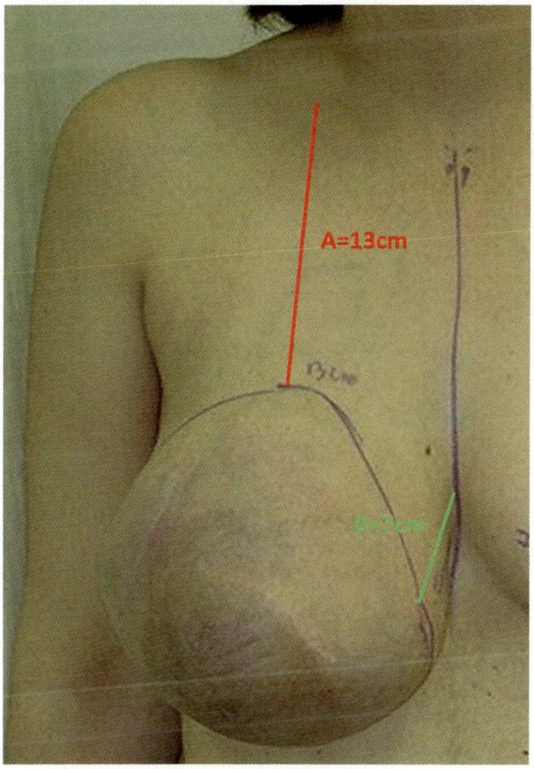


**Fig. 55.3** Operative Planning for delayed reconstruction: The vertical meridian is marked initially. The intersection of the vertical meridian with the existing scar is used as central point, and distances are measures to the four cardinal points: *red line*, or distance "*a*" is from the intersection to the mid clavicle; *blue line*, or distance "*b*" is from intersection to the lowest point of the desired inframammary fold; distance "*c*" to the medial cardinal point; and distance "*d*" to the lateral cardinal on the anterior axillary line (See Fig. 55.2)

to the vertical meridian is marked and distances to the cardinal points measured (Fig. 55.3).

## 55.3 Creation of a Template, Centering, and Transposition

### 55.3.1 Delayed Reconstruction and Asymmetrical Breasts

In delayed reconstruction, the intersection points of the mastectomy scar are transposed to the contralateral breast, and the medial and lateral endpoints of the existing scar mirrored on the contralateral side. A template of the original skin excision is recreated on the contralateral side (Fig. 55.4).

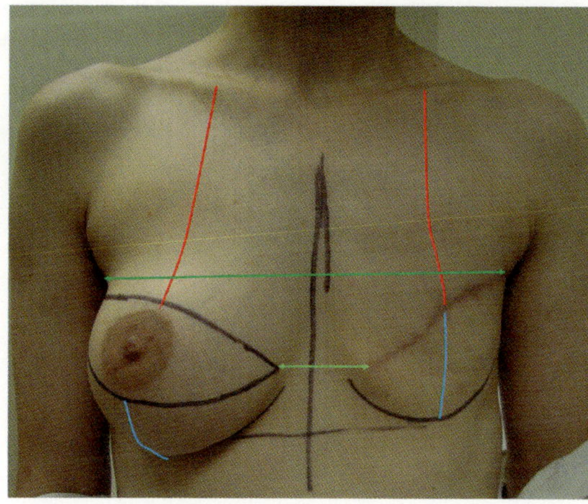

**Fig. 55.4** Operative planning for delayed reconstruction: Creation of a template. The contralateral "normal" breast is used as reference model. The meridians are traced on the contralateral breast. The medial and lateral ends of the existing mastectomy scar are transposed by symmetry on the normal side. Measurement "*a*" described in Fig. 55.3 is then used to mark a point along the superior vertical meridian, and similarly measurement "*b*" is used to mark a point along the inferior meridian. By joining the four points with a lenticular design, it is possible to recreate a template of the skin missing from the side to be reconstructed. This elliptical design is then transposed on the abdomen centered around the umbilicus where the nipple would be

When immediate reconstruction is performed in the setting of marked asymmetry in the mounds, a similar technique is used. The recreated template may be smaller or larger than the planned excision depending on the breast proportions (Fig. 55.5).

Next, the template sizing and centering is done by measuring the distance of the intersection points to the nipple on the contralateral breast. A template of cutout material is fabricated, with cardinal markings intersecting at the location of the nipple. The template is transposed face down to the abdomen, to produce a transposition of the contralateral template, and centered on the umbilicus. The orientation of the template depends on the planned rotation and inset of the abdominal flap, as discussed below. Generally, the shortest measurement is chosen to be placed above the umbilicus, in order to limit the superior extent of the flap harvest, and placement of the transverse abdominal scar (Fig. 55.6).

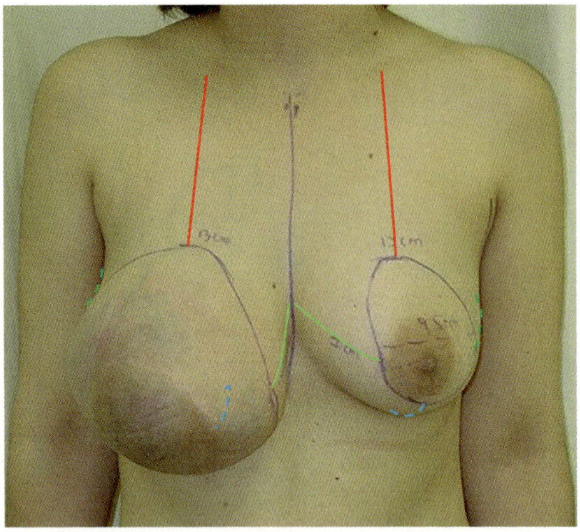

**Fig. 55.5** Operative Planning for immediate reconstruction: The cardinal distances to the planned resection line are transposed by symmetry to the contralateral "normal" breast. These points are joined, and the resulting template is usually ovoid. The resulting template is often different in size than the resection template due to normal asymmetry or tumor-induced asymmetry in breast size. In all cases, symmetry with the unoperated side is desirable, and that side, rather than the operated side, is used to create the template

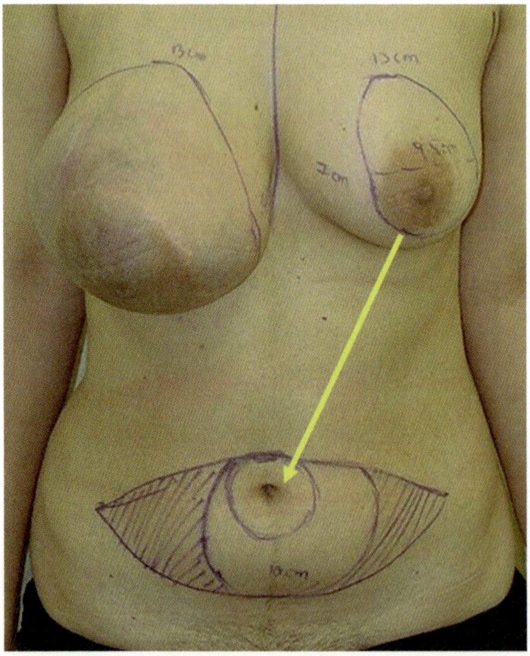

**Fig. 55.6** A mirror image of the template is transposed to the abdomen: This is often done by creating a cutout of the template, centered on the nipple, and placing it face down on the abdomen centered on the umbilicus. The reconstructive surgeon then decides on the rotation and inset on the abdominal flap (see text depending on ptosis, shape, etc.) and traces the outline of the skin paddle and subcutaneous tissues to be included in the flap design

### 55.3.2 Symmetrical Breasts in the Setting of Immediate Reconstruction

Most women will present with significant asymmetry, and the technique described above is chosen. In cases where breast are reasonably symmetrical preoperatively, the use of the contralateral breast as template is no longer needed. The planned resection is directly used as a template and transposed to the abdomen centered on the umbilicus. The distance to the cardinal points may be obtained to refine inset and shaping of the mound.

### 55.3.3 Skin-Sparing Mastectomy

In the setting of skin sparing mastectomy, a template for the skin excision is usually not required. However, a similar technique is employed to plan the distribution of the flap bulk around the everted umbilicus. The approximate size and distribution of the contralateral breast tissue is noted and transposed to the abdominal flap. The abdominal flap skin is deepithelialized centered on the umbilicus. The umbilicus and surrounding glabrous skin are preserved to be used as nipple-areola complex. Proper technique of deepithelialization is critical to preserve the subdermal plexus. Extensive striae make this difficult, and injury to the subdermal plexus may jeopardize the survival of the umbilical circumference.

### 55.3.4 Ptosis Grades 1–2

In such cases, the superior line of the mastectomy incision is usually at the superior edge of the areola. Subsequently, the periumbilical template usually sits in the same vertical orientation as the resection template. The bulk of the flap sits inferior to the nipple reconstruction, and either medial or lateral to the everted umbilicus depending on which pedicle is chosen. The abdominal flap rotation for a standard TRAM flap is zero for ipsilateral pedicles, or 90° in some cases. For DIEP/Free TRAM flaps, an ipsilateral inferior epigastric pedicle would require a microanastomosis to the long thoracic pedicle, and a contralateral pedicle may allow the use of the internal mammary pedicle depending on length. In all such cases, upper pole fullness is a challenge and is dependent on flap contouring and inset. The young patient with full upper poles should be informed that a subsequent revision, small implant, or fat transfer may be required secondarily.

### 55.3.5 Ptosis Grades 3

In such cases, the bulk of the breast tissue lies superior to the nipple, and inset of TRAM flaps is facilitated with a 180° rotation based on the contralateral superior epigastric pedicle. Likewise, inferior epigastric-based free flaps are rotated 180° and anastomosed to the internal mammary.

### 55.3.6 Sizing and Inset

Dissection of the abdominal flap proceeds in standard fashion. The umbilical stalk is detached from its fascial insertion on the linea alba, and care is made to preserve at least one periumbilical perforator on the side of the chosen pedicle. A safe amount of subcutaneous fat is preserved on the non-pedicle side of the umbilical stalk to ensure integrity of the subdermal plexus. The umbilicus is everted inside out and spontaneously assumes a nipple-like shape and projection. The superior third of the umbilical funnel usually flat tens out to form a surrounding disk of glabrous reflective skin, similar in texture to the areola. The projection of the everted umbilicus is 1–1.5 cm in 85% of cases and compares favorably to the projection of the native nipple. In rare instances of a highly projecting contralateral nipple, cartilage is harvested from the inferior ribs, or dermal allograft has been successfully used for auto-augmentation. The everted umbilicus leaves a hollowed-out cylinder in the subcutaneous tissues where the umbilical stalk used to lie. This space is approximated at multiple levels (dermal, fascia and deep fascia) with absorbable sutures to prevent spontaneous retraction of the everted umbilicus. In cases of auto-augmentation, transcutaneous loose horizontal mattress sutures are placed (Fig. 55.7).

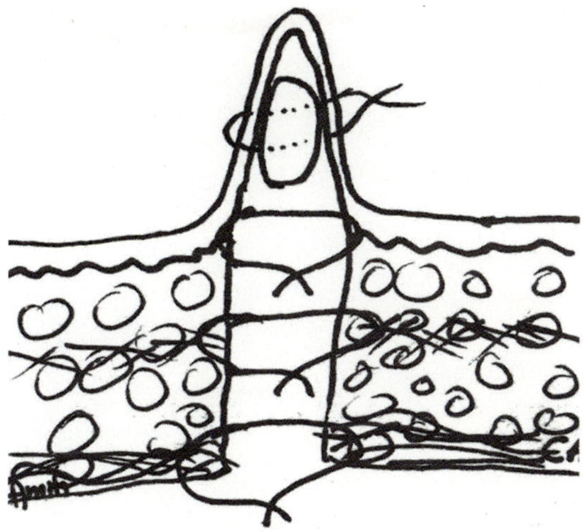

**Fig. 55.7** Everted umbilical funnel made into an extruded cone. Autograft or allograft can be used for augmentation in case a very large nipple is desired. It is however unnecessary in the vast majority of cases. The "dead space" left by the everted umbilicus is closed by several layers of resorbable suture in the deep dermis and subcutaneous fascias

The mastectomy specimen dimensions are obtained on the back table (radius along all four cardinal-meridians and thickness). These measurements, rather than weight of the specimen, are used to reconstruct a matching flap of abdominal tissues. Intraoperative ICG (indocyanine green) angiography is now used to assess viability of the flap. A template of the breast mound dimensions is marked on the viable portions of the abdominal flap, centered on the reconstructed nipple, using the measurements described above. Marginal deepithelialization around the skin paddle is done to the edges of the flap. In delayed reconstruction, the contralateral mound is used as template, with the patient lying supine, and the nipple areola manually centered on the mound if necessary. Measurements of the mound diameters are obtained in similar fashion and transposed to the abdominal flap centered on the umbilicus. The abdominal flap is contoured and suspended to emulate the contralateral mound. Typically, for patients with Grade 1–2 ptosis, the flap provides sufficient bulk to three quadrants, and the superior quadrant is reconstructed by folding the flap edges or sliding of the deeper planes (Fig. 55.8).

For patients with Grade 3 ptosis of the contralateral breast, the inferior quadrant is proportionately the smallest and is reconstructed by sliding/folding of the lateral edges (Fig. 55.9).

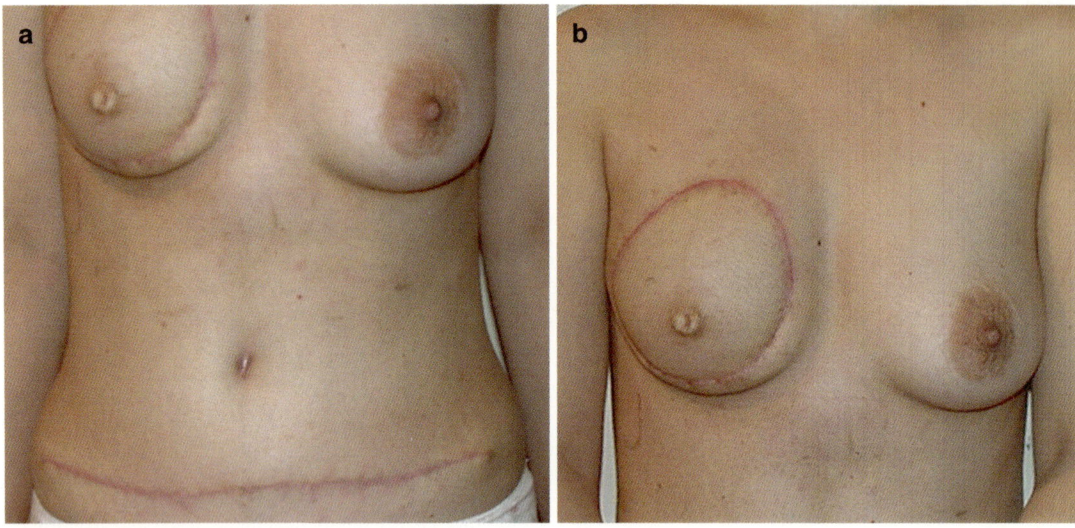


**Fig. 55.8** (**a**, **b**) Early results of immediate reconstruction in patient with Grade 1 ptosis. Note the natural-looking reconstructed umbilical depression, the higher location of the transverse abdominal donor scar, the satisfactory size and projection match for nipple size and location, and the glabrous smooth texture the skin immediately surrounding the everted umbilicus, comparing favorably with the areolar texture. Micropigmentation would improve the areola reconstruction

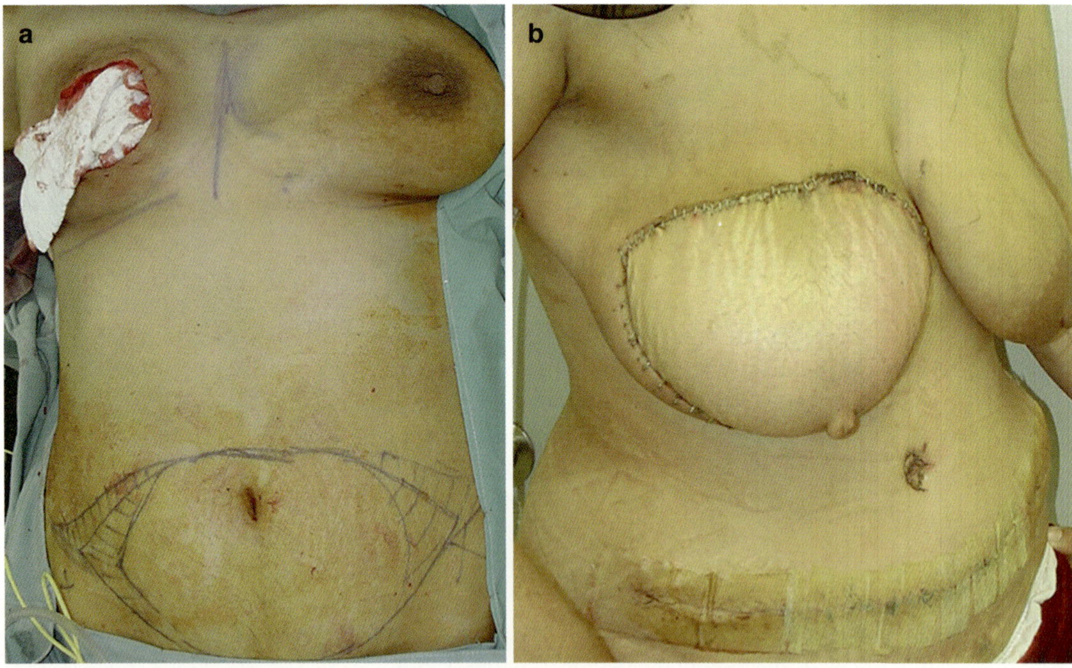


**Fig. 55.9** (**a**) Early result of immediate reconstruction in a patient with Grade 3 ptosis and heavy body habitus. Note size and centering of the abdominal template. (**b**) Postoperative with good size match of the breast mounds and good size and position match of the reconstructed nipple using the everted umbilicus

## References


1. El Amm CA, Sung JS, Sawan KT, Atiyeh BS, Workman MC. Immediate nipple reconstruction using the everted umbilicus. Plast Reconstr Surg. 2011;128(2):91e–2e.
2. De Cholnoky T. Breast reconstruction after radical mastectomy: formation of missing nipple by everted navel. Plast Reconstr Surg. 1966;38(6):577–80.

# 56 Reconstruction of the Nipple-Areolar Complex: An Algorithm for Decision-Making

Asmat H. Din and Jian Farhadi

## 56.1 Introduction

Reconstruction of the nipple-areolar complex (NAC) is most commonly undertaken as the final stage of breast reconstruction following mastectomy. This is due to the importance of adequate NAC positioning on an appropriately and symmetrically reconstructed breast mound.

For many patients this represents the completion point of their breast cancer treatment and as such has an attached substantial significance. The psychological implications of NAC reconstruction have been shown to be important and contribute to the patients' overall satisfaction with breast reconstruction, as well as more specifically their satisfaction with their nude appearance and sexual relations [1]. More rarely reconstruction may be required for congenital abnormalities, post burn injury or trauma, or following complications of breast surgery such as reduction mammoplasty.

The rates of breast cancer, and prophylactic mastectomies for those genetically at risk, are increasing [2]. This, as well as increased patient awareness of reconstructive options, has resulted in an increase in both breast and NAC reconstructions [3, 4]. Since the first account of nipple reconstruction in 1946 by Berson [5], there have been numerous techniques described as well as constant refinements to established procedures.

At this time the reconstructive surgeon has many different procedures available to them to reconstruct the NAC. This chapter aims to help the surgeon decide which type of technique may be most suitable in a particular situation, as well as addressing some technical considerations to optimise outcomes.

## 56.2 The Ideal Nipple-Areolar Complex Reconstruction

The goals for NAC reconstruction concentrate on achieving symmetry of the following characteristics:

1. Position
2. Size
3. Projection
4. Pigmentation
5. Shape
6. Texture

A.H. Din, M.A., M.B.B.S., M.R.C.S.
Department of Plastic Surgery, St Thomas' Hospital, Westminster Bridge Road, London SE1 7EH, UK
e-mail: asmatdin@hotmail.com

J. Farhadi, M.D. (✉)
Department of Plastic, Reconstructive and Aesthetic Surgery, University Hospital, Basel, Spitalstrasse 21, 4031 Basel, Switzerland

Department of Plastic and Reconstructive Surgery, St Thomas' Hospital, Westminster Bridge Road, London SE1 7EH, UK
e-mail: jian.farhadi@gstt.nhs.uk; jian@farhadi.com; office@farhadi.com


M.A. Shiffman (ed.), *Nipple-Areolar Complex Reconstruction*, https://doi.org/10.1007/978-3-319-60925-6_56

7. Sensate
8. Erectile
9. Lactiferous

The majority of advances in NAC reconstruction have led to the production of three-dimensional structures that aim to achieve the first six properties listed. The nipple is however a specialised structure comprised of smooth muscle and glandular ductal tissue, and as yet its variable consistency in the relaxed or erect condition and its specific sensation have not been attained [6].

## 56.3 Nipple Reconstruction

### 56.3.1 Nipple Sharing

In the case of unilateral nipple reconstruction, the contralateral nipple (with or without a part of the areola) can be partially harvested and used. Advocates of this technique point to a "like for like" match in terms of size, shape, projection, colour and texture [7]. The most common reasons for dissatisfaction following NAC reconstruction with a local flap are loss of projection and fading of tattoo [8]. These are avoided by use of sharing techniques. The major concern for both patients and surgeons is the potential to interfere with a healthy nipple. This risk of scarring, pain, loss of sensitivity, inability to breast feed as well as the potential loss of function of an erogenous structure have served to decrease the popularity of this method. Moreover, some patients will very reasonably refuse surgery on their 'healthy' breast. A number of studies point to a relatively low donor morbidity [7, 9, 10]; however, the risk of total desensitisation of the donor nipple was reported to be as high as 21% by Spear [7]. This represents a not insignificant risk. Interestingly 42% of nipple shares in one study showed erectile function at 6 months [11].

There are certain situations in which the nipple share technique may supersede others. Local flaps can struggle to achieve symmetry in cases of large well-projected contralateral nipples. In implant-based reconstructions with thin mastectomy skin flaps, local flaps may be contraindicated, especially if these tissues have been subjected to irradiation. Graft take in nipple sharing has not been shown to be significantly decreased in irradiated tissue [7, 11].

#### 56.3.1.1 Nipple Saving/Banking

First introduced in 1971 by Millard [12], this technique removed the entire NAC as a full thickness graft and transferred it to a distant site. Following reconstruction this 'banked' tissue was re-harvested and used as a composite graft to reconstruct the NAC. This procedure was largely abandoned when studied revealed the significant frequency of involvement of the NAC in breast cancer [13], followed by reports of cancerous cells spreading to inguinal lymph nodes when the tissue was banked in the groin [14, 15]. A modification of this technique saw the NAC examined by a pathologist before banking, but this suffered from poor outcomes [16]. NAC cryopreservation has also been utilised; however, results have been inconsistent [17].

### 56.3.2 Local Flaps

A great variety of local flaps have been described for nipple reconstruction. Specific techniques and modifications are discussed elsewhere in this book. Broadly local flaps can be separated into those that are centrally based and those based on single or multiple subdermal pedicles.

Local flaps allow for a relatively simple clinic-based reconstruction of the nipple. Their great benefit when used alone is the lack of a distant donor site, as well as a relatively low rate of complications. This results in a high degree of patient satisfaction.

The greatest limitation suffered by these reconstructions is a lack of long-lasting projection [8]. Loss of projection ranges from 40 to 75% in the reported literature [18]. Good comparative studies do not exist comparing relative loss of projection of different local flap types. Loss of projection is essentially influenced by two main factors: retraction forces of surrounding tissues and tissue contraction of the flap [6]. Retraction forces relate to the contractile elements of the surrounding tissue and the tension they have been put under. This is more true for centrally based flaps than those on a subdermal pedicle which have been freed from the underlying tissue and which usually have been sutured under minimal tension. All local flaps are subject to tissue contraction. This is related to a lack of three-dimensional tension, absence of normal structural support and the tendency of scars to contract. Flaps with more complicated designs may be subject to a greater degree of scar contracture. As such flaps have evolved to have simpler designs, to maximise blood flow through broad bases and to decrease retractional forces by largely being designed on the subdermal vascular plexus.

Local flaps for nipple reconstruction are based on a random vascular pattern, and as such their vascularity can be compromised by a number a factors. Poor design can relate to narrow pedicle bases, as well as to choice of axis of flap in relation to local scarring. If possible flaps should be designed so as to not include local scars as well as to ensure the base of flap is not immediately adjacent to scar. However, should ideal placement of the nipple mean that a scar crosses a limb of the flap then the flap can be designed including the scar, as in the vast majority of cases a subdermal plexus will have formed under the line of scarring. When performing a local flap reconstruction on an implant-based breast reconstruction, it can be necessary to place the nipple almost centrally over the mastectomy scar. In these cases double subdermal pedicle flaps are preferred whereby a flap is raised from either side of the mastectomy scar. This allows for a greater volume of tissue, ideal placement and decreased risk of insufficient vascularity as the mastectomy scar does not cross the base of the flap.

In general, local flaps are well tolerated for nipple reconstruction. A literature review of all described techniques by Sisti in 2016 [18] showed an overall complication rate of 7.9%, with a rate of total necrosis at 0.7% over 1498 reconstructions. Although they are suitable for most patients, particular care must be taken if they are to be made on thin mastectomy skin flaps with underlying implants that have been irradiated. In this setting the rate of complications dramatically increases, with significant risk of the underlying implant becoming exposed [19–22].

### 56.3.3 Nipple Augmentation

In an effort to address the relative lack of long-term projection, a number of autologous, allogenic and synthetic implant techniques have been described (Table 56.1).

The greatest quantity of evidence is available for autologous materials. Although they have a role in maintenance of nipple projection, the addition of donor sites can be problematic. Synthetic materials are the best at maintaining projection, but this comes at the cost of the highest rate of complications. These include extrusion and migration but also a higher tendency to total local flap or graft necrosis [18, 23]. The use of acellular dermal matrices (ADMs) may represent a compromise between the two previously described techniques. They solve the issue of donor-site morbidity whilst having a relatively low complication profile. Overall they are prone to loss of projection (around 45% [23]), but this can be easily accounted for in their design. They are likely to be of greatest use in breasts that have been reconstructed with implants that may not be suitable for local flaps or where local flaps would likely achieve poor projection. In these cases a small portion of the ADM used around the implant can be 'banked' at a distal site and grafted to the breast at a later time. Although

**Table 56.1** Different materials used in nipple augmentation [23]

| Autologous | Allogenic | Synthetic |
|---|---|---|
| Auricular cartilage | Acellular dermal matrix | Polyurethane |
| Costal cartilage | Lyophilized costal cartilage | Silicone |
| Labia minora | Extracellular matrix collagen | Teflon |
| Hallux toe pulp | | Artificial bone |
| Fat graft | | Calcium hydroxyapatite gel |
| Dermal graft | | |

there is some evidence for the use of AlloDerm (Lifecell Corp., Branchburg, N.J.), there is a relative paucity of publications using newer or thicker ADMs.

### 56.3.4 Areolar Reconstruction

#### 56.3.4.1 Grafting

Formerly a mainstay of areola reconstruction, often in combination with local flaps, full- or split-thickness grafts have been taken from a multitude of sites in attempts to achieve an appropriately pigmented and textured NAC. Despite numerous modifications in both donor site and technique, attempts to maintain areolar size and pigmentation remain unpredictable. Split-thickness skin grafts are prone to contracture, and so achieving symmetry in unilateral reconstruction can be difficult. If used in conjunction with a local flap, the contracture at the base of the flap may cause excessive loss of projection. Both hyper- and hypopigmentation of these grafts have been described, and certainly in unilateral cases, tattooing may be needed on top of the graft to achieve pigmentation matching. With the advances in tattooing, we do not advocate areolar grafting.

#### 56.3.4.2 Tattoo

Intradermal tattooing was first introduced in NAC reconstruction by Bunchman in 1974 [24]. These early tattoos suffered from an unnatural 'painted on' appearance. Since then there have been significant advances in the equipment and application of tattoos, resulting in the ability to create natural-looking, well-matched areolas that can create the optical allusion of a textured surface (thus mimicking Montgomery tubercles) [6, 25].

Tattoos can be used on their own to reconstruct the areola, or they can be used as an adjunct to other techniques to allow for best match of colour or to correct for discrepancies of size or position. When used independently they can be applied before or after nipple reconstruction. Advocates of tattooing prior to nipple reconstruction point to the difficulty in achieving uniform colour match when tattooing a projected local flap nipple reconstruction [26, 27]. However, raising a local flap on a circular base will distort the shape of the areola, and as such if this technique is to be employed, it requires careful and precise planning of the shape of the tattoo so as to decrease the chance of a loss of areolar symmetry. Tattooing post nipple reconstruction often takes more than visit to achieve an appropriate colour. It is our practice to wait 12 weeks post local flap nipple reconstruction before commencing tattooing, as like Spear [28] we believe it is best for the local flap to stabilise and contract to ensure accuracy of areolar markings. Tattooing has been reported to be performed at the time of local flap nipple reconstruction [29, 30]. This is advantageous to the patient as it decreases the number of visits they require; however, we are concerned that the additional dermal trauma of the tattooing may adversely affect the vascularity of our local flaps.

Tattooing is safe and inexpensive, with few risks of complications and high patient satisfaction [8, 28]. Tattoos are limited by their tendency to fade over time. This can be reasonably modelled, and as such a degree of overcompensation can be made at the time of the original tattoo to allow for fade [27, 31]. Achieving the best results from tattooing requires training and experience. In many centres it is performed by a specialist nurse, allowing a single practitioner to gain sufficient experience so as to improve their results. This also decreases the overall cost of the procedure and frees up a clinician's time [32].

Three-dimensional (3D) tattoo-only reconstruction of the NAC has recently been introduced [33]. This technique utilises the concepts of light and shadow to create an almost photo realistic nipple complete with Montgomery tubercles. Although the authors state that this can be achieved with conventional medical tattooing equipment, they suggest that the best results may be available through the use of professional tattoo artists. This offers an interesting alternative for difficult cases where irradiation and thin mastectomy skin flaps overlying an implant make other reconstructive options risky.

## 56.4 Patient Factors Affecting Choice of Reconstruction

The decision over which type of reconstruction to undertake must be tailored to the patient. It is no doubt easier to create symmetrical nipples in the case of bilateral reconstruction than it is to match an existing nipple, especially if it is large.

With autologous reconstruction of the breast mound, there is usually ample tissue of sufficient vascularity and quality such that a nipple may be best reconstructed with a local flap. Considerations have to be made with regard to the relative thickness of dermal tissue in different autologous reconstructions when planning local flaps. LD and SGAP flaps have a greater thickness of dermis than DIEP flaps. As the subdermal plexus must be included in the flap raise, this can lead to bulkier nipple reconstructions. Conversely the relative thin dermis of the TMG flap warrants the flap design to be larger for optimum maintenance of projection. Clinically this becomes problematic in the small breast reconstruction with a TMG flap. In these cases the use of a large local flap can lead to flattening of the breast mound around the NAC with an unacceptable loss of projection of the breast itself. In these often slim patients, fat grafting of the breast may not be an option to correct this.

Following irradiation local flaps still work well for autologous reconstructions. Only in cases where there has been severe skin damage related to radiotherapy would we consider alternate methods of reconstruction, and in these cases the safest would be 3D nipple-areolar tattooing.

Reconstruction of the breast mound with either an implant alone or with an expander and then an implant alters the characteristics of the overlying skin. In these cases the skin and subcutaneous layer over the implant may be overly thin for a local flap reconstruction. This can be compounded by radiotherapy, and studies have clearly shown an unacceptable rate of implant loss in this cohort [19, 21, 22]. We would consider local flap reconstruction to contra-indicted due to the risk of implant extrusion if there is any delayed healing or infection of the nipple reconstruction. If the implant is covered by an ADM, then an argument has been put forward that the chance of implant loss secondary to local flap reconstruction may be lower. However, as this has not been well demonstrated in the literature, we would still consider this approach to be of a higher risk.

Other patient factors including smoking, diabetes, age, body mass index (BMI) and implant volume have not been shown to be correlated to outcomes [21].

## 56.5 Other Considerations

NAC reconstruction has been undertaken at the time of breast reconstruction. The effects of postoperative radiotherapy, chemotherapy and general tissue healing do affect the shape and position of the breast mound reconstruction. As such it is our opinion that NAC reconstruction should be undertaken no sooner than 3 months following surgery, or completion of any adjuvant therapy, to allow the breast mound settle and permit optimal placement of the new NAC so as to achieve symmetry. Although it is unlikely in bilateral prophylactic mastectomy and breast reconstruction to require adjuvant therapy, there often remains a need to perform small symmetrising adjustments to the breast mound. In these cases we would also recommend NAC reconstruction as a final separate procedure.

In bilateral breast reconstruction, there is no template for the new NAC. One study of 600 breasts suggests that the average nipple projection is 0.9 cm, nipple diameter is 1.3 cm and areola diameter is 4 cm [34]. However, this study was in a Japanese population, and it highlights the problems with applying set measurements to a potentially heterogeneous population base. Rather than relying on idealised NAC measurements, reconstruction in bilateral cases must aim for symmetry and an aesthetically appropriate proportion to the underlying breast mound.

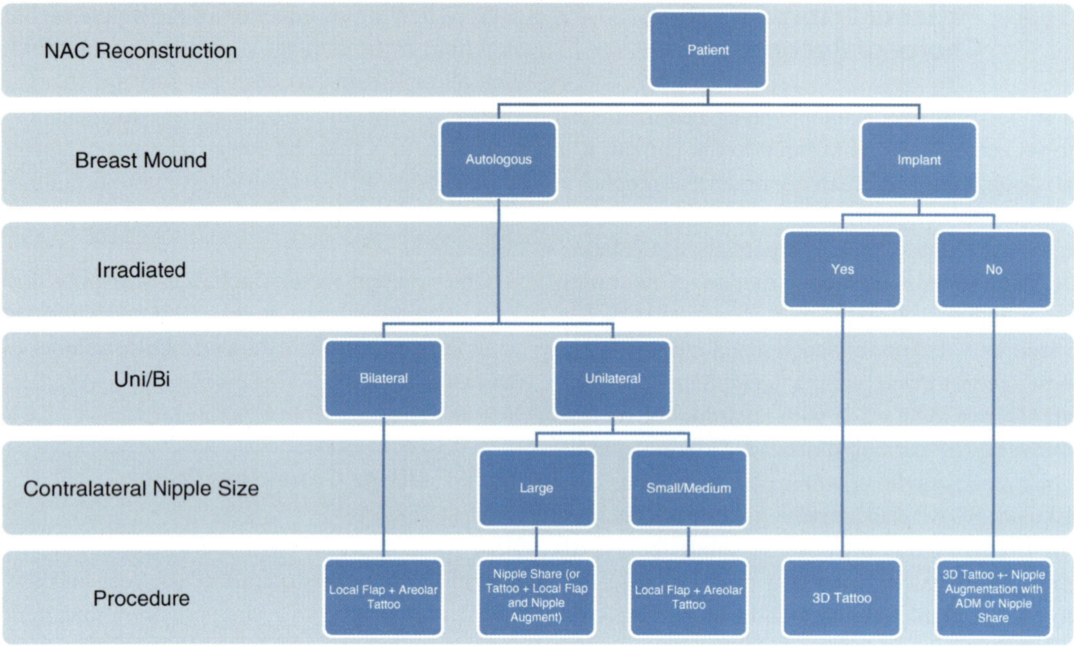


**Fig. 56.1** NAC reconstruction algorithm

## 56.6 Authors Preferred Technique

We have presented an algorithm relating the NAC reconstruction to help guide clinicians (Fig. 56.1). In the majority of autologous breast mound reconstructions, local flaps with tattooing of the areola can achieve excellent outcomes. Flap design must account for likely contraction and partial loss of projection. We use a modified arrow flap, where the cap component is raised intradermally to allow for a dermal base to be left on the breast mound for the whole reconstruction to sit on. This more stable support theoretically may reduce some of the potential projection loss. In implant-based reconstructions, we favour 3D NAC tattooing. This provides excellent aesthetic results whilst maintaining an absolute minimum of risk with regard to the breast reconstruction. As it is our practice to use ADMs in implant-based reconstructions, we have been offering patients who want some nipple projection banking of a roll of ADM in the groin for later grafting onto the breast and subsequent areola tattooing.

## References

1. Wellisch DK, Schain WS, Noone RB, Little JW III. The psychological contribution of nipple addition in breast reconstruction. Plast Reconstr Surg. 1987;80(5):699–704.
2. DeSantis C, Ma J, Bryan L, Jemal A. Breast cancer statistics, 2013. CA Cancer J Clin. 2014;64(1):52–62.
3. Albornoz CR, Bach PB, Mehrara BJ, Disa JJ, Pusic AL, McCarthy CM, Cordeiro PG, Matros E. A paradigm shift in U.S. Breast reconstruction: increasing implant rates. Plast Reconstr Surg. 2013;131(1):15–23.
4. Xie Y, Tang Y, Wehby GL. Federal health coverage mandates and health care utilization: the case of the Women's Health and Cancer Rights Act and use of breast reconstruction surgery. J Womens Health (Larchmt). 2015;24(8):655–62.
5. Berson MI. Construction of pseudoareola. Surgery. 1946;20(6):808.
6. Farhadi J, Maksvytyte GK, Schaefer DJ, Pierer G, Scheufler O. Reconstruction of the nipple-areola complex: an update. J Plast Reconstr Aesthet Surg. 2006;59(1):40–53.
7. Spear SL, Schaffner AD, Jespersen MR, Goldstein JA. Donor-site morbidity and patient satisfaction using a composite nipple graft for unilateral nipple reconstruction in the radiated and nonradiated breast. Plast Reconstr Surg. 2011;127(4):1437–46.

8. Goh SC, Martin NA, Pandya AN, Cutress RI. Patient satisfaction following nipple-areolar complex reconstruction and tattooing. J Plast Reconstr Aesthet Surg. 2011;64(3):360–3.
9. Haslik W, Nedomansky J, Hacker S, Nickl S, Schroegendorfer KF. Objective and subjective evaluation of donor-site morbidity after nipple sharing for nipple areola reconstruction. J Plast Reconstr Aesthet Surg. 2015;68(2):168–74.
10. Lee TJ, Noh HJ, Kim EK, Eom JS. Reducing donor site morbidity when reconstructing the nipple using a composite nipple graft. Arch Plast Surg. 2012;39(4):384–9.
11. Zenn MR, Garofalo JA. Unilateral nipple reconstruction with nipple sharing: time for a second look. Plast Reconstr Surg. 2009;123(6):1648–53.
12. Millard DR Jr, Devine J Jr, Warren WD. Breast reconstruction: a plea for saving the uninvolved nipple. Am J Surg. 1971;122(6):763–4.
13. Quinn RH, Barlow JF. Involvement of the nipple and areola by carcinoma of the breast. Arch Surg. 1981;116(9):1139–40.
14. Allison AB, Howorth MG Jr. Carcinoma in a nipple preserved by heterotopic auto-implantation. N Engl J Med. 1978;298(20):1132.
15. Rose JH Jr. Carcinoma in a transplanted nipple. Arch Surg. 1980;115(9):1131–2.
16. Lemperle G, Spitalny H. Reconstruction of the nipple and areola after radical mastectomy. Acta Chir Belg. 1980;79(2):155–7.
17. Nakagawa T, Yano K, Hosokawa K. Cryopreserved autologous nipple-areola complex transfer to the reconstructed breast. Plast Reconstr Surg. 2003;111(1):141–7.
18. Sisti A, Grimaldi L, Tassinari J, Cuomo R, Fortezza L, Bocchiotti MA, Roviello F, D'Aniello C, Nisi G. Nipple-areola complex reconstruction techniques: a literature review. Eur J Surg Oncol. 2016;42(4):441–65.
19. Momeni A, Ghaly M, Gupta D, Karanas YL, Kahn DM, Gurtner GC, Lee GK. Nipple reconstruction: risk factors and complications after 189 procedures. Eur J Plast Surg. 2013;36(10):633–8.
20. Momeni A, Ghaly M, Gupta D, Gurtner G, Kahn DM, Karanas YL, Lee GK. Nipple reconstruction after implant-based breast reconstruction: a "matched-pair" outcome analysis focusing on the effects of radiotherapy. J Plast Reconstr Aesthet Surg. 2013;66(9):1202–5.
21. Satteson ES, Reynolds MF, Bond AM, Pestana IA. An analysis of complication risk factors in 641 nipple reconstructions. Breast J. 2016;22(4):379–83.
22. Draper LB, Bui DT, Chiu ES, Mehrara BJ, Pusic AL, Cordeiro PG, Disa JJ. Nipple-areola reconstruction following chest-wall irradiation for breast cancer: is it safe? Ann Plast Surg. 2005;55(1):12–5.
23. Winocour S, Saksena A, Oh C, Wu PS, Laungani A, Baltzer H, Saint-Cyr M. A systematic review of comparison of autologous, allogeneic, and synthetic augmentation grafts in nipple reconstruction. Plast Reconstr Surg. 2016;137(1):14e–23e.
24. Bunchman HH 2nd, Larson DL, Huang TT, Lewis SR. Nipple and areola reconstruction in the burned breast. The "double bubble" technique. Plast Reconstr Surg. 1974;54(5):531–6.
25. Masser MR, Di Meo L, Hobby JA. Tattooing in reconstruction of the nipple and areola: a new method. Plast Reconstr Surg. 1989;84(4):677–81.
26. White CP, Gdalevitch P, Strazar R, Murrill W, Guay NA. Surgical tips: areolar tattoo prior to nipple reconstruction. J Plast Reconstr Aesthet Surg. 2011;64(12):1724–6.
27. Wong RK, Banducci DR, Feldman S, Kahler SH, Manders EK. Pre-reconstruction tattooing eliminates the need for skin grafting in nipple areolar reconstruction. Plast Reconstr Surg. 1993;92(3):547–9.
28. Spear SL, Arias J. Long-term experience with nipple-areola tattooing. Ann Plast Surg. 1995;35(3):232–6.
29. Eskenazi L. A one-stage nipple reconstruction with the "modified star" flap and immediate tattoo: a review of 100 cases. Plast Reconstr Surg. 1993;92(4):671–80.
30. Vandeweyer E. Simultaneous nipple and areola reconstruction: a review of 50 cases. Acta Chir Belg. 2003;103(6):593–5.
31. Levites HA, Fourman MS, Phillips BT, Fromm IM, Khan SU, Dagum AB, Bui DT. Modeling fade patterns of nipple areola complex tattoos following breast reconstruction. Ann Plast Surg. 2014;73(Suppl 2):S153–6.
32. Potter S, Barker J, Willoughby L, Perrott E, Cawthorn SJ, Sahu AK. Patient satisfaction and time-saving implications of a nurse-led nipple and areola reconstitution service following breast reconstruction. Breast. 2007;16(3):293–6.
33. Halvorson EG, Cormican M, West ME, Myers V. Three-dimensional nipple-areola tattooing: a new technique with superior results. Plast Reconstr Surg. 2014;133(5):1073–5.
34. Sanuki J, Fukuma E, Uchida Y. Morphologic study of nipple-areola complex in 600 breasts. Aesthet Plast Surg. 2009;33(3):295–7.

# 57 Nipple Reconstruction with Rolled Dermal Graft Support

Bien-Keem Tan, Weihao Liang, Preetha Madhukumar, and Benita K.T. Tan

## 57.1 Introduction

The reconstruction of the nipple-areolar complex is seen as the final step in breast reconstruction and makes the newly reconstructed breast complete aesthetically. A variety of techniques have been described for the reconstruction of the nipple. The long-term appearance of the reconstructed nipple is a significant factor in the patient's overall satisfaction with their breast reconstruction [1]. However, failure to maintain long-term projection remains a challenging problem when skin flaps are used to reconstruct the nipple. A significant loss of projection occurs during the first 3 months, before stabilizing by 1 year after reconstruction [2, 3]. Overall maintenance of nipple projection can be as low as 30% [4]. Some of the reasons for nipple flattening include external pressure and internal contractures within the nipple. However, the common underlying etiology is largely due to the absence of structural support internally.

To resist deformational forces causing nipple collapse, a pillar of tissue or implant can be used as an internal strut for structural support. Many authors have described the use of various materials to provide structural support. Autologous tissue such as cartilage [5, 6], fat [7], and bone [8], allografts such as acellular dermal matrices [9, 10], and even alloplastic materials such as hyaluronic acid [11], hydroxylapatite [12], and polytetrafluoroethylene [13] have been reported with variable success.

In this chapter, we describe using a tightly rolled dermal graft to create a graft with axial rigidity for nipple reconstruction. From our experience of 45 cases, this technique achieves long-lasting nipple projection with minimal donor site morbidity.

## 57.2 Surgical Technique (Fig. 57.1)

With the patient standing, the C-V flap [14] is marked using the contralateral breast as a reference for the nipple position and dimensions. If the

B.-K. Tan, FRCS, C.T.B.S. (✉) • W. Liang, M.R.C.S.
Department of Plastic, Reconstructive and Aesthetic Surgery, Singapore General Hospital,
Outram Rd, Singapore 169608, Singapore
e-mail: bienkeem@gmail.com; liangweihao82@gmail.com

P. Madhukumar, FRCS
Department of Surgical Oncology, National Cancer Center Singapore, Singapore, Singapore
e-mail: madhukumar.preetha@singhealth.com.sg

B.K.T. Tan, FRCS, Ph.D.
Department of General Surgery, Singapore General Hospital Academia, 20 College Road, Singapore 169856, Singapore

SingHealth Duke-NUS Breast Center, Singapore General Hospital, Singapore, Singapore
e-mail: benita.tan.k.t@singhealth.com.sg


M.A. Shiffman (ed.), *Nipple-Areolar Complex Reconstruction*,
https://doi.org/10.1007/978-3-319-60925-6_57

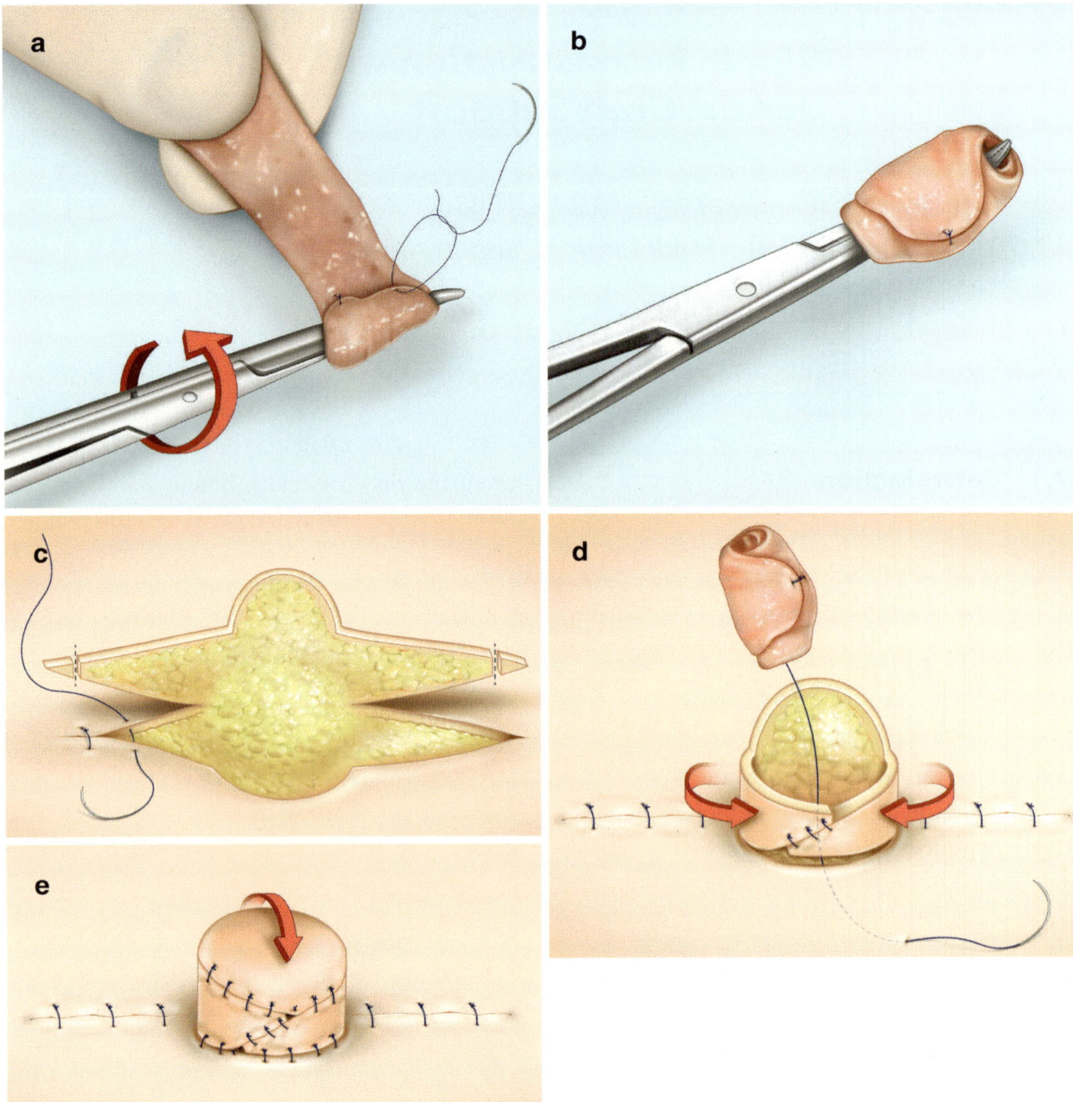


**Fig. 57.1** Operative technique of nipple reconstruction using a rolled dermal graft. (**a**) The dermal graft is rolled tightly, with the aid of an artery forceps clipped to one end of the graft. Sutures are placed at intervals to keep the roll compact and to prevent it from unraveling. (**b**) Appearance of dermal graft after rolling. (**c**) On the breast, the "C" and "V" flaps are elevated, and the "V" flap tips are blunted to prevent skin tip necrosis. (**d**) The rolled graft is threaded, in its erect position, into the trough formed by the V flaps. (**e**) The C flap is folded over and sutured to the V flaps

breast mound position is significantly different after breast reconstruction, the new nipple-areolar complex should be centered over the breast mound instead of mirroring its position to the opposite side. The orientation of the C-V flap can affect the shape of the central skin paddle which forms the future areola. In elliptical skin paddles, the C-V flap is orientated along the shorter axis of the ellipse. Closure of its donor site will "round" the ellipse allowing the scars to merge with the future areola margin.

Under local anesthesia, the "C" and "V" flaps are raised at the superficial subcutaneous level to preserve the subdermal plexus. The tips of the "V" flaps are blunted to avoid skin tip necrosis, and the donor sites are closed with subdermal Monocryl 5-0 and interrupted Ethilon 6-0 sutures (Ethicon Inc., Somerville, NJ, USA). The "V" flaps are then overlapped in a yin-yang fashion and sutured together using Monocryl 6-0 and Ethilon 7-0 sutures.

An ellipse of dermal graft, measuring approximately 3 × 1.5 cm, is harvested. It could be taken from the "dog-ear" portion of the previous TRAM incision or harvested from skin adjacent to scars. Care has to be taken to include mainly dermis and avoid scar tissue. The overlying epidermis is de-epithelialized very thinly with a size 10 blade to an approximate depth of 8/1000th in., thus preserving the maximal thickness of the dermis. Subcutaneous fat is not included as it resorbs and provides little rigidity to the construct.

The dermal graft is wound tightly around a pair of fine artery forceps, and interrupted Monocryl 6-0 sutures are placed at intervals to prevent the graft from unraveling. A 3-O Prolene suture (Ethicon Inc., Somerville, NJ, USA) is now tied to one end of the graft, and using the needle, the rolled dermal graft is inset in an erect position into the trough formed by the V flaps (Fig. 57.2). The C flap is then folded over as a roof over the construct and sutured to the V flaps with 7-0 Ethilon sutures. The entire nipple is lightly coated with Dermabond (Ethicon Inc., Somerville, NJ, USA) which is a cyanoacrylate adhesive. Once set, the glue becomes a well-molded transparent splint over the nipple (Fig. 57.3). We have observed that with the glue, the incidence of infection and tip necrosis has reduced because of its tension-relieving effect along the suture lines. In instances where the V and C flaps are too thick to be folded tightly, especially in LD flaps, they are loosely tagged, and any raw areas are grafted over with leftover de-epithelized skin.

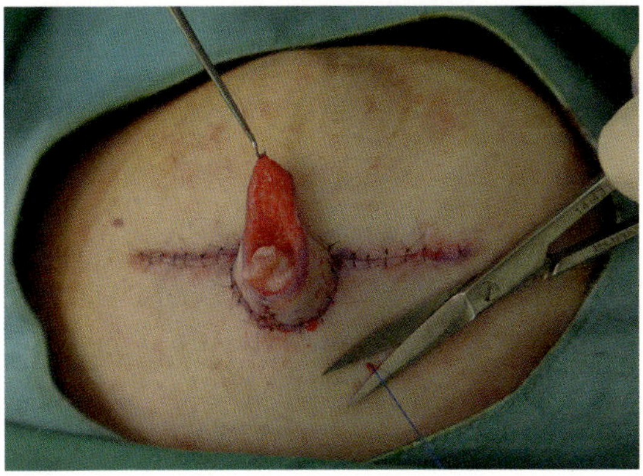

**Fig. 57.2** Slotting in the rolled dermal graft with the aid of a Prolene 3-0 retaining suture cut flushed with the skin

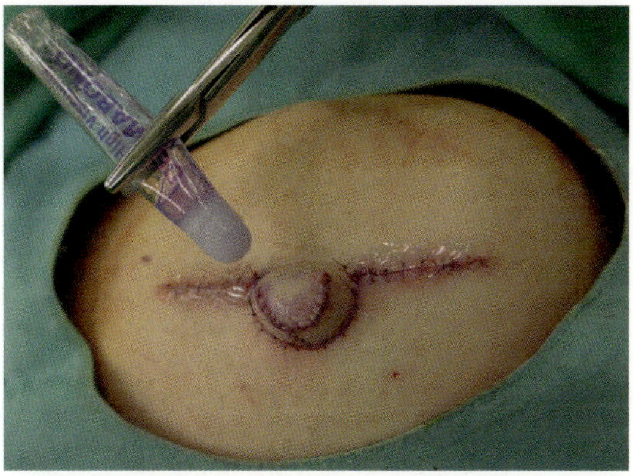

**Fig. 57.3** Cyanoacrylate glue is applied to create a molded splint over the construct

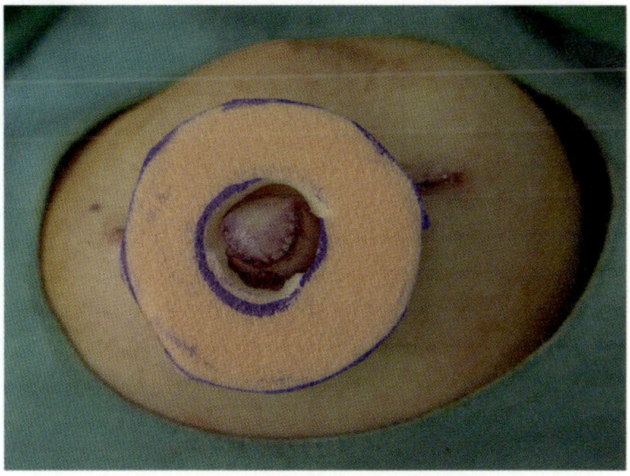

**Fig. 57.4** Stacked Allevyn sponge dressing is used to protect the nipple

Post-operatively, Allevyn (Smith & Nephew, London, UK) sponge dressings are cut into doughnut shapes and applied to splint the reconstructed nipple for 3–6 months (Fig. 57.4). This splinting is continued for a minimum of 3–6 months. The patient is advised to avoid tight-fitting brassiere. Tattooing of the nipple-areolar complex is performed 6 months after the wounds have fully healed.

## 57.3 Complications

In our series of 45 patients, there was one case of nipple necrosis. This was the result of excessive pressure from an overly large dermal graft. We would advise caution with tight-fitting dermal grafts. Three patients had minor wound dehiscence and exposure of the dermal graft. These healed with daily dressings.

## 57.4 Illustrative Cases

### 57.4.1 Case 1: Breast Cancer Reconstruction (Fig. 57.5)

A 45-year-old female with T2N1M0 invasive ductal carcinoma of the right breast underwent skin-sparing mastectomy and breast reconstruction with a free muscle-sparing TRAM flap.

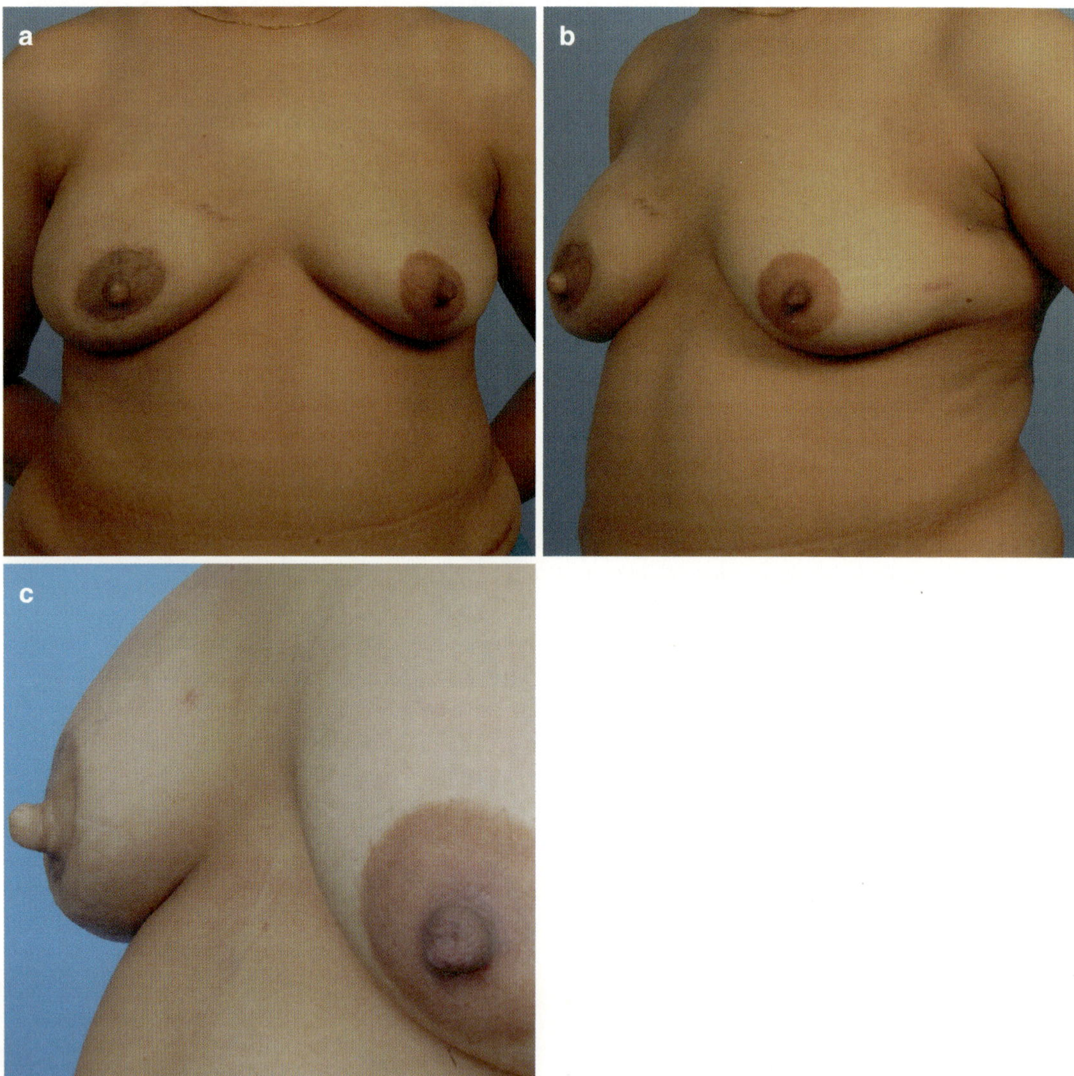


**Fig. 57.5** A 45-year-old female with T2N1M0 invasive ductal carcinoma of the right breast underwent skin-sparing mastectomy and breast reconstruction with a free muscle-sparing TRAM flap. Nipple reconstruction was performed 6 months post-operatively, followed by tattooing of the nipple-areolar complex. (**a–c**) One year post-operative. Her nipple projection was 0.8 cm

Nipple reconstruction was performed 6 months post-operatively, followed by tattooing of the nipple-areolar complex. The illustrations show the post-operative results at 1 year. Her nipple projection was 0.8 cm. Slight overcorrection of the nipple was achieved in anticipation of radiotherapy.

### 57.4.2 Case 2: Inverted Nipple Grade 3 (Fig. 57.6)

The rolled dermal graft is also useful for the severely retracted nipple in which the scarred and shortened lactiferous ducts make it impossible for the nipple to be pulled out physically. These are classified as Grade 3 inverted nipples. Grade 1 and 2 inverted nipples are those which evert with traction.

A 36-year-old female with a right inverted nipple from previous mastitis was referred for correction. A single 5 mm stab incision 3 mm beyond the nipple base was made, and through this incision, all retaining tissues were divided with a micro-knife under local anesthesia. Traction on the nipple with a temporary Prolene 3-0 stay suture maintained eversion and ensured the adequacy of the release. The resultant dead space was packed with a dermal graft harvested from skin adjacent to a previous scar in the groin. Care was taken not to devitalize the nipple, whose vascularity was solely dependent on the subdermal plexus as all deep tissues had been divided.

## 57.5 Discussion

The presence of thick, well-vascularized dermis is a key factor in maintaining of nipple projection. Nipples reconstructed from the thicker dermis of latissimus dorsi skin islands were more resistant to contractures than those reconstructed from the

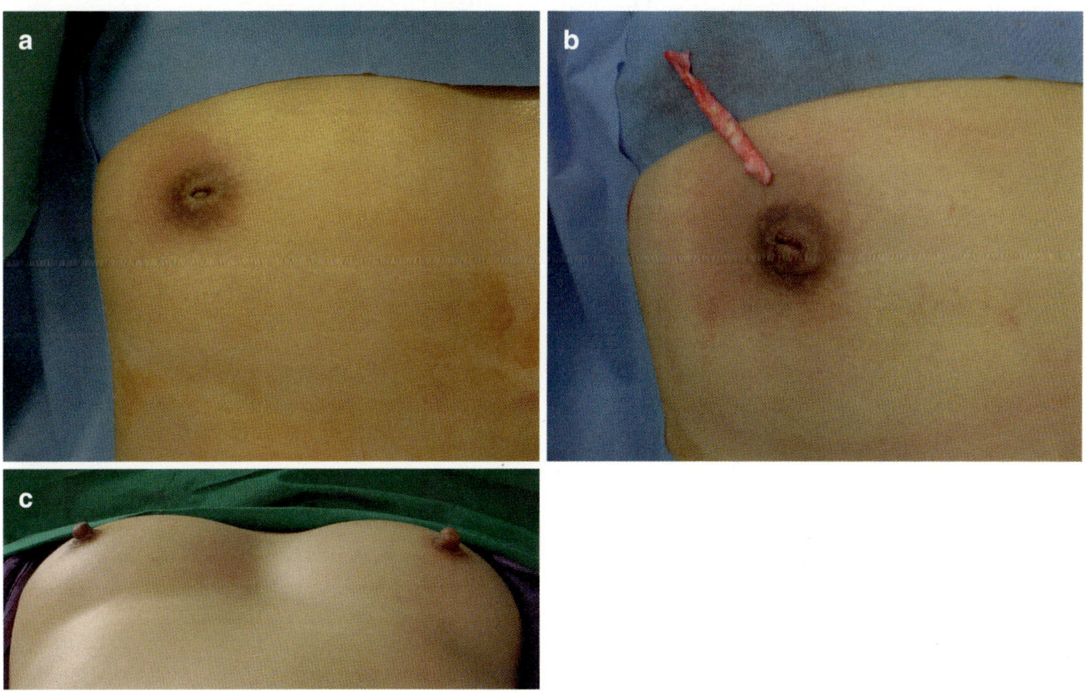


**Fig. 57.6** Correction of Grade 3 inverted nipple. (**a**) This 36-year-old female developed inverted nipple after mastitis. (**b**) Sharp release of all scarred ducts was accomplished through a 5 mm areolar incision. A strip of dermal graft was used to pack the resultant cavity and maintain projection. (**c**) Three months post-operative showing nipple projection and symmetry

thinner skin of the breast and abdomen [15]. Dermal grafts add to the dermal component of local skin flaps and being autologous, the risk of extrusion is negligible. Long-term histologic evaluation of dermal grafts revealed degeneration of epithelial remnants with eventual transformation of the implanted dermis into well-vascularized fibrous tissue [16]. Eo et al. [17] described the use of stacked dermal grafts at the base of the nipple to improve projection. In our technique, the dermal graft is rolled tightly to form a compact cylinder, providing axial rigidity to maintain nipple projection and shape. In our series, the maintenance of nipple projection (defined as the percentage of nipple height at 1 year post-operatively compared to at the time of surgery) was 69.6%, indicating slight graft shrinkage. A modest overcorrection helps compensate for this sequelae.

Other grafts, such as auricular cartilage [18], rib cartilage [5], and toe pulp [19], have been described. The drawback of these options is the need for an extra donor site. An exception is the rib cartilage, which can be harvested and banked when the internal mammary vessels are used as recipient vessels during breast reconstruction. Although rib cartilage is superior in maintaining nipple projection, the excessive rigidity it affords may not be desirable. Guerra et al. [5] reported 454 nipple reconstructions combining cartilage graft with a local arrow flap. Four percent of nipples in this study suffered cartilage graft loss due to graft exposure or flap ischemia.

Synthetic materials have also been used to augment nipple projection, and they include polytetrafluoroethylene implants [13], artificial bone [8], and semipermanent injectable fillers such as calcium hydroxylapatite [12]. Alloplastic materials are readily available and do not incur a donor site. However, these options have an increased risk of extrusion and may predispose the patient to infection and wound-healing complications. AlloDerm (LifeCell, Bridgewater, NJ, USA) has been used as an internal strut with favorable results [10, 20, 21] but is expensive.

**Acknowledgments** The authors thank Mr. Evan Lim of SingHealth Academy for the medical illustrations.

## References

1. Guyomard V, Leinster S, Wilkinson M. Systematic review of studies of patients' satisfaction with breast reconstruction after mastectomy. Breast. 2007;16(6):547–67.
2. Losken A, Mackay GJ, Bostwick J 3rd. Nipple reconstruction using the C-V flap technique: a long-term evaluation. Plast Reconstr Surg. 2001;108:361–9.
3. Few JW, Marcus JR, Casas LA, Aitken ME, Redding J. Long-term predictable nipple projection following reconstruction. Plast Reconstr Surg. 1999;104:1321–4.
4. Shestak KC, Gabriel A, Landecker A, Peters S, Shestak A, Kim J. Assessment of long-term nipple projection: a comparison of three techniques. Plast Reconstr Surg. 2002;110:780–6.
5. Guerra AB, Khoobehi K, Metzinger SE, Allen RJ. New technique for nipple areola reconstruction: arrow flap and rib cartilage graft for long-lasting nipple projection. Ann Plast Surg. 2003;50(1):31–7.
6. Cheng MH, Ho-Asjoe M, Wei FC, Chuang DC. Nipple reconstruction in Asian females using banked cartilage graft and modified top hat flap. Br J Plast Surg. 2003;56(7):692–4.
7. Bernard RW, Beran SJ. Autologous fat graft in nipple reconstruction. Plast Reconstr Surg. 2003;112(4):964–8.
8. Yanaga H. Nipple-areola reconstruction with a dermal fat flap: technical improvement from rolled auricular cartilage to artificial bone. Plast Reconstr Surg. 2003;112:1863–9.
9. Nahabedian MY. Secondary nipple reconstruction using local flaps and AlloDerm. Plast Reconstr Surg. 2005;115(7):2056–61.
10. Garramone CE, Lam B. Use of AlloDerm in primary nipple reconstruction to improve long-term nipple projection. Plast Reconstr Surg. 2007;119(6):1663–8.
11. Panettiere P, Marchetti L, Accorsi D. Filler injection enhances the projection of the reconstructed nipple: an original easy technique. Aesthet Plast Surg. 2005;29(4):287–94.
12. Evans KK, Rasko Y, Lenert J, Olding M. The use of calcium hydroxylapatite for nipple projection after failed nipple-areolar reconstruction: early results. Ann Plast Surg. 2005;55(1):25–9.
13. Wong RK, Wichterman L, Parson SD. Skin sparing nipple reconstruction with polytetrafluoroethylene implant. Ann Plast Surg. 2008;61(3):256–8.
14. Jones G, Bostwick J III. Nipple-areolar reconstruction. Oper Tech Plast Reconstr Surg. 1994;1:35–8.
15. Hammond DC, Khuthaila D, Kim J. The skate flap purse-string technique for nipple-areola complex reconstruction. Plast Reconstr Surg. 2007;120:399–406.
16. Davis RE, Guida RA, Cook TA. Autologous free dermal fat graft. Reconstruction of facial contour defects. Arch Otolaryngol Head Neck Surg. 1995;121:95–100.

17. Eo S, Kim SS, Da Lio AL. Nipple reconstruction with C-V flap using dermofat graft. Ann Plast Surg. 2007;58:137–40.
18. Tanabe HY, Tai Y, Kiyokawa K, Yamauchi T. Nipple-areola reconstruction with a dermal-fat flap and rolled auricular cartilage. Plast Reconstr Surg. 1997;100:431–8.
19. Klatsky SA, Manson PN. Toe pulp free grafts in nipple reconstruction. Plast Reconstr Surg. 1981;68:245–8.
20. Holton LH, Haerian H, Silverman RP, Chung T, Elisseeff JH, Goldberg NH, Slezak S. Improving long-term projection in nipple reconstruction using human acellular dermal matrix: an animal model. Ann Plast Surg. 2005;55:304–9.
21. Chen WF, Barounis D, Kalimuthu R. A novel cost-saving approach to the use of acellular dermal matrix (AlloDerm) in postmastectomy breast and nipple reconstructions. Plast Reconstr Surg. 2010;125:479–81.

# 58 A Modified Technique for Nipple-Areola Complex Reconstruction

Pier Camillo Parodi and Daria Almesberger

## 58.1 Introduction

Nipple-areola complex (NAC) reconstruction is the final step of the breast reconstructive ladder, in which a surgically created mound is transformed into an aesthetically pleasing breast, restoring the body image of breast cancer patients, who have undergone mastectomy [1]. Several authors have shown that recreation of the nipple-areola complex has a high correlation with overall patient satisfaction and acceptance of body image. Thus, completion of the breast reconstruction by creating a nipple-areola complex that matches the contralateral nipple in terms of size, shape, projection, and position adds significantly to the reconstructive result.

Correct location and an adequate size of the nipple-areola complex are mandatory for a beautiful breast. A nipple-areola complex is the key signature to the naturalness and attractiveness of the breast, highlighting the point of maximal anteroposterior projection and enhancing the conical shape of the breast [2].

Several techniques have developed over the past years in an effort to overcome the ongoing challenge of maintaining sustained nipple projection. This loss of projection is generally reported between 50 and 70% of initial height and is seen with both flap and implant breast reconstruction [1, 3]. Flattening of the nipple is the number one source of patient dissatisfaction, followed by color match, shape, size, texture, and position [2, 4].

Several techniques have been reported to overcome this complication, as composite nipple grafts, the star flap, the double-opposing tab design, the bell flap, the C-V flap, the skate flap, and other procedures including various materials and tissue-engineered structures between the skin flaps. Small pieces of dermal fat grafts, cartilage grafts, or AlloDerm may be placed and may contribute to both initial and long-term projection [1].

P.C. Parodi, M.D. (✉)
Department of Plastic Surgery-Academic Hospital, University of Udine, Piazzale S. Maria della Misericordia, 33100 Udine, Italy

Department of Medical, Experimental and Clinical Sciences—Plastic and Aesthetic Surgery, University of Udine, Piazzale S. Maria della Misericordia, 33100 Udine, Italy
e-mail: piercamillo.parodi@uniud.it

D. Almesberger, M.D.
Department of Plastic Surgery, University of Udine, Piazzale S. Maria della Misericordia, 33100 Udine, Italy
e-mail: daria_almes@yahoo.it


M.A. Shiffman (ed.), *Nipple-Areolar Complex Reconstruction*,
https://doi.org/10.1007/978-3-319-60925-6_58

## 58.2 Timing: Immediate or Delayed?

Because the reconstructed nipple is not easily moved, nipple reconstruction is usually reserved as the final step in breast reconstruction and could be critical for providing an aesthetically pleasing breast. In fact, patients with loss of the nipple and areola continue to experience psychological distress even long after breast mound reconstruction has taken place. Therefore, postponing NAC reconstruction in the final part of breast reconstruction could increase this psychological status.

The main problem in NAC reconstructions is the difficulty in determining the ideal position of the nipple-areola complex, when the effects of postoperative settling of the breast mound are unpredictable and the need for revision possible [1]. For these reasons, several authors prefer an immediate NAC reconstruction, rather than a delayed one, overcoming this argument with microsurgery. Craig [5] reported good outcomes with immediate nipple reconstruction, utilizing DIEP flap to recreate a natural-appearing and aesthetic nipple in select patients. He reported that nipple position relative to the flap breast mound has remained unchanged for up to 6 months.

On the contrary, a non-autologous reconstruction has unpredictable results.

The thickness of the skin envelope, the measure of the implant, and the postsurgical therapy play an important role in the final outcome. Therefore many surgeons prefer a delayed nipple reconstruction.

At our institution, patients reconstructed with flaps generally have the nipple created 3 months after the initial surgery. For patients with tissue expanders, nipple reconstruction may be performed at the time of exchange to implant or 3 months after the second stage has been completed. Anyway, timing of nipple-areola reconstruction depends, first, on the breast reconstruction technique (autologous or non-autologous techniques) used, on patient's postoperative therapy (radiotherapy), and, finally, on the NAC reconstruction technique we are intentioned to use.

## 58.3 Positioning of the Nipple

A nipple-areola complex is the key signature to the naturalness and attractiveness of the breast, highlighting the point of maximal anteroposterior projection and enhancing the conical shape of the breast [2]. Proper position and reasonable symmetry of the nipple on the breast are important.

Although the shape, projection, and contours of the nipple-areola complex differ significantly from patient to patient, aesthetic breasts consistently have nipple-areola complexes that reside at the point of the breast's maximal anteroposterior projection and either along the vertical meridian of the breast or slightly lateral to it [2].

A good breast reconstruction can become the worst reconstruction if the position and the shape of the nipple are asymmetric with the contralateral one. To obtain the most satisfactory result, it is important to involve always the patient in the decision of nipple placement. With the patient in the standing position, the surgeon should mark the new nipple in the same horizontal plane of the contralateral one. However, in unilateral cases, the ideal position on the reconstructed breast mound may not correlate with the nipple position on the contralateral breast.

In our department, once we have defined the best position on the breast mound, we used to provide the patient with an electrocardiograph sticker, thus to involve her in the last decision of the new nipple's location.

## 58.4 Radiation and Nipple Reconstruction

While nipple reconstruction is a safe procedure after implant-based breast reconstruction in patients without a history of radiotherapy, the presence of an irradiated field converts it to a high-risk one with a significant increase in postoperative complication rate.

The deleterious effects of radiotherapy, however, particularly in the context of implant-based breast reconstruction, are well documented [6–8]. The pathophysiologic basis for adverse effects seen after surgical interventions within an irradiated field is attributed to depletion of parenchymal and stem cells as well as progressive fibrosis, a disrupted normal wound healing, changes of vasculature, and fibroblast's and growth factor's function in wound healing [1, 8, 9]. The effects of radiotherapy furthermore appear to be relevant in patients in whom reconstruction with larger implants is planned and in those with particularly tenuous soft tissue envelope with thinner mastectomy skin flaps.

Anyway, the patient needs to be made aware that if larger implant volumes are necessary to achieve an aesthetically appealing result, the risk for developing complications is further augmented in the setting of radiation, in order to choose an autologous reconstruction instead of a non-autologous one.

## 58.5 Nipple Reconstruction Using the Fleur-De-Lis Flap Technique

Nipple-areola complex reconstruction is the last step in a breast reconstruction procedure. As reported above, numerous methods have been used for nipple reconstruction, all of which had the same drawback: a loss of nipple projection [10, 11]. Several techniques have been suggested to overcome this problem without satisfactory results [12–19]. The loss of nipple projection could be attributable to a fat component reabsorption of the local flaps commonly used for nipple reconstruction.

At this state, we tried to use a nipple-areola reconstruction technique that could provide the greater amount of dermal and dermocutaneous component.

The fleur-de-lis flap technique have revealed satisfactory outcomes in the majority of patients: it uses three dermocutaneous flaps with an added dermal component at the top of the flaps. The position and size of the new nipple is planned on the basis of the opposite nipple-areola complex (Fig. 58.1). The width of the central flap coincides with the diameter of the contralateral nipple, whereas the projection of the latter determines the length of the lateral flaps. Three elliptic dermocutaneous flaps are sculpted to form a clover leaf shape (Fig. 58.2). At the distal part of these flaps, three triangular dermo-adipose flaps are incised, leaving the skin intact. All the flaps then are raised, and the two lateral flaps are wrapped around to create the new nipple base, with the

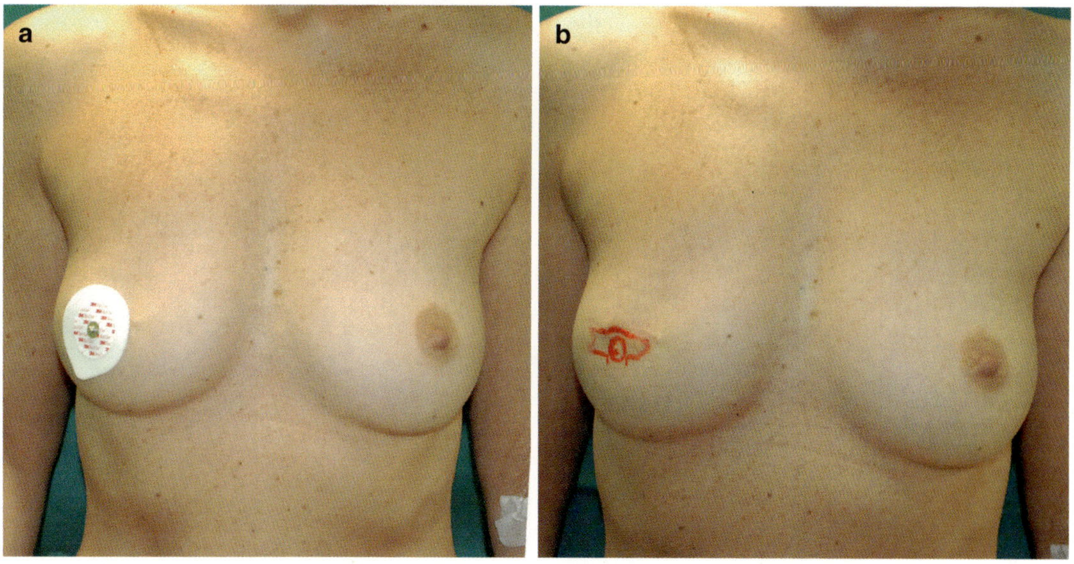


**Fig. 58.1** (**a**) Preoperative patient evaluation and accurate checking of nipple position with the aid of an electrocardiographic electrode. (**b**) Marking the flap

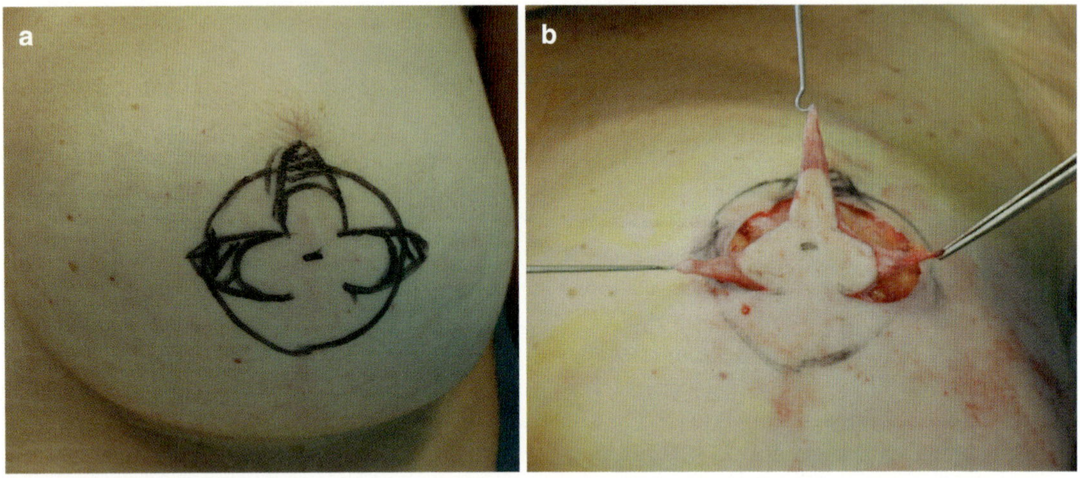


**Fig. 58.2** (**a**) Preoperative design of the nipple. In evidence, the triangular apex of the two lateral flaps. (**b**) Subsequently deepithelialized and raising the flap. The deepithelialized area is proportional to contralateral nipple dimensions

central flap sutured over them like a roof (Fig. 58.3). It is important not to make the cutaneous flaps excessively thin in the distal portion to avoid their devascularization.

The fleur-de-lis flap technique uses local flaps for nipple reconstruction, adding a dermal component at the top of dermocutaneous flaps. This additional component can avoid the need for nipple over-reconstruction, making possible an easy evaluation of its projection on the basis of the normal side (Figs. 58.4 and 58.5).

This procedure is a speedy and reliable method for reconstructing a natural-looking breast and for avoiding the loss of nipple projection; in fact,

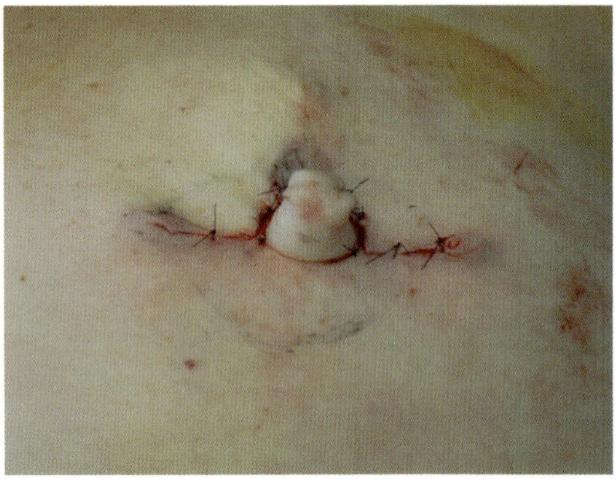

**Fig. 58.3** The new nipple after suturing of the three flaps

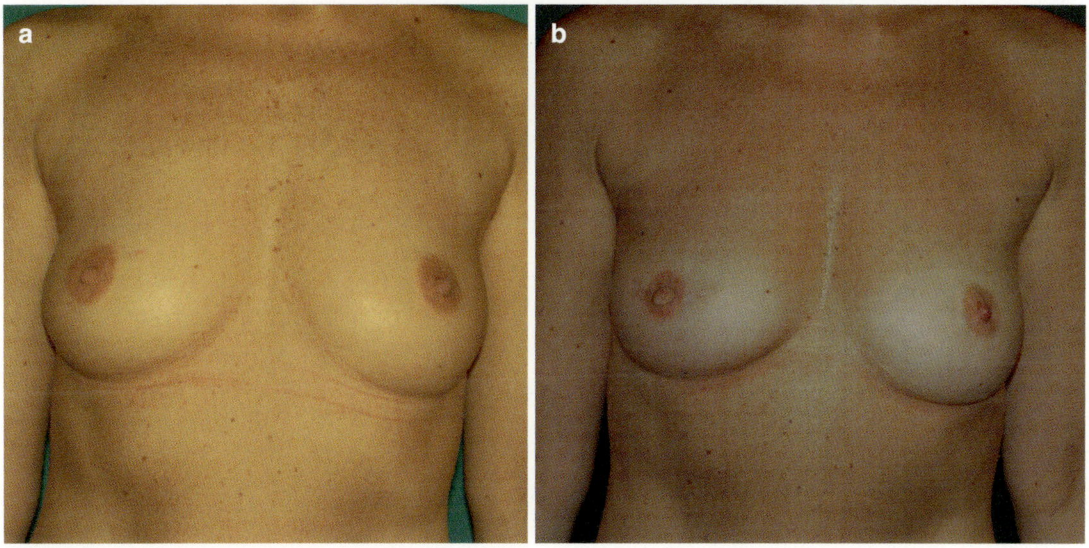


**Fig. 58.4** (**a**) Preoperative. (**b**) Postoperative

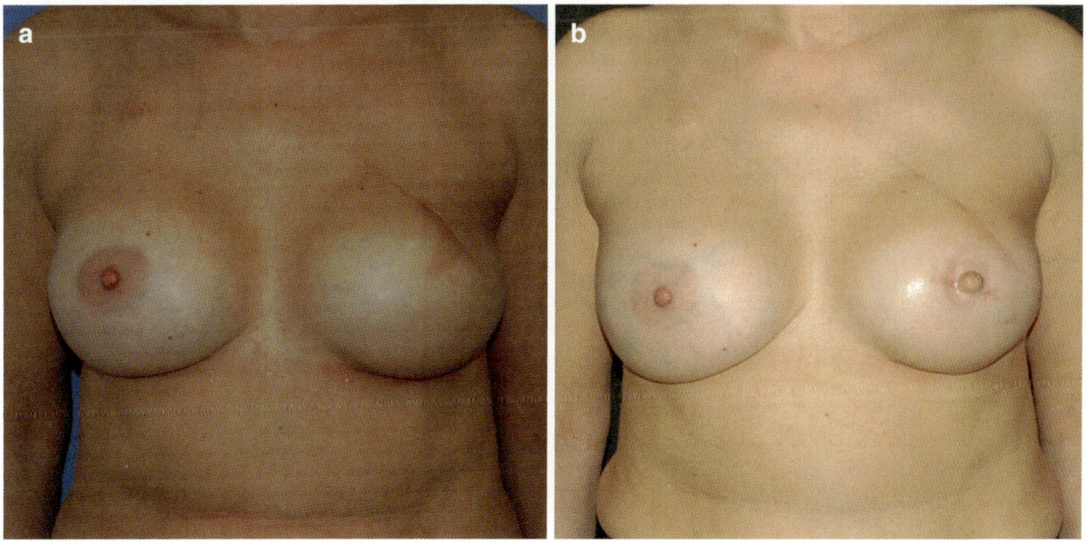


**Fig. 58.5** (**a**) Preoperative. (**b**) Postoperative

the peculiar design of the two lateral flaps with an added dermal component at the top of them, not influenced by reabsorption process, avoids nipple volume reduction.

## References


1. Spear SL, West JE. NAC reconstruction. In: Spear SL, Willey SC, Robb GL, Hammond DC, Nahabedian NY, editors. Surgery of the breast: principles and art. Philadelphia: Lippincott, Williams & Wilkins; 2011.
2. Blondeel PN, Hijjawi J, Depypere H, Roche N, Van Landuyt K. Shaping the breast in aesthetic and reconstructive breast surgery: an easy three-step principle. Plast Reconstr Surg. 2009;123(2):455–62.
3. Shestak KC, Gabriel A, Landecker A. Assessment of long-term nipple projection: a comparison of three techniques. Plast Reconstr Surg. 2002;110(3):780–6.
4. Jabor MA, Shayani P, Collis DR Jr, Karas T, Cohen BE. Nipple-areola reconstruction: satisfaction and clinical determinants. Plast Reconstr Surg. 2002;110(2):457–63.
5. Craig ES, Walker ME, Salomon J, Fusi S. Immediate nipple reconstruction utilizing the DIEP flap in areola-sparing mastectomy. Microsurgery. 2013;33(2):125–9.
6. Momeni A, Ghaly M, Gupta D, Karanas YL, Kahn DM, Gurtner GC, Lee GK. Nipple reconstruction: risk factors and complications after 189 procedures. Eur J Plast Surg. 2013;36(10):633–8.
7. Spear SL, Onyewu C. Staged breast reconstruction with saline-filled implants in the irradiated breast: recent trends and therapeutic implications. Plast Reconstr Surg. 2000;105:930–42.
8. Lin KY, Blechman AB, Brenin DR. Implant-based, two-stage breast reconstruction in the setting of radiation injury: an outcome study. Plast Reconstr Surg. 2012;129:817–23.
9. Delanian S, Lefaix JL. The radiation-induced fibroatrophic process: therapeutic perspective via the antioxidant pathway. Radiother Oncol. 2004;73:119–31.
10. Losken A, Mackay GJ, Bostwick J. Nipple reconstruction using the C-V flap technique: a long-term evaluation. Plast Reconstr Surg. 2001;108(2):361–9.
11. Lossing C, Brongo S, Holmström H. Nipple reconstruction with a modified S-flap technique. Scand J Plast Reconstr Surg Hand Surg. 1998;32(3):275–9.
12. Few JW, Marcus JR, Casas LA, Aitken ME, Redding J. Long-term predictable nipple projection following reconstruction. Plast Reconstr Surg. 1999;104:1321–4.
13. Gamboa-Bobadilla GM. Nipple reconstruction: the top hat technique. Ann Plast Surg. 2005;54:243–6.
14. Nahabedian MY. Secondary nipple reconstruction using local flaps and AlloDerm. Plast Reconstr Surg. 2005;115:2056–61.
15. Peled IJ. Purse-string suture for nipple projection. Plast Reconstr Surg. 1999;103:1480–2.
16. Vecchione TR. Reconstruction and/or salvage of nipple projection. Plast Reconstr Surg. 1986;78:679–83.
17. Yanaga H. Nipple–areola reconstruction with a dermal-fat flap: technical improvement from rolled auricular cartilage to artificial bone. Plast Reconstr Surg. 2003;112(7):1863–9.
18. Mohamed SA, Parodi PC. A modified technique for nipple-areola complex reconstruction. Indian J Plast Surg. 2011;44(1):76–80.
19. Germanò D, De Biasio F, Piedimonte A, Parodi PC. Nipple reconstruction using the fleur-de-lis flap technique. Aesthet Plast Surg. 2006;30(4):399–402.

# Nipple-Areola Reconstruction Using Local Flaps

# 59

Randall S. Feingold

## 59.1 Introduction

It is important to note the indications for impact and limitations of nipple-areola reconstruction. Nipple-areola reconstruction is indicated in post-mastectomy breast reconstruction when the nipple is resected in modified radical, skin-sparing, or areolar-sparing mastectomy approaches. Nipple reconstruction may even be necessary following unexpected nipple loss in nipple-areolar-sparing mastectomy, breast reduction, or mastopexy. The psychological impact of nipple loss is significant, and its contribution to a woman's sense of femininity, sensuality, and motherliness should not be underestimated (Fig. 59.1). While occasional breast reconstruction patients will initially question the necessity of nipple reconstruction, presentation of quality before-and-after images showing a breast mound with and without the restored nipple-areola will in most cases result in a woman's decision to undergo nipple reconstruction, albeit with a striking range of preference in nipple height. For those patients who suffer unexpected loss of nipple following breast reduction, mastopexy, or even gynecomastia surgery, the loss of the nipple-areola carries both psychological and potential medicolegal consequences. Thus, facility with nipple-areola reconstruction needs to be part of all breast plastic surgeon's skill sets. The deficiencies and limitations of nipple-areola reconstruction relate to the fact that the substrate used to create a nipple-areola does not truly replace "like tissue with like" insofar as there is the absence of contractile muscle in the reconstructed nipple mound and areola base. While some nipple-areola reconstructions gain tactile sensibility over time from the surrounding soft tissue envelope, it is not erotic sensation, nor is dynamic erectile function restored. Despite this, many patients are satisfied with nipple reconstruction.

## 59.2 Technique

### 59.2.1 Options in Technique

The skate flap of Little [1, 2], the triangular star flap of Spear [3], and the C-V flap [4, 5] are the most common flaps utilized for nipple reconstruction. The partial dermal thickness of the skate flap and the need for a full-thickness skin graft are disadvantages of this approach. The thinner flaps afford less volume, and while skin grafts can provide texture, partial or total skin graft loss can result in scars that mark the appearance of the result and are difficult to camouflage

R.S. Feingold, M.D.
Aesthetic Plastic Surgery, PC Great Neck Office, 833 Northern Boulevard, Suite 160, Great Neck, NY 11021, USA

Department of Surgery, Hofstra Northwell School of Medicine, Hempstead, NY, USA
e-mail: rfeingold@nybra.com


M.A. Shiffman (ed.), *Nipple-Areolar Complex Reconstruction*,
https://doi.org/10.1007/978-3-319-60925-6_59

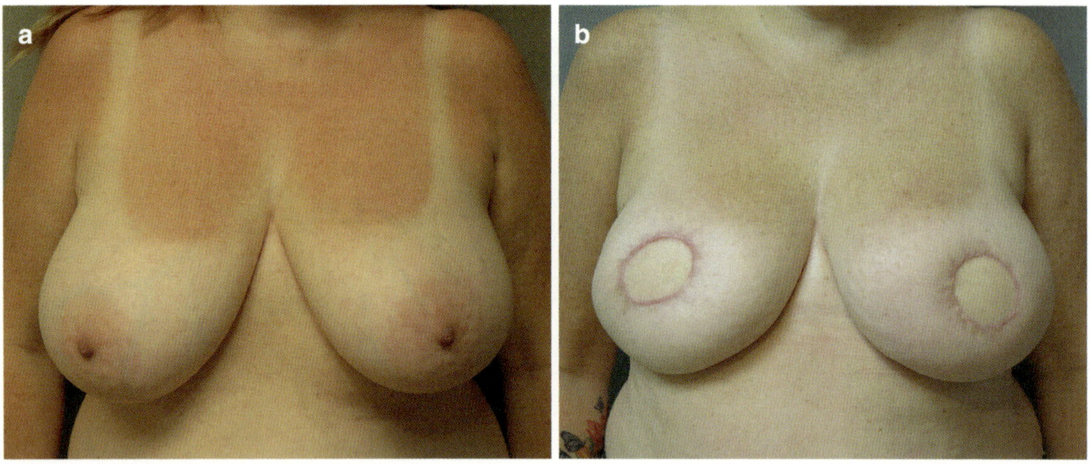


**Fig. 59.1** (**a**) Preoperative. (**b**) After skin-sparing mastectomy

with intradermal tattoo. The full-thickness flaps of the star flap and C-V flap provide greater bulk and avoid a skin graft donor site, but the midline vertical apposition of the flaps results in a linear contracture that directly opposes the desired nipple projection. Older graft techniques such as nipple-sharing from a remaining breast carry the risk of transferring tissue with oncogenic potential to the breast reconstruction [6] and are unappealing to most patients.

#### 59.2.1.1 Current Method

My current method of nipple-areola reconstruction utilizes a spiral wrap flap technique. This is a modification of and improvement over the star and C-V flaps, similar to the modified fishtail flap described by Jones [5]. This can be done whether the breast mound has been constructed with autologous tissue flaps alone, latissimus dorsi flaps over implants, or implants alone. In the case of skin-sparing mastectomies where the nipple-areola territory has been replaced with a skin island, it is best to have used a skin island of slightly oval shape, since the harvest of the nipple flaps forms the skin island and subsequent closure of the donor site will then result in a circular skin island. That will allow tattoo coverage of both the nipple and skin island to achieve a result that camouflages all surgical scars. The pattern is drawn upright before operative positioning and arm placement distorts the donor site. Two tapered rounded arms are drawn 180° off a central cap within a skin island or atop an implant reconstruction (Fig. 59.2). Incisions are made full thickness through the skin into the subcutaneous fat. In the case of autologous tissue breast mounds, a significant amount of fat may be included during elevation. In the case of implant-based breast mounds, thin tissue-expanded skin envelopes will contain little fat by comparison. A small amount of partial thickness pectoralis muscle may be included in the nipple flaps, without entry through the implant capsule. The nipple mound is then created before closure of the donor site. The flaps are rotated around each other in a spiral fashion first anchoring the base flap with a 4-0 chromic suture and then anchoring the other flap above it. Then the cap is anchored atop the upper flap. Interrupted 4-0 chromic completes all sutures lines. The height of the nipple is thus the additive height of each flap in its midportion, which is significantly higher than that achieved by suturing two flaps to each with a midline vertical apposition. Furthermore, the spiral orientation of the suture lines will not result in the linear contracture that a single vertical suture line would. Both of these features follow the principles achieved in the Z-plasty technique of relieving scar contracture by soft tissue lengthening and proper scar orientation. The donor site is then closed by 3-0 Vicryl deep dermal closure and 3-0 Monocryl subcuticular closure. In the case of an oval skin island donor

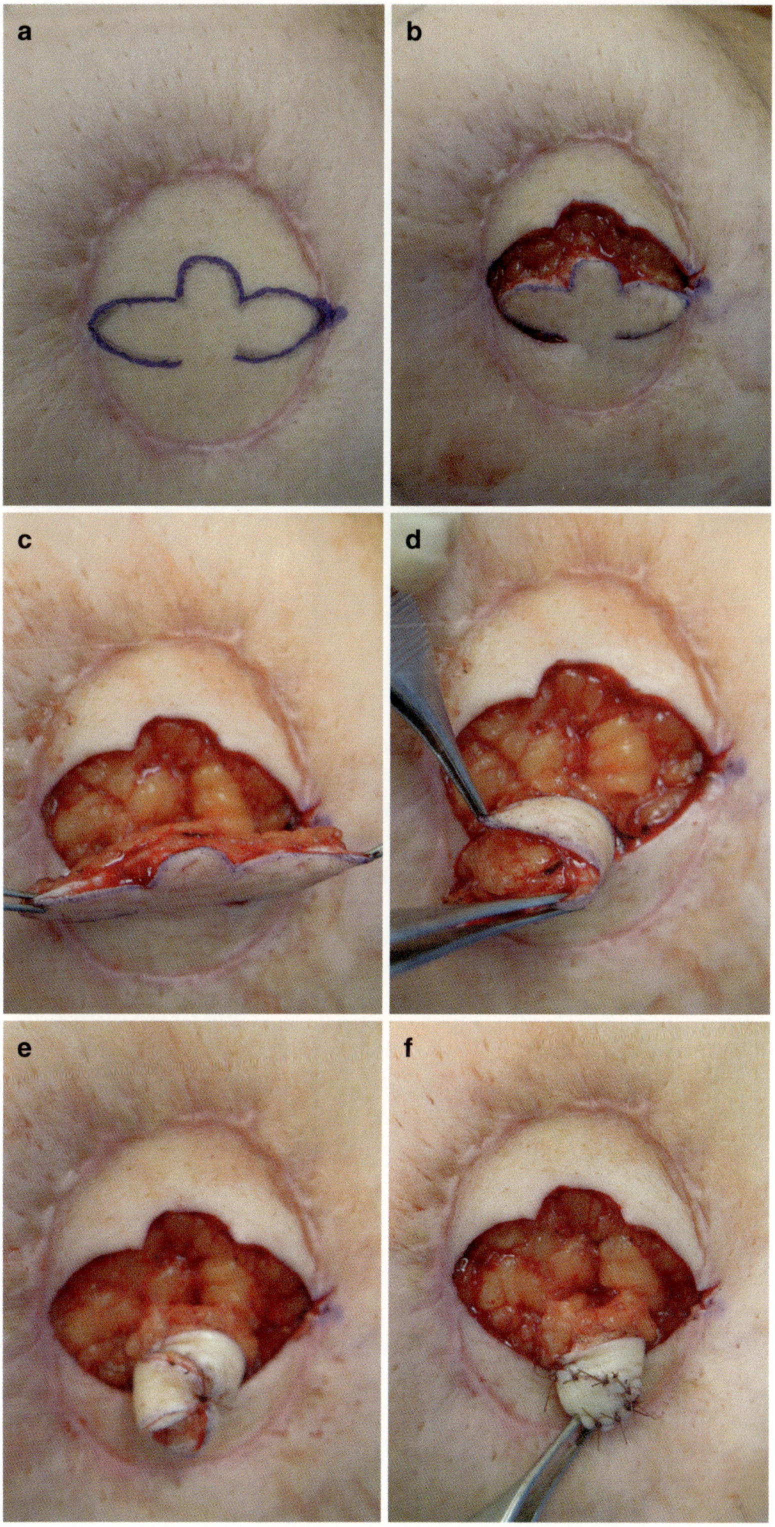


**Fig. 59.2** (**a**) Spiral wrap flap design. (**b**) Incision into subcutaneous flap. (**c**) Retention of fat on the surfaces of the flaps limbs. (**d**) First flap wrapped and anchored at the base. (**e**) Second flap wrapped and anchored atop the first flap. (**f**) Cap flap anchored. (**g**) All limbs sutured closed. (**h**) Donor site closed. (**i**) Completed nipple-areola on breast mound

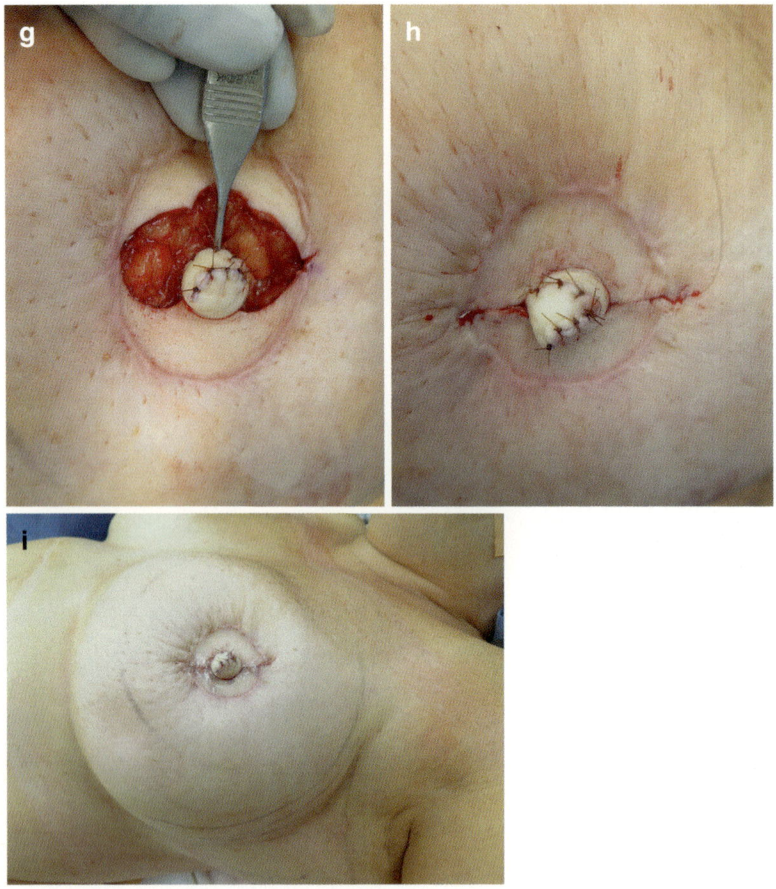


**Fig. 59.2** (continued)

site, the pattern is reduced to a circle. Direct closure can be performed when implants are utilized. Coverage with bacitracin and dry sterile dressing and application of a dermal sealant such as Dermabond are both acceptable. Moisturizer is encouraged after 1 week. Chromic suture remnants are generally resorbed by 4 weeks. Tattoo of the nipple mound and the areola territory is safely performed after 8 weeks. Since there is no contractile muscle in the nipple-areola reconstruction, generous size on the day of surgery is preferable even if the patient prefers a small nipple. If the nipple reconstruction is ultimately too long (Fig. 59.3), then revision by shortening at the tip or base can be done before or after the tattoo.

#### 59.2.1.2 Delay Procedure

Postradiation skin and thin tissue expansion envelopes pose additional challenges that may result in partial or total necrosis of nipple flaps. A two-stage or even three-stage nipple flap delay sequence may be performed depending on the circumstances. The pattern is designed in the same manner. First-stage delay procedure involves incision of the flaps through dermis into subcutaneous fat. The flaps can be sutured closed without elevation or elevated and then replaced for suture closure. One to two weeks are allowed to pass between stages. An optional intermediate stage to elevate and replace flaps that were only incised at first stage can be performed. Final stage involves re-incision, elevation, and spiral flap rotation to complete the nipple with closure of the donor site.

### 59.2.2 Management of Early and Late Nipple Failures

Despite careful technique and even with delay procedures, nipple flap necrosis or late flattening can occur. While diabetes, cigarette smoking, radiation, and thin skin may be predictors of skin flap necrosis or flattening, it can occur even in the absence of such risk factors. Early wound care consisting of topical cleaning, bacitracin, Silvadene, and sharp debridement will ultimately lead to secondary healing and wound closure. When faced with the types of healed nipples or those that have spontaneously flattened, secondary and even tertiary flap reconstruction with repeat spiral wrap technique can be quite successful. The pattern is drawn as to include the healed nipple remnant in the base of the three flaps, and elevation and spiral wrap performed in the usual fashion (Fig. 59.4). The scarred or flattened nipple remnant provides a stable base for additive tissue that results in taller and firmer results. This is also applicable to those patients who prefer very large nipples and demand additional reconstruction despite adequate projection or volume initially.

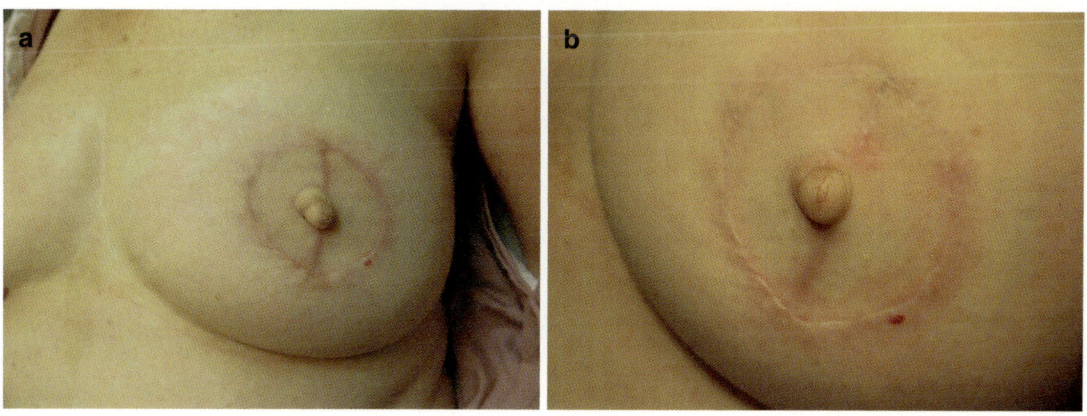


**Fig. 59.3** (**a**) Elongated nipple after spiral wrap. (**b**) Corrected nipple length

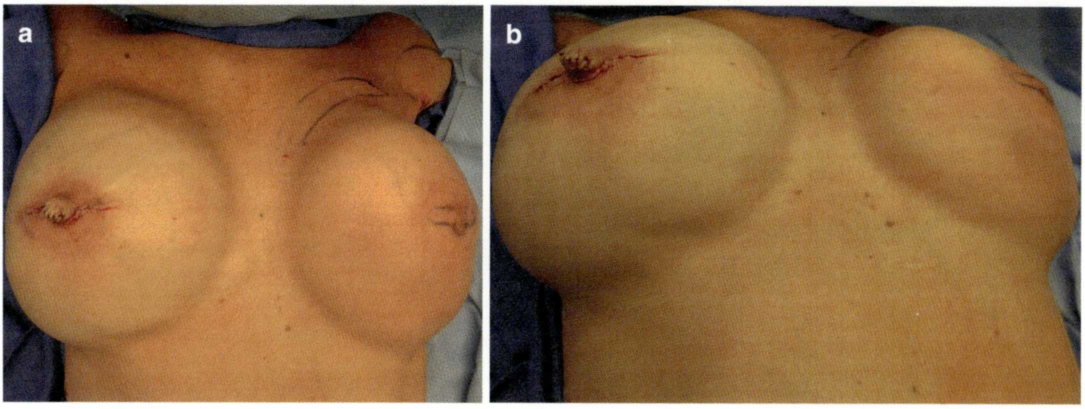


**Fig. 59.4** (**a**, **b**) Secondary nipple reconstruction with repeat spiral wrap on base of failed nipple

## 59.3 Discussion

While all methods of nipple-areolar reconstruction have some risk of early necrosis or late flattening, the spiral wrap method without grafts is as reliable as and more durable than other flap techniques. I have not found that insertion of AlloDerm or fat grafts substantially improves long-term nipple volume or projection. It has great versatility in many applications as shown below in results that are noted at least 1 year after nipple reconstruction. Supple nipples with excellent projection are seen in this tissue expander-implant patient who required two spiral wraps to achieve her goals (Fig. 59.5). Good nipple volume was maintained in this single-stage direct-to-implant patient (Fig. 59.6). The latissimus dorsi skin island over implant is an excellent substrate for natural appearing nipple-areolas (Fig. 59.7). Good symmetry has been achieved in these unilateral DIEP patients (Fig. 59.8). Outcomes in bilateral DIEP cases are quite good (Fig. 59.9).

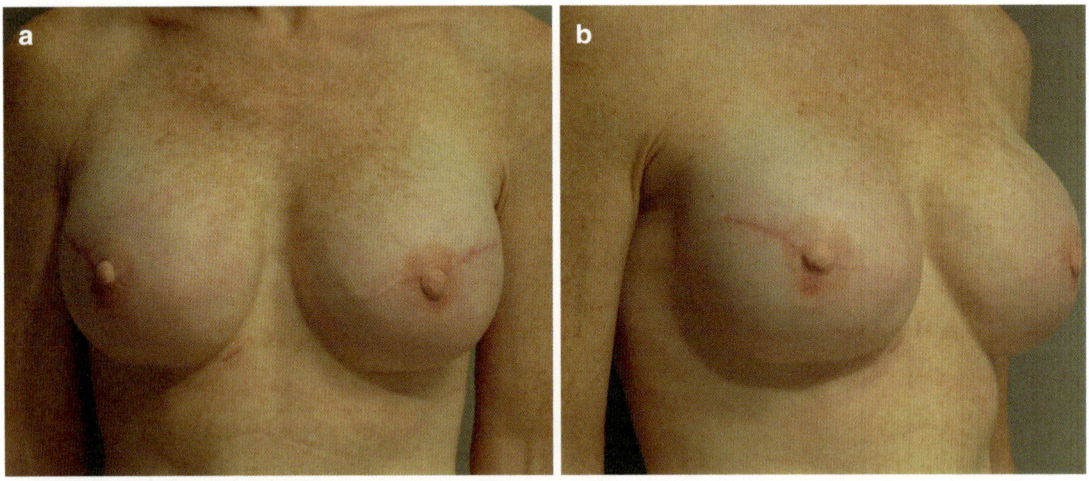


**Fig. 59.5** (**a**, **b**) Supple nipple projection on tissue expander patient

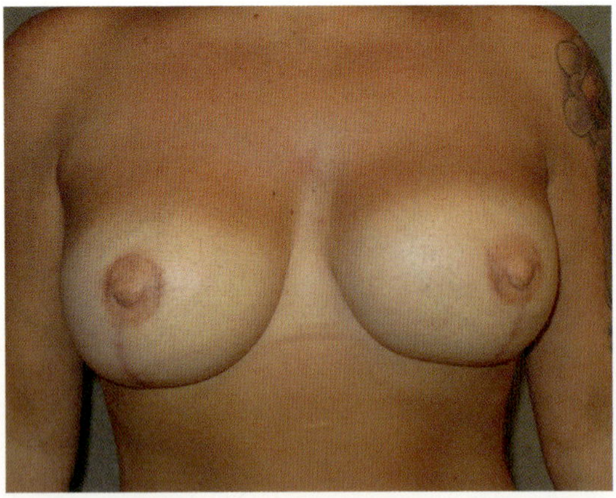

**Fig. 59.6** Good nipple volume on single-stage direct-to-implant patient

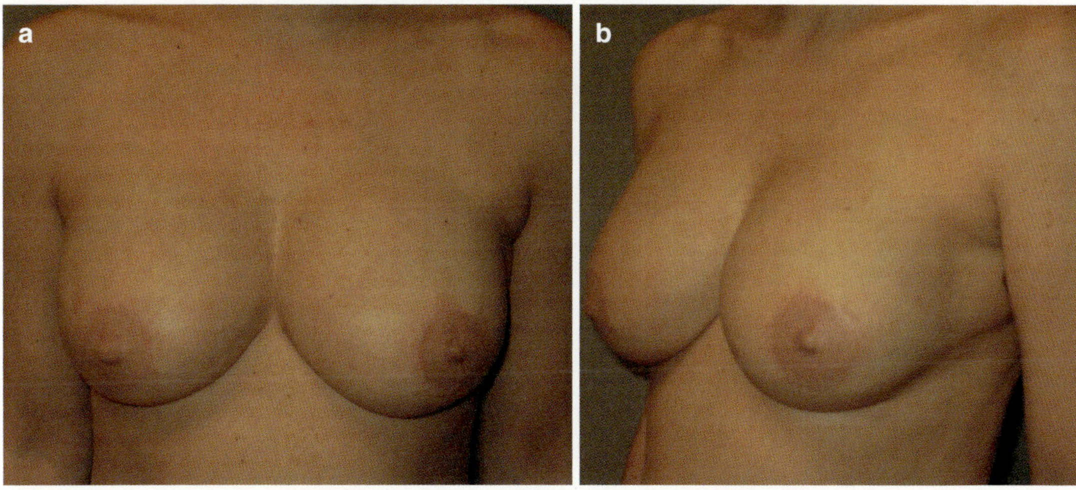


**Fig. 59.7** (**a**, **b**) Natural nipple-areola appearance on latissimus dorsi-implant patient

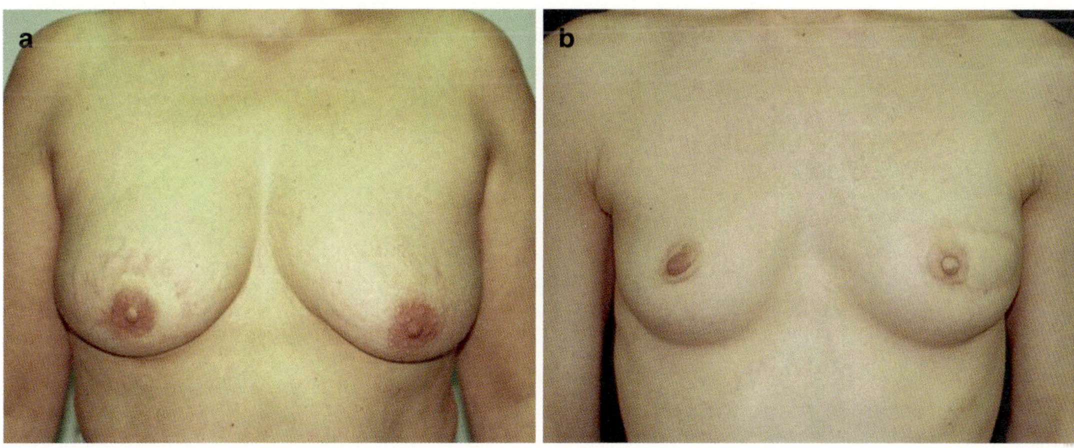


**Fig. 59.8** (**a**, **b**) Symmetric nipple-areola on a right unilateral DIEP patient

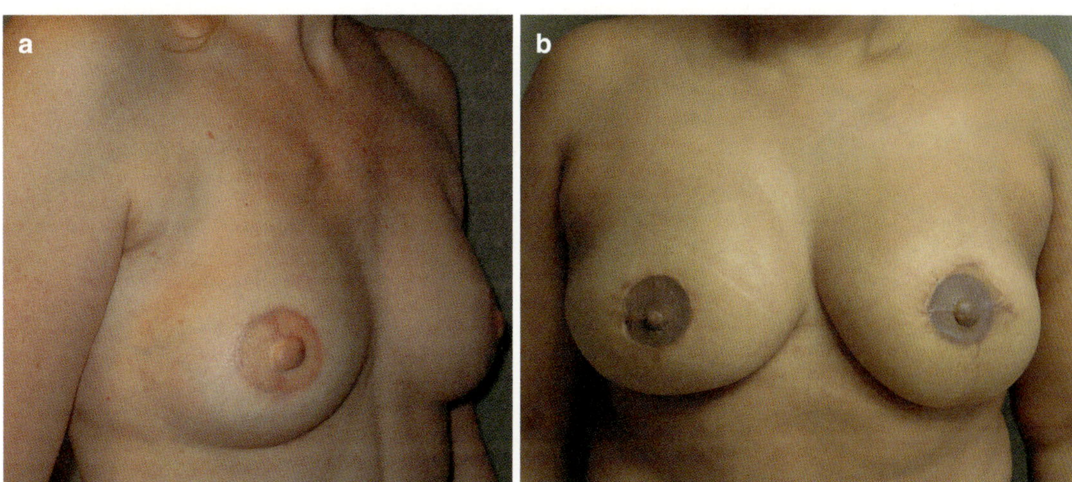


**Fig. 59.9** (**a**, **b**) Bilateral nipple-areola results in a DIEP patient

**Conclusions**

The spiral wrap flap technique is an excellent method of achieving nipple-areola reconstruction with good volume, projection, and durability, without tissue grafts or other donor sites. Like other techniques, revision may be required. It can be adapted in circumstances of radiation therapy and tissue-expanded skin and has great versatility in all types of breast reconstruction.

## References

1. Little JW III. Nipple-areola reconstruction. Clin Plast Surg. 1984;11:351–64.
2. Hammond D, Kuthaila D, Kim J. The skate flap purse-string technique for nipple areola complex reconstruction. Plast Reconstr Surg. 2007;120(2):399–406.
3. Shestak K, Gabriel A, Landecker A. Assessment of long-term nipple projection: a comparison of three techniques. Plast Reconstr Surg. 2002;110(3):780–6.
4. Losken A, Mackay G. Nipple reconstruction using the C-V flap technique: a long-term evaluation. Plast Reconstr Surg. 2001;108(2):361–9.
5. Jones G. Bostwick's plastic and reconstructive surgery. 3rd ed. St. Louis: Quality Medical Publishing; 2010. p. 1663–723.
6. Basu CB, Wahba M, Bullocks JM. Paget disease of a nipple graft following completion of a breast reconstruction with a nipple-sharing technique. Ann Plast Surg. 2008;60:144–5.

# Angel Flap for Nipple Reconstruction

# 60

Wendy W. Wong and Mark C. Martin

## 60.1 Introduction

Breast reconstruction is an important element of physical and psychological healing for women who have battled breast cancer. The creation of a nipple areolar complex (NAC) is the final stage in breast reconstruction. Procedures of this type are essential in giving a reconstructed mound the appearance of an actual breast. The resulting appearance of the reconstructed nipple can significantly contribute to a patient's overall satisfaction with the entire breast reconstruction. In evaluation of the breast, our eyes are naturally drawn to the NAC; for these reasons, it is imperative that reconstruction of this aspect provides a pleasing aesthetic outcome with consistent projection, minimal adjacent tissue distortion, and excellent symmetry.

W.W. Wong, M.D. (✉)
Department of Plastic Surgery, Loma Linda University, 11175 Campus Street, Suite 21126-CP, Loma Linda, CA 92354, USA

Gallery Plastic Surgery, 910 Major Sherman Lane, Suite 305, Monterey, CA 93940, USA
e-mail: galleryplasticsurgery@gmail.com

M.C. Martin, M.D., D.M.D.
Department of Plastic Surgery, Loma Linda University, 11175 Campus Street, Suite 21126-CP, Loma Linda, CA 92354, USA
e-mail: mcmartin@llu.edu

## 60.2 Ideal Nipple Reconstruction

The use of a variety of local tissue flaps has become the primary contemporary technique to reconstruct a nipple. Local flaps preclude the creation of an additional donor site, thereby minimizing perioperative discomfort and associated potential complications. While each local flap exhibits its own advantages, certain common limitations are ubiquitous. The loss of long-term projection is a common shortcoming seen with local flap techniques. Objective measures assessing long-term nipple projection in the literature are sparse, but some studies have cited a long-term loss of projection of 40% or more (Table 60.1) [1–19]. This problem has led many to advocate creating over-projection of the nipple to at least 150% of the contralateral side to allow for loss of projection. This technique is less than ideal, however, because it increases the necessary local tissue required, creating more distortion of the breast mound. Creating a nipple that over-projects also provides an inconsistent result and places a larger demand on the vascular pedicle which is already susceptible to necrosis. There remains a need to identify a simple and reliable method that can be used in all scenarios to create the necessary projection.

The ideal formula for nipple reconstruction would have good texture and shape, maintain long-term nipple projection, and have minimal donor site morbidity. To enhance reproducibility,


M.A. Shiffman (ed.), *Nipple-Areolar Complex Reconstruction*,
https://doi.org/10.1007/978-3-319-60925-6_60

**Table 60.1** Characteristics of the most commonly used flaps for nipple reconstruction

| Flap | Primary component of nipple core | Component of nipple foundation | Challenges with projection |
|---|---|---|---|
| Quadrapod flap [1] | Fat | Fat | Loss of projection |
| Cutaneous fat flap [2] | Fat | Fat | Not described for implant-based breast reconstruction |
| T-flap [3] | Fat | Fat | Decrease in nipple projection |
| Dermal fat flap [4] | Fat | Fat | Requires an additional donor site |
| Pinwheel flap [5] | Fat | Fat | Loss of projection |
| Buried dermal hammock [6] | Fat | Dermis | Inadequate projection |
| Skate flap [7] | Fat | Fat | 40% loss of projection [8] |
| | | | 75% loss of projection [9] |
| S-flap [10] | Fat and dermis | Fat | Contraction of nipple projection |
| Double-opposing tab flaps | Fat | Fat | 66% loss of projection [11] |
| | | | Inadequate projection (average = 2.43 mm) [12] |
| Star flap | Fat | Fat | Inadequate projection (average = 1.97 mm) [12] |
| | | | 77% loss of projection with implant-based breast reconstruction |
| | | | 64% loss of projection with autologous breast reconstruction |
| | | | 40% loss of projection [8] |
| H-flap | Fat | Fat | Decrease in nipple projection |
| Bell flap [16] | Fat | Fat | Unreliable vascular supply |
| | | | 70% loss of projection [8] |
| C-V flap [17] | Fat | Fat | Inadequate projection |
| Arrow flap [18] | Fat | Fat | 51% loss of projection |
| Dermofat graft with C-V flap [19] | Fat and dermis | Dermis | Unreliable vascular supply |

the design should be relatively simple with a short learning curve. When using local tissue, maintaining the base of the flap with an adequate width should be formed to avoid vascular compromise and necrosis. Incisions should be limited to minimize the use of local tissue, which can unaesthetically alter the overall breast shape. Ideal long-term results include adequate nipple projection, an aesthetically pleasing appearance, and satisfactory symmetry with the contralateral nipple. Efforts to fulfill the ideal formula for nipple reconstruction have led the senior author to develop the "angel flap," which is a modification of the skate flap.

## 60.3 Planning of the Nipple Flap

With the patient in a standing position, the new areolar location is determined with consideration of symmetry with the opposite nipple areolar complex if present. To involve the patient in the decision-making process, the patient is often given round electrocardiogram monitoring electrode adhesives and instructed to place them on their breast mound(s) where they think the reconstructed NAC should be. This is performed in front of a mirror in the privacy of a restroom. The patient is informed that their desired NAC position will be taken into account.

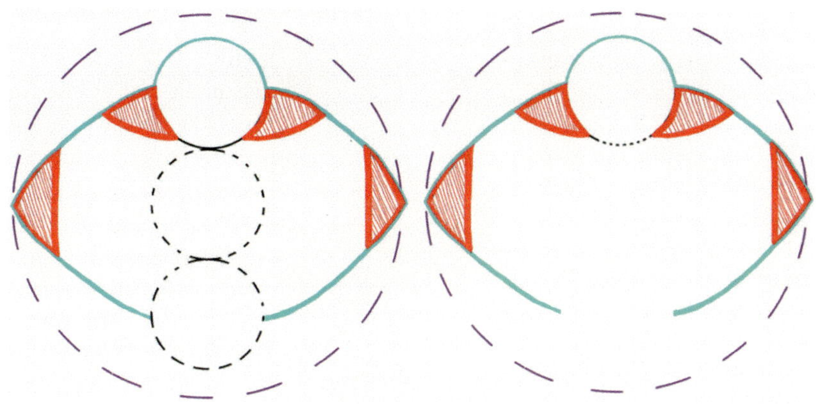

**Fig. 60.1** Design of the angel flap. (*Left*) Outline of the planned future areolar tattooing (*purple*). Depiction of the proposed regions for the incised edges of the flap (*blue*) and regions of de-epithelialization (*red*). (*Right*) The resulting "snow angel" appearance of the flap can be seen

The desired margins of the future circular areola(s) are then drawn to avoid extending incisions beyond the confines of this region. In unilateral reconstructions, the areolar diameter is created equal to the contralateral areola. In bilateral reconstructions, a metal cookie cutter of the desired size is used to guide the desired margins of the future areolas. A column of three circles of equal size is drawn to fit within the areolar marking (Fig. 60.1). The most superior circle will become the nipple tip of this inferiorly based flap, while the two inferior circles determine the nipple height. Next, a horizontal ellipse, extending from the lateral margins of the new areola, is drawn. The horizontal limbs of the ellipse bisect the midpoint of the superior and inferior circles. The planned flap has the shape reminiscent of a snow angel.

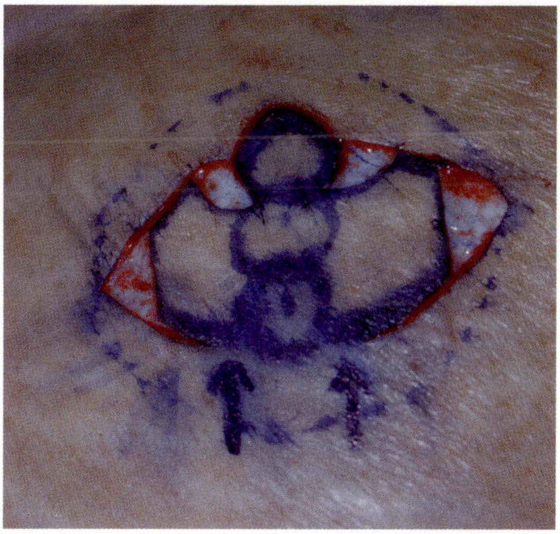

**Fig. 60.2** Angel flap design on a reconstructed breast mound. The de-epithelialization has been performed in the designated areas. The *arrows* indicate the pedicle that is to be preserved

## 60.4 Surgical Technique

Local anesthesia containing epinephrine is infiltrated, and four portions of the flap are de-epithelialized along its lateral "wing" and superior "head" portions as indicated in Fig. 60.1 and shown in Fig. 60.2. The flap is incised full thickness through the dermis, leaving an inferiorly based pedicle. Care must be taken to create upper and lower flap edges of equal length. The flap comprising the "wings" and "head" of the snow angel is elevated with approximately 2 mm of subcutaneous fat to ensure preservation of the subdermal plexus within it (Figs. 60.3 and 60.4). The lateral wings are brought together with the de-epithelialized portions conjoining and sutured together with 5-0 chromic sutures while inverting the de-epithelialized portions for support. The cylindrical core of the reconstructed nipple is composed of primarily dermis and also is made of a dermal

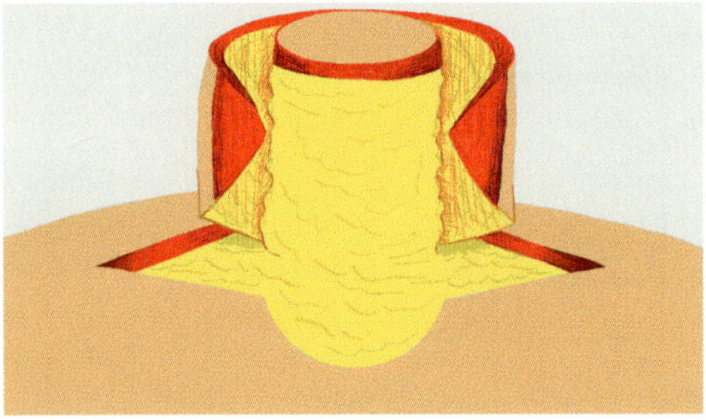

**Fig. 60.3** Elevation of the angel flap and formation of the nipple (view from inferior aspect of the breast)

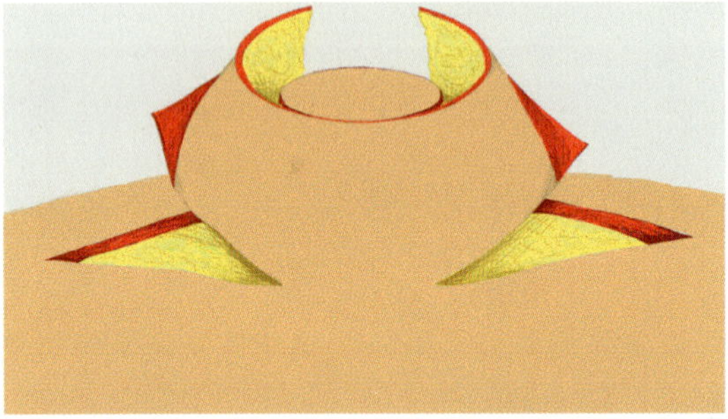

**Fig. 60.4** Elevation of the angel flap and formation of the nipple (view from superior aspect of the breast)

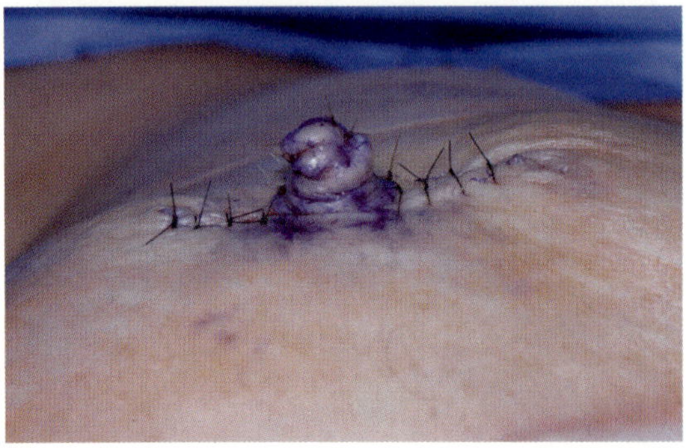

**Fig. 60.5** Immediate postoperative of a patient prior to placement of protective dressings

base (Fig. 60.5). The two de-epithelialized areas adjacent to the top of the nipple are tucked, which allow the edges of the nipple top to be approximated to the inferior aspect of the two de-epithelialized edges. The top of the nipple is laid onto the dermis-filled column and closed with absorbable 4-0 poliglecaprone sutures. The transverse incisions, still within the confines of the future areola, are approximated and sutured with 4-0 poliglecaprone sutures. A foam bolster is made and applied around the nipple to support the reconstruction. This also prevents contraction by avoiding anterior compressive forces from brassieres and clothing.

Postoperatively, patients are instructed to apply bacitracin ointment on the incisions and avoid pressure on the reconstructed nipple(s) until their follow-up visit. Approximately 8 weeks after this later, the appearance of an areola is tattooed around the reconstructed nipple.

## 60.5 Benefits of the Angel Flap

The design of the angel flap addresses the major problem of long-term diminished nipple projection associated with use of other local flaps. Flattening of the reconstructed nipple is thought to be multifactorial in etiology. One of such factors may be the centrifugal forces on the breast with the weight of the breast pushing against the reconstructed nipple base. Stress is placed on the minimal amount of dermal lining of the skin flaps, and local tissue loss through necrosis and atrophy leads to nipple contraction and subsequent flattening over time. Other local flaps may have a tenuous blood supply or lack of tissue of structural integrity. Flaps that create a nipple core and base of primarily fat rather than dense connective tissue make them susceptible to projection loss [20, 21]. Other techniques using various materials (e.g., cartilage grafts, buried dermal hammocks, acellular dermal matrix) have attempted to bolster the flaps to increase projection [22, 23]. However, if the base of the nipple is comprised primarily of fat, the tissue undergoes variable amount of necrosis, making any additional efforts to support the fat inconsequential. The current practice of using fat as the major component and structural support for nipple reconstruction may explain why flaps have unsuccessfully maintained long-term projection. The dermal foundation of the angel flap ameliorates this problem compared with these other methods. Long-lasting projection of the angel flap can be attributed to the longer height in the flap design and nipple core also being comprised primarily of dermis. This ultimately translates to high patient satisfaction (Figs. 60.6 and 60.7).

Another benefit of the angel flap is the design of the relatively wide base, which enhances vascularity and minimizes the potential of necrosis of the reconstructed nipple. A reliable blood supply is also necessary for viability of the dermal core. Lastly, keeping the entire design within the confines of the future areolar circumference prevents undesirable extension of scars past this margin. Keeping the transverse scars short minimizes the amount of local tissue necessary for reconstruction, thereby preserving the aesthetic shape of the breast mound. Natural appearing nipples are created with primary closure, precluding the need for skin grafts. The unpredictable pigmentation of skin grafts and additional donor sites are avoided.

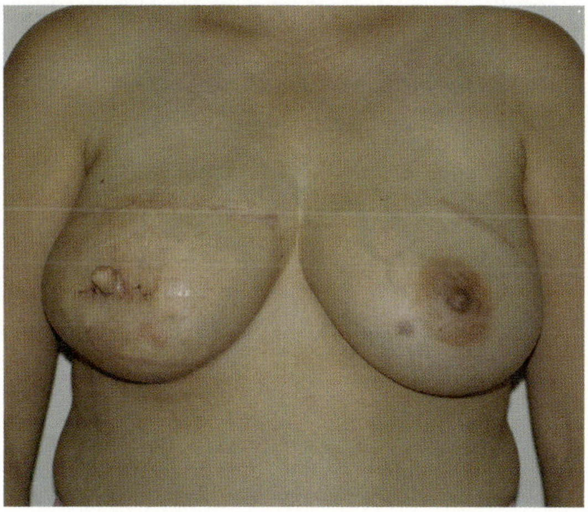

**Fig. 60.6** Three-week postoperative patient with good nipple projection following left nipple reconstruction with angel flap technique

The angel flap offers several essential benefits, one of which is long-lasting projection and preservation of overall breast mound aesthetics. We have had consistent, excellent results and high patient satisfaction in using this flap for nipple reconstruction.

## References


1. Little JW III, Munasifi T, McCulloch DT. One-stage reconstruction of a projecting nipple: the quadrapod flap. Plast Reconstr Surg. 1983;7:126–33.
2. Bosch G, Ramirez M. Reconstruction of the nipple: a new technique. Plast Reconstr Surg. 1984;73:977–81.
3. Chang WH. Nipple reconstruction with a T flap. Plast Reconstr Surg. 1984;73(1):140–3.
4. Hartrampf CR Jr. A dermal-fat flap for nipple reconstruction. Plast Reconstr Surg. 1984;73:982–6.
5. Cohen IK, Ward JA, Chandrasekhar B. The pinwheel flap nipple and barrier areola graft reconstruction. Plast Reconstr Surg. 1986;77:995–9.


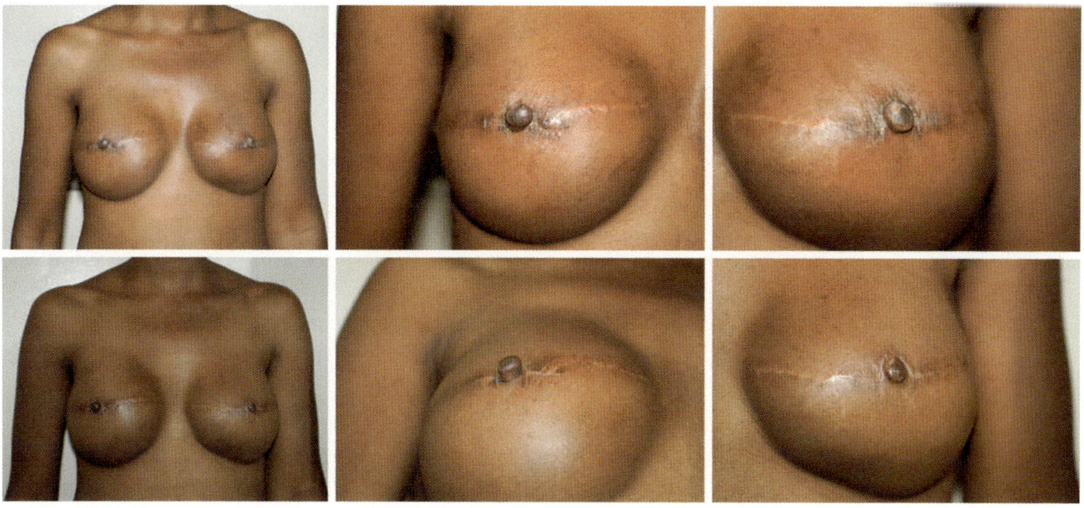

**Fig. 60.7** (*Top*) A patient showing typical results of the angel flap technique 4 weeks postoperatively. (*Bottom*) Twelve weeks postoperatively. Good nipple projection is seen with an overall pleasing aesthetic result

6. Mukherjee RP, Gottlieb V, Hacker L. Nipple-areolar reconstruction with the buried dermal hammock technique. Ann Plast Surg. 1987;3:421–3.
7. Little JW III. Nipple-areolar reconstruction. Clin Plast Surg. 1984;11:351–64.
8. Shestak KC, Gabriel A, Landecker A, Peters S, Shestak A, Kim J. Assessment of long-term nipple projection: a comparison of three techniques. Plast Reconstr Surg. 2002;110:780–6.
9. Zhong T, Antony A, Cordeiro P. Surgical outcomes and nipple projection using the modified skate flap for nipple-areolar reconstruction in a series of 422 implant reconstructions. Ann Plast Surg. 2009;623:591–5.
10. Cronin ED, Humphreys DH, Ruiz-Razura A. Nipple reconstruction: the S flap. Plast Reconstr Surg. 1988;81:783–7.
11. Kroll SS, Hamilton S. Nipple reconstruction with the double opposing-tab flap. Plast Reconstr Surg. 1989;84:520–5.
12. Kroll SS, Reece GP, Miller MJ, Evans GR, Robb GL, Baldwin BJ, Wang BG, Schusterman MA. Comparison of nipple projection with the modified double-opposing tab and star flaps. Plast Reconstr Surg. 1997;99:1602–5.
13. Anton LE, Hartrampf CR. Nipple reconstruction with local flaps: star and wrap flaps. Perspect Plast Surg. 1991;5:67–78.
14. Banducci DR, Le TK, Hughes KC. Long-term follow-up of a modified Anton-Hartrampf nipple reconstruction. Ann Plast Surg. 1999;43:467–70.
15. Hallock GG, Altobelli JA. Cylindrical nipple reconstruction using an H flap. Ann Plast Surg. 1993;30:23–6.
16. Eng J. Bell flap nipple reconstruction—a new wrinkle. Ann Plast Surg. 1996;36:485–8.
17. Losken GM, Bostwick J III. Nipple reconstruction using the C-V flap technique: a long-term evaluation. Plast Reconstr Surg. 2001;108:361–9.
18. Rubino CLD, Posadinu A. A modified technique for nipple reconstruction: the "arrow flap". Br J Plast Surg. 2003;56:247–51.
19. Eo SK, Da Lio AL. Nipple reconstruction with a C-V flap using dermofat graft. Ann Plast Surg. 2007;58:137–40.
20. Schwager RG, Smith JW, Gray GF, Goulian D Jr. Inversion of the human female nipple, with a simple method of treatment. Plast Reconstr Surg. 1974;54:564–9.
21. Pribaz JJ, Pousti T. Correction of recurrent nipple inversion with cartilage graft. Ann Plast Surg. 1998;40:14–27.
22. Brent B, Bostwick J. Nipple-areolar reconstruction with auricular tissues. Plast Reconstr Surg. 1977;60:353–61.
23. Garramone CE, Lam B. Use of AlloDerm in primary nipple reconstruction to improve long-term nipple projection. Plast Reconstr Surg. 2007;119:1663–8.

# Arrow Flap and Rib Cartilage Graft for Nipple-Areola Complex Restoration

# 61

Aldo B. Guerra, Stephen E. Metzinger, and Robert J. Allen

## 61.1 Introduction

Creation of the nipple-areola complex (NAC) is a fundamental step in the process of breast restoration after mastectomy [1]. The endpoint of the reconstructive process is often marked by the creation of the new nipple several months after the breast mound has been restored. Restoration of the nipple complex has been reported to increase the satisfaction rates with the appearance of the new breasts, improve self-esteem, and lead to other psychological benefits for cancer patients [2–5]. Over the years, many techniques have been developed using dermal flaps for nipple reconstruction [6–9]. Similarly, we have previously discussed the arrow flap as a successful method of NAC restoration [10].

A.B. Guerra, M.D. (✉)
Guerra Plastic Surgery Center, 8765 E. Bell Road, Suite 104, Scottsdale, AZ 85260, USA
e-mail: Drguerra@gmail.com

S.E. Metzinger, M.D.
Aesthetic Surgical Associates, 3223 8th Street, Suite 200, Metairie, LA 70002, USA
e-mail: Metzingermd@cox.net

R.J. Allen, M.D.
The Center for Microsurgical Breast Reconstruction, 2525 Severn Avenue, 4th Floor, Metairie, LA 70002, USA
e-mail: boballen@diepflap.com

We have also relied on autologous tissue reconstruction to restore a breast shape that feels, looks, and best resembles the native breast. The preferred methods include the use of deep inferior epigastric (DIEP) and gluteal artery perforator (GAP) flaps for breast reconstruction with microvascular anastomosis to the internal mammary vessels [11, 12]. In the process of recipient vessel exposure, a segment of rib cartilage requires removal, and this can be used to produce a more rigid and projecting nipple reconstruction when combined with appropriate soft tissue coverage.

The advantage of dermal skin flaps for nipple restoration is that many options are readily available to plastic surgeons in the newly reconstructed breasts, and these are relatively simple to construct with an appropriate design. A disadvantage of dermal flaps is that over time, nipple projection is lost, and this can lead to inconsistent results and increased patient dissatisfaction [13]. Achieving long-term nipple projection was therefore a motivating factor for the incorporation of a small but rigid cartilage graft to support our preferred dermal flap reconstruction technique. The rib cartilage graft provides a supporting scaffold to resist contractural forces in the soft tissue envelope that contribute to loss of neo-nipple projection over time.

The arrow flap is a random skin flap and receives its blood supply from the subdermal plexus of vessels of the newly reconstructed


M.A. Shiffman (ed.), *Nipple-Areolar Complex Reconstruction*,
https://doi.org/10.1007/978-3-319-60925-6_61

breast skin. The arrow flap has a reliable blood supply and can be combined with a rib cartilage graft to improve nipple projection. The closure of the vertical limb of the arrow flap occurs at 45° angles and resembles a W-plasty configuration, which redistributes the forces of contraction to minimize the risks of soft tissue collapse in the future.

In our hands, using the combination of an arrow flap with an underlying carved rib cartilage scaffold support, we have achieved an aesthetically pleasing nipple reconstruction that is highly gratifying over time.

## 61.2 Surgical Technique

### 61.2.1 Obtaining the Rib Cartilage Graft

The reconstruction of the nipple-areola complex (NAC) is delayed until after the initial breast reconstruction to allow for resolution of edema within the soft tissue flap. This technique of nipple restoration can be carried out with any soft tissue reconstruction, although we prefer to use perforator flaps with microvascular anastomosis to the internal mammary vessels for breast reconstruction. During the initial free tissue transfer, the internal mammary vessels are usually exposed by excision of the third rib cartilage at the costochondral junction to the sternochondral joint. To minimize the risks of pneumothorax and exposure of other underlying structures, the dissection of the rib cartilage is performed in a subperichondrial plane. Once the perichondrial plane is dissected anteriorly and the rib is exposed, a small segment of the costochondral junction is teased away with a rongeur. This is done carefully and under direct visualization to avoid penetrating below the plane of the posterior perichondrium. The surgeon can then introduce a blunt periosteal dissector to allow elevation of the rib cartilage. The cartilage is gently disarticulated from the sternochondral joint, removed as one intact piece and placed in a saline-soaked gauze until it is "banked" for later use in NAC reconstruction in a second stage procedure. With closure of the breast flap, the rib cartilage segment is placed between the deepithelialized breast flap and the chest wall skin, where it remains palpable until the second stage (Fig. 61.1). We make a routine to place the cartilage in the same position on the new breast where it can be readily localized at the time of nipple reconstruction.

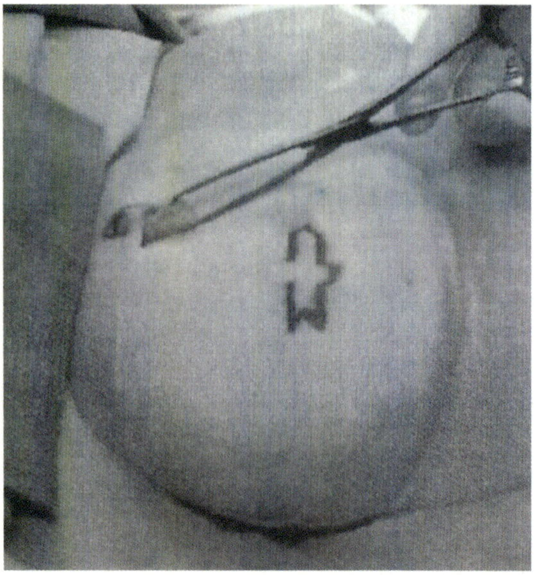

**Fig. 61.1** The banked rib cartilage segment is readied for nipple reconstruction

The rib cartilage segment can be sizeable, and so it is rare to observe resorption or warping of the cartilage graft in the months between reconstruction stages. Carving of the cartilage segment into the ideal shape is done with great care and begins by outlining with a surgical pen the desired thickness and level of projection (Fig. 61.2). The cartilage segment is then readily carved using a 15 blade. The first step involves removal of any remaining perichondrium along with the outer layer of cartilage to minimize the risks of warping [14]. Then, a relatively wide and stable base is planned out and carved with at least a 10 mm diameter. This stabilizing base has ranged from 10 to 15 mm in diameter. A projecting arm of cartilage is also carved in the center of the base which measures at least 15 mm in length (Fig. 61.3). The projecting arm of the cartilage can later be trimmed to the desired final projection based on the agreed upon plan with the patient.

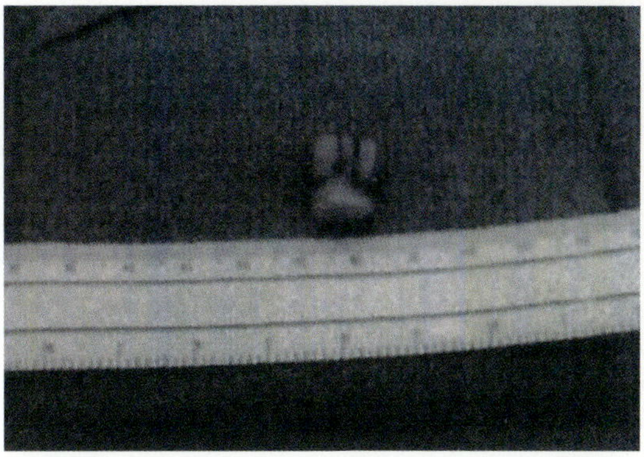

**Fig. 61.2** Carving of the cartilage segment begins by outlining with a surgical pen the desired thickness and level of projection

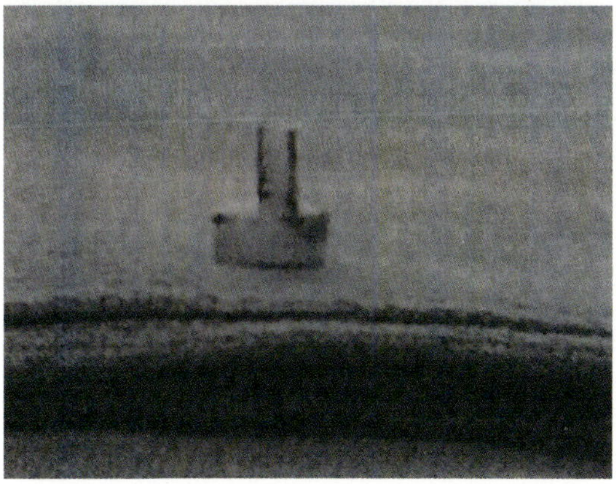

**Fig. 61.3** A wide and stable base is planned out and carved with at least a 10 mm diameter. A projecting arm of cartilage is also carved measuring at least 15 mm in length

### 61.2.2 Elevation of the Arrow Flap

Markings for the nipple-areola reconstruction are drawn on the breast with the patient in an upright position. We typically choose a point of greatest breast mound projection in the new breast. The arrow flap receives its blood supply from the dermal plexus of the newly reconstructed breast skin and is considered to be a random skin flap. The orientation of the base of the flap can face any direction, but for convenience and familiarity, we generally placed the base of the flap in a superior location (Fig. 61.4). The base of the flap must allow robust oxygen and nutrient delivery to the elevated component and should be at least 15 mm wide. The two lateral skin flaps, which will make up the cylindrical body of the new nipple and contribute to the level of nipple projection, are designed to be 20 mm in length. These lateral skin flaps resemble the shape of an arrow and is where the technique derives its name. The width of the lateral flaps can measure between 10 and 15 mm overall. The native opposite nipple complex can serve as a gauge for selecting the final flap width which will help to determine the level of projection on the newly reconstructed nipple. Because of the potential for skin flap contracture, the width of the lateral flaps should be designed at least 25% longer than desired. The "roof" of the new nipple complex is created by an extension of skin which lies directly opposite the flap base (Fig. 61.5). Since this segment of the flap is farthest from the base, it is critical to design the "roof" to an appropriate width (at least 10 mm) in order to achieve good oxygenation and healing while minimizing the risks of cartilage exposure.

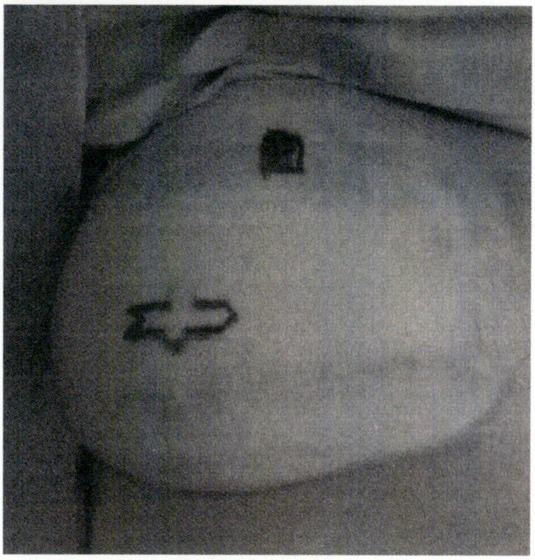

**Fig. 61.4** The orientation of the base of the flap can face any direction, but we generally placed the base of the flap in a superior location

Dissection begins by incising the skin and elevating the flap below the level of the subcutaneous fat plane. Leaving a small layer of fatty tissue on the underside of the flap will help preserve the dermal plexus. If the subdermal vessels that supply the flap are inadvertently exposed during dissection, conservative use of electrocautery

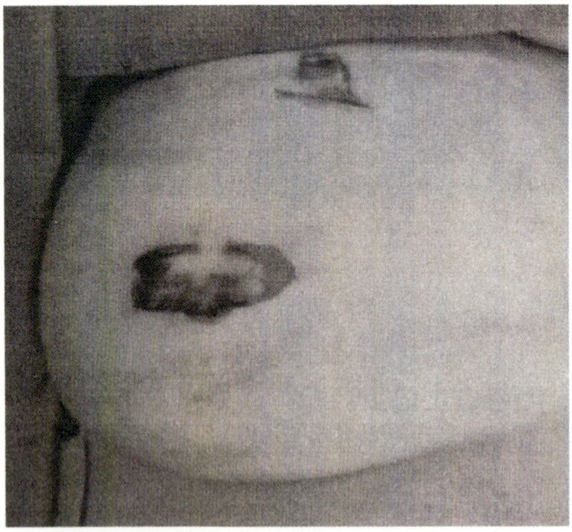

**Fig. 61.5** The "roof" of the new nipple complex is created by an extension of skin which lies opposite the flap base and is farthest from the base. A "roof" width design of at least 10 mm is needed to achieve good healing while minimizing the risks of cartilage exposure

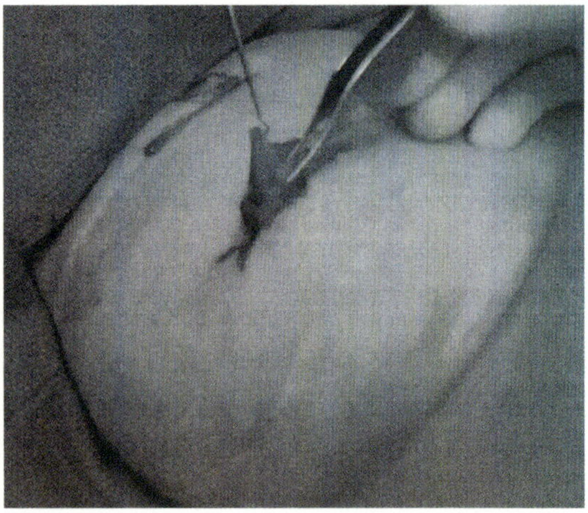

**Fig. 61.6** The carved cartilage is placed on the breast tissue at the level of the subcutaneous fatty component, and the skin flaps are then wrapped around the projecting cartilage arm

should be employed. As the dissection approaches the base of the flap, the plane of dissection is expanded to include more subcutaneous fatty tissue. The flap should always be handled with extreme care. This is especially important over the "roof" extension where the blood supply and oxygenation delivery can be tenuous. The donor site for the lateral flaps should be closed with two layers of suture before making an assessment of the arrow flap mobility. The ends of the flap should then be able to come together nicely without any tension and still offer plenty of space for the cartilage graft. Rarely, back cutting into the flap base is necessary to increase mobility and to allow the cartilage graft to be fully wrapped by tissue. This step should be done with extreme care to avoid compromising any vascularity.

Because the skin of the newly created breast is usually insensate, the procedure may be offered in an office setting using only local anesthesia for some patients. Because the arrow flap is a relatively small random flap, we routinely avoid using epinephrine for these cases. Intravenous sedation and general anesthesia are employed in cases involving our technique of nipple reconstruction with either donor site revisions, fat grafting, and/or when contralateral breast surgery are performed for symmetry in an operating room setting.

### 61.2.3 Developing the Cartilage-Arrow Flap Interaction

Creating the appropriate interaction between the soft tissue flap and the cartilage is another important step when using this technique. Once the arrow flap has been fully dissected, the carved cartilage graft is placed on the breast tissue at the level of the subcutaneous fatty component, and the skin flaps are then wrapped around the projecting cartilage arm (Fig. 61.6). The stabilizing wide base of the cartilage segment will therefore lie below the donor site and neo-nipple skin flap closure. This technique will give stability to the soft tissues as they project out from the breast mound. The arrow flap has a male end and a female end, and these ends of the flap fit ideally into each other at 45° angles. The final closure and position of the incision lines are able to break up any contractile forces by avoiding the formation of linear incisions on the vertical closure. Alternatively, the geometric final suture line of the arrow flap resembles a W-plasty configuration in the vertical limb of the newly reconstructed nipple. This is a straightforward soft tissue flap design and an elegant method to break up the potential for contractile forces which could later limit nipple projection (Fig. 61.7).

The "roof" segment of the arrow flap is then brought over the top of the neo-nipple and

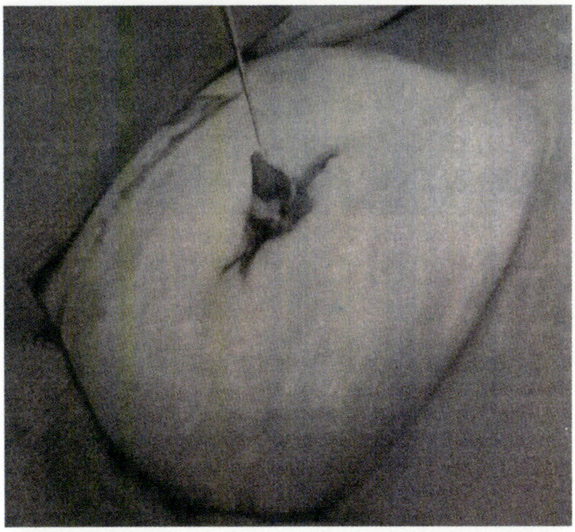

**Fig. 61.7** The arrow flap limbs fit ideally into each other at 45° angles. The final closure and position of the incision lines break up any contractile forces by avoiding the formation of linear incisions on the vertical closure

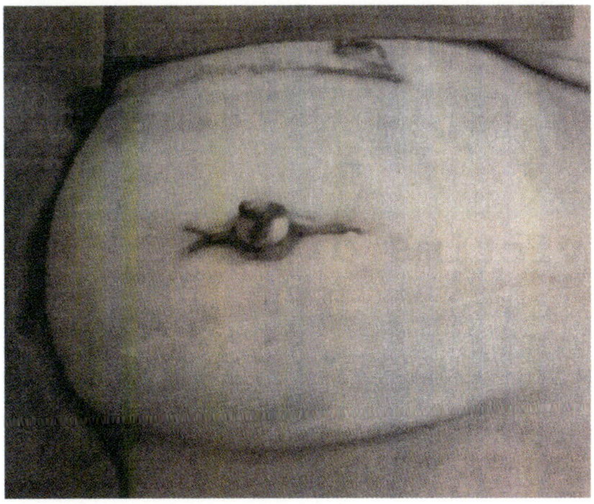

**Fig. 61.8** The "roof" segment of the arrow flap is then brought over the top of the neo-nipple and completely covers the cartilage graft

completely covers the cartilage graft (Fig. 61.8). It is necessary to sometimes trim the projecting cartilage arm in order to avoid generating too much pressure on the "roof" component and causing ischemia or necrosis. Skin closure on the neo-nipple is performed with simple, interrupted, absorbable, or nonabsorbable suture, depending on surgeon's preference.

Like other dermal flaps in the breasts, the dissection and elevation of the arrow flap is straightforward and reliable. However, complications have been observed including exposure and eventual loss of the cartilage graft in 18 out of 454 total breasts. When cartilage graft exposure was seen, it was associated with dehiscence of the skin flaps. Pressure from an inappropriately trimmed projecting cartilage arm was the most common cause of partial skin flap ischemia and eventual wound dehiscence. We also observed the less pliable skin found in the gluteal flap to be a contributing factor in wound dehiscence. Contour irregularities in the donor site for the cartilage graft are also problematic for patients with a low body mass index (BMI). Removing a smaller rib segment and avoiding the use of these techniques in patients with a BMI less than 19 can lead to less donor site morbidity. Additionally, fat grafting has emerged as a viable technique to camouflage contour irregularities at the donor site.

## 61.3 Discussion

Nipple-areola reconstruction is a key component of the breast reconstruction experience and plays a critical role in providing the breast with a natural appearance (Fig. 61.9). Multiple dermal flap techniques have been advanced to recreate this aesthetic focal point on the breast [15–18]. While initially successful at creating an aesthetic and projecting nipple complex, with time, shrinkage of the tissue and loss of projection occur. A study comparing normal nipples to inverted nipples suggests that a supportive network of connective tissue beneath the nipple is important in the maintenance of projection [19]. Histopathologic examinations comparing normal to inverted nipples demonstrated the connective tissue density of 8 mm in normal nipples, while inverted nipples had a density as low as 4 mm. To the authors, this was highly suggestive that normal nipple projection may be due to the presence of a greater bulk of dense connective tissue locally. In other words, a lack of adequate rigid connective tissue support locally underneath the nipple can be implicated in the loss of nipple projection [19]. Additionally, surgically created nipples also suffer from scar contracture with centrifugal forces acting on the new nipple to reduce projection further [20].

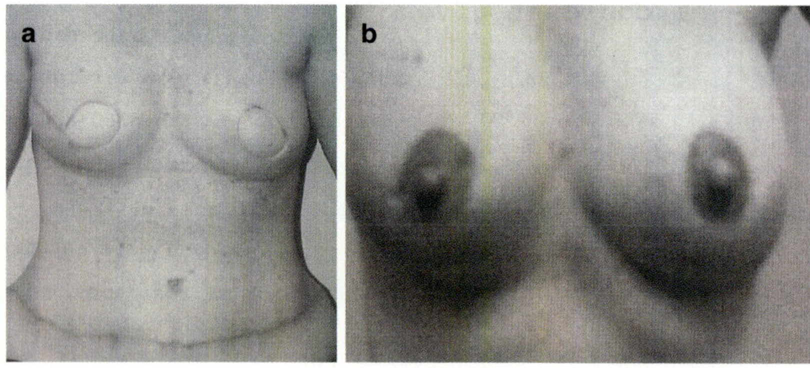

**Fig. 61.9** (**a**) Before nipple reconstruction with the arrow flap and carved rib cartilage technique. (**b**) Four years after nipple reconstruction using the arrow flap and carved rib cartilage technique

Based on these and our own observations, a logical conclusion was that replacement of this rigid tissue structure with an equally rigid scaffold would lead to lasting projection in reconstructed nipples [10]. This is supported by a recent systematic review comparing different methods used to increase nipple projection. In this review, the authors identified seven autologous graft types, five synthetic materials, and three allogenic materials used in nipple reconstruction [21]. Ear and rib cartilage, labia minora, dermal graft, fat graft, and toe pulp were some of the autologous options listed. On the other hand, the non-autologous list included acellular dermal matrix, lyophilized cartilage, silicone, polytetrafluoroethylene, hydroxylapatite, and other materials. The results of the review yielded a heterogeneity of materials used and inconsistent methodologies in the 31 publications which met the study criteria for quality and outcome measurement. They did conclude, however, that synthetic materials have higher complication rates, while allogenic and autologous grafts appear to have comparable nipple projection results [21]. Allogenic grafts can increase the material costs of surgery but may have less overall morbidity by bypassing a donor site.

Autologous grafts are attractive as they are readily available and typically associated with minimal donor site morbidity. Brent et al. [22] first reported the use of autologous ear cartilage in an effort to augment nipple projection. Rolled cartilage grafts combined with a bilobed and trilobed dermal flap technique were also reported in a previous publication [23]. The authors advocated the bilobed flap technique over the trilobed due to less issues with ischemia. Projection of the nipple was found to be improved with the rolled cartilage matrix support. Other investigators have reported long-lasting nipple projection with ear cartilage grafts for reconstructed breasts [24]. In the difficult recurrent inverted nipple, cartilage grafts worked well to supplement the lack of underlying support matrix and resulted in good overall projection [20]. The use of carved rib cartilage under a dermal flap was confirmed to improve the results of nipple projection in a prospective study involving 17 reconstructive patients [25]. The authors reported that 13 out of 17 patients judged their results to be very good with the average patient losing about 25% of the initial projection in the first postoperative year. Considering that isolated dermal flaps can show shrinkage in the range of 50–70% overall loss of projection, the authors felt that rib augmentation of nipple reconstruction to be a viable and reproducible option [13, 25].

We believe the design of a dermal flap used in nipple reconstruction should help to reduce the forces of wound contracture acting on the skin envelope [10]. These forces, over time, will create a dramatic contribution to the loss of nipple projection [16]. With the arrow flap, these intrinsic forces are redistributed into a W-shaped vertical incision when the male end of the flap is sutured in the female end of the flap (Fig. 61.10). There are no linear scars in the vertical vector of nipple projection, and instead, the new scar develops at the interface of the flap edges at 45° angles. This technique is similar to other well-established skin-fat flaps like the C-V flap [17]. We prefer to have areolar dermopigmentation performed once

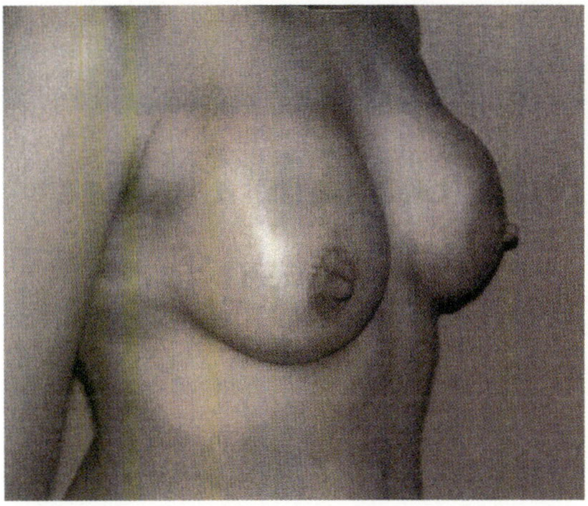

**Fig. 61.10** One year after nipple reconstruction using the arrow flap and carved rib cartilage technique. The DIEP flap was used to create the breast mound

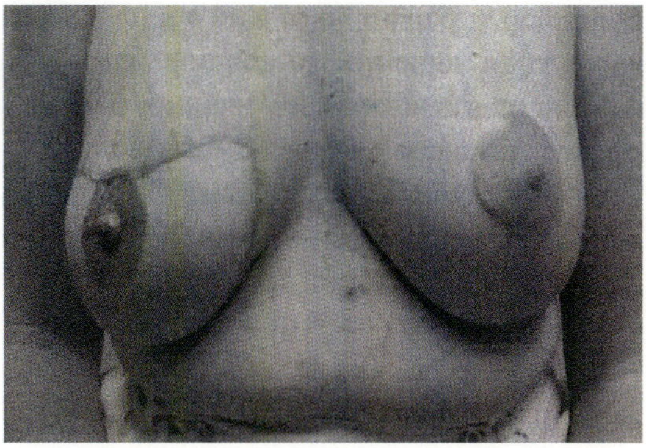

**Fig. 61.11** Results of nipple reconstruction using the arrow flap and carved rib cartilage technique. Excellent results from dermopigmentation and nipple projection is seen in the final result

the nipple has fully healed, and we make an effort to avoid skin graft reconstruction of the areola and having a second donor site [26].

The internal mammary vessels are the most common recipient blood vessels in free flap breast reconstruction. These vessels have extremely reliable anatomy and useable vessel diameter [27]. Using the internal mammary vessels routinely as recipients requires removal of rib cartilage to access their location [28]. With rib removal, there is always a risk the patient may develop a contour irregularity at the donor site. We recommend only removing the amount of rib necessary to carry out nipple reconstruction while appropriately accessing the vessels to accomplish microvascular anastomosis. We also find that thin patients with a BMI below 19 may be at higher risks of having contour problems in the donor region. Several strategies can work to reduce the risks of contour problems including replacing part of the rib or remnants of the rib in patients [29]. Remnants of rib not used for the nipple reconstruction may be cut into small pieces and placed in the rib space. The possibility of pneumothorax exists when positive pressure ventilation is used [30]. There is also an association between aesthetic and reconstructive breast surgery and the development of pneumothorax [31–33]. Removal of a cartilage graft should always be done carefully in order to reduce the risks of pneumothorax. Additionally, plastic surgeons should be well rehearsed in the techniques to diagnose, treat, and manage intraoperative pneumothorax.

Exposure of rib cartilage is usually noted in the early postoperative period and is a serious complication. Exposure of the cartilage usually implies the graft will eventually be lost, but some (two out 20) were saved with oral antibiotics, antibiotic irrigation, and flap re-advancement. The real determinant of cartilage graft loss is infection. Once the diagnosis of infection is made either by culture or clinical criteria, then the graft must be removed and will not be salvaged. Every attempt should be made during flap insetting to reduce pressure on the "roof" segment which can result in ischemia at the edges of the skin flap and increase the chance of cartilage exposure. Trimming more cartilage than necessary is a better alternative than exposure. We learned early that buttock skin is not as pliable leading to a greater risk of cartilage exposure when GAP flaps are used in breast reconstruction. We observed that 60% of documented exposures occurred with GAP flaps. Additionally, the dermis of GAP flaps is thicker, so a cartilage graft may not be necessary to obtain and maintain long-term projection. We no longer place cartilage for nipple reconstruction in gluteal flaps as a result of these lessons learned. DIEP flaps, on the other hand, continue to benefit from the rigidity that a cartilage graft can provide for nipple projection (Fig. 61.11).

## Conclusions

In order to establish improved results of nipple areola reconstruction, plastic surgeons have offered a myriad of techniques involving soft tissue flaps, with and without an underlying scaffold support. In the healthy nipple, normal projection is supported by a bulky underlying matrix of connective tissue. It makes sense, therefore, that our surgical options should attempt to replicate, with alternative materials, this supportive tissue matrix. The combination of a carved rib cartilage graft and an arrow flap, strategically designed to counter the effects of secondary wound contracture, is a viable alternative for nipple reconstruction in achieving long-term nipple projection. The arrow flap is similar to other random flaps and has a reliable blood supply. The flap dissection is straightforward, and its closure at 45° angles allows the scar to be broken into a W-configuration with diminution of wound contractile forces. With low donor-site morbidity, we advocate the use of rib cartilage grafts, which are routinely obtained during the breast reconstruction process and are banked until the time of nipple-areola reconstruction. Because loss of nipple projection over time continues to torment our efforts, this rigid autologous tissue scaffold is used as a substitute for the dense connective tissue normally found in the healthy and projecting nipple complex. We have shown that with our technique, restoration of an aesthetically pleasing breast is readily achievable, along with long-term maintenance of nipple projection.

## References


1. Little JW III. Nipple-areola reconstruction. Clin Plast Surg. 1984;11:351–64.
2. Yueh JH, Houlihan MJ, Slavin SA, Lee BT, Pories SE, Morris DJ. Nipple-sparing mastectomy: evaluation of patient satisfaction, aesthetic results, and sensation. Ann Plast Surg. 2009;62:586–90.
3. Alderman AK, Wilkins EG, Lowery JC, Kim M, Davis JA. Determinants of patient satisfaction in postmastectomy breast reconstruction. Plast Reconstr Surg. 2000;106:769–76.
4. Momoh AO, Colakoglu S, de Blacam C, Yueh JH, Lin SJ, Tobias AM, Lee BT. The impact of nipple reconstruction on patient satisfaction in breast reconstruction. Ann Plast Surg. 2012;69:389–93.
5. Wellisch DK, Schain WS, Noone RB, Little JW III. The psychological contribution of nipple addition in breast reconstruction. Plast Reconstr Surg. 1987;80:699–704.
6. Anton MR, Eskenazi LB, Hartrampf CR Jr. Nipple reconstruction with local flaps: star and wrap flaps. Perspect Plast Surg. 1991;5:67–74.
7. Eskenazi LB. A one-stage nipple reconstruction with the "modified star" flap and immediate tattoo: a review of 100 cases. Plast Reconstr Surg. 1993;92:671–80.
8. Hartampf CR Jr, Culbertson JH. A dermal-fat flap for nipple reconstruction. Plast Reconstr Surg. 1984;73:982–6.
9. Kroll SS, Hamilton S. Nipple reconstruction with the double-opposing tab flap. Plast Reconstr Surg. 1989;84:520–5.
10. Guerra AB, Khoobehi K, Metzinger SE, Allen RJ. New technique for nipple areola reconstruction: arrow flap and rib cartilage graft for long-lasting nipple projection. Ann Plast Surg. 2003;50:31–7.
11. Allen RJ, Treece P. Deep inferior epigastric perforator flap for breast reconstruction. Ann Plast Surg. 1994;32:32–8.
12. Allen RJ, Tucker C Jr. Superior gluteal artery perforator free flap for breast reconstruction. Plast Reconstr Surg. 1995;95:1207–12.
13. Schoeller T, Schubert HM, Pülzl P, et al. Nipple reconstruction using a modified arrow flap technique. Breast. 2006;15:762–8.
14. Gibson T, Davis WB. The distortion of autogenous cartilage grafts: its cause and prevention. Br J Plast Surg. 1958;10:257–98.
15. Broadbent TR, Woolf RM, Metz PS. Restoring the mammary areola by a skin graft from the upper inner thigh. Br J Plast Surg. 1977;30:220–2.
16. Bosch G, Ramirez M. Reconstruction of the nipple: a new technique. Plast Reconstr Surg. 1984;73: 977–81.
17. Jones G, Bostwick J III. Nipple-areola reconstruction. Oper Tech Plast Reconstr Surg. 1994;1:35–9.
18. Thomas SV, Gellis MB, Pool R. Nipple reconstruction with a new local tissue flap. Plast Reconstr Surg. 1996;97:1053–6.
19. Schwager RG, Smith JW, Gray GF, Goulian D Jr. Inversion of the human female nipple, with a simple method of treatment. Plast Reconstr Surg. 1974;54:564–9.
20. Pribaz JJ, Pousti T. Correction of recurrent nipple inversion with cartilage graft. Ann Plast Surg. 1998;40:14–7.
21. Winocour S, Saksena A, Oh C, Wu P, Laungani A, Baltzer H, Saint-Cyr M. A systematic review of comparison of autologous, allogenic, and synthetic augmentation grafts for nipple reconstruction. Plast Reconstr Surg. 2016;137:14e–23e.

22. Brent B, Bostwick J. Nipple-areola reconstruction with auricular tissues. Plast Reconstr Surg. 1977;60:353–61.
23. Tanabe HY, Tai YT, Kiyokawa K, Yamauchi T. Nipple-areola reconstruction with a dermal-fat flap and rolled auricular cartilage. Plast Reconstr Surg. 1997;100:431–8.
24. Collis N, Garrido A. Maintenance of nipple projection using auricular cartilage. Plast Reconstr Surg. 2000;105:2276–7.
25. Heitland A, Markowicz M, Koellensperger E, Allen R, Pallua N. Long-term nipple shrinkage following augmentation by an autologous rib cartilage transplant in free DIEP-flaps. J Plast Reconstr Aesthet Surg. 2006;59:1063–7.
26. Becker H. The use of intradermal tattoo to enhance the final result of nipple-areola reconstruction. Plast Reconstr Surg. 1986;77:673–6.
27. O'Neill AC, Hayward V, Zhong T, Hofer SO. Usability of the internal mammary recipient vessels in microvascular breast reconstruction. J Plast Reconstr Aesthet Surg. 2016;99:907–11.
28. Davidson JA. A technique to aid in rib cartilage excision for access to the internal mammary vessels. Plast Reconstr Surg. 2003;111:506–7.
29. Schoeller T, Schubert HM, Wechselberger G. Rib cartilage replacement to prevent contour deformity after internal mammary vessel access. J Plast Reconstr Aesthet Surg. 2008;61:464–6.
30. Fayman MS, Beeton A, Potgieter E. Barotrauma: an unrecognized mechanism for pneumothorax in breast augmentation. Plast Reconstr Surg. 2005;116:1825–6.
31. Mayridis S, Gnauk HG, Schumacher M, Wagner R. Bilateral pneumothoraces complicating reduction mammoplasty: a case report. BMC Surg. 2013;13:29.
32. Osborn JM, Stevenson TR. Pneumothorax as a complication of breast augmentation. Plast Reconstr Surg. 2005;116:1122–6.
33. Fayman MS. Air drainage: an essential technique for preventing breast augmentation-related pneumothorax. Aesthet Plast Surg. 2007;31:19–22.

# 62 Bell Flap Nipple-Areola Complex Reconstruction

John S. Eng

## 62.1 Introduction

The journey of a breast cancer patient, starting from the day of her original diagnosis until the day when she has completed all her pre- and postsurgical treatments, is an extraordinarily arduous trek. Their itineraries are replete with the ever-evolving treatment protocols of chemo-, hormonal, and radiation therapies at the outset, followed by a sequence of surgical procedures consisting of mastectomy, breast reconstruction, and nipple reconstruction. Anyone of these treatments come with its own unique complications, and some are even life-threatening. Although most complications associated with many current nipple reconstruction techniques are non-life-threatening, they can cause wound infection to both the surgical and skin graft donor sites leading to either total or partial loss of the nipple or color mismatch of the areola and, finally, unattractive results. Consequently, an unknown number of postmastectomy breast cancer patients, whether because of treatment fatigue, their aversion to the rigors of multiple surgeries, or inadequate insurance coverage, have decided to skip either the breast mound reconstruction and/or the nipple reconstruction after their mastectomies.

The name "BELL," as in bell flap, is an acronym made up of the initials of three surgeons: B is for Benelli [1], periareolar purse-string suture for areola definition; E is for Eng [2], boxing of the nipple an coning of the areola; and LL is for Little [3], the quadrapod flap—"inchworm" skin recruitment for nipple projection—whose ideas formed the backbone of this technique. The bell flap nipple reconstruction technique discussed here, which uses only local tattooed skin and its underlying subcutaneous tissue of a breast mound to build a properly pigmented three-dimensional nipple-areola complex in one single stage, under local or no anesthesia, and without skin graft, presents a simpler and gentler alternative to help many of these dispirited breast cancer patients to complete the final leg of their surgical journeys.

The basic concept and the structural design of the purse-string nipple reconstruction are borrowed directly from the ancient Chinese art of paper folding "折紙" (pronounced as *Zhe-Zhi* in Mandarin Chinese or *Ori-Gami* in Japanese). In paper folding, the artist uses a flat piece of paper, with or without ancillary cuttings, and folds it into the likeness of a three-dimensional object, such as a paper flower, crane, airplane, boat, etc. With the bell flap nipple reconstruction technique, a surgeon similarly cuts, folds,

J.S. Eng, M.D.
11118 Stephalee Lane, Rockville,
Maryland 20852, USA
e-mail: johnengmd@gmail.com


M.A. Shiffman (ed.), *Nipple-Areolar Complex Reconstruction*,
https://doi.org/10.1007/978-3-319-60925-6_62

and sutures a circular piece of skin and its underlying subcutaneous tissue on a breast mound to build the likeness of a nipple-areola complex. However, there is some big difference between these two activities, and that is, with the latter, the surgeon must ensure adequate blood supply to reach all the finished parts of the reconstructed nipple-areola complex for its immediate survival, healing, and longevity for years to come.

## 62.2 Surgical Technique

The design of the bell flap begins with the drawing of a circle having a diameter 20–25% larger than that of the opposite areola circle or that of a preplanned new areola circle on a predetermined location for the future nipple on a breast mound. Within this circle, a "bell"-shaped skin rotation flap, with a "bell handle," a "bell body," and a "bell bottom" (Fig. 62.1), is drawn from

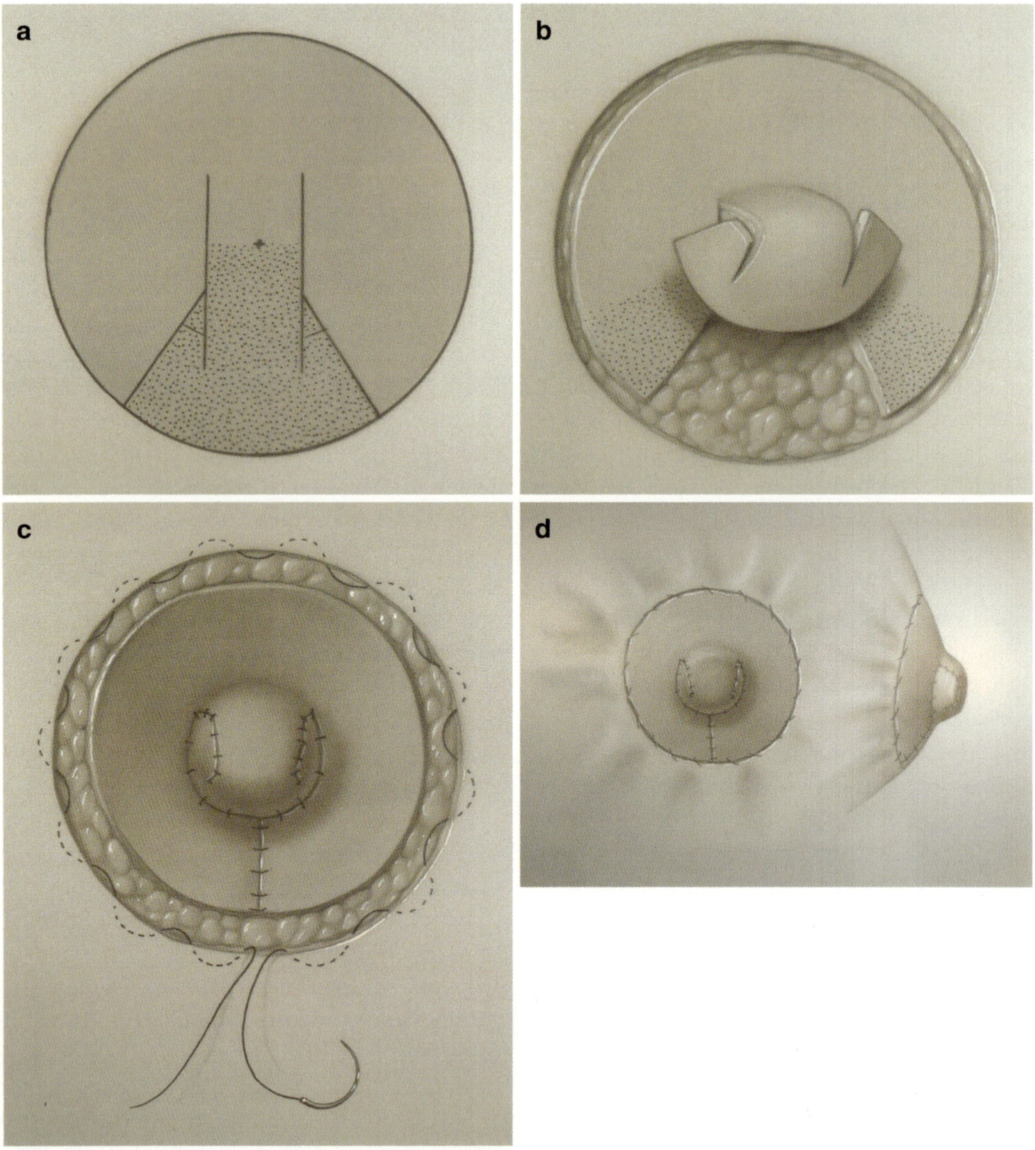


**Fig. 62.1** (**a**) Within a circle, a "bell"-shaped skin rotation flap, with a "bell handle," a "bell body," and a "bell-bottom," is incised, and the stippled area is undermined. (**b**) The small skin tips of the two triangular wing flaps are trimmed to form an inverted box, which will become the new nipple. (**c**) Temporarily converted into an inverted shallow cone. (**d**) A permanent purse-string suture is inserted into the dermis of the outer skin circle and is tightened reducing the diameter of the outer circle

the center of the circle to an arc at the rim of the circle, with the following obligatory and proportional dimensions. The width of the base or the origin of the bell "handle" at the center is equal to one fifth to one fourth the length of the diameter of the circle. The length of the bell flap, the "handle" plus the "body," starting from the small back cuts just past the center of the circle extending all the way to the rim is now equal to about 2.25 times the width of the base. The width of the bell's "bottom" at the rim is set at three times the width of the base. The "body" of the bell is formed by extending two lines from each side of the bell's "bottom" at the rim toward the middle half of the "handle." Because of this tapering effect, the final length to base ratio of the bell flap (in essence, a squatty but bottom-heavy random skin rotation flap), as interpreted in terms of the individual surface areas of the various parts, falls well within the golden ratio of length to width = 3 to 1 for the survival of most rotation flaps.

On the day of surgery and in a minor surgical treatment room, the above design is sketched onto the designated new nipple site on the breast mound. After sterile prep and drape, depending on the sensory status of the breast mound, the design is scratched deeply into the dermis with or without local anesthesia. The entire circle is tattooed with a preselected pigment. The bell flap is then incised around its "handle," "body," and "bottom," undermined (stippled area of the bell flap in Fig. 62.1), raised, boxed, and inset around the base of the pedicle at the center of the circle. The small skin tips of the two triangular wing flaps are trimmed to form an inverted box, which will become the new nipple. The rest of the tattooed skin and its subcutaneous fat inside the circle is circumferentially incised and released. By closing the defect previously vacated by the "body" of the bell flap, this skin-subcutaneous island flap is temporarily converted into an inverted shallow cone. A permanent purse-string suture is inserted into the dermis of the outer skin circle. As it is tightened, it reduces the diameter of the outer circle by 15–20% as originally planned, while the newly formed nipple-areola complex is squeezed well outside the breast mound. After inverting the flat cone and insetting it to the reduced outer skin circle, the result is a well-projecting, three-dimensional (in three tiers), and pigmented virtual nipple-areola complex. "Faux" glands of Montgomery are spotted with a high temperature cautery.

The surgical site is dressed with a piece of nonadherent liner gauze and a stack of 4 × 4's with a hole cut out in the middle to accommodate the new nipple. An optional outer waterproof barrier and a surgical brassiere complete the surgical bandaging before the patient is discharged.

## 62.3 Clinical Applications and Patient Cases

The bell flap nipple reconstruction technique has been proven to be rather versatile and capable of producing satisfactory nipple-areola complexes from a variety of existing but traumatized or newly reconstructed breast mounds as illustrated by the four following clinical examples.

### 62.3.1 Case 1

A 45-year-old was diagnosed with invasive lobular carcinoma of the right breast in 1991, treated with radiation and chemotherapy, followed by modified radical mastectomy in 1992 and TRAM flap breast reconstruction in 1993 (Fig. 62.2). In 1994, the patient underwent left breast reduction and right bell flap nipple reconstruction technique. The new nipple is seen at 1-week postoperative and at 1-year postoperative.

### 62.3.2 Case 2

A 45-year-old underwent left radical mastectomy for infiltrating ductal carcinoma in 1994 (Fig. 62.3). She had a left-sided TRAM flap breast mound reconstruction in 1996. In 1997, she underwent a left-sided bell flap nipple-areola complex reconstruction and breast mound scar revision as an outpatient. The nipple was seen 4 days postoperative with early lymphedema, at 7 days postoperative, and at 1 year postoperative. The new areola was undertattooed.

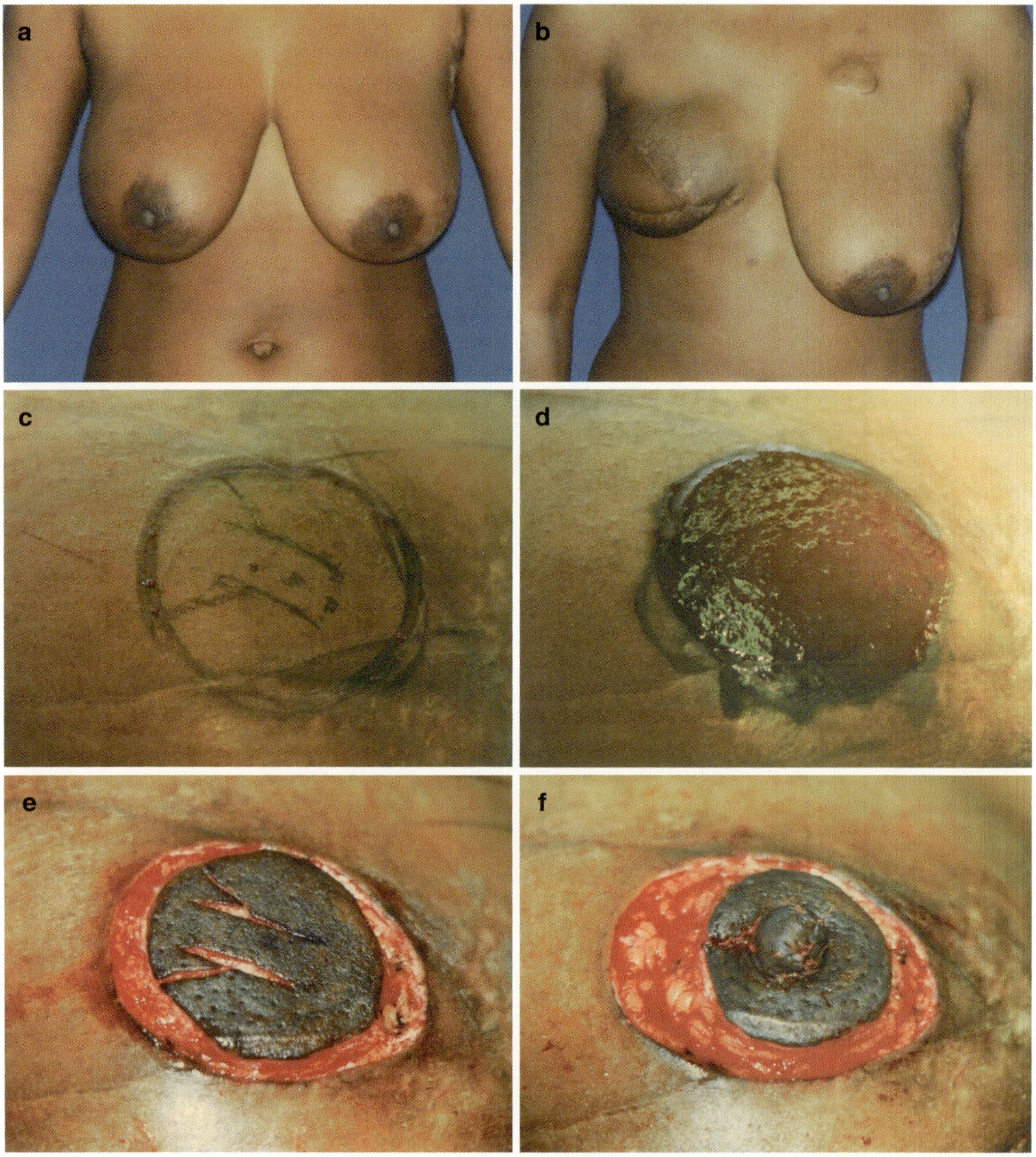


**Fig. 62.2** (**a**) Preoperative invasive lobular carcinoma of the right breast. (**b**) Postoperative following radical mastectomy and TRAM flap breast reconstruction. (**c–g**) Right bell flap nipple reconstruction. (**h**) One week postoperative. (**i–l**) New nipple after 1 year

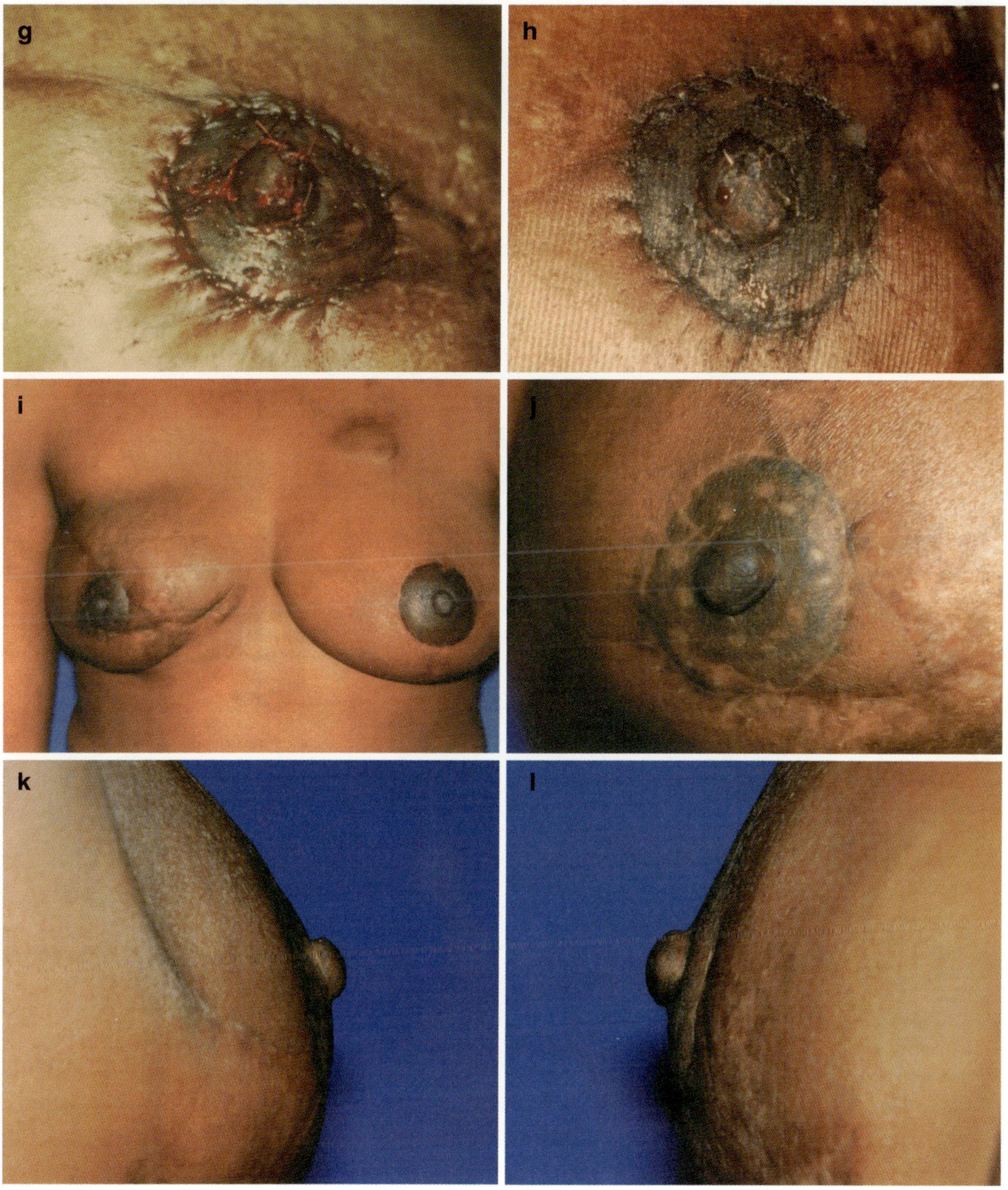


**Fig. 62.2** (continued)

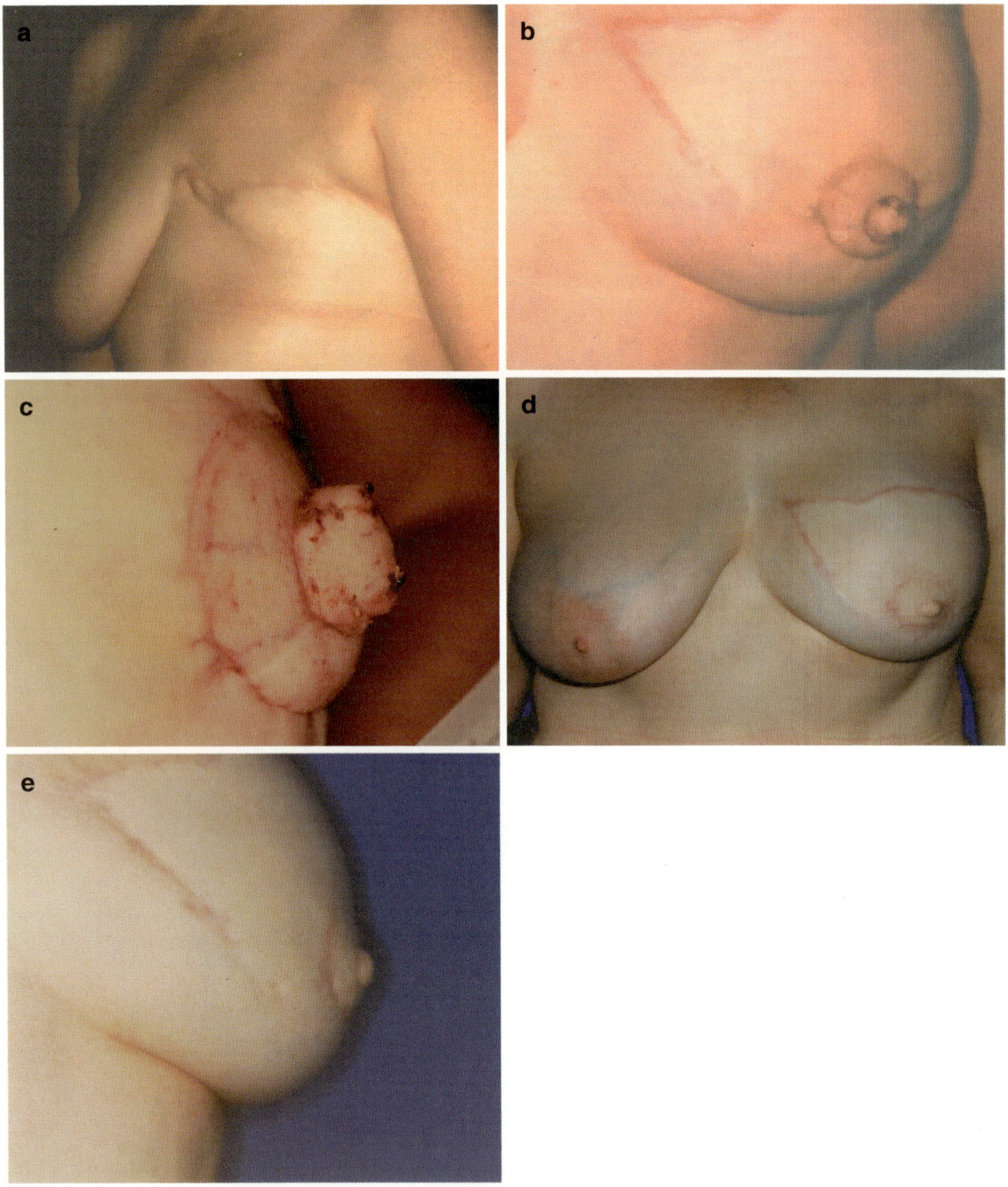


**Fig. 62.3** (**a**) After left radical mastectomy for infiltrating ductal carcinoma. (**b**) Four days postoperative after left-sided TRAM flap breast mound reconstruction. Note edema. (**c**) Seven days postoperative. (**d**, **e**) One year postoperative. New areola was undertattooed

### 62.3.3 Case 3

A 40-year-old underwent left subpectoral breast implant placement for breast mound reconstruction 1 year after modified radical mastectomy for infiltrating ductal carcinoma in 2002 (Fig. 62.4). Two years later in 2004, the patient underwent right breast mastopexy and left bell flap nipple reconstruction. Results at 4 months postoperative are shown. The patient declined

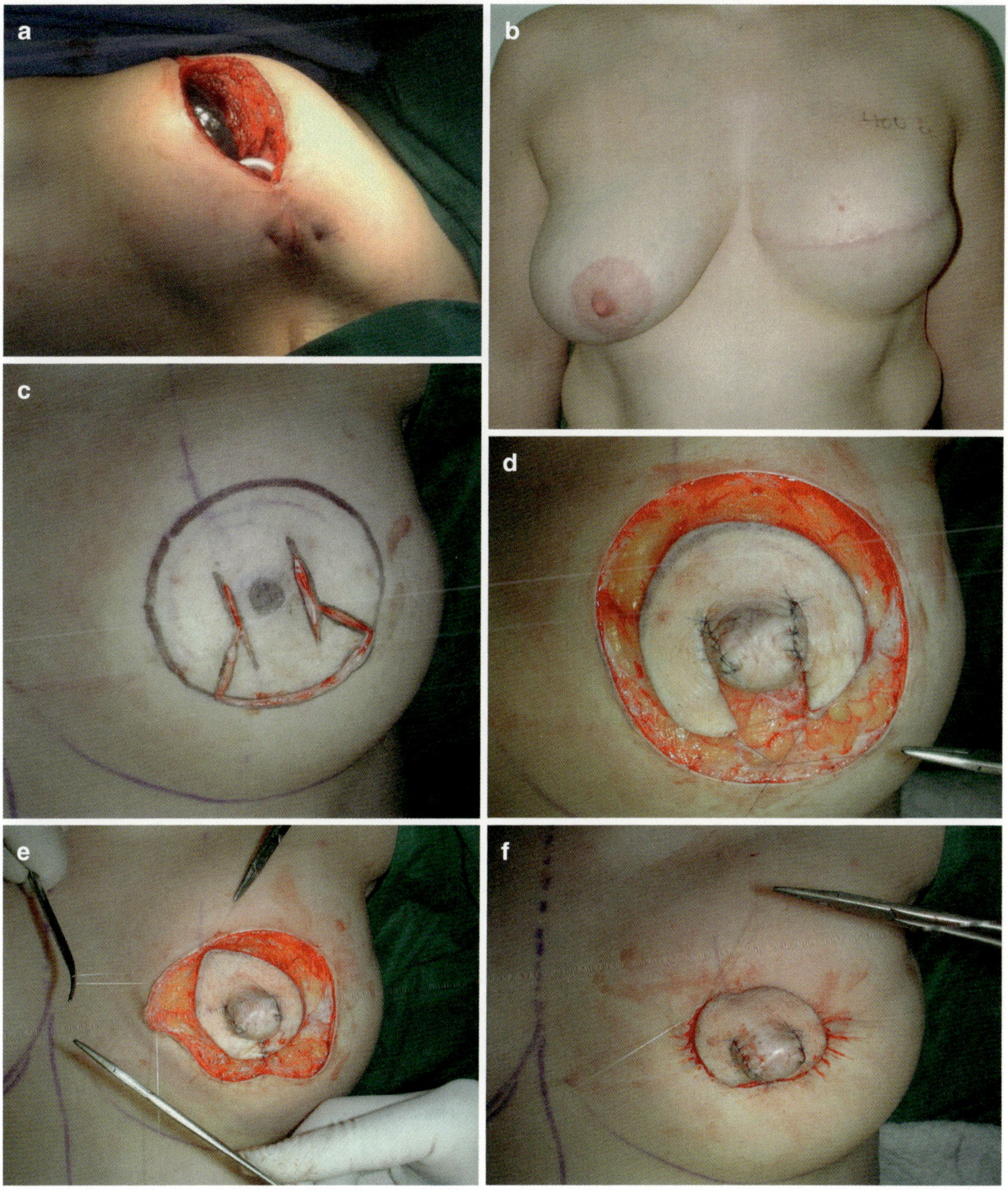

**Fig. 62.4** (**a**) The patient underwent left subpectoral breast implant placement for breast mound reconstruction 1 year after modified radical mastectomy for infiltrating ductal carcinoma. (**b–f**) She underwent right breast mastopexy and left bell flap nipple reconstruction. (**g**, **h**) Results at 4 months postoperative. The patient declined nipple tattooing but may do it later. Courtesy of Gaith Shubailat, M.D., Amman Jordan

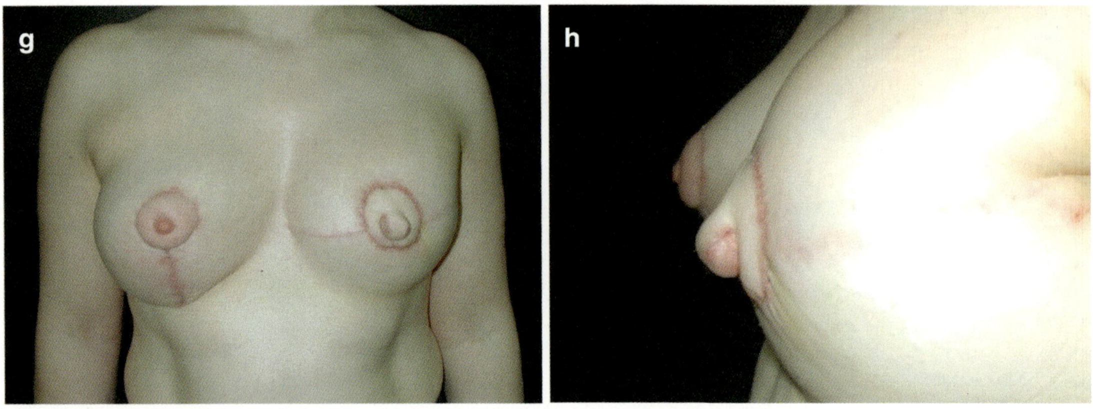


**Fig. 62.4** (continued)

nipple tattooing but may do it later. Additional significant shrinkage of the reconstructed nipple was expected.

Example III—bell flap nipple reconstruction on breast mound after modified radical mastectomy, followed by delayed subpectoral implant/expander placement for breast mound reconstruction.

### 62.3.4 Case 4

A 24-year-old underwent an unsuccessful breast reduction surgery with a malpositioned right nipple and a complete necrosis of the left nipple in 2004. A revision of the right breast and a bell flap nipple reconstruction with the existing scar were suggested to the patient, and the surgery was carried out in 2005 (Fig. 62.5). The patient understood that the scar tissue on her left breast, although supple and blenched well, might not produce a satisfactory outcome. She was willing to take that chance and consented to the surgery. The left breast was seen at 1 week postoperative and at 6 months postoperative.

## 62.4 Discussion

The bell flap nipple-areola complex reconstruction technique appears to be fairly straightforward and simple to perform "on paper." However, since, by definition, all traumatic and reconstructed breast mounds come with reduced axial and collateral blood supply, surgeons should pay special attention to the following technical hurdles uniquely germane to this technique to ensure successful outcomes:

1. Surgeons who are attempting the bell flap nipple reconstruction technique for the first time should come equipped with abundant prior experience in working with all types of rotation skin flap procedures. Novice surgeons with little to no prior experience in rotation flap surgeries should not try this technique as their initiative to flap surgeries. Surgeons who have little to no prior experience with skin tattooing should make an effort to learn it from other plastic surgeons who do or from commercial tattoo artists to ensure proper pigment match and retention. Alternatively, surgeons may have their patients tattooed by commercial tattoo artist well before or after the surgery to ensure better color retention.
2. Existing scar tissues on some breast mounds from previous surgical or traumatic events may crisscross the new incisions of the bell flap design (Fig. 62.2). But if the bell flap itself is placed on healthy and soft skin, most tissues trapped between the old scars and the new incisions can be tattooed and will survive as full-thickness skin grafts (Fig. 62.2). In rare situations, some scar tissue can encroach directly on the bell flap itself

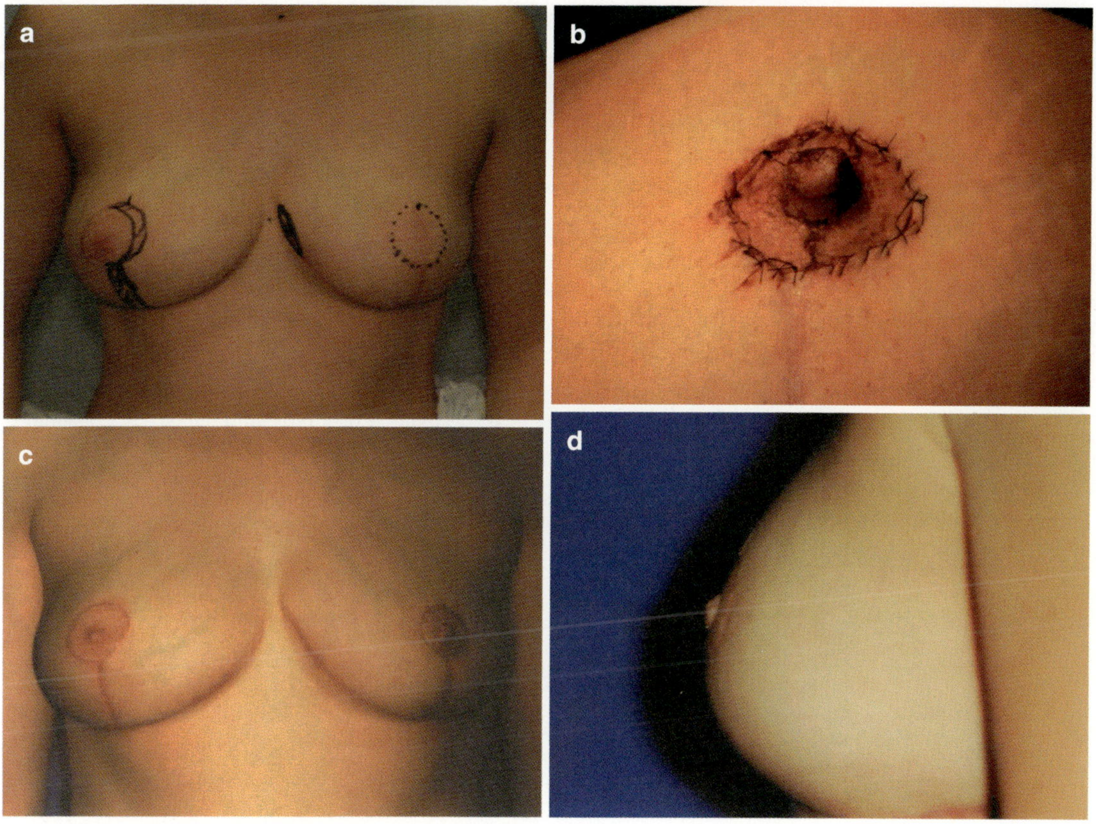


**Fig. 62.5** (**a**) This patient underwent an unsuccessful breast reduction surgery with malpositioned right nipple and a complete necrosis of the left nipple. Markings for reconstruction. (**b**) One week postoperatively after revision of the right breast and a bell flap nipple reconstruction with the existing scar. (**c**, **d**) Six months postoperative

(Fig. 62.5). But as long as esthetic scar is soft and appears to be well vascularized and in the absence of lymphatic congestion, it can be used to salvage a dismal situation as in Case 4, who was willing to take a chance with the bell flap technique but refused skin grafts from any sources.

3. The bell flap nipple reconstruction technique should not be attempted on breast mounds reconstructed using large implants or tissue expanders placed directly in a subcutaneous pocket. The thin skin flaps anterior to a large implant are stretched too thinly, and it may be impossible to predict the status of the blood supply needed to nourish the new nipple-areola. Any tissue loss will invariably lead to implant exposure. On the other hand, in breast mounds reconstructed with subpectoral placement of implants or expanders, a buffer of muscle and subcutaneous interface may provide a suitable environment for one to attempt such a reconstruction but only on a case-to-case basis (Fig. 62.4).
4. Since the blood supply to the bell flap is further diminished by the "boxing" and folding maneuvers of the rotation flap to form the nipple, which survives solely on a subcutaneous island flap, the final healed nipple-areola complex will undergo partial ischemic necrosis and shrink to approximately half of its size as compared to the one during the immediate postsurgical period (Fig. 62.3). Allowance must be made to compensate for this size reduction of the finished product.
5. As one might be tempted to "bulk up" the flaccid reconstructed nipple by this bell flap

nipple reconstruction or any other techniques, by injecting many of the currently available fillers [4], care must be taken to avoid using too large a bolus at the outset. Large boluses may produce excessive internal pressure leading to either partial or total necrosis of the nipple.

## Conclusions

The bell flap nipple reconstruction technique, as a simpler and less invasive surgical procedure, has the potential to produce a truly lifelike three-dimensional and properly pigmented nipple-areola complex on most existing but traumatized and reconstructed breast mounds in one single stage without skin grafts. Hopefully, it will encourage many more patients with breast cancer and other disfiguring diseases to complete their surgical journey and rehabilitation.

## References

1. Benelli L. A new periareolar mammoplasty: the "round block" technique. Aesthet Plast Surg. 1990;14:93–100.
2. Eng JS. Bell flap nipple reconstruction—a new wrinkle. Ann Plast Surg. 1996;36:485–8.
3. Little JW, Munasifi T, McCullough DT. One-stage reconstruction of a projecting nipple: the quadrapod flap. Plast Reconstr Surg. 1983;71:126–33.
4. Panettiere P, Marchetti L, Accorsi D. Filler injection enhances the projection of the reconstructed nipple: an original easy technique. Aesthet Plast Surg. 2005;4:287–94.

# The 'Cigar Roll' Flap for Nipple-Areola Complex Reconstruction

# 63

Benjamin Khoda and Simon Heppell

## 63.1 Introduction

Nipple-areola complex (NAC) reconstruction tends to be the final phase of postmastectomy reconstruction for many cancer patients. The objectives are to recreate a natural looking NAC, which transforms an amorphous breast mound into a more aesthetically realistic breast. Important features to achieve this are position, size, shape, colour, texture and projection.

Numerous techniques have been described reflecting the fact that no one technique is entirely satisfactory. Reconstruction techniques can involve nipple sharing, intradermal tattooing, local adipocutaneous flaps, distant tissue flaps and cartilage grafts. Common local flaps described include bell [1], skate flaps, star flaps [2], trilobed [3] and bilobed flaps and CV flap.

The most common problem following reconstruction is loss of projection. One study has found that the long-term reduction of nipple projection varied between 41 and 74% whilst using three popular techniques [5]. Projection tends to fail early and settle over time, as scars heal and the tissue softens and contract. Many surgeons have tried to overcome this problem by using different techniques including the use of cartilage grafts, AlloDerm and different dressings [4, 5].

We describe a novel method in NAC reconstruction called the 'cigar roll' technique. This local flap recreates an aesthetically pleasing NAC and has the benefit of no separate donor site morbidity, and we believe the deepithelialization confers the added benefit of long-term maintenance of projection.

## 63.2 Technique

Nipple position is marked preoperatively with the patient standing ensuring symmetry with the contralateral breast. The patient is asked to mark the nipple position whilst looking into the mirror. This position is then confirmed by markings from sternal notch to check that it matches the contralateral nipple. Skin and subcutaneous tissue is incised and the flaps are raised. One half of the flap is deepithelialized (Fig. 63.1). This is inset

B. Khoda, FRCS (Plast) (✉) • S. Heppell, FRCS (Plast)
Department of Plastic and Reconstructive Surgery, Queen Alexandra Hospital, Portsmouth, UK
e-mail: ben.khoda@yahoo.co.uk; simonheppell@me.com


M.A. Shiffman (ed.), *Nipple-Areolar Complex Reconstruction*,
https://doi.org/10.1007/978-3-319-60925-6_63

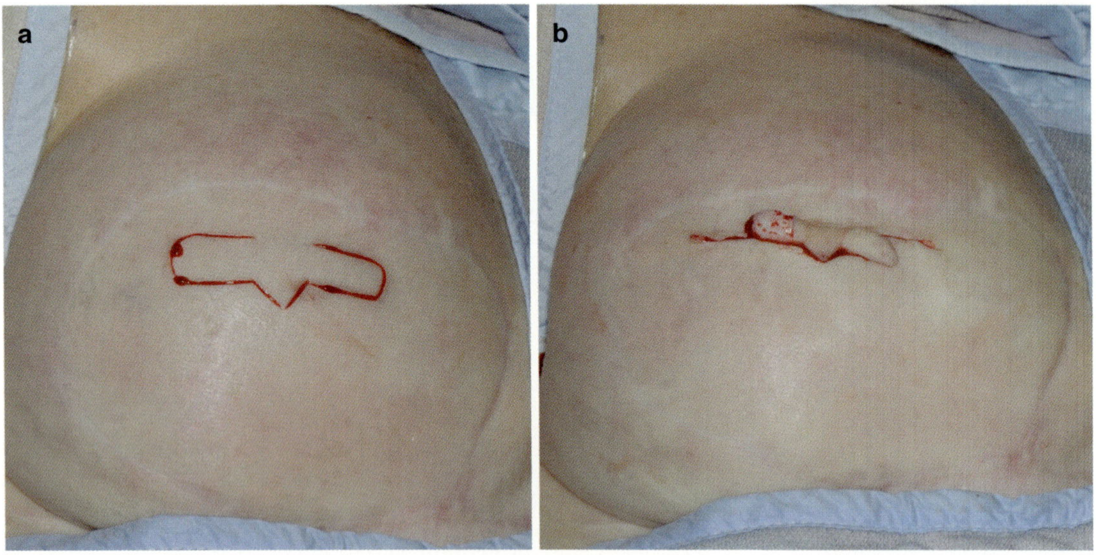


**Fig. 63.1** (**a**) Marking of flap. (**b**) Deepithelialization of one half of the flap

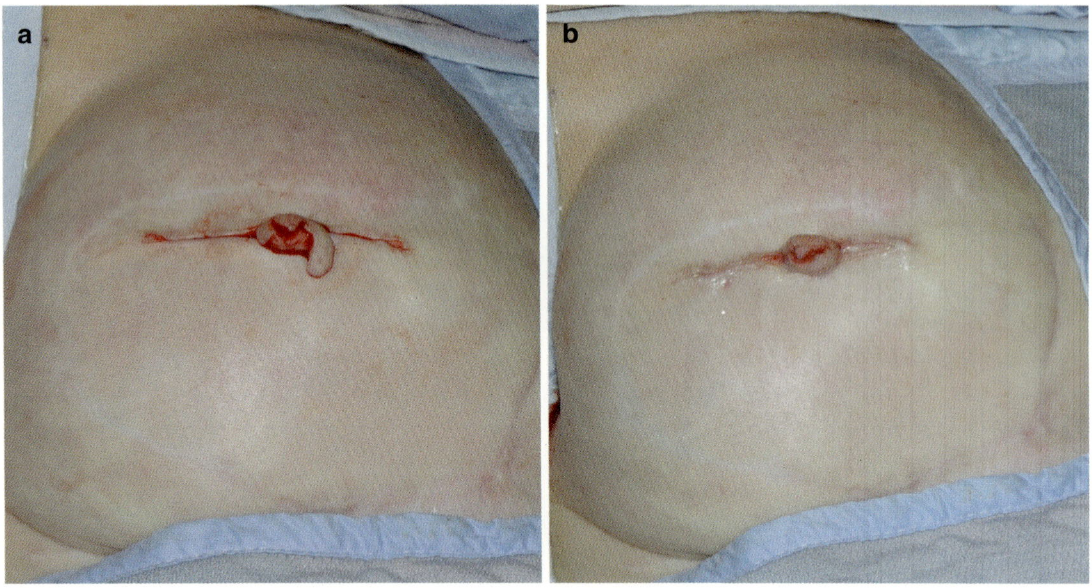


**Fig. 63.2** (**a**, **b**) Insetting of flap

into the new nipple-areola complex (Fig. 63.2). The opposing flap is then secured over creating a new nipple (Fig. 63.3). Donor site is sutured using 3-0 PDS (Ethicon) and 4-0 Monocryl (Ethicon), and the wound is sealed with Dermabond glue. Sponge and Jelonet dressing with Tegaderm are then applied. The dressings remain in situ for 10 days. Once the wound is healed, patients are offered tattooing on an outpatient basis.

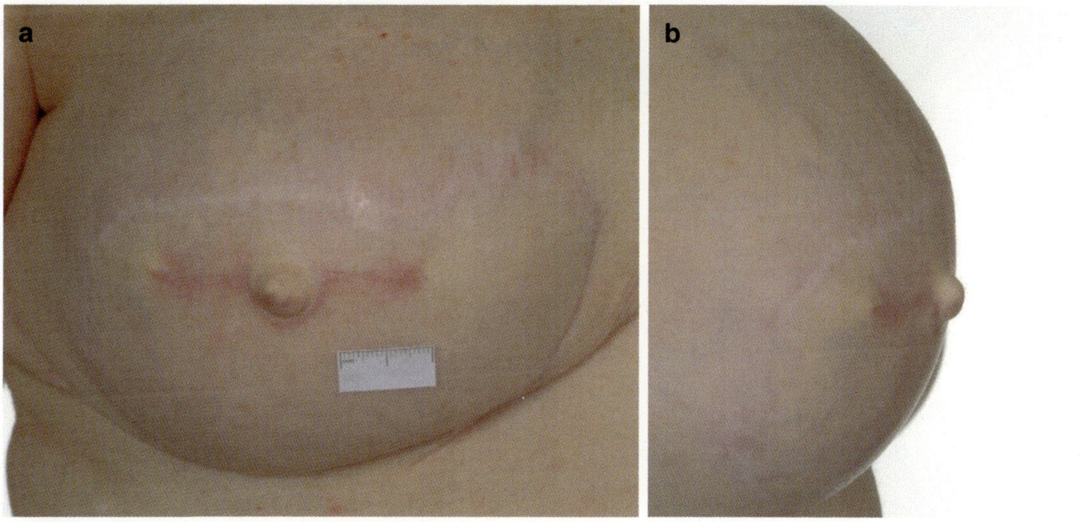

**Fig. 63.3** (**a**, **b**) Projection maintained at 6 months

## 63.3 Discussion

This technique has been used on more than 90 patients over the last 6 years, and the results are encouraging. Patients have been very pleased with the final product. Maintenance of projection has been consistently good at follow-up several months post-reconstruction. We have experienced seven complications (7%) in total. Two reconstructed nipples had partial flap necrosis, both healing by secondary intention and requiring no further surgical input. Two nipples (2%) showed loss of projection of which one was secondary to donor site wound dehiscence. They were both revised with satisfactory outcomes. Finally, one nipple was too large and this was subsequently revised.

**Conclusions**

The 'cigar roll' is a novel technique for nipple reconstruction, which has consistently shown good results. It is a simple, reproducible technique involving a local flap. The technique can be performed under local anaesthesia. Our experience has shown promising results with projection maintained at follow-up several months postoperatively, long after the time scale when projection tends to be lost.

## References

1. Eng JS. Bell flap nipple reconstruction—a new wrinkle. Ann Plast Surg. 1996;36:485–8.
2. Kroll SS, Reece GP, Miller MJ, Evans GR, Robb GL, Baldwin BJ, Wang BG, Schusterman MA. Comparison of nipple projection with the modified double opposing tab and star flaps. Plast Reconstr Surg. 1997;99:1602–5.
3. Shestak KC, Gabriel A, Landecker A, Peters S, Shestak A, Kim J. Assessment of long-term nipple projection: a comparison of three techniques. Plast Reconstr Surg. 2002;110:780–6.
4. Tanabe HY, Tai Y, Kiyokawa K, Yamauchi T. Nipple-areola reconstruction with a dermal-fat flap and rolled auricular cartilage. Plast Reconstr Surg. 1997;100(2):431–8.
5. Garramone CE, Lam B. Use of AlloDerm in primary nipple reconstruction to improve long-term nipple projection. Plast Reconstr Surg. 2007;119:1663–8.

# Nipple Reconstruction with C-V Flap Using Dermofat Graft

**64**

SuRak Eo and Andrew L. Da Lio

## 64.1 Introduction

Aesthetically satisfying nipple restoration plays an important role in postmastectomy breast reconstruction. Many techniques, such as the skate flap [1], star flap [1], C-V flap [2, 3], S-flap [4, 5], and double opposing tab flaps [6], are currently employed in nipple reconstruction. Recent additions to the repertoire of nipple reconstruction include a spiral flap made of residual scar tissue [7] and tissue engineering [8]. These last two procedures have an added advantage of minimizing donor site morbidity. The ideal method for nipple reconstruction would maintain long-term nipple projection, texture, color, and shape and have minimal donor site morbidity. Despite the plethora of techniques available, a simple and reliable method that maintains nipple projection remains elusive. In this chapter, we outline a simple technique that maintains long-term nipple projection. To this end, we have performed local C-V flaps augmented with autologous dermofat grafts harvested from excised breast tissues during breast mound revision.

S. Eo, M.D., Ph.D. (✉)
Department of Plastic and Reconstructive Surgery, Dongguk University Ilsan Hospital, Dongguk University Graduate School of Medicine, DongGukDae-Ro 27, IlSanDong-gu, GoYang-si, GyeongGi-do 10326, South Korea
e-mail: surakeo@yahoo.com

A.L. Da Lio, M.D.
UCLA Division of Plastic and Reconstructive Surgery, 200 UCLA Medical Plaza, Suite 465, Box 956960, Los Angeles, CA 90095-6960, USA
e-mail: ADalio@mednet.ucla.edu

## 64.2 Technique

Normal human nipples are made up of a dense connective tissue layer which surrounds numerous lactiferous ducts. This rigid connective tissue plays a major role in maintaining nipple projection [9]. Replacement of this rigid tissue with substitutes such as auricular cartilage [10–14], rib cartilage [15], contralateral nipple [16], toe pulp [17], and silicone aids in maintaining projection in the reconstructed nipple. But, it predisposes patients to additional donor site morbidity and/or the risk of foreign body reactions.

The method of autologous dermofat grafting has been well established. Furthermore, in comparison with alloplastic implants, dermofat grafts are a much safer alternative, with less potential for infection and rejection.

Nipple reconstructions on the majority are undertaken during breast mound revision, 3–6 months after breast reconstruction. In our patient population, all patients had history of


M.A. Shiffman (ed.), *Nipple-Areolar Complex Reconstruction*,
https://doi.org/10.1007/978-3-319-60925-6_64

breast cancer ablation and were reconstructed with either transverse rectus abdominis musculocutaneous (TRAM), deep inferior epigastric perforator (DIEP), or latissimus dorsi (LD) musculocutaneous flaps. Secondary breast mound revisions were needed for the correction of asymmetry and partial fat necrosis. These were corrected simply by excision and scar revision under general anesthesia. The nipples were reconstructed with excised autologous tissues simultaneously.

The position of the new nipple-areola complex was determined with the patient standing in front of a mirror. The diameter of the nipple was designed 15–20% larger than that of the desired one using C-V flaps (Fig. 64.1). The projection of the nipple was determined by the width of the V flap, and the diameter of the nipple depends based on the diameter of the C flap. In our design, we overcorrected nipple height (made 12–18 mm) to compensate for 25–50% decrease over time [18, 19]. The final nipple height was calculated to be 6–12 mm in height. The C-V flap could be oriented in any direction and was elevated to the thickness of the dermal fat to preserve the subdermal plexuses.

A dermofat graft with dimensions of 1 × 1 × 2 cm was harvested from the excised breast tissues (Fig. 64.1). This was then immediately placed at the center of the newly formed nipple with the dermal tissue laying in the deep aspect (Fig. 64.2). The C-V flap was sutured loosely with 4-0 chromic catguts, and donor site

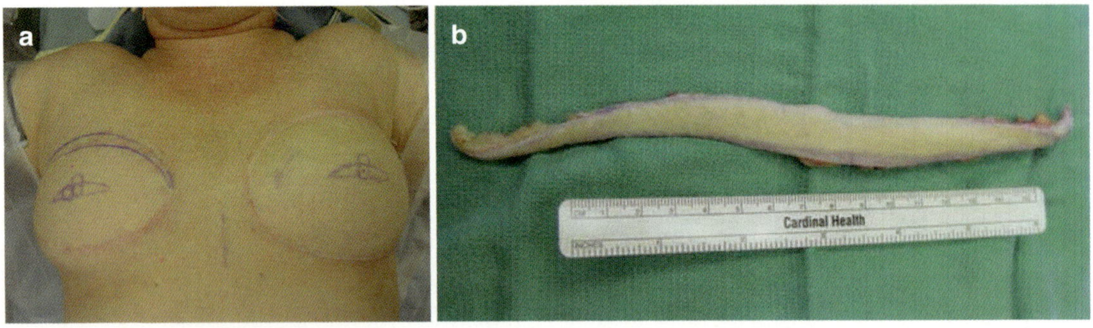


**Fig. 64.1** (**a**) Postoperative bilateral transverse rectus abdominis musculocutaneous (TRAM) free flap. C-V flaps were designed for nipple reconstruction on both breast mounds. (**b**) Scar tissue was excised with subcutaneous fat to reshape the left breast

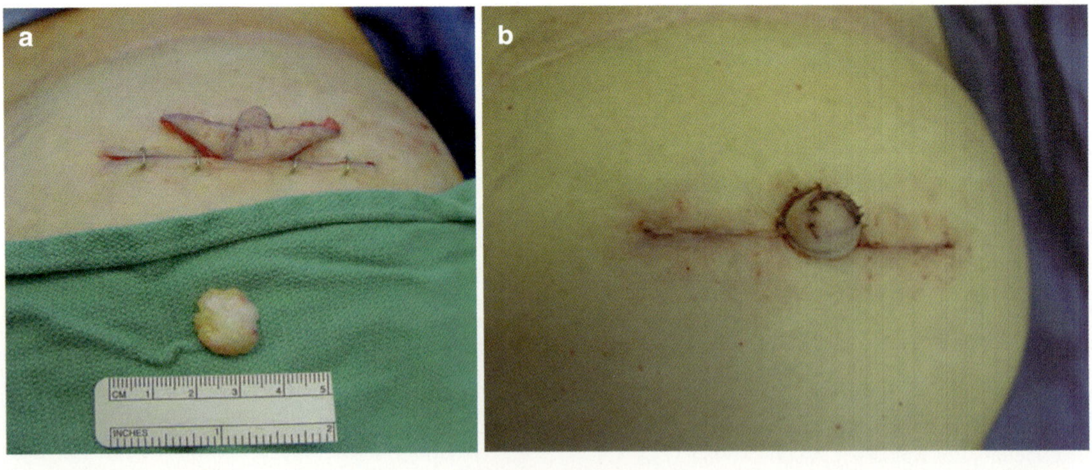


**Fig. 64.2** (**a**) The C-V flap was elevated on the left breast. And the 1 × 1 × 2 cm-sized dermofat graft was taken from the excised tissue. (**b**) Dermofat tissue was grafted under the C-V flap, dermis was positioned deeply, and the fat tissue oriented under the skin to minimize fat absorption

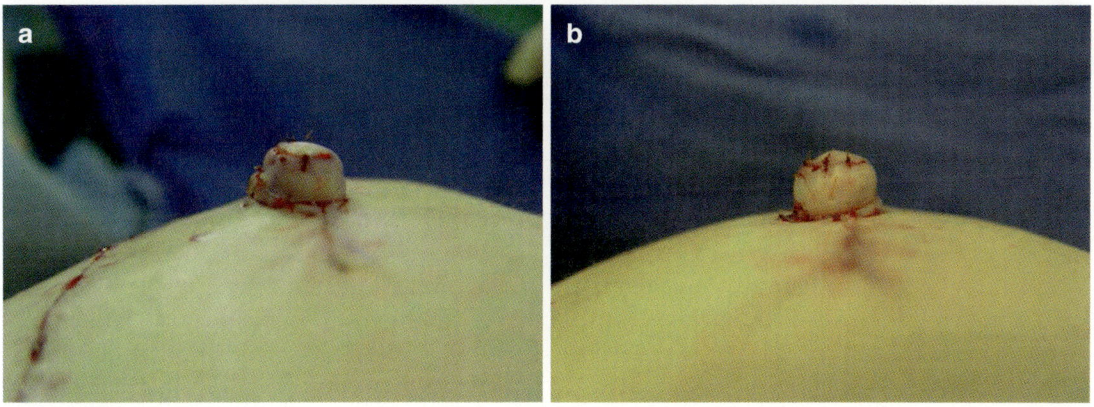


**Fig. 64.3** (**a**) Immediately postoperative showing a projecting nipple on left breast. (**b**) Immediate postoperatively showing a projecting nipple on the right breast

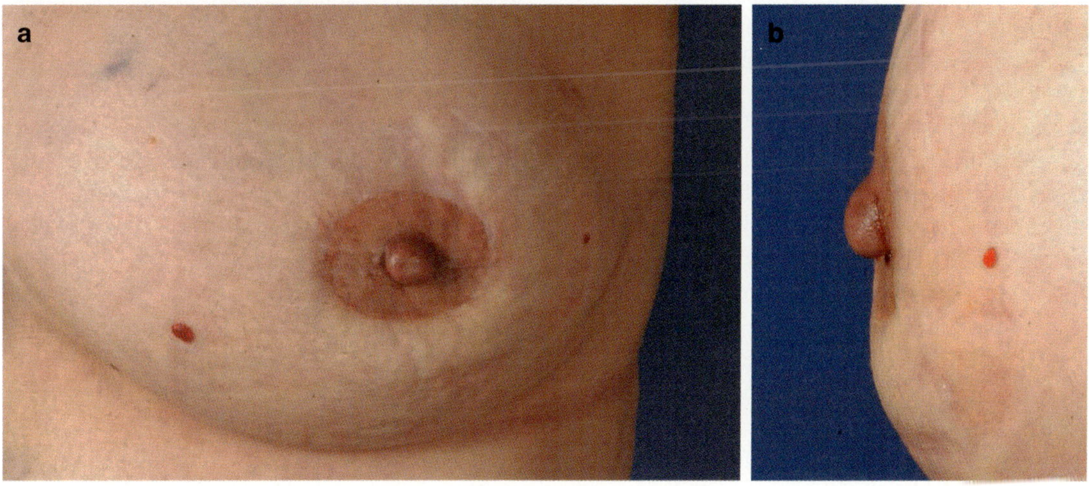


**Fig. 64.4** (**a**) Two years postoperatively of the left breast. (**b**) Good projection of the nipple can be seen of the left nipple

was closed primarily without tension in two layers using 4-0 Monocryl inverted dermal interrupted sutures and 4-0 Monocryl running subcuticular sutures (Fig. 64.3). Doughnut-shaped stent dressings made of cotton patches were maintained for 48 h to avoid direct pressure on the reconstructed nipple using folded cotton patches with central cutouts for the nipple. The areola was later tattooed in a separate office procedure.

All procedures were performed during the second stage (mound revisions) for breast reconstruction. The unfavorable length-to-width ratios of the C-V flaps (7 cm × 1.5 cm) did not adversely affect the flaps. Projection of the reconstructed nipple was well maintained, and the nipple qualitatively had a better shape and height with the dermofat graft as a sustaining strut (Fig. 64.4). Our patients have not only been satisfied but delighted with the three-dimensional projection of the nipple.

## 64.3 Discussion

The goals of nipple reconstruction are to achieve and maintain projection and symmetry while also providing for adequate color and texture match to the contralateral nipple [20]. The best time for nipple reconstruction is when the breast mound shape and position are well established. Another benefit to performing the nipple reconstruction during the second stage of breast reconstruction is the fact that the patient can be an active participant. She can guide the reconstructive surgeon as to the ideal location of the nipple [2]. In addition, patients with a long interval between the initial breast mound construction and nipple-areola reconstruction are reported to be less satisfied than those with shorter intervals between the procedures [21].

Local skin flaps such as skate flap [1], star flap [1, 22, 23], C-V flap [3], double opposing pennant and tab flap [24, 25], angel flap [26], Anton-Hartrampf star flap [22], fortified quadrapod flap [27], triple-V flap [28], bell flap [1, 29], S-flap [5], T-flap [30], H-flap [31], pinwheel flap [32], arrow flap [15], dermal-fat flap [10, 33], buried dermal hammock methods [34], and mushroom-shaped pedicle flap [35–37] with or without skin grafts have been the mainstay for nipple reconstructions [27]. With these methods, projection can be minimally improved by designing thicker and wider skin flaps. The dimensions of flap lengths and base diameters were shown to significantly affect long-term projection, and every increase of 1 cm led to a 0.16 cm increase in projection [1, 38]. Despite these efforts, all of these reconstructed nipple papules are infamous for their marked loss of projection: usually 25–50% and even up to 75% on scarred or grafted tissue [22, 25]. This occurs almost exclusively during the first 2–3 months postoperatively, and the height of the nipple eventually flattens as the scars soften over time [1]. This might be explained by the lack of natural anatomic infrastructure, centrifugal force under the reconstructed nipple, and wound contracture [34, 39].

To maintain long-term projection of reconstructed nipples, Cohen et al. [32] reported the barrier epithelial graft to prevent nipple retraction. Since then, others have inserted substances firmer than the surrounding soft tissues such as silicone, auricular cartilage [11], opposite nipple banking or sharing [16], earlobe tissue [12, 13], toe pulp [17], and subcutaneous inlay graft [13, 14, 40]. But, they are still complicated by multidirectional scars, foreign body reactions, additional donor site morbidity, and prolonged operation time.

According to Guerra et al. [15], the dermofat graft serves as the "irreducible" support and helps to break up the straight vertical scar that is placed on the nipple. Kroll [40] suggested that the best way to avoid flattening of the breast mound when reconstructing a nipple is to make the nipple not from the final mound but from tissue that was to be discarded as part of a breast mound revision. We followed this admonition and used the discarded dermofat tissue as internal splinting material for the nipple constructs. Our outlined method provides for greater long-term maintenance of nipple projection while minimizing donor site morbidity.

**Conclusions**

The goals of nipple reconstruction are adequate nipple projection and symmetry. The erect and protuberant nipple core seen immediately postoperatively falls victim to shrinkage and contraction, thus rendering a flattened nipple. Dermofat grafts harvested from excised tissue during mound revision were successfully utilized as internal struts for nipple papule projection. This technique is simple and permits greater freedom in choosing the final height of the nipple. Use of the C-V flap augmented with a dermofat graft results in an esthetically pleasing nipple that maintains long-term projection without any donor site morbidity.

## References

1. Shestak KC, Gabriel A, Landecker A, Peters S, Shestak A, Kim J. Assessment of long-term nipple projection: a comparison of three techniques. Plast Reconstr Surg. 2002;110(3):780–6.
2. Farhadi J, Maksvytyte GK, Schaefer DJ, Pierer G, Scheufler O. Reconstruction of the nipple-areola complex: an update. J Plast Reconstr Aesthet Surg. 2006;59(1):40–53.
3. Losken A, Mackay GJ, Bostwick J III. Nipple reconstruction using the C-V flap technique: a long-term evaluation. Plast Reconstr Surg. 2001;108(2):361–9.
4. Cronin ED, Humphreys DH, Ruiz-Razura A. Nipple reconstruction: the S flap. Plast Reconstr Surg. 1988;81(5):783–7.

5. Weiss J, Herman O, Rosenberg L, Shafir R. The S nipple-areola reconstruction. Plast Reconstr Surg. 1989;83(5):904–6.
6. Kroll SS, Hamilton S. Nipple reconstruction with the double-opposing tab flap. Plast Reconstr Surg. 1989;84(3):520–5.
7. Di Benedetto G, Sperti V, Pierangeli M, Bertani A. A simple and reliable method of nipple reconstruction using a spiral flap made of residual scar tissue. Plast Reconstr Surg. 2004;114(1):158–61.
8. Cao YL, Lach E, Kim TH, Rodríguez A, Arévalo CA, Vacanti CA. Tissue-engineered nipple reconstruction. Plast Reconstr Surg. 1998;102(7):2293–8.
9. Schwager RG, Smith JW, Gray GF, Goulian D Jr. Inversion of the human female nipple, with a simple method of treatment. Plast Reconstr Surg. 1974;54(5):564–9.
10. Yanaga H. Nipple-areolar reconstruction with a dermal-fat flap: technical improvement from rolled auricular cartilage to artificial bone. Plast Reconstr Surg. 2003;112(7):1863–9.
11. Collis N, Garrido A. Maintenance of nipple projection using auricular cartilage. Plast Reconstr Surg. 2000;105(6):2276–7.
12. Rose EH. Nipple reconstruction with four-lobe composite auricular graft. Ann Plast Surg. 1985;15(1):78–81.
13. Brent B, Bostwick J. Nipple-areola reconstruction with auricular tissues. Plast Reconstr Surg. 1977;60(3):353–61.
14. Tanabe HY, Tai Y, Kiyokawa K, Yamauchi T. Nipple-areolar reconstruction with a dermal-fat flap and rolled auricular cartilage. Plast Reconstr Surg. 1997;100(2):431–8.
15. Guerra AB, Khoobehi K, Metzinger SE, Allen RJ. New technique for nipple areola reconstruction: arrow flap and rib cartilage graft for long-lasting nipple projection. Ann Plast Surg. 2003;50(1):31–7.
16. Bhatty MA, Berry RB. Nipple-areolar reconstruction by tattooing and nipple sharing. Br J Plast Surg. 1997;50(5):331–4.
17. Klatsky SA, Manson PN. Toe pulp free grafts in nipple reconstruction. Plast Reconstr Surg. 1981;68(2):245–8.
18. Niechajev I, Sevćuk O. Long term results of fat transplantation: clinical and histologic studies. Plast Reconstr Surg. 1994;94(3):496–506.
19. Sawhney CP, Banerjee TN, Chakravarti RN. Behaviour of dermal fat transplants. Br J Plast Surg. 1969;22(2):169–76.
20. Bogue DP, Mungara AK, Thompson M, Cederna PS. Modified technique for nipple-areolar reconstruction: a case series. Plast Reconstr Surg. 2003;112(5):1274–8.
21. Jabor MA, Shayani P, Collins DR Jr, Karas T, Cohen BE. Nipple-areola reconstruction: satisfaction and clinical determinants. Plast Reconstr Surg. 2002;110(2):457–63.
22. Banducci DR, Le TK, Hughes KC. Long-term follow-up of a modified Anton-Hartrampf nipple reconstruction. Ann Plast Surg. 1999;43(5):467–9.
23. Eskenazi L. A one-stage nipple reconstruction with the "modified star" flap and immediate tattoo: a review of 100 cases. Plast Reconstr Surg. 1993;92(4):671–80.
24. Kroll SS, Reece GP, Miller MJ, Evans GR, Robb GL, Baldwin BJ, Wang BG, Schusterman MA. Comparison of nipple projection with the modified double-opposing tab and star flaps. Plast Reconstr Surg. 1997;99(6):1602–5.
25. Hugo NE, Sultan MR, Hardy SP. Nipple-areolar reconstruction with intradermal tattoo and double-opposing pennant flaps. Ann Plast Surg. 1993;30(6):510–3.
26. Wong WW, Hiersche MA, Martin MC. The angel flap for nipple reconstruction. Can J Plast Surg. 2013;21(1):e1–4.
27. Little JW III, Munasifi T, McCulloch DT. One-stage reconstruction of a projecting nipple: the quadrapod flap. Plast Reconstr Surg. 1983;71(1):126–33.
28. Klinger F, Caviggioli F, Vinci V, Forcellini D, Maione L, Lisa A, Klinger M. Triple-V flap: nipple reconstruction using a modified C-V flap technique for long-lasting improvement of projection. Eur J Plast Surg. 2013;36(11):689–92.
29. Eng JS. Bell flap nipple reconstruction-a new wrinkle. Ann Plast Surg. 1996;36(5):485–8.
30. Chang WH. Nipple reconstruction with a T flap. Plast Reconstr Surg. 1984;73(1):140–3.
31. Hallock GG, Altobelli JA. Cylindrical nipple reconstruction using an H flap. Ann Plast Surg. 1993;30(1):23–6.
32. Cohen IK, Ward JA, Chandrasekhar B. The pinwheel flap nipple and barrier areola graft reconstruction. Plast Reconstr Surg. 1986;77(6):995–9.
33. Temiz G, Yeşiloğlu N, Şirinoğlu H, Sarici M. A new modification of C-V flap technique in nipple reconstruction: rolled triangular dermal-fat flaps. Aesthet Plast Surg. 2015;39(1):173–5.
34. Mukherjee RP, Gottlieb V, Hacker L. Nipple-areolar reconstruction with buried dermal hammock technique. Ann Plast Surg. 1987;19(5):421–3.
35. Smith JW, Nelson R. Construction of the nipple with a mushroom-shaped pedicle. Plast Reconstr Surg. 1986;78(5):684–7.
36. Vecchione TR. Reconstruction and/or salvage of nipple projection. Plast Reconstr Surg. 1986;78(5):679–83.
37. Hobson MI, Williams N, Sharpe DT. The mushroom nipple-areolar reconstruction: a patient review. Ann Plast Surg. 1996;37(4):453.
38. Few JW, Marcus JR, Casas LA, Aitken ME, Redding J. Long-term predictable nipple projection following reconstruction. Plast Reconstr Surg. 1999;104(5):1321–4.
39. Bosch G, Ramirez M. Reconstruction of the nipple: a new technique. Plast Reconstr Surg. 1984;73(6):977–81.
40. Kroll SS. Integrated breast mound reduction and nipple reconstruction with the wraparound flap. Plast Reconstr Surg. 1999;104(3):687–93.

# C-Y Trilobed Flap for Improved Donor-Site Morbidity in Nipple-Areola Complex Reconstruction

**65**

Tulsi Roy, Daniel R. Butz, Zachary J. Collier, and David H. Song

## 65.1 Introduction

In addition to greater satisfaction with surgical outcomes, nipple-areola complex reconstruction provides numerous psychosocial benefits to patients and frequently represents the final aesthetic step in postmastectomy breast reconstruction [1]. Multiple techniques for reconstruction exist, including local flaps, skin grafts, 3D tattooing, and nipple augmentation with cartilage, hydroxyapatite, or acellular dermal matrix [2]. An ideal approach would be one that is technically facile, minimizes donor-site morbidity, reduces or conceals scarring, and reliably maintains nipple projection to provide an overall aesthetically pleasing and realistic outcome.

Trilobed flaps are dependable methods for nipple-areola complex reconstruction, particularly in conjunction with areolar tattooing. Trilobed flap-based reconstruction is versatile, and different "star" and "wrap" techniques are described in the literature, including skate, arrow, top-hat, and C-V flaps [3–7]. These flaps share a similar design: a vertical flap that acts as a cap and two lateral arm flaps that wrap around the base to provide nipple projection. Refinements of these techniques primarily focus on donor-site closure and the minimization of dog-ears [8]. However, these modifications frequently result in increasing the length of the final scar. The C-Y trilobed flap presented here is a facile and reproducible adaptation that preserves nipple projection provided by traditional trilobed flaps while obviating increased scar length.

## 65.2 Technique

With the patient in an upright position, the nipple position can be marked. The design itself can be modeled after the unaffected nipple-areola complex if available or drawn to create a nipple 1 cm in diameter. The base width of the flap is drawn 3 cm wide, and the lateral square flaps are each 1 × 1 cm (Fig. 65.1). The C flap extends inferiorly 1 × 1 cm from the central 1 cm segment of the inferior border [9].

In order to minimize thermal injury to the flaps, a no. 15 blade is used to incise and elevate the flaps. The lateral flaps are elevated with 1 mm of fat left on the dermis. At the central mound,

T. Roy, M.D. • D.R. Butz, M.D. • Z.J. Collier, B.A.
Department of Plastic Surgery, University of Chicago Medical Center, 5841 S. Maryland Avenue, Rm J641, MC 6035, Chicago, IL 60637, USA
e-mail: Tulsi.Roy@uchospitals.edu; Daniel.R.Butz@gmail.com; zjcollier@gmail.com

D.H. Song, M.D., M.B.A. (✉)
Section of Plastic and Reconstructive Surgery, Department of Surgery, The University of Chicago Medicine and Biological Sciences, 5841 South Maryland Avenue Room J641, MC 6035, Chicago, IL 60637, USA
e-mail: dsong@surgery.bsd.uchicago.edu


M.A. Shiffman (ed.), *Nipple-Areolar Complex Reconstruction*,
https://doi.org/10.1007/978-3-319-60925-6_65

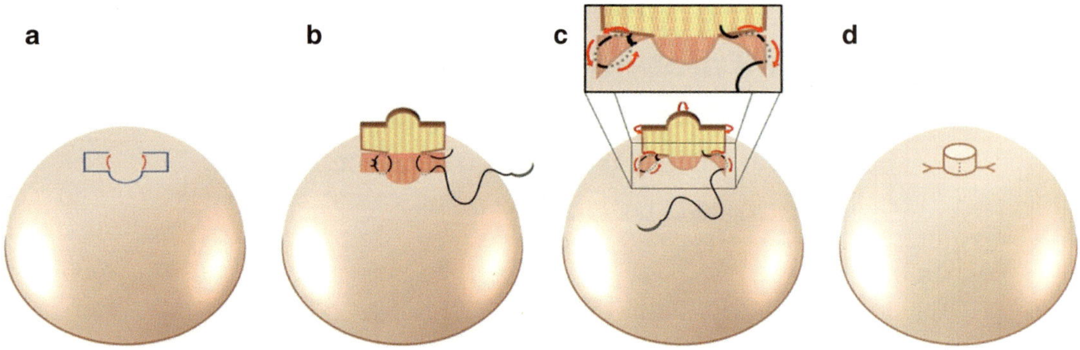


**Fig. 65.1** (**a**) The base width of the flap is drawn 3 cm wide, and the lateral square flaps are each 1 × 1 cm. (**b**) The flaps are raised, and the first two sutures are placed between the opposing medial corners to approximate the donor-site closure. (**c**) The remaining lateral donor sites are then approximated in a Y closure, using a triangular suture in superficial dermis extending from the superomedial edge to the lateral edge and then to the inferomedial edge. (**d**) The lateral flaps are approximated in the midline with suture, and a running suture is used to close the remaining incisions

the flap should be raised with approximately 5 mm of fat to provide bulk and protect the blood supply. 4-0 Maxon (Covidien, Mansfield, Mass.) is used for the deep dermal sutures. The first two sutures are placed between the opposing medial corners to approximate the donor-site closure (Fig. 65.1). The remaining lateral donor sites are then approximated in a Y closure, using a triangular suture in superficial dermis extending from the superomedial edge to the lateral edge and then to the inferomedial edge. The lateral flaps can then be approximated in the midline with deep dermal 4-0 Maxon suture. 5-0 Caprosyn (Covidien) is used in a running fashion to close remaining incisions. The nipple-areola complex is dressed with mupirocin ointment and Xeroform gauze. A hole is cut in a soft eye patch and placed around the Xeroform dressing. Two Tegaderm dressings (3M, St. Paul, Minn.) are placed over the Xeroform and eye patch to create a watertight seal and provide a padded buttress for preventing nipple compression. The dressing is removed in 1 week [9].

## 65.3 Discussion

The C-Y flap, as with other trilobed flaps, may be used with both autologous and implant-based breast reconstruction. The flap also provides many of the other benefits of trilobed flap reconstruction including simplicity of surgical technique and fast, reliable surgical outcomes with minimal donor-site morbidity. Similarly, the C-Y modification has a comparable rate of long-term loss of nipple projection to other trilobed flap-based reconstructive techniques, estimated to be 40–50% [10]. While loss of long-term projection proves to be a continuing challenge for nipple reconstruction [11], the literature suggests that this drawback may not have as significant an impact on patients' overall satisfaction with their breast reconstruction as previously thought [2].

The primary benefit of the C-Y modification is the reduction in donor-site scar length through a triangular closure that pulls the lateral incisions inward toward the nipple. This conceals the scars within the areolar tattoo. Furthermore, compared to linear closures, the small dog-ears resulting from this triangular Y closure may create a more realistic approximation of Montgomery tubercles and natural areolar texture in the final aesthetic result.

**Conclusions**

Trilobed flaps offer a basic and flexible method for nipple reconstruction. The C-Y modification's triangular closure of lateral donor sites facilitates a decreased scar length that can be concealed more easily within an areolar tattoo.

The C-Y modification, therefore, is an attractive option for local flap-based nipple reconstruction that minimizes donor-site morbidity and improves aesthetic outcomes while maintaining the ideal nipple projection and technical ease of the trilobed design.

## References


1. Wellisch DK, Schain WS, Noone RB, Little JW III. The psychological contribution of nipple addition in breast reconstruction. Plast Reconstr Surg. 1987;80(5):699–704.
2. Sisti A, Grimaldi L, Tassinari J, Cuomo R, Fortezza L, Bocchiotti MA, Roviello F, D'Aniello C, Nisi G. Nipple-areola complex reconstruction techniques: a literature review. Eur J Surg Oncol. 2016;42(4):441–65.
3. Eskenazi L. A one-stage nipple reconstruction with the "modified star" flap and immediate tattoo: a review of 100 cases. Plast Reconstr Surg. 1993;92:671–80.
4. Rubino C, Dessy LA, Posadinu A. A modified technique for nipple reconstruction: the 'arrow flap'. Br J Plast Surg. 2003;56(3):247–51.
5. Spyropoulou GA, Sterne GD. Algorithm for an aesthetically pleasing nipple-areola complex with the use of the C-V flap in cases of skin-sparing mastectomy and immediate reconstruction. Aesthet Plast Surg. 2009;33(2):240–2.
6. Hamori CA, LaRossa D. The top hat flap: for one stage reconstruction of a prominent nipple. Aesthet Plast Surg. 1998;22:142–4.
7. Hammond DC, Khuthaila D, Kim J. The skate flap purse-string technique for nipple-areola complex reconstruction. Plast Reconstr Surg. 2007;120:399–406.
8. Katerinaki E, Sircar T, Sterne GD. The C-V flap for nipple reconstruction after previous skin-sparing mastectomy and immediate breast reconstruction: refinements of donor-site closure. Aesthet Plast Surg. 2011;35(4):624–7.
9. Butz DR, Kim EK, Song DH. C-Y Trilobed flap for improved nipple-areola complex reconstruction. Plast Reconstr Surg. 2015;136(2):234–7.
10. Shestak KC, Gabriel A, Landecker A, Peters S, Shestak A, Kim J. Assessment of long-term nipple projection: a comparison of three techniques. Plast Reconstr Surg. 2002;110:780–6.
11. Farhadi J, Maksvytyte GK, Schaefer DJ, Pierer G, Scheufler O. Reconstruction of the nipple-areola complex: an update. J Plast Reconstr Aesthet Surg. 2006;59(1):40–53.

# The Skate Flap Purse-String Technique for Nipple-Areola Complex Reconstruction

66

Dennis Clyde Hammond and Eric Yu Kit Li

## 66.1 Introduction

Nipple-areola complex (NAC) reconstruction represents the last step in postmastectomy breast reconstruction, and it is well established that women who opt for this reconstruction have a higher degree of satisfaction with their final result [1–3]. Nearly universal to all techniques, however, is the loss of projection in reconstructed NACs over time [4]. In the pursuit of creating long-lasting NACs with adequate volume, numerous techniques have been attempted over the past four decades. In some, local flaps of various designs are harvested from the apex of the reconstructed breast to create the nipple. The challenge associated with these techniques is in harvesting large enough flaps to accomplish the goal of a projected nipple without excessively compromising the contour of the reconstructed breast after primary closure of the defect. Others have advocated the use of full-thickness skin grafts to provide coverage in the areas of the elevated flaps. These techniques face different problems, in that they require a second donor site, adequate graft take, and the grafted skin may not always optimally retain tattoo pigment.

We have previously described a technique for NAC reconstruction that attempts to resolve the aforementioned issues, described as the "skate flap purse-string nipple technique" [5]. The technique is a modification of the traditional skate flap that incorporates our purse-string techniques used in breast reduction and mastopexy [5–10]. Two rectangular flaps and a cap extension are used to reconstruct the nipple mound, two matching island flaps are used to reconstruct the areola, and the resulting peri-areolar defect is closed with a purse-string suture. This technique allows primary closure of all areas, and by advancing tissue from the entire periphery of the reconstructed areola, distortion to the overall breast contour is minimized. The skate flap purse-string technique can be ubiquitously applied to autologous breast reconstruction in either the immediate or delayed setting or also in implant-based techniques, provided the tissues have sufficient thickness and vascularity to allow such tissue rearrangement. In this chapter, we will elaborate on our technique.

D.C. Hammond, M.D. (✉)
Partners in Plastic Surgery of West Michigan, 4070 Lake Drive Suite 202, Grand Rapids, MI, USA

Department of Surgery, Michigan State University College of Human Medicine, East Lansing, MI, USA
e-mail: drhammond@pipsmd.com; hammonddc@aol.com

E.Y.K. Li, M.D.
Partners in Plastic Surgery of West Michigan, 4070 Lake Drive Suite 202, Grand Rapids, MI, USA
e-mail: yukit.li@medportal.ca


M.A. Shiffman (ed.), *Nipple-Areolar Complex Reconstruction*,
https://doi.org/10.1007/978-3-319-60925-6_66

## 66.2 Technique

The patient is marked in the upright position. A nipple with a desired diameter, usually 1 cm, is first marked at the most projecting portion of the breast mound. A modified skate flap pattern is then designed, such that the vertical length *P* is twice the final desired projection of the reconstructed nipple, taking into account likely postoperative contraction. The horizontal length *D* is the diameter of the areola and is generally designed greater than 4 cm to allow the skate flap wings to be approximated without tension. Next, the cap of the skate flap is designed as a hemi-oval, with a height that is approximately the same as the skate flap wings, to allow it to be folded down comfortably to create an aesthetically pleasing rounded tip. The design of the skate flap is best based inferiorly on the breast mound, so the elevated flap is hinged inferiorly. This nuance allows gravity to oppose the natural tendency of the reconstructed nipple mound to retract.

The inferior and superior areolar skin islands are designed last. From the center of the proposed nipple, a line equal in length to the radius of the areola ($D/2 = R$) is drawn extending inferiorly along the midline, concluding at the inferior margin of the inferior areolar island flap. Likewise, from the center of the cap flap, a line of the same length (*R*) is drawn extending superiorly along the midline, concluding at the superior margin of the superior areolar island flap. This superior extent, the aforementioned inferior extent, and the wings of the skate flap are then all joined together in a rounded arc, ultimately forming an elongated oval. Of note, the superior areolar island flap will be asymmetrically larger than its inferior counterpart since it is advanced around the reconstructed nipple before being approximated to each other. The final result upon closure is a circular areola (Fig. 66.1).

At the time of surgery, all marked areas are first incised in full-thickness fashion through the dermis. The skate flap is elevated in the subcutaneous plane, usually keeping 1–2 mm thickness of fat with the flap, toward its base, until it can be hinged 90° without any tethering. Of particular note, when elevating the cap portion of the skate flap, a small amount of dermis is intentionally left on the donor site. This tissue will act as a hammock to support and prevent

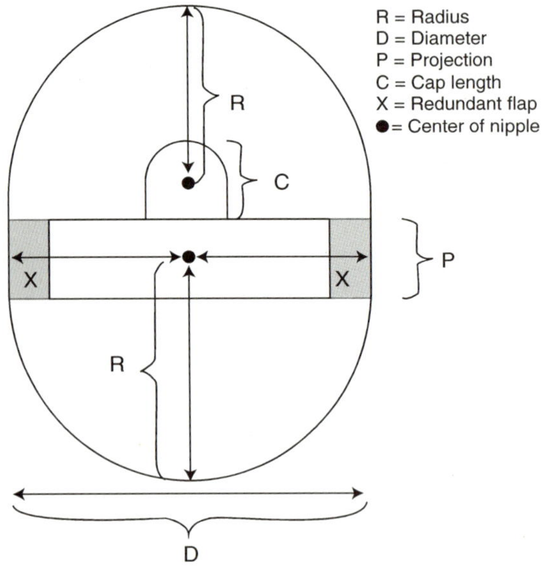


**Fig. 66.1** Preoperative markings of the skate flap purse-string technique

retraction of the reconstructed nipple mound. The thickness of the remainder of the skate flap can be altered depending on the skin thickness of the breast mound tissues. For example, in a latissimus dorsi skin island, less fat can be retained since back skin is thicker. Conversely, in a skin island of an abdominal-based flap, more fat is retained as the abdominal skin is thinner. Next, the inner edges of the areolar skin islands are elevated in the subcutaneous plane for a few millimeters, to facilitate their advancement toward the center. The wings of the skate flap are now trimmed as desired to create the ideal nipple circumference and volume.

Closure of the reconstructed NAC is first accomplished by approximating the wings of the skate flap with 5-0 absorbable gut sutures. The cap is then folded over and inset with the same sutures to create a rounded contour to the apex of the nipple. The two hemi-areolar skin islands are next advanced toward each other, around the reconstructed nipple, and approximated with inverted interrupted deep dermal 4-0 monofilament sutures. At this point, the reconstructed nipple fits into the hemi-oval defect left over from elevation of the cap, where it is also supported by the retained dermis at the base of the defect. Inset of the nipple and the two hemi-areolar flaps is completed with a simple running 5-0 absorbable gut suture (Fig. 66.2).

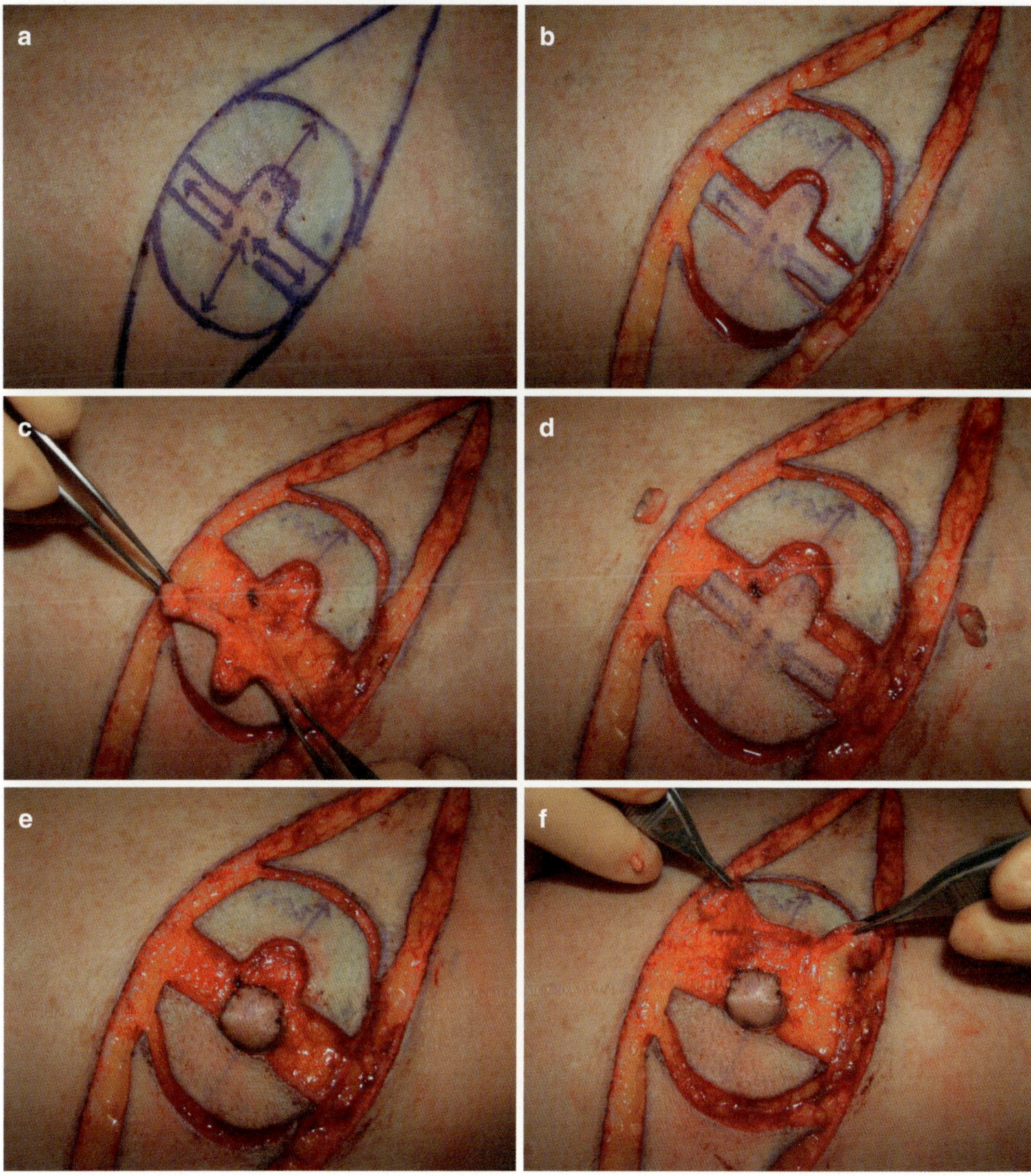


**Fig. 66.2** Technical steps for elevation of the modified skate flap and creation of the nipple mound. Preoperative markings of a patient in preparation for bilateral skin-sparing mastectomies and immediate breast reconstruction with pedicled latissimus dorsi musculocutaneous flaps. (**a**) Skate flaps have been designed on the skin paddles of the latissimus dorsi flaps based on their anticipated transposition to the chest. (**b**, **c**) The skate flap pattern is incised in full-thickness fashion and the skate flap raised. (**d**) Excess tissues from the wings of the skate flap are trimmed. (**e**) The nipple mound is first reconstructed, (**f**, **g**) followed by approximation of the areolar island flaps, which have been undermined slightly to facilitate their advancement. (**h**, **i**) The remainder of the latissimus dorsi flap is harvested and transposed to the chest, and the redundant skin paddle is removed. (**j**) The latissimus dorsi muscle and overlying fat provide volume to the breast mound underneath the mastectomy flaps, and the reconstructed NAC is inset into the skin-sparing mastectomy defect. Initial postoperative appearance

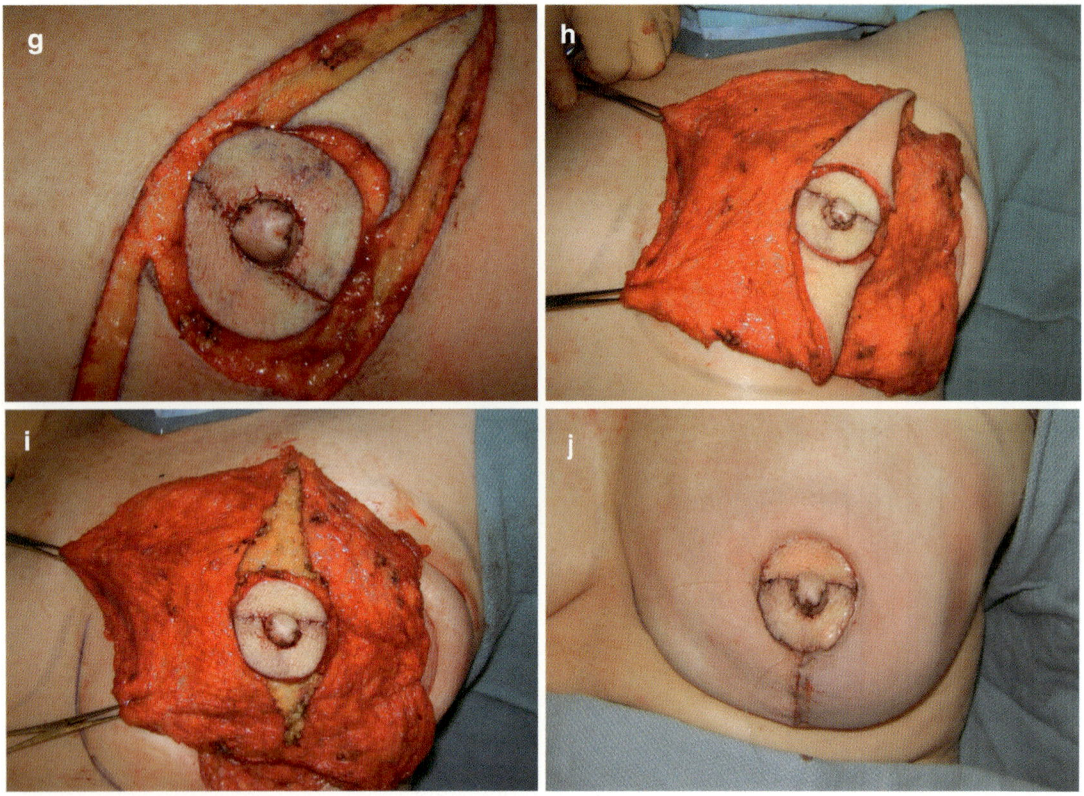


**Fig. 66.2** (continued)

At this point, the diameter of the peri-areolar defect is larger than the reconstructed areola, with the difference representing the "dog ear" associated with the design of this pattern. To control and securely close the peri-areolar defect, standard purse-string technique is applied. Eight evenly spaced cardinal points are marked on both the circular areola and the outer peri-areolar incision to guide suture placement. Next, the peripheral edges of the peri-areolar incision are elevated just below the dermis, extending out 1 cm. This will allow the edges to be later cinched down without tissue bunching. A 2-0 polytetrafluoroethylene (PTFE) or Teflon suture on a straight needle is used for the peri-areolar closure. This permanent monofilament suture is preferred by the authors due to the fact that it passes through the dermis with reduced friction and thus provides the surgeon with excellent control of the final size of the peri-areolar opening. Alternatively, a 2-0 Prolene suture on a straight needle can be used.

Irrespective of the suture chosen, the suture is passed, from deep to superficial on the medial dermal shelf of the outer peri-areolar incision, through the dermis of the corresponding cardinal point on the circular areola, inserted back into the outer dermal shelf, and then passed through the outer dermis to the next peri-areolar cardinal point. This weaving is repeated until the suture has passed completely around the peri-areolar defect, culminating in the appearance of a wagon wheel (Fig. 66.3). The free suture ends are then tightened to cinch down the outer peri-areolar incision to match the inner circular areola, followed by placement of 8–10 throws to secure a knot. If a mild pseudo-herniated result to the areola is desired, the cinching can be more aggressive to further reduce the peri-areolar defect. The knot complex is buried underneath the medial dermal shelf, and final peri-areolar closure is completed with a running subcuticular 4-0 monofilament suture. All incisions are then covered

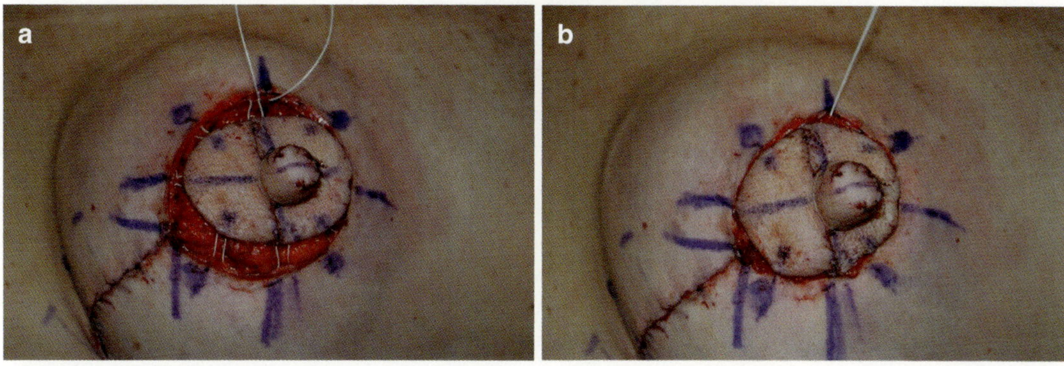


**Fig. 66.3** Purse-string technique for closure of the peri-areolar defect. (**a**) The purse-string technique is used to inset the reconstructed NAC. Note the eight evenly spaced cardinal points on both the circular areola and the outer peri-areolar incision to guide suture placement. (**b**) The free ends are tightened resulting in mild pseudo-herniation of the NAC

with Dermabond (Ethicon, Somerville, New Jersey) and clear adhesive semiocclusive dressings, which remain in place for 7–10 days. A cotton pad with a small cut out is applied to the reconstructed nipple for 4–6 weeks to protect it from pressure and shear. Finally, medical tattooing of the reconstructed NAC is completed at 3–6 months postoperatively.

## 66.3 Discussion

The skate flap purse-string nipple technique is a synergy of purse-string concepts initially described by Eng [11] and skate flap concepts initially described by Andersen and Menezes [12]. With this technique, the defect created from elevation of the skate flap is essentially redistributed to the peripheral peri-areolar area. By gathering tissues equally from the entire periphery, subsequent purse-string closure is able to minimize distortion to the overall reconstructed breast contour. Additional advantages include primary healing of all wounds and the avoidance of additional donor sites or scars beyond the reconstructed areola.

The skate flap purse-string nipple technique is applicable to a wide variety of breast reconstruction scenarios. In implant-based reconstructions, this technique can be used provided the native mastectomy flaps have sufficient thickness and vascularity to allow this tissue rearrangement. In autologous reconstructions, this technique can also be used in the immediate stage coinciding with flap inset (Fig. 66.4) or in a delayed fashion (Fig. 66.5) after settling of the reconstructed breast mound. Perhaps the most innovative use of this technique is in autologous reconstructions after skin-sparing mastectomy. If the orientation of the flap inset is predicted, the skate flap pattern can be expertly designed and created in the skin paddle of the flap (Fig. 66.4). This allows the NAC to be concurrently reconstructed with flap harvest and inset into the corresponding skin-sparing mastectomy defect, all in one procedure. We have done this on many occasions in immediate two-stage breast reconstructions with pedicled latissimus dorsi musculocutaneous flaps with great satisfaction.

Like other techniques, the skate flap purse-string technique is still susceptible to loss of nipple projection over time as the reconstructed nipple is not immune to the retractive forces of scar. However, this technique features three design elements that specifically counteract de-projection. The first is that height $P$ can be increased as deemed necessary to initially create an overcorrected projection without excessively compromising the contour of the reconstructed breast. For example, in nipples reconstructed from thinner abdominal skin, the initial projection can be made twice or more that of the contralateral nipple in anticipation of nipple mound contraction. For nipples reconstructed from

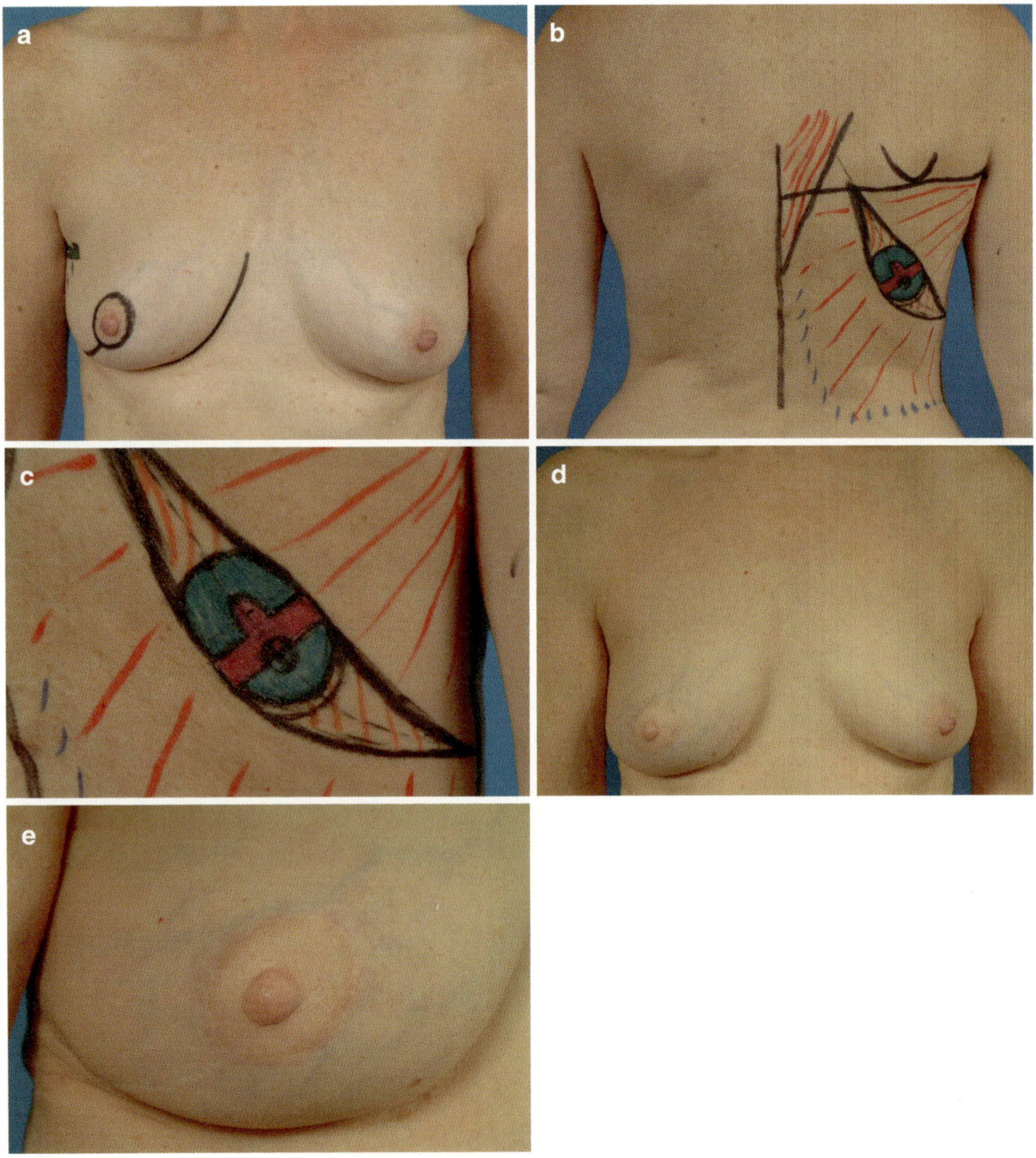

**Fig. 66.4** Use of the skate flap purse-string technique in conjunction with immediate breast reconstruction. (**a–c**) Preoperative markings of a patient in preparation for a right skin-sparing mastectomy, immediate breast reconstruction with a pedicled latissimus dorsi musculocutaneous flap, and immediate NAC reconstruction with the skate flap purse-string technique. (**d**, **e**) Six years postoperative

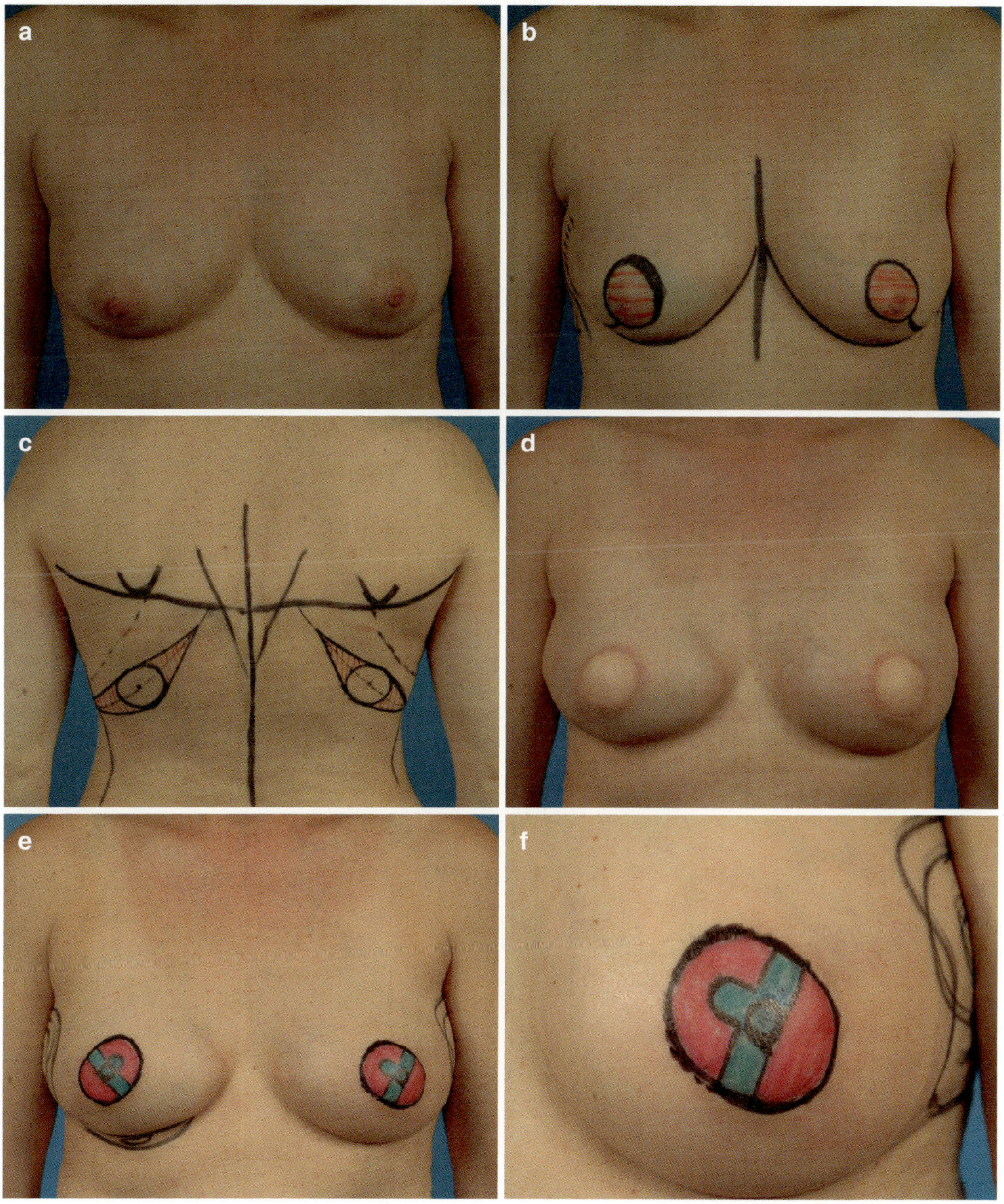


**Fig. 66.5** Use of the skate flap purse-string technique in conjunction with delayed breast reconstruction. (**a–c**) Preoperative markings of a patient in preparation for bilateral skin-sparing mastectomies and immediate breast reconstruction with pedicled latissimus dorsi musculocutaneous flaps. (**d**) Initial postoperative result. (**e**, **f**) Preoperative markings for delayed bilateral NAC reconstruction with the skate flap purse-string technique and fat grafting to the right breast 8 months after her initial surgery. (**g**) The skate flap pattern is first incised in full-thickness fashion and the skate flap raised. (**h**, **i**) The areolar island flaps have been undermined slightly to facilitate their advancement. (**j**, **k**) The nipple mound is reconstructed, followed by approximation of the areolar island flaps. (**k**, **l**) The purse-string technique is then used to cinch down the peri-areolar defect. (**m**, **n**) Reconstructed NAC after final closure. (**o**) One year postoperative. (**p**) Six years postoperative

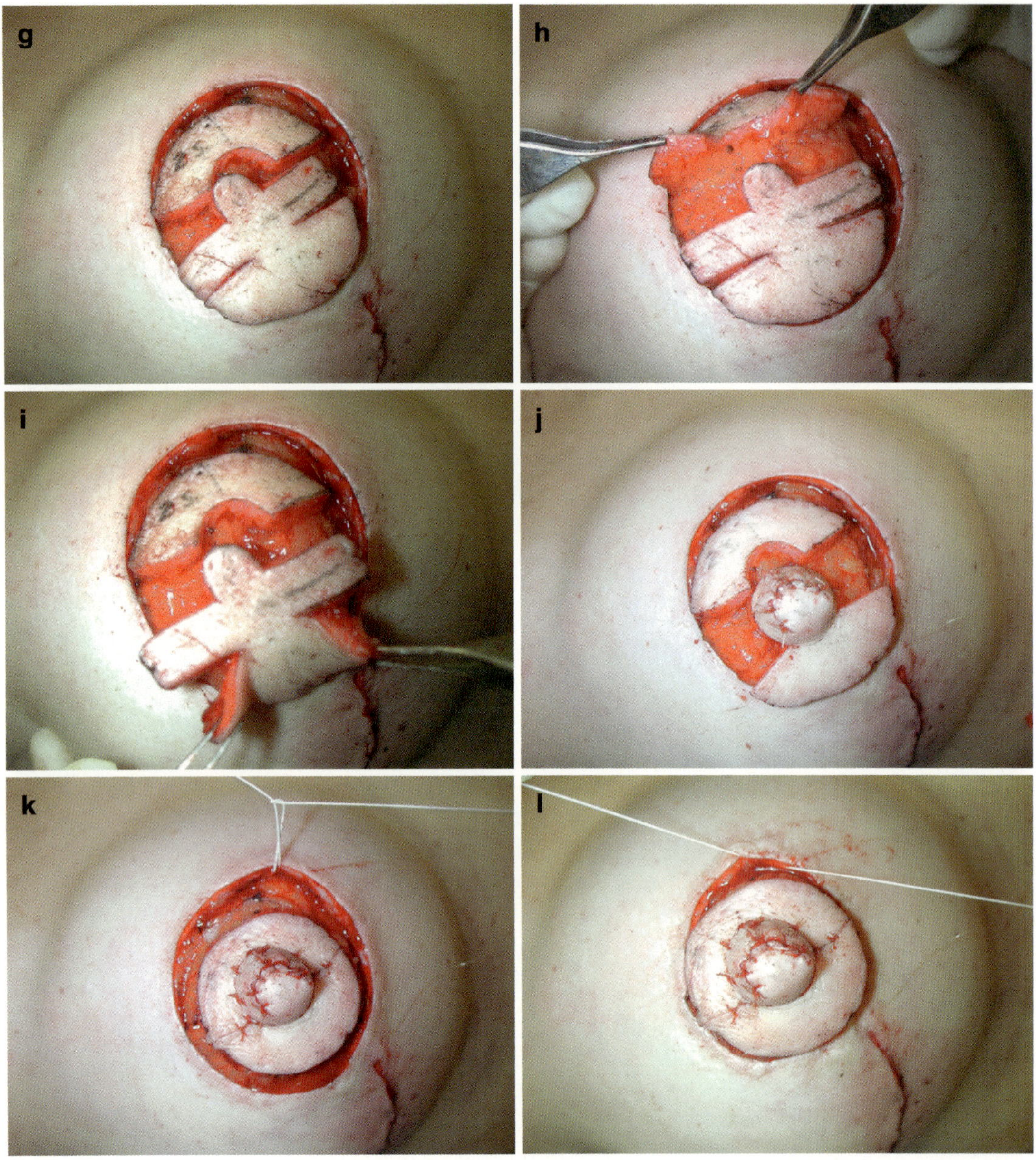


**Fig. 66.5** (continued)

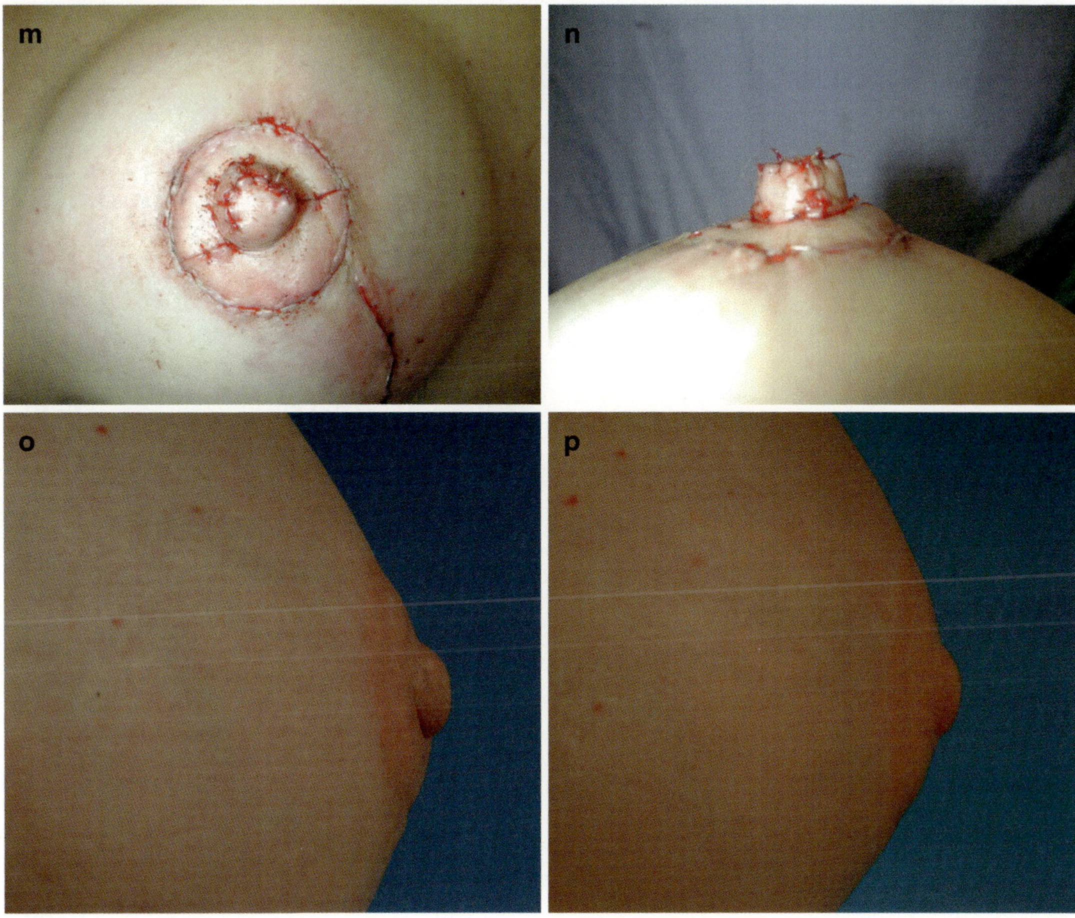


**Fig. 66.5** (continued)

thicker back skin, the height $P$ can be decreased slightly, and we recommend 1.5× the contralateral nipple height. The second element is that skate flap is based and hinged inferiorly, allowing gravity to oppose nipple mound retraction. Finally, the third element is the dermal hammock from the cap flap donor site which serves to suspend and support the reconstructed nipple above the breast mound.

In situations where a smaller diameter NAC is desired, the diameter $D$ of the skate flap can be made less than 4 cm. This, however, will shorten the skate flap wings. To avoid compromising the vascularity of the wing flaps once they are folded and approximated, it is best to extend the wings beyond the hemi-oval boundaries. This carries the final scar outside the reconstructed areola, but this is the necessary compromise. The remaining steps of the technique are the same.

Revisions, although uncommon, may sometimes be necessary. In the event of an excessively projected nipple, the skate flap can simply be reopened, shortened, and re-approximated as needed. If the final areolar shape is not circular, tattoos can be applied beyond the borders of the scars to create the desired areola shape and may also provide additional benefit in terms of camouflaging these scars.

## Conclusions

The skate flap purse-string nipple technique is a valuable and versatile method that uses efficient local tissue rearrangement to reconstruct the NAC and minimize distortion of the reconstructed breast contour. A nipple mound of adequate projection is created, and the reconstructed areola heals primarily, lending itself to more predictable tattooing. Disadvantages with other techniques, including additional donor sites, constricted breast contours, or scars beyond the reconstructed areola, are avoided. It is therefore highly recommended as a useful tool in the armamentarium of a reconstructive breast surgeon.

## References


1. Momoh AO, Colakoglu S, De Blacam C, Yueh JH, Lin SJ, Tobias AM, Lee BT. The impact of nipple reconstruction on patient satisfaction in breast reconstruction. Ann Plast Surg. 2012;69(4):389–93.
2. Wellisch DK, Schain WS, Noone RB, Little JW. The psychological contribution of nipple addition in breast reconstruction. Plast Reconstr Surg. 1987;80(5):699–704.
3. Yang JD, Ryu JY, Ryu DW, Kwon OH, Bae SG, Lee JW, Choi KY, Chung HY, Cho BC. Our experiences in nipple reconstruction using the Hammond flap. Arch Plast Surg. 2014;41(5):550–5.
4. Sisti A, Grimaldi L, Tassinari J, Cuomo R, Fortezza L, Bocchiotti MA, Roviello F, D'Aniello C, Nisi G. Nipple-areola complex reconstruction techniques: a literature review. Eur J Surg Oncol. 2016;42(4):441–65.
5. Hammond DC, Khuthaila D, Kim J. The skate flap purse-string technique for nipple-areola complex reconstruction. Plast Reconstr Surg. 2007;120(2):399–406.
6. Hammond DC. Short scar periareolar inferior pedicle reduction (SPAIR) mammaplasty. Plast Reconstr Surg. 1999;103(3):890–902.
7. Hammond DC. The short scar periareolar inferior pedicle reduction (SPAIR) mammaplasty. Semin Plast Surg. 2004;18(3):231–43.
8. Hammond DC. The SPAIR mammaplasty. Clin Plast Surg. 2002;29(3):411–21.
9. Hammond DC, Alfonso D, Khuthaila D. Mastopexy using the short scar periareolar inferior pedicle reduction technique. Plast Reconstr Surg. 2008;121(5):1533–9.
10. Hammond DC, Khuthaila D, Kim J. The interlocking Gore-Tex suture for control of areolar diameter and shape. Plast Reconstr Surg. 2007;119(3):804–9.
11. Eng JS. Bell flap nipple reconstruction—a new wrinkle. Ann Plast Surg. 1996;36(5):485–8.
12. Andersen JS, Menezes MJ. Purse-string reconstruction of nipple and areola. Presented at 56th Annual Meeting of the American Society of Plastic Surgeons: San Diego, California, 11–15 Oct 2013.

# Reconstruction of the Nipple-Areola Complex: How to Choose a Few, Among So Many Techniques

67

Jefferson Di Lamartine, Juldasio Galdino Jr., Leonardo David Pires Barcelos, and Leonardo Martins Costa Daher

## 67.1 Introduction

The reconstruction program of the nipple-areola complex (NAC) should neither be relegated to a third or fourth time of a breast reconstruction nor overlooked, for it is the finishing touch to a project that sometimes lasts for years, since the beginning of the breast cancer treatment. The proper NAC reconstruction is the ultimate step for patients in the struggle against breast cancer, due to its importance as an anatomical breast unit.

In 1949, Adams [1] pioneered the use of skin graft of the labia minora as donor area for NAC reconstruction. Other techniques using labia majora have been described but with disappointing results, due to inadequate color of the graft, in addition to the need for a donor area approach in which the residual deformity is a fact [2, 3]. In light-skinned patients, Brent and Bostwick [4] utilized skin grafting of the retroauricular region with good results, the rosy hue obtained in patients with little pigmentation of the NAC. The skin of the inguinoperineal region is best employed for reconstructions requiring darker pigmentation of the NAC [3, 5].

The so-called nipple banks were described by Millard et al. [6] in 1971. It consisted originally of the removal of the NAC and its transfer to the buttocks, groin, or abdomen in the form of graft during mastectomy. Later, during the reconstruction of the breast, the grafts were collected and used for NAC reconstruction. The findings of lymph node involvement with mammary cells in inguinal regions have raised concerns about the safety of this method.

The evolution of NAC reconstructions occurred in the past two decades, with the use of

J. Di Lamartine, M.D. (✉)
SCN Quadra 2, Torre A, Salas 1.121/1.123, 11o Andar, Shopping Liberty Mall, Brasília 70712-904, DF, Brazil

Di Lamartine Institute of Plastic Surgery—LTDA, Brasília, Brazil

Department of Plastic and Reconstructive Surgery, Daher Hospital, Brasília, Brazil
e-mail: jefferson@dilamartine.com.br

J. Galdino Jr., M.D.
SCN Quadra 2, Torre A, Salas 1.121/1.123, 11o Andar, Shopping Liberty Mall, Brasília 70712-904, DF, Brazil

Di Lamartine Institute of Plastic Surgery—LTDA, Brasília, Brazil
e-mail: juldasiojr@dilamartine.com.br

L.D.P. Barcelos, M.D. • L.M.C. Daher, M.D.
Department of Plastic and Reconstructive Surgery, Daher Hospital, Brasília, Brazil

SHIS, QI 07, Conjunto F, LagoSul, Brasília 71671-570, DF, Brazil
e-mail: ldpb1000@gmail.com; daher_leonardo@hotmail.com


M.A. Shiffman (ed.), *Nipple-Areolar Complex Reconstruction*, https://doi.org/10.1007/978-3-319-60925-6_67

local skin flaps, and that was the hallmark of evolutionary NAC reconstruction. The first technique was published by Berson [7] in 1946, in which he weaved three triangular skin flaps that would be elevated and sutured to form a nipple projection. In 1984, Little [8] created the skate flap, which became the most popular technique for NAC reconstruction (Fig. 67.1). The skate flap is a vertical dermofat graft flap that is elevated with both wings curled around a fat central nucleus to assure an adequate nipple projection. Dermopigmentation (tattoo) is used to obtain the NAC coloring. Several modifications have arisen from this technique, and among them is a quite efficient technique called double opposing flap described by Shestak and Nguyen [9] enabling NAC reconstruction with adequate diameter, good projection, and symmetry with the contralateral side, with the possibility of closing the donor area and all scars being contained within the topography of the reconstructed areola.

From the planning to the completion of a single or bilateral breast reconstruction, the objective should be the NAC reconstruction, so it is not improvised, because at the end of this meticulous process, the lack of planning implies unsatisfactory results though not that improvising based on technical principles which are not used in some cases according to the experience of each surgeon. Therefore, contrary to the expected, the NAC cannot be regarded as the last and most simple act of a breast reconstruction, because it gallantly concludes an excellent breast reconstruction or may devastate it when poorly planned.

The NAC reconstructions must be conceived in different types of breast reconstruction techniques, for these techniques present greater or lesser availability of tissue to be used in the preparation of the NAC. In cases utilizing distant flaps (TRAM and latissimus dorsi), such availability of tissues is greater than in the case of tissue expanders or local flaps.

Among the various existing techniques, the surgeon who works in this bright area of plastic surgery must know some of them so he is able to choose the most suitable for the resolution in most cases. Starting with the most simple of them, which is the free graft of papilla to the most complex ones. There is a variety of reasons and motives, as well as indications and contraindications for many of these techniques. One must also consider the need of single or bilateral reconstruction and the size of the NAC on the opposite side, the quality of the skin, treatment with radiotherapy or not, the presence or absence of scars and their disposition, among others. This way, as the surgeon dominates the techniques, he can adapt them to most cases with success and predictability of results, because the negligent planning of a NAC could harm an excellent reconstruction.

An important detail in the NAC reconstruction is whether or not it is necessary to approach that aggregate scars out of mammary topography, as, for example, the inguinal region, retroauricular region, and eyelids, among others. Often the approach to an area remote to the neo-nipple aims to obtain skin with the same color of the NAC on the opposite side; however, this can be obtained through dermopigmentation, which has become very safe and predictable nowadays, with the possibility of offering excellent results.

The ideal technique for NAC reconstruction should enable the works on any type of tissue, despite previous scars and radiotherapy, in addition to allowing that the limits of the new NAC do not exceed flap margins used in nipple reconstructions. Likewise, it is ideal that the approach of other areas of the body for the production of tissues is unnecessary, and in addition to the papilla, the reconstruction of a relief simulating the areola is possible. Losken et al. [10] (C-V flap), Anton et al. [11] (star flap), Eskenazi [12] (wrap flap), and Little [8] (skate flap) presented results in accordance with these characteristics. The double opposing flap, described by Shestak and Nguyen [9], ensures these principles and still adheres to an appointment that directs all phases of surgery and dictates the shape and the perimeter of the new NAC.

Following the evolution of the nipple reconstruction techniques, with various authors and mentioning one or two times at most, Hammond et al. [13] (Fig. 67.2) describe the possibility of reconstructing the NAC in first time plus a "double opposing flap-like" in that there is no need to

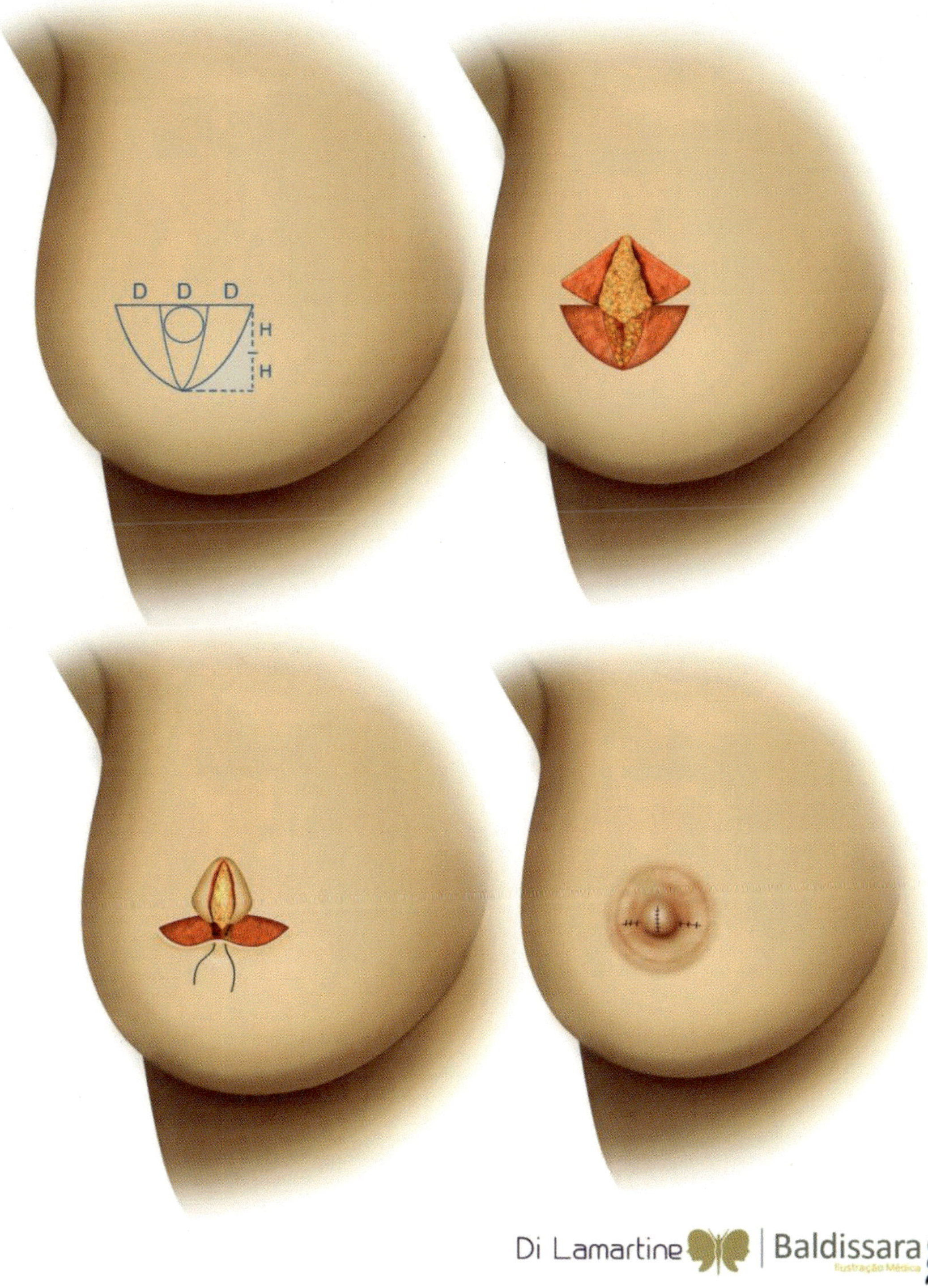


Fig. 67.1 Schematic drawing of the skate flap

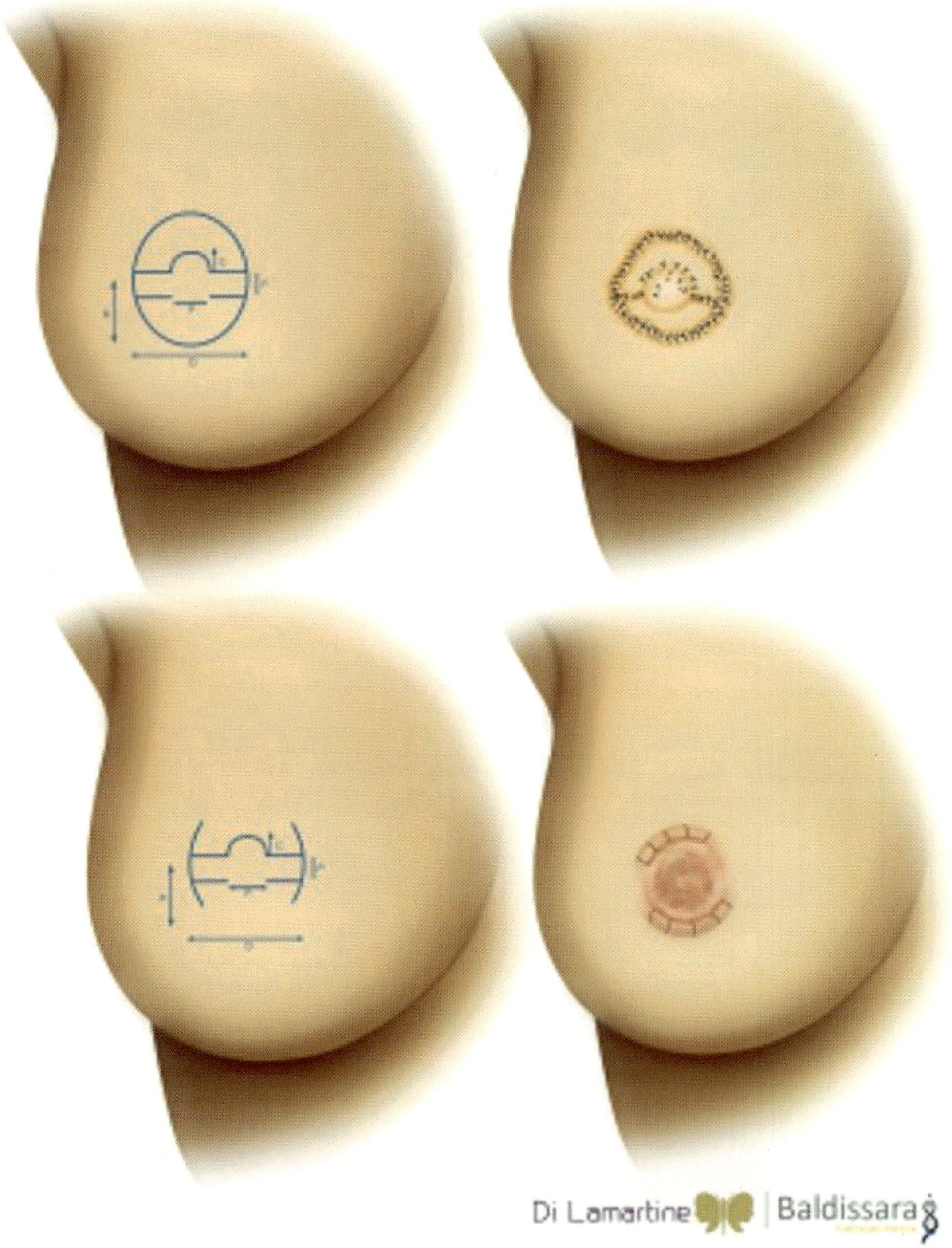


**Fig. 67.2** Comparison of the double opposing flap and the Hammond technique

use the entire incision in a circle as described by Shestak and Nguyen [9] but only part of it.

The comparison of the horizontal diameter (HD) and the nipple projection (NP) proposed by our team [14] for bilateral nipple reconstructions presented a higher similarity when compared to unilateral reconstructions. In bilateral reconstructions, the curves almost overlap, demonstrating similarity between the right and left breasts with regard to HD and NP.

According to Farhadi et al. [15], the NAC reconstruction should be deferred until the neo-nipple obtains stable configuration (usually from 4 to 6 months after breast reconstruction). In unilateral nipple reconstructions, the contralateral NAC should serve as a model; however, its position must be adapted to avoid residual breast asymmetries. The location of the NAC must be planned according to the anatomical references and aesthetic preferences of the patient in bilateral nipple reconstructions. Loss of projection of the reconstructed nipple should always be predicted due to scar retraction. Therefore, the programming of the new NAC should present a hypercorrection ranging from 25 to 50% of the desired result [9].

The goals of NAC reconstruction are:

1. Good correlation position of the reconstructed nipple with the contralateral nipple
2. Adequate and sustainable projection of the nipple resembling the opposite nipple
3. Same skin tonality and color between the two sides

## 67.2 Technique

Among all the techniques employing flaps for NAC reconstruction, the technique described by Shestak and Nguyen [9], called double opposing flap (DOF), enables the reconstruction with the appropriate diameter, good projection, and symmetrical to the contralateral, with the possibility of closing the donor area in addition to maintaining all the scars in the topography of the new reconstructed nipple. A detail of this technique is that it allows the creation of a NAC with relief in relation to the adjacent skin, which mimics the natural look of an areola and nipple.

The DOF, as most local flaps, must be performed after obtaining the neo-nipple projection stability, usually in the second or third times of breast reconstructions, although it can be done in the first time. In unilateral nipple reconstructions with the goal of better symmetrization, one should initially study the position of the contralateral nipple, the diameter of the base and projection, and the horizontal and vertical measures of the areola and nipple.

Two important details in the planning of the NAC reconstruction and aiming at preserving more subcutaneous tissue (TCSC) in the projection of the new NAC are:

1. Not using the same mastectomy scar at the time of exchanging the expander for prosthetics, in case it is in the projection of the NAC to be reconstructed.
2. Preserving more subcutaneous tissue (SCT) enables fat grafting in that area, postponing NAC reconstruction to a third time. We highlight the singular importance of fat grafting in nipple reconstructions as described by various authors [16–18]. In addition to aggregating substrate to cover the implants, such procedure would invigorate the skin on the irradiated breasts and recover the SCT [15, 17, 18].

Given the predictability and security offered by the DOF, we elected it in our routine as the preferred technique in most NAC reconstructions, for in addition to the excellent attributes described by the creator of the technique, we find enough security in its confection, even in cases of several scars and radiotherapy. The important detail of this technique is the two sessile flaps providing perfusion capability of the entire new areola and nipple (Fig. 67.3).

We incorporated some modifications in our series regarding the flap design with the purpose of that after all the sutures are made, its format is indeed round and keep the nipple in the center (Fig. 67.3) [14]. The way we idealize, the oval design allows us to achieve a circular NAC, and the nipple is centered, which did not occur with the original design, so that there was need for dermopigmentation exceeding the limits of the scars with demerit in the result. Whenever the flaps show shortage of SCT, we added fibrous

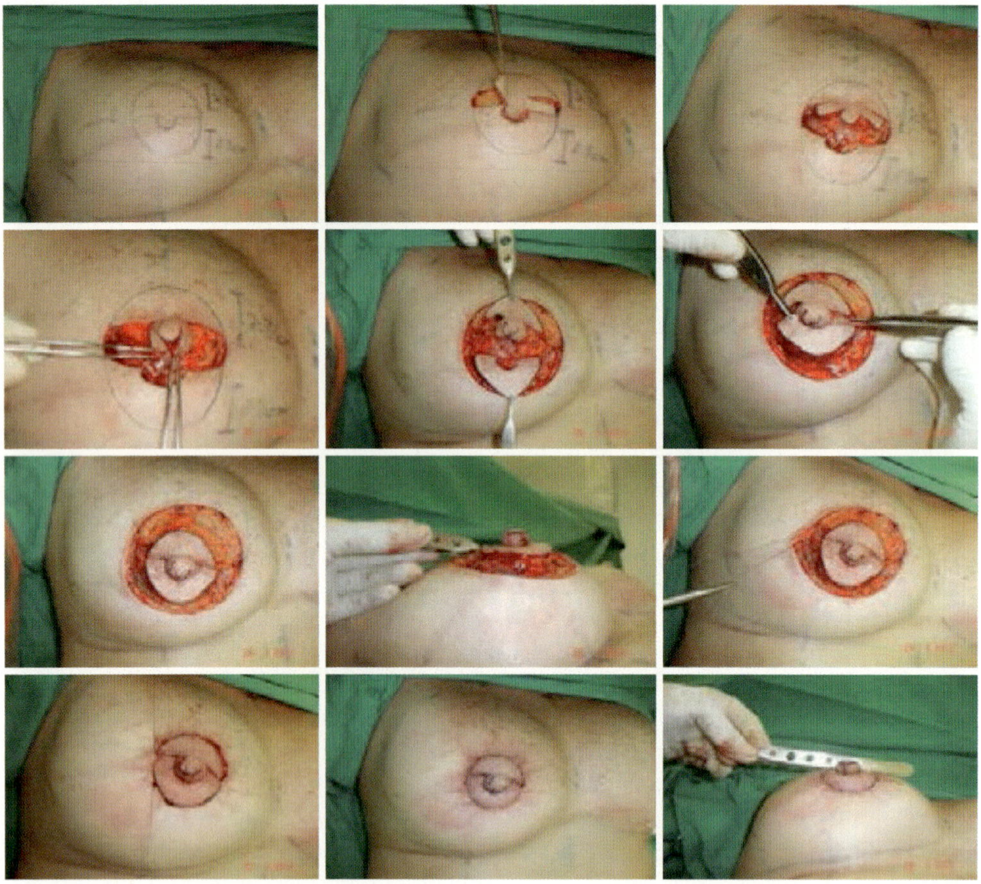

**Fig. 67.3** Surgery technique demonstrating the oval design, the flap dissection, the synthesis between the various segments, the round block suture with Nylon® 3/0 or 2/0, and the result with good projection

tissue grafts or dermis (deepithelialized) inside the nipple to ensure an increase and better long-term maintenance of the NAC projection.

The flap is designed with the nipple located at the point of greatest projection of the neo-nipple, whereas the opposite areola in cases of unilateral reconstruction. The width of the base of the opposite nipple and its projection determine the size of the flap made. In the case of bilateral reconstructions, this measure must be individualized, but most of the time their dimensions must be between 10 and 12 mm. The widths of the side extensions determine the nipple projection. The length of the side extensions must be between 20 and 22 mm, and may reach 30 mm (Fig. 67.4) [14].

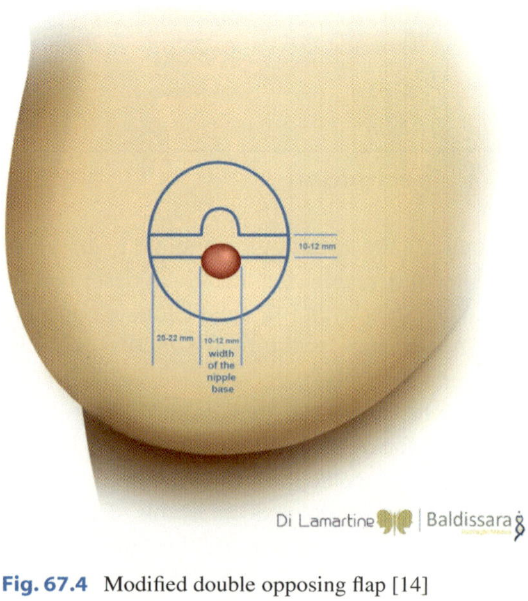


**Fig. 67.4** Modified double opposing flap [14]

The areola on the opposite side must be carefully analyzed and their diameters registered. The reconstruction of NAC must be planned to introduce measures 20–25% larger in relation to the opposite side for symmetry regarding the contralateral at the end of the whole process of scarring and remodeling. A round block suture is performed to equalize its dimensions and promote the reconstructed NAC overlapping in relation to neo-nipple skin (Fig. 67.5). After 3–4 months, the diameter of the reconstructed NAC should resemble the opposite side, so that the

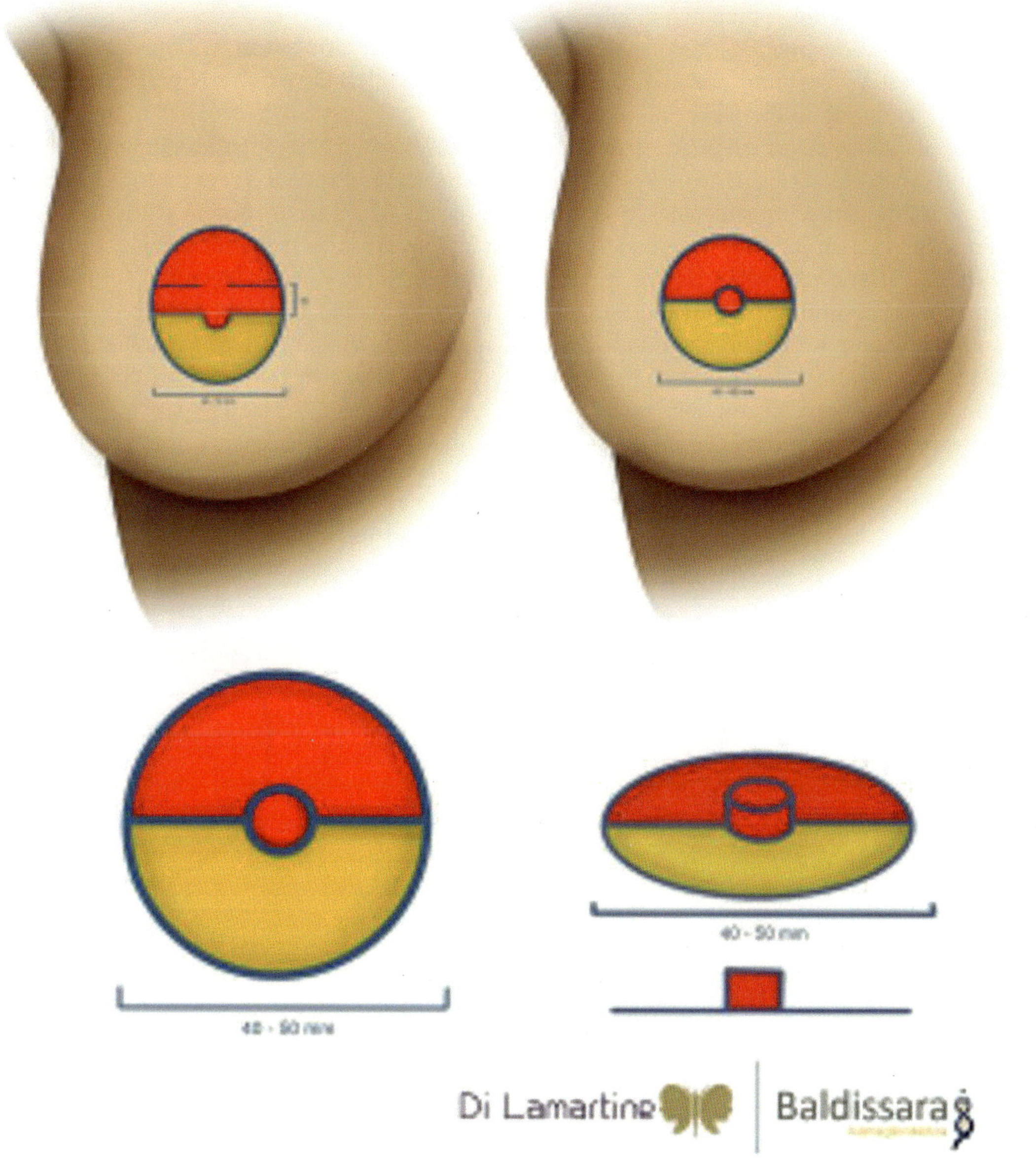


**Fig. 67.5** (**a**) Round block. (**b**) Round block and unloading the skin excess at topography of T of Pitanguy (**c**) immediate post operative (**d**) marking of surgery (**e**) pos operative front photo (**f**) pos operative 3/4 photo

dermopigmentation does not exceed the borders of the scars. Sometimes the round block suture produces a skin wrinkle, and this can be easily solved using the mastectomy scars or even unloading this excess skin in the topography of the vertical branch of the inverted T of Pitanguy [19]. This tactic is also efficient due to improving breast projection, while only the DOF sometimes combines with flattening of the neo-nipple.

In bilateral reconstructions, areolar measures must be about 40–50 mm, and the placement must vary according to the perspective of better blood supply to the elevated flap and with greater availability of the skin (Fig. 67.6).

For learning curve in residencies or specialization in plastic surgery, the technique can be performed with the exceeding tissues in reconstruction of flaps, similarly to those performed by the reconstruction technique with the TRAM (Fig. 67.7).

One of the NAC reconstructions will demonstrate the following experience of our service and how we face adversities like the scars on previous mammoplasties, the mastectomy scars, and the scarcity of adipose tissue under the skin (SCT), adverse effects of radiotherapy, and the deletion of previously reconstruction nipples and others.

## 67.3 Cases/Situations

### 67.3.1 Reconstructions with Opposite Nipple Grafts

In cases where the opposite nipple shows sufficient size to donate tissue to the side to be reconstructed, the reconstruction with the opposite nipple graft is an excellent technique with good predictability of results. As a rule, the graft to be removed should represent 60% of the donating nipple with the purpose of obtaining similar nipples, because the graft will suffer atrophy. The graft deployment in the neo-nipple can be made with a small transverse incision or a cross incision,

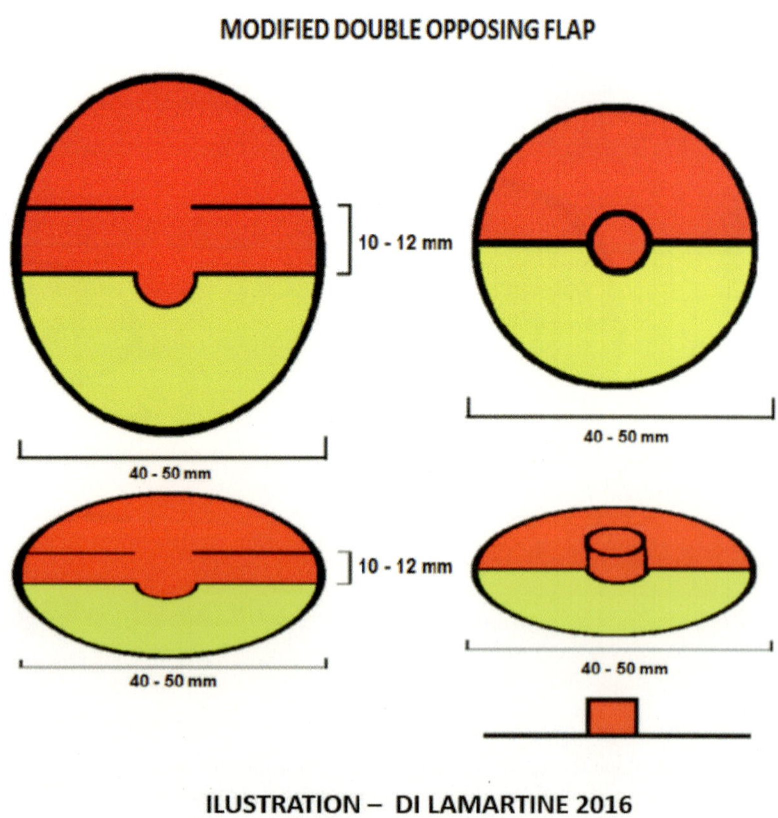


**Fig. 67.6** Tactic for the circular format of double opposing flap

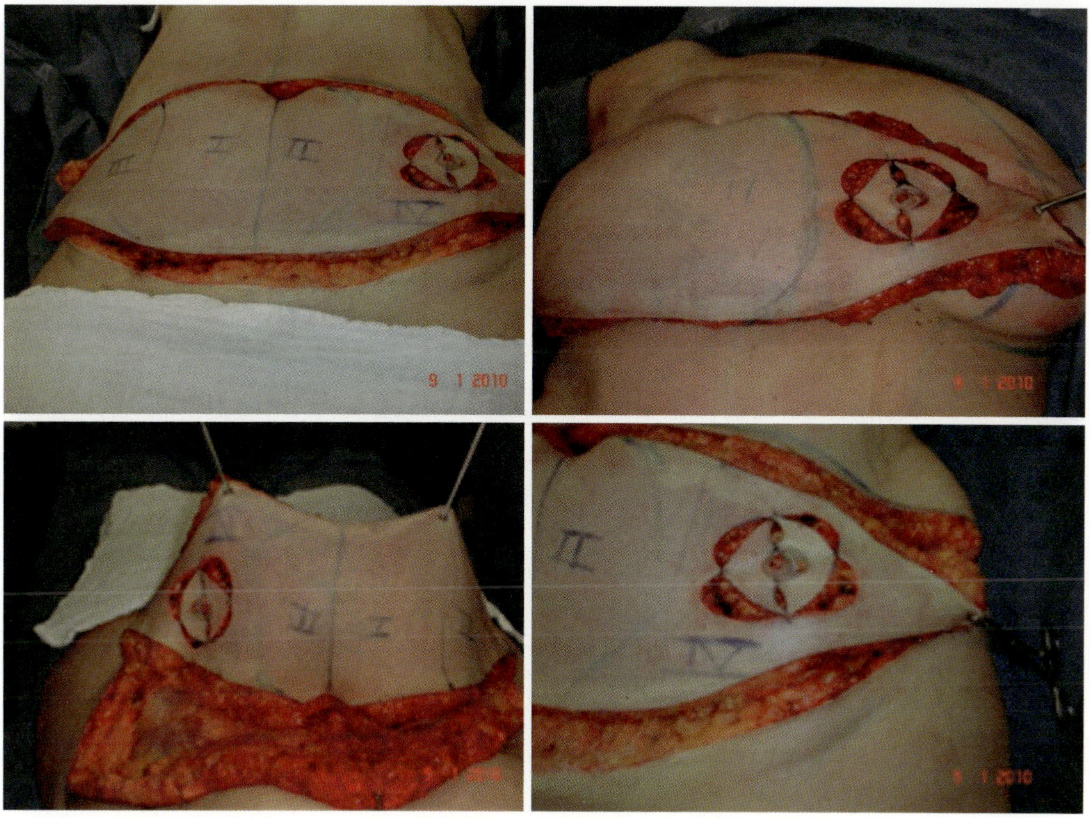

**Fig. 67.7** Turning in flap fragments of TRAM flaps on the right rectus abdominis, zone IV

always seeking the best bed for graft integration. The patching must immobilize the graft, similarly to Brown patching [20]. We currently use a sterile gauze bandage attached to the skin with a sterile plastic film such as the Tegaderm Pad®, Derm®, or other similar that are left in place for about 7 days.

In Fig. 67.8, we have the case of a patient once subjected to quadrantectomy and radiotherapy who had a new cancer (invasive ductal carcinoma at the junction of the medial quadrants) 10 years later. The immediate reconstruction of the right breast was made with temporary expander in two times. By virtue of having the donating nipple on the left side and due to the lack of skin in the right neo-nipple, we opted for graft reconstruction of the nipple. Note that there is maintenance of the result after 2 years and that the dermopigmentation enhances the reconstruction.

After removing the bandage, there is always a crust over the grafted nipple that should not be removed surgically before 3–4 weeks under risk of removal of viable tissue and thus harming the projection and the final volume of the grafted nipple. In most cases, the dermopigmentation is made in both NACs, since it is difficult to achieve color similarity with the non-amputee nipple, and it should be performed by professionals with adequate training and technique, with medicinal use inks [21, 22].

It is currently possible to use 3D dermopigmentation without rebuilding the NAC in cases where the patient does not want reconstruction or it is contraindicated for some clinical or surgical comorbidity. After approximately 2–3 years, the re-pigmentation of the NAC may be necessary due to partial loss of coloring [21, 22].

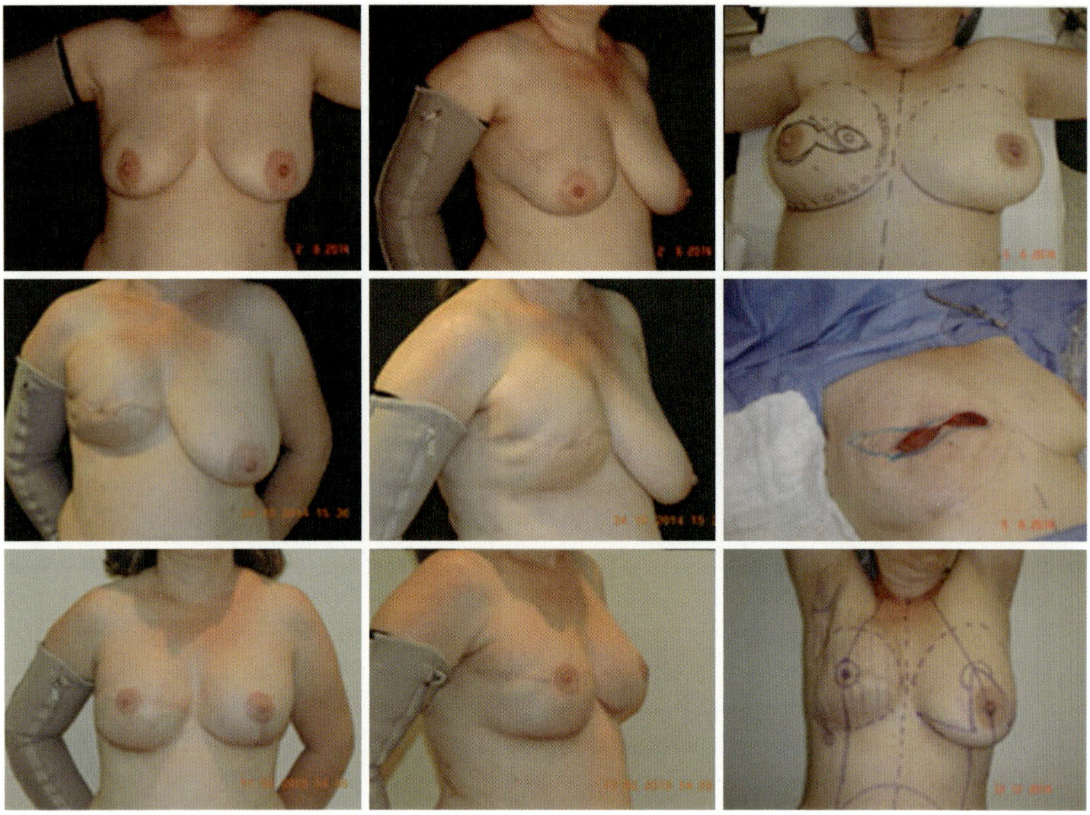

**Fig. 67.8** (*Top*) Preoperative. (*Middle*) Pre-reconstruction. (*Bottom*) Post-reconstruction with lymphedema in right upper limb, sequel of the quadrantectomy and radiotherapy

A regulated professional is required to perform the dermopigmentation under our guidance, through the marking of the position and desired dimensions, in addition to regional anesthetic blocking of lidocaine 0.5% with vasoconstrictor (1:200,000) for greater patient comfort.

In the next case (Fig. 67.9), we present a case of late breast reconstruction with latissimus dorsi muscle associated with silicone implant in which the opposite nipple was sufficient to be a donor with approximately 60% of its volume to be grafted on the opposite side.

### 67.3.2 C-V Type Flap Reconstructions or Fish-Tail or Skate Flap

In cases where the mastectomy scar is close to or exactly the projection of the new NAC, traditional flaps such as the fish-tail, skate flap, or similar [23] can be used because the refinement of incisions and the skin accommodation can be made on the previous scar (Fig. 67.10).

### 67.3.3 Reconstruction with Double Opposing Flap in Cases with Permanent Expanders in Bilateral Mastectomies Without Radiotherapy

In nipple reconstructions with tissue expanders, there is naturally a decreased thickness of the SCT caused by the pressure exerted by the centrifugal form expander pressing the skin. In Fig. 67.11 there is a case of bilateral mastectomy, where one of the NACs has been preserved, but after the expansion conclusion of Becker 50

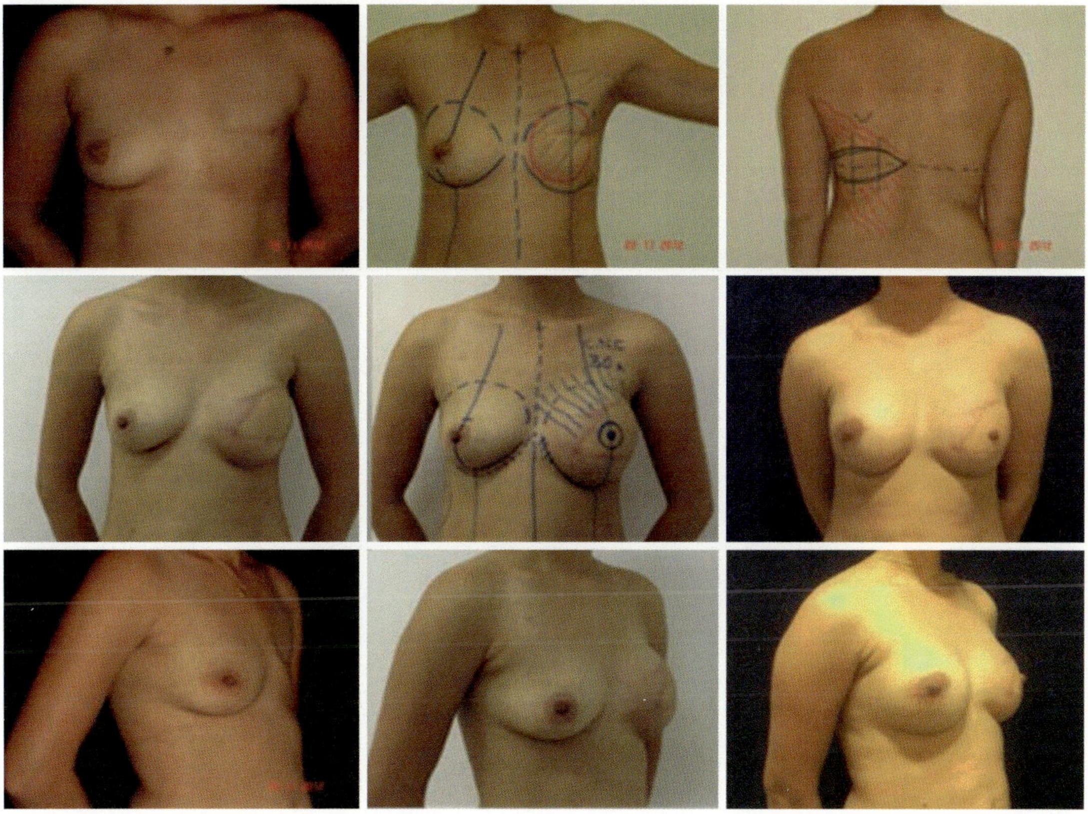

**Fig. 67.9** (*Top, middle, bottom*) Late reconstruction with latissimus dorsi in two stages. NAC rebuilt with nipple graft

expanders to 450 mL, the eccentricity of the remaining NAC hampered its migration to the proper position. For this reason and wishes of the patient, the NAC was removed and the DOF reconstruction planned on both sides. Note that after 15 months, both reconstructed NACs maintain the projection.

In this case the another important data is that although the preparation of round block suture, we accommodated the skin incisions on mastectomy scars. Note also that in addition to the maintenance of an acceptable nipple projection, there is a relief bordering the areolas of neighboring skin (Fig. 67.11).

### 67.3.4 Reconstruction with DOF in Cases with Unilateral Temporary Tissue Expanders Without Radiotherapy and Mastopexy with Opposite Breast Prosthesis

In the immediate temporary mammary tissue expander reconstructions in that there is no need for radiotherapy, the unwanted outcomes are diminished. In Fig. 67.12 the NAC's reconstruction is planned in a third time associated with refinement and fat grafting. In planning for this surgery, the surgeon performs the mastectomy

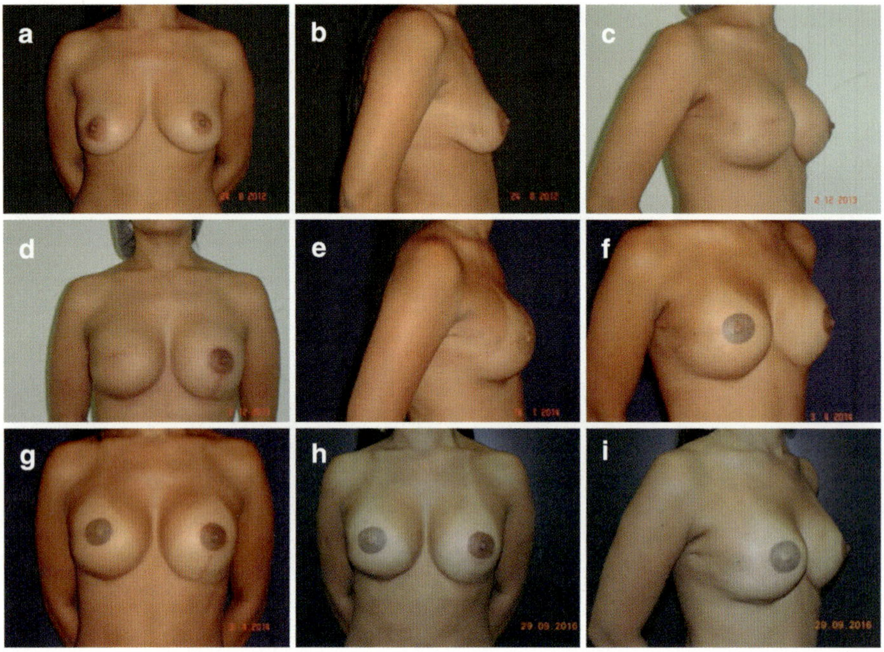

**Fig. 67.10** (**a**, **b**) Preoperative. (**c**, **d**) Postmastectomy with scar. (**e–g**) NAC reconstructed with C-V flap. (**h**, **i**) Three years postoperative. Notice the depigmentation of the NAC but maintaining reasonable projection

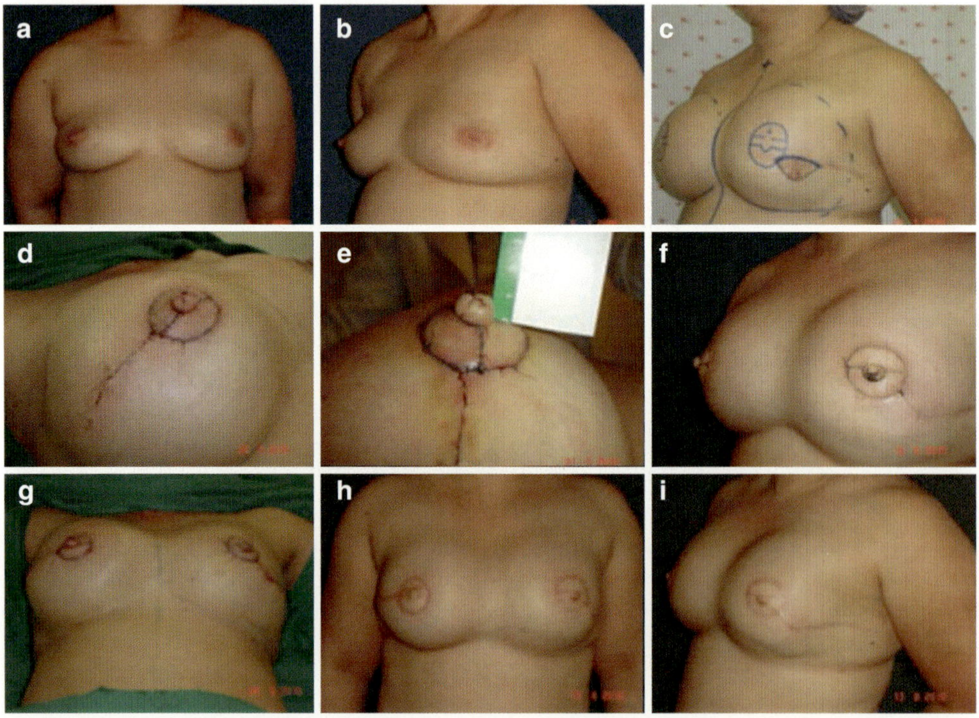

**Fig. 67.11** (**a**, **b**) Preoperative. (**c**) Planning of flaps. (**d–g**) Bilateral reconstruction with Becker 50 and bilateral DOF and the skin after a round block suture using the mastectomy scar. (**h**, **i**) Postoperative

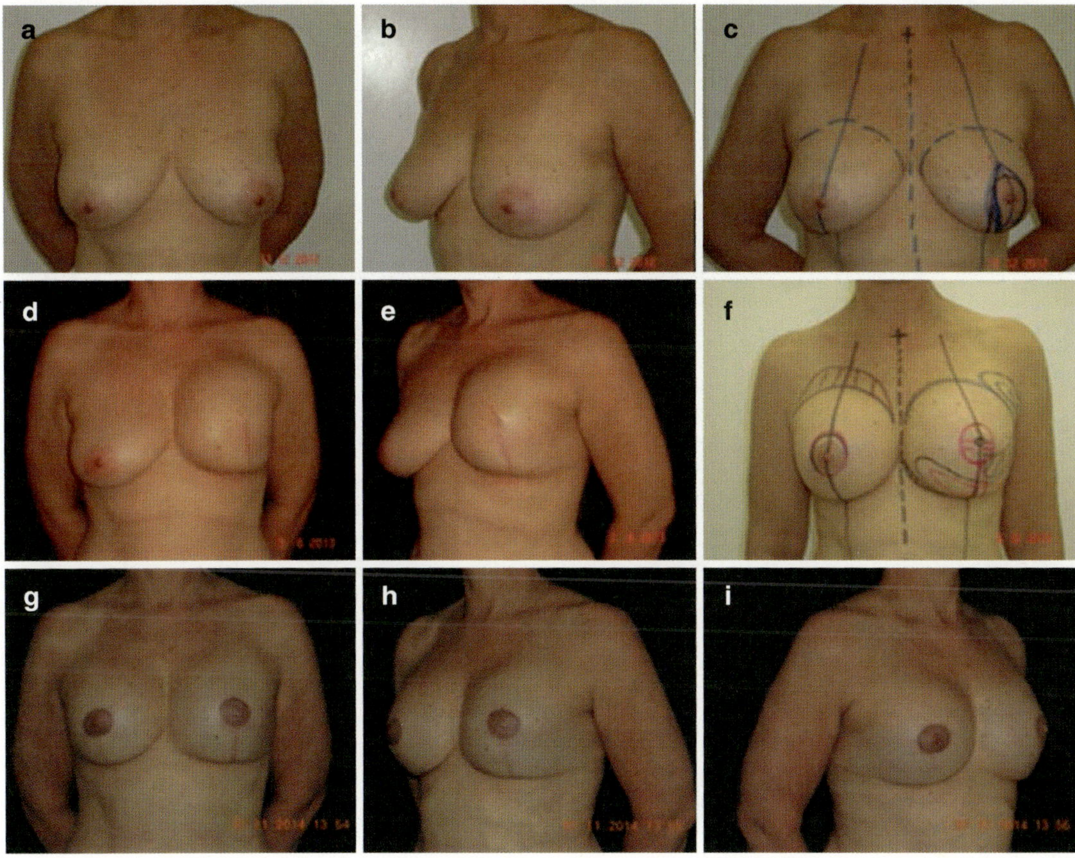

**Fig. 67.12** (**a**, **b**) Preoperative. (**c**) Marking. (**d**, **e**) Immediate temporary expander after mastectomy. (**f**) Marking for reconstruction with DOF. (**g**–**i**) Reconstruction completed

through a vertical incision at the end of the reconstruction to resemble a reduction mammaplasty in relation to scars for being better accepted when compared to transverse, radiated, or oblique incisions. During mammary symmetrization (second time), a broad tissue resection (partial adenomastectomy) of the opposite breast is performed so that the implant is always placed in retro muscle plan, to achieve greater similarity between the breasts in the following aspects: volume, mobility of the implant, position of the submammary fold, flap, and texture. In the third time, in addition to the NAC reconstruction, the position of the areola (Fig. 67.12) is adjusted besides the liposuction/fat grafting.

### 67.3.5 Reconstruction with the DOF with Unilateral Temporary Tissue Expanders with Radiotherapy

Figure 67.13 is a case of left breast reconstruction immediately followed by radiotherapy sessions. Note as the treatment effect of adjuvant radiotherapy is deleterious to the skin, a new approach after 6–8 months with the lipofilling increases the thickness of the covering and improves its quality. In this case, the NAC reconstruction was scheduled to be held in the third stage after the improvement in form, texture, and vitality of irradiated skin. The choice

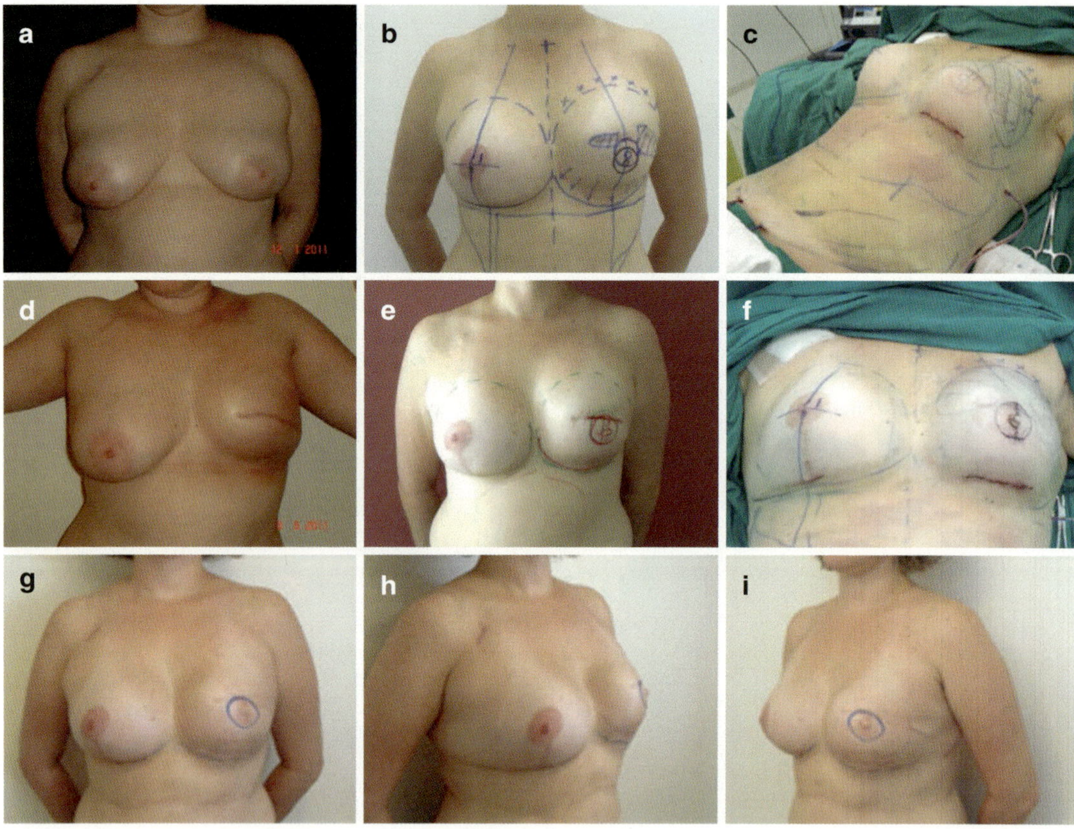


**Fig. 67.13** (**a**) Preoperative. (**b**) Marking for mastectomy. (**c, d**) Postoperative. (**e**) Marking for third stage NAC reconstruction with the technique of Hammond. (**f**) Third stage with refinements, height adjustment of the implant on the left side and the NAC reconstruction. (**g–i**) Planning of position and diameter for dermopigmentation

for incision in the right submammary groove for exchanging the expander for the silicone implant spares new aggression in future NAC area, allowing the lipofilling in this region in the second time. During symmetrization, a partial adenomastectomy with placement of silicone implant in the retro plan muscle of the opposite nipple was performed, so the breasts have the same texture and shape for prevention of the phenomenon known as double bubble. The NAC reconstruction was Hammond's modified technique.

### 67.3.6 Reconstruction with the DOF in Cases with the Use of Latissimus Dorsi and Implants

Figure 67.14 shows the reconstruction with the DOF after mastectomy and reconstruction with latissimus dorsi. In this case the island of skin of the latissimus dorsi has been initially made with the oval shape because DOF needs it as noted. It is relevant to note that in the reconstruction with latissimus dorsi, chances of NAC reconstructions

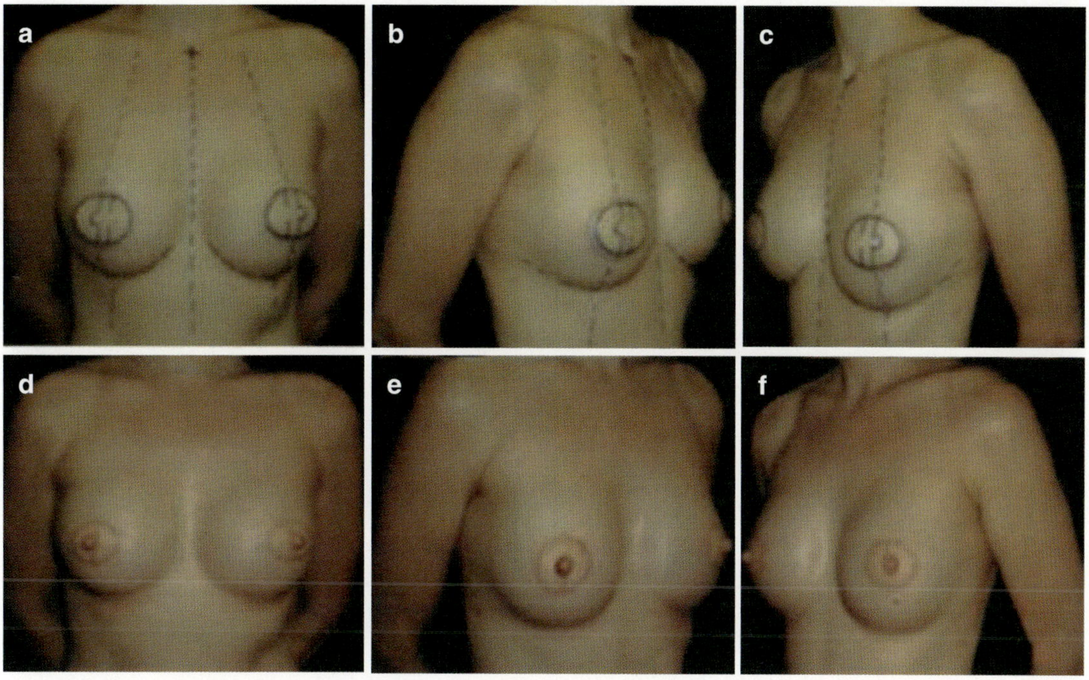


**Fig. 67.14** (**a–c**) Preoperative marking. (**d–f**) Reconstruction with bilateral DOF

are more fruitful and efficient due to the skin of the back be thicker, which implies a nipple with longer-lasting projection.

### 67.3.7 Reconstruction with the DOF in Cases with the Use of the TRAM (Transverse Rectus Abdominis Muscle) Flap

Figure 67.15 shows reconstruction with the DOF after mastectomy and reconstruction with the Transverse Rectus Abdominis Myocutaneous (TRAM) flaps. The DOF was used as a saving measure after a NAC necrosis on bilateral nipple-sparing mastectomy. After the NAC right necrosis, a reconstruction with grafts of half the papilla from the opposite side and skin grafting of inguinal region for resolution of the case was conducted. Good integration occurred from skin grafting; however, papilla grafts were not successful. In these situations the DOF is an interesting asset due to its attributes and predictability of results. Therefore, the DOF in addition to being an excellent technique for primary NAC reconstructions also serves as a rescue technique for its versatility when other techniques have failed.

## 67.4 Specific Cases

In some cases of NAC reconstruction, for whatever reason, we have to do something innovative or totally remake the NAC. We may consider the cases below in this category. In several cases, the DOP can be replaced or performed as a rescue maneuver.

### 67.4.1 Partial Necrosis of the DOF

In this case, we had partial necrosis of DOF, but we did nothing more than waiting for a better

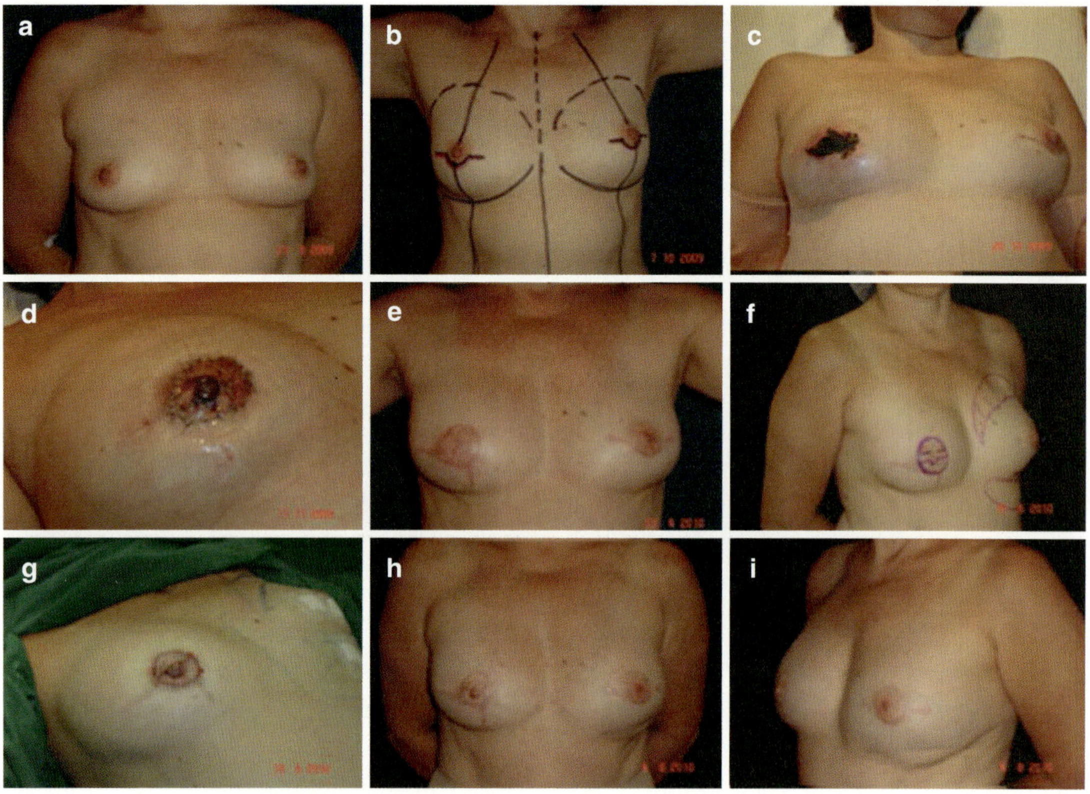

**Fig. 67.15** (**a**) Preoperative. (**b**) Marking for nipple-sparing mastectomy. (**c**) Necrosis of flap. (**d**, **e**) Rescue technique after graft failure. (**f**) Marking for DOF. (**g**) Postoperative. (**g–i**) Final result

opportunity to debride a fragment without harming the NAC (Fig. 67.16).

### 67.4.2 Venous Clogging or Poor Blood Supply

This patient had performed strict radiotherapy, and we were able to perceive poor tissue perfusion evidence in one of the DOF fins (Fig. 67.17). We opted for aborting the sutures and performing them a few days later. After some days, we performed the sutures at the doctor's office under local anesthesia. After this case, we aborted the vasoconstrictor in infiltration solution during the NAC reconstruction, or most of the times, we do not perform infiltration when the surgery is done under general anesthesia.

### 67.4.3 NAP Larger than the Patient Wishes

Sometimes the NAC reconstruction can be higher or larger than the natural condition before the mastectomy and could result in patient dissatisfaction. In some cases, the NAC could be smooth and empty, and patient may request a filling. Whenever the NAC is large enough, the solution lies in reducing part of flaps or filling them with a piece of scar or fibrosis (Fig. 67.18). In this case (the bilateral *latissimus dorsi* flap), initially we need to decrease the NAC using a Pitanguy model for resection under local anesthesia. After several months, the patient requested breast reduction, and we needed to move up the NAC. In order to solve similar cases, we treat the NACs like a natural nipple.

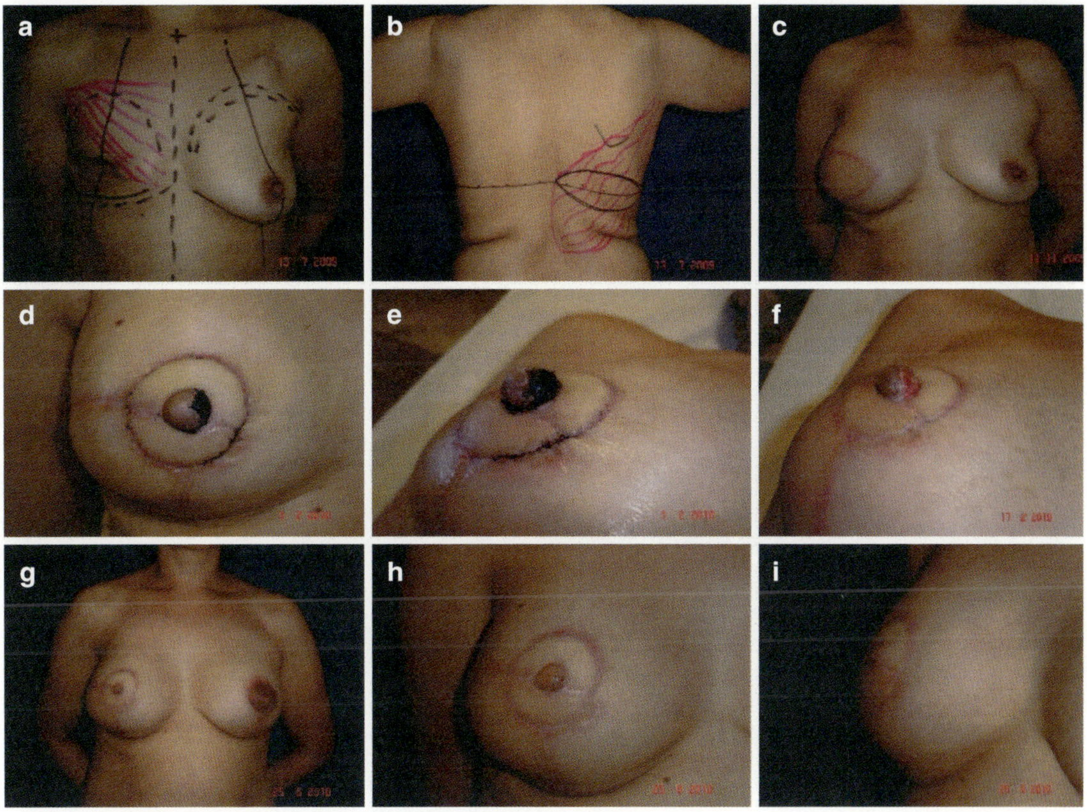

**Fig. 67.16** Partial necrosis of double opposing flap (DOF). (**a**, **b**) Preoperative marking. (**c**) Postoperative after double opposing flap. (**d**, **e**) Nipple necrosis. (**f**) After debriding a fragment. (**g–i**) Postoperative

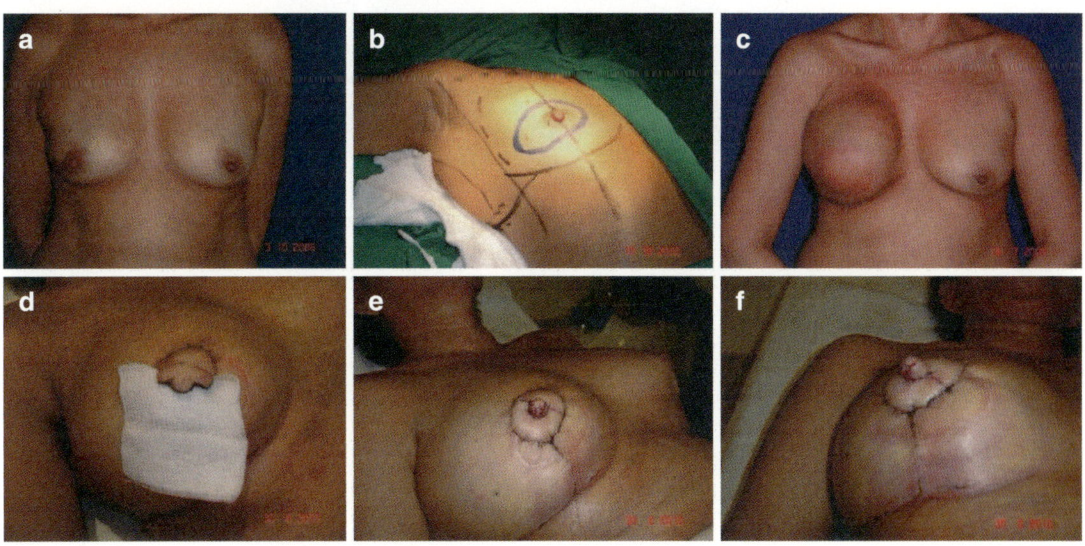

**Fig. 67.17** Radiotherapy can cause poor tissue perfusion evidence. (**a**) Preoperative. (**b**) Marking. (**c**) Postoperative double opposing flap. (**d**) Poor tissue perfusion in one fin of the double opposing flap. (**e**, **f**) Postoperative after suturing

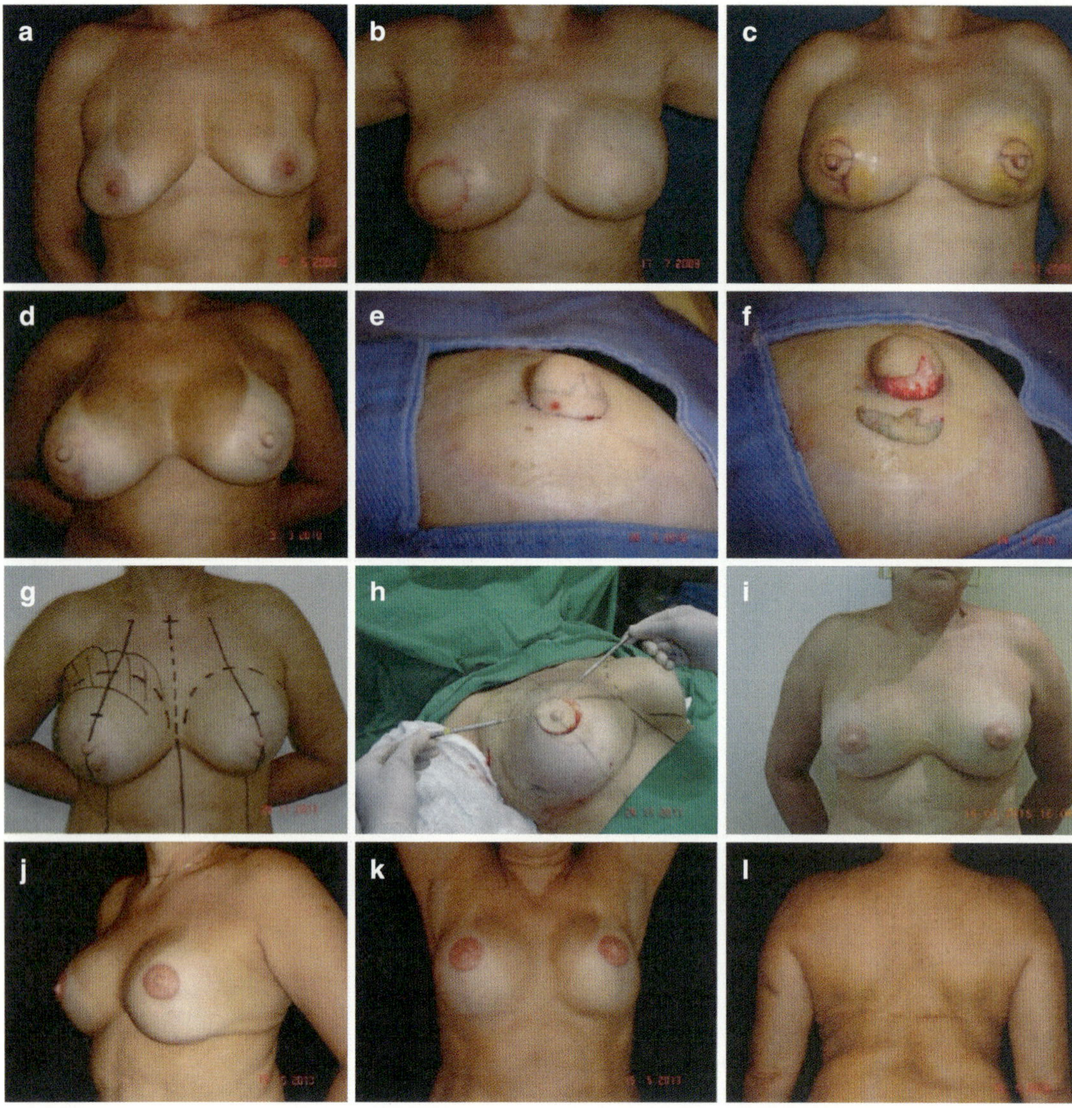


**Fig. 67.18** DOF can move up like a natural nipple. (**a**) Preoperative. (**b**) After latissimus dorsi flap bilaterally. (**c**) Reconstruction nipple. (**d**) Postoperative. (**e**, **f**) Nipple decreased. (**g**) Marking. (**h**) Breast reduction and nipple moved up. (**i**) Immediately postoperative. (**j–l**) Final result

## Conclusions

The loss of projection and the final result of the confections of papilla are related to a number of reasons: reduced subcutaneous tissue, poor flap planning, natural process of wound contraction, tissue memory, increase of the internal (strained sutures) or external pressure (e.g., the pressure made by the use of the bra), prior infection, and radiation. Therefore, the main challenge is to rebuild a papilla able to overcome these local obstacles and natural tendencies [1–18].

In order to achieve graceful results in nipple reconstructions and including the NAC reconstruction, the surgeon should be aware of some of the several available techniques and filter those with greater and better odds and perspectives for good results.

## References


1. Adams WM. Labial transplant for correction of loss of the nipple. Plast Reconstr Surg. 1949;4(3):295–8.
2. Cronin TD, Upton J, McDonough JM. Reconstruction of the breast after mastectomy. Plast Reconstr Surg. 1977;59(1):1–14.
3. Broadbent TR, Woolf RM, Metz PS. Restoring the mammary areola by a skin graft from the upper inner thigh. Br J Plast Surg. 1977;30(3):220–2.
4. Brent B, Bostwick J. Nipple-areola reconstruction with auricular tissues. Plast Reconstr Surg. 1977;60(3):353–61.
5. Gruber RP. Nipple-areola reconstruction: a review of techniques. Clin Plast Surg. 1979;6(1):71–83.
6. Millard DR Jr, Devine J Jr, Warren WD. Breast reconstruction: a plea for saving the uninvolved nipple. Am J Surg. 1971;122(6):763–4.
7. Berson MI. Construction of pseudoareola. Surgery. 1946;20(6):808.
8. Little JW III. Nipple-areola reconstruction. Clin Plast Surg. 1984;11(2):351–64.
9. Shestak KC, Nguyen TD. The double opposing periareola flap: a novel concept for nipple-areola reconstruction. Plast Reconstr Surg. 2007;119(2):473–80.
10. Losken A, Mackay GJ, Bostwick J III. Nipple reconstruction using the C-V flap technique: a long-term evaluation. Plast Reconstr Surg. 2001;108(2):361–9.
11. Anton M, Eskenazi LB, Hartrampf CR Jr. Nipple reconstruction with local flaps: star and wrap flaps. Perspect Plast Surg. 1991;5(1):67–78.
12. Eskenazi L. A one-stage nipple reconstruction with the "modified star" flap and immediate tattoo: a review of 100 cases. Plast Reconstr Surg. 1993;92(4): 671–80.
13. Hammond DC, Khuthaila D, Kim J. The skate flap purse-string technique for nipple-areola complex reconstruction. Plast Reconstr Surg. 2007;120(2):399–406.
14. Lamartine JD, Cintra Junior R, Daher JC, Cammarota MC, Galdino J, Pedroso DB, Cintra RH. Reconstrução do complexo areolopapilar com double opposing flap. Rev Bras Cir Plast. 2013;28(2):233–40.
15. Farhadi J, Maksvytyte GK, Schaefer DJ, Pierer G, Scheufler O. Reconstruction of the nippleareola complex: an update. J Plast Reconstr Aesthet Surg. 2006;59(1):40–53.
16. Toledo LS, Mauad R. Fat injection: a 20-year revision. Clin Plast Surg. 2006;33(1):47–53.
17. Illouz YG, Sterodimas A. Autologous fat transplantation to the breast: a personal technique with 25 years of experience. Aesthet Plast Surg. 2009;33(5):706–15.
18. Spear SL, Wilson HB, Lockwood MD. Fat injection to correct contour deformities in the reconstructed breast. Plast Reconstr Surg. 2005;116(5):1300–5.
19. Pitanguy I. Mammaplastia - Estudo de 245 casos consecutivos de mamaplastia e apresentação de técnica pessoal. Rev Bras Cir. 1961;42:201–20.
20. Mehta HK. A new method of full-thickness skin graft fixation. Br J Plast Surg. 1985;38:125–8.
21. Spear SL, Convit R, Little JW III. Intradermal tattoo as an adjunct to nipple-areola reconstruction. Plast Reconstr Surg. 1989;83(5):907–11.
22. Bhatty MA, Berry RB. Nipple-areolar reconstruction by tattooing and nipple sharing. Br J Plast Surg. 1997;50(5):331–4.
23. Tostes ROG, Araujo Silva KD, Guedes de Andrade JCC Jr, Castro Ribeiro GV, Machado Rodrigues RB. Reconstrução do mamilo por meio da técnica do retalho C-V: contribuição à técnica. Rev Bras Cir Plást. 2005;20(1):36–9.

# The Diamond Double-Opposing V–Y Flap: A Reliable, Simple, and Versatile Technique for Nipple Reconstruction

68

Ginger Slack and Malcolm Lesavoy

## 68.1 Introduction

In the United States, breast cancer is the most commonly diagnosed cancer among women. In 2015, about 246,600 cases of breast cancer were diagnosed [1]. After an arduous physical and emotional journey in the battle against breast cancer, the final surgical procedure for breast reconstruction for many women is nipple reconstruction. Studies have supported improved emotional satisfaction with a nipple reconstruction [2–4].

The nipple is an essential defining component to restore the semblance and appearance of a natural breast. Aesthetically, there is significant variation in dimension, texture, and color across ethnic groups and among individuals. Generally, a normal areola diameter is 4.2–5 cm. The projection or height of the nipple should be around ½–¼ of the areolar diameter or 1–1.6 cm. The nipple should be located in the center of the breast mound; however, occasionally, it is slightly off of the center.

The first described nipple reconstruction was performed in the 1940s by Adams [5]. There are many techniques described in the literature on how to perform this procedure [5–13]. Nipple reconstructions can be performed as tattoos, skin grafts, prosthetic implants, or local flaps. Skin graft techniques include contralateral nipple full-thickness grafts and areolar split-thickness skin grafts from either the areola, groin, or labia minora.

In the United States, the preferred technique is the use of a local flap for the nipple followed by tattooing of the areola. The use of local dermal flaps is most common, due to the ease of the procedure, minimal donor-site morbidity, and the ability to tailor this tissue in the mastectomy skin envelope. The negative aspects of local dermal flaps include the addition of further scars on the breast, although minimal, and the challenge of incorporating preexisting scars for nipple reconstruction.

The star flap [6] is a commonly used technique that raises a crane (bird)-shaped dermal flap whose two arms wrap around each other while the third flap rests on the folded arms (Fig. 68.1). The bell flap [7] elevates a cone-shaped superiorly based flap, while the central flap is folded on itself, and the donor area is closed with advancement of the adjacent flaps in a circular shape (Fig. 68.2). The skate (fish) flap [8] is a dermal flap in the shape of a semicircle with a superiorly based central pedicle where the lateral arms wrap around the center of the flap (Fig. 68.3). The double-opposing tab flap [9] is a dermoglandular flap (Fig. 68.4). The C–V flap [10, 11] is similar to the star flap (Fig. 68.5). The

G. Slack (✉)
Department of Plastic and Reconstructive Surgery, UCLA Medical Center, 200 UCLA Medical Plaza, Suite 465, Los Angeles, CA 90095-6960, USA
e-mail: gslack@mednet.ucla.edu

M. Lesavoy, M.D.
Department of Plastic and Reconstructive Surgery, David Geffen School of Medicine at UCLA, Los Angeles, CA 90095, USA
e-mail: drlesavoy@aol.com


M.A. Shiffman (ed.), *Nipple-Areolar Complex Reconstruction*, https://doi.org/10.1007/978-3-319-60925-6_68

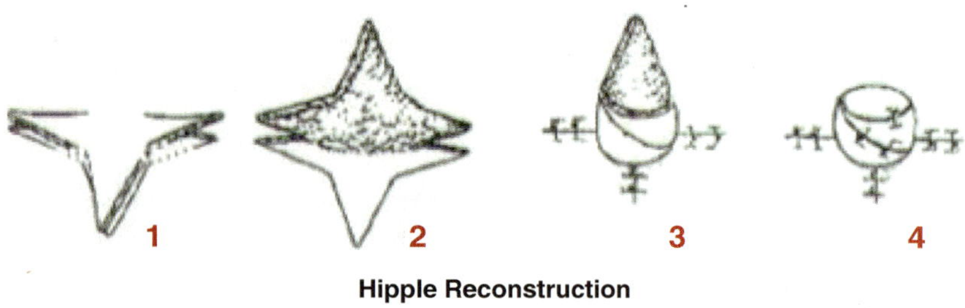


**Fig. 68.1** (*1–4*) Star flap schematic [6]

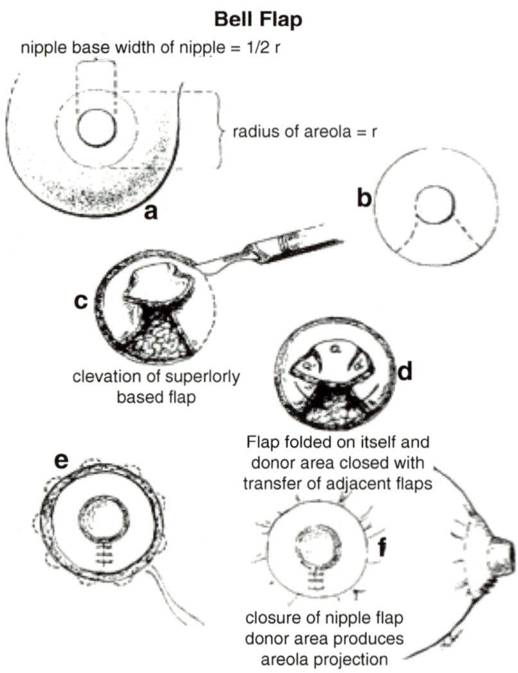


**Fig. 68.2** (**a–d**) Bell flap schematic [7]

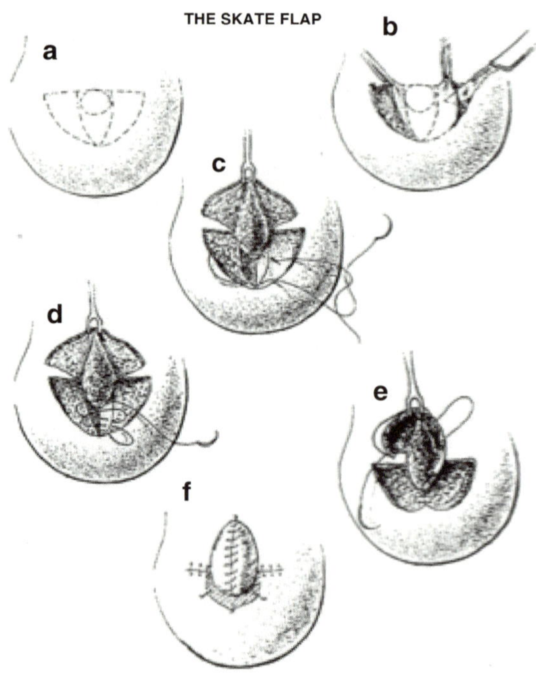


**Fig. 68.3** (**a–f**) Skate flap schematic [7, 8]

spiral flap [12] spirals a thin ellipse dermal flap around itself to create projection (Fig. 68.6).

We present the double-opposing diamond V–Y flap as a reliable and versatile technique for nipple reconstruction. This technique is based with a simple design, a subcutaneous pedicle, which has a more reliable blood supply than a dermal pedicle and can allow versatile incorporation of previous scars if needed. It is simple to perform, reproducible, and easy to teach.

## 68.2 Surgical Technique

Candidates for nipple reconstruction are patients who have undergone a skin-sparing mastectomy or total mastectomy followed by either implant based or autologous reconstruction and have completed all stages of the breast mound reconstruction. All modifications of the shape, size, and positioning of the breast mound should be completed prior to nipple reconstruction. The nipples define the center of the breast, and its position should be determined after any mound modification. When the patient is satisfied with their breast mounds, ideally 3 months following the last breast procedure is allowed to pass to allow for reduction in edema and settling of implants, if present. At this point, she can be scheduled for nipple reconstruction.

In the preoperative area, the patient and surgeon together pick the nipple position. Using round electrocardiographic leads and a mirror, the patient is told to place the leads in the desired

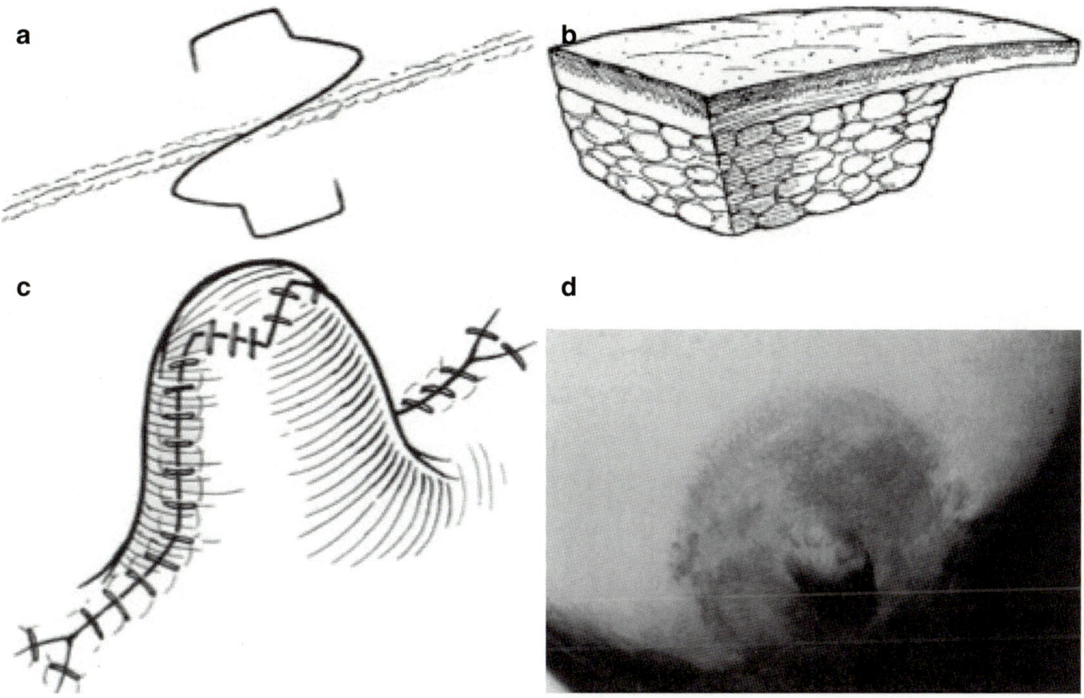

**Fig. 68.4** (**a**–**d**) Double-opposing tab flap schematic and result [9]

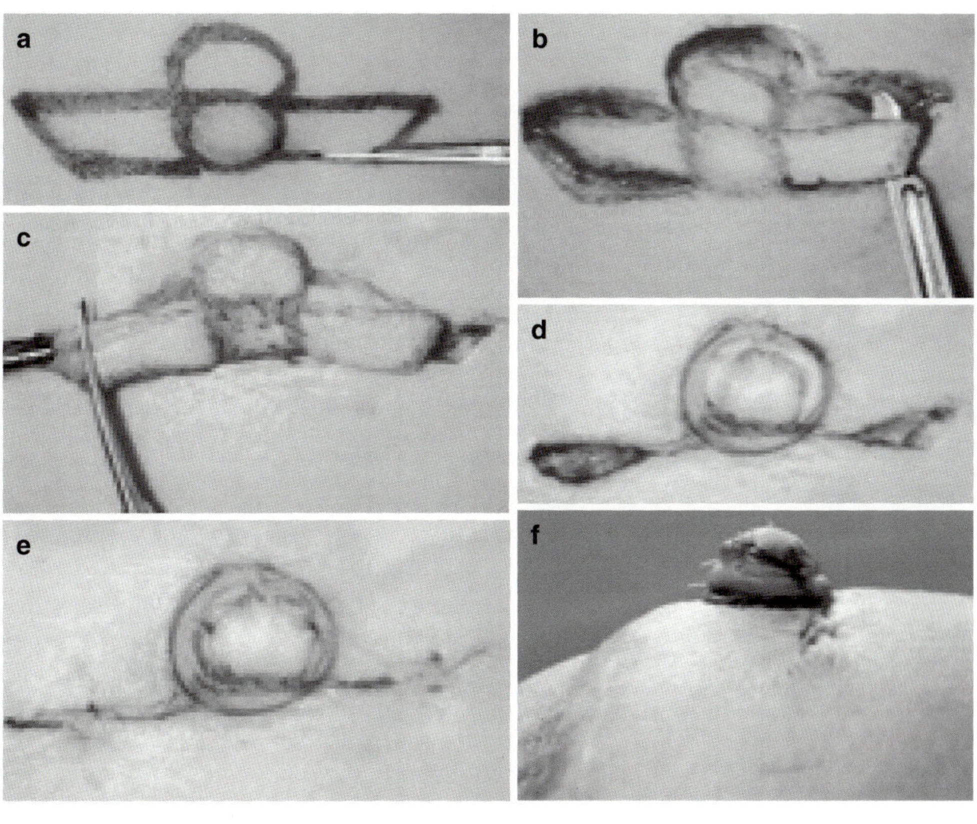

**Fig. 68.5** (**a**–**f**) The C–V flap. Source: C–V flap [10]

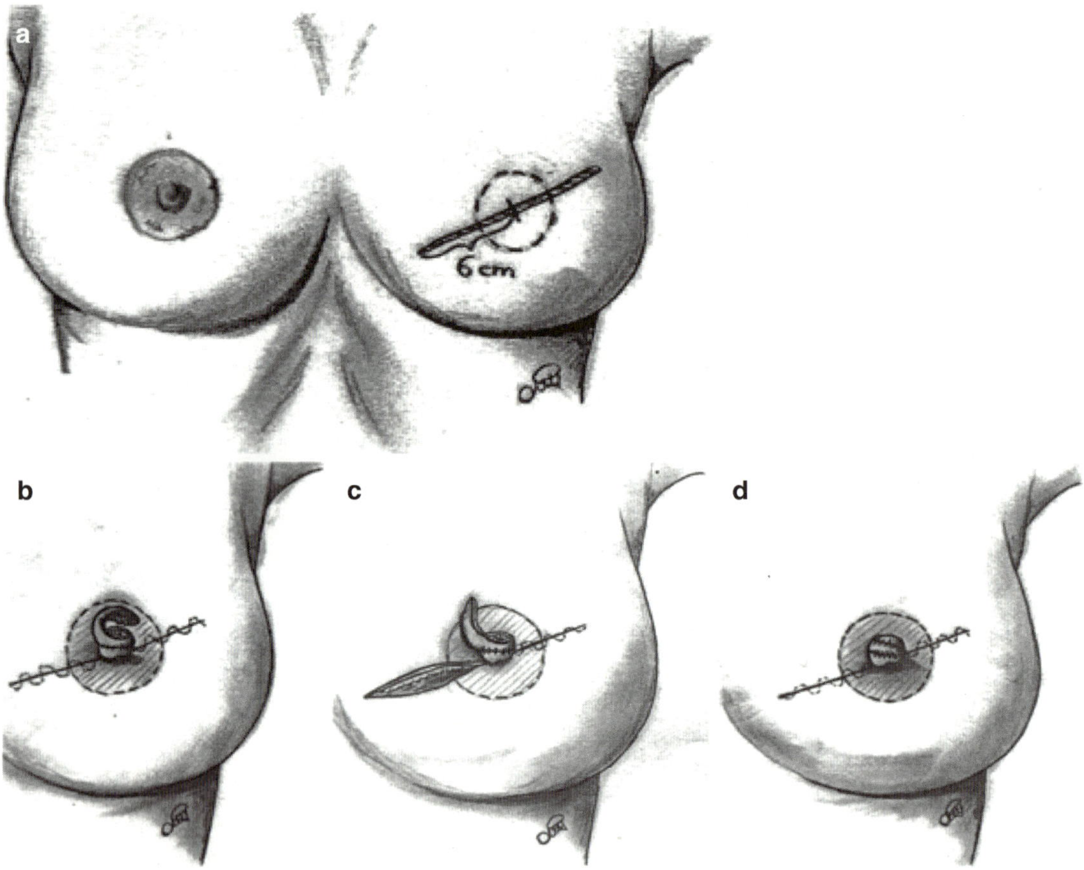


**Fig. 68.6** (**a**–**d**) Spiral flap schematic [13]

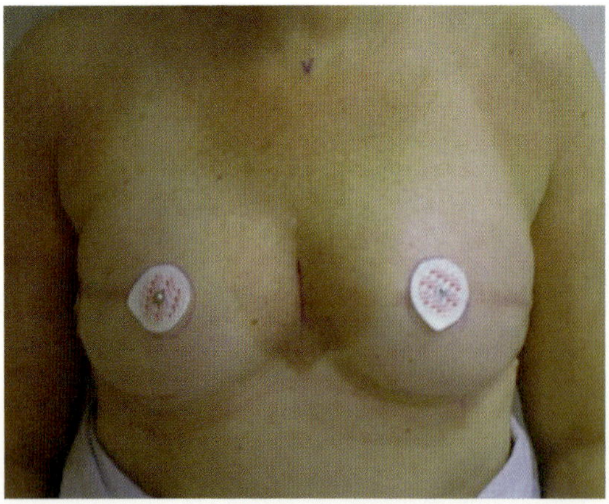

**Fig. 68.7** In the preoperative area, EKG pads are used to estimate the desired nipple position allowing the patient and surgeon to confirm the optimal positioning on the breast mound

nipple position while the patient is upright (Fig. 68.7). It is important that this view is from the view of the mirror, rather than the downward gaze on her breasts. The surgeon can confirm the position based on symmetry with the contralateral breast, if present, and offer suggestions based on aesthetics and measurements. In most cases, the nipples should be on the central vertex of the breast mound, and an equilateral triangle should be formed by the three points of the sternal notch and the bilateral nipples. The nipple position should be approximately at the level of the mid-humerus, although notably there are variations in higher or lower breasts. The outline of the electrocardiographic leads can be marked onto the patient as a general guideline and the full diamond-shaped flap markings performed when the patient is on the operating table (Fig. 68.8).

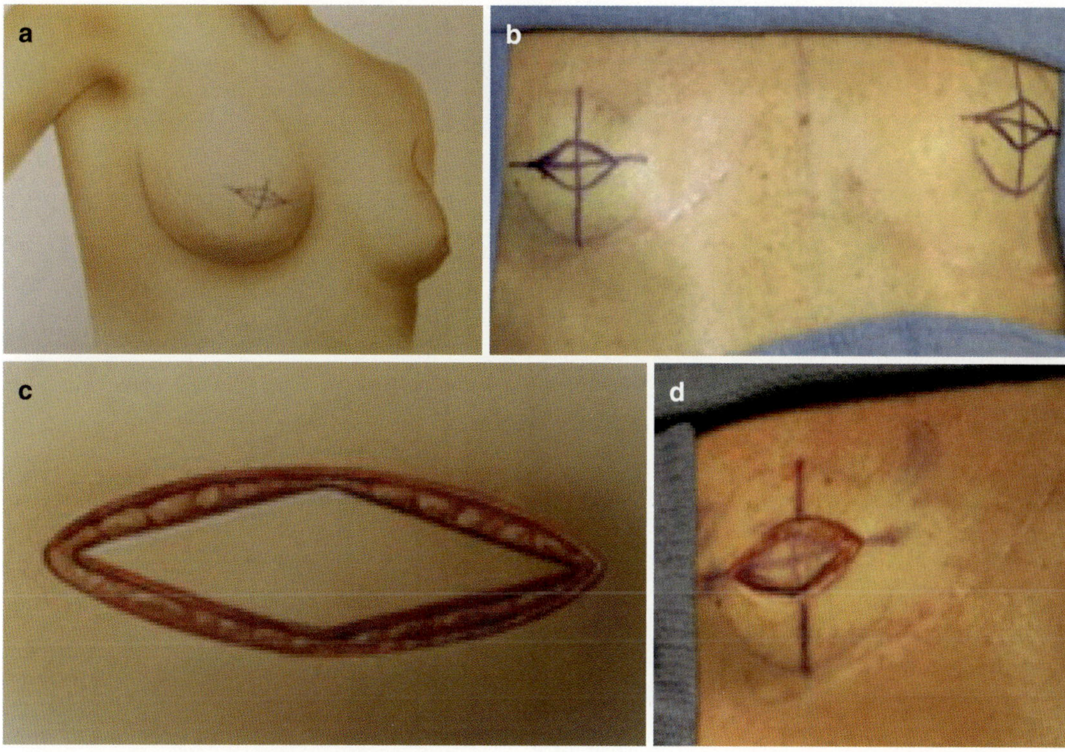


**Fig. 68.8** (**a**) Diamond island flap placement. (**b**) Flap marked on patient. (**c**) Full-thickness skin incision of the diamond island flap. (**d**) Incision on patient

If needed, the previous mastectomy scars are incorporated into the diamond limbs so that they can be closed in the same fashion. However, technically, the mastectomy scars can be disregarded in this methodology as the diamond flap has a subcutaneous pedicle. This is in contrast to the dermatocutaneous flaps where scars going through the design will interrupt the dermal pedicle's vascularity and thus can be compromised. The double-opposing diamond flap has a subcutaneous pedicle and is reliable even based on a scar.

The procedure is done with local anesthesia in an office setting procedure room. A diamond skin design is centered over the apex of the new nipple position. The long axis of the diamond is generally oriented horizontally. It can be in line with the previous mastectomy scars, as previously mentioned, if the scars happen to be where the neo nipple is planned. Full-thickness incisions through the skin and dermis are made along the diamond pattern. The horizontal length of the diamond is approximately 4 cm, leaving 1 cm + centrally and 1 cm + for the medial and lateral limbs. The lateral and medial limbs (1 cm±) are elevated at the subcutaneous level, leaving the central third (diameter of 1 cm±) subcutaneous pedicle intact. This is the blood supply to the reconstructed nipple. This central third pedicle needs to be a minimum of 1 cm in diameter (Fig. 68.9). The flap edges are undermined conservatively laterally and medially away from the pedicle to allow for enough laxity for rotation and closure of the limbs to meet each other (Fig. 68.10). The medial and lateral limb tips are sutured to each other to cover the central subcutaneous pedicle and tubularize the diamond. The medial and lateral donor incisions are closed in a V–Y fashion. The Y portion of the closure is inset at the base of the nipple. The end result is a nipple with good projection and a pair of horizontal linear incisions on each side of the nipple. For postoperative management, an antibiotic ointment is placed over the nipple and 2 × 2

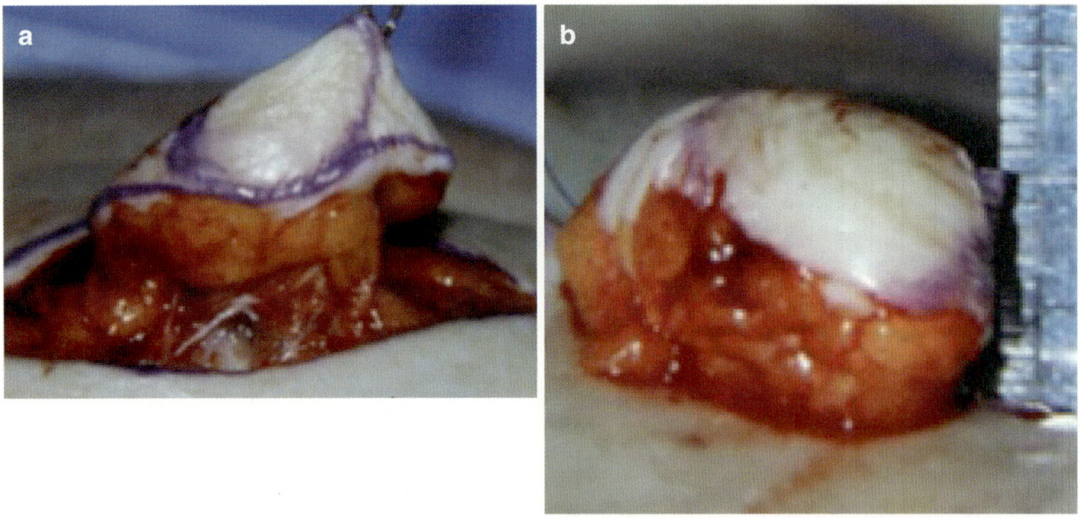


**Fig. 68.9** (**a**, **b**) The central pedicle is one-third of the flap diameter. In order for there to be sufficient blood supply and projection, the author has found this should be a minimum of 1 cm diameter

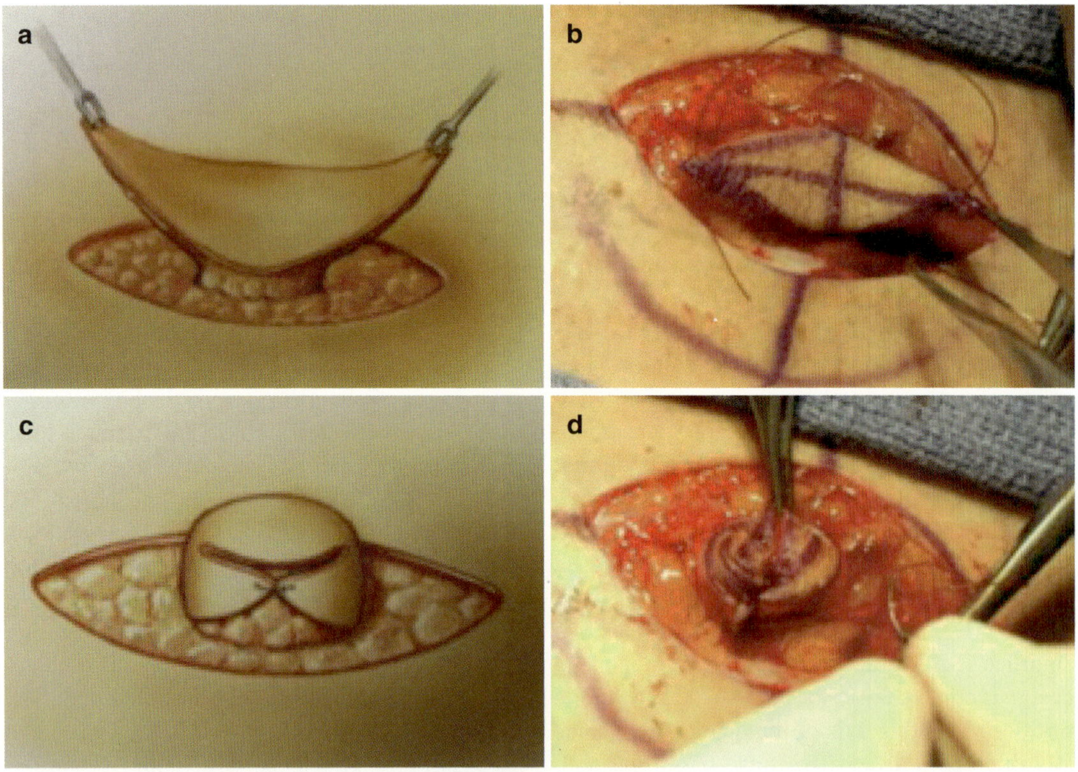


**Fig. 68.10** (**a**) Elevation of the corners of the flap, with care taken to preserve the central subcutaneous pedicle of at least 1 cm. (**b**) Elevation of flap on patient. (**c**, **d**) Medial rotation of the flap limbs with a central suture. Subcutaneous donor site left open to demonstrate the size of the original flap before rotation

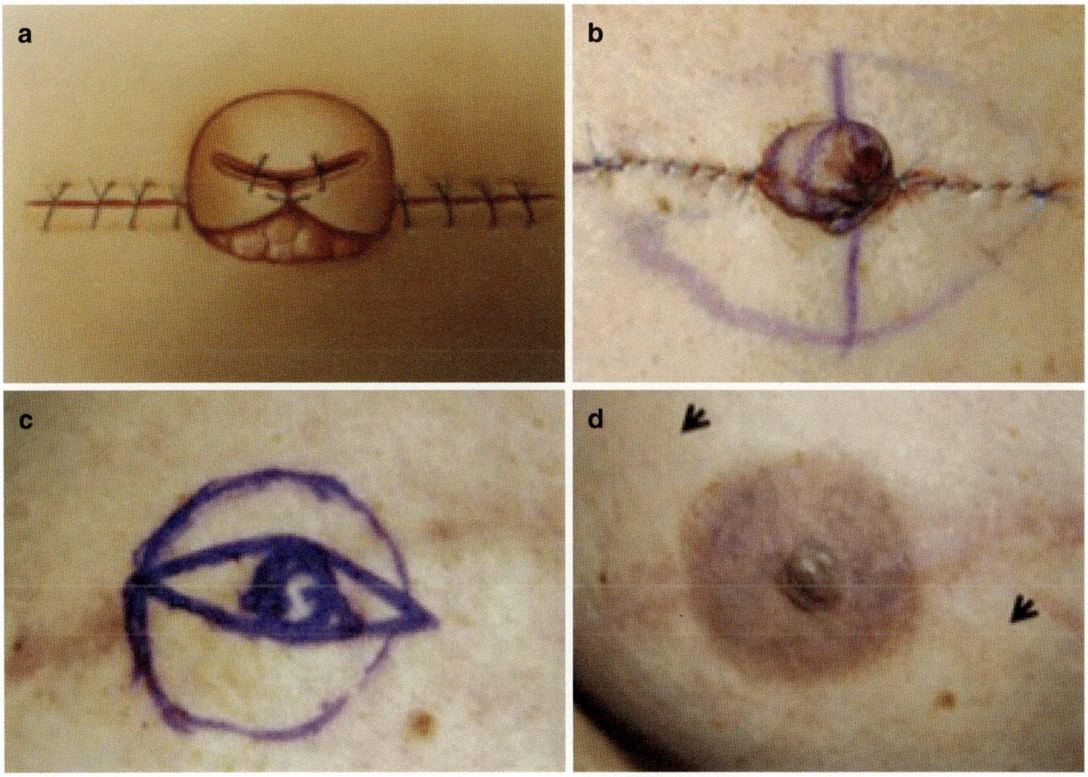


**Fig. 68.11** (**a**, **b**) V–Y closure of the donor site limbs. (**c**) Patient marked with previously healed transverse mastectomy scar with diamond flap design. Note that the direction of the diamond island limbs is opposite the previous mastectomy scars. (**d**) Once healed, the donor site scars are discreet. Arrows show direction of flap design

gauze with central holes to protect the nipple from compression. The dressing stays in place for 5 days and sutures are removed at follow-up. When the incisions are healed, areolar tattooing is performed for appropriate pigmentation (Fig. 68.11).

## 68.3 Results

The senior author (ML) has used this flap for nipple reconstruction for the past 22 years with excellent results. Approximately 50 nipple reconstructions were performed. Forty-five were completing alloplastic-based reconstructions, and five were on autologous breast reconstructions. Two nipple reconstructions (4%) had early complications of partial flap loss and healed secondarily with debridement and wound care. The same flap design was re-elevated after the wounds were healed. These complications were early in the design of this flap and attributed to over dissection of the central subcutaneous pedicle. The technique was then modified to retain a minimum of 1 cm diameter of subcutaneous pedicle for the minimum flap pedicle required for vascularity. Since this technique has been subscribed, there have been no other early complications. Nipple projection has been studied as well, and roughly 80% of projection is maintained after 1 year [12–14]. Donor sites are imperceptible after tattooing (Fig. 68.12). The author has applied this technique in both female and male patients with excellent results (Fig. 68.13).

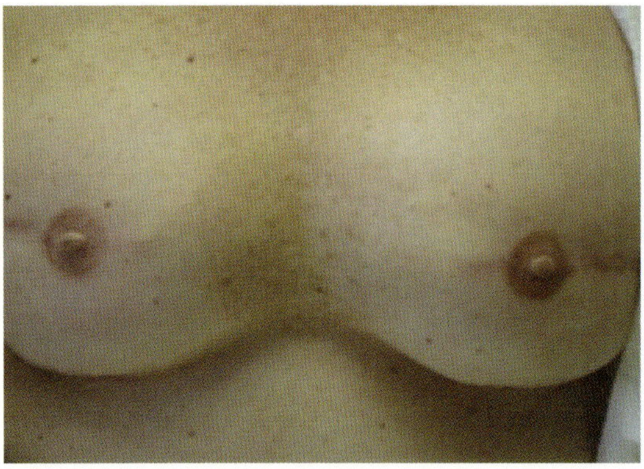

**Fig. 68.12** Postoperative result of island flap nipple reconstruction after areola tattooing (bilateral alloplastic breast reconstruction) after 8 years

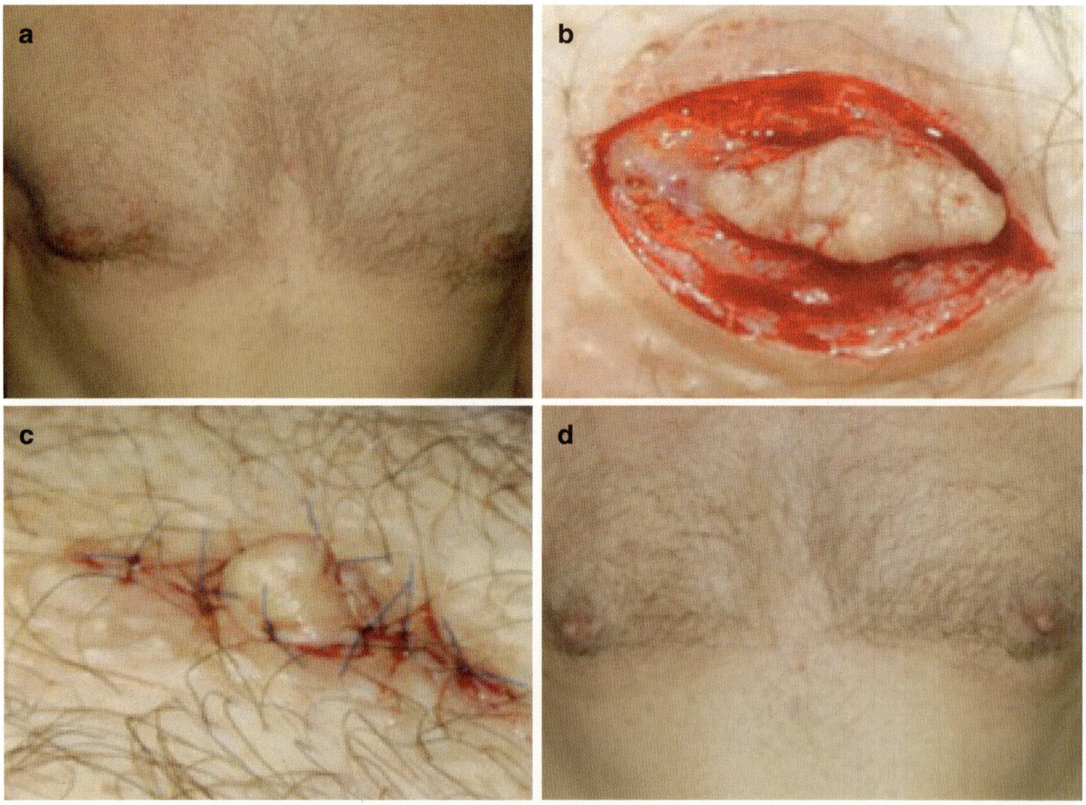

**Fig. 68.13** (**a**) Preoperative male patient. (**b**) Flap. (**c**) Closure. (**d**) Two-year postoperative

## Conclusions

We believe that this is the optimal technique for nipple reconstruction as the subcutaneous pedicle is a reliable blood supply, easy design, and ability to incorporate adjacent scars for optimal aesthetics. This technique can be used in nipple reconstruction, unilateral or bilateral, alloplastic or autologous, female or male, with excellent aesthetic results.

## References


1. Breascancer.org. US breast cancer statistics. 2016. http://www.breastcancer.org/symptoms/understand_bc/statistics. Accessed 8 Dec 2016.
2. Lipa JE, Addison PD, Neligan PC. Patient satisfaction following nipple reconstruction incorporating autologous costal cartilage. Can J Plast Surg. 2008;16:85–8.
3. Wellisch DK, Schain WS, Noone RB, Little JW III. The psychological contribution of nipple addition in breast reconstruction. Plast Reconstr Surg. 1987;80:699–704.
4. Jabor MA, Shayani P, Collins D Jr, Karas T, Cohen BE. Nipple areola reconstruction: satisfaction and clinical determinants. Plast Reconstr Surg. 2002;110:457–63.
5. Adams WM. Free transplantation of the nipples and areola. Surgery. 1944;15:186–95.
6. Anton MA, Hartrampf CR Jr. Nipple reconstruction with the star flap. Plast Surg Forum. 1990;13:100–3.
7. Shestak KC, Gabriel A, Landecker A, Peters S, Shestak A, Kim J. Assessment of long-term nipple projection: a comparison of three techniques. Plast Reconstr Surg. 2002;110:780–6.
8. Little JW. Nipple-areola reconstruction. Clin Plast Surg. 1984;11:351–64.
9. Kroll SS. Nipple reconstruction using the double-opposing tab flap. Plast Reconstr Surg. 1999;104:511–4.
10. Losken A, Mackay GJ, Bostwick J. Nipple reconstruction using the C-V flap technique: a long-term evaluation. Plast Reconstr Surg. 2001;108:361–9.
11. Eo S, Kim SS, Da Lio AL. Nipple reconstruction with C-V flap using dermofat graft. Ann Plast Surg. 2007;58:137–40.
12. Lesavoy M, Liu TS. The diamond double-opposing V-Y flap: a reliable, simple, and versatile technique for nipple reconstruction. Plast Reconstr Surg. 2010;125(6):1643–8.
13. Di Benedetto G, Sperti V, Pierangeli M, Bertani A. A simple and reliable method of nipple reconstruction using a spiral flap made of residual scar tissue. Plast Reconstr Surg. 2004;114:158–61.
14. Cheng MH, Rodriguez ED, Smartt JM, Cardenas-Mejia A. Nipple reconstruction using the modified top hat flap with banked costal cartilage graft. Ann Plast Surg. 2007;59:621–8.

# A Simple and Reliable Method of Nipple Reconstruction Using a Spiral Flap Made of Residual Scar Tissue

69

Matteo Torresetti, Alessandro Scalise, and Giovanni Di Benedetto

## 69.1 Introduction

Several conditions can lead to loss of the nipple-areola complex (NAC), such as cancer excision, posttraumatic or burn deformities, congenital absence (athelia, amastia), or complications from breast surgery (reduction mammaplasty).

In the cases of breast cancer, recreation of a soft, ptotic, aesthetically pleasing breast mound, similar to the natural breast, represents the ultimate goal of postmastectomy breast reconstruction. Recreation of the NAC is an integral part of this task, and it has been strongly associated with a higher overall patient satisfaction with significant psychosocial benefits for women, including acceptance of body image, sense of completeness, and an improved perception of symmetry. Therefore, every patient should be fully counseled about the potential benefits that NAC reconstruction could have on all forms of breast reconstruction [1].

NAC reconstruction is often considered as a mark for completion of the breast reconstructive process. Despite recent trends in selected patients advocated for nipple-sparing mastectomies and immediate nipple reconstructions in order to alleviate the delay, NAC reconstruction is often secondarily required. Therefore, many variables that may determine the timing to completion of the reconstructive process must be considered, such as the type of breast reconstruction, surgeon preference, presence of complications, and need for postoperative chemotherapy or radiation therapy [2].

Ideal reconstruction of the NAC usually requires symmetry in position, size, shape, texture, pigmentation, and permanent projection. In the cases of unilateral reconstruction, the contralateral NAC serves as a template. If bilateral reconstruction is necessary, the plastic surgeon should use standard values to create the new NAC [3]. Diminution of volume and projection is a common drawback encountered in a reconstructed nipple, due to an unavoidable process of contraction of the skin, with a reported shrinkage rate of about 40–60% in the long term [4]. Therefore, loss of projection should always be anticipated, and overcorrection of 25–50% of the desired result is advisory in NAC reconstruction with local flaps. Furthermore, the type of previous breast reconstruction is another important factor to consider in patient selection. Indeed patients with implant-based reconstruction usually have a thin, expanded skin-subcutaneous tissue base with a centrally placed mastectomy scar, while in autologous reconstruction patients will typically have an

M. Torresetti, M.D. (✉) • A. Scalise, M.D.
G. Di Benedetto, M.D., Ph.D.
Department of Plastic and Reconstructive Surgery, Marche Polytechnic University Medical School, Regional Hospital, Via Conca 71, 60020 Ancona, Italy
e-mail: torresetti.matteo@gmail.com; alescalise1@gmail.com; dibenplast@hotmail.com


M.A. Shiffman (ed.), *Nipple-Areolar Complex Reconstruction*, https://doi.org/10.1007/978-3-319-60925-6_69

elliptical- or circular-shaped scar. These variables should be always considered in the preoperative planning, as thin flaps can potentially decrease nipple projection and poorly located scars may preclude the use of certain flap techniques [3].

Although loss of projection is the most frequent complication, further problems could be observed after NAC reconstruction such as nipple necrosis, tip loss, wound infection, and wound breakdown. Rare cases of implant exchange or removal due to severe wound infection or tissue loss have been also described. A recent investigation described an analysis of complication risk factors in nipple reconstructions. While chest-wall irradiation was associated with a higher rate of projection-related complications, hypertension and diabetes seems to be related with wound healing delays. Interestingly, smoking was not identified as an independent variable associated with higher complication rates. Therefore, those individuals with a history of radiation and medical problems should be informed about these risks [5].

To date, various techniques have been described in the current available literature. Several categories of reconstructive methods could be distinguished: local flaps (centrally based flaps, subdermal pedicle, and pull-out/purse-string flap techniques), flaps with autologous graft augmentation (auricular and costal cartilage graft, fat graft, composite nipple graft, labia minora, hallux toe pulp, dermal graft), flaps with allograft augmentation (acellular dermal matrices, lyophilized costal cartilage, extracellular matrix collagen), and flaps with alloplastic augmentation (polyurethane-coated silicone gel implant, calcium hydroxyapatite gel, hydroxyapatite-tricalcium-phosphate ceramic, hyaluronic acid, artificial bone, polytetrafluoroethylene) [3, 6].

A literature review recently investigated that local flaps are the most frequently described technique for nipple reconstruction and seems to be more safe and reliable then grafts, even if the loss of projection remains an important drawback of this method [7]. Among currently available flaps, we usually perform NAC reconstruction by using a spiral flap made of preexisting mastectomy scar tissue. The preliminary results of this technique were already reported in 2004 [8].

## 69.2 Surgical Technique

We usually perform NAC reconstruction on an outpatient basis as a secondary procedure, after mastectomy and immediate reconstruction, mostly using an adjustable expander/prosthesis, but we have performed it as a single-stage procedure. A full-thickness skin graft harvested from the inguinal crease is usually adopted for areola restoration, as its characteristics of color matching, texture, wrinkled surface, and distinct pigmentation make it more suitable than other alternative methods such as tattooing.

Preoperative planning and marking of the new NAC is mandatory in order to obtain satisfactory results. The patient is marked in the upright position, and the symmetrical placement of the new nipple site is chosen by the surgeon and the patient. Accurate measurements from fixed landmark points such as suprasternal notch, midline, midclavicular line, and inframammary fold are taken. The new position usually falls on the breast meridian lines on a well-reconstructed breast mound. Furthermore, the patient's desired size, volume, and position of the nipple should be also taken into consideration. Finally, the direction of the mastectomy scars on the breast mound that may lie directly near or in the selected position for nipple placement should be also evaluated.

Once the new position of the NAC has been chosen, we usually start by drawing a circle at the center of the breast mound, thus resembling the neo-areola. This circle is mostly located on the central portion of the previous mastectomy scar, which has to be used as the donor site for the neo-nipple. The part of the residual scar located medially to the circle is drawn like an arrow approximately 3–5 cm in length and 1–1.5 cm in width (Fig. 69.1). If the medial length of the scar is not enough, some millimeters of healthy skin could be used to obtain the desired length to create the neo-nipple. The operation is usually performed under local anesthesia; we prefer using no epinephrine to enable adequate intraoperative assessment of flap viability.

Skin incisions are made through the epidermis, dermis, and subcutaneous fat from medial to lateral, taking care to leave a wide base (about 2 cm in width) at the center of the previously drawn neo-areola. A meticulous deepithelialization of the circular area surrounding the flap is then performed (Fig. 69.1). The flap is raised by dissection in the deep subcutaneous plane with a variable amount of fat. As the base is approached, the plane of dissection is deepened to include more subcutaneous tissue; muscle strips can be also included, depending on the projection and thickness of the contralateral normal nipple. Finally

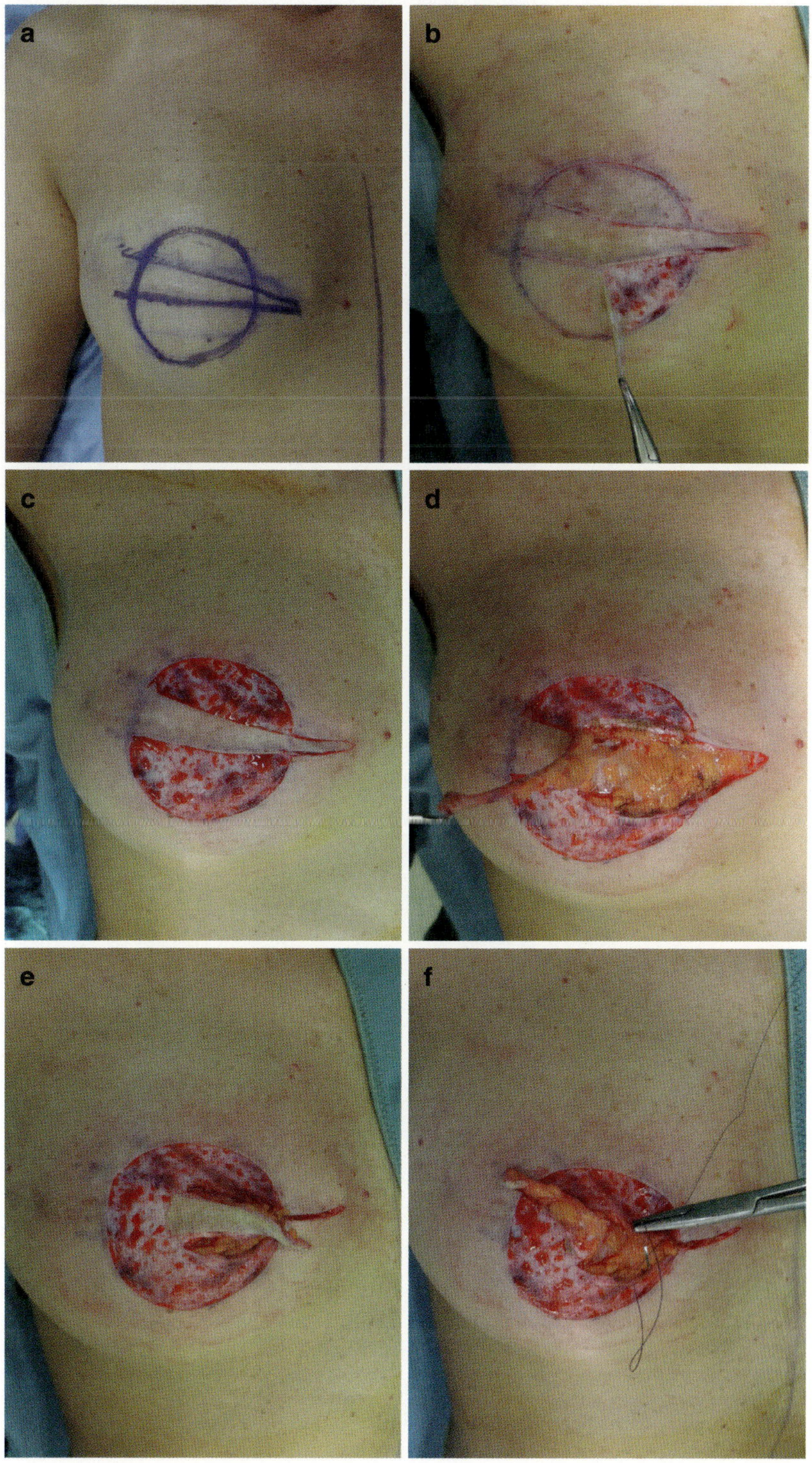


**Fig. 69.1** (**a**) Pre-operative planning and marking of the new NAC. (**b**, **c**) Meticulous deepithelization of the circular area surrounding the flap. (**d**) Flap raising by dissection in the deep subcutaneous plane with a variable amount of fat. (**e**) Deepithelization of the flap base. (**f**) Donor-site defect is primarily closed with Vicryl 3–0 interrupted sutures. (**g**, **h**) The flap is then carefully twisted in a spiral way on its main axis and sutured, to resemble a snail, with Nylon 5/0 interrupted stitches. (**i**) A meshed full-thickness skin graft is placed to restore the areola. (**j**) Application of a polyurethane foam dressing in a donut shape. (**k**) The tip of the reconstructed nipple is then anchored with 4/0 nylon stitches to a 5 mL syringe that was previously cut

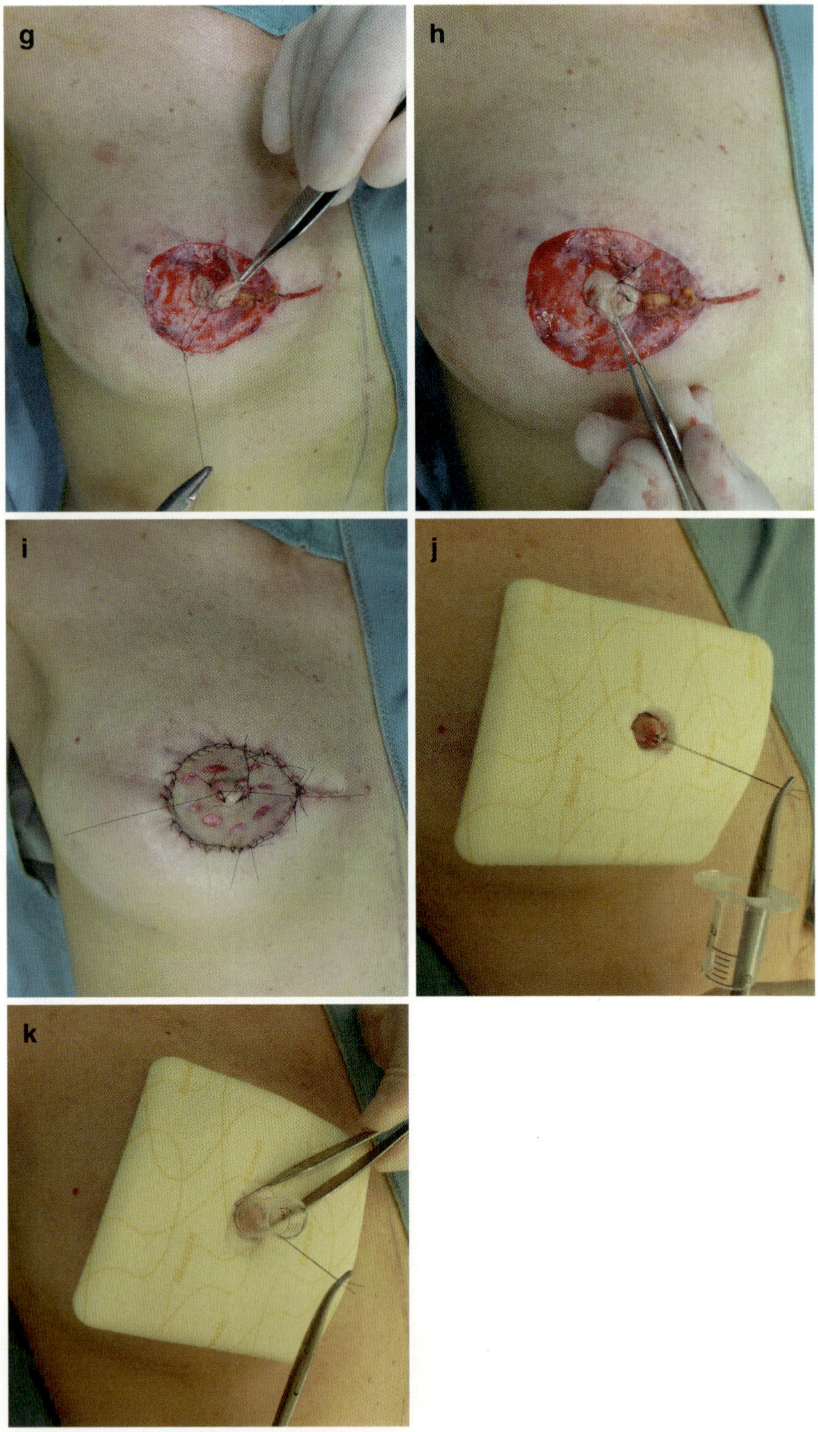


**Fig. 69.1** (continued)

the flap base is deepithelialized as well. The donor-site defect at the apex of the arrow is subsequently primarily closed in a linear fashion with Vicryl 3–0 interrupted sutures. The flap is then raised and must be handled with extreme care. Therefore, it is then carefully twisted in a spiral way on its main axis approximately three times and sutured, to resemble a snail, with nylon 5/0 interrupted sutures. Excessive twisting or skin overtightening should be avoided in order to preserve its viability and blood supply. The neo-nipple will have an over-projection of approximately 60% compared with the contralateral healthy nipple, thus preventing the subsequent wound contracture and shrinkage of tissues that are responsible for loss of projection. Finally, a meshed full-thickness skin graft harvested from the inguinal crease is placed to restore the areola. Postoperative care includes application of a polyurethane foam dressing in a donut shape, to support the take of the skin graft. The tip of the reconstructed nipple is then anchored with 4/0 nylon stitches to a 5 ml syringe that was previously cut. This syringe is applied for approximately 3 weeks, and it is able to maintain the position and projection of the nipple and allows to clean the surgical site, thus minimizing the risk of infection.

## 69.3 Discussion

The nipple-areola complex is the primary landmark of the breast. Its anatomy is really variable in dimension, texture, projection, and color across ethnic groups and among individuals. The normal projection of a normal nipple is usually ≥1 cm, with a diameter of 4–7 mm, while areolar diameter is approximately 4.2–4.5 cm [3].

Several methods have been proposed for nipple reconstruction. The ideal reconstructed nipple should provide sustained projection, the fewest complications, and high levels of patient satisfaction. As postoperative shrinkage of the reconstructed nipple remains an important limitation for most of the techniques, thus maintaining projection represents an ongoing challenge among plastic surgeons. Recently a systematic review studied the efficacy, projection, and complication rate of different techniques that are currently used in order to improve the projection of the neo-nipple. This review suggests that synthetic materials have the least loss of projection but with a higher incidence of complications secondary to migration and exposure. Acellular dermal matrices have yielded promising results with a low incidence of complications and no donor-site morbidity; nevertheless, their use poses a greater financial problem on patients [6, 9]. Therefore, a literature review recently investigated that local flaps are the most frequently used technique for the nipple reconstruction, even if the loss of projection often remains unpredictable [7].

Challenges with many local flaps design may be the adequate matching of their geometric patterns and the need to incorporate them into often unpredictable breast scars. Sometimes, the choice results in the sacrifice of creating an additional scar to achieve optimal nipple position, thus abandoning the use of previous scars. The use of avascular scar tissue as a free graft harvested from a linear fragment of mastectomy scar, in combination with the healthy skin of a local flap, has been already proposed [10]. Nevertheless, the use of an adjacent mastectomy preexisting scar as donor-site for flaps harvesting has been avoided for many years due to the fear of flap ischemia and necrosis [11, 12].

The senior author (Di Benedetto G.) [8] has been using the above-described technique for NAC reconstruction for the past 12 years, with excellent results in terms of both projection and donor-site morbidity (Figs. 69.2, 69.3, 69.4, and 69.5). In the last decade, several authors reported satisfactory results by using a similar technique. Lesavoy and Liu [11] described in 2010 the diamond double-opposing V–Y flap, this reliable technique showed good results allowing the incorporation of prior mastectomy scars into the flap limbs if they are in the appropriate location. Gurunluoglu et al. [12] described in 2012 a star flap technique incorporating a previous scar, and no significant vascular compromise was reported, with acceptable nipple projection and volume. Riccio et al. [13] reported in 2015 a V–Y advancement flap which incorporates a previous wise pattern mastectomy or mammaplasty scar into the newly reconstructed nipple, thereby decreasing new scar formation on the breast and leading to favorable cosmetic result.

In our opinion, this flap seems to have several important benefits. First, the use of scar tissue and healthy skin together is associated with, in our experience, the advantage of providing lower tissue shrinkage compared with other methods,

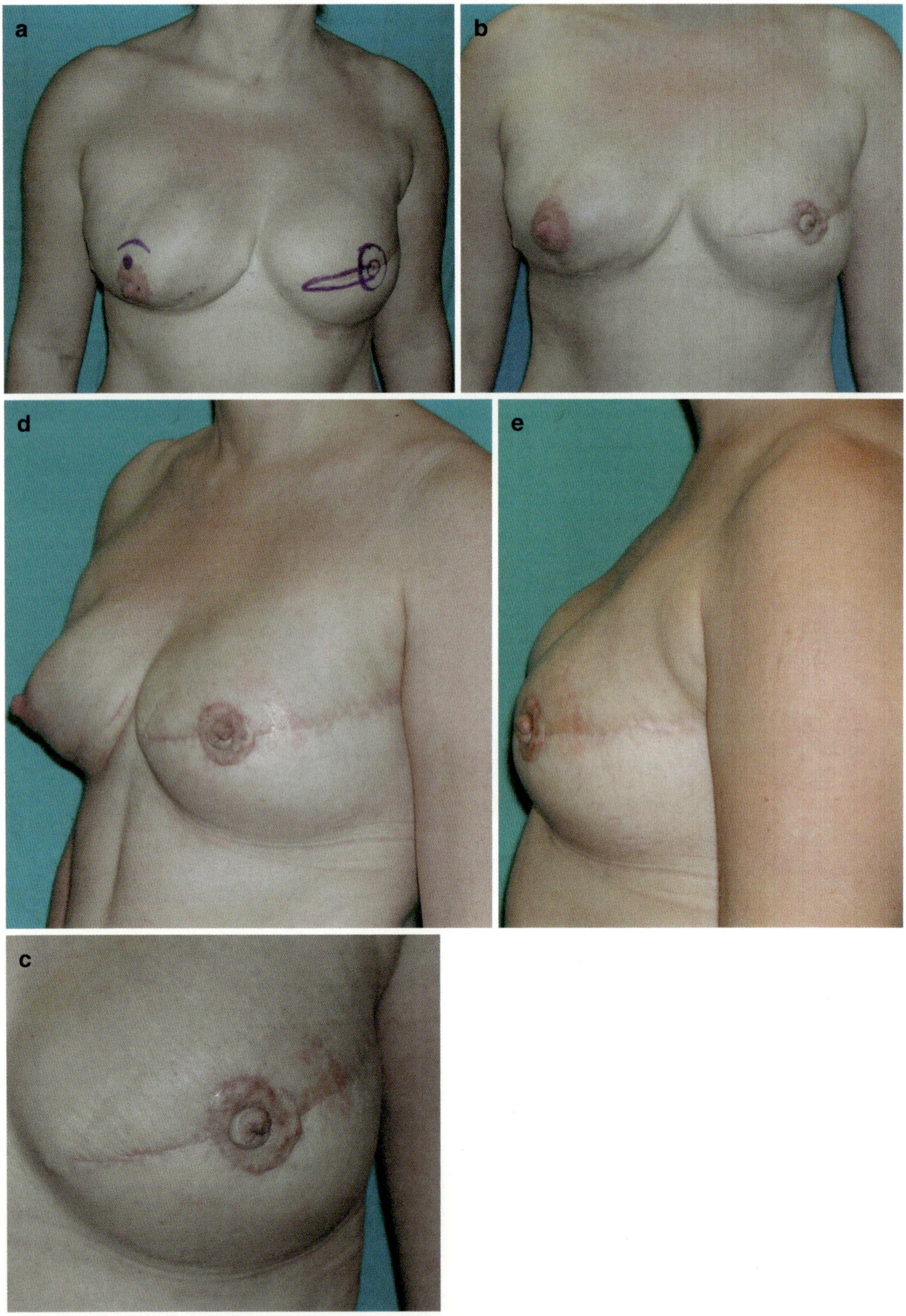


**Fig. 69.2** A 47-year-old woman presented with invasive breast carcinoma of the left breast following right mastectomy and immediate breast reconstruction. (**a**) Preoperative planning and marking of the left NAC reconstruction and contralateral symmetrization; (**b–e**) eight months postoperatively, the reconstructed nipple is symmetrical and maintained good projection with satisfactory color and texture distinction of the nipple-areola complex

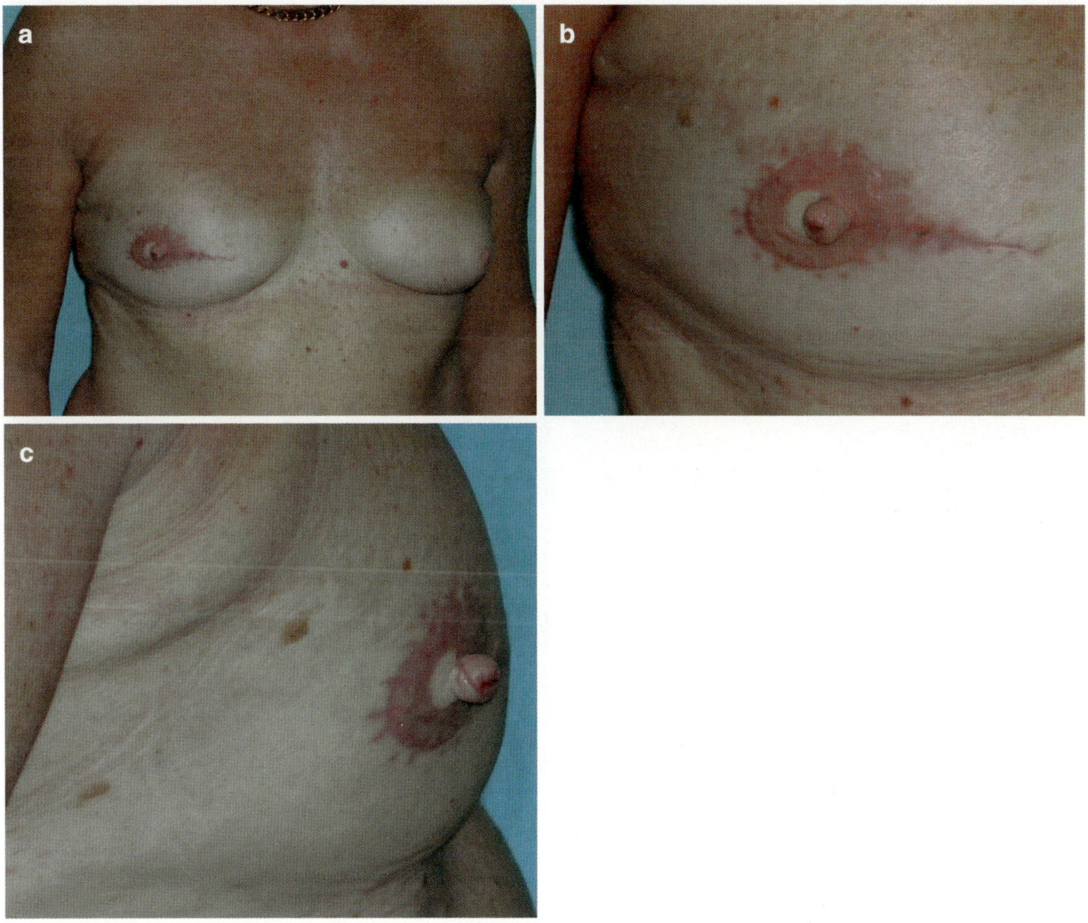


**Fig. 69.3** A 64-year-old woman after right breast reconstruction with prosthesis. (**a–c**) Two months after NAC reconstruction

although in the preoperative planning we always consider an over-projection of the neo-nipple in the range of 50–60%. Second, this flap requires no complicated flap designs and related multidirectional scars. Third, this method allows to use scar tissue that would otherwise have been thrown away, thus avoiding the creation of additional scars. Fourth, no allogenic or synthetic augmentation grafts are necessary in order to obtain long-term nipple projection; nevertheless, it is important to stress that the flap base has to be wide enough, because flap width is the most important factor for obtaining acceptable long-lasting projection. Five, a short learning curve for this flap is needed due to the simplicity and reliability of this technique.

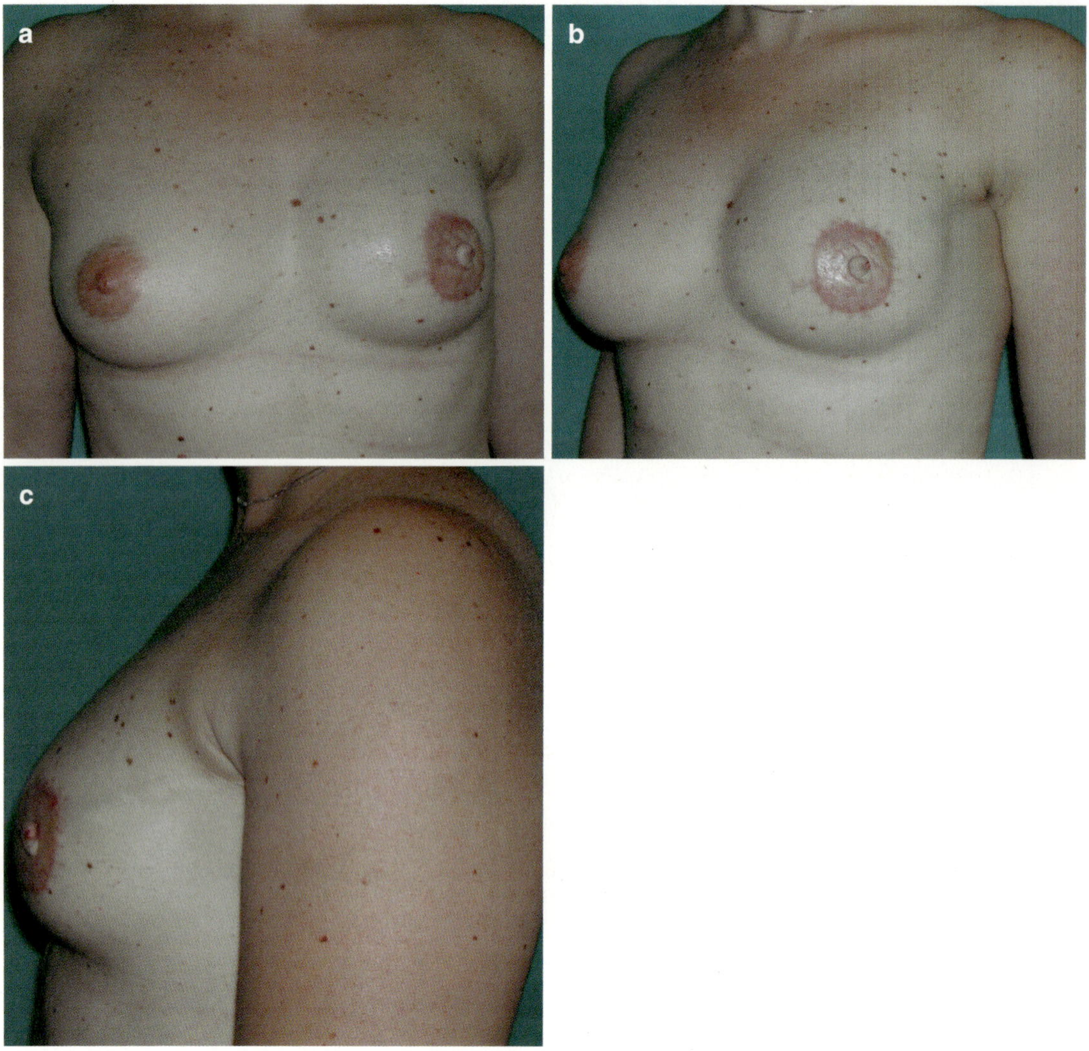

**Fig. 69.4** A 51-year-old woman after left breast reconstruction with prosthesis. (**a**–**c**) Three months postoperatively after NAC reconstruction, with excellent symmetry in terms of projection and color matching

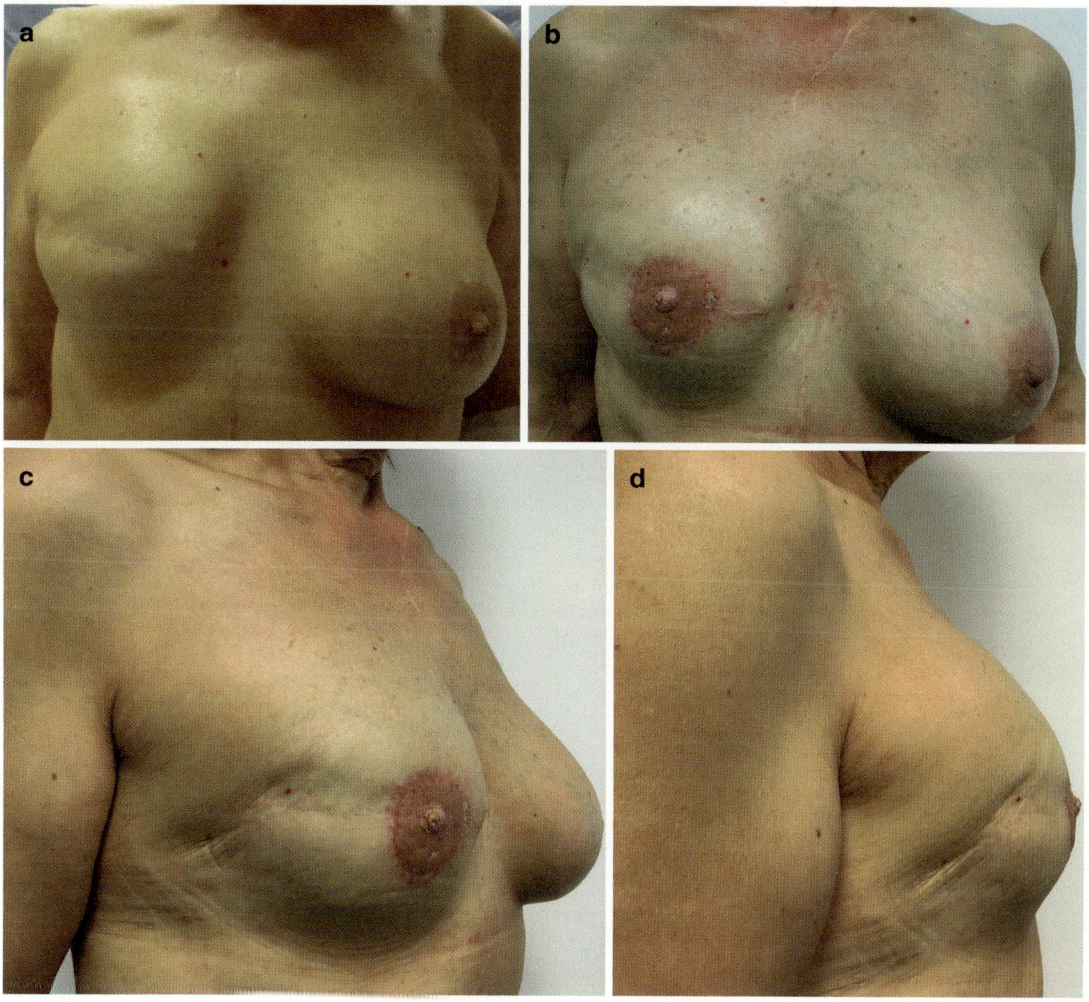


**Fig. 69.5** A 56-year-old woman after right breast reconstruction with prosthesis. (**a**) Preoperative. (**b–d**) One month postoperatively after NAC reconstruction, with good symmetry in terms of projection

## Conclusions

Although several techniques have been proposed over the years to restore nipple integrity, the main problem remains the degree of shrinkage in nipple projection after reconstruction. We propose a new, simple, and reliable method of nipple reconstruction in which the residual mastectomy scar is used to reconstruct a neo-nipple. The nipple thus obtained will have an overprojection of approximately 60%, compared with the opposing normal nipple, to make up for the shrinkage of tissue. Simplicity, reliability, good projection, and reduction in the donor site morbidity are the main points of this technique.

Our long clinical experience and the satisfactory results that we obtained in a large number of patients represent an important reassurance about the long-term reliability of this technique, which could be therefore considered as a valid option in autologous nipple reconstruction.

## References


1. Momoh AO, Colakoglu S, de Blacam C, Yueh JH, Lin SJ, Tobias AM, Lee BT. The impact of nipple reconstruction on patient satisfaction in breast reconstruction. Ann Plast Surg. 2012;69(4):389–93.
2. Losken A, Duggal CS, Desai KA, McCullough MC, Gruszynski MA, Carlson GW. Time to completion of nipple reconstruction: what factors are involved? Ann Plast Surg. 2013;70(5):530–2.
3. Nimboriboonporn A, Chuthapisith S. Nipple-areola complex reconstruction. Gland Surg. 2014;3(1):35–42.
4. Shestak KC, Gabriel A, Landecker A, Peters S, Shestak A, Kim J. Assessment of long-term nipple projection: a comparison of three techniques. Plast Reconstr Surg. 2002;110(3):780–6.
5. Satteson ES, Reynolds MF, Bond AM, Pestana IA. An analysis of complication risk factors in 641 nipple reconstructions. Breast J. 2016;22(4):379–83.
6. Winocour S, Saksena A, Oh C, Wu PS, Laungani A, Baltzer H, Saint-Cyr M. A systematic review of comparison of autologous, allogeneic, and synthetic augmentation grafts in nipple reconstruction. Plast Reconstr Surg. 2016;137(1):14e–23e.
7. Sisti A, Grimaldi L, Tassinari J, Cuomo R, Fortezza L, Bocchiotti MA, Roviello F, D'Aniello C, Nisi G. Nipple-areola complex reconstruction techniques: a literature review. Eur J Surg Oncol. 2016;42(4):441–65.
8. Di Benedetto G, Sperti V, Pierangeli M, Bertani A. A simple and reliable method of nipple reconstruction using a spiral flap made of residual scar tissue. Plast Reconstr Surg. 2004;114(1):158–61.
9. Garramone CE, Lam B. Use of AlloDerm in primary nipple reconstruction to improve long-term nipple projection. Plast Reconstr Surg. 2007;119(6):1663–8.
10. Gullo P, Buccheri EM, Pozzi M, De Vita R. Nipple reconstruction using a star flap enhanced by scar tissue: the Regina Elena cancer institute experience. Aesthet Plast Surg. 2011;35(5):731–7.
11. Lesavoy M, Liu TS. The diamond double-opposing V–Y flap: a reliable, simple, and versatile technique for nipple reconstruction. Plast Reconstr Surg. 2010;125(6):1643–8.
12. Gurunluoglu R, Shafighi M, Williams SA, Kimm GE. Incorporation of preexisting scar in the star-flap technique for nipple reconstruction. Ann Plast Surg. 2012;68(1):17–21.
13. Riccio CA, Zeiderman MR, Chowdhry S, Wilhelmi BJ. Review of nipple reconstruction techniques and introduction of V to Y technique in a bilateral wise pattern mastectomy or reduction mammaplasty. Eplasty. 2015;6(15):e11.

# Breast Reconstruction Under Local Anesthesia: Second-Stage Implant Exchange, Nipple Flap Reconstruction, and Nipple Flap Tattoo

70

Dimitri J. Koumanis and Jessie Bujouves

## 70.1 Introduction

Each year in the latter part of this decade, more than 90,000 patient women underwent breast reconstruction. Of all those women, over two-thirds were implant-based reconstruction. Possibly two-thirds of these patients were also postmastectomy breast reconstruction patients [1, 2].

Implant-based reconstruction is strictly performed in three stages in our practice. The first stage is the tissue expander and acellular dermal matrix sling procedure performed immediately after the mastectomies. The second-stage reconstruction involves the removal of the tissue expander with a small incision, replacement with a permanent silicone gel implant, and possible revisions of the breast flaps breast flaps if needed. Finally, the third stage involves nipple flap reconstruction. Patients typically wait a few months post surgeries before undergoing medical tattooing of the areola and nipple to give it a three-dimensional look. Over 200,000 women received a diagnosis of breast cancer in 2011 according to one study, and approximately 96,000 women who underwent breast reconstruction had tissue expander and implant reconstruction [3].

There are studies that show that patients who undergo reconstruction have a better body image compared with those who forego reconstruction [4–6]. It has also been shown that breast reconstruction after mastectomy offers a significant psychosocial benefit to women [7–10]. Elder and colleagues reported that women's self-image scores were equal to those of the normal population 1 year after breast reconstruction surgery and recovery [11].

Although the mastectomy portion of breast reconstruction requires general anesthesia, the second stage is more amendable to local anesthetic settings. This can be performed in select patients with small incisions as will be described in this chapter. In fact, there are some practices that have successfully performed breast augmentation with a local anesthetic in an office-based surgery setting, which is more involved compared to second-stage breast implant reconstruction [12].

Reconstruction of the nipple-areola complex is most frequently associated with breast cancer reconstruction. Nipple reconstruction is the most amenable part of the reconstruction process to be performed under local anesthetic and even more so in an office-based setting. Although NAC reconstruction is the simplest of the three stages of breast reconstruction, the psychological

D.J. Koumanis, M.D. (✉)
Capital Area Plastic Surgery of New York, 377 Church Street, Saratoga Springs, NY 12866, USA
e-mail: jkoumanis@yahoo.com

J. Bujouves, BSc
262 Callaway Rd, London, ON, Canada, N6G 0M3
e-mail: jessbujouves@gmail.com


M.A. Shiffman (ed.), *Nipple-Areolar Complex Reconstruction*, https://doi.org/10.1007/978-3-319-60925-6_70

impact is quite significant. Some studies have shown that the final NAC reconstruction leads to greater overall satisfaction, improved sexual behavior, and body self-image [13].

Presently there is no standard technique to nipple-areola reconstruction. Current literature illustrates the vast number of NAC techniques performed by surgeons, highlighting the available options for this type of reconstruction. A recent review article attempted a classification of techniques for NAC reconstruction. The article found 75 papers from 1946 to 2015 with different techniques. The nipple was predominantly reconstructed using local flaps and approximate 50 articles [14]. Nipple-areolar reconstruction was first described and documented by Adams in 1949 [15] with the areola being historically reconstructed on the nonoperative side with sharing techniques and grafting from other sites.

Reconstruction of the nipple flap itself has been achieved through various methods including centrally based flaps, subdermal pedicle flaps, grafting, internal nipple prostheses, and autogenous implants [16, 17]. The areola reconstruction in complement to the nipple reconstruction has also historically been carried out with multiple techniques including local flaps, skin grafts, and medical tattooing alone [13, 18–22].

Although skin grafting in conjunction with areolar tattooing can provide an aesthetically successful result, it does require a skin graft to be harvested which in turn produces an additional donor site wound. As an alternative, in our practice, we use a simple star flap procedure in combination with 3D areolar tattooing to produce an equally aesthetically pleasing result without the need for a donor wound site.

Local anesthetic as an alternative to general or monitored anesthesia care (MAC) [23] has been utilized in the past three decades and provides many benefits over general anesthesia to the patient. Although general anesthesia has been proven to be reasonably safe, several of the health risks associated with general anesthesia-NAC are present with the use of local anesthesia. In addition, if second-stage breast reconstruction with tissue expander exchange to permanent breast implant and NAC reconstruction are performed in outpatient settings under no sedation, patients are permitted to go home immediately following the procedure. Conversely, general anesthesia or MAC procedures require the patients to remain in a post anesthesia care unit to recover from the anesthetic gases. Sometimes these patients also needed to be admitted for postoperative nausea or other sequelae associated with general anesthesia or deep sedation. Due to ever-rising healthcare costs, the need for reducing surgical costs will only become more important in the near future [23]. In a small series conducted by our practice, we showed that possibly $2000 can be saved on average in this clinical scenario [24].

In second- and third-stage breast reconstruction, more specifically tissue expander exchange to permanent breast implant and nipple-areola complex reconstruction, it is feasible for both of these procedures to be performed under local anesthesia and to maintain successful and reliable results. The treatment goals for restoring the female's breast and body image should be carefully planned. Special considerations should be made for position, size, shape, texture, projection, scar position, and symmetry when planning each stage of the reconstruction. Breast reconstruction is a very important part of the healing process for women undergoing breast cancer surgery and mastectomy. Research has shown that it exudes a positive influence on the overall recovery course of these women after mastectomy for breast cancer [24, 25].

## 70.2 Second-Stage Reconstruction: Tissue Expander Exchange to Permanent Silicone Breast Implant

### 70.2.1 The Preoperative Plan

At this stage, the patient's breast tissue expander is fully expanded and ready to exchange for a more permanent silicone gel implant. In our study, we almost exclusively use silicone gel implants instead of saline implants for reconstruction unless there is a contraindication.

Studies have shown that women undergoing silicone breast implant reconstruction view the result more favorable when compared to saline implants [26].

Timing between each stage of breast reconstruction is of utmost importance. Variables including radiation, chemotherapy, wound complications, infections, etc., have all been shown to contribute to the variability of waiting periods between each stage of the implant reconstruction. In fact, a recent study even argued against starting tissue expansion after the first stage too early. The current conventional approach was initiation of expansion at approximately 14 days postoperatively. The authors discovered that by waiting 6 weeks before starting expansion, a Velcro affect in relation to capsular contracture was reduced in association with certain types of tissue expanders [27]. The most significant issue in relation to implant reconstruction is radiation. Radiation is known to cause capsular contractures significantly in breast implant reconstruction along with soft tissue discoloration, increased chance of infection, and ultimately reconstruction failure [28–30]. The optimal time period between last radiation treatment and tissue expander exchange has been debated in the past. Cordeiro et al. [28] looked at their data using a multivariable analysis for 1143 patients in their own practice. The authors concluded that 6 months is the optimal time postradiation to perform an implant exchange. Reconstructive failure rates were less for radiation during tissue expander versus after final implant exchange, 18.1% versus 12.4%, respectively. This corroborated previous studies demonstrating even higher failure rates between the two groups [31]. Both studies disagreed on timing of radiation, after tissue expansion or following permanent implant exchange, and the effect on aesthetic outcome. Codeiro et al. [28] found that aesthetic outcome was improved when patients were radiated after tissue expander exchange in comparison to after the final permanent implant procedure.

Although nipple flap reconstruction is almost always amenable to local anesthetic techniques, this stage of tissue exchange to a permanent implant (with possible flap or breast pocket revisions) requires more scrutiny when stratifying patients to undergo the procedure with local anesthetic. The surgeon must calculate anesthetic dosing in relation to the amount of dissection and revision of the breast flaps required and the patient's potential discomfort and anxiety. If the dissection is to be large enough, thereby putting the lidocaine calculations at unsafe dosing, we obviously perform the procedure under general anesthesia. However, if it is an issue of anxiety or the patient shows apprehension, then we add intravenous (IV) sedation with monitored anesthesia care performed by the anesthesiologist.

The patient is marked in the preoperative holding area with a surgical marker. An existing scar is used to make the incision, and generally the scar is excised with 1 mm margins in order to provide clean tissue for subsequent closure. If the patient's breast has been radiated, then a separate incision is made in the inferolateral inframammary fold as described by Nahabedian [32]. By avoiding reentry into a previously radiated scar, the incidence of incisional dehiscence based on mechanical factors was reduced significantly.

Patients are given one dose of prophylactic antibiotics covering gram-positives, unless the patient had a previous infection in which case the choice of antibiotics is directed by previous cultures. Recently we have adjusted our protocol and practice and have continued antibiotics for a total of 24 h. Previous studies analyzed the literature for antibiotic regimens using one dose preoperatively, 24 h, and greater than 24 h. There was no significant difference in infection rates between 24 h and greater than 24 h of antibiotic use [1, 33]. Conversely, there was an article associated with higher infection rate with only administration of one preoperative dose of antibiotic [34].

Recently after reviewing the evidence, we have adjusted our protocol and practice and have continued antibiotics for a total of 24 h based on the evidence to date including a randomized controlled study [35]. This protocol is applied to all stages of breast implant reconstruction procedures including the final stage of nipple flap reconstruction.

### 70.2.2 The Procedure

The patient is placed on the operative room table in the supine position with her arms extended and wrapped with gauze around the arm boards to facilitate sitting the patient up and checking for symmetry during the procedure. A chlorhexidine preparation is used to sterilize the skin, and if the procedure requires only a small incision and simple exchange for tissue expander to a permanent implant, a measured amount of 1% lidocaine with 1: 100,000 epinephrine mixture is injected into this incision line. Lidocaine and epinephrine solution is also injected deeper as the surgeon dissects down toward the capsule and acellular dermal junction or near the muscle. If concomitant larger flap revisions of the breasts are required, intravenous sedation and/or intercostal blocks can be injected, as described in a recent study [12].

The intercostal blocks are injected into the third to seventh intercostal spaces with 1% lidocaine and 0.25% bupivacaine with 1:100,000 epinephrine in an equal parts mixture. This lidocaine and bupivacaine mixture is injected at the mid-axillary line and the lateral border of the sternum if needed. Due to the added toxicity of both mixtures, the dose calculation remains at 4 mg/kg, residing at the lower end for safe dosing (Fig. 70.1).

The breast pocket is entered at the junction of the acellular dermal capsule in the pectoralis muscle if the tissue expander occurred under the pectoralis major muscle. This junction is easily identified in the preoperative holding area or on the table if the patient is awake by asking them to flex the pectoralis major muscle. However, as described before, if the breast was radiated, then an incision along the inferolateral inframammary fold is implemented.

The most minimal incision is used in order to remove the tissue expander from the pocket with a #15 scalpel blade over suction. This incision will be kept at a minimum for insertion of a silicone gel implant. The size of the silicone gel implants is ascertained by the total office measurements of tissue expansion and verified using silicone gel sizers. In our practice, a Keller funnel is utilized to introduce the implant into the breast pocket. The Keller funnel has standardized markings that presents a specific diameter opening of the funnel and allows us to use a smaller incision per implant size (Figs. 70.2 and 70.3). The end of the funnel is cut with straight Mayo scissors according to the size that is needed to fill the breast pocket appropriately. The use of the Keller funnel has shown to decrease bacterial loads in breast implant cases [24]. In a separate study, triple antibiotic solution such as Ancef 1 g, 50,000 units bacitracin, and gentamicin 80 mg in

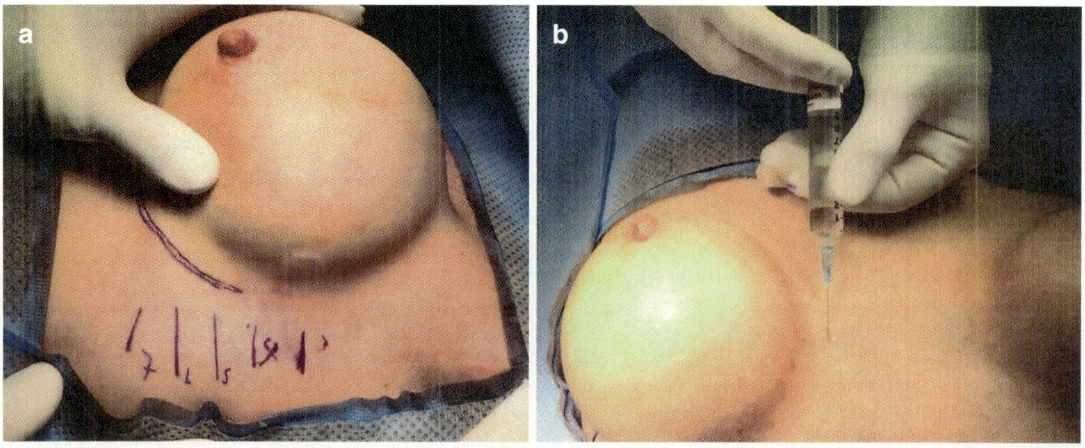


**Fig. 70.1** (**a**) Injection of 1:1 local anesthetic solution of 1% lidocaine and 0.25% bupivacaine with 1:100,000 epinephrine, 2 mL in each intercostal space from lateral ribs 3–7. (**b**) The lateral margin of the sternum is also injected

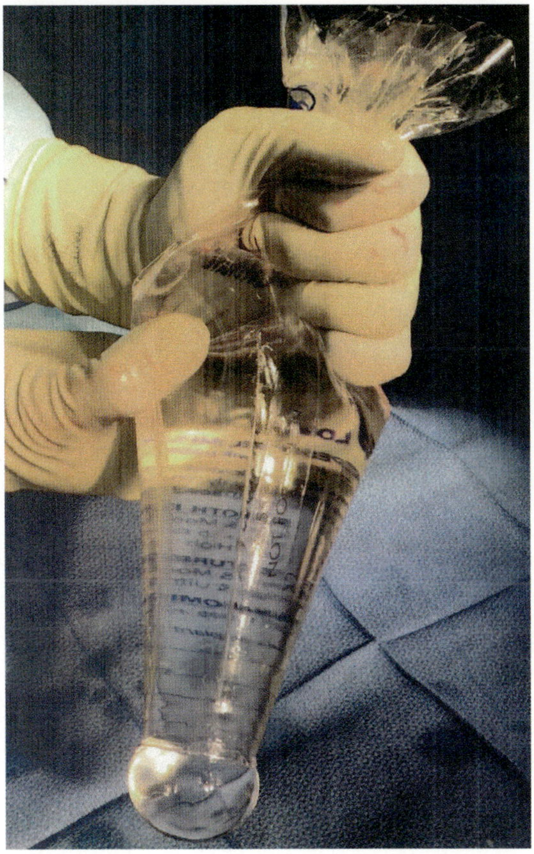

**Fig. 70.2** Close-up of Keller funnel with silicone gel breast implant

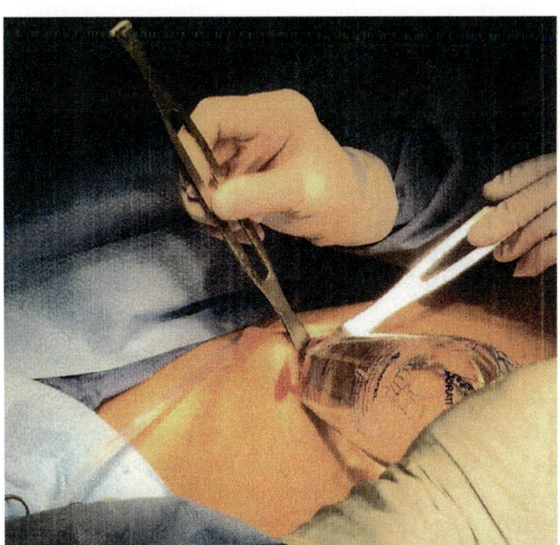

**Fig. 70.3** Insertion of silicone gel implant into small incision and breast pocket using the Keller funnel

500 mL of sterile normal saline was used to irrigate the pocket, bathe the implants, and reduce bacterial load and in turn reduce capsular contracture rates [36]. Along with changing our gloves, re-prepping the skin with chlorhexidine before implant insertion, triple antibiotic solution for the Keller funnel, and a minimum touch technique, we aim at reducing infection.

The final step involves closing the incision in a multilayer fashion and putting on sterile steri-strips and sterile gauze.

## 70.3 Nipple-Areola Reconstruction

### 70.3.1 The Preoperative Plan

The nipple-areola complex (NAC) is an important aesthetic landmark of the breast. Therefore, it is an essential component of the breast reconstruction process. Many women in our practice state they felt complete once the nipple-areola flap reconstruction was completed. This sentiment is supported by research representing psychological impact and contribution in breast reconstruction [13, 37]. Several techniques have been described in nipple reconstruction including nipple sharing techniques, local dermal flaps, and grafts [38–41]. A thorough review of the numerous flap and projection techniques for nipple-areolar reconstruction was recently published [14]. However, there exists no definitive study on the most optimal technique for NAC reconstruction, and thus the choice is usually directed by the surgeon's familiarity and previous successes with a particular approach. In our practice, we invariably perform the modified star flap as described by several investigators over the years [42, 43]. It has offered consistent results and satisfactory outcomes and circumvents the need for any skin or tissue grafts and the morbidity associated with these methods. The star flap is a procedure that is easily carried out with local anesthesia, avoiding the higher costs and potential morbidities such as nausea and vomiting associated with it. Before making the final decision to perform the procedure under local anesthetic, we consider the patient's anxiety toward the procedure and the needle, and if present, intravenous sedation is added to the anesthetic plan. Additionally, a neurological assessment of the anterior skin of the breast mound is performed evaluating for light touch, pressure, and pain. Frequently, patients experience little sensation in this area due to the previous mastectomy and reconstructive procedures.

The operative plan for the modified star flap begins with several key measurements based on specific anatomic points. Key measurements include the suprasternal notch, the midclavicular line, and inframammary fold and are all marked when placing a nipple into position (Fig. 70.4). Most of the nipple measurements are within the meridian of the breast and form the shape of an equilateral triangle in relation to the sternal notch and the nipples on each side with the line connecting both nipples on a horizontal [44]. Measurements are taken so that the nipples look as symmetrical as possible within their respective positions on each breast mound. The patient is also involved in the final decision of the nipple position by asking her to look into the mirror with us and comment on the placement of the circles we have drawn. If the case is unilateral, the native nipple is used as a reference point. We typically perform a mastopexy for reduction symmetry operations in the second stage of an implant breast reconstruction when we perform

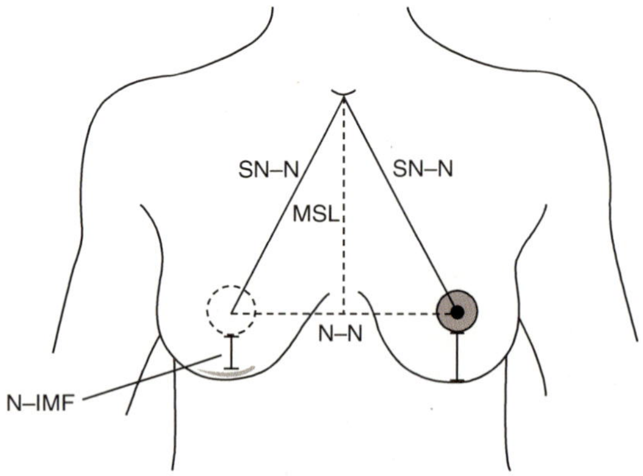


**Fig. 70.4** Key markings from sternal notch to each nipple (SN–N), nipple to nipple (N–N), nipple to inframammary fold (N–IMF) and mid-sternal line (MSL)

the exchange from tissue expander to permanent implant. Therefore, the native nipple has already settled to a more stable position providing more accurate comparison when performing our nipple flap reconstruction during this final stage.

The three limbs of the flap are then designed, with the lateral and medial limbs having 2 cm lengths and a 1.5 cm width at their bases. The inferior limb is drawn shorter to about 1.5 cm, with the width of approximately 2 cm at the base (Fig. 70.5). The inferior limb can become a superior limb in certain cases, depending on the direction of the blood supply to the flap. As described by Gurunluoglu et al. [45], the horizontal and vertical scar are incorporated into the flap design so that the limb making up the superior cap of the nipple is the one that may cross a previous scar. For example, vertical scar incorporation means that the star flap was designed laterally or medially and an inferior based or superior based flap in relation to a horizontal mastectomy scar.

## 70.3.2 Patient Positioning and Procedure

The patient lies down on the table in the supine position, and the skin is prepared with a 4% chlorhexidine skin preparation. Once our sterile field is secured, the operation begins. A single preoperative prophylactic dose of intravenous antibiotic is given due to the reconstruction being associated with an implant.

Local anesthetic of 1% lidocaine with 1:100,000 epinephrine mixture is drawn into a mL syringe. If the patient has sensation to the skin involved in the surgery, we add 1 mL of bicarbonate for every 9 mL of lidocaine drawn into our syringe. We usually inject the patient right before scrubbing our hands to allow the epinephrine at least 9 minutes to take full effect. Additionally, the nipple flap surgery encompasses only a small surface area with little local anesthetic used, and therefore we add 0.25% bupivacaine with 1:100,000 epinephrine mixture at the end of the procedure for longer-acting analgesia. However, if we are performing larger breast flap revisions at the same time as the

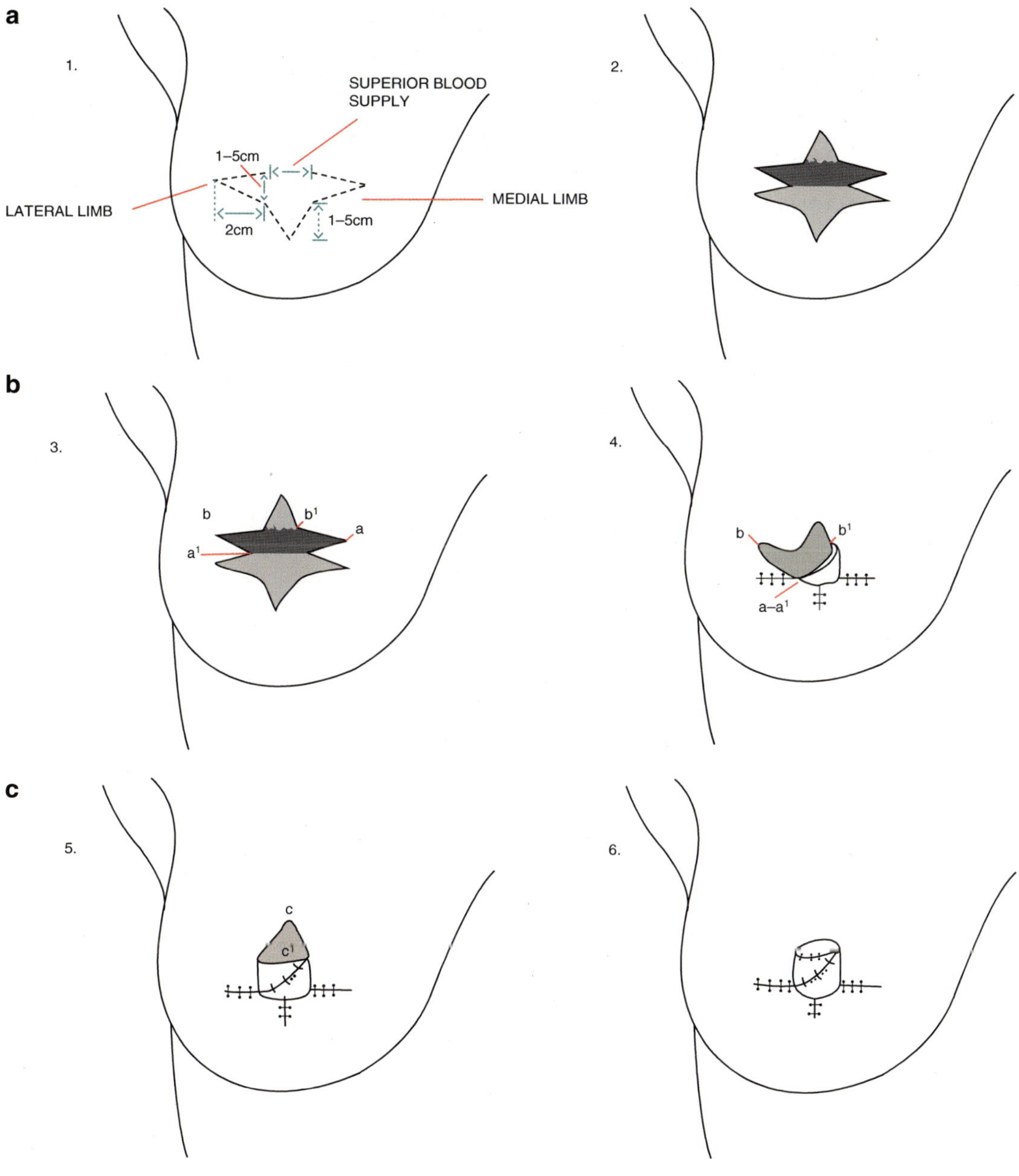


**Fig. 70.5** (**a–c**) Creation of Star Flap for nipple reconstruction

nipple flap reconstructions, we do not use bupivacaine because of its lower lethal dose calculations compared with lidocaine (maximum dose 2–3 mg per kg bupivacaine with epinephrine versus 5–7 mg of 1% lidocaine with epinephrine). Additionally, animal studies have shown that mixing the two local anesthetics, bupivacaine and lidocaine, contributes to an additive toxicity making calculations of toxic levels even more difficult [46]. Cardiotoxicity related to bupivacaine is a serious and life-threatening side effect and generally unresponsive to resuscitation efforts according to some animal studies [47, 48]. Therefore, we prefer the use of lidocaine over bupivacaine in procedures requiring large volumes of anesthetic. It is also beneficial to carry intralipid within the facility when using bupivacaine as a local anesthetic. Intralipid is a lipid emulsion of fat emulsion used intravenously as a cardioprotective agent in the treatment of ischemic reperfusion injury [49] and in the treatment of severe cardiotoxicity from intravenous overdose of bupivacaine [50, 51]. If our calculations are anywhere near toxic doses of local anesthetic, we plan the case for general anesthesia.

The skin incisions are made with a #15 scalpel blade and are raised with sufficient subcutaneous fat and thickness. The subcutaneous thickness should be greatest near the base of the pedicle. The medial and lateral flaps form the cylindrical base of the flap and are created with an interdigitating pattern whereby the inferior limb makes up the superior cap of the flap. We used a combination of 5–0 chromic sutures and 4–0 chromic sutures to sew the limbs together depending on the thickness of the flaps. The donor site is then undermined full thickness just above the pectoralis muscle fascia, and the defect is closed in two layers with 3–0 Monocryl for the deep dermal stitches and a combination of running and interrupted 4–0 nylon sutures to close the skin defect as needed. The interrupted 4–0 nylon sutures are used to reinforce areas near the base of the flap to close the skin around it. The skin at the base of the flap is secured to the skin of the donor breast tissue with multiple interrupted 5–0 chromic sutures. We then dress the flap with bacitracin ointment and single strips of Xeroform one layer thick. We cover the nipple with a nipple protective cup if available as the outer dressing. If nipple protective cups are not available, then lose 4 × 4 gauze dressings with light tape is put on the most outer layer being careful not to compress the flap. We direct the patient to sleep supine in order to keep any pressure away from the flaps for approximately 2–3 weeks. Keeping our dressing light has not increased any complications, including infection.

Approximately 3–6 months after the nipple reconstruction is complete, the patient's flaps and incisions are ready for nipple and areolar tattooing (Fig. 70.8).

## 70.4 Nipple-Areola Tattooing

After 3–6 months have elapsed since the previous nipple flap reconstruction, the patient is brought to the office to evaluate the scars and readiness for nipple and areola tattooing. We use a professional medical tattoo artist to perform the tattoos. The tattoo artist is capable of recreating small three-dimensional nuances of the female nipple and areola including the areolar glands and the traditional nature of areola tissue to regular skin. As discussed earlier, there are many variations and flap designs for nipple reconstruction. One of the major difficulties is maintaining projection especially in thin or irradiated skin and soft tissue [17, 52–54]. At the same time, too much projection can be embarrassing for the patient, and, therefore, the surgeon and the medical tattoo artist should work together in communication to maximize results. A recent paper discussed nipple-areola complex tattoos by using lighter ink for the nipple compared to the areola and a darker rim that is thicker inferiorly [22]. This gives the nipple-areola complex a three-dimensional appearance including tattooing of Montgomery glands. medical tattoo artist utilizes the base of fundamentals of tattooing which have been ignored in traditional nipple-areola complex tattooing. Medical practitioners use pigments based on vegetable oil and metal salts and are mixed very thin limiting the choices available and decreasing the longevity of results. To prevent fading over time, our medical tattoo artist uses professional tattoo pigments and a color wheel to provide color match and improve pigment retention [22]. The cost of three-dimensional nipple-areola complex tattoos varies by artist and location, but our patients currently pay approximately $400 for a unilateral tattoo and $600 for a bilateral tattoo. Many of the insurance companies will reimburse some or all of the tattoo procedure [22]. A satisfactory outcome can be obtained with three-dimensional tattooing techniques of the nipple-areola complex, obviating the need for full-thickness skin grafts and the associated added incisions and morbidities associated with it.

## 70.5 Discussion

Surgical complications for implant breast reconstruction include infection, scarring, hematoma, flap necrosis, and capsular contracture. Although it is considered a clean elective procedure, breast reconstruction infection rates can exceed 20%, attributed to the presence of prosthetic devices and drains. Preventative measures taken to avoid infection include strict aseptic techniques, the use of antibiotics, decreasing operating room traffic, and the Keller Funnel. The Keller Funnel is a medical device resembling a Baker's Funnel. It is of medical-grade vinyl in a clear conical shape with an interior hydrophilic coating which creates a slick surface that allows the implants to easily pass through a smaller hole or incision. The function of the device is to reduce the amount of handling and skin contact between the implant, the surgeon, and the patient. The no-touch technique is intended to limit the potential for breast pocket contamination. Bacterial contamination was significantly reduced with the Keller Funnel compared with standard digital insertion techniques [55]. Although the cause is not entirely clear, there is a correlation between capsule contracture and bacterial infection [36, 56]. Adams et al. [36] conducted a study of optimal broad-spectrum antibiotic coverage for the organisms that are most frequently encountered during implant contracture and infection. The original analysis established that a combination of povidone-iodine, gentamicin, and cefazolin provided optimal coverage. However, due to FDA disapproval of using povidone-iodine against implant devices, the regimen was changed to bacitracin, gentamicin, and cefazolin mixture. This mixture has been credited to reduce the clinical incidence of capsular contracture compared with other published reports [56].

A discussion of anesthetic complications is obviously relevant to this article. General anesthesia affects the entire body and presents potential for multiple complications, although it is generally safe. Complications include potential for aspiration, increased blood pressure, allergic reaction, damage to the teeth and lips, increased heart rate, laryngeal swelling, nausea and vomiting, infection, myocardial infarction, cerebrovascular accident, delirium, malignant hyperthermia, systemic toxicity, and, even rarely, death. Locally infiltrative anesthetics, however, are distributed only to the operative location, alleviating most of the potential risks associated with general anesthesia or anesthesia involving deep conscious sedation. Risks associated with local anesthesia are minimal; however, its ability to cross the blood-brain barrier presents an absorption risk that can, in rare cases, lead to serious systemic reactions. In the presence of toxic levels, respiratory arrest, cardiac arrhythmia, coma, hypotension, and systemic collapse are possible. Preventive measures can be achieved through proper calculation, suggested dosing, heart rate, blood pressure and electrocardiogram monitoring, and frequent syringe aspiration for blood before injection. Also, an initial test or sample dose may be performed on a patient who has never received local anesthetic in the past. If symptoms of systemic toxicity develop, local anesthetic injections should be stopped immediately and ventilation with oxygen should be maintained to resist hypoxemia, hypercarbia, and acidosis because the presence of these increases in systemic toxicity [54, 57–59].

Regarding the safety and efficacy of breast surgery, Colque and Eisemann [12] were able to show that the operation of breast augmentation (with our without mastopexy) can be performed successfully with a lidocaine/bupivacaine solution using intercostal blocks and surgeon-directed sedation. In the breast augmentation-only group ($N = 132$), the average 1% lidocaine/0.25% bupivacaine with 1:100,000 epinephrine mixture injected was 79.6 mL (range 25–120 mL), and, in the breast augmentation/mastopexy group, it was 90.9 mL (range 45–144 mL). Minor side effects associated with the IV sedation medicine included slight nausea (between 10% and 12.5%) across both groups, but there were no deaths and no hospital admissions. There were no serious complications in either group, underscoring the safety and efficacy of this approach. Average operating room time was 63.8 min in the breast augmentation-only group and 134.7 min in the breast augmentation/mastopexy group. The investigators avoided the use of propofol as a sedative and the need for anesthesiologist or nurse anesthetist. This cost reduction is significant for the patient.

In the recent article by the present authors, a cost analysis of our nipple-areola reconstruction under general versus local anesthetic was undertaken. Cost variables included operating room time, recovery room (PACU), pharmacy, medical supplies, and anesthesia fees. We showed savings of approximately $2143 US dollars when the surgeon chose local anesthetic versus a general anesthetic. [24]

**Conclusions**

Breast reconstruction can be performed safely with local anesthesia providing the patient with minimal discomfort and minimal complications while reducing healthcare costs. Star flap method, out of all stages of breast implant reconstruction, is the most amenable to local anesthetic techniques due to its minimalist approach. The star flap method in conjunction with tattoo successfully provides optimal aesthetic results without the need for an additional donor site. During the second stage, tissue expander to silicone implant exchange, the use of triple antibiotic irrigation as well as the Keller Funnel is recommended to decrease both infection and capsular contracture. All other operative settings, including sterility and sound operative surgical techniques, should be mainstay of any practice. Minimizing complications and maximizing results while reducing costs are imperative in today's healthcare environment and its associated rising costs.

## References


1. Phillips BT, Bishawi M, Dagum AB, Khan SU, Bui DT. A systematic review of antibiotic use and infection in breast reconstruction: what is the evidence? Plast Reconstr Surg. 2013;131(1):1–13.
2. Bogue DP, Mungara AK, Thompson M, Cederna PS. Modified technique for nipple-areolar reconstruction: a case series. Plast Reconstr Surg. 2003;112(5):1274–8.
3. Huber KM, Zemina KL, Tugertimur B, Killebrew SR, Wilson AR, DallaRosa JV, Prabhakaran S, Dayicioglu D. Outcomes of breast reconstruction after mastectomy using tissue expander and implant reconstruction. Ann Plast Surg. 2016;76(Suppl 4):S316–9.
4. Nicholson RM, Leinster S, Sassoon EM. A comparison of the cosmetic and psychological outcome of breast reconstruction, breast conserving surgery and mastectomy without reconstruction. Breast. 2007;16(4):396–410.
5. Draper LB, Bui DT, Chiu ES, Mehrara BJ, Pusic AL, Cordeiro PG, Disa JJ. Nipple-areola reconstruction following chest-wall irradiation for breast cancer: is it safe? Ann Plast Surg. 2005;55(1):12–5.
6. Disa JJ, McCarthy CM, Mehrara BJ, Pusic AL, Hu QY, Cordeiro PG. Postmastectomy reconstruction: an approach to patient selection. Plast Reconstr Surg. 2009;124(1):43–52.
7. Dean C, Chetty U, Forrest AP. Effects of immediate breast reconstruction on psychosocial morbidity after mastectomy. Lancet. 1983;1(8322):459–62.
8. Stevens LA, McGrath MH, Druss RG, Kister SJ, Gump FE, Forde KA. The psychological impact of immediate breast reconstruction for women with early breast cancer. Plast Reconstr Surg. 1984;73(4):619–28.
9. Wellisch DK, Schain WS, Noone RB, Little JW III. Psychosocial correlates of immediate versus delayed reconstruction of the breast. Plast Reconstr Surg. 1985;76(5):713–8.
10. Rosenqvist S, Sandelin K, Wickman M. Patients' psychological and cosmetic experience after immediate breast reconstruction. Eur J Surg Oncol. 1996;22(3):262–6.
11. Elder EE, Brandberg Y, Björklund T, Rylander R, Lagergren J, Jurell G, Wickman M, Sandelin K. Quality of life and patient satisfaction in breast cancer patients after immediate breast reconstruction: a prospective study. Breast. 2005;14(3):201–8.
12. Colque A, Eisemann ML. Breast augmentation and augmentation-mastopexy with local anesthesia and intravenous sedation. Aesthet Surg J. 2012;32(3):303–7.
13. Yang JD, Ryu JY, Ryu DW, Kwon OH, Bae SG, Lee JW, Choi KY, Chung HY, Cho BC. Our experiences in nipple reconstruction using the Hammond flap. Arch Plast Surg. 2014;41(5):550–5.
14. Sisti A, Grimaldi L, Tassinari J, Cuomo R, Fortezza L, Bocchiotti MA, Roviello F, D'Aniello C, Nisi G. Nipple-areola complex reconstruction techniques: a literature review. Eur J Surg Oncol. 2016;42(4):441–65.
15. Adams WM. Labial transplant for correction of loss of the nipple. Plast Reconstr Surg. 1949;4(3):295–8.
16. Farhadi J, Maksvytyte GK, Schaefer DJ, Pierer G, Scheufler O. Reconstruction of the nipple-areola complex: an update. J Plast Reconstr Aesthet Surg. 2006;59(1):40–53.
17. Zhong T, Antony A, Cordeiro P. Surgical outcomes and nipple projection using the modified skate flap for

nipple-areolar reconstruction in a series of 422 implant reconstructions. Ann Plast Surg. 2009;62(5):591–5.
18. Berson MI. Construction of pseudoareola. Surgery. 1946;20(6):808.
19. Barton FE Jr. Latissimus dermal-epidermal nipple reconstruction. Plast Reconstr Surg. 1982;70(2):234–7.
20. Silversmith PE. Nipple reconstruction by quadrapod flaps. Plast Reconstr Surg. 1983;72(3):422.
21. Chang WH. Nipple reconstruction with a T flap. Plast Reconstr Surg. 1984;73(1):140–3.
22. Halvorson EG, Cormican M, West ME, Myers V. Three-dimensional nipple-areola tattooing: a new technique with superior results. Plast Reconstr Surg. 2014;133(5):1073–5.
23. McKay DR. Costs of regional and general anesthesia: what the plastic surgeon needs to know. Clin Plast Surg. 2013;40(4):529–35.
24. Koumanis DJ, Colque A, Eisemann ML, Smith J. Breast surgery under local anesthesia: second-stage implant exchange, nipple flap reconstruction, and breast augmentation. Clin Plast Surg. 2013;40(4):583–91.
25. Mohamed SA, Parodi PC. A modified technique for nipple-areola complex reconstruction. Indian J Plast Surg. 2011;44(1):76–80.
26. Macadam SA, Ho AL, Cook EF Jr, Lennox PA, Pusic AL. Patient satisfaction and health-related quality of life following breast reconstruction: patient-reported outcomes among saline and silicone implant recipients. Plast Reconstr Surg. 2010;125(3):761–71.
27. Paek LS, Giot JP, Tétreault-Paquin JO, St-Jacques S, Nelea M, Danino MA. The impact of postoperative expansion initiation timing on breast expander capsular characteristics: a prospective combined clinical and scanning electron microscopy study. Plast Reconstr Surg. 2015;135(4):967–74.
28. Cordeiro PG, Albornoz CR, McCormick B, Hudis CA, Hu Q, Heerdt A, Matros E. What is the optimum timing of postmastectomy radiotherapy in two-stage prosthetic reconstruction: radiation to the tissue expander or permanent implant? Plast Reconstr Surg. 2015;135(6):1509–17.
29. Krueger EA, Wilkins EG, Strawderman M, Cederna P, Goldfarb S, Vicini FA, Pierce LJ. Complications and patient satisfaction following expander/implant breast reconstruction with and without radiotherapy. Int J Radiat Oncol Biol Phys. 2001;49(3):713–21.
30. Motwani SB, Strom EA, Schechter NR, Butler CE, Lee GK, Langstein HN, Kronowitz SJ, Meric-Bernstam F, Ibrahim NK, Buchholz TA. The impact of immediate breast reconstruction on the technical delivery of postmastectomy radiotherapy. Int J Radiat Oncol Biol Phys. 2006;66(1):76–82.
31. Nava MB, Pennati AE, Lozza L, Spano A, Zambetti M, Catanuto G. Outcome of different timings of radiotherapy in implant-based breast reconstructions. Plast Reconstr Surg. 2011;128(2):353–9.
32. Nahabedian MY. Minimizing incisional dehiscence following 2-stage prosthetic breast reconstruction in the setting of radiation therapy. Gland Surg. 2013;2(3):133–6.
33. Phillips BT, Fourman MS, Bishawi M, Zegers M, O'Hea BJ, Ganz JC, Huston TL, Dagum AB, Khan SU, Bui DT. Are prophylactic postoperative antibiotics necessary for immediate breast reconstruction? Results of a prospective randomized clinical trial. J Am Coll Surg. 2016;222(6):1116–24.
34. Clayton JL, Bazakas A, Lee CN, Hultman CS, Halvorson EG. Once is not enough: withholding postoperative prophylactic antibiotics in prosthetic breast reconstruction is associated with an increased risk of infection. Plast Reconstr Surg. 2012;130(3):495–502.
35. Phillips BT, Halvorson EG. Antibiotic prophylaxis following implant-based breast reconstruction: what is the evidence? Plast Reconstr Surg. 2016;138(4):751–7.
36. Adams WP Jr, Conner WC, Barton FE Jr, Rohrich RJ. Optimizing breast pocket irrigation: an in vitro study and clinical implications. Plast Reconstr Surg. 2000;105(1):334–8.
37. Delay E, Mojallal A, Vasseur C, Delaporte T. Immediate nipple reconstruction during immediate autologous latissimus breast reconstruction. Plast Reconstr Surg. 2006;118(6):1303–12.
38. Bhatty MA, Berry RB. Nipple-areola reconstruction by tattooing and nipple sharing. Br J Plast Surg. 1997;50(5):331–4.
39. Losken A, Mackay GJ, Bostwick J III. Nipple reconstruction using the C-V flap technique: a long-term evaluation. Plast Reconstr Surg. 2001;108(2):361–9.
40. Kroll SS, Reece GP, Miller MJ, Evans GR, Robb GL, Baldwin BJ, Wang BG, Schusterman MA. Comparison of nipple projection with the modified double-opposing tab and star flaps. Plast Reconstr Surg. 1997;99(6):1602–5.
41. Lesavoy M, Liu TS. The diamond double-opposing V Y flap: a reliable, simple, and versatile technique for nipple reconstruction. Plast Reconstr Surg. 2010;125(6):1643–8.
42. Shestak KC, Gabriel A, Landecker A, Peters S, Shestak A, Kim J. Assessment of long-term nipple projection: a comparison of three techniques. Plast Reconstr Surg. 2002;110(3):780–6.
43. Anton MA, Eskenazi LB, Hartrampf CR Jr. Nipple reconstruction with local flaps: star and wrap flaps. Semin Plast Surg. 1991;5(1):67–78.
44. Mathes SJ, Ueno CM. Reconstruction of the nipple areola complex. In: Mathes SJ, Hentz VR, editors. Plastic surgery. Philadelphia, PA: Saunders Elsevier; 2006. p. 791–818.
45. Gurunluoglu R, Shafighi M, Williams SA, Kimm GE. Incorporation of a preexisting scar in the star-flap technique for nipple reconstruction. Ann Plast Surg. 2012;68(1):17–21.
46. Mets B, Janicki PK, James MF, Erskine R, Sasman B. Lidocaine and bupivacaine cardiorespiratory toxicity is additive: a study in rats. Anesth Analg. 1992;75(4):611–4.

47. Albright GA. Cardiac arrest following regional anesthesia with etidocaine or bupivacaine. Anesthesiology. 1979;51(4):285–7.
48. Marx GF. Cardiotoxicity of local anesthetics–the plot thickens. Anesthesiology. 1984;60(1):3–5.
49. Li J, Iorga A, Sharma S, Youn JY, Partow-Navid R, Umar S, Cai H, Rahman S, Eghbali M. Intralipid, a clinically safe compound, protects the heart against ischemia-reperfusion injury more efficiently than cyclosporine-a. Anesthesiology. 2012;117(4):836–46.
50. Picard J, Meek T. Lipid emulsion to treat overdose of local anaesthetic: the gift of the glob. Anaesthesia. 2006;61(2):107–9.
51. Weinberg GL, VadeBoncouer T, Ramaraju GA, Garcia-Amaro MF, Cwik MJ. Pretreatment or resuscitation with a lipid infusion shifts the dose-response to bupivacaine-induced asystole in rats. Anesthesiology. 1998;88(4):1071–5.
52. Richter DF, Reichenberger MA, Faymonville C. Comparison of the nipple projection after reconstruction with three different methods. Handchir Mikrochir Plast Chir. 2004;36(6):374–8.
53. Jabor MA, Shayani P, Collins DR Jr, Karas T, Cohen BE. Nipple-areola reconstruction: satisfaction and clinical determinants. Plast Reconstr Surg. 2002;110(2):457–63.
54. Boccola MA, Savage J, Rozen WM, Ashton MW, Milner C, Rahdon R, Whitaker IS. Surgical correction and reconstruction of the nipple-areola complex: current review of techniques. J Reconstr Microsurg. 2010;26(9):589–600.
55. Moyer HR, Ghazi B, Saunders N, Losken A. Contamination in smooth gel breast implant placement: testing a funnel versus digital insertion technique in a cadaver model. Aesthet Surg J. 2012;32(2):194–9.
56. Adams WP Jr, Rios JL, Smith SJ. Enhancing patient outcomes in aesthetic and reconstructive breast surgery using triple antibiotic breast irrigation: six-year prospective clinical study. Plast Reconstr Surg. 2006;117(1):30–6.
57. Van Laeken N, Genoway K. Nipple reconstruction using a two-step purse-string suture technique. Can J Plast Surg. 2011;19(2):56–9.
58. Mulroy MF. Systemic toxicity and cardiotoxicity from local anesthetics: incidence and preventive measures. Reg Anesth Pain Med. 2002;27(6):556–61.
59. Barash PG, Cullen BF, Stoelting RK, editors. Clinical anesthesia. 4th ed. Philadelphia: Lippincott Williams & Wilkins; 2001. p. 459–62.

# Nipple Reconstruction Using the Modified Top Hat Flap with Banked Costal Cartilage

# 71

Neil S. Sachanandani and Ming-Huei Cheng

## 71.1 Introduction

The challenge of nipple reconstruction in the Asian population is to create a well-projected nipple with a relatively small areolar footprint. This necessitates a technique that minimizes lengthy scars and subsequently limits the amount of areolar tattooing required. While trying to achieve the ideal result for our patient population, another major issue encountered is the loss of projection that typically occurs within the first the 2 months following the initial reconstruction. Approximately 50% of the projection of traditional nipple reconstruction is lost during this time period. In our opinion, soft tissue alone is not enough to provide durability to the reconstructed nipple's projection, and therefore we utilize the readily-available costal cartilage graft for underlying support. In this chapter, we describe the technique for nipple reconstruction that is utilized in our hospital.

N.S. Sachanandani, M.D. (✉)
Division of Reconstructive Microsurgery, Department of Plastic and Reconstructive Surgery, Chang Gung Memorial Hospital, No. 199, Dunhua North Road, Songshan, Taipei, Taiwan
e-mail: neilsacha@gmail.com

M.-H. Cheng, M.D., MBA (✉)
Department of Plastic and Reconstructive Surgery, Chang Gung Memorial Hospital, College of Medicine, Chang Gung University, Kwei-Shan, Tao-Yuan, Taiwan
e-mail: minghueicheng@gmail.com

## 71.2 Technique

During autologous breast reconstruction, we routinely remove third costal cartilage for recipient vessel exposure of the internal mammary vessels. Instead of discarding this tissue, we save it and utilize it for a staged nipple reconstruction. Nipple reconstruction is typically undertaken at a time point approximately at 3 months following reconstruction of the breast mound and not prior to the completion of chemotherapy/radiotherapy.

A 10 mm segment of rib cartilage is harvested and banked during the initial reconstruction. We are careful to include a cuff of perichondrium with the cartilage segment to help promote vascular ingrowth during the final placement. During the first stage reconstruction, the cartilage graft is stored in damp saline gauze during the operation until banked at an inconspicuous location near the surgical incision. This helps prevent desiccation of the cartilage graft. In the setting of an autologous reconstruction, this is usually placed at the 6 o'clock position at the junction of the flap and the native skin envelope. During implant-based reconstruction, the fourth rib cartilage is utilized for a more concealed effect, and this is banked in a pre-pectoral position at either the 3 o'clock or the 9 o'clock positions, for the right or left breast, respectively.

During the nipple reconstruction procedure, the ideal nipple position is marked while the patient is standing. This is represented in


M.A. Shiffman (ed.), *Nipple-Areolar Complex Reconstruction*,
https://doi.org/10.1007/978-3-319-60925-6_71

Fig. 71.1 by the dashed circle connecting points a, a', b', and b. The height of the nipple is designed to be 20% greater than the contralateral nipple to account for postoperative loss of projection. It is important to note that the nipple height corresponds to the width of the "wings" in the marking of the top hat flap. The previously banked cartilage graft is retrieved (Fig. 71.2). Our current design of the cartilage graft is to shape the graft as a disk with pillar design. This is a 10 mm diameter disk with 3 mm height. The central pillar is approximately 7 mm tall. The flap is elevated with a layer of subcutaneous flap in order to provide tissue bulk and maximize vascularity by preserving the subdermal plexus (Fig. 71.3). The cartilage graft is placed as a strut under the top hat flap and is secured with 3–0 PDS suture to the dermis (Fig. 71.4). The roof of the flap and the ends of the wings are sutured together utilizing 5–0 nylon suture effectively wrapping the cartilage construct. This results in a pleasing shape of the reconstructed nipple (Fig. 71.5). Antibiotic ointment and light dressing are applied.

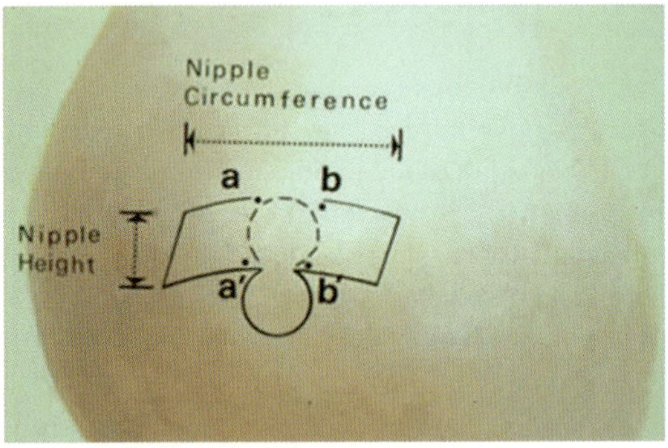


**Fig. 71.1** Markings of the modified top hat flap, the new nipple will be located in the circle a–a'–b'–b, with height and circumference corresponding to the width and length of the wing flaps, respectively

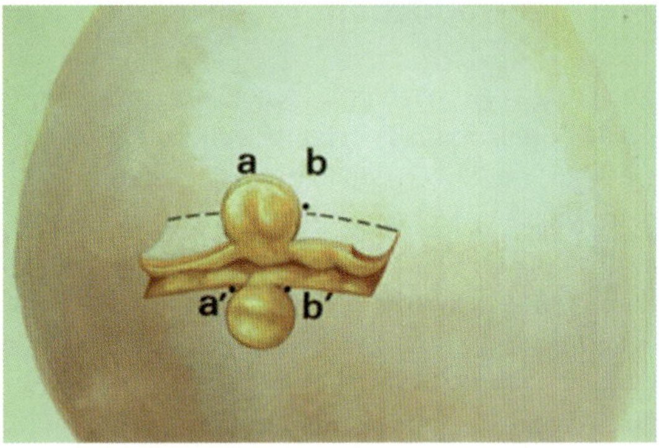


**Fig. 71.3** The flap is elevated with subcutaneous fat attached to the flap. The a-b curve is preserved, and no incision is placed there in order to preserve the circulation

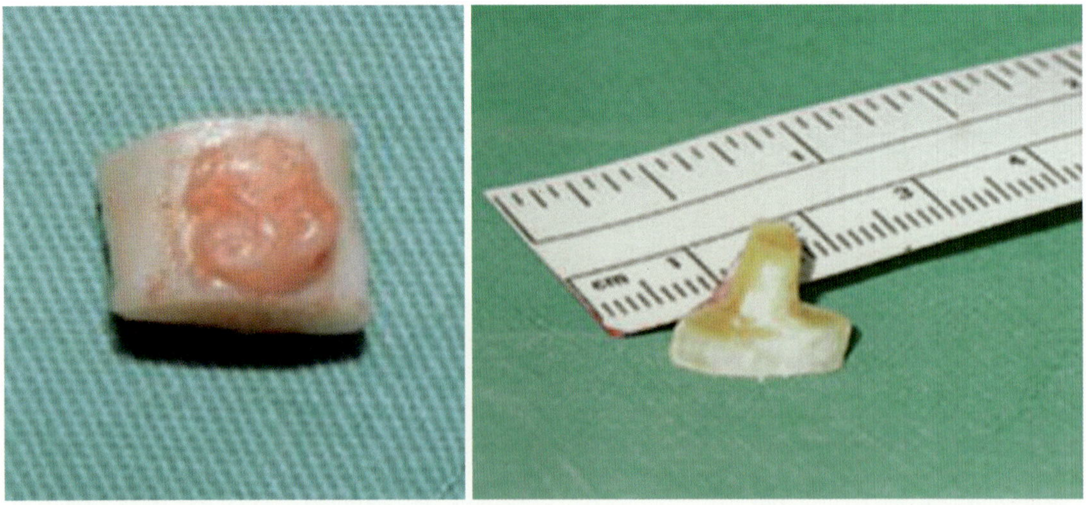

**Fig. 71.2** (*Left*) Banked cartilage has been retrieved with preservation of the perichondrium. (*Right*) The cartilage graft is sculpted into a disk shape with a central pillar

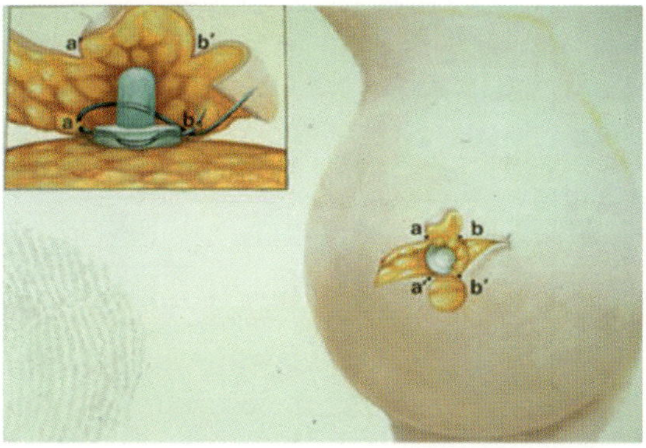


**Fig. 71.4** (*Left* and *right*) The cartilage graft is secured to the subcutaneous tissue of the flap with PDS suture and the wings wrap the cartilage strut

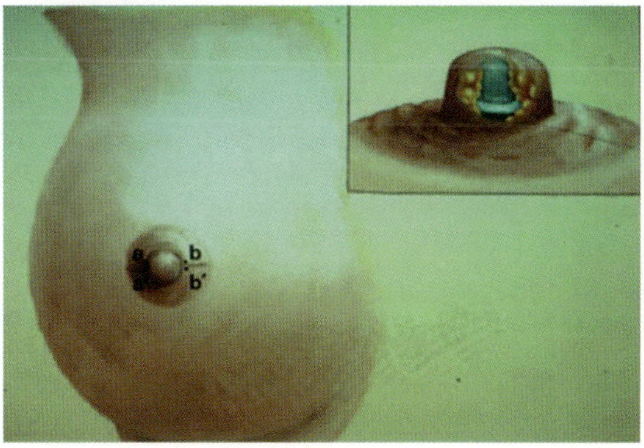


**Fig. 71.5** (*Left* and *right*) The wound closure ensures that the a and a' points approximate and the b and b' points approximate. The cartilage graft is wrapped and contained within the designed flap and will maintain the nipple projection

## 71.3 Outcomes

We have retrospectively reviewed 58 of our patients that underwent this nipple reconstruction technique with a mean follow-up of 44.9 months. The average loss of nipple projection was approximately 26.1% during this period of follow-up. The overall complication rate was 12.1% (seven cases) with a surgical revision rate of 8.6% (five cases). Early complication with partial loss of the wing flap margins in two patients healed uneventfully with appropriate projection in the long term. Two patients that had costal cartilage graft exposure required local V–Y advancement flaps to heal their wounds. Three patients in long-term follow-up needed surgical intervention for inversion or tilting of the costal cartilage graft and had repositioning performed to restore the nipple height. Also, it should be noted that none of our patients had complaints regarding discomfort involving the banked cartilage graft.

Although the top hat flap can be either superiorly or inferiorly based, we prefer to use a superiorly based flap to conceal the scars of the reconstructed nipple. The flap design is versatile and can be adapted to the specific clinical situation.

## 71.4 Illustrative Case

A 49-year-old woman with previous implant-based reconstruction presented for completion of nipple reconstruction. The modified top hat flap technique was employed to reconstruct the nipple-areolar complex (Fig. 71.6). After the nipple reconstruction was fully healed, tattooing of the nipple-areolar complex was utilized to provide a realistic hue to the reconstructed nipple. A pleasing, symmetric result was achieved.

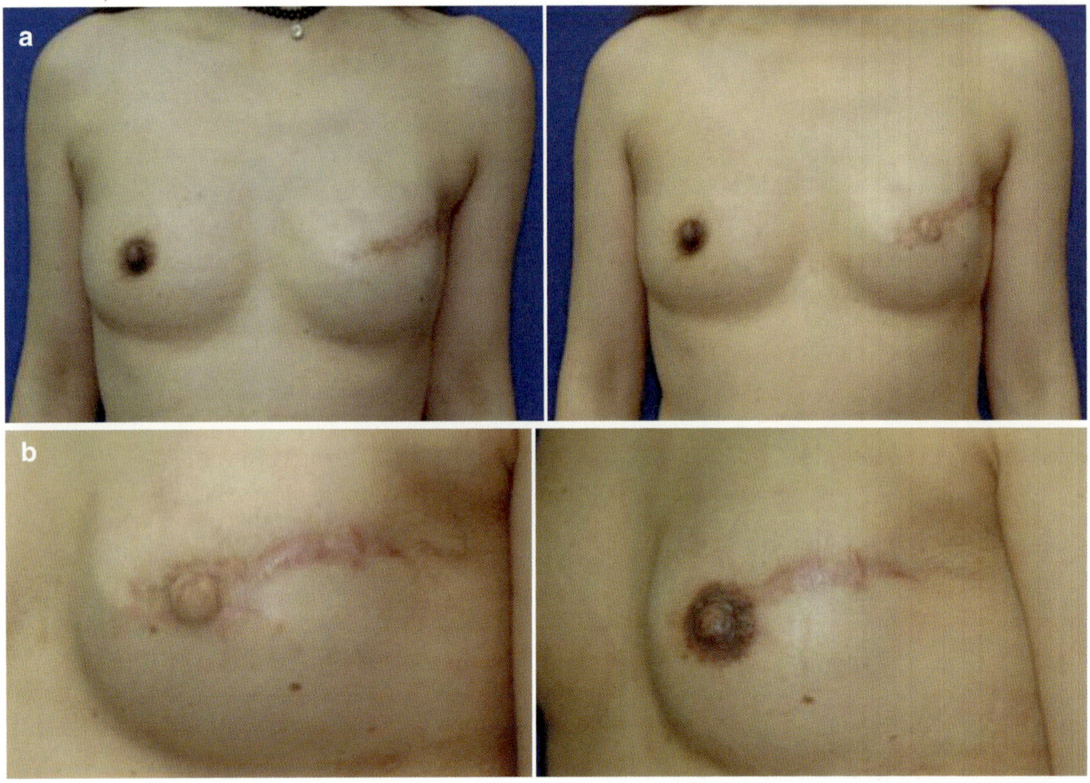


**Fig. 71.6** (**a**) (*Left*) Preoperative patient with implant-based reconstruction prior to nipple reconstruction. (*Right*) Patient after nipple reconstruction is performed. (**b**) (*Left*) Nipple reconstruction prior to nipple-areolar complex tattoo. (*Right*) Nipple reconstruction after completion of the nipple-areolar complex tattoo

## Conclusions

We have described the technique of nipple reconstruction that is utilized at Chang Gung Memorial Hospital. This technique provides a durable result with appropriate nipple projection in a small areolar footprint. The technique does not require excessive donor site morbidity or the use of alloplastic materials, is easy to perform, and has an acceptable complication profile which can be readily managed.

# Nipple-Areola Complex Reconstruction

# 72

Diego Schavelzon, Guillermo Blugerman, and Victoria Schavelzon

## 72.1 Introduction

Many techniques have been described for the reconstruction of the nipple-areola complex after the total mastectomy. Finding one that suits our patients is a challenge for plastic surgeons.

There are a few techniques utilized:

1. Inserting tissues that are firmer than surrounding structures as cartilage, fibrocartilage, or Silastic®
2. Transposing other structures projected from other parts of the body such as portion of the contralateral nipple, ball of the thumb, dermis, or earlobe [1]
3. Using local flaps [2–4]

All these techniques are affected by the skin cover and its tension. The skin as well as the clothes [2] flattens the projected structure.

The present technique was described by Smith and Nelson in 1986 [5]. The aim was to produce a structure that maintains the projection on the surface tissue of the skin. The objectives are contrast pigmentation between nipple and areola, contrast in texture, three-dimensional relationship between those structures, and good vertical projection from the flat areola.

D. Schavelzon, M.D. • G. Blugerman, M.D. (✉)
V. Schavelzon, M.D.
B&S Centro de Excelencia en Cirugia Plástica, Laprida 1579, C1425EKK Buenos Aires, Argentina
e-mail: schavelzon@centrosbys.com; blugerman@centrosbys.com; draschavelzon@centrosbys.com

## 72.2 Technique

Mark a circular island flap (Fig. 72.1). Raise partial thickness skin graft leaving a central base of a quarter the size of the whole nipple-areola complex (NAC) attached (Fig. 72.2). The central stalk, remains in the position of the future NAC. This structure will be the areola, and the center of the nipple with its base will maintain the vascularity. The base must be a quarter of the areola designed and large enough to ensure vascularization of the nipple. A needle is placed through the flaps (Fig. 72.3), and a suture is passed through the needle (Fig. 72.4). This procedure is reversed, and the suture is passed back through the needle and tied (Fig. 72.5). The open areas of the flaps (Fig. 72.6) are then sutured closed. The skin that is exposed outside the stalk will shrink with the process of scar it and retraction to be the nipple in the new location that will be the size of the contralateral nipple (Fig. 72.7).

The size of the base depends on skin type and condition. It will be larger or smaller depending on whether it received radiotherapy or not, has a split-thickness skin, or if the skin has a scar through it. These factors determine the size of attachment to


M.A. Shiffman (ed.), *Nipple-Areolar Complex Reconstruction*,
https://doi.org/10.1007/978-3-319-60925-6_72

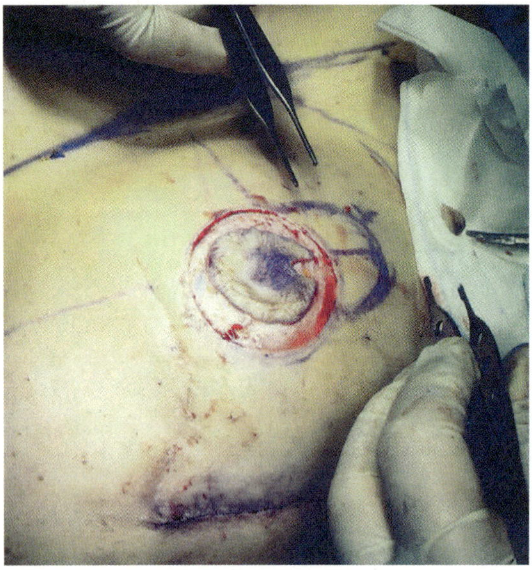

**Fig. 72.1** Flaps raised and central stalk is in position for the new NAC

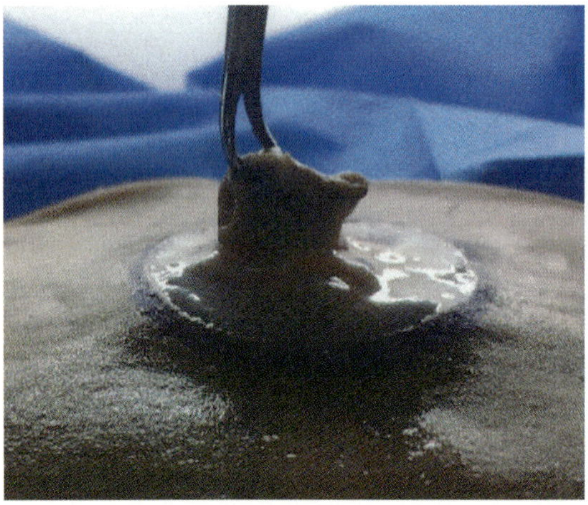

**Fig. 72.2** Raise partial thickness skin graft leaving a central base of a quarter the size of the whole nipple-areola complex (NAC) attached

the base in order to ensure proper circulation on this segment. The size of the nipple-areola complex is based on the contralateral complex.

Areola reconstruction is recreated by taking a full-thickness graft skin below the inguinal crease [6]. It should be similar to the size of the partial thickness graft elevated for the reconstruction of the nipple. All remaining fat should be taken off. The inguinal graft covers the bloody area around the nipple, and the nipple

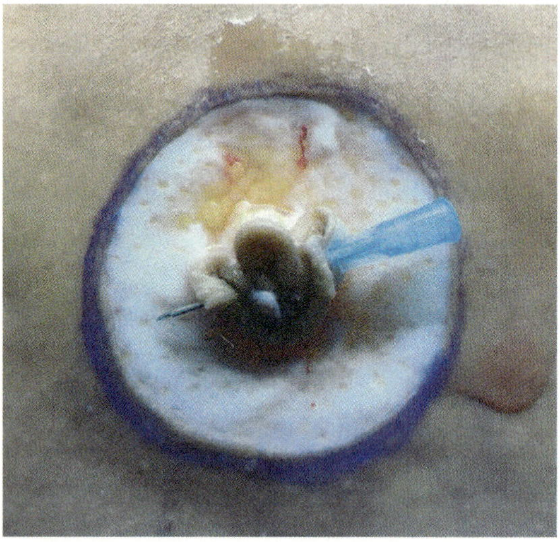

**Fig. 72.3** Needle passed through the raised flaps

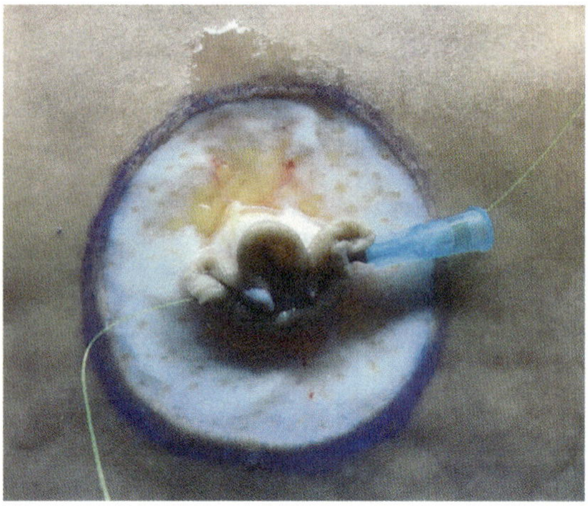

**Fig. 72.4** Suture passed through needle

also is sutured around the periphery of the new areola. Once the suturing is completed, a small incision is created in the center of the graft just large enough to permit delivery of the dermal-epidermal flap stalk through the opening. Nothing more needs to be done to the raw surface of the new nipple. The groin wound is closed. The nipple gradually contracts down over a 2- or 3-month period giving progressively more forward projection to the new nipple and wrinkling of the skin.

Once the suture on the periphery of the areola is finished, a dressing is placed over the groin graft enclosing the nipple with a similar size of

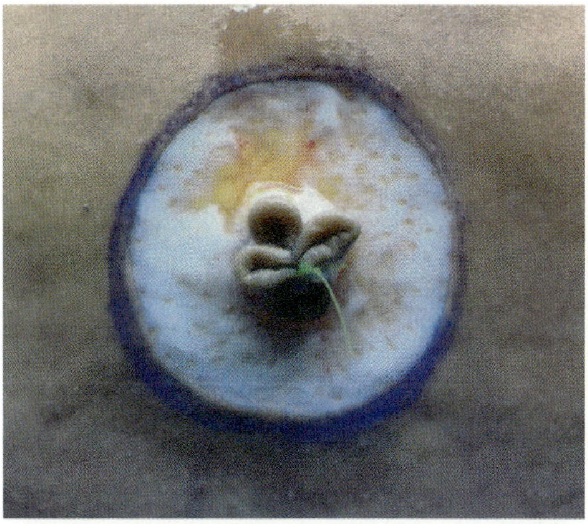

Fig. 72.5 Result after suture tied

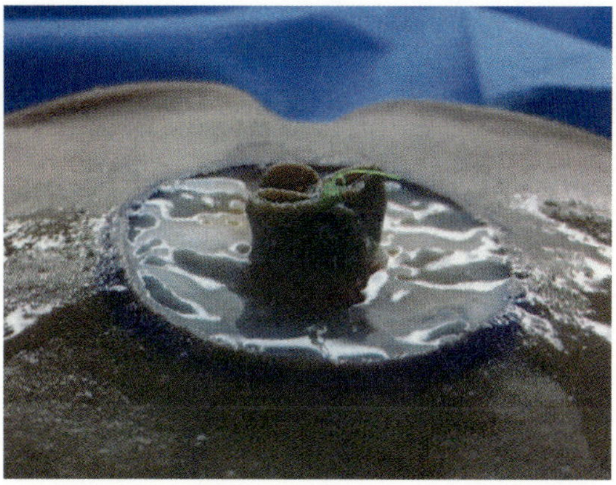

Fig. 72.6 Open areas of the flaps are sutured closed

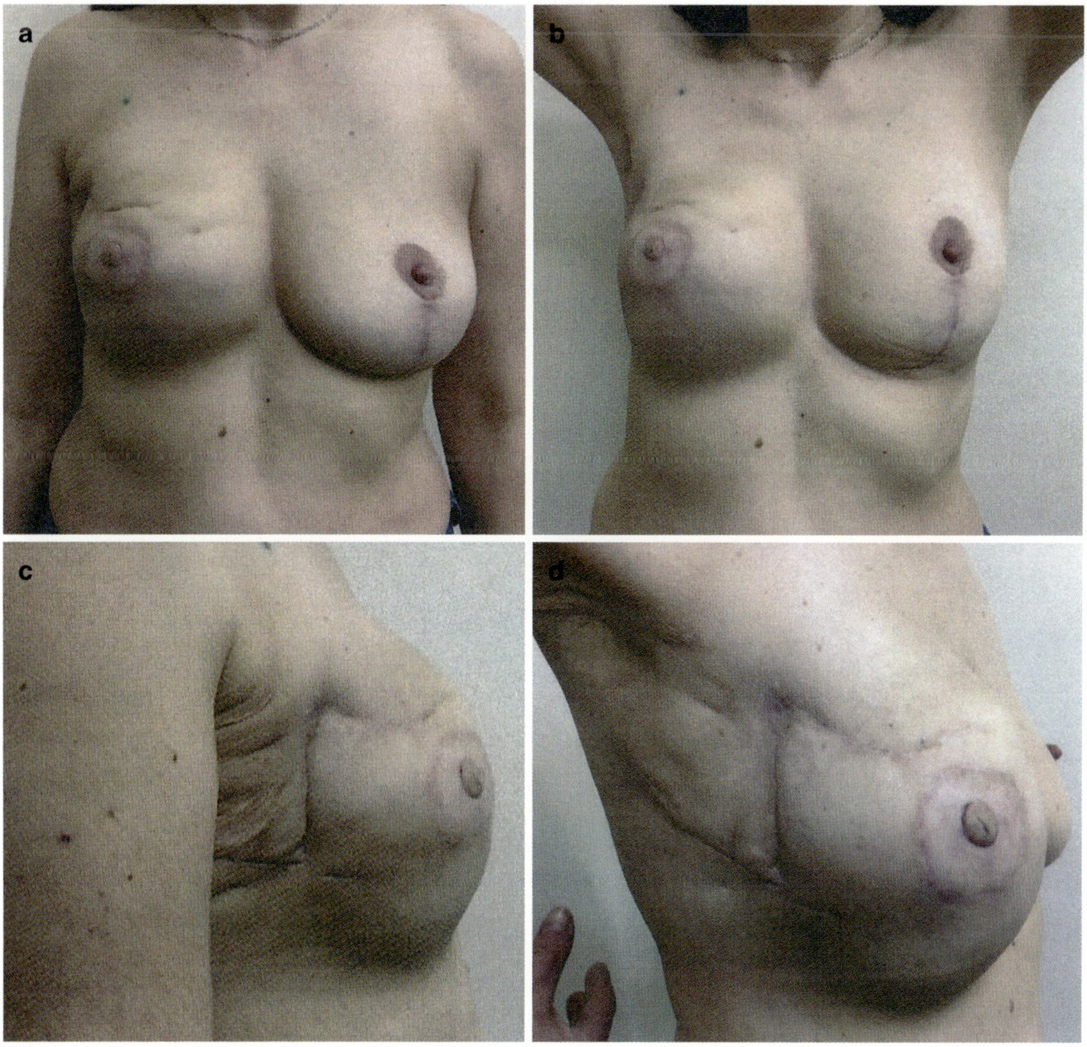


Fig. 72.7 (**a**–**d**) Postoperative result

the structures to not affect irrigation: a soft and bulky dressing is left for 7 days.

The new nipple is checked to show good definition. The projection remains and presents a satisfactory three-dimensional perception. The nipple maintains better projection with the groin graft.

If the skin is nearer to the desired color by the patient, you can place a small segment of the contralateral nipple skin. Preserving vascularization of the nipple prevents a second operation.

## References

1. Brent B, Bostwick J. Nipple-areola reconstruction with auricular tissues. Plast Reconstr Surg. 1977;69:353–61.
2. Bosch G, Ramirez M. Reconstruction of the nipple: a new technique. Plast Reconstr Surg. 1984;73:977–81.
3. Muruci D, Dantas JJ, Nogueira LR. Reconstruction of the nipple areola complex. Plast Reconstr Surg. 1978;61:558–60.
4. Hartrampf CR, Culbertson JH. A dermal-fat flap for nipple reconstruction. Plast Reconstr Surg. 1984;73:982–6.
5. Smith JW, Nelson R. Construction of the nipple with a mushroom-shaped pedicle. Plast Reconstr Surg. 1986;78(5):684–7.
6. Broadbent TR, Woolf RM, Metz PS. Restoring the mammary areola by a skin graft from the upper inner thigh. Br J Plast Surg. 1977;30:220–2.

# 3D Bioprinting in Nipple-Areola Complex Reconstruction

73

Michael P. Chae, David J. Hunter-Smith, Sean V. Murphy, and Warren Matthew Rozen

## 73.1 Introduction

Nipple-areola complex (NAC) constitutes an important landmark on a breast, and, as a result, it is not difficult to appreciate the devastation induced by the loss of NAC from breast cancer treatment and the significance of NAC reconstruction to these patients. Due to increasing population, the prevalence and incidence of breast cancer continue to rise, and one in eight women in the Unites States is expected to be diagnosed with breast cancer in their lifetime [1]. In order to achieve cure, an increasing number of women are opting for mastectomy early [2], and evidences demonstrate that postmastectomy breast reconstruction significantly improves the psychosexual well-being [3–5].

Recently, the rate of nipple-sparing mastectomy (NSM) has increased dramatically, spurred on by a perceived notion that it preserves the integrity of the body, improves cosmesis, and reduces psychological distress surrounding the loss of breasts [6–8]. Interestingly, numerous publications report minimally increased oncological risk from NSM compared to the traditional radical mastectomy or skin-sparing mastectomy (SSM) [9–13]. However, currently there is lack of a large-scale prospective data and a reliable national guideline to enable clinicians to offer appropriate type of mastectomy [8]. Encouragingly, recent studies demonstrate that SSM provides a similar rate of overall satisfaction as NSM [14, 15]. Furthermore, NSM is associated with an increased rate of nipple necrosis and loss [16, 17]. Therefore, combining SSM with subsequent NAC reconstruction would most reliably achieve complete oncological control and an aesthetically pleasing outcome [14, 18].

NAC reconstruction is generally performed 4–6 months postmastectomy, depending on the type of breast reconstruction, surgeon's experience, presence of complications, and postoperative chemotherapy or radiotherapy

M.P. Chae, M.B.B.S., B.Med.Sc. (✉)
Department of Plastic and Reconstructive Surgery, Frankston Hospital, Peninsula Health, 2 Hastings Road, Frankston, VIC 3199, Australia
e-mail: mpc25@me.com

D.J. Hunter-Smith, M.B.B.S., M.P.H., F.R.A.C.S., F.A.C.S. • W.M. Rozen, M.B.B.S., B.Med.Sc., M.D., Ph.D., F.R.A.C.S.
Department of Surgery, School of Clinical Science at Monash Health, Monash University, Level 5, E Block, Monash Medical Centre, 246 Clayton Road, Clayton, VIC 3168, Australia

Department of Plastic and Reconstructive Surgery, Frankston Hospital, Peninsula Health, 2 Hastings Road, Frankston, VIC 3199, Australia

S.V. Murphy, Ph.D.
Wake Forest Institute for Regenerative Medicine, Wake Forest University School of Medicine, Winston-Salem, NC, USA


M.A. Shiffman (ed.), *Nipple-Areolar Complex Reconstruction*,
https://doi.org/10.1007/978-3-319-60925-6_73

[19]. A number of studies have reported statistically significant improvement in psychological well-being and patient satisfaction following a NAC reconstruction [20–23]. Reconstructive options range from local flaps with tattooing and pigmented skin grafts to local flaps with autologous, allograft, or alloplastic graft augmentation [18, 24]. However, current reconstructive techniques have inconsistent long-term outcomes regarding maintenance of the neo-nipple projection, color, size, shape, and texture, leading to polarizing patient satisfaction [25]. To this effect, the novel regenerative medicine technology, three-dimensional (3D) bioprinting, which combines tissue engineering with 3D printing platform, has been touted as a potential solution. In this review, we discuss the current medical application of 3D bioprinting and its use in NAC reconstruction so far.

## 73.2 3D Bioprinting

### 73.2.1 Background

3D bioprinting describes a method of creating individualized 3D tissue constructs from traditional tissue engineering by incorporating the novel 3D printing technology, which has become more affordable and easy to use in recent times (Table 73.1) [26].

**Table 73.1** Summary of 3D bioprinting techniques

| Bioprinting techniques | Mechanism | Advantages | Disadvantages | Clinical application |
|---|---|---|---|---|
| Inkjet | Thermal | High resolution | Exposure to high heat (300°C) | Skin [111] |
| | | Low cost | | |
| | | High speed | Absolute requirement for biological material to be liquid | |
| | | Biocompatibility | | Cartilage [112] |
| | Acoustic | High resolution | Cell lysis at 15–25 kHz | |
| | | Low cost | | |
| | | High speed | Absolute requirement for biological material to be liquid | Bone [113] |
| | | Biocompatibility | | |
| Microextrusion | Pneumatic | Affordable | Lower spatial control | Aortic valve [121] |
| | | Simpler components | Low cell viability | |
| | | Viscous biologic material | Low resolution | |
| | | | Slow speed | Blood vessels [122] |
| | Mechanical | Affordable | Sophisticated components | |
| | | Superior spatial control | Low cell viability | Ovarian cancer model [123] |
| | | Viscous biologic material | Low resolution | |
| | | | Slow speed | |
| Laser-Assisted | LIFT | Compatibility with range of viscosity, resolution, and speed | Slow print speed | Skin [133] |
| | | | | Skull defect [134] |
| ITOP | Pneumatic | Microchannel formation | Limited accessibility | Mandibular bony defect [84] |
| | | Microscale nozzle | | Ear cartilage [84] |
| | | Produce well-vascularized, human-scale tissue construct | | Skeletal muscle [84] |

*LIFT* laser-induced forward transfer, *ITOP* integrated tissue organ printer

**Table 73.2** Summary of 3D-bioprinted or tissue-engineered NAC reconstructions

| Type | Company | Technique | Reference |
|---|---|---|---|
| Synthetic scaffold | N/A | Pluronic® F-127 seeded with porcine chondrocytes, secured with purse-string suture | [228] |
| Decellularized allograft scaffold | NovoThelium LLC | Decellularized donor NAC scaffold seeded with autologous nipple cells | [229] |
| 3D-bioprinted NAC graft | TeVido BioDevices LLC | Cellatier™ | [230] |
| | | 3D-bioprinted pigmented autologous skin graft overlying volume-stable adipose tissue | |

*N/A* not applicable

### 73.2.2 Tissue Engineering

Tissue engineering utilizes cells, biomaterials, and biologically active factors to produce a biological tissue that matures into functional, vascularized tissue upon implantation in vivo (Table 73.2) [27]. The cells are obtained by culturing and expanding the primary cells from a small biopsy of the desired tissue [28–33]. The biomaterial and the growth factors must provide a controlled gradient in mechanical properties and cellular signaling, respectively, for optimal cell growth in vitro [34]. Given that the maximum nutrient diffusion distance for cells to survive without vascularity is only 100–200 μm [35], manufacturing a well-vascularized, complex tissue in a clinically suitable size using conventional laboratory techniques has been challenging [27, 36]. The addition of angiogenic growth factors may be helpful [34, 37, 38], but ultimately a 3D scaffold with interconnected pores to enable vascularity is required.

Early researchers used decellularization technique, where the cellular component of a donor tissue is removed either mechanically or chemically while retaining its mechanical properties and is repopularized with desired culture cells [39]. These constructs elicit minimal host immune response [40, 41], and the donor extracellular matrix (ECM) is gradually replaced by ECM excreted by the implanted cells [42]. However, allogeneic donor tissues are rare, and autologous options may lead to potential donor site morbidity. As a result, various methods of fabricating synthetic material-based scaffolds have been described, such as 3D fiber deposition [43], particulate-leaching technique [44], and electrospinning [45]. In comparison, 3D printing can additionally produce fine-scale internal porous structures with desired complexity [46–48] that facilitate nutrient and oxygen diffusion [49–51] and the creation of patient-specific composite tissue constructs [26, 52–56].

## 73.3 3D Printing

3D printing, also known as rapid prototyping or additive manufacturing, describes a process by which a 3D construct derived from a computer-aided design (CAD) is built in a layer-by-layer fashion [57–60]. One of the major advantages of 3D printing is its convenience in building custom designs with complex geometries in comparison to the traditional manufacturing process [61–63]. 3D printing has been utilized in industrial designs for decades; however, it has only been adapted for medical application in the last decade [64].

Imaging data from routine computed tomography (CT) or magnetic resonance imaging (MRI) scans can be converted into a CAD file using a variety of 3D software programs, such as 3D Slicer (Surgical Planning Laboratory; Boston, MA, USA). The file is subsequently manufactured into 3D object using a 3D printer, such as a fused filament fabrication (FFF) printer, where a melted filament of thermoplastic material is deposited on to a build plate in a layer-by-layer fashion [65]. This technology has been applied clinically, for use in breast reconstruction (Fig. 73.1), with 3D

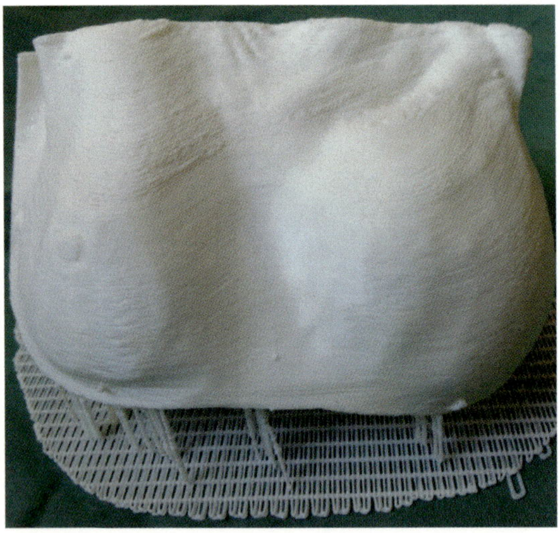

**Fig. 73.1** A 3D-printed haptic, tactile biomodel of breasts, produced from routine CT data. Printing performed using Cube 2 printer (3D Systems, Rock Hill, SC, USA) and white polylactic acid (PLA) filaments [231]. Reproduced with permission

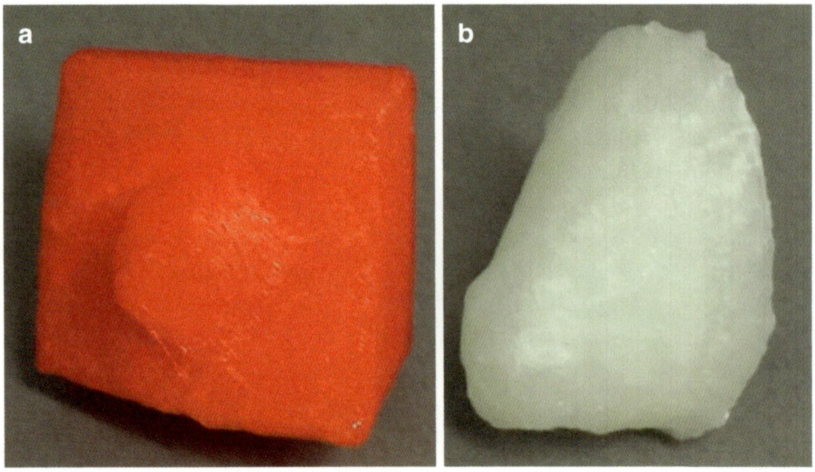


**Fig. 73.2** 3D-printed models of nipples scanned using (**a**) CT scans in supine position and (**b**) MRI scans in prone position with back extended 45 degrees. *CT* computed tomography; *MRI* magnetic resonance imaging

printing used to model breasts for volume and shape assessment. The same technology can be applied specifically to nipple and areolar reconstruction for shape and size assessment (Fig. 73.2), as a primary model and for planning.

Aided by expiration of key patents in early 2000s, FFF 3D printers have become readily available, and this technology has been adopted in 3D bioprinters.

## 73.4 3D Bioprinting Composition

A 3D bioprinter typically consists of a structural scaffold, cell carrier, and cells.

### 73.4.1 Scaffold

The scaffold provides a 3D structure to support tissue growth, mimic ECM and local microenvironment, and induce tissue formation. The external shape of the scaffold is based on the CT/MRI-derived CAD file of the desired organ or tissue, while the internal porous architecture must be based on vascularization and support oxygen diffusion gradient [66]. In addition, synthetic polymers used by 3D bioprinters can be incorporated with biologically active domains to enhance tissue regeneration in vivo [31, 67–69], such as cell-adhesion peptides [70], silk functionalized with titanium-binding peptides [71], collagen [72], and growth factors [73]. One of the most commonly used polymers for 3D-bioprinted scaffold is polycaprolactone (PCL) [74, 75]. PCL has a low melting temperature (60°C) and cools rapidly upon deposition, making it cell compatible [74]. It also has a relatively long degradation period (1.5–2 years), deeming it durable and becomes completely excreted from the body, hence, its biocompatibility [75]. One of its main disadvantages is its flexibility and inability to provide mechanical strength. To this effect, Pluronic® F-127 (BASF SE; Ludwigshafen, Germany) polymer, composed of hydrophobic polypropylene glycol and hydrophilic polyethylene glycol, can provide mechanical strength and also extrudes easily from a nozzle [76]. Furthermore, it is rapidly degradable and can be washed out immediately once printing is complete. Its main disadvantage is poor cell compatibility [77].

### 73.4.2 Cell Carrier

A cell carrier, also known as hydrogel, should protect the cells from physical stress during printing, contain appropriate cell-specific signaling cues, possess negligible cytotoxicity, and provide adequate mechanical support [78, 79]. A variety of both natural and synthetic cell carriers have been reported, such as alginate [48, 80–83], fibrin [48, 80–82, 84], gelatin [84], hyaluronic acid [84], glycerol [84], and Pluronic® F-127 Derby, 2012 #2409} [80–82]. Fibrin can provide stability to the hydrogel and enhances cell adhesion and proliferation. Hyaluronic acid and glycerol can improve uniform cell dispersion and prevent nozzle clogging.

### 73.4.3 Cells

Typically, stem cells, such as mesenchymal stem cells (MSC), are deposited by a 3D bioprinter so that the final construct can differentiate and mature inside an ex vivo or an in vivo bioreactor [85–89]. Cells can be classified into autologous or allogeneic. Despite its indisputable advantage, autologous stem cells can be difficult to culture and expand in vitro to a sufficient number for clinical application [90, 91]. This can be partly addressed by including the use of precursor and progenitor cells [92]. Furthermore, MSCs are difficult to maintain in culture and attach to 3D-printed scaffolds [93]. In contrast, allogeneic stem cells can be stored and accessed readily when needed. However, there is a risk of graft-versus-host disease and subsequent graft failure.

## 73.5 3D Bioprinting Techniques

3D bioprinting techniques can be broadly classified by their mechanism of cell deposition into inkjet [55, 94–96], microextrusion [97–99], or laser-assisted bioprinting [100–102]. Integrated tissue organ printer (ITOP) is a novel 3D bioprinting technique that simultaneously deposits cell-laden hydrogel and synthetic biodegradable polymer in microextrusion fashion using a pneumatic pressure controller [84].

### 73.5.1 Inkjet Bioprinting

Inkjet bioprinting is the earliest described technique where either thermal [96] or acoustic [103–105] forces are used to eject drops of liquid on to a scaffold. Electrically heated thermal printheads can produce localized temperature increase to 200–300°C for a short duration (2 ms) but produce only 4–10°C rise in the overall temperature [106]. Despite some studies demonstrating minimal impact on the stability of biological molecules, such as DNA [103, 104], there still remains a potential risk using thermal inkjet bioprinters to exposing cell and the tissue construct to heat and mechanical stress. Acoustic waves created by piezoelectric crystal break liquid into regular droplets [107]. Pulse, duration, and amplitude of the sound wave can be adjusted to alter the size of droplets and rate of ejection. The major disadvantage of using acoustic forces lies with the potential risk of cell damage and lysis from 15 to 25 kHz frequencies emitted by the piezoelectric crystals [108]. In summary, despite their low cost, high resolution, high speed, and biocompatibility, both thermal and acoustic inkjet bioprinting are limited by its requirement of the biological material to be in liquid form. This limitation can be potentially addressed by immediately curing the material with chemical, pH, or ultraviolet [109, 110]. However, this increases the printing time significantly and introduces chemical modifications leading to cell damage. To date, inkjet 3D bioprinters have been utilized to fabricate functional skin [111], cartilage [112], and bone [113] only in preclinical models.

### 73.5.2 Microextrusion Bioprinting

Microextrusion bioprinters are the most common and affordable bioprinters used in research [66]. In comparison to an inkjet bioprinter that extrudes liquid droplets, a microextrusion bioprinter ejects microbeads of a material, such as hydrogel, biocompatible copolymers, and cell spheroids, using pneumatic [76, 110, 114, 115] or mechanical [116, 117] dispensing systems. Pneumatic printers are built with simpler components, but mechanical dispensers provide a greater spatial control. Major advantages of microextrusion printers include their compatibility with materials with a wide range of fluid properties, such as viscosity [53], and the ability to deposit very high cell densities, such as tissue spheroids that can self-assemble directly into complex structures [118, 119]. One of the major disadvantages of microextrusion technique is its relatively low cell viability rate (40–86%) [115, 120], low print resolution, and speed [113]. To date, microextrusion technology has been used to fabricate the aortic valves [121], the blood vessels [122], and in vitro ovarian cancer model [123] in preclinical studies.

### 73.5.3 Laser-Assisted Bioprinting

Laser-assisted bioprinting (LAB) is the least commonly used technique and relies on the principle of laser-induced forward transfer (LIFT) [124, 125]. In a LIFT system, a pulsed laser beam is directed on to the laser-energy-absorbing layer (e.g., gold or titanium) over a "ribbon" containing the donor transport system. The laser induces formation of a high-pressure bubble that propels biological material containing cells forward toward a scaffold. Microscale resolution of LAB means that, in addition to cells [126], it can be used to deposit peptides [127] and DNAs [128]. One of the main advantages of LAB technology is its flexibility, as it is compatible with a wide range of viscosity, resolution (i.e., single cell per drop to $10^8$ cell per ml), and speed (i.e., 5 kHz to 1600 mm/s) [102]. Moreover, this technique has a negligible effect on cell viability and function [129–131]. A major drawback is its slow print speed due to the requirement of rapid gelation of the deposited material due to its high resolution [132]. In preclinical studies, LAB has been used to create a small cellularized skin construct [133] and a skull defect [134].

### 73.5.4 Integrated Tissue Organ Printer (ITOP)

Integrated tissue organ printer (ITOP) is an innovative bioprinting technique, developed by Kang et al., which consists of a multimaterial-dispensing printer system controlled by a custom-designed microscale nozzle motion program enabling simultaneous deposition of both cell-laden hydrogel and synthetic biodegradable polymer to deliver a human-scale tissue construct [84]. Despite its relatively high resolution, inkjet bioprinting is limited by its requirement of liquid hydrogel that results in low structural integrity and mechanical strength. Microextrusion method utilizes viscous fluid and can produce more stable 3D constructs, but the generated shear stress reduces cell viability, printing resolution, speed, and size. LAB technique requires rapid gelation of hydrogels to achieve its very high resolution, leading to low flow rates.

ITOP deposits PCL-based scaffolds in various designs that provide mechanical strength to the construct and also forms networks of microchannels that facilitate cell nutrient and oxygen diffusion. However, the bulk of mechanical stability is provided by Pluronic® F-127 hydrogel extruded from a separate nozzle that acts as an outer sacrificial support layer. The composite hydrogel system in ITOP consists of fibrinogen, gelatin, hyaluronic acid, and glycerol in disparate concentrations optimized for each target tissue. The nozzle motion program is customized based on the printing pattern and the fabrication condition (i.e., scan speed, temperature, material information, and air pressure). Once the printing is completed, thrombin is added to cross-link fibrinogen into stable fibrin, while the other hydrogels, including Pluronic® F-127, are washed out. Using 3T3 fibroblast cell model, authors demonstrate ≥95% cell viability at 6 days and persistent tissue growth at 15 days.

As a result, ITOP can manufacture well-vascularized, human-scale, complex shape, structurally stable tissue constructs. Using human amniotic fluid-derived stem cells, authors have demonstrated its application in constructing a human mandibular bony defect in vitro and successfully implanted an ITOP-printed skull defect in rodents. Using rabbit chondrocytes, authors have built a human ear-shaped cartilage and demonstrated viability at 1 month after implantation in preclinical models. Furthermore, the authors have fabricated functional 15 × 5 × 1 mm rodent skeletal muscle tissue.

## 73.6 3D-Bioprinted Medical Applications

Encouraged by its increasing accessibility and rapid improvements in the last decade, clinicians have expanded the application of 3D bioprinting to various human tissues in increasing engineering complexity: flat tissues, tubular structures, hollow viscus, and complex solid organs.

### 73.6.1 Flat Tissues

Earliest attempts in tissue engineering have been spent to regenerate flat tissue types that are predominantly populated by a single cell type, such as the integument and cornea.

#### 73.6.1.1 Integument

Tissue-engineered skin has received numerous attentions due to its potential utility in the management of severe burn injury and chronic wound healing [135]. Researchers have developed method of harvesting autologous skin cells that harvested in the operating room and either immediately "sprayed-on" the area of need [136, 137] or expanded ex vivo and then implanted in the future [138, 139]. Despite their early commercial success, wide-scale adoption of tissue-engineered skin has been limited by their cost and accessibility [140, 141]. Furthermore, future consideration for improvements may include reconstituting the skin adnexa, such as hair follicle, pigment, and secretory glands.

#### 73.6.1.2 Cornea

Cornea plays an important role in light refraction for vision via its maintenance of shape, organization of highly aligned collagen matrix, and active secretion of aqueous humor. As such, corneal damage from injury can lead to vision loss. Currently, gold standard treatment of corneal blindness is transplantation; however, there is a worldwide significant shortage of donor tissue. Fagerholm et al. have developed a tissue-engineered biosynthetic corneal implant that mimics corneal ECM and showed improved vision at 24 months [142, 143].

### 73.6.2 Tubular Structures

Tubular anatomical structures generally consist of two different cell types arranged in a circular, bilayered manner, where the inner layer lined by endothelial or epithelial cells provides a function barrier and the outer layer lined by smooth muscle or connective tissue provides structural support. Their main function is acting as a conduit for air or fluid, such as the urethra and blood vessels.

#### 73.6.2.1 Urethra

Current surgical management of urethral defects and permanent strictures caused by traumatic injury or oncological clearance likely requires complex autologous reconstructive surgery that results in significant donor site morbidity [144–146]. Raya-Rivera et al. [29] developed a tissue-engineered urethra by seeding biodegradable polyglycolic acid (PGA)/polylactic-co-glycolic acid (PLGA) scaffolds with autologous urethral muscle and epithelial cells and showed successful functional outcome in five patients at 6-year follow-up.

#### 73.6.2.2 Blood Vessels

Shin'oka et al. [147] have constructed a pulmonary artery by seeding biodegradable collagen and synthetic scaffold with autologous cells from peripheral vein biopsy and successfully transplanted in a 4-year-old girl with total right pulmonary artery occlusion at 7-month follow-up. L'Heureux et al. [148] have used a sheet of autologous fibroblasts and endothelial cells wrapped around a stainless steel cylinder to fabricate a vascular graft for ten patients requiring hemodialysis for the management of end-stage renal disease. More recently, Dahl et al. [149] have developed a vessel allograft by seeding smooth cells on a tubular PGA scaffold and then inducing it acellular by washing away cells with detergents. This method allowed the authors to store the allografts long term and showed successful implantation in preclinical animal models.

### 73.6.3 Hollow Viscus

Similar to tubular structures, hollow viscus structures, such as bladder and vagina, consist of inner and outer layers of cells for functional and structure capacity, respectively. However, hollow viscus comprises at least two cell different cell types and requires more complex scaffold design for regenerative therapy due to its wider functional parameters, higher metabolic requirements, and more intricate intracellular and inter-organ interactions [90, 150, 151].

#### 73.6.3.1 Bladder

Researchers at Wake Forest (Winston-Salem, NC, USA) have harvested and ex vivo expanded autologous urothelial and smooth cells from bladder biopsy that they have seeded on to image-derived patient-specific bladder-shaped biodegradable polymer scaffold. Their initial study in animal models [152] was successfully translated in seven patients with myelomeningocele [28].

#### 73.6.3.2 Vagina

De Filippo et al. [153] have seeded PGA/PLGA scaffolds with rabbit epithelial cells and maintained its perfusion in a bioreactor before successfully transplanting as total vaginal replacement in animal models. Clinical trials involving human participants are currently ongoing (COFEPRIS HIM87120BSO).

### 73.6.4 Complex Solid Organs

In comparison to the previous tissue types, a solid organ undoubtedly commands the highest level of complexity. Tissue engineering or 3D bioprinting a solid organ requires precise organization of multiple, disparate cell types, integration with surrounding tissues, incorporation of vascular networks, and gradients of biologically active factors [154]. As a result, despite a wide range of organs being studied in regenerative medicine, only a small number of studies have been translated to human studies. Furthermore, cells harvested from solid organs of diseased patients for ex vivo expansion and autologous implantation may also be affected by the disease; the density of stem and progenitor cells may be compromised [155]. Hence, in recent times, researchers have focused on developing targeted 3D-bioprinted solid organ regenerative solutions for specific clinical indications.

#### 73.6.4.1 Soft Tissues

Numerous regenerative efforts have been made to build the breasts, kidneys, penis, heart, liver, and functional pancreatic islets. However, currently these studies are limited to preclinical animal models, most commonly using decellularization techniques, and have not been translated in humans yet.

#### 73.6.4.2 Breast

Earlier studies where breast-shaped polymer scaffolds were implanted in animal models without cells were filled with nonspecific fibrovascular tissue due to lack of adipogenic stimulus [156, 157]. Lin et al. seeded human adipose tissue-derived mesenchymal stem cells on to synthetic polymer scaffold and successfully grew vascularized adipose tissue in animal models [158]. Similarly, Chhaya et al. seeded human umbilical cord perivascular stem cells to patient-specific 3D-printed polymer scaffolds derived from 3D laser scanning and implanted them successfully in animal models after ex vivo maturation [159]. Current limitations in wide-scale production of 3D-bioprinted breast tissue are due to the cost related to scaling up tissue culture to complex Good Manufacturing Practice (GMP)-certified laboratory [160–164] and difficulty vascularizing a clinical relevant volume of breast tissue (>75 ml) using current techniques. Introduction of ITOP this year that facilitates construction of well-vascularized large-volume tissue in breast reconstruction appears promising [84].

##### 73.6.4.3 Kidney

Lanza et al. [165] built miniature kidney structures by seeding bovine renal cells on to collagen-coated biodegradable scaffolds in animal studies. Orlando et al. [166] used decellularized porcine kidney to yield an ECM-based scaffold that was implanted in pigs showing successfully integration with native tissue.

##### 73.6.4.4 Penis

Chen et al. implanted a decellularized rabbit penis, repopulated with corpora cavernosa penile muscle and endothelial cells in animals, and demonstrated successful function outcome [167].

**Heart**

Ott et al. [168] perfused a decellularized rodent heart with endothelial cells and neonatal cardiac cells and showed successful function outcome in animal models.

##### 73.6.4.5 Liver

Baptista et al. [169] repopulated decellularized animal livers with human fetal hepatocytes and human umbilical vein endothelial cells and implanted successfully in animal models.

### 73.6.5 Pancreatic Islet Replacement

De Carlo et al. [170] were able to regenerate insulin-producing pancreatic islets in animal models by implanting decellularized rodent pancreatic scaffolds.

#### 73.6.5.1 Bones and Cartilages

Most studies aimed at regenerating bones have focused on treating mandibular defects created from traumatic injury or oncological resection [84, 171–173]. Warnke et al. reported an interesting technique where a patient-specific design, ceramic scaffold seeded with bone marrow-derived mesenchymal stem cells is implanted in patient's latissimus dorsi, so that the patient is acting as their own bioreactor [174, 175]. More evidence in large-scale randomized clinical trials remains to be seen. Similarly, efforts to construct tissue engineered [171–173, 176] or 3D bioprinted [84] have not yet been translated in prospective human trials.

## 73.7 Nipple-Areola Complex Reconstruction

### 73.7.1 Background

An ideal NAC reconstruction must achieve symmetry in nipple position, size, shape, texture, and pigmentation and additionally offer lasting projection [24]. To date, an exhaustive list of surgical techniques has been described, local flap, skin graft, nipple tattooing, local flap with autologous, allograft, or alloplastic graft augmentation.

### 73.7.2 Local Flap

First described by Berson in 1946 [177], local flaps are the most commonly used surgical technique in immediate and delayed nipple reconstruction, and unsurprisingly, an astonishing number of techniques and their modifications have been reported in the literature. The details and clinical outcomes following each approach are covered in more details in the current book and are beyond the scope of the current book chapter. Currently, two modifications of Little's skate flap [178], Anton's star flap [179], and Jones' C–V flap [180] are the most commonly used local techniques due to their reliability, easy to perform, and well described [181–187].

### 73.7.3 Skin Graft

First skin graft using pigmented skin from labia minora was described by Adams in 1949 [188]. Since then, skin graft from other hyperpigmented cutaneous locations [189] and contralateral nipple graft [190] has been reported. Similarly, detailed descriptions of these grafts are discussed elsewhere in this book. In summary, skin grafts alone have been unreliable due to fading of pigmentation with time [191] and loss of projection at 3–6 months [192].

### 73.7.4 Tattooing

In order to address loss of pigmentation with time, adjuvant tattooing by nursing practitioners or professional tattoo artists have accompanied other traditional surgical approaches [179, 181, 193–197]. Tattooing is associated with minimal complication rate (1.6%) and high patient satisfaction rate (>90%) [196, 198–202]. Recently, 3D tattooing techniques have also been described where depth is created on a 2D chest wall [203]. This work is also described in more detail elsewhere in the current book.

### 73.7.5 Local Flap with Graft Augmentation

In order to enhance and maintain adequate nipple projection, augmentation with various autologous, allograft, and alloplastic grafts to existing local flap approaches has been described.

#### 73.7.5.1 Autologous Grafts

Historically, augmentation with autologous cartilage graft has been well described due to their longevity without pedicled blood supply.

#### 73.7.5.2 Costal Cartilage

Early studies utilized costal cartilage harvested when preparing the internal mammary artery recipient site during free flap breast reconstruction for immediate NAC reconstruction and demonstrated excellent long-term projection [195]. However, this approach was associated with a relatively high rate of complication (4%), such as graft exposure and skin flap ischemia. In later studies, clinicians "banked" the cartilage graft in the abdominal wall that was used in delayed NAC reconstruction [204–208]. As a result, the authors generally reported a reduced rate of complications and reasonable long-term projection (up to 8.5 mm at 45 months).

#### 73.7.5.3 Auricular Cartilage

Using auricular cartilage graft was first described by Brent in 1977 [209]. Tanabe et al. [210] rolled the graft and wrapped inside a bilobed flap surrounded by skin graft, showing moderate success. More recently, Collis et al. [193] utilized the cartilage harvested from the posterior extension of the sharp fold in the upper conchal fossa palpable in the postauricular sulcus, which reduced scarring of the donor site and maintained nipple projection at 2 years. Later, Norton et al. [211] described a "hamburger" technique where a punch biopsy is used to harvest conchal cartilage discs and stack them. Jones et al. [212] reported in a long-term study using the stacked conchal cartilage discs only modest nipple projection at 2 years (mean of 3.3 mm), despite low complication rate. Furthermore, in general, auricular cartilage has been relatively unpopular due to potential risk of donor site morbidity.

#### 73.7.5.4 Allograft Materials

In search of a more permanent augmentative material, clinicians have investigated allograft materials, such as acellular dermal matrix (ADM) and biologic collagen cylinders.

##### Acellular Dermal Matrix (ADM)

AlloDerm (LifeCell Corp, Branchburg, NJ, USA) is a cadaveric split-thickness dermal graft with low antigenicity [213, 214] and fast host integration (7 days) [215]. Garramone et al. [198]

implanted 1.5 × 4.5 cm piece of AlloDerm in 30 NAC reconstructions and demonstrated 47–56% rate of projection at 12 months [198]. Interestingly, Rao et al. [216] used ADM as an onlay graft for areola reconstruction and demonstrated high graft take rate but did not use it to provide nipple projection.

**Biologic Collagen Cylinder**

Tierney et al. [217] reported the use of Biodesign Nipple Reconstruction Cylinder (NRC; Cook Inc., Bloomington, IN, USA) in 115 nipple reconstructions. NRC is created by rolling ECM collagen derived from porcine small intestine submucosa and adhesive glycoprotein as scaffold. The study reports low complication rate (3.5%) and modest sustained nipple projection of 3–5 mm at 6-month follow-up. It remains to be validated and demonstrated effective in a multicenter randomized clinical trial.

#### 73.7.5.5 Alloplastic Materials

Similarly, numerous inert, biocompatible alloplastic materials have been used, such as silicone rod, Artecoll injection, and artificial bones.

**Silicone Rod**

Jankau et al. report good projection from using silicone rod for augmentation in 30 NAC reconstructions [218, 219]. Interestingly, however, the study found that all ten silicone rods used in combined tissue expander and latissimus dorsi free flap reconstructions lead to overlying skin necrosis leading to material removal.

**Artecoll Injection**

Polymethyl methacrylate is an inert, nonbiodegradable poly(methyl methacrylate) microspheres suspended in a partially denatured bovine collagen, marketed as Artecoll by Artes Medical (San Diego, CA, USA) and Canderm Pharma Inc. (Saint-Laurent, Canada) [220]. Artecoll is injected subcutaneously as a delayed secondary procedure after the primary nipple reconstruction. While the bovine collagen will be degraded in 3 months and replaced by autologous collagen, the synthetic microspheres are too large for degradation by macrophages and provide nipple projection. At 9 months, the authors report a modest nipple projection (2.93 mm) but statistically significant ($P < 0.001$) improvement.

**Artificial Bone**

Ceratite (Chugai Medical Device, Tokyo, Japan) is a composite material of 20% tricalcium phosphate and 80% hydroxyapatite [221]. The material was initially developed for use in craniomaxillofacial reconstruction [222]. In 100 NAC reconstructions over 8 years, the authors report good projection in all patients from the clinician's subjective assessment and a low complication rate (5%) [221]. Radiesse™ (Bioform Inc., Franksville, WI, USA) is composed of calcium hydroxylapatite that was used in six patients with relatively modest improvements [223]. It has an added disadvantage of remaining radiopaque in mammograms and interfering with breast cancer screening [224].

## 73.8 3D-Bioprinted Nipple-Areola Complex

### 73.8.1 Background

Despite improvement in local flap techniques and availability of advanced materials, an ideal NAC reconstructive option has eluded clinicians historically. Current reconstructive techniques lead to loss of nipple projection in 40–75% overall in long term [18], ultimately result in loss of pigmentation [191], and do not have significant impact on patient satisfaction. Furthermore, there are no significant differences between various local flap designs, and large-scale studies report an overall complication rate of all current reconstructive approaches up to 10% [195, 225–227].

To this effect, 3D bioprinting can be useful, since novel 3D bioprinters like ITOP printers produce well-vascularized, sustainable, human-scale tissue constructs that integrate well with surrounding structures.

### 73.8.2 Tissue-Engineered NAC

#### 73.8.2.1 Synthetic Scaffold

In a preclinical animal study, Cao et al. [228] demonstrated the utility of seeding biocompatible Pluronic F-127 with porcine chondrocytes and implanting them into desired shape using purse-string suture technique. The authors report satisfactory nipple projection, size, and shape at 10 weeks. Interestingly, this technique has not been reinvestigated since 1998.

#### 73.8.2.2 Decellularized Allograft Scaffold

Recently, a biotechnology company, called NovoThelium LLC, has been launched based on patent-pending technology where decellularized NAC scaffold from donor tissues is seeded with patient's nipple cells obtained at mastectomy [229]. The allograft scaffold is matured in an ex vivo bioreactor before being implanted on to a thick, deepithelialized dermal base as a delayed procedure. The major advantage of utilizing decellularized allograft is the preservation of intrinsic NAC cell signaling cues that submicron level tissue architecture. However, the company does not explain the potential risk of harvesting nipple cells from patients undergoing breast cancer treatment and how oncogenic cells will be removed and controlled. Preclinical studies are underway.

## 73.9 3D-Bioprinted NAC Graft

In 2011, TeVido BioDevices LLC biotechnology company was set up to market and produce 3D-bioprinted NAC graft based on their patent-pending technique, called Cellatier™ [230]. The company aims to manufacture autologous NAC graft with pigmented skin layer, supported by volume-stable, patient-specific design adipose tissue base. Since commencement, TeVido has generated immense media attention and has secured large funds from National Science Foundation (Arlington, VA, USA) and raised crowdfunding from Indiegogo (San Francisco, CA, USA). Currently, preclinical in vitro and animal studies are underway.

**Conclusions**

Nipple-areola complex (NAC) constitutes an important landmark on a breast, and its loss due to breast cancer treatment can be devastating. Evidences demonstrate significant improvement in psychosexual well-being, and patient satisfaction can be achieved following a successful NAC reconstruction. Various reconstructive options have been reported historically. However, they are all associated with inconsistent long-term outcomes regarding maintenance of the neo-nipple projection, color, size, shape, and texture, leading to polarizing patient satisfaction rates. To this effect, novel regenerative medicine technology, three-dimensional (3D) bioprinting, which combines the conventional tissue engineering with 3D printing platform, has been touted as a potential solution. Recently, TeVido BioDevices company has begun developing an entirely 3D-printed NAC graft, but the results are currently limited to preclinical studies.

## References

1. DeSantis C, Ma J, Bryan L, Jemal A. Breast cancer statistics, 2013. CA Cancer J Clin. 2014;64:52–62.
2. Shons AR, Mosiello G. Postmastectomy breast reconstruction: current techniques. Cancer Control. 2001;8:419–26.
3. Zhong T, Hu J, Bagher S, Vo A, O'Neill AC, Butler K, Novak CB, Hofer SO, Metcalfe KA. A comparison of psychological response, body image, sexuality, and quality of life between immediate and delayed autologous tissue breast reconstruction: a prospective long-term outcome study. Plast Reconstr Surg. 2016;138:772–80.
4. Duraes EF, Durand P, Duraes LC, Orra S, Moreira-Gonzalez A, Sousa JB, Djohan RS, Zins J, Bernard S, Schwarz GS. Comparison of preoperative quality of life in breast reconstruction, breast aesthetic and non-breast plastic surgery patients: a cross-sectional study. J Plast Reconstr Aesthet Surg. 2016;69(11):1478–85.
5. Ng SK, Hare RM, Kuang RJ, Smith KM, Brown BJ, Hunter-Smith DJ. Breast reconstruction post mastectomy: patient satisfaction and decision making. Ann Plast Surg. 2016;76(6):640–4.
6. Didier F, Arnaboldi P, Gandini S, Maldifassi A, Goldhirsch A, Radice D, Minotti I, Ballardini B, Luini A, Santillo B, Rietjens M, Petit JY. Why

do women accept to undergo a nipple sparing mastectomy or to reconstruct the nipple areola complex when nipple sparing mastectomy is not possible? Breast Cancer Res Treat. 2012;132:1177–84.
7. Peled AW, Wang F, Foster RD, Alvarado M, Ewing CA, Sbitany H, Esserman LJ. Expanding the indications for total skin-sparing mastectomy: is it safe for patients with locally advanced disease? Ann Surg Oncol. 2016;23:87–91.
8. Sisco M, Kyrillos AM, Lapin BR, Wang CE, Yao KA. Trends and variation in the use of nipple-sparing mastectomy for breast cancer in the United States. Breast Cancer Res Treat. 2016;160:111–20.
9. Amanti C, Vitale V, Lombardi A, Maggi S, Bersigotti L, Lazzarin G, Nuccetelli E, Romano C, Campanella L, Cristiano L, Bartoloni A, Argento G. Importance of perforating vessels in nipple-sparing mastectomy: an anatomical description. Breast Cancer. 2015;7:179–81.
10. Shimo A, Tsugawa K, Tsuchiya S, Yoshie R, Tsuchiya K, Uejima T, Kojima Y, Shimo A, Hayami R, Nishikawa T, Yabuki Y, Kawamoto H, Sudo A, Fukuda M, Kanemaki Y, Maeda I. Oncologic outcomes and technical considerations of nipple-sparing mastectomies in breast cancer: experience of 425 cases from a single institution. Breast Cancer. 2015;23(6):851–60.
11. De La Cruz L, Moody AM, Tappy EE, Blankenship SA, Hecht EM. Overall survival, disease-free survival, local recurrence, and nipple-areolar recurrence in the setting of nipple-sparing mastectomy: a meta-analysis and systematic review. Ann Surg Oncol. 2015;22:3241–9.
12. Ou KW, Yu JC, Ho MH, Chiu WK, Ou KL, Chen TM, Chen SG. Oncological safety and outcomes of nipple-sparing mastectomy with breast reconstruction: a single-centered experience in Taiwan. Ann Plast Surg. 2015;74(Suppl 2):S127–31.
13. Adam H, Bygdeson M, de Boniface J. The oncological safety of nipple-sparing mastectomy–a Swedish matched cohort study. Eur J Surg Oncol. 2014;40:1209–15.
14. van Verschuer VM, Mureau MA, Gopie JP, Vos EL, Verhoef C, Menke-Pluijmers MB, Koppert LB. Patient satisfaction and nipple-areola sensitivity after bilateral prophylactic mastectomy and immediate implant breast reconstruction in a high breast cancer risk population: nipple-sparing mastectomy versus skin-sparing mastectomy. Ann Plast Surg. 2016;77:145–52.
15. Krajewski AC, Boughey JC, Degnim AC, Jakub JW, Jacobson SR, Hoskin TL, Hieken TJ. Expanded indications and improved outcomes for nipple-sparing mastectomy over time. Ann Surg Oncol. 2015;22:3317–23.
16. Cho JW, Yoon ES, You HJ, Kim HS, Lee BI, Park SH. Nipple-areola complex necrosis after nipple-sparing mastectomy with immediate autologous breast reconstruction. Arch Plast Surg. 2015;42:601–7.
17. Bingol UA, Cinar C. Skin necrosis in a patient with factor v leiden mutation following nipple sparing mastectomy. Plast Reconstr Surg Glob Open. 2015;3:e529.
18. Sisti A, Grimaldi L, Tassinari J, Cuomo R, Fortezza L, Bocchiotti MA, Roviello F, D'Aniello C, Nisi G. Nipple-areola complex reconstruction techniques: a literature review. Eur J Surg Oncol. 2016;42:441–65.
19. Losken A, Duggal CS, Desai KA, McCullough MC, Gruszynski M, Carlson GW. Time to completion of nipple reconstruction: what factors are involved? Ann Plast Surg. 2013;70:530–2.
20. Wellisch DK, Schain WS, Noon RB, Little JW III. The psychological contribution of nipple addition in breast reconstruction. Plast Reconstr Surg. 1987;80:699–704.
21. Delay E, Mojallal A, Vasseur C, Delaporte T. Immediate nipple reconstruction during immediate autologous latissimus breast reconstruction. Plast Reconstr Surg. 2006;118:1303–12.
22. Chattopadhyay D, Gupta S, Jash PK, Murmu MB, Gupta S. Skin sparing mastectomy with preservation of nipple areola complex and immediate breast reconstruction in patients with breast cancer: a single centre prospective study. Plast Surg Int. 2014;2014:589068.
23. Momoh AO, Colakoglu S, de Blacam C, Yueh JH, Lin SJ, Tobias AM, Lee BT. The impact of nipple reconstruction on patient satisfaction in breast reconstruction. Ann Plast Surg. 2012;69:389–93.
24. Nimboriboonporn A, Chuthapisith S. Nipple-areola complex reconstruction. Gland Surg. 2014;3:35–42.
25. Jabor MA, Shayani P, Collins DR Jr, Karas T, Cohen BE. Nipple-areola reconstruction: satisfaction and clinical determinants. Plast Reconstr Surg. 2002;110:457–63.
26. Murphy SV, Atala A. 3D bioprinting of tissues and organs. Nat Biotechnol. 2014;32:773–85.
27. Atala A, Kasper FK, Mikos AG. Engineering complex tissues. Sci Transl Med. 2012;4:160rv112.
28. Atala A, Bauer SB, Soker S, Yoo JJ, Retik AB. Tissue-engineered autologous bladders for patients needing cystoplasty. Lancet. 2006;367:1241–6.
29. Raya-Rivera A, Esquiliano DR, Yoo JJ, Lopez-Bayghen E, Soker S, Atala A. Tissue-engineered autologous urethras for patients who need reconstruction: an observational study. Lancet. 2011;377:1175–82.
30. Raya-Rivera AM, Esquiliano D, Fierro-Pastrana R, López-Bayghen E, Valencia P, Ordorica-Flores R, Soker S, Yoo JJ, Atala A. Tissue-engineered autologous vaginal organs in patients: a pilot cohort study. Lancet. 2014;384:329–36.
31. Amini AR, Laurencin CT, Nukavarapu SP. Bone tissue engineering: recent advances and challenges. Crit Rev. Biomed Eng. 2012;40:363–408.
32. Bichara DA, O'Sullivan NA, Pomerantseva I, Zhao X, Sundback CA, Vacanti JP, Randolph MA. The tissue-engineered auricle: past, present, and future. Tissue Eng Part B Rev. 2012;18:51–61.

33. Ostrovidov S, Hosseini V, Ahadian S, Fujie T, Parthiban SP, Ramalingam M, Bae H, Kaji H, Khademhosseini A. Skeletal muscle tissue engineering: methods to form skeletal myotubes and their applications. Tissue Eng Part B Rev. 2014;20:403–36.
34. Lee YB, Polio S, Lee W, Dai G, Menon L, Carroll RS, Yoo SS. Bio-printing of collagen and VEGF-releasing fibrin gel scaffolds for neural stem cell culture. Exp Neurol. 2010;223:645–52.
35. Jain RK, Au P, Tam J, Duda DG, Fukumura D. Engineering vascularized tissue. Nat Biotechnol. 2005;23:821–3.
36. Mikos AG, Herring SW, Ochareon P, Elisseeff J, Lu HH, Kandel R, Schoen FJ, Toner M, Mooney D, Atala A, Van Dyke ME, Kaplan D, Vunjak-Novakovic G. Engineering complex tissues. Tissue Eng. 2006;12:3307–39.
37. Lee W, Debasitis JC, Lee VK, Lee JH, Fischer K, Edminster K, Park JK, Yoo SS. Multi-layered culture of human skin fibroblasts and keratinocytes through three-dimensional freeform fabrication. Biomaterials. 2009;30:1587–95.
38. Boland T, Xu T, Damon B, Cui X. Application of inkjet printing to tissue engineering. Biotechnol J. 2006;1:910–7.
39. Dahms SE, Piechota HJ, Dahiya R, Lue TF, Tanagho EA. Composition and biomechanical properties of the bladder acellular matrix graft: comparative analysis in rat, pig and human. Br J Urol. 1998;82:411–9.
40. Chen F, Yoo JJ, Atala A. Acellular collagen matrix as a possible "off the shelf" biomaterial for urethral repair. Urology. 1999;54:407–10.
41. Probst M, Dahiya R, Carrier S, Tanagho EA. Reproduction of functional smooth muscle tissue and partial bladder replacement. Br J Urol. 1997;79:505–15.
42. Brown BN, Valentin JE, Stewart-Akers AM, McCabe GP, Badylak SF. Macrophage phenotype and remodeling outcomes in response to biologic scaffolds with and without a cellular component. Biomaterials. 2009;30:1482–91.
43. Moroni L, de Wijn JR, van Blitterswijk CA. 3D fiber-deposited scaffolds for tissue engineering: influence of pores geometry and architecture on dynamic mechanical properties. Biomaterials. 2006;27:974–85.
44. Kretlow JD, Mikos AG. Founder's award to Antonios G. Mikos, ph.D., 2011 society for biomaterials annual meeting and exposition, Orlando, Florida, April 13–16, 2011: bones to biomaterials and back again–20 years of taking cues from nature to engineer synthetic polymer scaffolds. J Biomed Mater Res A. 2011;98:323–31.
45. Tan JY, Chua CK, Leong KF. Fabrication of channeled scaffolds with ordered array of micro-pores through microsphere leaching and indirect rapid prototyping technique. Biomed Microdevices. 2013;15:83–96.
46. Hutmacher DW. Scaffolds in tissue engineering bone and cartilage. Biomaterials. 2000;21:2529–43.
47. Hollister SJ. Porous scaffold design for tissue engineering. Nat Mater. 2005;4:518–24.
48. Derby B. Printing and prototyping of tissues and scaffolds. Science. 2012;338:921–6.
49. Cabodi M, Choi NW, Gleghorn JP, Lee CS, Bonassar LJ, Stroock AD. A microfluidic biomaterial. J Am Chem Soc. 2005;127:13788–9.
50. Ling Y, Rubin J, Deng Y, Huang C, Demirci U, Karp JM, Khademhosseini A. A cell-laden microfluidic hydrogel. Lab Chip. 2007;7:756–62.
51. Stachowiak AN, Bershteyn A, Tzatzalos E, Irvine DJ. Bioactive hydrogels with an ordered cellular structure combine interconnected macroporosity and robust mechanical properties. Adv Mater. 2005;17:399–403.
52. Mironov V, Visconti RP, Kasyanov V, Forgacs G, Drake CJ, Markwald RR. Organ printing: tissue spheroids as building blocks. Biomaterials. 2009;30:2164–74.
53. Jones N. Science in three dimensions: the print revolution. Nature. 2012;487:22–3.
54. Ferris CJ, Gilmore KG, Wallace GG, In het Panhuis M. Biofabrication: an overview of the approaches used for printing of living cells. Appl Microbiol Biotechnol. 2013;97:4243–58.
55. Xu T, Zhao W, Zhu JM, Albanna MZ, Yoo JJ, Atala A. Complex heterogeneous tissue constructs containing multiple cell types prepared by inkjet printing technology. Biomaterials. 2013;34:130–9.
56. Durmus NG, Tasoglu S, Demirci U. Bioprinting: functional droplet networks. Nat Mater. 2013;12:478–9.
57. Chae MP, Rozen WM, McMenamin PG, Findlay MW, Spychal RT, Hunter-Smith DJ. Emerging applications of bedside 3D printing in plastic surgery. Front Surg. 2015;2:25.
58. Chae MP, Hunter-Smith DJ, Rozen WM. Image-guided 3D-printing and haptic modeling in plastic surgery. In: Saba L, Rozen WM, Alonso-Burgos A, Ribuffo D, editors. Imaging in plastic surgery. London, UK: CRC Taylor and Francis Press; 2014.
59. Gerstle TL, Ibrahim AM, Kim PS, Lee BT, Lin SJ. A plastic surgery application in evolution: three-dimensional printing. Plast Reconstr Surg. 2014;133:446–51.
60. Goiato MC, Santos MR, Pesqueira AA, Moreno A, dos Santos DM, Haddad MF. Prototyping for surgical and prosthetic treatment. J Craniofac Surg. 2011;22:914–7.
61. Levy GN, Schindel R, Kruth JP. Rapid manufacturing and rapid tooling with layer manufacturing (LM) technologies, state of the art and future perspectives. CIRP Ann-Manuf Techn. 2003;52:589–609.
62. Sealy W. Additive manufacturing as a disruptive technology: how to avoid the pitfall. Am J Eng Technol Res. 2011;11:86–93.
63. Hoy MB. 3D printing: making things at the library. Med Ref Serv Q. 2013;32:93–9.
64. Klein GT, Lu Y, Wang MY. 3D printing and neurosurgery--ready for prime time? World Neurosurg. 2013;80:233–5.

65. Crump SS. Apparatus and method for creating three-dimensional objects. 1992; US Patent No. 5,121,329: June 9.
66. Peltola SM, Melchels FP, Grijpma DW, Kellomaki M. A review of rapid prototyping techniques for tissue engineering purposes. Ann Med. 2008;40:268–80.
67. Fong EL, Watson BM, Kasper FK, Mikos AG. Building bridges: leveraging interdisciplinary collaborations in the development of biomaterials to meet clinical needs. Adv Mater. 2012;24:4995–5013.
68. Lu L, Zhu X, Valenzuela RG, Currier BL, Yaszemski MJ. Biodegradable polymer scaffolds for cartilage tissue engineering. Clin Orthop Relat Res. 2001;(391 Suppl):S251–70.
69. Butler DL, Goldstein SA, Guldberg RE, Guo XE, Kamm R, Laurencin CT, McIntire LV, Mow VC, Nerem RM, Sah RL, Soslowsky LJ, Spilker RL, Tranquillo RT. The impact of biomechanics in tissue engineering and regenerative medicine. Tissue Eng Part B Rev. 2009;15:477–84.
70. Silva NA, Cooke MJ, Tam RY, Sousa N, Salgado AJ, Reis RL, Shoichet MS. The effects of peptide modified gellan gum and olfactory ensheathing glia cells on neural stem/progenitor cell fate. Biomaterials. 2012;33:6345–54.
71. Vidal G, Blanchi T, Mieszawska AJ, Calabrese R, Rossi C, Vigneron P, Duval JL, Kaplan DL, Egles C. Enhanced cellular adhesion on titanium by silk functionalized with titanium binding and RGD peptides. Acta Biomater. 2013;9:4935–43.
72. Engelhardt EM, Micol LA, Houis S, Wurm FM, Hilborn J, Hubbell JA, Frey P. A collagen-poly(lactic acid-co-varepsilon-caprolactone) hybrid scaffold for bladder tissue regeneration. Biomaterials. 2011;32:3969–76.
73. Phipps MC, Xu Y, Bellis SL. Delivery of platelet-derived growth factor as a chemotactic factor for mesenchymal stem cells by bone-mimetic electrospun scaffolds. PLoS One. 2012;7:e40831.
74. Serrano MC, Pagan R, Vallet-Regi M, Peña J, Rámila A, Izquierdo I, Portolés MT. In vitro biocompatibility assessment of poly(epsilon-caprolactone) films using L929 mouse fibroblasts. Biomaterials. 2004;25:5603–11.
75. Sun H, Mei L, Song C, Cui X, Wang P. The in vivo degradation, absorption and excretion of PCL-based implant. Biomaterials. 2006;27:1735–40.
76. Chang CC, Boland ED, Williams SK, Hoying JB. Direct-write bioprinting three-dimensional biohybrid systems for future regenerative therapies. J Biomed Mater Res B Appl Biomater. 2011;98:160–70.
77. Lippens E, Swennen I, Girones J, Declercq H, Vertenten G, Vlaminck L, Gasthuys F, Schacht E, Cornelissen R. Cell survival and proliferation after encapsulation in a chemically modified Pluronic(R) F127 hydrogel. J Biomater Appl. 2013;27:828–39.
78. Schuurman W, Khristov V, Pot MW, van Weere PR, Dhert WJ, Malda J. Bioprinting of hybrid tissue constructs with tailorable mechanical properties. Biofabrication. 2011;3:021001.
79. Shim JH, Lee JS, Kim JY, Cho DW. Bioprinting of a mechanically enhanced three-dimensional dual cell-laden construct for osteochondral tissue engineering using a multi-head tissue/organ building system. J Micromech Microeng. 2012;22:085014.
80. Fedorovich NE, De Wijn JR, Verbout AJ, Alblas J, Dhert WJ. Three-dimensional fiber deposition of cell-laden, viable, patterned constructs for bone tissue printing. Tissue Eng Part A. 2008;14:127–33.
81. Jakab K, Neagu A, Mironov V, Markwald RR, Forgacs G. Engineering biological structures of prescribed shape using self-assembling multicellular systems. Proc Natl Acad Sci U S A. 2004;101:2864–9.
82. Landers R, Hubner U, Schmelzeisen R, Mulhaupt R. Rapid prototyping of scaffolds derived from thermoreversible hydrogels and tailored for applications in tissue engineering. Biomaterials. 2002;23:4437–47.
83. Joddar B, Garcia E, Casas A, Stewart CM. Development of functionalized multi-walled carbon-nanotube-based alginate hydrogels for enabling biomimetic technologies. Sci Rep. 2016;6:32456.
84. Kang HW, Lee SJ, Ko IK, Kengla C, Yoo JJ, Atala A. A 3D bioprinting system to produce human-scale tissue constructs with structural integrity. Nat Biotechnol. 2016;34:312–9.
85. Brivanlou AH, Gage FH, Jaenisch R, Jessell T, Melton D, Rossant J. Stem cells. Setting standards for human embryonic stem cells. Science. 2003;300:913–6.
86. Condic ML, Rao M. Regulatory issues for personalized pluripotent cells. Stem Cells. 2008;26:2753–8.
87. Hochedlinger K, Jaenisch R. Nuclear transplantation, embryonic stem cells, and the potential for cell therapy. N Engl J Med. 2003;349:275–86.
88. Bae H, Puranik AS, Gauvin R, Edalat F, Carrillo-Conde B, Peppas NA, Khademhosseini A. Building vascular networks. Sci Transl Med. 2012;4:160ps123.
89. Lovett M, Lee K, Edwards A, Kaplan DL. Vascularization strategies for tissue engineering. Tissue Eng Part B Rev. 2009;15:353–70.
90. Cilento BG, Freeman MR, Schneck FX, Retik AB, Atala A. Phenotypic and cytogenetic characterization of human bladder urothelia expanded in vitro. J Urol. 1994;152:665–70.
91. Zhang YY, Ludwikowski B, Hurst R, Frey P. Expansion and long-term culture of differentiated normal rat urothelial cells in vitro. In Vitro Cell Dev Biol Anim. 2001;37:419–29.
92. Caplan AI, Correa D. The MSC: an injury drugstore. Cell Stem Cell. 2011;9:11–5.
93. Lam MT, Longaker MT. Comparison of several attachment methods for human iPS, embryonic and adipose-derived stem cells for tissue engineering. J Tissue Eng Regen Med. 2012;6(Suppl 3):s80–6.
94. Klebe RJ. Cytoscribing: a method for micropositioning cells and the construction of two- and three-dimensional synthetic tissues. Exp Cell Res. 1988;179:362–73.

95. Xu T, Jin J, Gregory C, Hickman JJ, Boland T. Inkjet printing of viable mammalian cells. Biomaterials. 2005;26:93–9.
96. Cui X, Boland T, D'Lima DD, Lotz MK. Thermal inkjet printing in tissue engineering and regenerative medicine. Recent Pat Drug Deliv Form. 2012;6:149–55.
97. Cohen DL, Malone E, Lipson H, Bonassar LJ. Direct freeform fabrication of seeded hydrogels in arbitrary geometries. Tissue Eng. 2006;12:1325–35.
98. Iwami K, Noda T, Ishida K, Morishima K, Nakamura M, Umeda N. Bio rapid prototyping by extruding/aspirating/refilling thermoreversible hydrogel. Biofabrication. 2010;2:014108.
99. Shor L, Guceri S, Chang R, Gordon J, Kang Q, Hartsock L, An Y, Sun W. Precision extruding deposition (PED) fabrication of polycaprolactone (PCL) scaffolds for bone tissue engineering. Biofabrication. 2009;1:015003.
100. Barron JA, Wu P, Ladouceur HD, Ringeisen BR. Biological laser printing: a novel technique for creating heterogeneous 3-dimensional cell patterns. Biomed Microdevices. 2004;6:139–47.
101. Guillemot F, Souquet A, Catros S, Guillotin B, Lopez J, Faucon M, Pippenger B, Bareille R, Rémy M, Bellance S, Chabassier P, Fricain JC, Amédée J. High-throughput laser printing of cells and biomaterials for tissue engineering. Acta Biomater. 2010;6:2494–500.
102. Guillotin B, Souquet A, Catros S, Duocastella M, Pippenger B, Bellance S, Bareille R, Rémy M, Bordenave L, Amédée J, Guillemot F. Laser assisted bioprinting of engineered tissue with high cell density and microscale organization. Biomaterials. 2010;31:7250–6.
103. Okamoto T, Suzuki T, Yamamoto N. Microarray fabrication with covalent attachment of DNA using bubble jet technology. Nat Biotechnol. 2000;18:438–41.
104. Goldmann T, Gonzalez JS. DNA-printing: utilization of a standard inkjet printer for the transfer of nucleic acids to solid supports. J Biochem Biophys Methods. 2000;42:105–10.
105. Xu T, Kincaid H, Atala A, Yoo JJ. High-throughput production of single-cell microparticles using an inkjet printing technology. J Manuf Sci Eng. 2008;130:021017.
106. Cui X, Dean D, Ruggeri ZM, Boland T. Cell damage evaluation of thermal inkjet printed Chinese hamster ovary cells. Biotechnol Bioeng. 2010;106:963–9.
107. Tekin E, Smith PJ, Schubert US. Inkjet printing as a deposition and patterning tool for polymers and inorganic particles. Soft Matter. 2008;4:703–13.
108. Tasoglu S, Demirci U. Bioprinting for stem cell research. Trends Biotechnol. 2013;31:10–9.
109. Murphy SV, Skardal A, Atala A. Evaluation of hydrogels for bio-printing applications. J Biomed Mater Res A. 2013;101:272–84.
110. Khalil S, Sun W. Biopolymer deposition for freeform fabrication of hydrogel tissue constructs. Mater Sci Eng C. 2007;27:469–78.
111. Skardal A, Mack D, Kapetanovic E, Atala A, Jackson JD, Yoo J, Soker S. Bioprinted amniotic fluid-derived stem cells accelerate healing of large skin wounds. Stem Cells Transl Med. 2012;1:792–802.
112. Cui X, Breitenkamp K, Finn MG, Lotz M, D'Lima DD. Direct human cartilage repair using three-dimensional bioprinting technology. Tissue Eng Part A. 2012;18:1304–12.
113. De Coppi P, Bartsch G Jr, Siddiqui MM, Xu T, Santos CC, Perin L, Mostoslavsky G, Serre AC, Snyder EY, Yoo JJ, Furth ME, Soker S, Atala A. Isolation of amniotic stem cell lines with potential for therapy. Nat Biotechnol. 2007;25:100–6.
114. Fedorovich NE, Swennen I, Girones J, Moroni L, van Blitterswijk CA, Schacht E, Alblas J, Dhert WJ. Evaluation of photocrosslinked Lutrol hydrogel for tissue printing applications. Biomacromolecules. 2009;10:1689–96.
115. Chang R, Nam J, Sun W. Effects of dispensing pressure and nozzle diameter on cell survival from solid freeform fabrication-based direct cell writing. Tissue Eng Part A. 2008;14:41–8.
116. Jakab K, Damon B, Neagu A, Kachurin A, Forgacs G. Three-dimensional tissue constructs built by bioprinting. Biorheology. 2006;43:509–13.
117. Visser J, Peters B, Burger TJ, Boomstra J, Dhert WJ, Melchels FP, Malda J. Biofabrication of multimaterial anatomically shaped tissue constructs. Biofabrication. 2013;5:035007.
118. Marga F, Jakab K, Khatiwala C, Shepherd B, Dorfman S, Hubbard B, Colbert S, Gabor F. Toward engineering functional organ modules by additive manufacturing. Biofabrication. 2012;4:022001.
119. Mironov V, Kasyanov V, Markwald RR. Organ printing: from bioprinter to organ biofabrication line. Curr Opin Biotechnol. 2011;22:667–73.
120. Smith CM, Stone AL, Parkhill RL, Stewart RL, Simpkins MW, Kachurin AM, Warren WL, Williams SK. Three-dimensional bioassembly tool for generating viable tissue-engineered constructs. Tissue Eng. 2004;10:1566–76.
121. Duan B, Hockaday LA, Kang KH, Butcher JT III. Bioprinting of heterogeneous aortic valve conduits with alginate/gelatin hydrogels. J Biomed Mater Res A. 2013;101:1255–64.
122. Norotte C, Marga FS, Niklason LE, Forgacs G. Scaffold-free vascular tissue engineering using bioprinting. Biomaterials. 2009;30:5910–7.
123. Xu F, Celli J, Rizvi I, Moon S, Hasan T, Demirci U. A three-dimensional in vitro ovarian cancer coculture model using a high-throughput cell patterning platform. Biotechnol J. 2011;6:204–12.
124. Bohandy J, Kim B, Adrian F. Metal deposition from a supported metal film using an excimer laser. J Appl Phys. 1986;60:1538–9.
125. Barron JA, Ringeisen BR, Kim H, Spargo BJ, Chrisey DB. Application of laser printing to mammalian cells. Thin Solid Films. 2004;453:383–7.
126. Ringeisen BR, Kim H, Barron JA, Krizman DB, Chrisey DB, Jackman S, Auyeung RY, Spargo

BJ. Laser printing of pluripotent embryonal carcinoma cells. Tissue Eng. 2004;10:483–91.
127. Chrisey DB. Materials processing: the power of direct writing. Science. 2000;289:879–81.
128. Colina M, Serra P, Fernandez-Pradas JM, Sevilla L, Morenza JL. DNA deposition through laser induced forward transfer. Biosens Bioelectron. 2005;20:1638–42.
129. Hopp B, Smausz T, Kresz N, Barna N, Bor Z, Kolozsvári L, Chrisey DB, Szabó A, Nógrádi A. Survival and proliferative ability of various living cell types after laser-induced forward transfer. Tissue Eng. 2005;11:1817–23.
130. Gruene M, Deiwick A, Koch L, Schlie S, Unger C, Hofmann N, Bernemann I, Glasmacher B, Chichkov B. Laser printing of stem cells for biofabrication of scaffold-free autologous grafts. Tissue Eng Part C Methods. 2011;17:79–87.
131. Koch L, Kuhn S, Sorg H, Gruene M, Schlie S, Gaebel R, Polchow B, Reimers K, Stoelting S, Ma N, Vogt PM, Steinhoff G, Chichkov B. Laser printing of skin cells and human stem cells. Tissue Eng Part C Methods. 2010;16:847–54.
132. Guillotin B, Guillemot F. Cell patterning technologies for organotypic tissue fabrication. Trends Biotechnol. 2011;29:183–90.
133. Michael S, Sorg H, Peck CT, Koch L, Deiwick A, Chichkov B, Vogt PM, Reimers K. Tissue engineered skin substitutes created by laser-assisted bioprinting form skin-like structures in the dorsal skin fold chamber in mice. PLoS One. 2013;8:e57741.
134. Keriquel V, Guillemot F, Arnault I, Guillotin B, Miraux S, Amédée J, Fricain JC, Catros S. In vivo bioprinting for computer- and robotic-assisted medical intervention: preliminary study in mice. Biofabrication. 2010;2:014101.
135. O'Connor NE, Mulliken JB, Banks-Schlegel S, Kehinde O, Green H. Grafting of burns with cultured epithelium prepared from autologous epidermal cells. Lancet. 1981;1:75–8.
136. Gerlach JC, Johnen C, Ottomann C, Bräutigam K, Plettig J, Belfekroun C, Münch S, Hartmann BV. Method for autologous single skin cell isolation for regenerative cell spray transplantation with non-cultured cells. Int J Artif Organs. 2011;34:271–9.
137. Wood FM, Giles N, Stevenson A, Rea S, Fear M. Characterisation of the cell suspension harvested from the dermal epidermal junction using a ReCell(R) kit. Burns. 2012;38:44–51.
138. Carsin H, Ainaud P, Le Bever H, et al. Cultured epithelial autografts in extensive burn coverage of severely traumatized patients: a five year single-center experience with 30 patients. Burns. 2000;26:379–87.
139. Centanni JM, Straseski JA, Wicks A, Hank JA, Rasmussen CA, Lokuta MA, Schurr MJ, Foster KN, Faucher LD, Caruso DM, Comer AR, Allen-Hoffmann BL. StrataGraft skin substitute is well-tolerated and is not acutely immunogenic in patients with traumatic wounds: results from a prospective, randomized, controlled dose escalation trial. Ann Surg. 2011;253:672–83.
140. Bottcher-Haberzeth S, Biedermann T, Reichmann E. Tissue engineering of skin. Burns. 2010;36:450–60.
141. Langer A, Rogowski W. Systematic review of economic evaluations of human cell-derived wound care products for the treatment of venous leg and diabetic foot ulcers. BMC Health Serv Res. 2009;9:115.
142. Fagerholm P, Lagali NS, Merrett K, Jackson WB, Munger R, Liu Y, Polarek JW, Söderqvist M, Griffith M. A biosynthetic alternative to human donor tissue for inducing corneal regeneration: 24-month follow-up of a phase 1 clinical study. Sci Transl Med. 2010;2:46ra61.
143. Fagerholm P, Lagali NS, Carlsson DJ, Merrett K, Griffith M. Corneal regeneration following implantation of a biomimetic tissue-engineered substitute. Clin Transl Sci. 2009;2:162–4.
144. Palmer DA, Marcello PW, Zinman LN, Vanni AJ. Urethral reconstruction with rectal mucosa graft onlay: a novel, minimally invasive technique. J Urol. 2016;196:782–6.
145. Lv X, Xu YM, Xie H, Feng C, Zhang J. The selection of procedures in one-stage urethroplasty for treatment of coexisting urethral strictures in anterior and posterior urethra. Urology. 2016;93:197–202.
146. Bayramicli M, Akdeniz ZD. Urethra reconstruction with lateral pectoral flap in female-to-male transsexual patients. J Plast Reconstr Aesthet Surg. 2016;69(11):1558–60.
147. Shin'oka T, Imai Y, Ikada Y. Transplantation of a tissue-engineered pulmonary artery. N Engl J Med. 2001;344:532–3.
148. L'Heureux N, McAllister TN, de la Fuente LM. Tissue-engineered blood vessel for adult arterial revascularization. N Engl J Med. 2007;357:1451–3.
149. Dahl SL, Kypson AP, Lawson JH, et al. Readily available tissue-engineered vascular grafts. Sci Transl Med. 2011;3:68ra69.
150. Scriven SD, Booth C, Thomas DF, Trejdosiewicz LK, Southgate J. Reconstitution of human urothelium from monolayer cultures. J Urol. 1997;158:1147–52.
151. Soler R, Fullhase C, Atala A. Regenerative medicine strategies for treatment of neurogenic bladder. Therapy. 2009;6:177–84.
152. Oberpenning F, Meng J, Yoo JJ, Atala A. De novo reconstitution of a functional mammalian urinary bladder by tissue engineering. Nat Biotechnol. 1999;17:149–55.
153. De Filippo RE, Bishop CE, Filho LF, Yoo JJ, Atala A. Tissue engineering a complete vaginal replacement from a small biopsy of autologous tissue. Transplantation. 2008;86:208–14.
154. Pashuck ET, Stevens MM. Designing regenerative biomaterial therapies for the clinic. Sci Transl Med. 2012;4:160sr164.
155. Cuomo AV, Virk M, Petrigliano F, Morgan EF, Lieberman JR. Mesenchymal stem cell concentration and bone repair: potential pitfalls from bench to bedside. J Bone Joint Surg Am. 2009;91:1073–83.

156. Lokmic Z, Thomas JL, Morrison WA, Thompson EW, Mitchell GM. An endogenously deposited fibrin scaffold determines construct size in the surgically created arteriovenous loop chamber model of tissue engineering. J Vasc Surg. 2008;48:974–85.
157. Findlay MW, Dolderer JH, Trost N, Craft RO, Cao Y, Cooper-White J, Stevens G, Morrison WA. Tissue-engineered breast reconstruction: bridging the gap toward large-volume tissue engineering in humans. Plast Reconstr Surg. 2011;128:1206–15.
158. Lin SD, Wang KH, Kao AP. Engineered adipose tissue of predefined shape and dimensions from human adipose-derived mesenchymal stem cells. Tissue Eng Part A. 2008;14:571–81.
159. Chhaya MP, Melchels FP, Holzapfel BM, Baldwin JG, Hutmacher DW. Sustained regeneration of high-volume adipose tissue for breast reconstruction using computer aided design and biomanufacturing. Biomaterials. 2015;52:551–60.
160. Reichert JC, Cipitria A, Epari DR, Saifzadeh S, Krishnakanth P, Berner A, Woodruff MA, Schell H, Mehta M, Schuetz MA, Duda GN, Hutmacher DW. A tissue engineering solution for segmental defect regeneration in load-bearing long bones. Sci Transl Med. 2012;4:141ra193.
161. Rohner D, Hutmacher DW, Cheng TK, Oberholzer M, Hammer B. In vivo efficacy of bone-marrow-coated polycaprolactone scaffolds for the reconstruction of orbital defects in the pig. J Biomed Mater Res B Appl Biomater. 2003;66:574–80.
162. Schantz JT, Lim TC, Ning C, et al. Cranioplasty after trephination using a novel biodegradable burr hole cover: technical case report. Neurosurgery. 2006;58:ONS-E176.
163. Rai B, Oest ME, Dupont KM, Ho KH, Teoh SH, Guldberg RE. Combination of platelet-rich plasma with polycaprolactone-tricalcium phosphate scaffolds for segmental bone defect repair. J Biomed Mater Res A. 2007;81:888–99.
164. Stevens MM, Marini RP, Schaefer D, Aronson J, Langer R, Shastri VP. In vivo engineering of organs: the bone bioreactor. Proc Natl Acad Sci U S A. 2005;102:11450–5.
165. Lanza RP, Chung HY, Yoo JJ, Wettstein PJ, Blackwell C, Borson N, Hofmeister E, Schuch G, Soker S, Moraes CT, West MD, Atala A. Generation of histocompatible tissues using nuclear transplantation. Nat Biotechnol. 2002;20:689–96.
166. Orlando G, Farney AC, Iskandar S, Mirmalek-Sani SH, Sullivan DC, Moran E, AbouShwareb T, De Coppi P, Wood KJ, Stratta RJ, Atala A, Yoo JJ, Soker S. Production and implantation of renal extracellular matrix scaffolds from porcine kidneys as a platform for renal bioengineering investigations. Ann Surg. 2012;256:363–70.
167. Chen KL, Eberli D, Yoo JJ, Atala A. Bioengineered corporal tissue for structural and functional restoration of the penis. Proc Natl Acad Sci U S A. 2010;107:3346–50.
168. Ott HC, Matthiesen TS, Goh SK, Black LD, Kren SM, Netoff TI, Taylor DA. Perfusion-decellularized matrix: using nature's platform to engineer a bioartificial heart. Nat Med. 2008;14:213–21.
169. Baptista PM, Siddiqui MM, Lozier G, Rodriguez SR, Atal A, Soker S. The use of whole organ decellularization for the generation of a vascularized liver organoid. Hepatology. 2011;53:604–17.
170. De Carlo E, Baiguera S, Conconi MT, Vigolo S, Grandi C, Lora S, Martini C, Maffei P, Tamagno G, Vettor R, Sicolo N, Parnigotto PP. Pancreatic acellular matrix supports islet survival and function in a synthetic tubular device: in vitro and in vivo studies. Int J Mol Med. 2010;25:195–202.
171. Fedorovich NE, Schuurman W, Wijnberg HM, Prins HJ, van Weeren PR, Malda J, Alblas J, Dhert WJ. Biofabrication of osteochondral tissue equivalents by printing topologically defined, cell-laden hydrogel scaffolds. Tissue Eng Part C Methods. 2012;18:33–44.
172. Xu T, Olson J, Zhao WX, Atala A, Zhu JM, Yoo JJ. Characterization of cell constructs generated with inkjet printing technology using in vivo magnetic resonance imaging. J Manuf Sci Eng Trans ASME. 2008;130:021013.
173. Zhao W, Xu T, Aboushwareb T, Atala A, Yoo J. In vivo generation of functional tissues using the inkjet printing technology for reconstructive surgery. J Am Coll Surg. 2010;211:S87.
174. Warnke PH, Springer IN, Wiltfang J, Acil Y, Eufinger H, Wehmöller M, Russo PA, Bolte H, Sherry E, Behrens E, Terheyden H. Growth and transplantation of a custom vascularised bone graft in a man. Lancet. 2004;364:766–70.
175. Warnke PH, Wiltfang J, Springer I, Acil Y, Bolte H, Kosmahl M, Russo PA, Sherry E, Lützen U, Wolfart S, Terheyden H. Man as living bioreactor: fate of an exogenously prepared customized tissue-engineered mandible. Biomaterials. 2006;27:3163–7.
176. Malafaya PB, Silva GA, Reis RL. Natural-origin polymers as carriers and scaffolds for biomolecules and cell delivery in tissue engineering applications. Adv Drug Deliv Rev. 2007;59:207–33.
177. Berson MI. Construction of pseudoareola. Surgery. 1946;20:808.
178. Little JW III, Spear SL. The finishing touches in nipple-areolar reconstruction. Perspect Plast Surg. 1988;2:1–22.
179. Anton LE, Hartrampf CR. Nipple reconstruction with local flaps: star and wrap flaps. Perspect Plast Surg. 1991;5:67–78.
180. Jones G, Bostwic J. Nipple-areolar reconstruction. Oper Tech Plast Reconstr Surg. 1994;1:35–8.
181. Mori H, Hata Y. Modified C–V flap in nipple reconstruction. J Plast Reconstr Aesthet Surg. 2008;61:1109–10.
182. Brackley PT, Iqbal A. Enhancing your C-V flap nipple reconstruction. J Plast Reconstr Aesthet Surg. 2009;62:128–30.

183. El-Ali K, Dalal M, Kat CC. Modified C-V flap for nipple reconstruction: our results in 50 patients. J Plast Reconstr Aesthet Surg. 2009;62:991–6.
184. Witt P, Dujon DG. The V-V flap--a simple modification of the C-V flap for nipple reconstruction. J Plast Reconstr Aesthet Surg. 2013;66:1009–10.
185. Elizabeth Clark S, Turton E. The CC-V flap: a novel technique for augmenting a C-V nipple reconstruction using a free dermal graft. World J Plast Surg. 2014;3:8–12.
186. Salgarello M, Cavalcanti P, Barone-Adesi L. Atypical patterns in C-V flap nipple reconstruction: a customisation of the C-V flap. J Plast Reconstr Aesthet Surg. 2014;67:1598–9.
187. Temiz G, Yesiloglu N, Sirinoglu H, Sarici M. A new modification of C-V flap technique in nipple reconstruction: rolled triangular dermal-fat flaps. Aesthet Plast Surg. 2015;39:173–5.
188. Adams WM. Labial transplant for correction of loss of the nipple. Plast Reconstr Surg. 1949;4:295–8.
189. Gruber RP. Nipple-areola reconstruction: a review of techniques. Clin Plast Surg. 1979;6:71–83.
190. Millard DR Jr. Nipple and areola reconstruction by split-skin graft from the normal side. Plast Reconstr Surg. 1972;50:350–3.
191. Dean NR, Neild T, Haynes J, Goddard C, Cooter RD. Fading of nipple-areolar reconstructions: the last hurdle in breast reconstruction? Br J Plast Surg. 2002;55:574–81.
192. Haslik W, Nedomansky J, Hacker S, Nickl S, Schroegendorfer KF. Objective and subjective evaluation of donor-site morbidity after nipple sharing for nipple areola reconstruction. J Plast Reconstr Aesthet Surg. 2015;68:168–74.
193. Collis N, Garrido A. Maintenance of nipple projection using auricular cartilage. Plast Reconstr Surg. 2000;105:2276–7.
194. Bernard RW, Beran SJ. Autologous fat graft in nipple reconstruction. Plast Reconstr Surg. 2003;112:964–8.
195. Guerra AB, Khoobehi K, Metzinger SE, Allen RJ. New technique for nipple areola reconstruction: arrow flap and rib cartilage graft for long-lasting nipple projection. Ann Plast Surg. 2003;50:31–7.
196. Gamboa-Bobadilla GM. Nipple reconstruction: the top hat technique. Ann Plast Surg. 2005;54:243–6.
197. Hammond DC, Khuthaila D, Kim J. The skate flap purse-string technique for nipple-areola complex reconstruction. Plast Reconstr Surg. 2007;120:399–406.
198. Garramone CE, Lam B. Use of AlloDerm in primary nipple reconstruction to improve long-term nipple projection. Plast Reconstr Surg. 2007;119:1663–8.
199. Zenn MR, Garofalo JA. Unilateral nipple reconstruction with nipple sharing: time for a second look. Plast Reconstr Surg. 2009;123:1648–53.
200. Wong WW, Hiersche MA, Martin MC. The angel flap for nipple reconstruction. Can J Plast Surg. 2013;21:e1–4.
201. Grosdidier A, Lebeau J, Ochala C, Payan R, Bettega G. "double flag" flap nipple reconstruction. Clinical evaluation on 70 cases. Ann Chir Plast Esthet. 2014;59:123–9.
202. Yang JD, Ryu JY, Ryu DW, Kwon OH, Bae SG, Lee JW, Choi KY, Chung HY, Cho BC. Our experiences in nipple reconstruction using the Hammond flap. Arch Plast Surg. 2014;41:550–5.
203. Halvorson EG, Cormican M, West ME, Myers V. Three-dimensional nipple-areola tattooing: a new technique with superior results. Plast Reconstr Surg. 2014;133:1073–5.
204. Cheng MH, Ho-Asjoe M, Wei FC, Chuang DC. Nipple reconstruction in Asian females using banked cartilage graft and modified top hat flap. Br J Plast Surg. 2003;56:692–4.
205. Heitland A, Markowicz M, Koellensperger E, Allen R, Pallua N. Long-term nipple shrinkage following augmentation by an autologous rib cartilage transplant in free DIEP-flaps. J Plast Reconstr Aesthet Surg. 2006;59:1063–7.
206. Cheng MH, Rodriguez ED, Smartt JM, Cardenas-Mejia A. Nipple reconstruction using the modified top hat flap with banked costal cartilage graft: long-term follow-up in 58 patients. Ann Plast Surg. 2007;59:621–8.
207. Lipa JE, Addison PD, Neligan PC. Patient satisfaction following nipple reconstruction incorporating autologous costal cartilage. Can J Plast Surg. 2008;16:85–8.
208. Mori H, Uemura N, Okazaki M. Nipple reconstruction with banked costal cartilage after vertical-type skin-sparing mastectomy and deep inferior epigastric artery perforator flap. Breast Cancer. 2015;22:95–7.
209. Brent B, Bostwick J. Nipple-areola reconstruction with auricular tissues. Plast Reconstr Surg. 1977;60:353–61.
210. Tanabe HY, Tai Y, Kiyokawa K, Yamauchi T. Nipple areola reconstruction with a dermal-fat flap and rolled auricular cartilage. Plast Reconstr Surg. 1997;100:431–8.
211. Norton S, Akhavani MA, Kang N. The 'hamburger' technique for harvesting cartilage grafts in nipple reconstruction. J Plast Reconstr Aesthet Surg. 2007;60:957–9.
212. Jones AP, Erdmann M. Projection and patient satisfaction using the "hamburger" nipple reconstruction technique. J Plast Reconstr Aesthet Surg. 2012;65:207–12.
213. Breuing KH, Warren SM. Immediate bilateral breast reconstruction with implants and inferolateral AlloDerm slings. Ann Plast Surg. 2005;55:232–9.
214. Nahabedian MY. Secondary nipple reconstruction using local flaps and AlloDerm. Plast Reconstr Surg. 2005;115:2056–61.
215. Wong AK, Schonmeyr B, Singh P, Carlson DL, Li S, Mehrara BJ. Histologic analysis of angiogenesis and lymphangiogenesis in acellular human dermis. Plast Reconstr Surg. 2008;121:1144–52.

216. Rao SS, Seaman BJ, Davison SP. The acellular dermal matrix onlay graft for areolar reconstruction. Ann Plast Surg. 2014;72:508–12.
217. Tierney BP, Hodde J, Changkuo DI. Biologic collagen cylinder with skate flap technique for nipple reconstruction. Plast Surg Int. 2014;2014:194087.
218. Jankau J, Jaskiewicz J, Ankiewicz A. A new method for using a silicone rod for permanent nipple projection after breast reconstruction procedures. Breast. 2011;20:124–8.
219. Jankau J. Use of silicone rod for permanent nipple projection after breast reconstruction procedures. In: Shiffman MA, editor. Breast reconstruction: art, science and new clinical techniques. Berlin: Springer; 2016. p. 987–93.
220. McCarthy CM, VanLaeken N, Lennox P, Scott AM, Pusic AL. The efficacy of Artecoll injections for the augmentation of nipple projection in breast reconstruction. Eplasty. 2010;10:e7.
221. Yanaga H. Nipple-areola reconstruction with a dermal-fat flap: technical improvement from rolled auricular cartilage to artificial bone. Plast Reconstr Surg. 2003;112:1863–9.
222. Nishiyama T, Nakajima T, Yoshimura Y, Nakanishi Y. Utilizing solid models for preoperative shaping of HAP-TCP ceramic bone substitute: application for craniomaxillofacial surgery. Eur J Plast Surg. 1994;17:173.
223. Evans KK, Rasko Y, Lenert J, Olding M. The use of calcium hydroxylapatite for nipple projection after failed nipple-areolar reconstruction: early results. Ann Plast Surg. 2005;55:25–9.
224. Holbrook A, Lee S, Soo MS. Mammographic appearance of calcium hydroxylapatite (RadiesseTM) injected into the breast for nipple reconstruction. Breast J. 2013;19:104–13.
225. Germano D, De Biasio F, Piedimonte A, Parodi PC. Nipple reconstruction using the fleur-de-lis flap technique. Aesthet Plast Surg. 2006;30:399–402.
226. Cronin TD, Upton J, McDonough JM. Reconstruction of the breast after mastectomy. Plast Reconstr Surg. 1977;59:1–14.
227. Gruber RP. Method to produce better areolae and nipples on reconstructed breasts. Plast Reconstr Surg. 1977;60:505–13.
228. Cao YL, Lach E, Kim TH, Rodriguez A, Arevalo CA, Vacanti C. A. Tissue-engineered nipple reconstruction. Plast Reconstr Surg. 1998;102:2293–8.
229. Cerqueira B, Cornell L. NovoThelium LLC. Tissue engineered nipples for breast reconstruction. http://www.novothelium.com. Accessed 23 Oct 2016.
230. Bosworth L, Collins S, Boland T. TeVido BioDevices. http://tevidobiodevices.com/. Accessed 23 Oct 2016.
231. Chae MP, Hunter-Smith DJ, Spychal RT, Rozen WM. 3D volumetric analysis for planning breast reconstructive surgery. Breast Cancer Res Treat. 2014;146:457–60.

# Part X

# Complications

# Nipple-Sparing Mastectomy and Nipple Ischemia

# 74

Yan T. Ortiz-Pomales and Grant W. Carlson

## 74.1 Introduction

Nipple-sparing mastectomy (NSM) has become an accepted approach in selected cases of breast cancer and prophylactic mastectomy. NSM and immediate breast reconstruction (IBR) is growing in popularity because of increased patient satisfaction and perceived aesthetic benefits [1, 2]. Various surgical techniques have been described, and nipple ischemia has been a common complication. Lemaine et al. studied mastectomy skin flap necrosis in 175 operated breasts (skin sparing mastectomy (SSM) 103 and NSM 72) [3]. They found that NSM was more likely to have any degree of mastectomy skin flap necrosis (67% vs. 20%). This difference was attributed solely to the incidence of nipple-areola complex (NAC) ischemia. Potential risk factors for nipple ischemia after nipple-sparing mastectomy are reviewed in this chapter.

Y.T. Ortiz-Pomales, M.D.
Division of Plastic Surgery, Emory University School of Medicine, Atlanta, GA 30319, USA
e-mail: ortizpomales@gmail.com

G.W. Carlson, M.D. (✉)
Division of Plastic Surgery, Emory University School of Medicine, Atlanta, GA 30319, USA

Winship Cancer Institute,
1365C Clifton Road, Atlanta, GA 30322, USA
e-mail: grant_carlson@emory.org

## 74.2 Perfusion of the Nipple-Areolar Complex

The main blood supply to the nipple-areolar complex (NAC) comes from branches of the internal mammary and lateral thoracic vessels [4]. The second intercostal perforator off the internal mammary artery is the most prominent vessel supplying the NAC [5]. This emphasizes the importance of its preservation during NSM. It exits the pectoralis major muscle outside of the breast parenchyma. Stolier et al. [6] noted that in their experience, the third and fourth intercostal perforators frequently penetrate the breast parenchyma making preservation more difficult.

This pattern of vascularity has also been confirmed through laser Doppler and fluorescein flowmetry studies, as well as newer infrared technology using indocyanine green dye [4]. It is important to point out that attempts at preserving these perforating vessels should be made during flap dissection to reduce the risk of NAC ischemia.

Screening modalities to predict risks for nipple ischemia have been proposed. A study by Wapnir et al. [7] found that intraoperative imaging of nipple perfusion patterns was predictive of ischemia complications in NSM using indocyanine green and infrared camera technology. In their study, they discovered that there was


M.A. Shiffman (ed.), *Nipple-Areolar Complex Reconstruction*,
https://doi.org/10.1007/978-3-319-60925-6_74

a 71% rate of ischemia complication in patients with a pattern of arterial blood inflow to the NAC that was predominantly from the underlying breast tissue, rather than from the surrounding skin or a combination of both. They concluded that the anatomic configuration of the blood supply to the NAC might be helpful in determining ischemia and help guide clinical decision-making.

## 74.3 Risks Factors of Nipple Necrosis in NSM

There is significant variability in the reported incidence of nipple ischemia following NSM. Most series report an ischemia rate of 10–15%, but study reports range from 0% to 48% [8–16]. The lack of standardization of surgical technique and the lack of a clear definition for nipple necrosis have made these studies difficult to compare for adequate determination of the true incidence of nipple necrosis with this procedure. As a consequence, strict independent risk factors that could help classify patients based on risk for proper preoperative counseling need to be explored (Table 74.1).

### 74.3.1 Morphological Factors

The volume and degree of ptosis of the breast increase the length of the remaining skin envelope from the thoracic wall increasing the potential risks of poor vascularization to the NAC [17, 18]. Reconstructing these breasts with larger volume implants and autologous tissue creates pressure on the skin flaps, further reducing skin perfusion [14, 19, 20]. Gould et al. [21] found partial or total nipple necrosis in 20% of 113 cases of NSM and IBR. Larger breasts (C cup or larger) were associated with higher rates of nipple necrosis (34% for C cup, 6% for A and B cup; $p = 0.003$).

**Table 74.1** Risk factors for nipple ischemia after nipple-sparing mastectomy

| Risk factors |
|---|
| Morphological factors (breast size, ptosis) [14, 17–21] |
| Periareolar incision [8, 14, 22, 23] |
| Oncologic resection [7, 10, 13, 24] |
| Radiation [23, 25] |
| Tobacco use [2, 8, 14] |
| Autologous reconstruction [14] |

### 74.3.2 Incisions

The nipple-sparing mastectomy technique preserves the skin and the nipple-areolar complex, and once the breast parenchyma has been excised, the NAC is dependent on the subdermal plexus that forms an anastomotic network from the medial and lateral sides.

A periareolar incision disrupts this network, reducing its blood supply. This has been shown experimentally in a perfusion study examining radial and periareolar incisions in the pig model using infrared fluorescence imaging [26]. The use of skin retractors along the areolar margin during flap elevation may also play a role in ischemia seen with these incisions.

Algaithy et al. [8] prospectively studied 50 consecutive mastectomies, 40 for oncological resection, and 10 prophylactic and identified young age, periareolar incisions, tobacco use, and a flap thickness less than 5 mm as risks factors for nipple necrosis in NSM. Carlson et al. [22] prospectively evaluated 71 consecutive NSM, all with duct excision from the undersurface of the nipple on the ipsilateral side of the cancerous lesion, and determined that operations for cancer and periareolar incisions predispose the nipple to ischemia. This group did not find a direct correlation between smoking and the risk of nipple necrosis.

Garwood et al. [14] showed that incisions extending around more than 30% of the areola circumference were an independent risk factor for necrosis. Komorowski et al. [27] showed that vascular complications were dramatically reduced when choosing the inframammary fold (IMF) or lateral incisions over the periareolar approach. Accordingly, with growing experience, the inframammary fold or radial incisions are preferred over the periareolar approach.

### 74.3.3 Oncological Resection

The low locoregional recurrence rates in patients who have undergone NSM make it a safe and sound surgical treatment from the oncological standpoint, but the management of the nipple after NSM is still controversial and far from standardized among surgeon, and clearly this technical aspect of this procedure is a significant independent risk factor for complications such as nipple ischemia. Some surgeons recommend excising the central core of the nipple in an attempt to remove as much ductal tissue as possible [10, 13, 24]. Others advocate leaving a 5-mm-thick portion of glandular tissue in an attempt to improve viability [28]. Rusby et al. [29] studied the vascular anatomy of the nipple papilla and determined that leaving a 3-mm-rim of nipple preserves 66% of nipple vessels. In some studies, nipples in breasts containing cancer were treated by nipple inversion and excision of the central ducts without ischemic threat given that at least 50% of the blood supply to the nipple-areolar complex is located at the periphery of the nipple [22]. In prophylactic cases, a thin rim of breast tissue was left under the nipple. The sub-areolar tissue preservation in non-oncologic cases undoubtedly accounted for cancer surgery being an independent risk factor for nipple ischemia after NSM, with an adjusted odds ratio of 10.5 ($p = 0.007$) [7].

#### 74.3.3.1 Radiation

Radiotherapy (RT) both prior RT and postmastectomy radiotherapy (PMRT) increases the complication rates including implant loss and skin and nipple necrosis after NSM and IBR. In a recent retrospective analysis of 982 NSMs by Tang et al. [25], it was found that both preoperative and post-mastectomy radiation increased the nipple lose rate compared to the non-radiated group (4.3 vs. 4.1 and 0.9%, $p = 0.04, 0.02$, respectively). Colwell et al. [23] in their review of 500 NSMs found a nipple necrosis rate of 4.4%. Logistic regression analysis found that preoperative RT and periareolar incisions were positive predictors of NAC necrosis. Inframammary fold incisions were a negative predictor of NAC necrosis.

### 74.3.4 Tobacco Use

Nicotine in cigarette smoke is a direct cutaneous vasoconstrictor and indirectly inhibits capillary blood flow by releasing catecholamines. There is a large body of evidence showing that tobacco smoking increases the risk of native skin flap necrosis after SSM [12, 30, 31]. Studies have shown that it increases skin flap and nipple necrosis after mastectomy [2, 8, 14]. Many consider active tobacco smoking as a relative contraindication to NSM.

### 74.3.5 Tumescent Solution

The use of dilute lidocaine and epinephrine solution facilitates sharp skin flap development and avoids excessive electrocautery during NSM. It is especially useful in minimal access incisions like the IMF. There are conflicting reports as to its impact on skin and NAC viability, but its use clearly makes clinical assessment of more difficult [2, 32, 33].

## 74.4 Nipple Necrosis and Postoperative Care

The management of NAC necrosis depends on its depth and extent and the type of reconstruction performed. Skin necrosis after expander reconstruction should be managed aggressively to prevent implant exposure and the development of infection necessitating implant removal. It has been suggested to perform a delayed-immediate reconstruction after NSM in patients with questionable skin flap viability [34]. In cases of autologous reconstruction, it has been suggested to bank the autologous tissue under the native skin flap until potential areas of ischemia declare themselves [35].

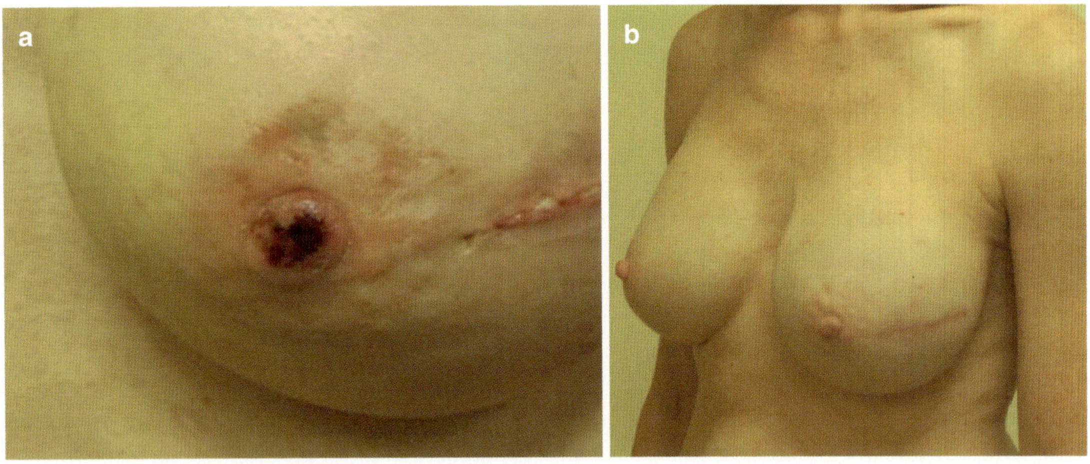

**Fig. 74.1** (**a**) Superficial necrosis of the nipple after NSM via a radial incision and tissue expander reconstruction. (**b**) Healing by secondary intention after local wound care

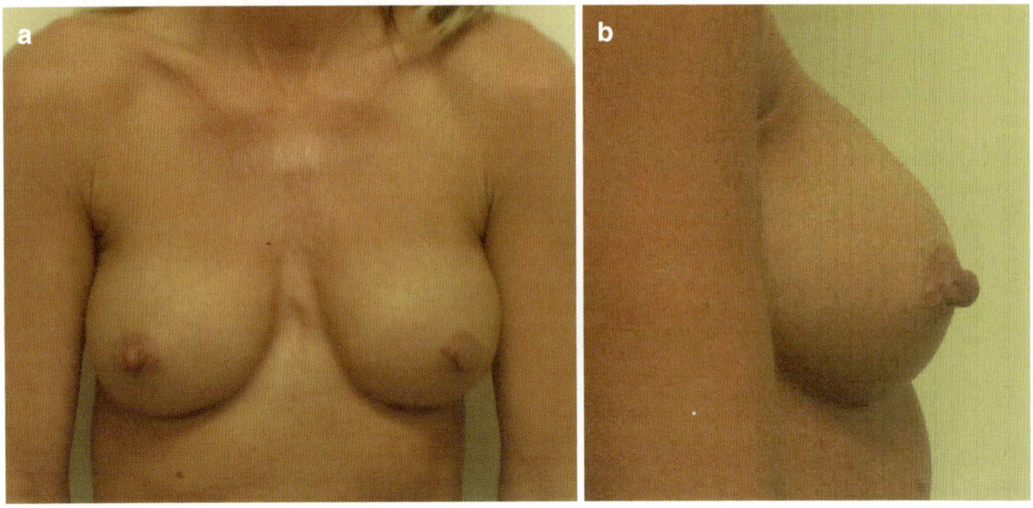

**Fig. 74.2** (**a**, **b**) A 41-year-old with a history of submuscular breast augmentation with 375 mL submuscular implants

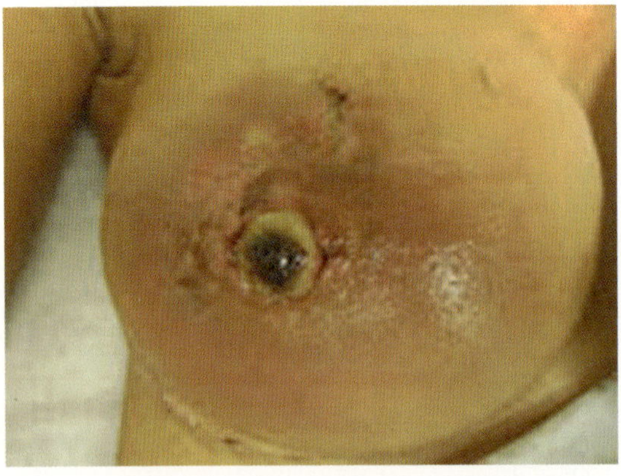

**Fig. 74.3** Postoperative appearance of partial skin and NAC necrosis after NSM and immediate tissue expander reconstruction via an IMF incision

Postoperative NAC ischemia can generally be managed conservatively with local wound care and partial deflation of the tissue expander to reduce tension of the skin flaps (Fig. 74.1). Dent et al. [36] reviewed their experience with 318 NSM via IMF incisions and immediate implant reconstruction. Nipple ischemia occurred in 65 cases (20.4%): partial necrosis 44 (13.8%) and full-thickness necrosis 21 (6.6%). All cases of partial thickness loss resolved with conservative treatment, as did 81% of full-thickness losses.

Full-thickness nipple ischemia may result in loss of nipple projection or complete nipple loss (Figs. 74.2, 74.3, 74.4, 74.5, and 74.6). A simple

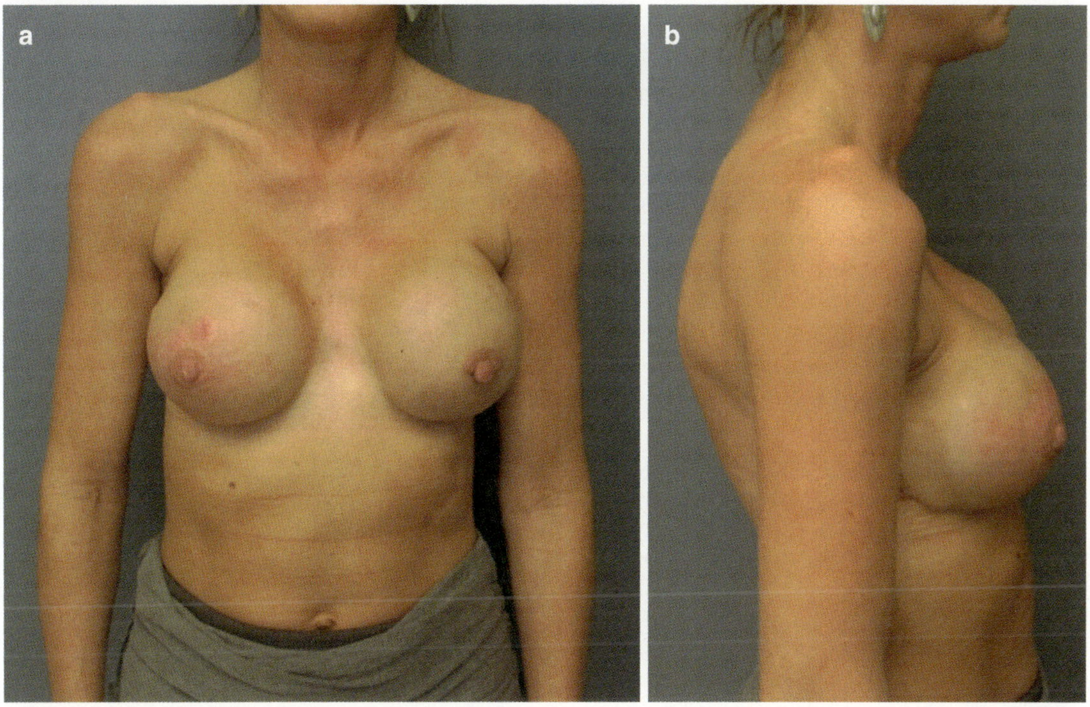

**Fig. 74.4** (**a**, **b**) After the areas of necrosis were treated with topical antibiotics. Note the loss of nipple projection

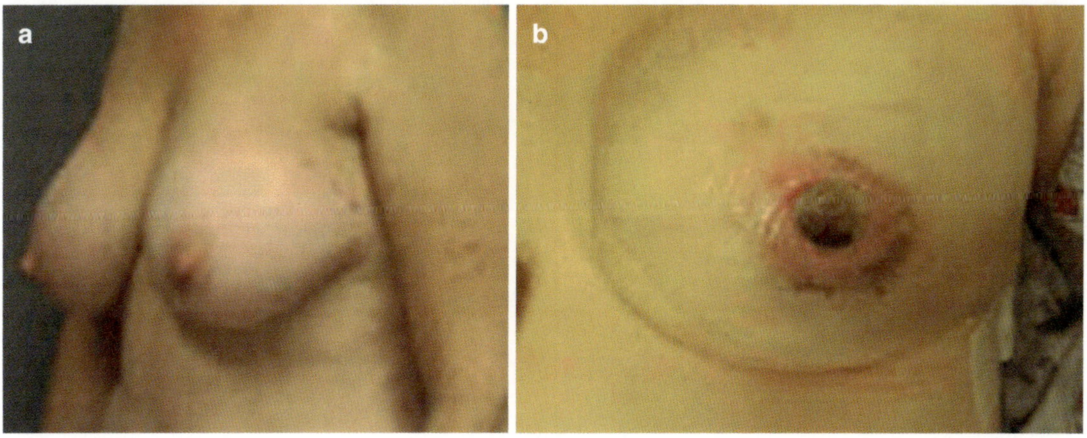

**Fig. 74.5** (**a**) A 49-year-old with left breast cancer. Note the grade I breast ptosis. (**b**) Postoperative appearance of the left breast after NSM and tissue expander reconstruction filled with 500 mL of saline

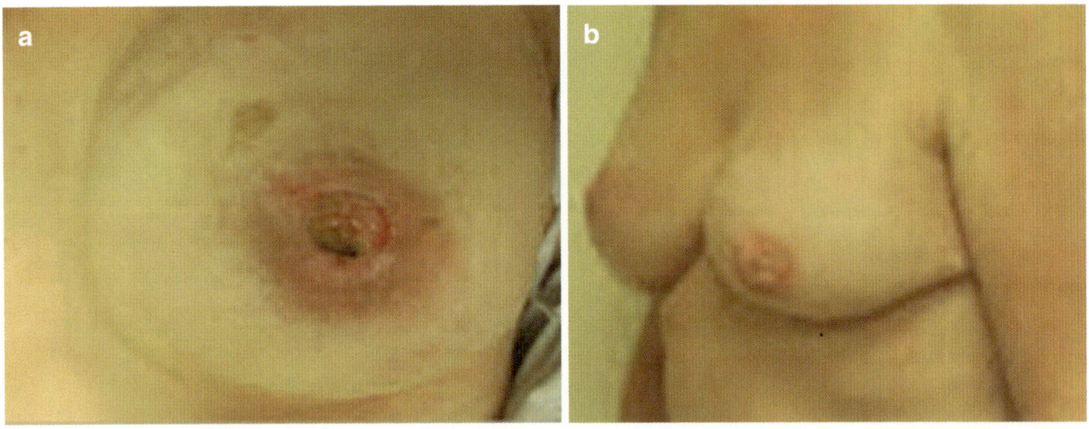

**Fig. 74.6** (**a**) Progressive healing of the partial thickness necrosis. (**b**) Postoperative after implant exchange. Note the total loss of nipple height

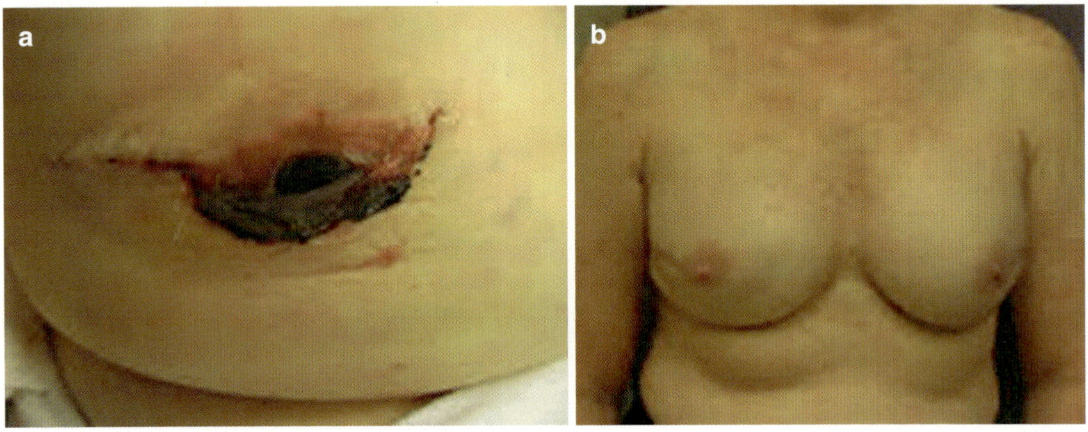

**Fig. 74.7** (**a**) Full-thickness nipple necrosis after NSM via a periareolar incision with lateral extension. (**b**) Right nipple reconstruction with free nipple graft from left breast

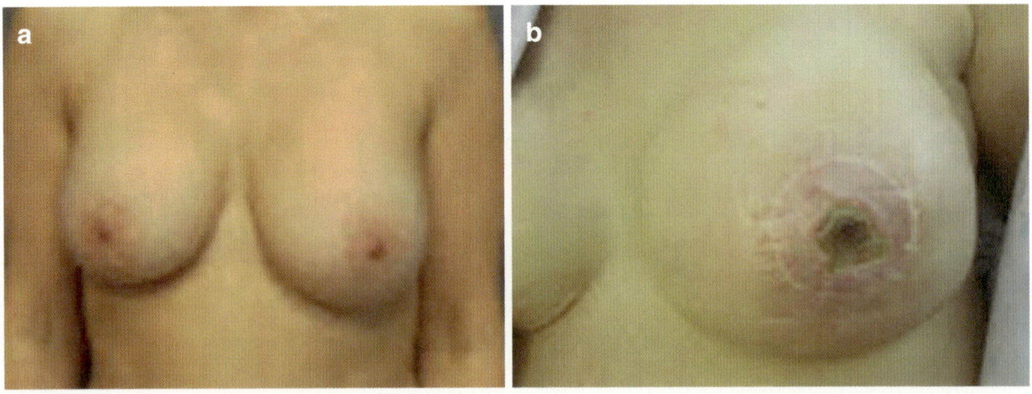

**Fig. 74.8** (**a**) A 42-year-old with diffuse DCIS of the left breast. She has a history of bilateral augmentation/mastopexy with 375 mL submuscular implants 5 years prior to diagnosis. (**b**) Postoperative appearance of left breast after NSM and tissue expander reconstruction with 400 mL of saline

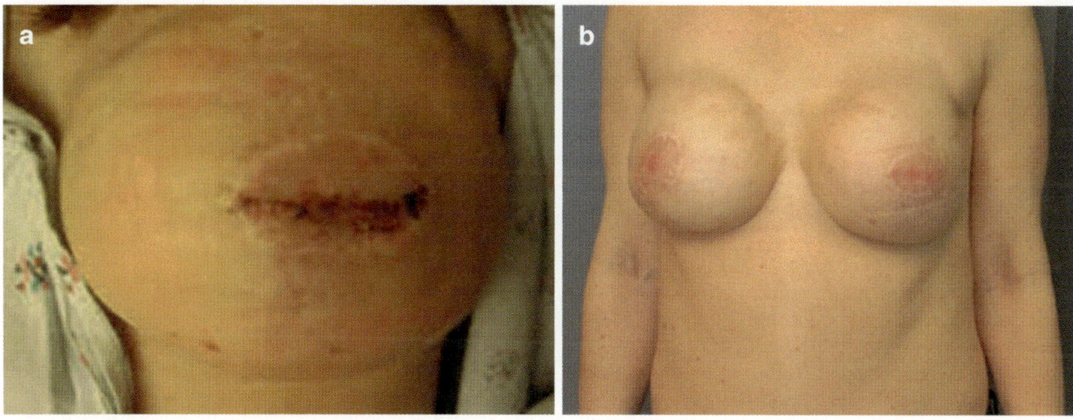


**Fig. 74.9** (**a**) Postoperative after resection of necrotic nipple and linear closure. (**b**) Preoperative appearance prior to implant exchange

option to correct this deformity is a free nipple graft from the opposite breast (Fig. 74.7). Isolated nipple necrosis can be reconstructed with a C-V flap of remaining areola, but areolar necrosis necessitates a skate flap [37]. Rarely, full-thickness necrosis may necessitate aggressive operative intervention to prevent implant exposure (Figs. 74.8 and 74.9).

## 74.5 Preventive Measures to Avoid NAC Ischemia

Patient selection is the most important measure to prevent NAC ischemia. As discussed, specific risk factors including large breast volume, breast ptosis, periareolar incisions, previous radiation, and tobacco use must be recognized (Table 74.1). Surgical delay of the NAC in high-risk patients prior to NSM has been described [38]. Jensen et al. [38] performed surgical delay by undermining the NAC 7–21 days prior to mastectomy in patients considered at high risk of nipple necrosis. There was no nipple ischemia in 31 cases of NSM. Martinez et al. [39] described surgical delay in 20 patients. In the first stage by undermining the NAC, raising breast flaps and placing silicone sheeting in the dissected pocket. Two weeks later, NSM was successfully performed without complications.

Most recently, a randomized placebo-controlled trial was performed to examine the impact of topical nitroglycerin on mastectomy flap necrosis after IB [40]. The study was stopped at the fist interim analysis of the initial 165 patients (SSM 121, NSM 44) enrolled due to an 18.5% reduction rate ($p = 0.006$) in mastectomy flap necrosis on patients who received the ointment.

**Conclusions**

Nipple-sparing mastectomy is a safe surgical option for oncological resection of breast cancers and for prophylactic mastectomies. It provides another option for patients seeking immediate reconstruction with high satisfaction rates and aesthetic results. Although the risk of nipple-areola complex ischemia is a concern with this particular technique, the rates are low and acceptable. As discussed, specific risk factors of NAC ischemia include large breast volumes, breast ptosis, periareolar incisions, radiation, tobacco use, and autologous reconstruction. There are intraoperative modalities with infrared technology that may elucidate information about blood supply patterns that could put patients at risk for developing nipple ischemia. In the event of partial nipple necrosis, conservative management usually yields great outcomes.

## References


1. Didier F, Radice D, Gandini S, Bedolis R, Rotmensz N, Maldifassi A, Santillo B, Luini A, Galimberti V, Scaffidi E, Lupo F, Martella S, Petit JY. Does nipple preservation in mastectomy improve satisfaction with cosmetic results, psychological adjustment, body image and sexuality? Breast Cancer Res Treat. 2009;118(3):623–33.
2. Moyer HR, Ghazi B, Daniel JR, Gasgarth R, Carlson GW. Nipple-sparing mastectomy: technical aspects and aesthetic outcomes. Ann Plast Surg. 2012;68(5):446–50.
3. Lemaine V, Hoskin TL, Farley DR, Grant CS, Boughey JC, Torstenson TA, Jacobson SR, Jakub JW, Degnim AC. Introducing the SKIN score: a validated scoring system to assess severity of mastectomy skin flap necrosis. Ann Surg Oncol. 2015;22(9):2925–32.
4. van Deventer PV. The blood supply to the nipple-areola complex of the human mammary gland. Aesthet Plast Surg. 2004;28(6):393–8.
5. Palmer JH, Taylor GI. The vascular territories of the anterior chest wall. Br J Plast Surg. 1986;39(3):287–99.
6. Stolier AJ, Levine EA. Reducing the risk of nipple necrosis: technical observations in 340 nipple-sparing mastectomies. Breast J. 2013;19(2):173–9.
7. Wapnir I, Dua M, Kieryn A, Paro J, Morrison D, Kahn D, Meyer S, Gurtner G. Intraoperative imaging of nipple perfusion patterns and ischemic complications in nipple-sparing mastectomies. Ann Surg Oncol. 2014;21(1):100–6.
8. Algaithy ZK, Petit JY, Lohsiriwat V, Maisonneuve P, Rey PC, Baros N, Lai H, Mulas P, Barbalho DM, Veronesi P, Rietjens M. Nipple sparing mastectomy: can we predict the factors predisposing to necrosis? Eur J Surg Oncol. 2011;38(2):125–9.
9. Ashikari RH, Ashikari AY, Kelemen PR, Salzberg CA. Subcutaneous mastectomy and immediate reconstruction for prevention of breast cancer for high-risk patients. Breast Cancer. 2008;15(3):185–91.
10. Caruso F, Ferrara M, Castiglione G, Trombetta G, De Meo L, Catanuto G, Carillio G. Nipple sparing subcutaneous mastectomy: sixty-six months follow-up. Eur J Surg Oncol. 2006;32(9):937–40.
11. Crowe JP Jr, Kim JA, Yetman R, Banbury J, Patrick RJ, Baynes D. Nipple-sparing mastectomy: technique and results of 54 procedures. Arch Surg. 2004;139(2):148–50.
12. Davies K, Allan L, Roblin P, Ross D, Farhadi J. Factors affecting post-operative complications following skin sparing mastectomy with immediate breast reconstruction. Breast. 2010;20(1):21–5.
13. Garcia-Etienne CA, Borgen PI. Update on the indications for nipple-sparing mastectomy. J Support Oncol. 2006;4(5):225–30.
14. Garwood ER, Moore D, Ewing C, Hwang ES, Alvarado M, Foster RD, Esserman LJ. Total skin-sparing mastectomy: complications and local recurrence rates in 2 cohorts of patients. Ann Surg. 2009;249(1):26–32.
15. Petit JY, Veronesi U, Rey P, Rotmensz N, Botteri E, Rietjens M, Garusi C, De Lorenzi F, Martella S, Bosco R, Manconi A, Luini A, Galimberti V, Veronesi P, Ivaldi GB, Orecchia R. Nipple-sparing mastectomy: risk of nipple-areolar recurrences in a series of 579 cases. Breast Cancer Res Treat. 2009;114(1):97–101.
16. Regolo L, Ballardini B, Gallarotti E, Scoccia E, Zanini V. Nipple sparing mastectomy: an innovative skin incision for an alternative approach. Breast. 2008;17(1):8–11.
17. Chirappapha P, Petit JY, Rietjens M, De Lorenzi F, Garusi C, Martella S, Barbieri B, Gottardi A, Andrea M, Giuseppe L, Hamza A, Lohsiriwat V. Nipple sparing mastectomy: does breast morphological factor related to necrotic complications? Plast Reconstr Surg Glob Open. 2014;2(1):e99.
18. Rusby JE, Gui GP. Nipple-sparing mastectomy in women with large or ptotic breasts. J Plast Reconstr Aesthet Surg. 2010;63(10):e754–5.
19. Basta MN, Gerety PA, Serletti JM, Kovach SJ, Fischer JP. A systematic review and head-to-head meta-analysis of outcomes following direct-to-implant versus conventional two-stage implant reconstruction. Plast Reconstr Surg. 2015;136(6):1135–44.
20. Gdalevitch P, Ho A, Genoway K, Alvrtsyan H, Bovill E, Lennox P, Van Laeken N, Macadam S. Direct-to-implant single-stage immediate breast reconstruction with acellular dermal matrix: predictors of failure. Plast Reconstr Surg. 2014;133(6):738e–47e.
21. Gould DJ, Hunt KK, Liu J, Kuerer HM, Crosby MA, Babiera G, Kronowitz SJ. Impact of surgical techniques, biomaterials, and patient variables on rate of nipple necrosis after nipple-sparing mastectomy. Plast Reconstr Surg. 2013;132(3):330e–8e.
22. Carlson GW, Chu CK, Moyer HR, Duggal C, Losken A. Predictors of nipple ischemia after nipple sparing mastectomy. Breast J. 2014;20(1):69–73.
23. Colwell AS, Tessler O, Lin AM, Liao E, Winograd J, Cetrulo CL, Tang R, Smith BL, Austen WG Jr. Breast reconstruction following nipple-sparing mastectomy: predictors of complications, reconstruction outcomes, and 5-year trends. Plast Reconstr Surg. 2014;133(3):496–506.
24. Crowe JP, Patrick RJ, Yetman RJ, Djohan R. Nipple-sparing mastectomy update: one hundred forty-nine procedures and clinical outcomes. Arch Surg. 2008;143(11):1106–10.
25. Tang R, Coopey SB, Colwell AS, Specht MC, Gadd MA, Kansal K, McEvoy MP, Merrill AL, Rai U. Nipple-sparing mastectomy in irradiated breasts: selecting patients to minimize complications. Ann Surg Oncol. 2015;22(10):3331–7.
26. Ashitate Y, Lee BT, Ngo LH, Laurence RG, Hutteman M, Oketokoun R, Lunsford E, Soo Choi H, Frangioni JV. Quantitative assessment of nipple perfusion with near-infrared fluorescence imaging. Ann Plast Surg. 2013;70(2):149–53.

27. Komorowski AL, Zanini V, Regolo L, Carolei A, Wysocki WM, Costa A. Necrotic complications after nipple- and areola-sparing mastectomy. World J Surg. 2006;30(8):1410–3.
28. Petit JY, Veronesi U, Orecchia R, Luini A, Rey P, Intra M, Didier F, Martella S, Rietjens M, Garusi C, DeLorenzi F, Gatti G, Leon ME, Casadio CV. Nipple-sparing mastectomy in association with intra operative radiotherapy (ELIOT): a new type of mastectomy for breast cancer treatment. Breast Cancer Res Treat. 2006;96(1):47–51.
29. Rusby JE, Brachtel EF, Taghian A, Michaelson JS, Koerner FC, Smith BL. George Peters award. Microscopic anatomy within the nipple: implications for nipple-sparing mastectomy. Am J Surg. 2007;194(4):433–7.
30. Carlson GW, Styblo TM, Lyles RH, Jones G, Murray DR, Staley CA, Wood WC. The use of skin sparing mastectomy in the treatment of breast cancer: the Emory experience. Surg Oncol. 2003;12(4):265–9.
31. Hultman CS, Daiza S. Skin-sparing mastectomy flap complications after breast reconstruction: review of incidence, management, and outcome. Ann Plast Surg. 2003;50(3):249–55.
32. Chun YS, Verma K, Rosen H, Lipsitz SR, Breuing K, Guo L, Golshan M, Grigorian N, Eriksson E. Use of tumescent mastectomy technique as a risk factor for native breast skin flap necrosis following immediate breast reconstruction. Am J Surg. 2011;201(2):160–5.
33. Vinton AL, Traverso LW, Jolly PC. Wound complications after modified radical mastectomy compared with tylectomy with axillary lymph node dissection. Am J Surg. 1991;161(5):584–8.
34. Zenn MR. Staged immediate breast reconstruction. Plast Reconstr Surg. 2015;135(4):976–9.
35. Park SW, Lee TJ, Kim EK, Eom JS. Managing necrosis of the nipple-areola complex in breast reconstruction after nipple-sparing mastectomy: immediate nipple-areola complex reconstruction with banked skin. Plast Reconstr Surg. 2014;133(1):73e–4e.
36. Dent BL, Small K, Swistel A, Talmor M. Nipple-areolar complex ischemia after nipple-sparing mastectomy with immediate implant-based reconstruction: risk factors and the success of conservative treatment. Aesthet Surg J. 2014;34(4):560–70.
37. Dent BL, Chao JW, Eden DJ, Stone BV, Swistel A, Talmor M. Nipple resection and reconstruction after attempted nipple-sparing mastectomy. Ann Plast Surg. 2016;78(1):28–34.
38. Jensen JA, Lin JH, Kapoor N, Giuliano AE. Surgical delay of the nipple-areolar complex: a powerful technique to maximize nipple viability following nipple-sparing mastectomy. Ann Surg Oncol. 2012;19(10):3171–6.
39. Martinez CA, Reis SM, Sato EA, Boutros SG. The nipple-areola preserving mastectomy: a multistage procedure aiming to improve reconstructive outcomes following mastectomy. Plast Reconstr Surg Glob Open. 2015;3(10):e538.
40. Gdalevitch P, Van Laeken N, Bahng S, Ho A, Bovill E, Lennox P, Brasher P, Macadam S. Effects of nitroglycerin ointment on mastectomy flap necrosis in immediate breast reconstruction: a randomized controlled trial. Plast Reconstr Surg. 2015;135(6):1530–9.

# Nipple Reconstruction: Risk Factors and Complications

75

Gabrielle B. Davis, Travis Miller, and Gordon Lee

## 75.1 Introduction

The final stage of breast reconstruction consists of recreation of the nipple-areolar complex (NAC). The goals of NAC reconstruction emphasize the creation of an aesthetically pleasing appearance incorporating nipple projection and natural pigmentation. Nipple projection has traditionally been achieved utilizing local flaps or skin grafts and pigmentation through nipple tattooing. While nipple reconstruction is associated with improved psychological well-being and patient satisfaction, it is not without inherent risks [1–3]. The utilization of local tissue in the setting of thin, fibrotic skin, as in previous radiation exposure, can lead to nipple necrosis, tip loss, delayed wound healing, and surgical site infections. In cases of implant-based reconstruction, infections resulting in implant exposure or extrusion can necessitate the removal of the implant. These reported complications may explain the fact that only 50% of women will undergo nipple reconstruction. Furthermore, rates of postoperative nipple projection loss range from 26.1% to 75% with revision rates from 2% to 8.6% [2]. The loss of projection with time correlates to decreased patient satisfaction. Techniques of NAC reconstruction are constantly evolving in order to combat this problem. However, one must understand that there is a fine balance in enhancing longevity of projection while minimizing complications.

## 75.2 Anatomy of the Nipple-Areolar Complex

To successfully address the challenges of the reconstructive process of the nipple, it is integral to have a thorough understanding of the native anatomy. The NAC is located at the most projecting portion of the breast mound. The nipple itself may project over 1 cm, and the diameter is approximately 4–7 mm. The surrounding areola consists of pigmented skin and is on average 4.2–4.5 cm in diameter. The areola is made up of keratinized stratified epithelium, which contains lactiferous sinus openings, sebaceous glands, and Montgomery glands (which are specialized glands intermediate in nature between sebaceous and lactiferous glands and are thought to secrete lipoid fluid and olfactory stimuli for neonatal appetite). The nipple and areola have a network of connecting myoepithelial cells surrounding lactiferous sinus openings. Smooth muscle fibers are also arranged circumferentially and radially to the connective tissue of the areola and are

G.B. Davis, M.D., M.S. (✉) • T. Miller, M.D.
G. Lee, M.D.
Division of Plastic Surgery, Department of Surgery, Stanford University, 770 Welch Road, Suite 400, Palo Alto, CA 34304, USA
e-mail: gabriel7@stanford.edu; travismi@stanford.edu; glee@stanford.edu


M.A. Shiffman (ed.), *Nipple-Areolar Complex Reconstruction*,
https://doi.org/10.1007/978-3-319-60925-6_75

responsible for nipple erection [4]. The blood supply to the nipple, as with the breast parenchyma, is redundant and rich. The internal mammary perforators, lateral thoracic perforators, and intercostal perforators all supply the subdermal plexus of the nipple. The innervation of the nipple is primarily through the lateral cutaneous branch of the fourth intercostal nerve via two branches. One branch passes superficial to the breast parenchyma and the other branch passes through the retromammary space. The third and fifth intercostal nerves may provide some sensory innervation as well [4].

Statistical analyses for the dimensions of the breast suggest that the "ideal" distance from the sternal notch to the nipple and from the midclavicular line is each 19–21 cm. The distance from the nipple to the inframammary fold is 5–7 cm, and the distance from the nipple to the midline is 19–21 cm [5–8]. In determining proper placement for the reconstructed nipple, the NAC is ideally placed at the point of maximal projection; however, symmetry with the contralateral side should be used primarily to guide placement. In bilateral reconstruction, standardized values can aid in determining nipple size and location. These measurements offer guidelines, but ultimately surgical efforts must be tailored to individual patient preference and proportionality. No amount of measurements is a substitute for gross visualization of the breast and identifying the "right spot" for the nipple.

## 75.3 History of Nipple-Areolar Reconstruction

Initial techniques were introduced in the 1940s utilizing the contralateral nipple and distant tissue. Adams described the use of the contralateral NAC as a composite graft, and the technique of nipple sharing was later refined by Millard in the 1970s [9, 10]. Adams [11] also described the use of grafts from the labia minora, but due to donor site morbidity, this technique did not gain wide popularity. Other grafts including toe pulp, auricular cartilage, and mucous membranes were also attempted over the years, but again donor site morbidity prevented these grafts from achieving wide use [12, 13]. Nipple banking provided an option for the nipple to be "saved" for later use on a distant part of the body. However the oncologic safety of this method was questionable, with some reports of cancer being transplanted with the banked nipple, leading to the abandonment of this technique [14]. A new paradigm was introduced in the 1980s with introduction of the use of local flaps [15–17]. These flaps allowed the use of tissue rearrangement to make the projection of the neonipple, allowing primary closure of the flap. These flaps eliminated the issue of distant donor site morbidity in reconstructing the nipple projection. Newer techniques incorporate augmentation of existence of flaps or grafts using autologous, allogeneic, or synthetic tissue. Augmented tissue is positioned as an internal strut providing support to the overlying tissue to withstand internal contractive and external compressive forces thought to contribute to projection loss. Areolar reconstruction was initially accomplished by free grafts from pigmented areas of the body. Nipple tattooing however has become the most universal form of restoration of the pigmented portion of the areola without undue donor site morbidity of grafting. The first use of tattooing for NAC reconstruction was reported by Rees in 1975 [18], who tattooed redundant skin of the contralateral, intact breast of a patient and later transferred the pigmented skin as a free graft. Becker then reported the use of tattooing neonipples created from local flaps in the 1980s, and Spear subsequently popularized the technique [19, 20].

## 75.4 Techniques of Nipple Reconstruction and Outcomes

### 75.4.1 Local Flaps

Flap-based nipple reconstruction employs random pattern flaps with blood supply from the subdermal plexus. The basic principles of flap creation, such as designing wide-based pedicles away from existing scars, are critical for optimal outcomes. Numerous techniques have been described for flap-based nipple reconstruction, and among the most popular are the skate, star, and C–V flap. The skate flap was described by Little in 1984, and many derivatives have since been proposed. It was traditionally paired with a skin graft to provide both nipple and areolar reconstruction. The desired diameter of the areola is determined and marked. A line is drawn horizontally across the uppermost marked areola at the 12 o' clock position. This line is split into thirds and a semicircular line is drawn inferior from the base line. The inner and outer thirds of the semicircle will make the nipple sidewall and the central portion the most projected portion of the nipple. A superior semicircle is also drawn from this line and the skin deepithelialized to create a donut-shaped defect in which a skin graft will be placed to create the areola. The skate flap gives one of the highest early projection distances of local flaps, with up to >9 mm after 6 months [21]. The star flap is a derivative of the skate flap and was first described by Anton 1991 [22]. The star flap allows for primary closure of the donor site, in contrast to the original skate flap. However, the star flap provides less projection immediately and long term, with one study showing only 1.97 mm mean projection after 2 years [23]. The design of the flap is based on three wings. The two outer wings are elevated in a subdermal plane, and the central wing is elevated with subcutaneous fat to form the nipple core. The two outer wings are folded over the other to form the lower base of the flap [22]. The sites from which the wings are harvested are then closed primarily, forming a T-shaped scar. In a series of 422 nipple reconstructions using the skate flap technique, a 7.2% complication rate was noted. Skin donor site dehiscence was the most common complication followed by partial take of the skin graft [24]. Satteson et al. [2] found a 2.95 greater odds ratio of complications with the use of the skate flap vs. the star flap in over 400 patients undergoing nipple reconstructions. They postulated that harvesting of the skin graft, particularly from the groin, leads to a higher risk of infectious complications. The C–V flap has a similar design to the star flap with two triangular-shaped "Vs" that will be the base of the nipple, emanating from a central "C"-shaped core (Figs. 75.1, 75.2, and 75.3). The "C" will become the cap of the nipple. The width of the

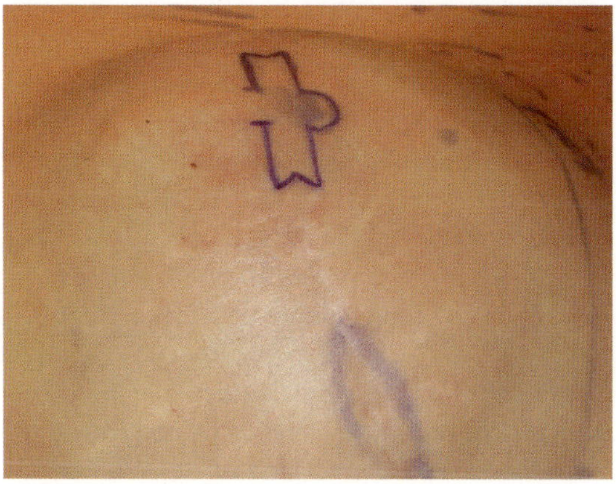

**Fig. 75.1** Modification of the C–V flap

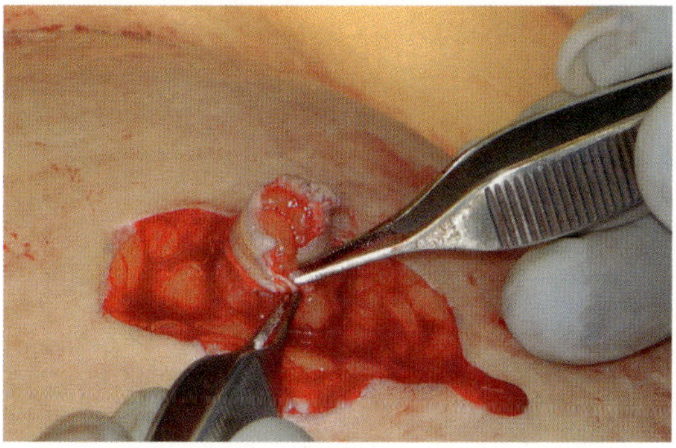

**Fig. 75.2** The ends of the flap interdigitate to aid in projection

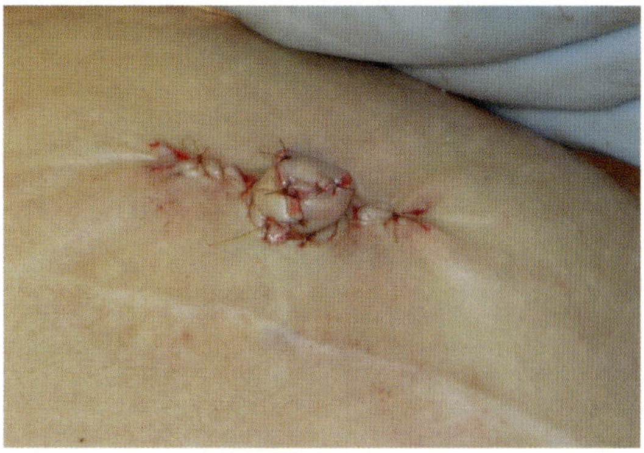

**Fig. 75.3** Outcome after flap inset

sides will determine the height of the nipple and length the diameter. The flap can then be closed primary as a V to Y advancement, creating two linear scars. In a review of 252 nipple reconstructions utilizing the C–V technique in patients undergoing autologous, hybrid, and implant-based reconstruction, the overall complication rate was 4%. The complications reported included tip necrosis in 3.2% and dehiscence in 0.8% of their patient population. 1.6% of patients underwent revision surgery for the loss of projection. Hybrid procedures were associated with the highest rates of complications followed by implant based, and autologous reconstructions had the lowest complication rates [25]. Overall there are limited comparative studies in the literature to determine the superiority between flap-based reconstruction techniques.

### 75.4.2 Graft-Based Nipple Reconstruction and Nipple Sharing

Skin graft nipple reconstruction, once popular in the origins of NAC reconstruction, is now of limited use. Donor site morbidity secondary to harvesting the graft from pigmented sites, often insensitive areas including the labia minora, labia majora, and inner thigh, is undesirable to most patients. In addition, there are unpredictable rates of graft take that are dependent on often tenuous recipient sites as well as patient comorbidities. Composite nipple grafting, however, is now becoming more popularized as it provides the most optimal aesthetic outcomes in matching color and texture, in addition to providing reliable long-term projection. Appropriate candidates for nipple sharing must have a nipple projection of at least 8 mm. The distal 50% of the contralateral nipple is removed, and thus the patient must be amenable to decrease the size of their native nipple. The harvested tip is inset on the deepithelialized recipient bed. Skin grafting has been described to create the areola; however, most women elect for nipple tattooing. The major complications associated with nipple sharing are loss of sensation and erectile function of the native nipple. Modifications of this technique reported to decrease sensation loss include harvesting a wedge of the superior or superomedial rim to preserve the lateral cutaneous branch of the fourth intercostal nerve. In addition, one can harvest a circular rim of tissue at the periphery of the areola to construct the contralateral nipple. This technique preserves the lactiferous ducts and thus the ability to breastfeed. Other complications reported with this technique are chronic pain, asymmetry, and scar formation in the donor nipple [26]. While over half of women will experience an initial decrease in the donor nipple sensation, sensation typically improves with time. Zenn and Garofalo [27] reviewed outcomes in 57 patients who underwent contralateral nipple grafting, and while a majority of patients reported a "change" in sensation, the majority of patients were happy with the final appearance.

### 75.4.3 Nipple Augmentation

Some advocate the use of autologous, allogeneic, or synthetic tissue to augment local flaps. Autologous tissue utilized includes dermal grafts, fat, cartilage, and bone. Autologous tissue harvest is dependent on abundance and ease of harvest while limiting donor site morbidity [26]. Fat harvested by liposuction for fat grafting in revisional breast surgery can also be injected at the base of the reconstructed nipple. Adequate amounts of fat must be injected to account for predictable losses from reabsorption. However, one must be cautious of placing undue pressure on the flap and in turn compromising blood supply. It is recommended to inject no more than 1–2 mL of fat for the purposes of nipple reconstruction [28]. In addition, incorporating too much adipose tissue leads to migration of fat resulting asymmetry. To date there is limited literature on long-term outcomes of this technique. Cartilage, shaped in a cylindrical construct, can provide support and prevent collapse of the overlying skin flap. Small fragments of cartilage placed underneath the projected areola can also recreate the texture of Montgomery tubercles. Studies cite stable long-term projection with only a 4% rate of cartilage loss [29]. The rib cartilage from an initial flap-based breast reconstruction can be banked in subcutaneous tissue for anticipated nipple reconstruction for several months [30]. No significant resorption or warping of the cartilage has been reported with banking. Dermal grafts can be harvested from the breast or abdominal tissue during revision procedures, such as dog-ear excision. Similar to the cartilage, a cylindrical construct can be made with the dermis, and it is placed at the base of the reconstructed flap. Maintenance in long-term projection is reported to be over 70% in autologous-based reconstruction and over 60% in implant based without any significant increase in complication rates [31].

Allogeneic tissue used for augmentation includes acellular dermal matrices and ECM components in the form of fillers. Acellular dermal matrices have been proven to be advantageous in implant-based breast reconstruction by providing soft tissue coverage and reinforcement of the implant. Over time the matrices presumably become vascularized and may play a protective role in radiated tissues. Allogeneic augmentation with ADM provides reliable long-term projection with low complication rates and no donor site morbidity. In a series of 30 patients, ADM maintains 56% of projection in autologous reconstructions and 47% in implant-based reconstructions over 12 months. No complications were noted in this series [32]. Unfortunately, there is no clear evidence of improved outcomes compared to dermal flaps, and the radioprotective effects have not been evaluated with respect to nipple reconstruction. Therefore, substantial cost of these materials limits its applicability. Evans utilized injectable calcium hydroxyapatite in cellulose gel (Radiesse™) to augment reconstructed nipples, with most patients satisfied with improvement in nipple appearance [33]. Panettiere et al. [34] have utilized hyaluronic acid for augmentation, also with durable results, though the trial reported a false-positive result on a PET scan with respect to cancer recurrence.

Silicone or synthetic polymers such as polyurethane and polytetrafluoroethylene have also been utilized in nipple augmentation. Hillock advocated the use of a silicone "gumdrop"-shaped implant for nipple fabrication as a salvage-type procedure, reporting good projection after a year in two patients [35]. However, high complication rates have been reported with silicone augmentation with a 30% rate of nipple necrosis and silicone exposure [36]. The use of artificial bone substance (Certatite™) has also been proposed [37, 38]. In a systematic review comparing modalities of nipple augmentation, synthetic components provided the most sustainable projection over time at the consequence of having the highest complication rates specifically with respect to migration and extrusion [26].

### 75.4.4 Nipple Tattooing and 3D Nipple Tattooing

Nipple tattooing was initially considered an adjunct to flap- or graft-based nipple reconstruction to create natural pigmentation of the NAC. It is now being offered as the sole modality of nipple reconstruction in patients without sufficient skin for flap-based nipple reconstruction and women that do not desire a graft-based reconstruction. Early nipple tattooing was one dimensional, applying a single set of colors and the use of concentric circles. 3D nipple tattooing is a relatively new technique, which creates an optical illusion of projection with shadowing and highlights (Figs. 75.4, 75.5, 75.6, and 75.7). It was initially performed by tattoo artists but is

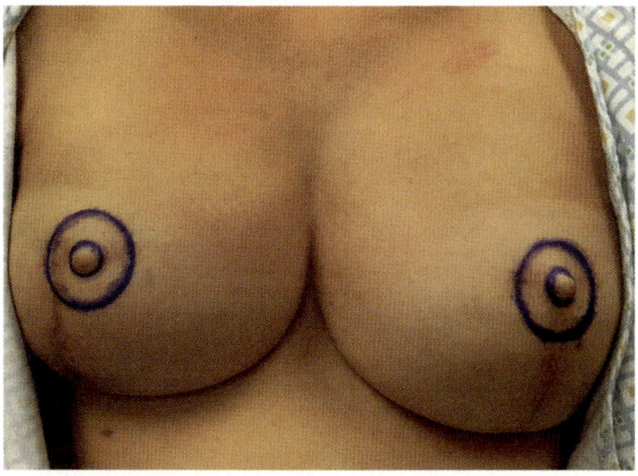

**Fig. 75.4** Bilateral nipple reconstruction with markings for nipple-areolar tattooing

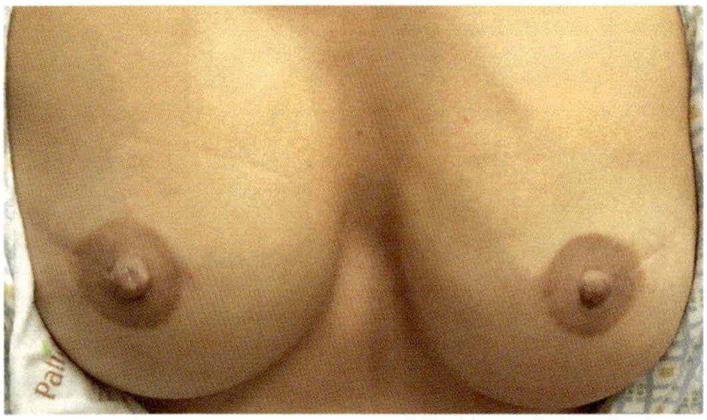

**Fig. 75.5** Bilateral nipple reconstruction after nipple tattooing

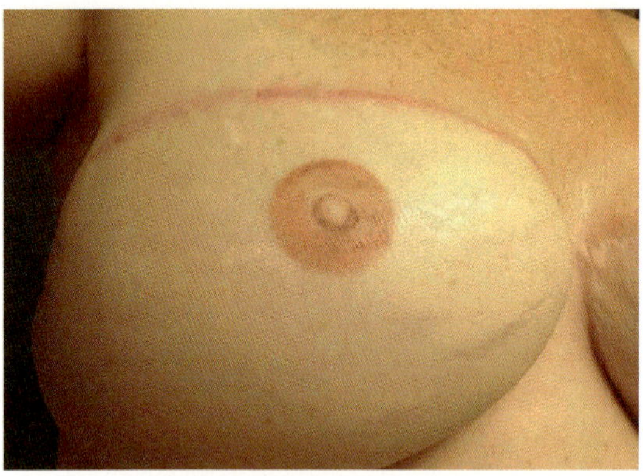

**Fig. 75.6** 3D nipple tattooing

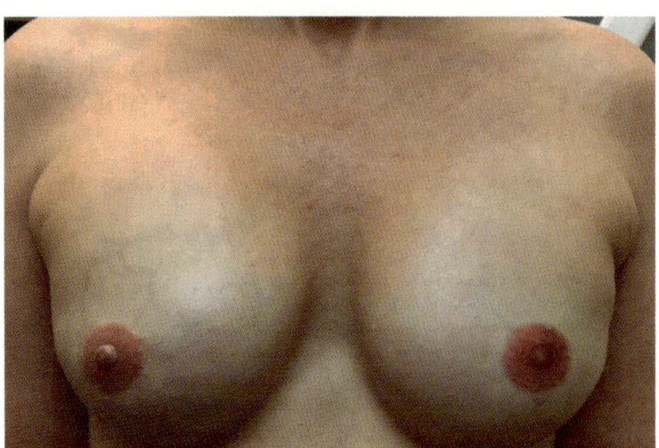

**Fig. 75.7** Unilateral nipple reconstruction with 3D nipple tattooing

now proving to be a valuable skillset used by healthcare providers. Complications associated with nipple tattooing include allergic reaction to the ink, inappropriate color matching, and fading of the tattoo over time. Most patients will require repeat sessions to maintain optimal results. There are recommended shades of ink dependent on the Fitzpatrick scale, but the ink used ultimately depends on the contralateral nipple as well as the patient's preference. Nipple tattooing is typically performed as a separate procedure after NAC reconstruction. While there have been reports of single-stage NAC reconstructions, it is associated with a 17% complication rate [39]. The majority of complications were irregular dye uptake, which may be related to increase inflammatory reaction and macrophage degradation associated with combined procedures.

### 75.4.5 Timing of Nipple Reconstruction

Timing of the NAC reconstruction is critical as adjuvant therapies may change breast dimensions that may lead to asymmetry of a previously reconstructed nipple. Most advocate nipple-areolar reconstruction to be performed 6 weeks to 3 months after breast mound reconstruction and adjuvant treatment [40]. This allows for the reconstructed breast mound to reach its final position for optimal nipple placement. Nipple reconstruction at the time of the breast mound reconstruction is associated with better outcomes in autologous versus implant-based reconstruction. Williams et al. [41] found that immediate nipple reconstruction in the setting of free TRAM resulted in similar complication rates and patient satisfaction as delayed nipple reconstruction. Immediate nipple reconstruction in the setting of implant-based reconstruction leads to an increase in complication rates secondary to paucity of the skin, thin skin envelope, and compressive forces from the implant, placing it at a higher risk for vascular compromise. It is currently advocated that immediate nipple reconstruction should only be attempted in the setting of autologous breast reconstruction.

## 75.5 Outcomes

In a literature review of over 2000 nipple-areolar reconstructions, local flaps had an overall complication rate of 7.9% with no significant difference noted between techniques. Skin graft-based reconstruction was associated with the highest complication rate of 46.9%. Allogeneic and autologous augmentation complication rates were 5.3%. Nipple tattooing for areolar reconstruction had a complication rate of 1.6% compared to 10.1% of areolar reconstruction with skin grafting. Composite nipple grafting was not included in this analysis [42]. In our series we found a total complication rate of 13.2% for nipple reconstruction in the setting of implant-based reconstruction. We found no correlation with implant fill volume and the incidence of complications. Prior radiation exposure to the breast was the only risk factor identified, increasing the complication rate by eightfold [43]. In another series performed at our institution, a "matched-pair" analysis was utilized comparing complication rates in patients undergoing bilateral nipple reconstruction after unilateral radiation therapy. We found a sevenfold increase risk of complications on the radiated side [44]. Satteson et al. [2] reviewed 641 nipple reconstructions and found that implant-based reconstruction and radiotherapy were independent risk factors for complications. Interestingly, patient comorbidities including hypertension, diabetes, BMI, and smoking status in addition to implant volume were not found to be significant risk factors. Tissue expansion causes thinning of the dermis, which attenuates the blood supply in the subdermal plexus. The subdermal plexus is the sole blood supply to the nipple flap or graft. Radiation adds a second insult with progressive fibrosis, depletion of resident stem cells, and impaired vascularity. Therefore, one must proceed with caution when performing nipple reconstruction in the face of prior radiation and implant-based breast reconstruction. For tissues that are atrophic and fibrotic and, hence, are at increased risk of wound complications, there should be a strong consideration for performing areolar tattooing alone.

The long-term projection for nipple reconstruction is also dependent on the immediate postoperative care. Over a period of 6 months and beyond, it is not uncommon for nipple reconstructions to lose up to 70% of projection immediately postoperatively. This is thought to be due in part to contractile forces on the wound. There is some evidence that specialized nipple guards applied postoperatively mitigate some contractile forces and may also protect the healing neonipple leading to more durable results. In a randomized trial, Asteame Nipple Guard™ was compared to dry gauze dressing for 6 weeks postoperatively with the device arm of the study showing decreased loss of nipple projection at 6 months (46.6% projection loss in the experiment group versus 71.8% in the control) [45].

## Conclusions

Many techniques have been described in the literature for nipple reconstruction with no sole optimal method achieving pleasing aesthetics while limiting morbidity. It is difficult to compare outcomes between techniques as most studies are underpowered and do not control for patient comorbidities. General principles can be applied to maximize outcomes such as minimizing tension, designing the pedicle away from existing scars, and providing a wide base to the pedicle to allow adequate blood supply. Loss of projection with time is inevitable and related to wound contracture and external pressure applied. Judicious postoperative care is warranted with prevention of compression with lose fitting clothing to protective dressings and nipple guards. Initial over-projection must also be considered to account for later losses. NAC reconstruction is the final stage of breast reconstruction and correlates significantly with patient satisfaction. In this competitive healthcare market, patient satisfaction is critical, and it is important that the patient understands all possible risks and complications. Nonetheless, breast reconstruction is a multidisciplinary process in which all aspects of breast cancer treatment contribute to the final outcome. Therefore, optimal care is dependent on clear communication between the breast surgeon, medical oncologist, reconstructive team, and the patient.

## References


1. Momoh AO, Colakoglu S, de Blacam C, Yueh JH, Lin SJ, Tobias AM, Lee BT. The impact of nipple reconstruction on patient satisfaction in breast reconstruction. Ann Plast Surg. 2012;69:389–93.
2. Satteson ES, Reynolds MF, Bond AM, Pestana IA. An analysis of complication risk factors in 641 nipple reconstructions. Breast J. 2016;22(4):379–83.
3. Wei CH, Scott AM, Price AN, Miller HC, Klassen AF, Jhanwar SM, Mehrara BJ, Disa JJ, McCarthy C, Matros E, Cordeiro PG, Sacchini V, Pusic AL. Psychosocial and sexual well-being following nipple-sparing mastectomy and reconstruction. Breast J. 2016;22:10–7.
4. Grotting JC, Neligan PC. Plastic surgery. In: Breast, vol. vol. 5. Philadelphia: Elsevier Health Sciences; 2012.
5. Penn J. Breast reduction. Br J Plast Surg. 1955;7:357–71.
6. Liu Y-J, Thomson JG. Ideal anthropomorphic values of the female breast: correlation of pluralistic aesthetic evaluations with objective measurements. Ann Plast Surg. 2011;67:7–11.
7. Tepper OM, Unger JG, Small KH, Feldman D, Kumar N, Choi M, Karp NS. Mammometrics: the standardization of aesthetic and reconstructive breast surgery. Plast Reconstr Surg. 2010;125:393–400.
8. Westreich M. Anthropomorphic breast measurement: protocol and results in 50 women with aesthetically perfect breasts and clinical application. Plast Reconstr Surg. 1997;100:468–79.
9. Adams W. Free transplantation of the nipples and areola. Surgery. 1944;15:186–69.
10. Millard DRJ. Nipple and areola reconstruction by split-skin graft from the normal side. Plast Reconstr Surg. 1972;50:350–3.
11. Adams WM. Labial transplant for correction of loss of the nipple. Plast Reconstr Surg. 1949;4:295–8.
12. Brent B, Bostwick J. Nipple-areola reconstruction with auricular tissues. Plast Reconstr Surg. 1977;60:353–61.
13. Klatsky SA, Manson PN. Toe pulp free grafts in nipple reconstruction. Plast Reconstr Surg. 1981;68:245–8.
14. Cucin RL, Gaston JP. Case report: implantation of breast cancer in a transplanted nipple: a plea for preoperative screening. CA Cancer J Clin. 1981;31:281–3.
15. Chang WH. Nipple reconstruction with a T flap. Plast Reconstr Surg. 1984;73:140–3.
16. Hartrampf CRJ, Culbertson JH. A dermal-fat flap for nipple reconstruction. Plast Reconstr Surg. 1984;73(6):982.
17. Muruci A, Dantas JJ, Noguerira LR. Reconstruction of the nipple-areola complex. Plast Reconstr Surg. 1978;61:558–60.
18. Rees TD. Reconstruction of the breast areola by intradermal tattooing and transfer. Case report. Plast Reconstr Surg. 1975;55:620–1.
19. Becker H. The use of intradermal tattoo to enhance the final result of nipple-areola reconstruction. Plast Reconstr Surg. 1986;77:673–6.
20. Spear SL, Convit R, Little JW III. Intradermal tattoo as an adjunct to nipple-areola reconstruction. Plast Reconstr Surg. 1989;83:907–11.
21. Richter DF, Reichenberger MA, Faymonville C. Comparison of the nipple projection after reconstruction with three different methods. Handchir Mikrochir Plast Chir. 2004;36(6):374–8.
22. Anton M, Eskenazi LB, Hartrampf CR Jr. Nipple reconstruction with local flaps: star and wrap flaps. Perspect Plast Surg. 1991;5(1):67–78.
23. Kroll SS, Reece GP, Miller MJ, Evans GRD, Robb GL, Baldwin BJ, Wang BG, Schusterman MA. Comparison of nipple projection with the modified double-opposing tab and star flaps. Plast Reconstr Surg. 1997;99:1602–5.
24. Zhong T, Antony A, Cordeiro P. Surgical outcomes and nipple projection using the modified skate flap for nipple-areolar reconstruction in a series of 422 implant reconstructions. Ann Plast Surg. 2009;62(5):591.
25. Otterburn DM, Sikora KE, Losken A. An outcome evaluation following postmastectomy nipple reconstruction using the C-V flap technique. Ann Plast Surg. 2010;64:574–8.
26. Winocour S, Saksena A, Oh C, Wu PS, Laungani A, Baltzer H, Saint-Cyr M. A systematic review of comparison of autologous, allogeneic, and synthetic augmentation grafts in nipple reconstruction. Plast Reconstr Surg. 2016;137:14e–23e.
27. Zenn MR, Garofalo JA. Unilateral nipple reconstruction with nipple sharing: time for a second look. Plast Reconstr Surg. 2009;123:1648–53.
28. Bernard RW, Beran SJ. Autologous fat graft in nipple reconstruction. Plast Reconstr Surg. 2003;112:964–8.
29. Guerra AB, Khoobehi K, Metzinger SE, Allen RJ. New technique for nipple areola reconstruction: arrow flap and rib cartilage graft for long-lasting nipple projection. Ann Plast Surg. 2003;50:31–7.
30. Heitland A, Markowicz M, Koellensperger E, Allen R, Pallua N. Long-term nipple shrinkage following augmentation by an autologous rib cartilage transplant in free DIEP-flaps. J Plast Reconstr Aesthet Surg. 2006;59:1063–7.
31. Chia HL, Wong M, Tan BK. Nipple reconstruction with rolled dermal graft support. Arch Plast Surg. 2014;41:158–62.
32. Garramone CE, Lam B. Use of AlloDerm in primary nipple reconstruction to improve long-term nipple projection. Plast Reconstr Surg. 2007;119:1663–8.
33. Evans KK, Rasko Y, Lenert J, Olding M. The use of calcium hydroxylapatite for nipple projection after failed nipple-areolar reconstruction: early results. Ann Plast Surg. 2005;55:25–9.
34. Panettiere P, Marchetti L, Accorsi D. Filler injection enhances the projection of the reconstructed nipple: an original easy technique. Aesthet Plast Surg. 2005;29:287–94.

35. Hallock GG. Polyurethane nipple prosthesis. Ann Plast Surg. 1990;24:80–5.
36. Jankau J, Jaśkiewicz J, Ankiewicz A. A new method for using a silicone rod for permanent nipple projection after breast reconstruction procedures. Breast. 2011;20:124–8.
37. Wong RK, Wichterman L, Parson SD. Skin sparing nipple reconstruction with polytetrafluoroethylene implant. Ann Plast Surg. 2008;61:256–8.
38. Yanaga H. Nipple-areola reconstruction with a dermal-fat flap. Plast Reconstr Surg. 2003;112:1863–9.
39. Liliav B, Loeb J, Hassid VJ, Antony AK. Single-stage nipple-areolar complex reconstruction technique, outcomes, and patient satisfaction. Ann Plast Surg. 2014;73(5):492–7.
40. Nahabedian MY. Nipple reconstruction. Clin Plast Surg. 2007;34:131–7.
41. Williams EH, Rosenberg LZ, Kolm P, de la Torre JI, Fix RJ. Immediate nipple reconstruction on a free TRAM flap breast reconstruction. Plast Reconstr Surg. 2007;120:1115–24.
42. Sisti A, Grimaldi L, Tassinari J, Cuomo R, Fortezza L, Bocchiotti MA, Roviello F, D'Aniello C, Nisi G. Nipple-areola complex reconstruction techniques: a literature review. Eur J Surg Oncol. 2016;42:441–65.
43. Momeni A, Ghaly M, Gupta D, Karanas YL, Kahn DM, Gurtner GC, Lee GK. Nipple reconstruction: risk factors and complications after 189 procedures. Eur J Plast Surg. 2013;36:633–8.
44. Momeni A, Ghaly M, Gupta D, Gurtner G, Kahn DM, Karanas YL, Lee GK. Nipple reconstruction after implant-based breast reconstruction: a "matched-pair" outcome analysis focusing on the effects of radiotherapy. J Plast Reconstr Aesthet Surg. 2013;66:1202–5.
45. Rosing JH, Momeni A, Kamperman K, Kahn D, Gurtner G, Lee GK. Effectiveness of the Asteame Nipple Guard in maintaining projection following nipple reconstruction: a prospective randomised controlled trial. J Plast Reconstr Aesthet Surg. 2010;63:1592–6.

# 76 Managing Necrosis of the Nipple-Areolar Complex Following Reduction Mammaplasty and Mastopexy

Neal Handel and Sara Yegiyants

## 76.1 Introduction

Nipple-areolar complex ischemia may be due to arterial insufficiency but more commonly is caused by venous congestion [1]. Venous congestion can occur for a variety of reasons: inadequate preservation of venous drainage, long pedicles, kinking or compression of the pedicle, and excessively tight skin closure or a hematoma. Clinical signs of venous congestion include excessively brisk capillary refill, dark rapid bleeding on pinprick, and cyanosis and edema of the nipple. Systemic factors such as obesity, diabetes, and cigarette smoking may also increase the risk of ischemia.

The risk of nipple-areolar ischemia is also increased with large volume tissue resection, in transposition of the nipple-areolar complex to long distances (more than 15 cm) [2], and in cases where secondary mastopexy is performed in previously augmented patients [3].

The manifestations of NAC ischemia run the spectrum from spontaneous, completely reversible nipple congestion (Fig. 76.1) to total loss of the nipple (Fig. 76.2) with extensive necrosis of subadjacent breast tissue (Fig. 76.3). The appropriate response to nipple ischemia depends upon the severity of circulatory compromise. The guiding principle is to avoid aggressive surgical therapy as long as possible to give the injured tissues the best possible chance to recover spontaneously.

The objectives of this chapter are to explain the mechanisms of injury that result in ischemia of the NAC, to offer recommendations about the management of this complication, and to illustrate reconstructive techniques that can be used to correct deformities arising from necrosis of the NAC. With these goals in mind, the remainder

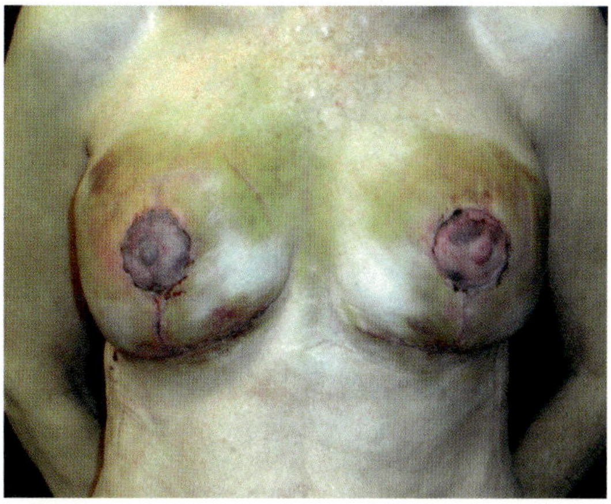

**Fig. 76.1** Reversible ischemia of the right NAC 48 h after reduction mammaplasty

N. Handel, M.D.
225 W. Pueblo St., Suite A, Santa Barbara, CA 93105, USA

Division of Plastic Surgery, Geffen School of Medicine at UCLA, Los Angeles, CA, USA
e-mail: info@drhandel.com

S. Yegiyants, M.D. (✉)
225 W Pueblo St, Santa Barbara, CA 93105, USA
e-mail: syegiyants@yahoo.com


M.A. Shiffman (ed.), *Nipple-Areolar Complex Reconstruction*,
https://doi.org/10.1007/978-3-319-60925-6_76

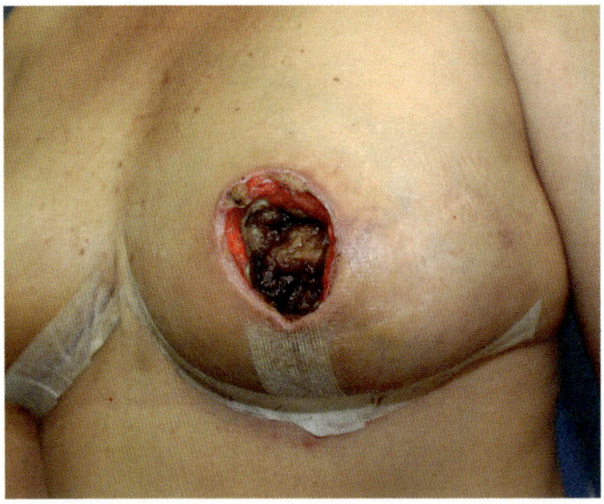

**Fig. 76.2** Complete necrosis of the left NAC 10 days post reduction mammaplasty

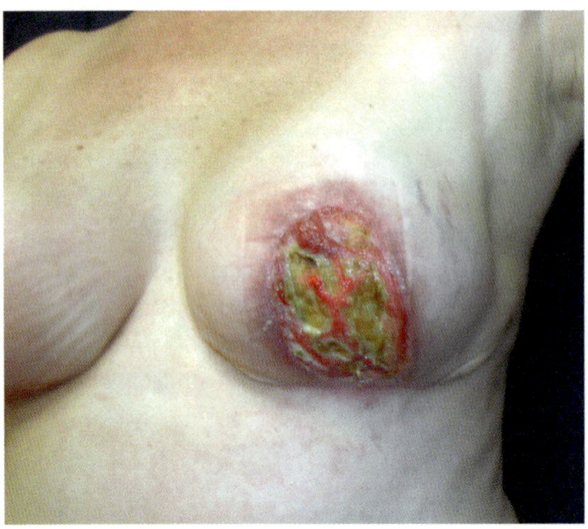

**Fig. 76.3** Total loss of the NAC and extensive fat necrosis of subadjacent breast tissue

of this chapter is divided into three sections: (1) prevention of ischemia of the nipple-areolar complex, (2) management of the ischemic nipple, and (3) reconstruction after ischemic necrosis of the nipple and areola.

## 76.2 Preventing Ischemia of the Nipple-Areolar Complex

Preventing ischemic complications is greatly preferable to treating a necrotic nipple and areola. When performing reduction mammaplasty or mastopexy, care must be taken to select the operation that will likely produce the best outcome with the least risk of complications.

Understanding the vascular anatomy of the breast is paramount in preserving the arterial inflow and the essential venous drainage network of the nipple-areolar complex. Cadaveric dissection studies have shown that the most reliable blood supply to the nipple-areolar complex is from the internal thoracic-anterior intercostal system, supplying the NAC from medio-inferior aspect. An additional collateral system composed of lateral thoracic and other minor contributors supplies the NAC from superolateral aspect [1]. Venograms of the breast have shown an extensive network of veins draining the NAC with the most reliable patterns located in superomedial/medial and inferior pedicles [4].

A wide variety of techniques have been described for transferring the nipple in breast reduction and mastopexy. Nipple transposition can be carried on an inferior pedicle, superior pedicle, and superomedial or central pedicles. The reported rates of nipple necrosis vary with the use of different pedicles ranging from 0.8% to 2.3% (0.8% with inferior pedicle, 2.1% total nipple necrosis with the use of superodermal pedicle, and 2.3% with superolateral pedicle) [1]. However, there are no randomized controlled trials comparing NAC necrosis rate for the different techniques.

In recent years, short-scar techniques including the vertical pattern [5] and SPAIR technique [6] have been introduced. Because there are so many possible combinations of skin pattern and vascular pedicle, it is difficult to objectively compare one technique to another. In a recent "matched cohort" study [7], the authors compared superomedial pedicle vertical scar breast reduction to inferior pedicle wise-pattern reduction and found there was no significant difference in complications between these two techniques. It is likely that adherence to the basic principles of plastic surgery is more critical than the particular surgical technique selected. Regardless of which approach is chosen, the surgeon must be careful to maintain a pedicle of adequate thickness, be cognizant of the length to width ratio of the pedicle, prevent kinking the blood supply when insetting the flap, and avoid excessively tight skin closure.

One group of patients especially at risk for ischemic complications of the NAC is previously augmented women with ptosis who present for mastopexy. These patients are at increased risk of circulatory compromise because of the inevitable changes in breast anatomy and physiology caused by implants. In many augmented patients, the soft tissue envelope surrounding the implant becomes attenuated. Most of the thinning and atrophy caused by implants occurs in the inferior pole of the breast. It is important to take this into account when selecting which pedicle to use in patients undergoing secondary mastopexy. A conventional wise-pattern skin excision coupled with an inferior pedicle may be prone to ischemia because of thinning of the tissues of the inferior pole. In such cases, it may be prudent to preserve a superior pedicle as well (as in a traditional McKissock reduction mammaplasty) to ensure adequate arterial perfusion and sufficient venous drainage. Vertical mastopexy techniques are applicable in previously augmented patients; however, vertical techniques that depend on an inferior pedicle, such as the short-scar periareolar-inferior pedicle reduction (or SPAIR) mammaplasty may be relatively contraindicated. Procedures that incorporate a superior pedicle (Lassus [8], Lejour [9], Hall-Findlay [10]) are probably safer in terms of preserving circulation to the nipple and areola.

When selecting the specific mastopexy operation for correction of ptosis in the augmented patient, there is a wide spectrum of procedures from which to choose. These include crescent nipple lift, periareolar mastopexy, vertical lift, and finally the conventional wise-pattern mastopexy. In general, the least aggressive mastopexy that will achieve the desired result is preferred. In secondary mastopexy patients, it is also critical to consider the effect of prior skin incisions on the blood supply of the nipple and the skin flaps and to avoid insertion of excessively large implant, which may cause compression of the vascular pedicle and lead to venous congestion.

## 76.3 Managing Ischemia of the Nipple-Areolar Complex

When circulatory compromise of the nipple and areola is recognized early, either in the operating room or in the immediate postoperative period, urgent steps should be undertaken to reduce permanent tissue loss. Recognition of irreversible ischemia of the nipple may be hard to determine by clinical criteria alone. Intravenous fluorescein has been used to assess viability of the nipple [11]. Indocyanine green videofluorography [12] is a newer technique that can be used to evaluate NAC viability intraoperatively. Advantages of this technique include repeated use during the same operation and ability to evaluate both the arterial microcirculation and venous outflow. Intraoperative detection of NAC nonviability is an indication to convert to a full-thickness graft. In cases where there is irreversible ischemia of the nipple, conversion of the nipple from a pedicle flap to a full-thickness graft can result in a satisfactory aesthetic outcome [13]. If it is elected to convert to a graft, it is crucial that the recipient site have an excellent blood supply.

Conversion of the nipple to a graft is indicated only dire cases. Usually when ischemia of the nipple is identified early, conservative measures are effective in reversing or at least ameliorating the problem (Fig. 76.4). Release of the dermal and subdermal sutures around the periphery of the areola may result in dramatic improvement in venous drainage with transformation of tissues from a violaceus hue to a pink color within a matter of minutes. The application of Nitro-Bid® (Nitroglycerin Ointment USP, 2%) may help by causing vasodilation and promoting drainage of blood. Steroids, such as a Medrol Dosepak® (methylprednisolone), have also been recommended to reduce local tissue swelling and promote venous drainage. Leeches can also be used to improve venous drainage [14]. Consideration should also be given to the use of hyperbaric oxygen therapy [15]. The mechanism of action of hyperbaric oxygen therapy is to increase tissue oxygen tension, which results in production of reactive oxygen species and reactive nitrogen species that promote neovascularization and improve postischemic tissue survival [16].

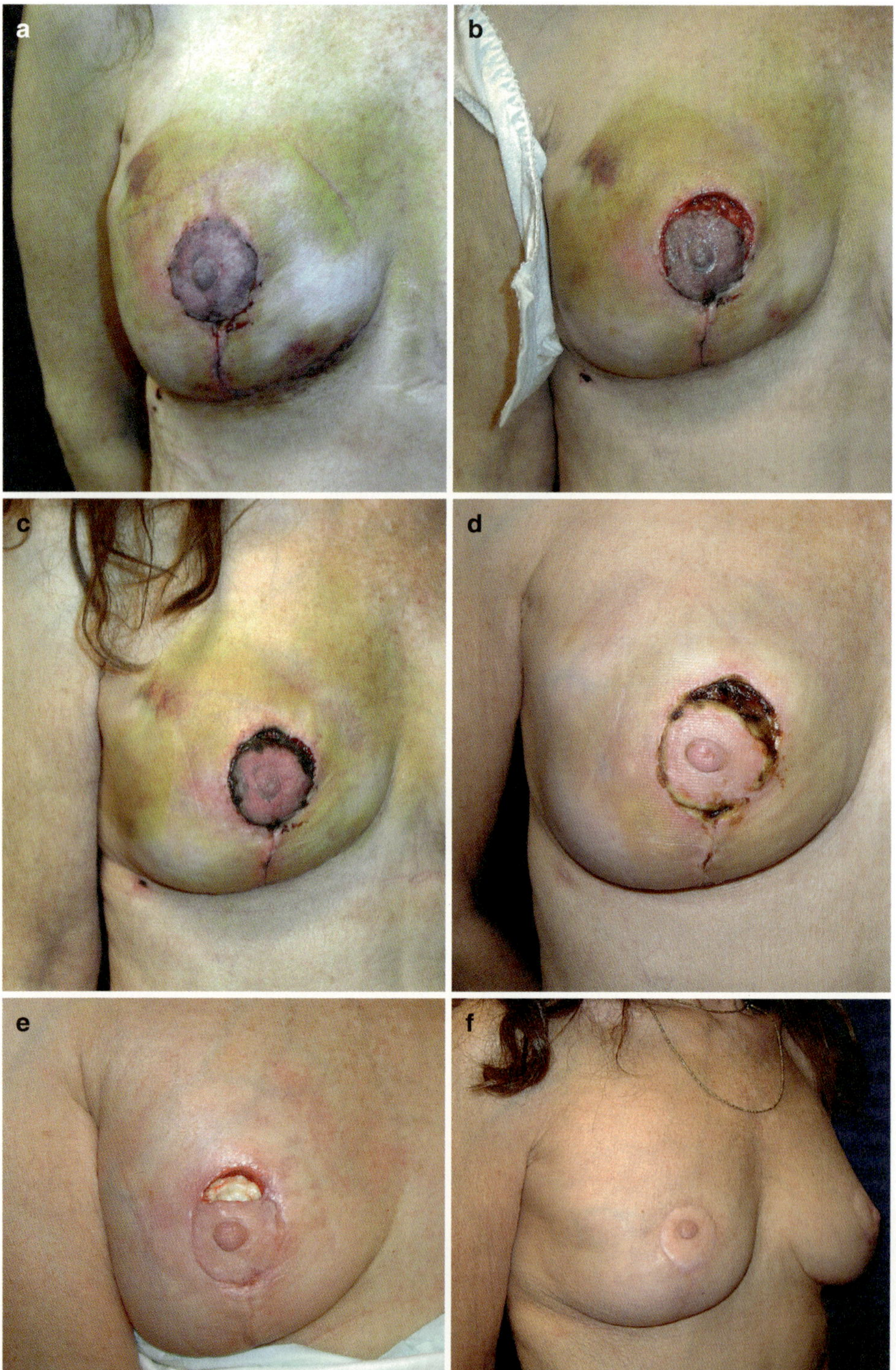


**Fig. 76.4** (**a**) Venous congestion of NAC 48 h after reduction mammaplasty. (**b**) Appearance of NAC 72 h postoperative after removal of skin and subdermal sutures. (**c**) Improved appearance of NAC at postoperative day (POD) #7. (**d**) Further improvement in circulation at POD #10. (**e**) Fat necrosis of underlying breast tissue treated by surgical debridement and delayed primary closure. (**f**) 18 months postoperative

The guiding principle in surgical management of ischemic complications of the nipple-areolar complex is to avoid aggressive treatment until the tissues have demarcated. It is often difficult early in the acute phase to gauge which tissues will ultimately prove viable and which tissues will necrose (Fig. 76.5). During the interim, it is advisable to maintain patients on oral antibiotics to reduce the risk of infection. A wide variety of antimicrobials are available and include drugs such as Penicillin VK 500 mg Q6H or cephalexin 500 mg Q6H. Consideration should be given to adding Bactrim DS BID to the regimen as prophylaxis against methicillin-resistant staphylococcus aureus. In addition to systemic antibiotics, topical antimicrobials may be used to further reduce the chance of secondary infection. Several topical agents are commonly used for this purpose, such as Neosporin® (neomycin-polymyxin B-bacitracin) triple antibiotic ointment or Silvadene® (1% silver sulfadiazine) cream.

Once the tissues have demarcated, a decision can be made about appropriate surgical management. If the area of nonviable tissue is limited (partial loss of nipple, subtotal loss of areola), allowing the necrotic tissues to slough and the resulting defect to heal by secondary intention may be the most prudent approach. If the amount of necrotic tissue is more sizeable, debridement and delayed primary closure may be indicated (Fig. 76.6). Regardless of whether the defect is allowed to close spontaneously or is closed surgically, there

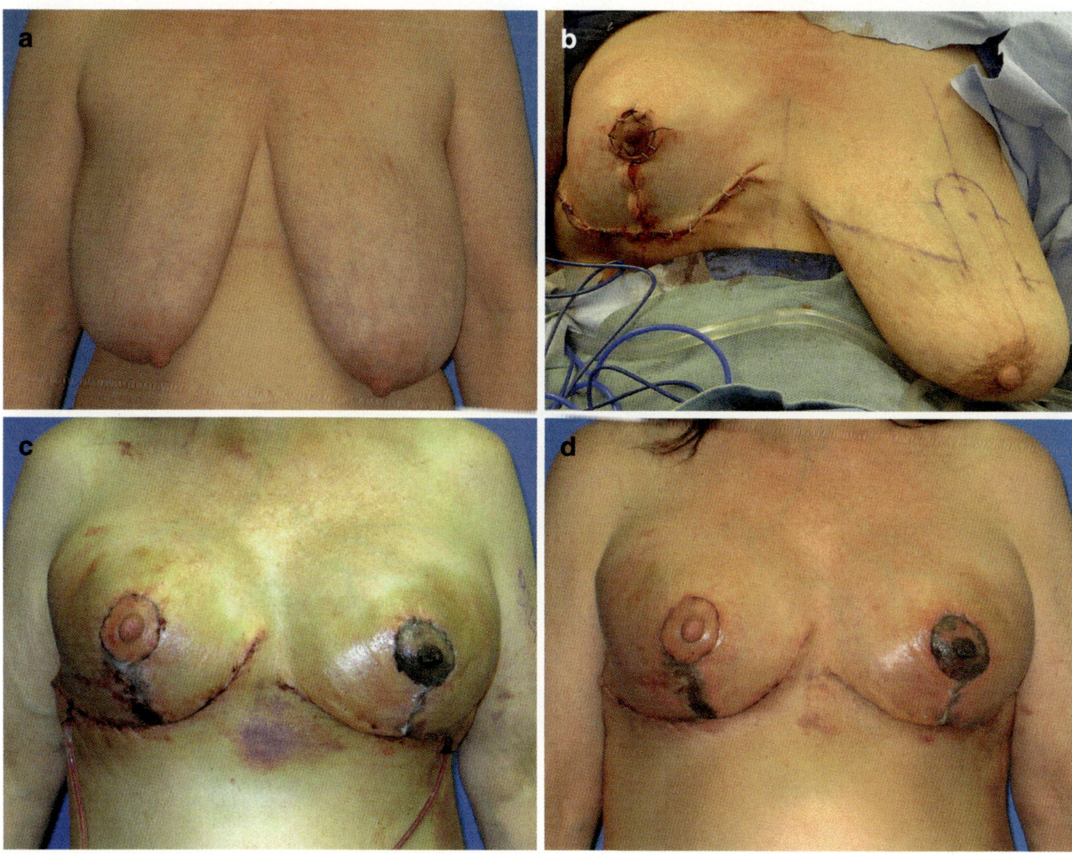


**Fig. 76.5** (**a**) Preoperative patient with extremely pendulous breasts. (**b**) Intraoperatively after reduction of the right breast performed with central pedicle and wise skin excision (nipple elevated approx. 20 cm). (**c**) Appearance on POD #2. (**d**) Appearance on POD #5. (**e**) Appearance on POD #9. (**f**) Appearance at 2 weeks. (**g**) Appearance at 3 weeks. (**h**) Appearance at 5 weeks. (**i**) Appearance at 2 months. (**j**) Appearance at 3 months. (**k**) Appearance at 4 months. (**l**) Appearance at 2 years. Patient was offered further reconstruction of left NAC but declined additional surgery. (**m**) Appearance at 7 years without reconstruction

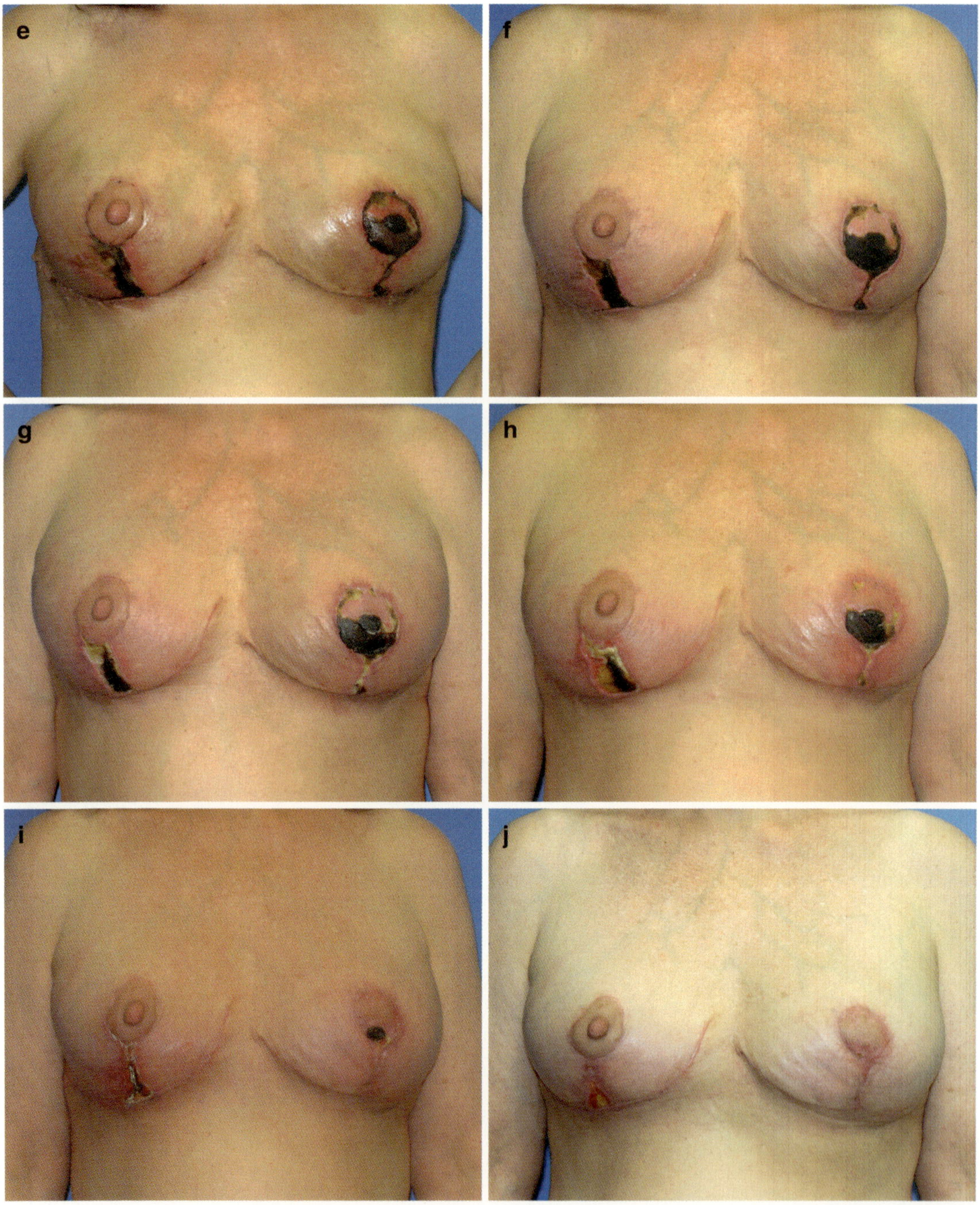


Fig. 76.5 (continued)

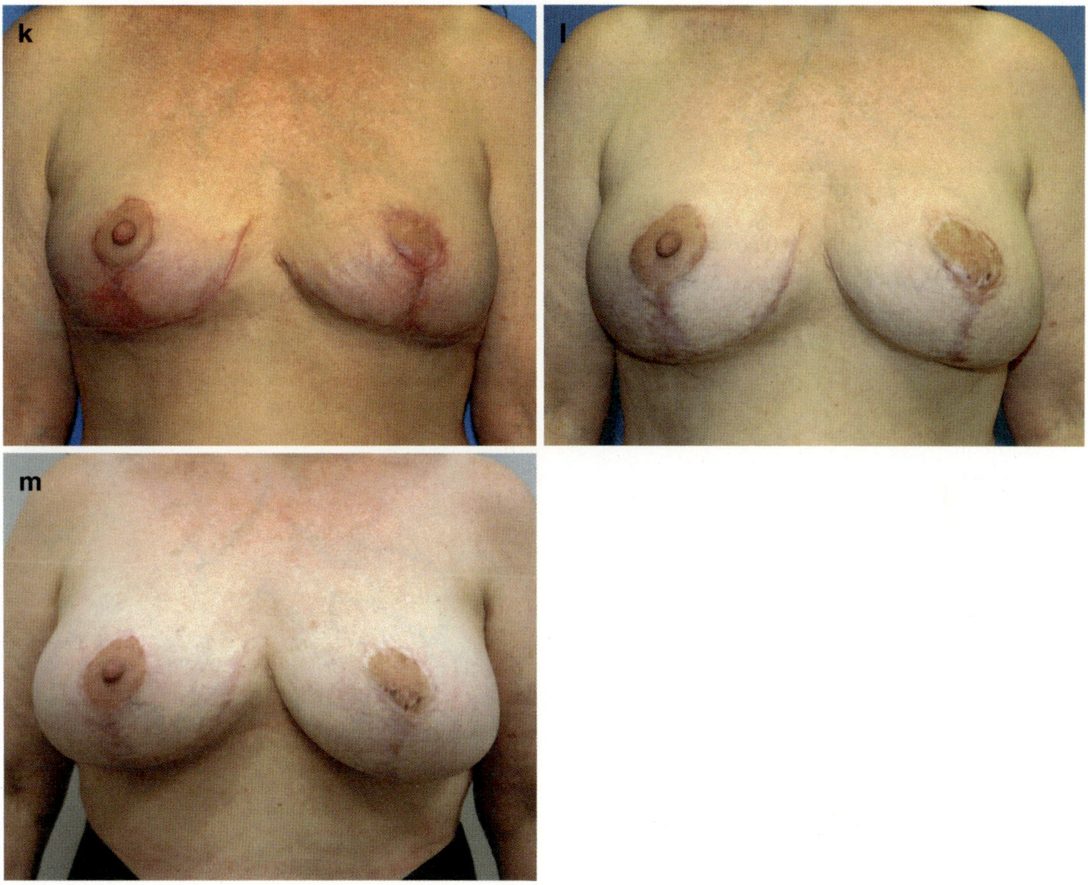

**Fig. 76.5** (continued)

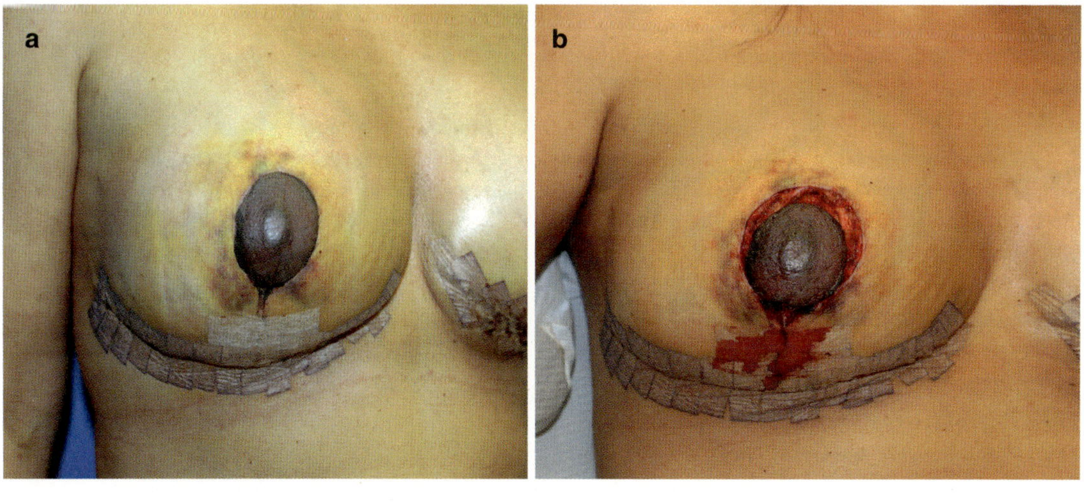

**Fig. 76.6** (**a**) Impaired circulation of right NAC 5 days post reduction mammaplasty. (**b**) Immediately following removal of skin and subdermal sutures *color* of NAC improved. (**c**) Nitroglycerine ointment applied to ischemic NAC. (**d**) Despite conservative measures, NAC undergoes complete necrosis by POD #10. (**e**) Appearance shortly after debridement of all nonviable tissue and closure of defect

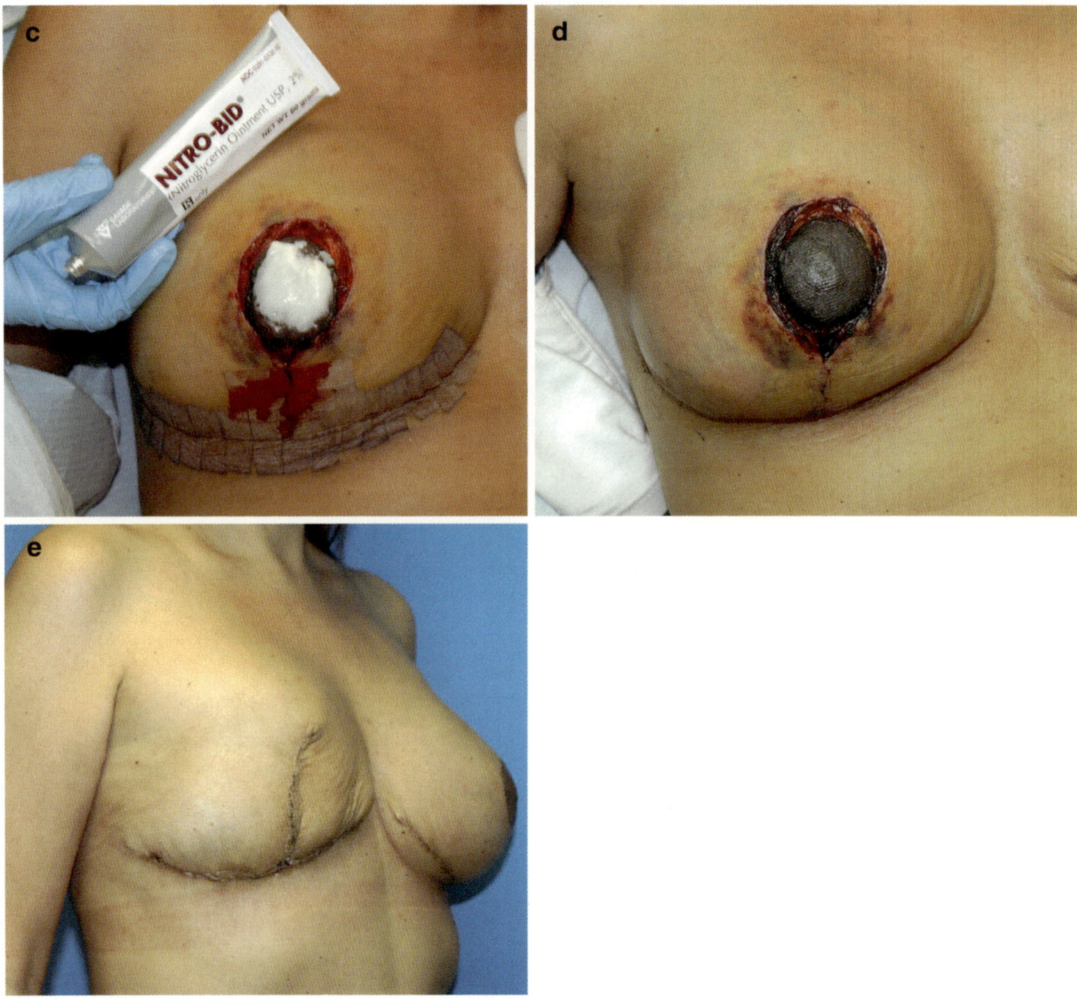


**Fig. 76.6** (continued)

should be a delay before any reconstructive procedure is attempted. It is critical to give the injured tissues time to "recover" before proceeding with further intervention. A waiting period of 3 to 6 months is usually adequate to allow for resolution of inflammation, improvement in local circulation, and maturation and softening of scar tissue.

## 76.4 Reconstruction of the Necrotic Nipple and Areola

The appropriate reconstructive procedure depends upon the nature of the deficit. In some cases, the amount of "missing" tissue is negligible, which facilitates reconstruction. For example, if only a portion of the areola is absent, it may be possible to reconstruct the defect with a full-thickness graft from the contralateral areola. Likewise, if the areola is intact but part of or even the entire nipple has been lost, a composite graft from the opposite nipple may be indicated (assuming there is adequate tissue for "sharing"). In some cases, there is residual nipple and/or areola, but the degree of tissue damage or tissue loss is so extensive that best approach is to discard the remaining tissue and perform de novo nipple-areolar reconstruction. In such cases, or when the NAC has been completely lost, there are many excellent techniques for recreating a natural-appearing nipple.

A variety of operations have been described for reconstruction of the nipple. Composite grafts, such as the pulp of the toe [17] or the earlobe, have been used to reconstruct the missing nipple. However, even when these grafts take successfully, they do not match the texture or pigmentation of a normal nipple. Composite grafts from the contralateral nipple can yield an excellent aesthetic result provided there is adequate nipple on the intact side to serve as a donor site. More commonly, the nipple is reconstructed with local tissues. These procedures typically consist of some type random flap, which is elevated and rotated or folded to create a projecting structure of the desired size and shape. Among the operations that have been described are the star flap [18, 19], the double-opposing tab flap [20], and the double-opposing periareolar flap [21]. Most of these techniques are derivatives of the "skate" flap [22], which has proven to be a safe and reliable technique for reconstruction of the nipple [23].

It is critical to remember that reconstruction of the nipple in patients who have suffered ischemic necrosis of the native NAC differs substantially from reconstruction of the nipple in mastectomy patients. Patients who have lost their NAC as a result of ischemic complications are more likely to have scarred, poorly vascularized tissues at the site of the proposed reconstruction. When planning nipple reconstruction, it is important to consider the quality of the local tissues in designing pedicles to ensure the best chance of flap survival (Figs. 76.7 and 76.8).

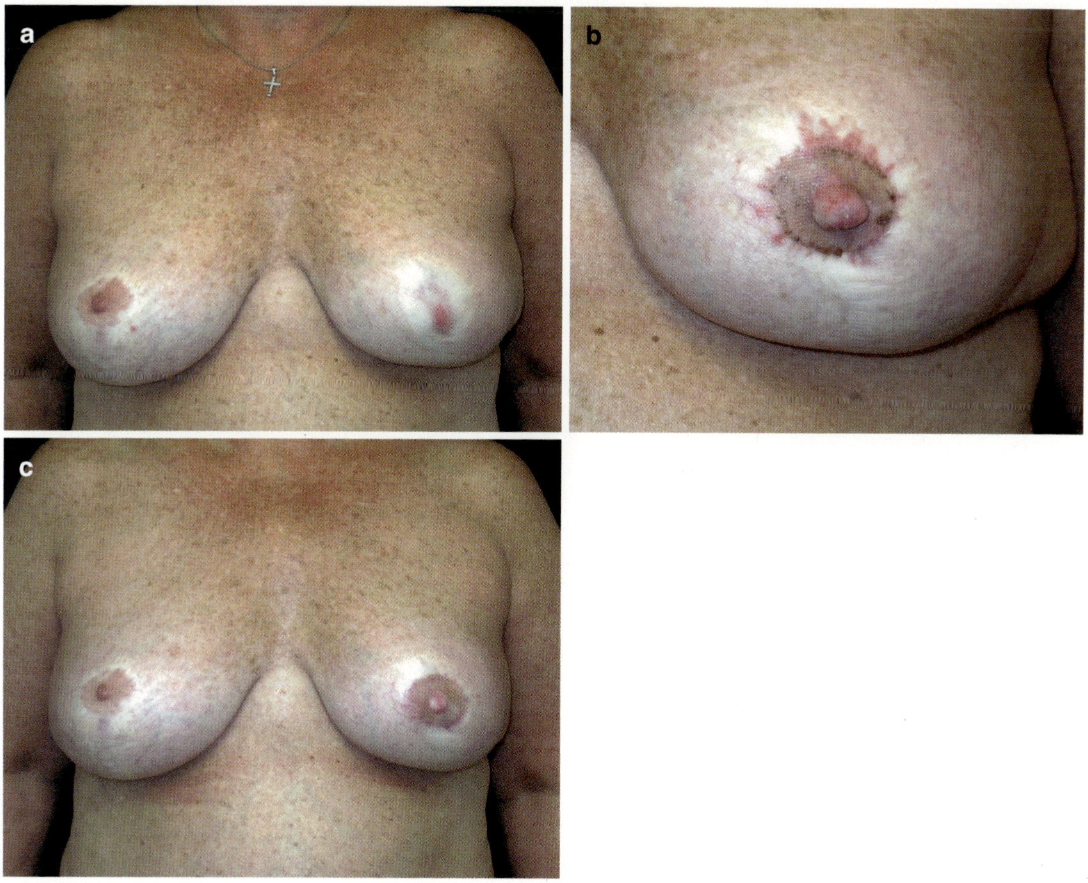

**Fig. 76.7** (**a**) Patient referred for reconstruction of left NAC lost following reduction mammaplasty. (**b**) Appearance of reconstructed NAC 3 weeks postoperative. Nipple was reconstructed with a modified skate flap and areola from full-thickness skin graft from the upper inner thigh. (**c**) One year following reconstruction, there has been some loss of projection of the reconstructed nipple which is typical in these cases

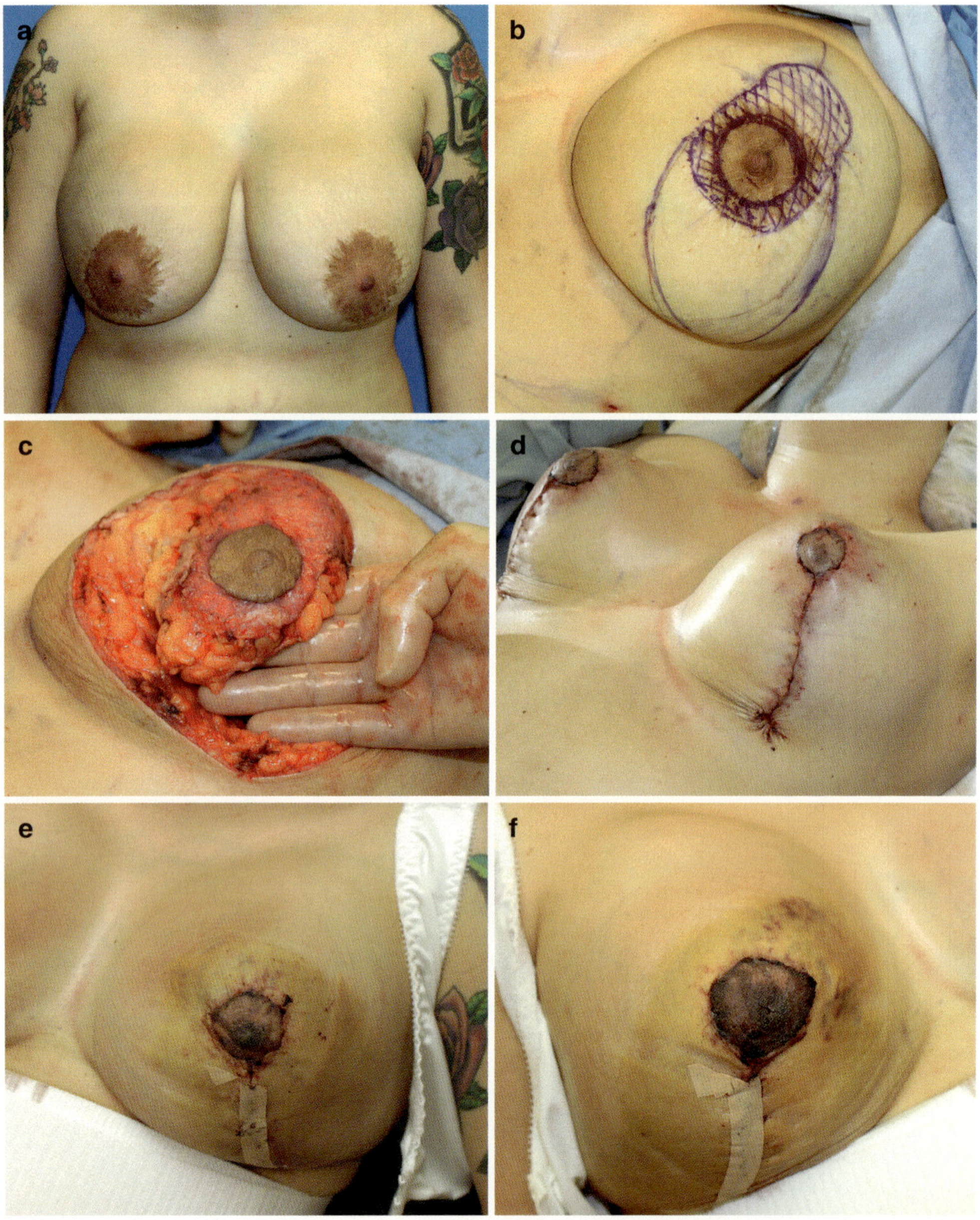


**Fig. 76.8** (**a**) A 23-year-old woman who previously had bilateral augmentation mammaplasty and circumareolar mastopexy presents with dissatisfaction due to persistent breast ptosis and disfigured NACs. (**b**) Design for vertical mastopexy with superior pedicle for transposition of nipple. (**c**) Intraoperative after nipple has been mobilized. Note relatively short distance nipple needs to be raised and thick (3 cm) superior pedicle. (**d**) Appearance of the breast at completion of procedure. Both NACs appear viable. (**e**, **f**) Appearance 4 days postoperative. Significant venous congestion of NACs, *right side* worse than *left side*, dermal sutures released and nitroglycerine paste applied. (**g**, **h**) Appearance ten days postoperative with necrotic eschar separating revealing partial survival of areola bilaterally. (**i**, **j**) Appearance 24 days postoperative. Central band of tissue on *left side* has survived, but only tiny amount of tissue on *right side* is viable. (**k**) Six weeks postoperative. Open areas characterized by healthy granulation tissue. Patient undergoes delayed primary closure of wounds bilaterally. (**l**) By 4 months after delayed closure, both breasts have healed. (**m**) At 6 months, tissues have softened and scars have matured; patient is ready for reconstruction. (**n**, **o**) Three months following bilateral NAC reconstruction. Nipple has been created using a modified skate flap with care taken to incorporate residual pigmented tissue into reconstructed papilla; areolas have been reconstructed from full-thickness skin grafts from the upper inner thigh

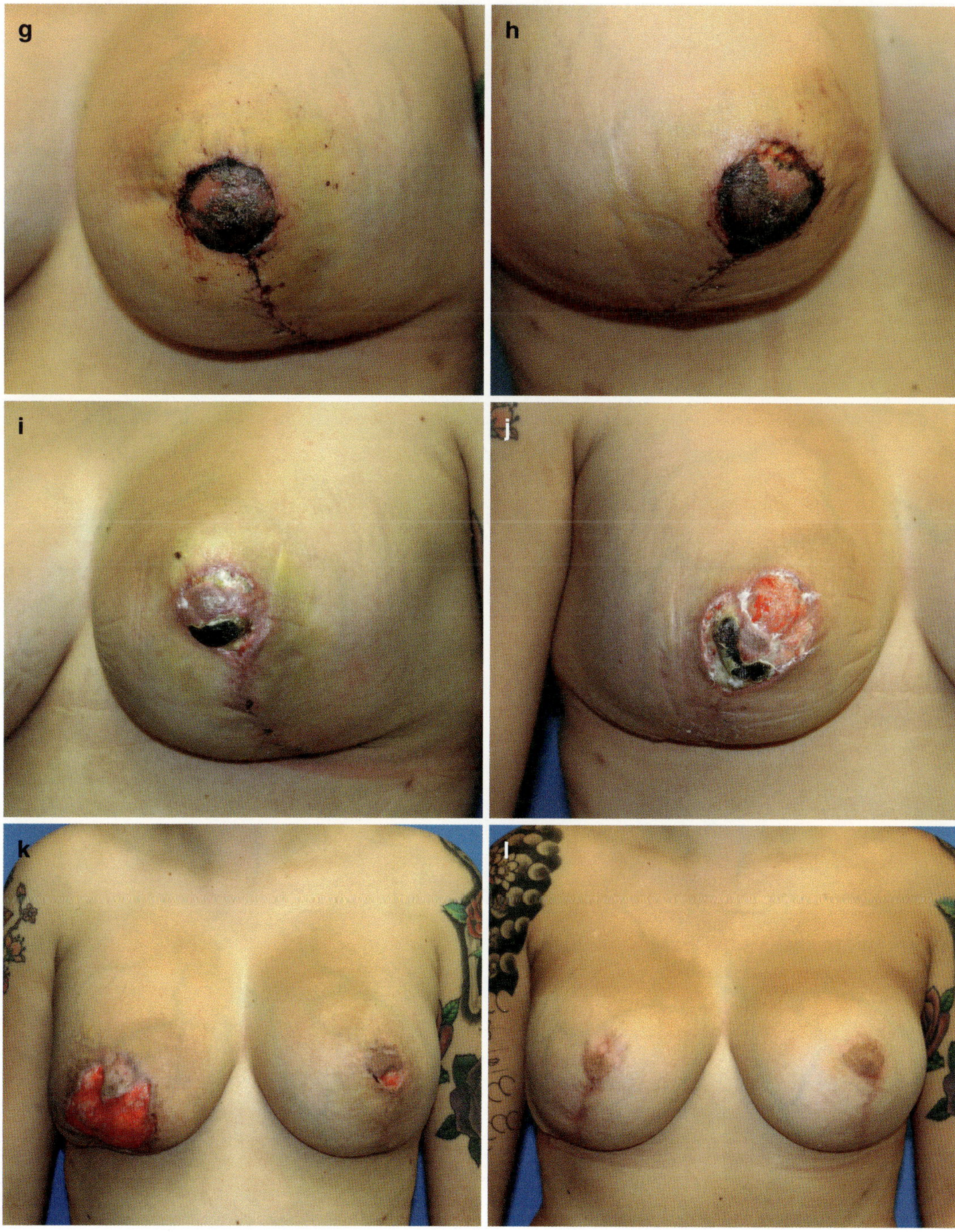


**Fig. 76.8** (continued)

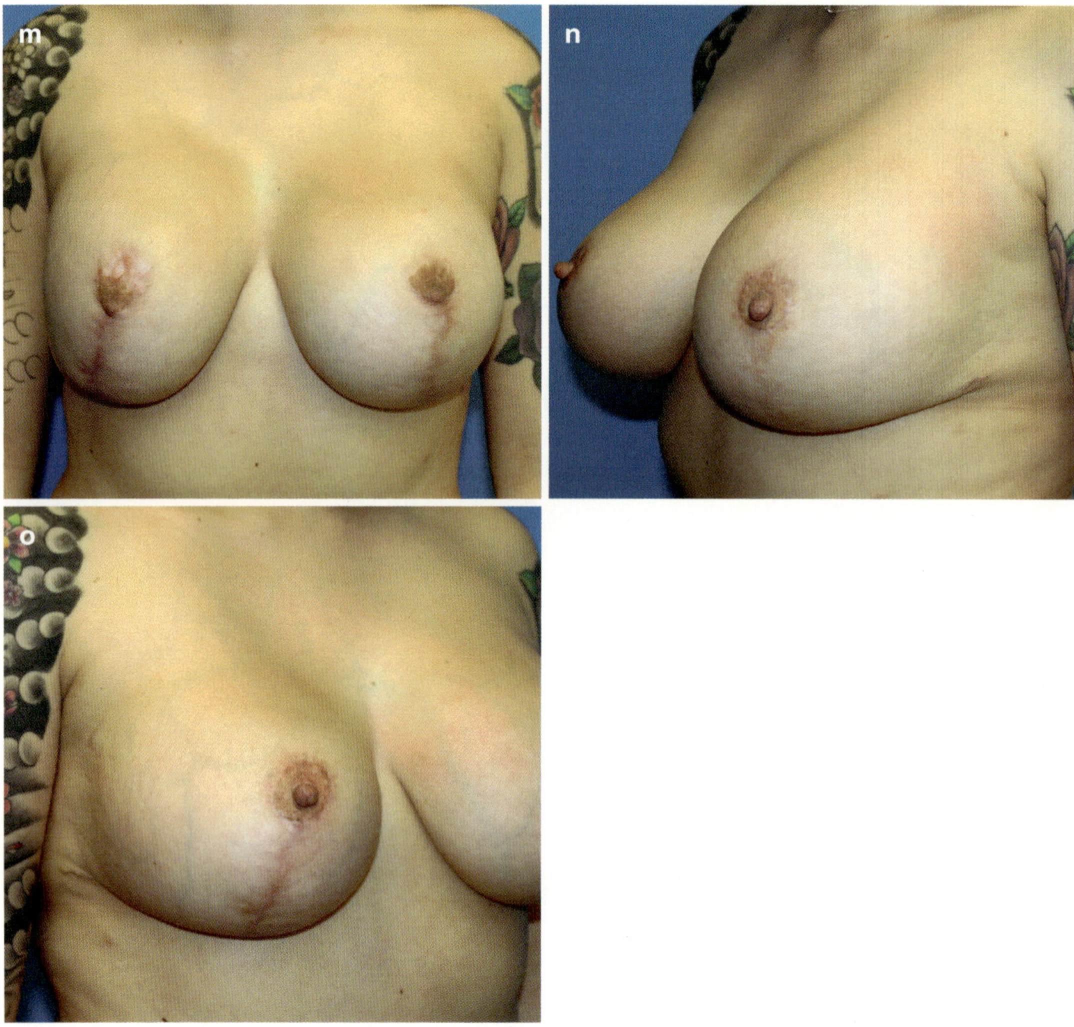


**Fig. 76.8** (continued)

With regard to reconstruction of the areola, the most natural-appearing areola is created using a full-thickness skin graft from the contralateral breast. The feasibility of using the opposite areola as a donor site depends of course upon how much tissue is available for harvesting. Fortunately, the areola tends to be a very "elastic" structure, and if a washer-shaped piece of pigmented skin is harvested from the periphery of the intact areola, the residual pigmented skin will usually stretch enough so the donor areola maintains a reasonable size. Other sites that have been used for areolar reconstruction include full-thickness grafts from the labia minora and the upper inner thigh. While the early results of these grafts are often very pleasing, there is a tendency for the grafted skin to lose pigmentation over time. Frequently after an interval of 2–3 years following reconstruction, the pigmentation has completely faded, and the only indication of areolar reconstruction is a circular scar around the periphery of the reconstructed nipple. For this reason, intradermal tattooing has gained great popularity for areolar reconstruction. Tattooing can be employed either with or without preliminary skin grafting [24]. The tattooed areola may also fade over time, but "touch-up" tattooing is a relatively easy way to restore the desired pigmentation.

Necrosis of all or part of the NAC after reduction mammaplasty or mastopexy is a devastating complication. It is not only disappointing for patients but also can be disheartening for the surgeon. However, with properly timed and well-executed reconstructive procedures, it is possible in most cases to restore a very natural-appearing nipple-areolar complex.

## References

1. van Deventer PV, Page BJ, Graewe FR. The safety of pedicles in breast reduction and mastopexy procedures. Aesthet Plast Surg. 2008;32:307–12.
2. Gravante G, Araco A, Sorge R, et al. Postoperative wound infections after breast reductions: the role of smoking and the amount of tissue removed. Aesthet Plast Surg. 2008;32:25–31.
3. Handel N. Secondary mastopexy in the augmented patient: a recipe for disaster. Plast Reconstr Surg. 2006;118(7 Suppl):152S–63S.
4. le Roux CM, Pan WR, Matousek SA. Preventing venous congestion of the nipple-areola complex: an anantomical guide to preserving essential venous drainage networks. Plast Reconstr Surg. 2011;127(3):1073–9.
5. Hall-Findlay EJ. Vertical breast reduction with a medially based pedicle. Aesthet Surg J. 2002;22:185–94.
6. Hammond DC. Short scar periareolar inferior pedicle reduction (SPAIR) mammaplasty. Plast Reconstr Surg. 1999;103:890–901.
7. Antony AK, Yegiyants SS, Danielson KK, et al. A matched cohort study of superomedial pedicle vertical scar breast reduction (100 breasts) and traditional inferior pedicle Wise-pattern reduction (100 breasts): an outcomes study over 3 years. Plast Reconstr Surg. 2013;132(5):1068–76.
8. Lassus C. A technique for breast reduction. Int Surg. 1970;53(1):69–72.
9. Lejour M. Vertical mammaplasty. Plast Reconstr Surg. 1993;92(5):985–6.
10. Hall-Findlay EJ. A simplified vertical reduction mammaplasty: shortening the learning curve. Plast Reconstr Surg. 1999;104(3):748–59.
11. Singer R, Krant SM. Intravenous fluorescein for evaluating the dusky nipple-areola during reduction mammaplasty. Plast Reconstr Surg. 1981;67(4):534–5.
12. Murray JD, Jones GE, Elwood T. Fluorescent intraoperative tissue angiography with indocyanine green: evaluation of nipple-areola vascularity during breast reduction surgery. Plast Reconstr Surg. 2010;126(1):33e–4e.
13. Wray RC, Luce EA. Treatment of impending nipple necrosis following reduction mammaplasty. Plast Reconstr Surg. 1981;68(2):242–4.
14. Pannucci CJ, Nelson JA, Chung CU, Fischer JP, et al. Medicinal leeches for surgically uncorrectable venous congestion after free flap breast reconstruction. Microsurgery. 2014;34(7):522–6.
15. Friedman HI, Fitzmaurice M, Lefaivre JF, et al. An evidence-based appraisal of the use of hyperbaric oxygen on flaps and grafts. Plast Reconstr Surg. 2006;117(7 Suppl):175S–90S.
16. Thom SR. Hyperbaric oxygen: its mechanisms and efficacy. Plast Reconstr Surg. 2011;127(Suppl 1):131S–41S.
17. Klatsky SA, Manson PN. Toe pulp free grafts in nipple reconstruction. Plast Reconstr Surg. 1981;68(2):2458.
18. Sierakowski A, Niranjan N. Star flap with a dermal platform for nipple reconstruction. J Plast Reconstr Aesthet Surg. 2011;64(2):e55–6.
19. Eskenazi L. A one-stage nipple reconstruction with the "modified star" flap and immediate tattoo: a review of 100 cases. Plast Reconstr Surg. 1993;92(4):671–80.
20. Kroll SS, Reece GP, Miller MJ, et al. Comparison of nipple projection with the modified double-opposing tab and star flaps. Plast Reconstr Surg. 1997;99:1602–5.
21. Shestak KC, Nguyen TD. The double opposing periareola flap: a novel concept for nipple-areola reconstruction. Plast Reconstr Surg. 2007;119(2):473–80.
22. Little JW. Nipple areolar reconstruction. In: Cohen M, editor. Mastery of plastic and reconstructive surgery, vol. II. Boston: Little, Brown; 1994.
23. Hammond DC, Khuthaila D, Kim J. The skate flap purse-string technique for nipple-areola complex reconstruction. Plast Reconstr Surg. 2007;120(2):399–406.
24. Becker H. The use of intradermal tattoo to enhance the final result of nipple-areola reconstruction. Plast Reconstr Surg. 1986;77(4):673–5.

# 77 High-Grade and Recurrent Inverted Nipple: An Effective Surgical Treatment for the Most Challenging Cases

Roberto Bracaglia and Marco D'Ettorre

## 77.1 Introduction

The inverted nipple was first described by Cooper [1] in 1840. It is generally considered a congenital malformation; however, specific causes may be responsible for it, leading to an acquired condition: breast carcinoma, mastitis, macromastia, trauma, and breast surgery. Congenital inverted nipple may result from anatomically too short and fibrotic ducts. Although not uncommon, its prevalence varies between 1.77% and 10%, most of which cases (from 73% to 96.23%) are umbilicated (nipple can be pulled out without exerting undue pressure), more rarely invaginated (from 3.77% to 26%), and not extractable [2–5]. Moreover, it is a bilateral occurrence in the majority of the cases. In addition to unaesthetic appearance, it comes along with disturbances concerning function (breast feeding is seriously compromised) and psychology.

R. Bracaglia, M.D.
Bracaglia Aesthetic Center for Plastic Surgery and Aesthetic Medicine, Casa di Cura Villa Stuart – EUROSANITÁ SPA, Via Trionfale, 5952, 00135 Rome, Italy
e-mail: info@bracaglia.it

M. D'Ettorre, M.D. (✉)
Plastic Surgery Institute,
Viale di Villa Pamphili 85, 00152 Rome, Italy
e-mail: marco.dettorre@outlook.com

In 1999, Han and Hong [6] classified inverted nipples into three grades, which helps in achieving proper treatment: in grade I, the nipple can easily be pulled out manually and maintains its projection without traction. In grade II, the nipple can be pulled out manually but retracts when released. In grade III, there are retracting forces beneath the nipple, with remarkable fibrosis and lactiferous ducts seriously shortened. Although both conservative and surgical treatments have been described for the correction of inverted nipples, nonsurgical approaches are unlikely to solve the most severe cases.

## 77.2 Technique [5]

Our technique was conducted on 29 patients with congenital inverted nipple between 2000 and 2015: 18 patients (36 nipples) having severe inverted nipple (grade III) and 11 patients (19 nipples) presenting with relapses. The average age of patients was 39 years (range, 25–49), and they were followed up for a mean period of 2.7 years (range, 6 months to 3 years). All the patients were informed that surgical division of the ducts would have precluded their future ability to breastfeed.

Our technique can be performed under local anesthesia. However, in case of correction during breast augmentation, with periareolar access, a general anesthesia is preferable.

First of all, a periareolar access is defined in the lower pole. A primary blunt dissection with


M.A. Shiffman (ed.), *Nipple-Areolar Complex Reconstruction*,
https://doi.org/10.1007/978-3-319-60925-6_77

scissors is helpful to reach and isolate the inverted nipple, which is completed afterwards by ducts and fibrous tissue cut (Fig. 77.1) eliciting irreversible cessation of lactation. Temporary traction sutures (alternatively, Gillies hooks) are exploited to achieve nipple disinvagination, and transfixed 2U sutures at 3 and 9 o'clock are placed and tightened at the base to maintain eversion (Fig. 77.2). The "dead space" obtained beneath the nipple is filled in by a sculpted dermoglandular monolobed flap. If a major tissue gap is located under the nipple, even two separate monolobed flaps, overturned and sutured medially, can be defined (Fig. 77.3). The donor-site area is closed with a 3/0 Vicryl (Ethicon, Inc., Somerville, NJ) and the skin with Ethilon 6/0 (Ethicon, Inc., Somerville, NJ) (Fig. 77.4), and a doughnut-type dressing was placed to compress the surrounding areola.

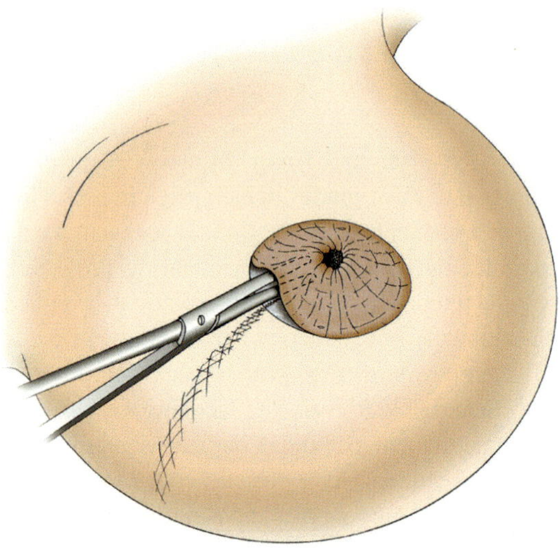

**Fig. 77.1** Ducts and fibrous tissue are cut with scissors in order to obtain a complete isolation of the inverted nipple [5]. [Bracaglia R, Tambasco D, Gentileschi S and D'Ettorre M. Recurrent inverted nipple. A reliable technique for the most difficult cases. Ann Plast Surg 2012;69(1):24–6. http://journals.lww.com/annalsplasticsurgery]

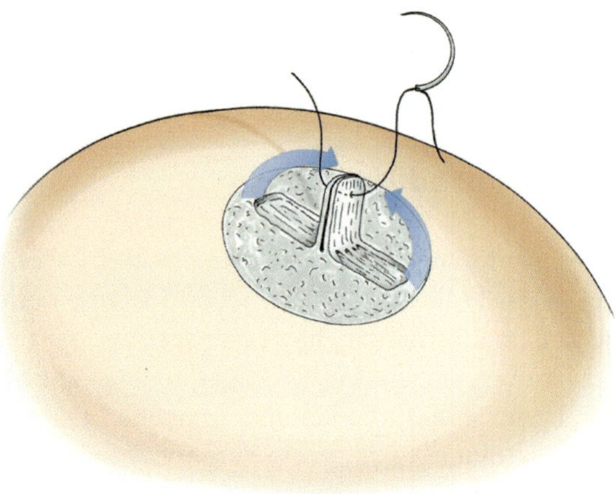

**Fig. 77.3** The "dead space" obtained beneath the nipple is filled in by a sculpted dermoglandular monolobed flap or two monolobed flaps, overturned and sutured medially [5]. [Bracaglia R, Tambasco D, Gentileschi S and D'Ettorre M. Recurrent inverted nipple. A reliable technique for the most difficult cases. Ann Plast Surg 2012;69(1):24–6. http://journals.lww.com/annalsplasticsurgery]

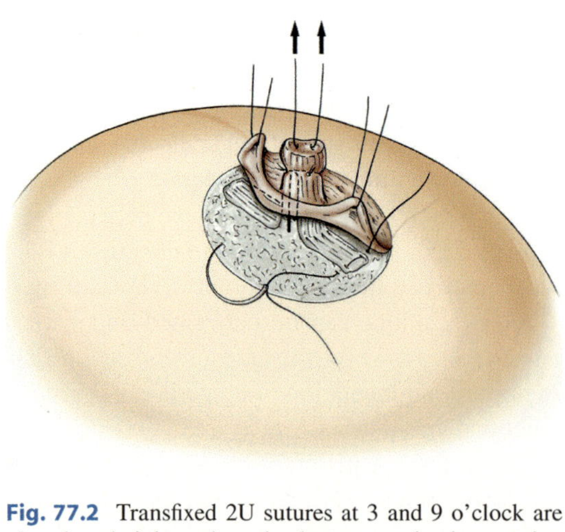

**Fig. 77.2** Transfixed 2U sutures at 3 and 9 o'clock are placed and tightened at the base to maintain eversion [Bracaglia R, Tambasco D, Gentileschi S and D'Ettorre M. Recurrent inverted nipple. A reliable technique for the most difficult cases. Ann Plast Surg 2012;69(1):24–6. http://journals.lww.com/annalsplasticsurgery] [5]

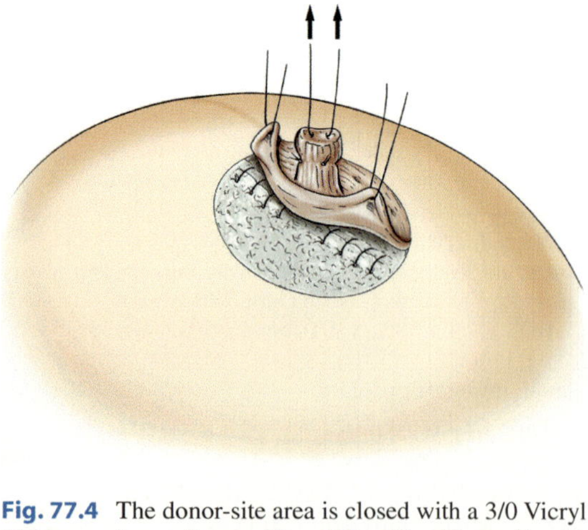

**Fig. 77.4** The donor-site area is closed with a 3/0 Vicryl (Ethicon, Inc., Somerville, NJ) [5]. [Bracaglia R, Tambasco D, Gentileschi S and D'Ettorre M. Recurrent inverted nipple. A reliable technique for the most difficult cases. Ann Plast Surg 2012;69(1):24–6. http://journals.lww.com/annalsplasticsurgery]

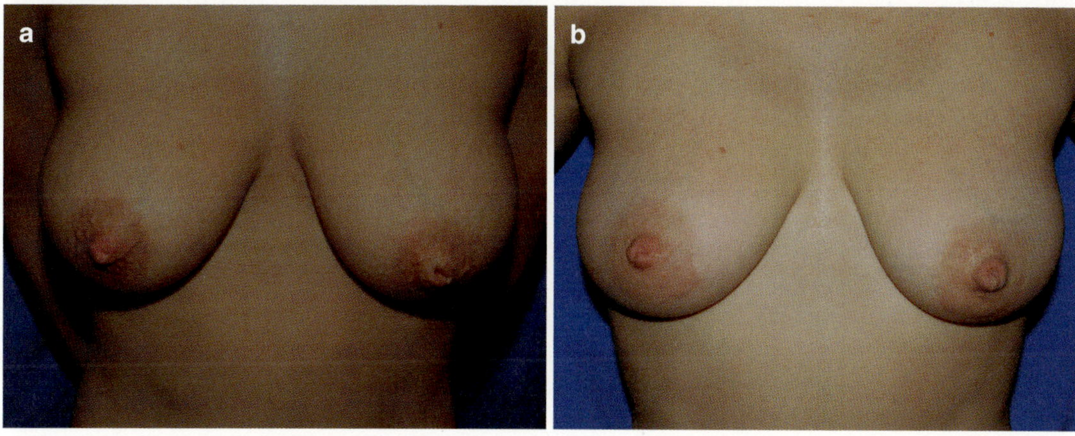


**Fig. 77.5** (**a**) Preoperative 36-year-old patient. (**b**) Two years postoperative after surgical procedure. Amelioration of preoperative condition and stability of the results are obtained

In two cases, our technique was ineffective. One case of temporary loss of sensitivity (absence of contractile response upon brush stimulation) was noticed, but none of the patients showed major complications (necrosis, infection, hematoma, and permanent numbness), relapses, or pathological scarring at follow-up. In our series, the shape and the projection after the procedures were evaluated as stable and satisfactory by the patients without any protective devices use (Fig. 77.5). Our technique showed absolute reliability in the most difficult cases, where less invasive approaches may be ineffective: grade III and relapses.

## 77.3 Discussion

The modern tendency is always to perform min-invasive procedures in order to preserve anatomical structures. This is extremely remarkable in order to minimize annoyances to the patients. However, there must be consciousness about the fact that effectiveness is the goal to achieve. Thus, although it is certainly important to minimize postsurgical disturbances to the patients, it is even more crucial to provide them with effective results, really eradicating the problems. Furthermore, it is always advisable to perform overcorrection of inverted nipple, in order to minimize the risk of future recurrence, which should be avoided with any efforts.

Both conservative and surgical treatments have been described for the correction of inverted nipples [7, 8]. For example, years ago McGeorge [7] proposed its “Niplette,” a negative pressure system with a plastic device to be collocated on the inverted nipple to facilitate its correction. Scholten [9] introduced a piercing method to evert the nipple in pregnant women to be removed 3 months prior to the birth. He reported lactation preservation and eversion maintained up to 1 year post-breastfeeding. However, these methods can be beneficial for, or applicable to, reversible, grade I cases only. In addition to that, sometimes they may lead to infections, for example, due to secretion leakage, elicited by negative pressure.

The only effective treatment for grade II or III cases is surgical, due to the high recurrence risk, responsible for patients’ and doctors’ frustrations. The main drawback following a more invasive procedure is loss of lactation function. However, in grade III inversion, where the nipple cannot be everted even after mechanical traction, lactation is usually already compromised [5]. Despite this, surgical methods that preserve lactation function have been described and include suturing techniques, dermal flaps, and dermis analogs.

In reference to the first group, Kolker and Torina [10] suggested the release of fibroductal structures with an 18-gauge needle passed through a limited access and closure with sequential reinsertion of suture through suture exit points. Cabalag et al. [11] proposed the use of a microknife to divide the ducts and the fibrous tissue plus transverse to longitudinal skin closure. According to the authors, however, these techniques are inadequate to correct relapse or grade III cases: the amount of soft tissue beneath the nipple may be insufficient, the postsurgical fibrosis can be conspicuous, and the short-scar incision may not allow an easy identification of the right surgical plane. Peeters et al. [12] proposed the PDS sheet, a synthetic absorbable implant causing foreign-body capsule formation. Despite its potential usefulness, it is a prosthetic material, thus possibly eliciting excessive scarring fibrosis.

Furthermore, Karacaoglu [13] described the "antenna flap": dermoadipose flaps generated within the area of deepithelization of mastopexy. It is an effective and innovative technique, whose limit however is represented by the necessity of being performed during a mastopexy. Durgun et al. [14] recently proposed a technique based on two areola dermal flaps plus traction (through a device obtained by 50 mL syringe), kept on site for 21 days. Despite potential effectiveness and referred preservation of lactation, its main drawback is possible decubitus elicitation.

Finally, techniques involving multiple and complex flaps [15] have been also suggested, but they are less easily repeatable and less safe (e.g., due to abnormal vascular supply) and can create evident linear scarring toward the areola or reduced nipple size [16].

The aforementioned surgical treatments are, in our opinion, certainly a valid solution for grade II cases, also providing patients with the possibility to breast feed afterwards. By contrast, our technique has demonstrated to be easily repeatable and effective in the most severe cases, whose priority is not represented by preservation of lactation. This is the reason why, differently from the past, we perform this approach in the most difficult and challenging cases only, opting for less invasive methods in lower grades [17].

### Conclusions

Inverted nipple is a not so uncommon malformation prsenting both congenitally, mainly, and as an acquired condition.

Over the years, many treatment strategies have been proposed; however, there is still an open debate about which is the best correction method. Of course, conservative approaches are preferable in case of mild deformities (grade I). Surgical techniques, even though are usually responsible for cessation of lactation, are the only effective treatment in grade II and III malformations. Our technique, although it is not the best in terms of invasiveness, has proved to be effective, leads to stable results, and prevents recurrences, which is the greatest concern in the most severe cases and relapses, where it finds its main field of application.

## References


1. Cooper AP. Anatomy of the breast. London: Longmans; 1840. p. 1–89.
2. Schwager RC, Smith JW, Gray GF, Goulian D Jr. Inversion of the human female nipple, with a simple method of treatment. Plast Reconstr Surg. 1974;54(5):564–9.
3. Crestinu JM. Inverted nipple: the new method of correction. Aesthet Plast Surg. 1989;13(3):189–97.
4. Park HS, Yoon CH, Kim HJ. The prevalence of congenital inverted nipple. Aesthet Plast Surg. 1999;23(2):144–6.
5. Bracaglia R, Tambasco D, Gentileschi S, D'Ettorre M. Recurrent inverted nipple. A reliable technique for the most difficult cases. Ann Plast Surg. 2012;69(1):24–6.
6. Han S, Hong YG. The inverted nipple: its grading and surgical correction. Plast Reconstr Surg. 1999;104(2):389–95.
7. McGeorge DD. The "Niplette": an instrument for the nonsurgical correction of inverted nipples. Br J Plast Surg. 1994;47(1):46–9.
8. Min KH, Park SS, Heo CY, Min KW. Scar-free technique for inverted-nipple correction. Aesthet Plast Surg. 2010;34(1):116–9.
9. Scholten E. A contemporary correction of inverted nipples. Plast Reconstr Surg. 2001;107(2):511–3.
10. Kolker AR, Torina PJ. Minimally invasive correction of inverted nipple. Ann Plast Surg. 2009;62(5):549–53.
11. Cabalag MS, Chui HK, Tan BK. Correction of inverted nipple using a microknife and transverse to

longitudinal skin closure. J Plast Reconstr Aesthet Surg. 2010;63(8):e627–30.
12. Peeters G, Decloedt J, Nagels H, Cambier B. Treatment of the severe or recurrent inverted nipple by interposition of a resorbable polydioxanone sheet. J Plast Reconstr Aesthet Surg. 2010;63(2):e175–6.
13. Karacaoglu E. Correction of recurrent grade III inverted nipple with antenna dermoadipose flap: case report. Aesthet Plast Surg. 2009;33(6):843–8.
14. Durgun M, Özakpinar HR, Selçuk CT, Sarici M, Ceran C, Seven E. Inverted nipple correction with dermal flaps and traction. Aesthet Plast Surg. 2014;38(3):533–9.
15. Kim JT, Lim YS, Oh JG. Correction of inverted nipples with twisting and locking principles. Plast Reconstr Surg. 2006;118(7):1526–31.
16. Burm JS, Kim YW. Correction of inverted nipples by strong suspension with areola-based dermal flaps. Plast Reconstr Surg. 2007;120(6):1483–6.
17. Bracaglia R, Fortunato R, Falasca D, Di Giulio G. Introflexed nipple surgical reconstruction: our experience. Riv Ital Chir Plastica. 1993;25(Suppl 1):167–71.

# Part XI

# Outcomes and Satisfaction

# Single-Stage Reconstruction of the Nipple-Areolar Complex: Outcomes and Patient Satisfaction

78

Emilie C. Robinson, Vicky Kang, Andrea B. McNab, and Anuja K. Antony

## 78.1 Introduction

Nipple-areolar complex (NAC) reconstruction completes the reconstructive process of the postmastectomy breast. Although many methods exist, the objectives are the same: create a realistic and aesthetically pleasing nipple-areolar complex and achieve high patient satisfaction. The psychological benefits of nipple-areolar reconstruction are well established, with patients completing breast reconstruction, demonstrating increased patient satisfaction [1, 2]. A challenge remains with the potential for patients to fatigue toward the end of the long reconstructive process and fail to complete nipple reconstruction. Techniques that reduce the number of procedures benefit the patient and may have an economic impact on overall healthcare costs.

Reconstruction of the nipple-areolar complex is most commonly performed in two stages, first with reconstruction of the nipple by local flaps (with or without augmentation using biologic tissues), followed by tattooing of the nipple and areola after the neo-nipple has healed [3]. NAC reconstruction using local flaps and skin grafting from the inner thigh, labia, or groin has also been described but has the added disadvantage of donor-site morbidity. Implementation of an effective single-stage technique affords the opportunity to reduce patient fatigue and improve overall patient satisfaction with the breast construct. The focus of this chapter will be on simple and effective methods for single-stage NAC reconstruction.

## 78.2 Nipple-Areolar Complex Reconstruction and Patient Satisfaction

A key determinant of success in breast reconstruction is patient satisfaction; reconstruction of the nipple-areolar complex is no exception. In fact, the completion of the NAC reconstruction itself is an independent predictor of increased patient satisfaction. In 2010, Buck et al. [1] published results of an investigation into cosmetic outcomes at various stages in the breast

E.C. Robinson, M.D. (✉)
Department of General Surgery, Rush University Medical Center, 1725 West Harrison Street Suite, 425 Chicago, IL 60612, USA
e-mail: emilie_c_robinson@rush.edu

V. Kang, B.S.
Rush University Medical Center, 1725 West Harrison Street #425, Chicago, IL 60612, USA
e-mail: vicky_kang@rush.edu

A.B. McNab, M.D. • A.K. Antony, M.D., M.P.H.
Department of Plastic and Reconstructive Surgery, Rush University Medical Center, 1725 West Harrison Street, Suite #425, Chicago, IL 60612, USA
e-mail: andrea_b_mcnab@rush.edu; anuja_k_antony@rush.edu


M.A. Shiffman (ed.), *Nipple-Areolar Complex Reconstruction*,
https://doi.org/10.1007/978-3-319-60925-6_78

reconstruction process. These were based on a questionnaire, in which the patient rated her level of satisfaction with breast reconstruction in intimate, social, and professional settings. This study demonstrated that women's responses were significantly higher after completion of NAC reconstruction compared with women who completed only breast mound reconstruction. Additional studies have demonstrated the profound benefit of NAC reconstruction on a woman's sexual health; in particular, completion of the reconstruction facilitates the assimilation of the reconstructed breast into the patient's own body image [2, 4]. These studies serve to further validate clinical practice as nipple-areolar complex reconstruction is a critical step in achieving successful postmastectomy reconstruction and a substantial contributor to overall satisfaction.

Among women who complete NAC reconstruction, an important prognosticator of patient satisfaction is the length of time needed to complete reconstruction. Jabor et al. [5] demonstrated that patients had significantly lower satisfaction with a longer interval between breast mound and nipple-areolar reconstruction, even after the NAC reconstruction was complete. It is intuitive that a more efficient reconstructive pathway would be preferable to patients; however, the authors further hypothesize that the delay in NAC reconstruction allows time for patients to adapt and accept the less complete breast reconstruction. This may mean that the nipple reconstruction has a decreased benefit gain and becomes a less powerful influence on overall satisfaction. It follows that as more time elapses between breast reconstruction and NAC reconstruction, women become less likely to undergo additional operations to complete the process and may end up settling on an incomplete reconstruction. Single-stage NAC reconstruction lessens the patient burden by reducing the number of procedures and consolidating the creation of the nipple and the tattooing into a single operation. To this end, single-stage reconstruction demonstrates distinct advantages over two-stage reconstruction, by eliminating the waiting period between nipple reconstruction and tattooing, shortening the total duration of reconstruction by several months.

In addition to the timing and efficiency of the reconstructive steps, further determinants of satisfaction with nipple-areolar complex reconstruction are aesthetic parameters, the most influential of which are projection and color match [5]. The single-stage technique offers many advantages over the two-stage technique with respect to the tattoo process, which may allow for superior color matching and more effective dye implantation and uptake. The details of these advantages are discussed in a later section of the chapter.

## 78.3 Historical Concerns

The traditional two-stage approach to nipple-areolar complex reconstruction was founded on the belief that completed wound healing of the reconstructed nipple is necessary prior to tattooing. This was borne out of concerns for the potential risk of contamination from the unsterile tattoo dye when used on fresh incisions. The fear is amplified in the setting of an implant, where the consequences of an infection are disastrous. The two-stage approach is further supported by concerns for vascular compromise to the flap from immediate tattooing. Neither of the complication has been substantiated in the literature, and numerous studies have demonstrated the single-stage approach to be safe and effective [6–10].

In a review of five studies on the single-stage technique, all using varying methods of combining local flap nipple creation with tattooing, complication rates were consistently low [6–10]. Liliav et al. [7] demonstrated in a study of 29 cases that there were no cases of infection or necrosis; only one case (3.4%) of dehiscence required subsequent revision. All patients demonstrated high patient satisfaction via survey analysis. Børsen-Koch et al. [10] did not experience any complications requiring surgical intervention in 28 cases but had one case (3.6%) of wound infection and one case (3.6%) of partial necrosis which was treated conservatively. Eskenazi [6] conducted 100 simultaneous nipple and areola reconstructions and had no infections and only one case (1%) of partial necrosis which underwent surgical correction. Hugo et al. [8] in a review of 102 single-stage reconstructions and Vandeweyer [9] in a review of 50 reconstructions both reported no incidence of major complications, including infection or necrosis. The successful results throughout these studies serve to address historical arguments for the two-stage technique and validate the single-stage approach as a viable alternative.

## 78.4 Alternative Techniques of Areolar Reconstruction

Skin grafting is an alternative technique for areolar reconstruction and, like tattooing, can be performed in combination with local flaps for a single-stage reconstruction of both the nipple and areola. The principle is to create an areola that appears distinct from the surrounding skin, either by texture or pigmentation. The contour of the full-thickness skin graft in contrast to normal skin creates the appearance of an areola, and grafting creates a textured surface that resembles the Montgomery tubercles of the natural areola. The effect is enhanced by utilizing donor sites with increased pigmentation, such as the groin, inner thigh, or labia [11]. Overall, the graft technique has demonstrated higher rates of local complications compared to tattooing and carries an added risk of donor-site morbidity such as wound dehiscence [12]. Cases of nipple necrosis and rejection of the graft compromise the aesthetic outcome and require additional procedures for revision, which delays completion of the reconstructive process [11].

Another alternative to surgical reconstruction of the nipple instead utilizes three-dimensional tattooing for the nipple and areola. This relatively new technique capitalizes on the principles of light and shadow in two dimensions to create depth and the illusion of projection of a nipple [13]. In 2014, the three-dimensional tattooing technique was described utilizing variations in tattoo color to create dimensionality to the nipple-areolar construct. The nipple is designed with a light inner circle lined inferiorly with a dark border to create the appearance of shadow. Standard medical tattooing equipment can be used for a satisfactory result, but professional tattooing equipment and a tattoo artist can produce a superior result, with improved color match and pigment retention [13]. Though this technique cannot produce true nipple projection, it may be a reasonable option for women who do not wish to undergo another surgical procedure or may be poor candidates for nipple flap elevation.

## 78.5 Single-Stage Nipple-Areolar Complex Reconstruction Surgical Technique

This chapter discusses simultaneous nipple and areolar reconstruction utilizing local skin flaps and intradermal tattooing for the nipple and areola performed in a single operation, a technique that has demonstrated successful results in both implant-based and autologous tissue reconstruction. For a unilateral reconstruction, care is taken at every phase to match the features of the contralateral native nipple; this includes size, projection, color, and positioning on the breast. Tattoo colors are selected preoperatively and should consist of pigments two to three shades darker than the final desired color, as the colors will fade over time. An example of early fading is demonstrated in Fig. 78.1. Generally, two pigments are selected, a darker shade for the nipple and a lighter shade for the areola.

The position of the nipple is determined by the patient and the surgeon collaboratively with visual placement of EKG lead(s) (or circular self-adhesive products), most preferably along or bordering the mastectomy scar to camouflage it. The markers are placed with the patient upright, and the desired position is confirmed with the patient prior to final marking. In unilateral reconstructions, symmetry with the contralateral side can be done with measurements from the sternal notch, inframammary fold, and midsternal line. Repositioning can be carried out until satisfactory location is acquired, and once confirmed, the markers are traced with a marking pen. The layout for the local nipple flap is then drawn within the areolar markings (typically with the base of the pedicle along the mastectomy scar). This

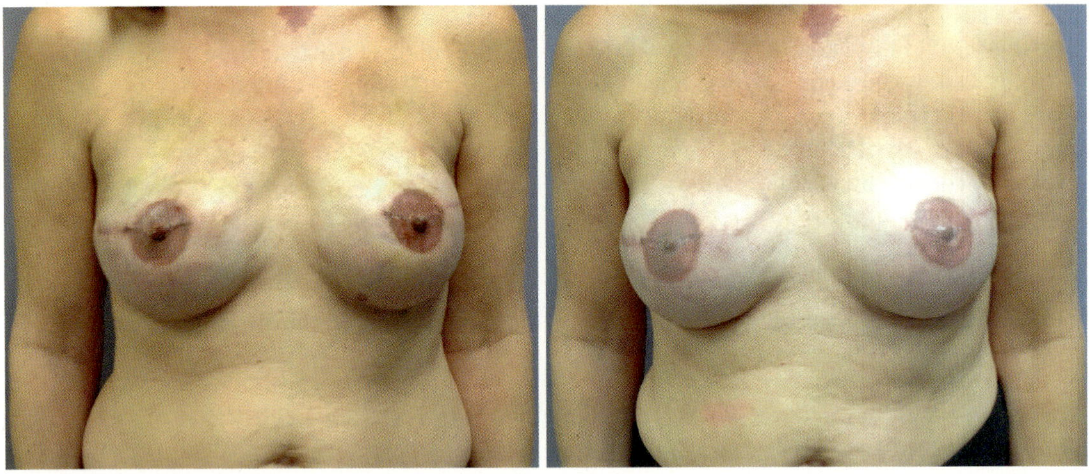

**Fig. 78.1** (*Left*) Bilateral single-stage NAC reconstruction at 1 week postoperatively. (*Right*) Three months postoperatively, demonstrating pigment fading

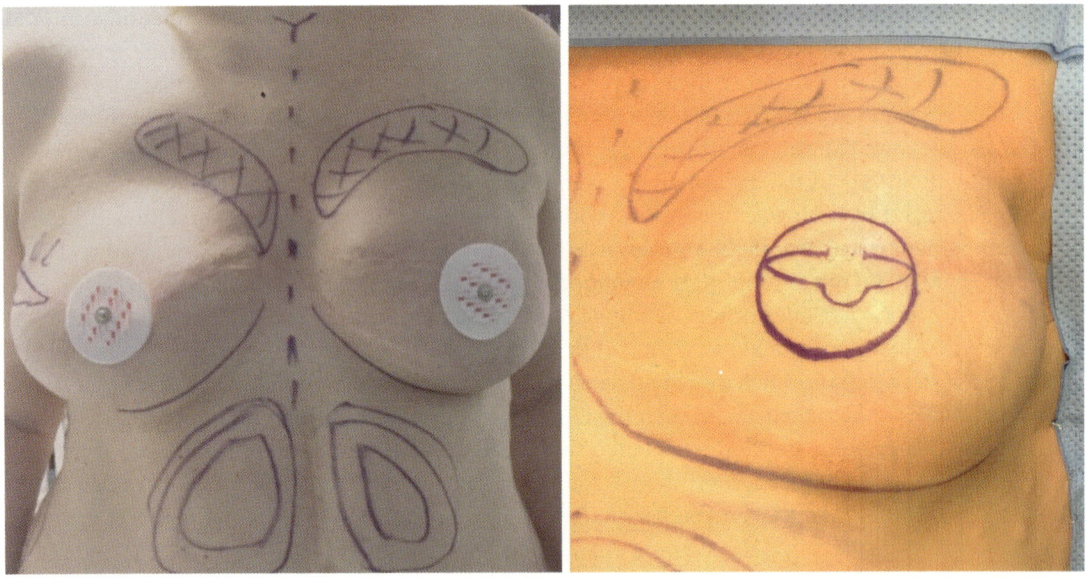

**Fig. 78.2** (*Left*) Placement of EKG leads for position of nipple-areolar complex in bilateral reconstruction. This patient has additional preoperative markings for a revision to the right breast and liposuction of the upper abdomen and fat grafting to bilateral upper poles. (*Right*) Marking for C-V flap with 1 cm pedicle base

ensures the incisions and subsequent scarring from elevation of the flap are camouflaged within the areola (Fig. 78.2) [7].

Though many patterns for local flaps have been described, the majority utilize the same basic technique: a base with two lateral wings to construct the walls of the nipple and a tab to form the roof. The long axis of this flap, a line through the center of the two lateral wings, as well as the direction of the nipple, can be oriented in any direction necessary to best avoid preexisting scars. Our preference is orientation of the long axis of the flap along the mastectomy flap scar. It is the width of the wings that determines the height of the nipple [6]. Long term, some degree of loss of nipple projection is inevitable

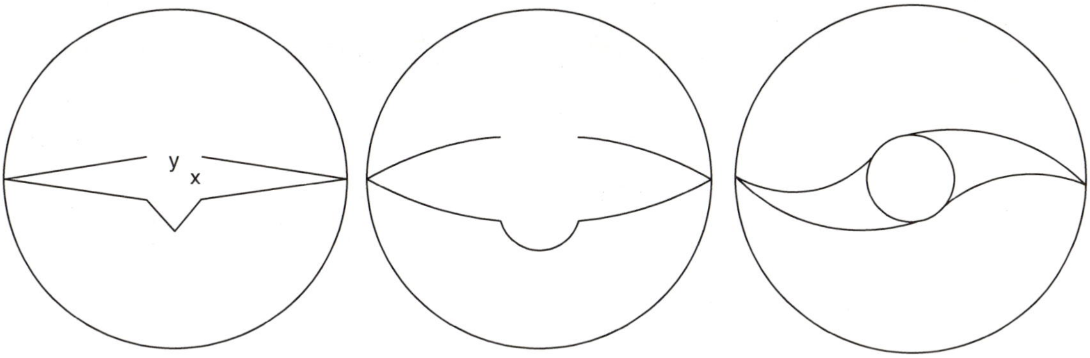


**Fig. 78.3** (*Left*) Star flap, the width of the wings "x" corresponds to the height of the reconstructed nipple; the length of the base "y" determines the diameter of the nipple; these basic principles apply to the majority of flap designs. (*Middle*) C-V flap, first described by Jones in 1994 [12]. (*Right*) Propeller flap, this technique has maximal benefit when reconstructing a smaller areola because by curving the wings, a longer length can be achieved while remaining within the border of the areola [17]

due to contraction during wound healing. A literature review of nipple-areolar complex reconstructions published by Sisti et al. [12] in 2016 demonstrated loss of projection ranged from 40% to 75% of the immediate postoperative height. Some authors advocate for adjusting the height of the flap to account for this eventual loss [6]. Our preference is the addition of an allograft material to enhance the nipple projection if the donor fat or tissue is inadequate. The size of the base of the flap will correspond to the size of the nipple and is typically around 1 cm in diameter. Three representative flap designs are demonstrated in Fig. 78.3. Our technique incorporates the use of the CV flap.

The initial step of the operation is to tattoo the flap with the darker of the two pigments (Fig. 78.4); the tattoo is extended 1–2 mm beyond the markings for the flap to ensure that no subsequent tattooing is needed on the incision edges [7]. The perimeter of the flap is then incised, and the wings are raised as skin flaps in the dermal plane and deepened toward the base to include subcutaneous fat. This adds more bulk to the base of the nipple and results in better projection. The donor sites for the wings are closed in a linear fashion on either side of the nipple, typically in two layers with interrupted Vicryl (Ethicon) sutures for the dermis and interrupted chromic sutures for the epidermis

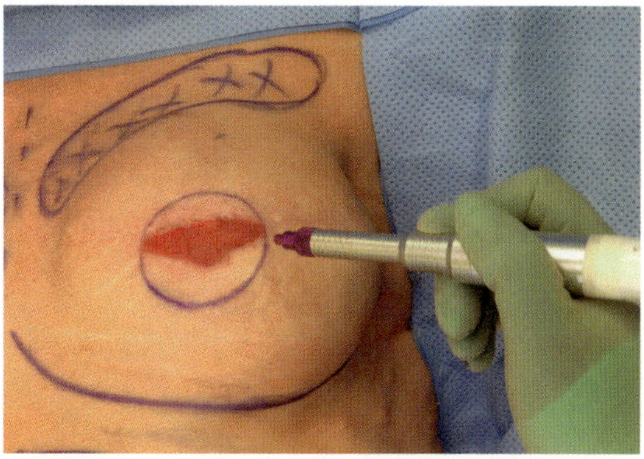

**Fig. 78.4** Tattooing of the flap with the darker pigment, 1–2 mm outside the perimeter of the flap

(Fig. 78.5). Properly placed sutures and well-tied knots at these sites ensure the closure will withstand trauma from subsequent tattooing of the areola. The wings of the flap are wrapped around to form the vertical walls of the nipple. The lower wing is set into the base with chromic sutures, the flaps are sutured together, and the top of the flap is folded over and closed to form the tip of the nipple [6, 7]. A variation of this flap technique was described by Hugo et al. in 1993 [8] and involves complete detachment of the nipple flap from the surrounding skin. The authors propose this method allows for greater projection of the nipple beyond the level of the skin, and though the flaps are

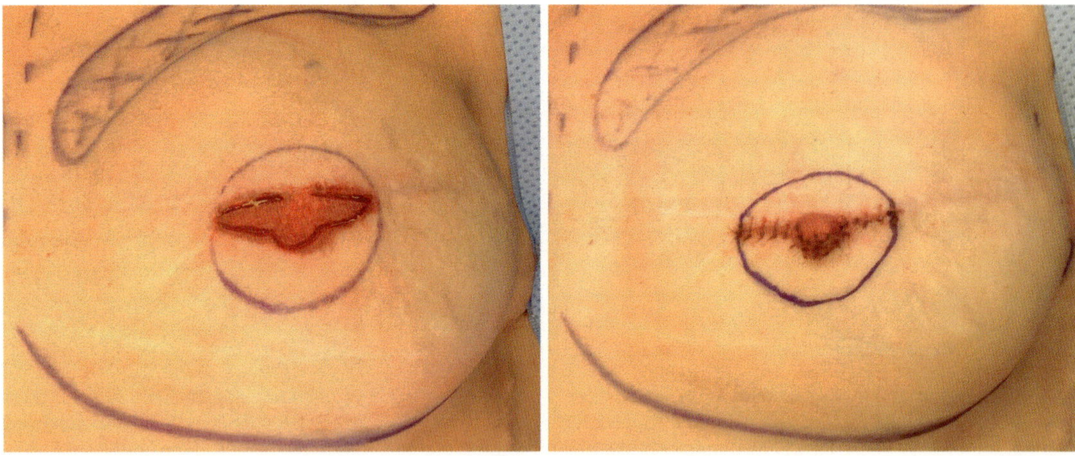

**Fig. 78.5** (*Left*) Incision of the flap prior to elevation, note the tattoo extends beyond the incision. (*Right*) Closure of the wings of the flap. Note the now oval shape of the areolar markings

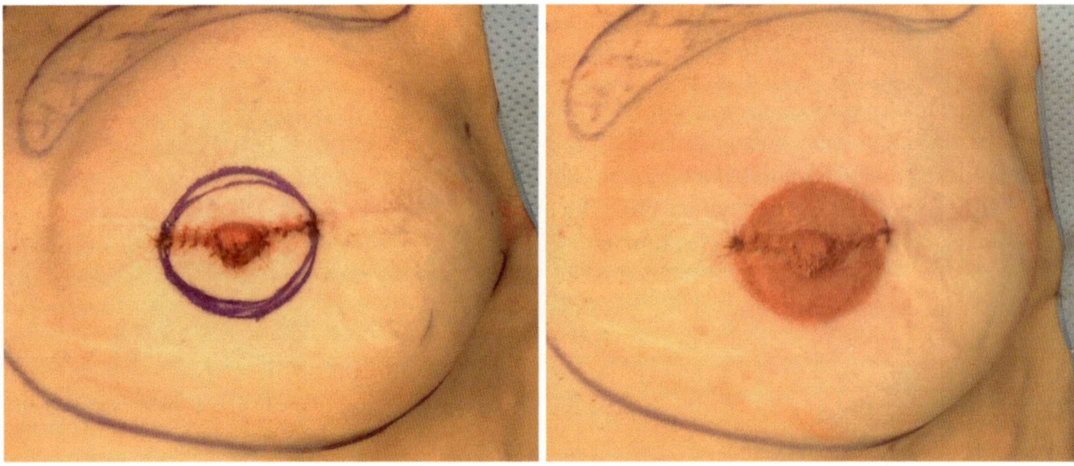

**Fig. 78.6** (*Left*) Areolar outline is remarked to establish circular shape. (*Right*) Areola is tattooed

vascularized only by the underlying fat, there were no cases of flap necrosis in the 102 reconstructions analyzed. Most surgeons however employ a pedicled local flap based on 1 cm skin attachment. Nipple projection can further be augmented using an autograft of chondral or auricular cartilage or a cylinder of allograft material, such as acellular dermal matrix. This is placed inside the walls of the nipple prior to the closure of the tip. The circular outline of the areola must be redrawn after closure of the wings as this will pull in the edges and create an oval (Fig. 78.6). The areola is tattooed with the lighter of the two pigments, or a blend of the two, and is done so that the pigment fades slightly toward the periphery and the edges of the areolar are slightly blurred, creating a more natural appearance (Figs. 78.6 and 78.7).

A slight alternative to this technique has been described by several authors and involves tattooing of the entire complex prior to elevation of the graft. In this modification, either the starting areolar shape is oval which will be pulled into a circular shape with closure of the wing sites

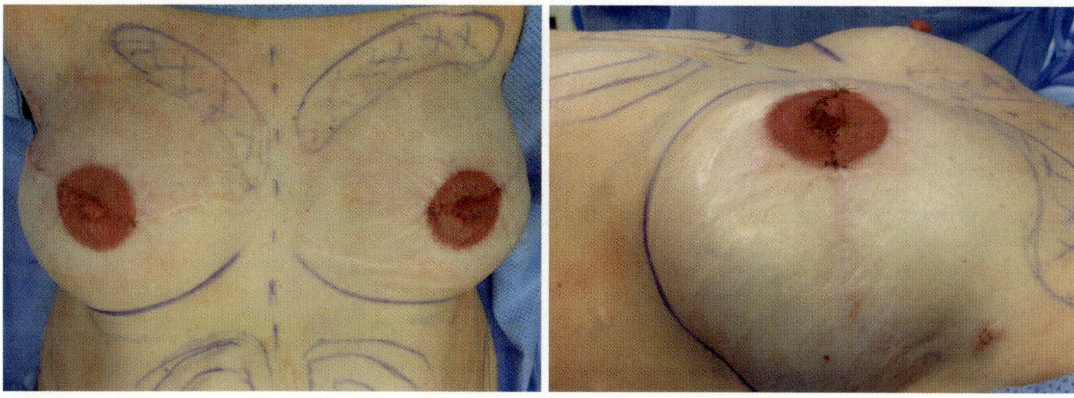

**Fig. 78.7** (*Left*) Completed reconstruction of bilateral nipple-areolar complex with revision and mastopexy on the *right* and fat grafting to bilateral upper poles. (*Right*) Lateral view demonstrates good nipple projection

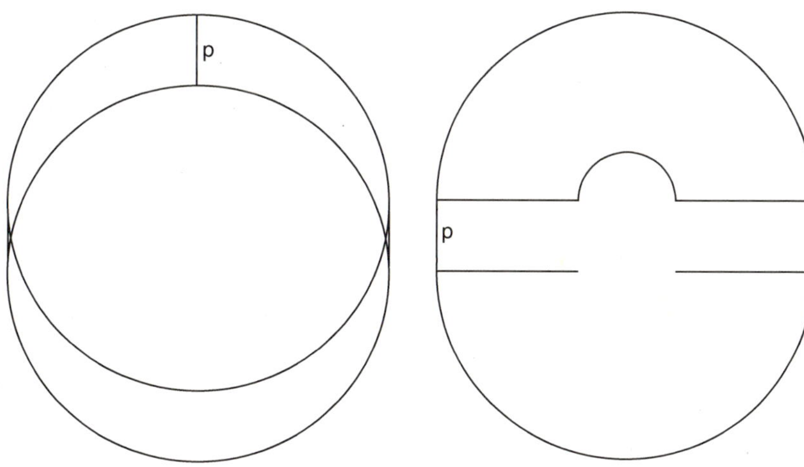


**Fig. 78.8** (*Left*) Flap design as described by Børsen-Koch et al. [10]; two circles are marked that correspond to the desired diameter of the areola; the circles are offset by a length, "p" that will correspond to the height of the reconstructed nipple. (*Right*) This entire shaped is tattooed and then a flap is raised as a C-V or C-U flap

(Fig. 78.8) or the areolar outline is tattooed again after the closure to reestablish the proper shape [9, 10]. This technique avoids tattooing over the freshly closed incisions of the flap wings, as some authors suggest the trauma from the tattoo process and contact with the tattoo needle compromises the integrity of the stitches and the closure [9].

After completion of the reconstruction, a postoperative dressing is applied with bacitracin ointment, Xeroform (Kendall/Covidien) gauze, and eye pads with center cutout to avoid pressure on the nipple. Patients are followed in the clinic postoperatively and, depending on the surgeon, may be advised to wear nipple protectors for up to six weeks after the reconstruction to preserve projection of the nipple [7].

## 78.6 Advantages

An advantage of single-stage nipple-areolar complex reconstruction is the proposed improved quality of pigmentation achieved by the tattoo process. In two-stage reconstruction, the nipple and surrounding areola are tattooed 4–6 months after the reconstruction. This is disadvantageous both because the uptake of dye in the resultant scar tissue may be more irregular and because tattooing the mobile, three-dimensional structure of the nipple is more difficult [14]. The former point is emphasized by observation of tattooing of the nipple-areolar complex on breasts with implant-based reconstruction, where a mastectomy scar across the breast leads to unpredictable uptake of ink and irregular pigmentation [7]. Single-stage reconstruction obviates the challenges posed by the two-stage reconstruction by allowing for tattooing the skin on a flat surface and prior to the formation of scar tissue.

While comparative studies between the two-stage and one-stage techniques have not been published, the available literature on the single-stage method demonstrates effective reconstruction with little need for tattoo revision. Evolving technology to more objectively analyze color match between the neo-nipple and native contralateral nipple in unilateral reconstruction involves the use of color-matching software [15, 16]. In the absence of this technology, rates of tattoo revisions can be employed as a surrogate for the ability of tattoo to achieve a satisfactory result. Børsen-Koch et al. [10] published preliminary results on the introduction of the single-stage technique at two institutions in 2013 which included a tattoo revision rate of 14.3% at 3-month follow-up. Though not a discrete statistical analysis, this study compared two-stage reconstructions that were performed at the same institutions prior to the implementation of the single-stage nipple reconstruction and found revision rates largely equivocal at 17.9%. Several articles discussing results of single-stage reconstruction quote rates of tattoo revision ranging from 3% to 14.3%, which fairs well in comparison to two-stage nipple-areolar reconstructions ranging from 2.5% to 18% [3, 6, 7, 9, 10, 14, 15]. One study cited re-tattoo rate of 40% among single-stage reconstructions, though re-tattooing was both to darken the areola and camouflage scars [8]. This likely resulted from initial color choice without consideration for the tattoo pigment's tendency to fade and was likely not influenced by the tattoo method employed. Further insight could be gained by a study specifically aimed to compare single-stage and two-stage techniques.

## 78.7 Patient Satisfaction

In all studies reviewed, patient satisfaction was uniformly high. Our study explicitly surveyed patients postoperatively and found 100% of patients surveyed were "very satisfied." Other studies in the literature state consistent high levels of satisfaction throughout patients, though this was not formally evaluated. In conjunction with low incidence of complications and improved ease of tattooing, single-stage nipple-areolar complex reconstruction offers a more timely and efficient reconstructive option with excellent aesthetic outcomes for women after mastectomy, allowing shorter duration of reconstruction and a more expedient return to normal life.

## References

1. Buck D, Shenaq D, Heyer K, Kato C, Kim J. Patient-subjective cosmetic outcomes following the varying stages of tissue expander breast reconstruction: the importance of completion. Breast. 2010;19(6):521.
2. Wellisch DK, Schain WS, Noone RB, Little JW 3rd. The psychological contribution of nipple addition in breast reconstruction. Plast Reconstr Surg. 1987;80(5):699–704.
3. Goh SC, Martin NA, Pandya AN, Cutress RI. Patient satisfaction following nipple areolar complex reconstruction and tattooing. J Plast Reconstr Aesthet Surg. 2011;64(3):360–3.
4. Schain WS, Wellisch DK, Pasnau RO, Landsverk J. The sooner the better: a study of psychological factors in women undergoing immediate versus delayed breast reconstruction. Am J Psychiatry. 1985;142:40–6.
5. Jabor MA, Shayani P, Collins DR Jr, Karas T, Cohen BE. Nipple-areola reconstruction: satisfaction and clinical determinants. Plast Reconstr Surg. 2002;110(2):457–63. 464-5
6. Eskenazi L. A one-stage nipple reconstruction with the "modified star" flap and immediate tattoo: a review of 100 cases. Plast Reconstr Surg. 1993;92(4):671–80.
7. Liliav B, Loeb J, Hassid VJ, Antony AK. Single-stage nipple-areolar complex reconstruction technique, outcomes, and patient satisfaction. Ann Plast Surg. 2014;73(5):492–7.
8. Hugo NE, Sultan MR, Hardy SP. Nipple-areola reconstruction with intradermal tattoo and double-opposing pennant flaps. Ann Plast Surg. 1993;30(6):510–3.

9. Vandeweyer E. Simultaneous nipple and areola reconstruction: a review of 50 cases. Acta Chir Belg. 2003;103(6):593–5.
10. Børsen-Koch M, Bille C, Thomsen JB. Promising results after single-stage reconstruction of the nipple and areola complex. Dan Med J. 2013;60(10):A4674.
11. Zhong T, Antony A, Cordeiro P. Surgical outcomes and nipple projection using the modified skate flap for nipple-areolar reconstruction in a series of 422 implant reconstructions. Ann Plast Surg. 2009;62(5):591–5.
12. Sisti A, Grimaldi L, Tassinari J, Cuomo R, Fortezza L, Bocchiotti MA, Roviello F, D'Aniello C, Nisi G. Nipple-areola complex reconstruction techniques: a literature review. Eur J Surg Oncol. 2016;42(4):441–65.
13. Halvorson EG, Cormican M, West ME, Myers V. Three-dimensional nipple-areola tattooing: new technique with superior results. Plast Reconstr Surg. 2014;133:1073.
14. Spear SL, Arias J. Long-term experience with nipple-areola tattooing. Ann Plast Surg. 1995;35(3):232–6.
15. El-Ali K, Dalal M, Kat CC. Tattooing of the nipple-areola complex: review of outcome in 40 patients. J Plast Reconstr Aesthet Surg. 2006;59:1052–7.
16. Levites HA, Fourman MS, Phillips BT, Fromm IM, Khan SU, Dagum AB, Bui DT. Modeling fade patterns of nipple areola complex tattoos following breast reconstruction. Ann Plast Surg. 2014;73(Suppl 2):S153–6.
17. Teimourian B, Duda G. The propeller flap: a one-stage procedure for nipple-areola reconstruction. Aesthet Plast Surg. 1994;18(1):81–4.

# Analyzing Patient Preference for Nipple-Areola Complex Reconstruction Using Utility Outcome Studies

79

Ahmed M.S. Ibrahim, Frank H. Lau, Hani H. Sinno, Bernard T. Lee, and Samuel J. Lin

## 79.1 Introduction

Breast reconstruction following mastectomy is a process that can entail numerous surgeries with multiple revisions to address shape and symmetry [1–3]. This can be especially challenging in patients who have dealt with the mental burden of a cancer diagnosis and subsequent treatment [1]. Ultimately, the goal of surgery is the creation of an aesthetically pleasing breast which closely resembles its natural configuration [2]. Reconstruction of the nipple-areola complex (NAC) is a fundamental component of this process and is often the final step [4, 5]. Furthermore, patients correlate this stage with the completion of treatment. Despite the simplicity of this surgery, it can have a great effect on a patient's self-esteem [6, 7]. Moreover, it may result in increased overall satisfaction, nude appearance, and sexual behavior [6, 8].

Numerous techniques attempt to enhance nipple reconstruction [4]. As a result, different approaches have been described to retain nipple projection and shape over time. Despite this, none report consistent outcomes [4, 9–17]. Even the most popular flaps result in loss of nipple projection 70% of the time in the first three postoperative years [14]. In unilateral reconstruction, matching the color of the areola to that of the other side can also be challenging. Intradermal tattooing is one of the most common solutions but has a tendency to reduce nipple projection and fade over time [4, 18].

In the face of these shortcomings, women will still opt to proceed with nipple reconstruction to restore a more natural appearance of the breast [4]. This is in spite of the paucity of evidence in the literature looking at patient preferences for NAC reconstruction. The few studies reporting on patient satisfaction have produced conflicting outcomes [4, 8, 18–21]. Some have shown improved satisfaction rates [4, 8, 18, 20], while others have either reported increased satisfaction with breast mound reconstruction only or discontent with NAC reconstruction in general, especially in younger patient populations [19, 21].

A.M.S. Ibrahim, M.D., Ph.D. (✉) • F.H. Lau, M.D.
Division of Plastic and Reconstructive Surgery, Louisiana State University Health Sciences Center, 1542 Tulane Avenue, New Orleans, LA 70112, USA
e-mail: aibra1@lsuhsc.edu; flau@lsuhsc.edu

H.H. Sinno, M.D.
Division of Plastic Surgery, McGill University, Montreal, QC, Canada, H3A 0G4
e-mail: hanisinno@gmail.com

B.T. Lee, M.D., M.B.A., M.P.H.
S.J. Lin, M.D., M.B.A.
Division of Plastic and Reconstructive Surgery, Beth Israel Deaconess Medical Center, Harvard Medical School, 110 Francis Street, Lowry Suite 5A, Boston, MA 02215, USA
e-mail: blee3@bidmc.harvard.edu; sjlin@bidmc.harvard.edu


M.A. Shiffman (ed.), *Nipple-Areolar Complex Reconstruction*, https://doi.org/10.1007/978-3-319-60925-6_79

Utility outcome studies permit the objective standardization of the health state preference of a health condition or disease state [22]. They range from 0 (death) to 1 (perfect health); as such, a numeric value can be assigned to different health states [23]. They are validated preference-based measures employed to assist in surgical decision making by providing a quantitative metric of the risk benefit/ratio for a range of conditions [23–34]. Furthermore, they are a recognized means of forming comparisons in health economics and research pertaining to individual health states [35, 36]. Utility indices were first introduced into the Plastic Surgery literature by Kerrigan et al. [23, 37] who measured the health state preferences in women with breast hypertrophy. It has since been used for numerous health states within the specialty [2, 22, 30–34, 38–40]. In this chapter, the use of utility outcome studies for analyzing patient preferences for NAC reconstruction based on a previously published study by the authors will be described [2].

## 79.2 Technique

### 79.2.1 Recruitment of Study Participants

Online ads were posted on the websites www.kijiji.ca and www.craigslist.org for a period of 1 year to recruit prospective participants from the general population. This was supplemented by enlisting medical students at McGill University (Montreal, Quebec). Of note, participation in this study was voluntary. All study participants were asked to complete an online survey which included an anonymous demographic questionnaire, a health state questionnaire, and utility assessment. To prevent multiple entries by a single participant entry, it was made obligatory that a valid email address be entered at the conclusion of the online survey. No one under the age of 18 years was included in this study. An electronic consent form was signed by all volunteers prior to their participation in this study.

### 79.2.2 Exclusion and Inclusion Criteria

To ensure that study participants were able to comprehend the nature of this study, they were asked to compare monocular blindness (having a higher utility score or health state closer to perfect health) and binocular blindness (having a lower utility score or a health state closer to death). Those that rated monocular blindness as having a lower utility score (closer to death) were excluded from participation in this study. To guarantee simplicity of the online survey, a five-point Likert scale was used to measure its ease of understanding.

### 79.2.3 Participant Demographics

A total of 118 prospective volunteers were enrolled in this study. One hundred three participants (87%) were able to comprehend the nature of this study, that is, they rated binocular blindness as being lower than monocular blindness and were included. A majority of study subjects were Caucasian (62.1%), female ($n$ = 81 females versus $n$ = 22 males) with an average age of 24.7 ± 8.2 years [2].

### 79.2.4 Basic Principles of Utility Outcome Indices

To ascertain the utility outcome scores and thereby objectifying the burden of a particular health state, different tests have been designed [23, 35–37]. Three validated health state preference instruments were employed for the measurement of utility scores for nipple-areola complex (NAC) reconstruction. These included standard gamble (SG), visual analogue scale (VAS), and time trade-off (TTO) [37, 41, 42]. The purpose of employing all three of these tools is to reduce the inherent deficiencies of any single test, decreasing bias and increasing reliability [22].

Study participants were shown a photograph of a patient who underwent breast reconstruction without right NAC reconstruction (Fig. 79.1). In the standard gamble (Fig. 79.2), they were given two choices and asked to pick one: in this case, either opt to remain in the given health state (breast reconstruction without NAC reconstruction) or gamble (undergo NAC reconstruction) with the probability of success (perfect health) or failure (death). Success and failure rates were then alternated until the participant became indifferent about whether to take a gamble or stay in the given health state. Standard gamble was calculated as:

$$\text{Utility health state} = \left(1.00 - \text{risk of death at the point of indifference}\right) \div 100$$

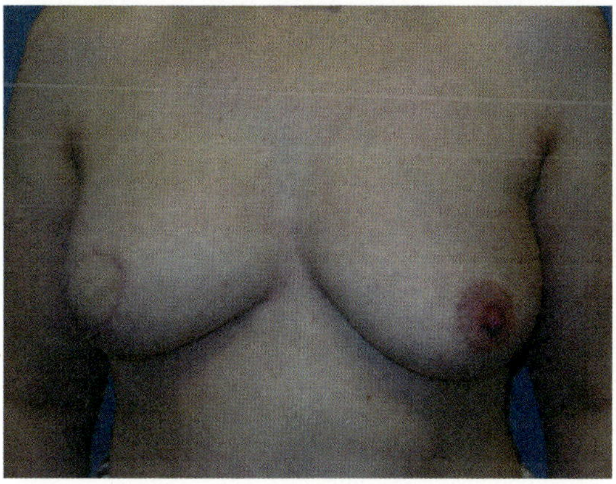

**Fig. 79.1** Patient without reconstructed NAC following breast reconstruction shown to prospective participants [2]. Reprinted with permission

To determine the subject's point of indifference, a bisecting search routine algorithm was employed. In the algorithm, a total of six iterations are utilized [37, 43]. In the event that a participant refuses to accept a 1% possibility of death, the test prompts them to answer whether they would be willing to accept any risk of death. Statements posed to the study participant are purposely phrased in terms of the probability of living in perfect health to eliminate the biasing effect of phrasing a question in terms of the chance of death [44]. To aid in the participant's comprehension of life years remaining, visual aids in the form of "smiley faces" and "Xs" are used [37].

In the visual analogue scale (Fig. 79.3), the study participant was asked to assign a value to the given health state (breast reconstruction without NAC reconstruction) on a scale of 0 (death) to 100 (perfect health). This is then calculated as:

$$\text{Utility health state} = \text{score} \div 100$$

In time trade-off (Fig. 79.4), the study participants were given the choice between living a specified number of years in the given health state (breast reconstruction without NAC reconstruction) or selecting to "trade-off" life years to attain perfect health (undergo NAC reconstruction). Similar to standard gamble, a bisecting search routine algorithm is employed to systematically

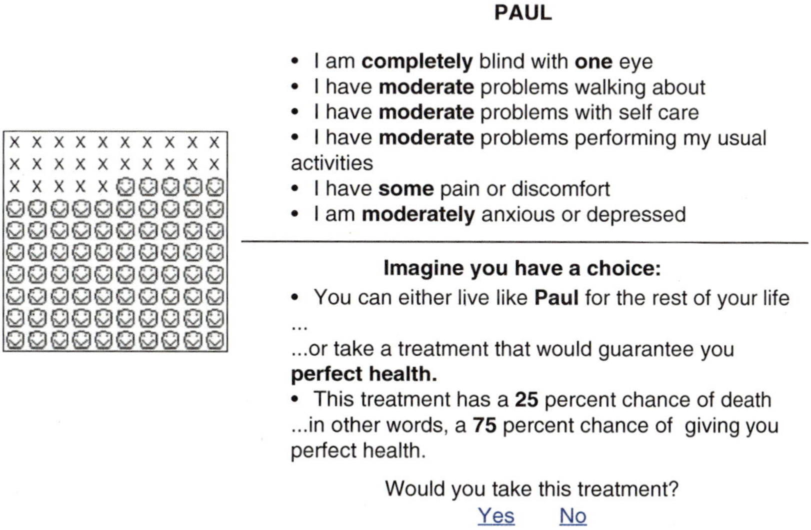


**Fig. 79.2** Utility assessment of standard gamble for monocular blindness [22]. Reprinted with permission

**Fig. 79.3** Utility assessment through a visual analogue scale for blindness [22]. Reprinted with permission

- I am **completely** blind with **one** eye
- I have **moderate** problems walking about
- I have **moderate** problems with self care
- I have **moderate** problems performing my usual activities
- I have **some** pain or discomfort
- I am **moderately** anxious or depressed

Imagine you are like **Paul**, completely blind in one eye. Rate your health state on the scale below from 0 (death) to 100 (perfect health):

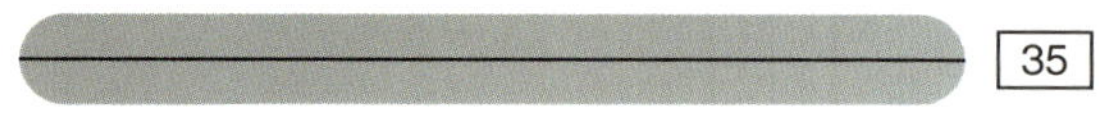


Click Below when you are finished

Next

**Fig. 79.4** Utility assessment time trade-off of survey for monocular blindness [22]. Reprinted with permission

**PAUL**

- I am **completely** blind with **one** eye
- I have **moderate** problems walking about
- I have **moderate** problems with self care
- I have **moderate** problems performing my usual activities
- I have **some** pain or discomfort
- I am **moderately** anxious or depressed

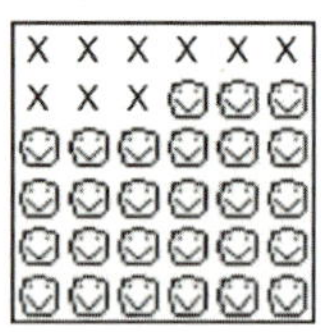


**Imagine you have a choice:**

- You can either live like Paul for the rest of your 36 years of life...
- ...or take a treatment that would guarantee you perfect health but you will lose **9** year of your life ...in other words you would live in perfect health for **27** years.

Would you take this treatment?

Yes No

alternate the number of years traded-off until the indifference point of the study participant is obtained. It is calculated as:

$$\text{Utility} = \left(\begin{array}{l}\text{number of years specified} \\ \text{in the described health state} - \\ \text{number of years traded} \\ \text{off at the indifference point}\end{array}\right) \div \text{number of years specified in the described health stage}$$

Once again, visual aid tools are used to ease the subject's comprehension of percentage of perfect health.

### 79.2.5 Statistical Analysis

SPSS for Windows, PASW Statistics 18, Release 18.0.0 (SPSS, Inc., Chicago, IL) was used for statistical analysis. To obtain mean utility scores and to compare continuous variables, independent and paired $t$-tests were done. To compare categorical variables, Chi-squared or Fisher's exact test was done. A linear regression model was used to measure each of the utility outcome measures (SG, TTO, and VAS) using age, sex, race, and education as independent predictors. Statistical significance was assigned to a value of $p < 0.05$.

#### 79.2.5.1 Utility Outcome Scores for Nipple-Areola Complex Reconstruction

Utility outcome measures for SG, VAS, and TTO for breast reconstruction without NAC reconstruction (0.92 ± 0.11, 0.84 ± 0.18, and 0.92 ± 0.11, respectively) were significantly different ($p < 0.001$) from those of monocular blindness

(0.85 ± 0.18, 0.60 ± 0.20, and 0.84 ± 0.17, respectively) and binocular blindness (0.66 ± 0.25, 0.32 ± 0.19, and 0.64 ± 0.27, respectively) [2]. These correlate to an 8% chance of death in order to obtain perfect health and a willingness to sacrifice 2.8 years of life when choosing to undergo NAC reconstruction. Study participants with a higher income (>$10,000) were more willing to gamble (SG $p = 0.015$) and risk (VAS $p = 0.049$) to attain perfect health (NAC reconstruction). Furthermore, based on linear regression analyses, having a medical education (including members of the general population with a medical background) impacted utility scores. Medical education was directly proportional to the SG and TTO scores ($p < 0.05$). No statistically significant differences in utility outcome scores were observed with gender (SG, $p = 0.616$, VAS, $p = 0.422$; TTO, $p = 0.152$) and being Caucasian (SG, $p = 0.989$, VAS, $p = 0.739$; TTO, $p = 0.596$) [2].

## 79.3 Discussion

In the current competitive healthcare marketplace, patient satisfaction has become an essential metric of quality of care [4, 45]. This is reinforced by the myriad of studies focused on gaining a better understanding of patient satisfaction in those undergoing breast reconstruction [46–50]. Despite this, there are only a few studies that have attempted to investigate the importance of nipple reconstruction in this patient population but with inconsistency in their outcomes [4, 8, 20, 21]. Although the result of nipple-areola complex (NAC) reconstruction may be more aesthetically pleasing [51], one study reports that this can be attributed to the plastic surgeon's own concept of naturalness and beauty rather than the patient's opinion [19]. To the contrary, Momoh et al. [4] found that patients who underwent nipple reconstruction had significantly higher general and aesthetic satisfaction scores. This notion is reinforced by Goh et al. [18] who reported that NAC reconstruction and tattooing were important to 96% of women with 93% stating that they would choose to undergo the procedure again. Timing of NAC reconstruction may also affect patient satisfaction as demonstrated by Losken et al. [3] who suggested that the greater the time interval from breast reconstruction to NAC reconstruction, the lower the satisfaction.

Among the various articles focused on patient satisfaction and quality of life for breast and NAC reconstruction, none had addressed the impact of living with breast reconstruction without NAC reconstruction, or NAC deformity, and the utility of undergoing NAC reconstruction until our previously published report [2]. The utility of NAC deformity was found to be comparable to other aesthetically comprised conditions including massive weight loss requiring a body contouring procedure [32], arm laxity needing a brachioplasty [52], thigh laxity necessitating a thigh lift [53], nasal deformity after primary rhinoplasty requiring revision [30], and aging neck calling for rejuvenation [33]. However, they were found to be higher than the respective scores for bilateral mastectomy [54], unilateral mastectomy [39], mastopexy for breast ptosis [40], and facial disfigurement requiring facial transplantation (Table 79.1) [34]. What this means is that if faced with choice of having to undergo NAC reconstruction, our participant population would be willing to take a similar theoretical risk on NAC reconstruction as they would for a body contouring procedure, brachioplasty, thigh lift, revision rhinoplasty, or a neck rejuvenation procedure. However, they would be willing to give up more, that is, take a greater risk to address unilateral mastectomy or bilateral mastectomy warranting breast reconstruction, breast ptosis needing mastopexy, and facial disfigurement necessitating facial transplantation. Therefore, the higher the utility score, the less morbid the condition from the perspective of the surveyed participant population and the lower the willingness to risk morbidity/mortality as well as number of years that a participant would be willing to sacrifice to obtain "perfect health."

A higher income was found to be a significant predictor for willingness to have the procedure done and attain the desired health state (reconstructed NAC). This may perhaps suggest that for these individuals there is more importance or value on one's body image and hence the

**Table 79.1** Comparison of utility scores for NAC deformity to other conditions

| Plastic surgical conditions | Visual analogue scale (VAS) | Time trade-off (TTO) | Standard gamble (SG) |
|---|---|---|---|
| NAC deformity [2] | 0.84 ± 0.18 | 0.92 ± 0.11 | 0.92 ± 0.11 |
| Aesthetic nasal deformity after primary rhinoplasty requiring revision [30] | 0.80 ± 0.13 | 0.90 ± 0.12 | 0.91 ± 0.13 |
| Massive weight loss requiring a body contouring procedure [32] | 0.79 ± 0.13 | 0.89 ± 0.12 | 0.89 ± 0.15 |
| Aging neck needing rejuvenation [33] | 0.89 ± 0.07 | 0.94 ± 0.08 | 0.95 ± 0.10 |
| Arm laxity needing brachioplasty [51] | 0.80 ± 0.14 | 0.91 ± 0.12 | 0.94 ± 0.10 |
| Thigh laxity necessitating thigh lift [52] | 0.77 ± 0.15 | 0.90 ± 0.11 | 0.89 ± 0.14 |
| Facial disfigurement requiring facial transplantation [34] | 0.46 ± 0.02 | 0.68 ± 0.03 | 0.66 ± 0.03 |
| Unilateral mastectomy [38] | 0.75 ± 0.17 | 0.87 ± 0.15 | 0.86 ± 0.18 |
| Breast ptosis needing mastopexy [39] | 0.80 ± 0.14 | 0.87 ± 0.18 | 0.90 ± 0.14 |
| Bilateral mastectomy [53] | 0.70 ± 0.18 | 0.85 ± 0.16 | 0.86 ± 0.17 |

completeness of all stages of breast reconstruction including NAC reconstruction compared to their lower-income counterparts. Having a medical background also correlated to an increased willingness to undergo NAC reconstruction. This result can perhaps be linked to the fact that this subgroup of participants may have a better understanding of the risks and benefits synonymous with this procedure. No significant differences were observed in utility outcomes within ethnic groups and among the different genders. Although the process of breast and NAC reconstruction following mastectomy may be more of a relevant issue for women, the purpose of this investigation was to obtain data on population preferences as a whole and to observe any variations. This finding may be attributed to similarities in the perception of living with NAC deformity among men and women.

This analysis is not without its limitations. As previously reported [2], these include sampling bias, that is, the extent to which this participant population is representative of the general population as a whole. To reduce the effects of this bias, data was not just ascertained from women undergoing breast or NAC reconstruction. Further studies may investigate the utility scores within this subset of patients prior to and following NAC reconstruction [2]. Similarly, plastic surgeons were not surveyed to abolish the inherent bias placed on the value of NAC reconstruction as well as conflict of interest with regard to financial compensation for this procedure. The question remains, should utility scores be obtained from a sample of the general population or patients living with the specific health states? To date there is still an ongoing debate [37]. The panels on cost-effectiveness in health and medicine recommend that utility outcomes be performed on a sample from the general public [55] although a questionnaire aimed at the general public might not adequately be able to capture the influence of the described health state on those affected. Obtaining utility scores from the affected patient population offers the distinct advantage of understanding the psychological and physical impact that a disease state or condition has on these individuals. However, studies have demonstrated that patients living with these health states become accustomed and therefore less bothered by their condition [22]. One study showed that patients with facial disfigurement adjust to their appearance to the extent that they would be willing to give up less to correct their deformity [56]. One could also make the argument that health states involving infants such as cleft lip and palate are at the discretion of family members. With that said, family members may be less willing to proceed with a corrective procedure to avoid even minimal short-term morbidity to their child. This reinforces the notion that assessment of utility scores should be from a neutral sample of the general population.

Another concern is the notion that absence of the NAC may not be a disease state. Furthermore, no standard definition was used for NAC reconstruction, for example, true reconstruction in the operating room versus tattooing in clinic which may have affected participant responses especially those without a medical background. These issues may have been overcome by our large sample size ($n = 103$) and subgroup analysis excluding patients who could not comprehend the nature of the study.

## Conclusions

Utility outcome studies can be used to objectively assess the health state burden of living without the presence of a nipple-areola complex in a reconstructed breast. Patient preferences can be ascertained using these indices with the current data indicating that the general population would be prepared to risk an 8% chance of death in order to obtain perfect health and a willingness to sacrifice 2.8 years of life when choosing to undergo NAC reconstruction. Furthermore, patients choosing to undergo NAC reconstruction would be as willing to take a similar theoretical risk as in previously reported aesthetically comprised conditions.

## References


1. Jenkins M, Patel S. Assessment of risk factors associated with nipple reconstruction. Breast J. 2016;22:377–8.
2. Ibrahim AM, Sinno HH, Izadpanah A, et al. Nipple-areolar complex reconstruction following postmastectomy breast reconstruction: a comparative utility assessment study. Plast Reconstr Surg Glob Open. 2015;3:e380.
3. Losken A, Duggal CS, Desai KA, McCullough MC, Gruszynski MA, Carlson GW. Time to completion of nipple reconstruction: what factors are involved? Ann Plast Surg. 2013;70:530–2.
4. Momoh AO, Colakoglu S, de Blacam C, et al. The impact of nipple reconstruction on patient satisfaction in breast reconstruction. Ann Plast Surg. 2012;69:389–93.
5. Craig ES, Walker ME, Salomon J, Fusi S. Immediate nipple reconstruction utilizing the DIEP flap in areolasparing mastectomy. Microsurgery. 2013;33: 125–9.
6. Sisti A, Grimaldi L, Tassinari J, et al. Nipple-areola complex reconstruction techniques: a literature review. Eur J Surg Oncol. 2016;42:441–65.
7. Yang JD, Ryu JY, Ryu DW, et al. Our experiences in nipple reconstruction using the hammond flap. Arch Plast Surg. 2014;41(5):550.
8. Wellisch DK, Schain WS, Noone RB, Little JW 3rd. The psychological contribution of nipple addition in breast reconstruction. Plast Reconstr Surg. 1987;80:699–704.
9. Shestak KC, Nguyen TD. The double opposing periareola flap: a novel concept for nipple-areola reconstruction. Plast Reconstr Surg. 2007;119:473–80.
10. Weiss J, Herman O, Rosenberg L, Shafir R. The S nipple-areola reconstruction. Plast Reconstr Surg. 1989;83:904–6.
11. Chang WH. Nipple reconstruction with a T flap. Plast Reconstr Surg. 1984;73:140–3.
12. Kroll SS. Nipple reconstruction with the double-opposing tab flap. Plast Reconstr Surg. 1999;104:511–4; discussion 5–7.
13. Eo S, Kim SS, Da Lio AL. Nipple reconstruction with C-v flap using dermofat graft. Ann Plast Surg. 2007;58:137–40.
14. Schoeller T, Schubert HM, Pulzl P, Wechselberger G. Nipple reconstruction using a modified arrow flap technique. Breast. 2006;15:762–8.
15. Germano D, De Biasio F, Piedimonte A, Parodi PC. Nipple reconstruction using the fleur-de-lis flap technique. Aesthetic Plast Surg. 2006;30:399–402.
16. Gamboa-Bobadilla GM. Nipple reconstruction: the top hat technique. Ann Plast Surg. 2005;54:243–6.
17. Rubino C, Dessy LA, Posadinu A. A modified technique for nipple reconstruction: the 'arrow flap'. Br J Plast Surg. 2003;56:247–51.
18. Goh SC, Martin NA, Pandya AN, Cutress RI. Patient satisfaction following nipple-areolar complex reconstruction and tattooing. J Plast Reconstr Aesthet Surg. 2011;64(3):360.
19. Jabor MA, Shayani P, Collins DR Jr, Karas T, Cohen BE. Nipple-areola reconstruction: satisfaction and clinical determinants. Plast Reconstr Surg. 2002;110:457–63; discussion 64–5.
20. Asplund O. Nipple and areola reconstruction. A study in 79 mastectomized women. Scand J Plast Reconstr Surg. 1983;17:233–40.
21. Andrade WN, Baxter N, Semple JL. Clinical determinants of patient satisfaction with breast reconstruction. Plast Reconstr Surg. 2001;107:46–54.
22. Sinno H, Dionisopoulos T, Slavin SA, Ibrahim AM, Chung KC, Lin SJ. The utility of outcome studies in plastic surgery. Plast Reconstr Surg Glob Open. 2014;2:e189.
23. Kerrigan CL, Collins ED, Kneeland TS, et al. Measuring health state preferences in women with breast hypertrophy. Plast Reconstr Surg. 2000;106:280–8.
24. Liem YS, Bosch JL, Hunink MG. Preference-based quality of life of patients on renal replacement therapy: a systematic review and meta-analysis. Value Health. 2008;11:733–41.

25. Lara AM, Wakholi BN, Kasirye A, et al. Utility assessment of HIV/AIDS-related health states in HIV-infected Ugandans. AIDS. 2008;22(Suppl 1):S123–30.
26. Coffey JT, Brandle M, Zhou H, et al. Valuing health-related quality of life in diabetes. Diabetes Care. 2002;25:2238–43.
27. Smith KJ, Roberts MS. Quality-of-life utility values for erectile function and sildenafil treatment. Clin Drug Investig. 2005;25:99–105.
28. Schmidlin M, Fritsch K, Matthews F, Thurnheer R, Senn O, Bloch KE. Utility indices in patients with the obstructive sleep apnea syndrome. Respiration. 2010;79:200–8.
29. Sinno H, Izadpanah A, Tahiri Y, et al. The impact of living with severe lower extremity lymphedema: a utility outcomes score assessment. Ann Plast Surg. 2014;73(2):210–4.
30. Sinno H, Izadpanah A, Thibaudeau S, et al. The impact of living with a functional and aesthetic nasal deformity after primary rhinoplasty: a utility outcomes score assessment. Ann Plast Surg. 2012;69(4):431.
31. Sinno H, Thibaudeau S, Izadpanah A, et al. Utility outcome scores for unilateral facial paralysis. Ann Plast Surg. 2012;69:435–8.
32. Sinno H, Thibaudeau S, Tahiri Y, et al. Utility assessment of body contouring after massive weight loss. Aesthetic Plast Surg. 2011;35:724–30.
33. Sinno HH, Ibrahim AM, Izadpanah A, et al. Utility outcome assessment of the aging neck following massive weight loss. Otolaryngol Head Neck Surg. 2012;147:26–32.
34. Sinno HH, Thibaudeau S, Duggal A, Lessard L. Utility scores for facial disfigurement requiring facial transplantation [outcomes article]. Plast Reconstr Surg. 2010;126:443–9.
35. Torrance GW, Feeny D. Utilities and quality-adjusted life years. Int J Technol Assess Health Care. 1989;5:559–75.
36. Read JL, Quinn RJ, Berwick DM, Fineberg HV, Weinstein MC. Preferences for health outcomes. Comparison of assessment methods. Med Decis Making. 1984;4:315–29.
37. Chang WT, Collins ED, Kerrigan CL. An Internet-based utility assessment of breast hypertrophy. Plast Reconstr Surg. 2001;108:370–7.
38. Sinno H, Izadpanah A, Tahiri Y, et al. The impact of living with severe lower extremity lymphedema: a utility outcomes score assessment. Ann Plast Surg. 2014;73:210–4.
39. Sinno H, Izadpanah A, Vorstenbosch J, et al. Living with a unilateral mastectomy defect: a utility assessment and outcomes study. J Reconstr Microsurg. 2014;30:313–8.
40. Ibrahim AM, Sinno HH, Izadpanah A, et al. Mastopexy for breast ptosis: utility outcomes of population preferences. Plast Surg (Oakv). 2015;23:103–7.
41. Torrance GW. Measurement of health state utilities for economic appraisal. J Health Econ. 1986;5:1–30.
42. Stevens KJ, McCabe CJ, Brazier JE. Mapping between Visual Analogue Scale and Standard Gamble data; results from the UK Health Utilities Index 2 valuation survey. Health Econ. 2006;15:527–33.
43. Boyd NF, Sutherland HJ, Heasman KZ, Tritchler DL, Cummings BJ. Whose utilities for decision analysis? Med Decis Making. 1990;10:58–67.
44. McNeil BJ, Pauker SG, Sox HC Jr, Tversky A. On the elicitation of preferences for alternative therapies. N Engl J Med. 1982;306:1259–62.
45. Williams B. Patient satisfaction: a valid concept? Soc Sci Med. 1994;38:509–16.
46. ES H, Pusic AL, Waljee JF, et al. Patient-reported aesthetic satisfaction with breast reconstruction during the long-term survivorship Period. Plast Reconstr Surg. 2009;124:1–8.
47. Alderman AK, Wilkins EG, Lowery JC, Kim M, Davis JA. Determinants of patient satisfaction in postmastectomy breast reconstruction. Plast Reconstr Surg. 2000;106:769–76.
48. Saulis AS, Mustoe TA, Fine NA. A retrospective analysis of patient satisfaction with immediate post-mastectomy breast reconstruction: comparison of three common procedures. Plast Reconstr Surg. 2007;119:1669–76; discussion 77–8.
49. Yueh JH, Slavin SA, Adesiyun T, et al. Patient satisfaction in postmastectomy breast reconstruction: a comparative evaluation of DIEP, TRAM, latissimus flap, and implant techniques. Plast Reconstr Surg. 2010;125:1585–95.
50. Craft RO, Colakoglu S, Curtis MS, et al. Patient satisfaction in unilateral and bilateral breast reconstruction [outcomes article]. Plast Reconstr Surg. 2011;127:1417–24.
51. Didier F, Arnaboldi P, Gandini S, et al. Why do women accept to undergo a nipple sparing mastectomy or to reconstruct the nipple areola complex when nipple sparing mastectomy is not possible? Breast Cancer Res Treat. 2012;132:1177–84.
52. Ibrahim AM, Sinno HH, Izadpanah A, et al. Population preferences of undergoing brachioplasty for arm laxity. Ann Plast Surg. 2014;73(Suppl 2):S149–52.
53. Izadpanah A, Sinno H, Vorstenbosch J, Lee BT, Lin SJ. Thigh laxity after massive weight loss: a utilities outcomes assessment. Ann Plast Surg. 2013;71:304–7.
54. Sinno H, Izadpanah A, Thibaudeau S, Christodoulou G, Lin SJ, Dionisopoulos T. An objective assessment of the perceived quality of life of living with bilateral mastectomy defect. Breast. 2013;22:168–72.
55. Weinstein MC, Stason WB. Foundations of cost-effectiveness analysis for health and medical practices. N Engl J Med. 1977;296:716–21.
56. Barker JH, Furr A, Cunningham M, et al. Investigation of risk acceptance in facial transplantation. Plast Reconstr Surg. 2006;118:663–70.

# 80 How Long Does the Nipple Projection Last After Reconstruction Using Purse-String Technique?

Yoko Katsuragi-Tomioka and Masahiro Nakagawa

## 80.1 Introduction

Nipple-areola reconstruction (NAR) is the tip procedure in breast reconstruction, especially having emotional influence for the patients. Numerous techniques have been reported so far. Here we will share our experience using Hammond flap and will give a discussion especially focusing on the projection after long follow-up with each technique.

## 80.2 Technique

Hammond et al. [1] reported the skate flap purse-string technique for nipple-areola complex reconstruction in 2007. As compared with other techniques, such as the star flap, skate flap, double-opposing tab flap, and others, this method has a great advantage that it does not produce a scar outside the areola, because the donor for the flap is closed with two island flaps using the circling purse-string technique. It neither disturbs the shape of the breast that is usually inevitable by simple closure of the local flap donor in other techniques. We report here the results of a retrospective study to determine how the projection lasts after reconstruction by this method [2].

Between August of 2004 and April of 2009, 16 female patients underwent nipple-areola complex reconstruction using this technique at the Shizuoka Cancer Center. The women were aged 32–64 years (average, 49 years). Six patients underwent breast reconstruction with autologous tissue, and ten received implants.

The areola diameter was designed to be equal to that of the opposite areola, which ranged from 27 to 34 mm (average, 31 mm), and the height of the flap was designed to be 10–17 mm (average, 11 mm) (Fig. 80.1). Other procedures were as described in the first report by Hammond et al. [1].

The projection of the nipple tended to shrink with time (Fig. 80.2). In patients followed up for more than 12 months, the average size of the projection was 2.3 mm (32% of that of the opposite nipple), and in patients followed up for more than 24 months, the average was 1.9 mm (27% of that of the opposite nipple). There was no difference in the degree of shrinkage between patients who underwent autologous reconstruction and those who received implants [2].

Y. Katsuragi-Tomioka, M.D. (✉)
M. Nakagawa, M.D., Ph.D.
Division of Plastic and Reconstructive Surgery|,
Shizuoka Cancer Center Hospital,
Shimonagakubo 1007, Naga-Izumi, Shizuoka
411-8777, Japan
e-mail: yoko1031prs@gmail.com; yoko-prs@umin.ac.jp; m.nakagawa@scchr.jp


M.A. Shiffman (ed.), *Nipple-Areolar Complex Reconstruction*,
https://doi.org/10.1007/978-3-319-60925-6_80

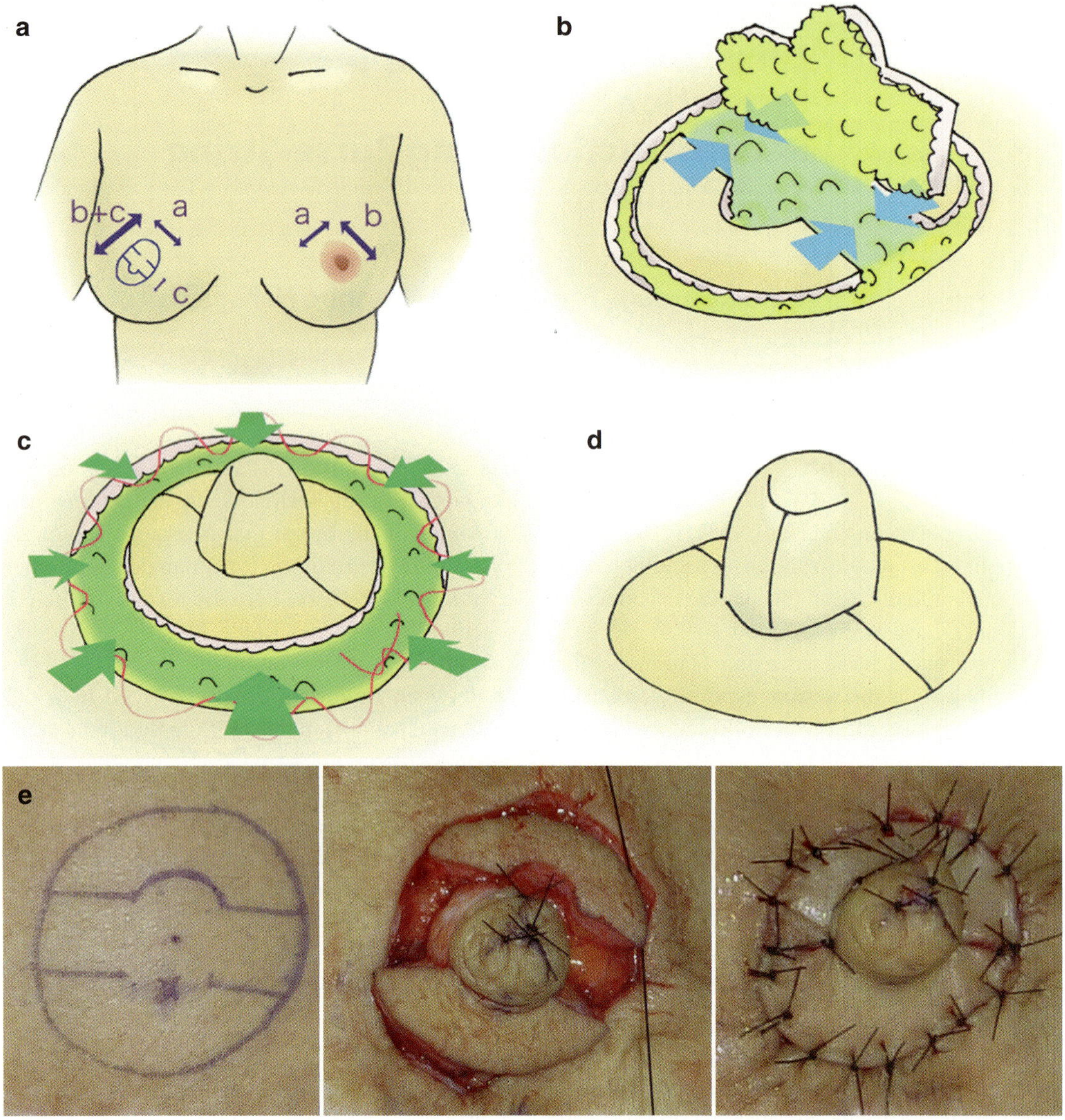


**Fig. 80.1** Procedure of modified skate flap purse-string technique. (**a**) Many areolas are not in precise *circle* but are *elliptic*. Since the height of the reconstructed nipple tends to shrink from half to one thirds, authors recommend to design the flap height 10–15 mm (**c**), according to the desired height. Either *circle* or *elliptic* areola can be designed by adding this height to the minor (**a**) or longer (**b**) axis. (**b**) The modified skate flap is raised at the subcutaneous plane. The donor of the skate flap (area in *blue*) will be covered by the two island flaps. (**c**) The circular gap (area in *green*) will be covered by the surrounding skin, which is gathered by purse-string technique (*red string*). This is the reason why this technique does not influence the shape of the reconstructed breast. (**d**) Scar does not exceed the outline of the areola, which is another advantage of this technique. (**e**) Procedure on a patient

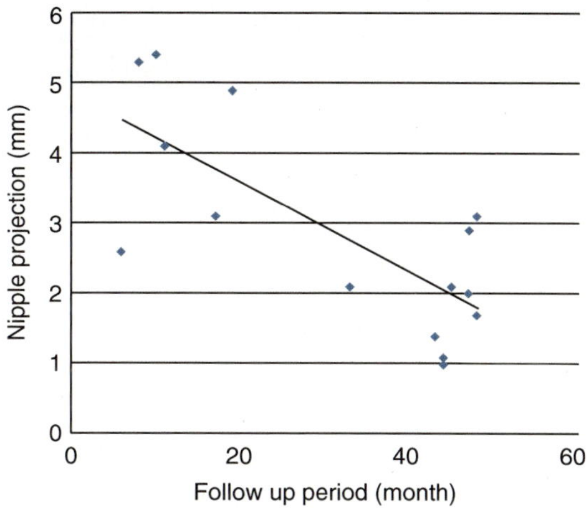


**Fig. 80.2** (*Left*, *middle*, *right*) Nipple projection is unlikely to be maintained much in long-term follow-up. There was no difference in shrinkage rate between patients with autologous reconstruction and those with implants

## 80.3 Discussion

The modified skate flap purse-string technique was useful in both autologous/implant groups, with minimum donor sacrifice and inconspicuous scarring. The use of this technique does not affect the shape of the reconstructed breast and enables reconstruction of not only circular areolas but also oval areolas; however, further improvements still need to be devised for the reconstruction of nipples with greater height.

Past reports show variations in the projection of the reconstructed nipple depending on the technique used and the length of follow-up after surgery. Zhong et al. [3] reported that with the nipples reconstructed with the modified skate flap, the mean projection was 2.5 mm (range: 1–4 mm) at a median follow-up of 44 months. In other studies in which the mean follow-up period or minimum follow-up period was longer than 2 years, Few et al. reported that the residual projection was 41% after reconstruction with the star flap as compared with the intraoperative projection [4], and Kroll [5] reported a projection of 2.43 mm after reconstruction using the double-opposing tab flap method and of 1.96 mm after using the star flap method.

To maintain better projection of the reconstructed nipple, usage of cartilage or allografts is reported. Tanabe et al. reported that the remaining projection was 94.6% 1–3 years after reconstruction using a bilobed flap with concha cartilage storing [6]. Another technique reported by Mori et al. was to use the dermis of the DIEP to support costal cartilage after skin-sparing mastectomy (SSM) [7]. Their technique was to bank the costal cartilage. Then, with SSM and the costal cartilage, immediate reconstruction using DIEP and at the nipple-areolar complex (NAR) the costal cartilage was fixed on the dermal base of the buried DIEP flap, which prevented sinking of the cartilage. At a mean follow-up of 12.6 months, 59% of the nipple projection was maintained [7]. Garramone and Lam [8] reported that the use of AlloDerm with a modified star flap improved long-term nipple projection and also that there was a significant difference in the remaining projection between the subjects undergoing reconstruction with transverse rectus abdominis musculocutaneous flaps and those receiving implants.

Winocour et al. [9] made a great systematic review. According to their study, each final/initial nipple projection was 3.3 mm/6.4 mm with auricular cartilage, 5.2 mm/9.4 mm with acellular dermal matrix, 4.1 mm/6.4 mm with composite tissue, 3.5 mm/5.6 mm with contralateral breast tissue, 7.0 mm/9.9 mm with costal cartilage, 8.0 mm/11.5 mm with rolled dermal fat, 4.0 mm/6.5 mm with ECM collagen cylinder, 9.4 mm/15.0 mm with fat grafts, 5.6 mm/6.6 mm with labia minora, 8.0 mm/8.0 mm with polyurethane prosthesis, and 12.9 mm/16.7 mm with silicone rods [9]. They concluded that synthetic materials have higher complication rates and allogeneic grafts have nipple projection comparable to that of autologous grafts. Sisti et al. [10] also made a literature review, finding that flaps appear to be more reliable (complication rate 10.1%) than grafts (complication rate 46.9%) in nipple reconstruction.

In our study, there were no significant differences between the patients undergoing autologous breast reconstruction and those receiving implants. On the other hand, Gilleard reported that the nipples reconstructed on implant-only breast mounds maintained projection to a greater extent than those reconstructed on purely autologous tissue [11]. They commented the possibility that the implant provides a more solid foundation for the flap, which is a very reasonable explanation.

For patients who can accept sacrificing half of the height of the prominent nipple, nipple sharing is a viable option [12]. It is particularly beneficial for patients with large contralateral nipples, providing good color and texture match for the nipple and also the opportunity to reduce the size of the donor nipple. The donor-site morbidity might be the main concern for the patients; many concerns remain to cut the healthy nipple. Haslik [13] has reported that after a mean follow-up period of 21 ± 12 months, nipple sharing led to a projection of 3.0 mm (2.0–3.0) for the reconstructed nipple and 4.5 mm (4.0–5.0) for the donor. Furthermore they evaluated the sensitivity in the donor nipple: decreasing from 1.2 g/mm$^2$ (0.8–1.6) to 1.8 g/mm$^2$ (0.8–4.8) which was insignificantly ($p = 0.054$, $N = 26$). It was notable that 88% of their patients were "very satisfied" or "somewhat satisfied," which would encourage patients and surgeons to undergo nipple sharing.

Focusing on the postoperative care to maintain nipple projection, direct pressure must be avoided. Dressing is another factor that influences the lasting projection; Salgarello et al. [14] suggest using silicone nipple shield for over a month. Doughnut-shaped dressings made from sponges or cotton are also commonly used [6, 15–17]. Rosing et al. [17] reported the effectiveness of the Asteame Nipple Guard TM; the mean decrease in nipple projection at 6 months was 46.6% while that of the control group was 71.8% ($p < 0.05$).

As the psychology contribution is reported by Wellisch et al. [18], the final appearance of the NAC has an important role for breast reconstruction patients. Momoh et al. [19] reported that patients' satisfaction was greater when NAR was followed after breast reconstruction, and furthermore, Jabor et al. [20] reported that the main point of patient dissatisfaction with NAR is inadequate nipple projection. Further studies with high-level evidence are needed to determine the gold standard for nipple reconstruction, since projection, color, texture, and sensitivity are all essential factors for better matching NAR.

## Conclusions

The Hammond flap gives minimal distortion of the contour of the breast by using a purse-string technique of the donor defect. It is usable after both autologous reconstruction and expander/implant reconstruction. The donor scar does not exceed from the areola; also the areola can be reconstructed in an oval shape, which is seen in many contralateral breasts.

Postoperative care to avoid direct pressure can improve the projection in the long term. Loss of height is seen in all autologous NAR; so far the evidence level of the outcome assessment is low in this area.

## References

1. Hammond DC, Khuthaila D, Kim J. The skate flap purse-string technique for nipple-areola complex reconstruction. Plast Reconstr Surg. 2007;120:399–406.
2. Katsuragi Y, Kayano S, Koizumi T, Matsui T, Nakagawa M. How long does the nipple projection last after reconstruction using the skate flap purse-string technique? Plast Reconstr Surg. 2011;127:149e–51e.
3. Zhong T, Antony A, Cordeiro P. Surgical outcomes and nipple projection using the modified skate flap for nipple-areolar reconstruction in a series of 422 implant reconstructions. Ann Plast Surg. 2009;62:591–5.
4. Few JW, Marcus JR, Casas LA, Aitken ME, Redding J. Long-term predictable nipple projection following reconstruction. Plast Reconstr Surg. 1999;104:1321–4.

5. Kroll SS, Reece GP, Miller MJ, Evans GR, Robb GL, Baldwin BJ, Schusterman MA. A comparison of nipple projection with the modified double-opposing tab and star flaps. Plast Reconstr Surg. 1997;99:1602–5.
6. Tanabe HY, Tai Y, Kiyokawa K, Yamauchi T. Nipple-areola reconstruction with a dermal-fat flap and rolled auricular cartilage. Plast Reconstr Surg. 1997;100:431–8.
7. Mori H, Uemura N, Okazaki M. Nipple reconstruction with banked costal cartilage after vertical-type skin-sparing mastectomy and deep inferior epigastric artery perforator flap. Breast Cancer. 2012;22: 95–7.
8. Garramone CE, Lam B. Use of AlloDerm in primary nipple reconstruction to improve long-term nipple projection. Plast Reconstr Surg. 2007;119:1663–8.
9. Winocour S, Saksena A, Oh C, Wu PS, Laungani A, Baltzer H, Saint-Cyr M. A systematic review of comparison of autologous, allogeneic, and synthetic augmentation grafts in nipple reconstruction. Plast Reconstr Surg. 2016;137:14e–23e.
10. Sisti A, Grimaldi L, Tassinari J, Cuomo R, Fortezza L, Bocchiotti MA, Roviello F, D'Aniello C, Nisi G. Nipple-areola complex reconstruction techniques: a literature review. Eur J Surg Oncol. 2016;42:441–65.
11. Gilleard O, Bowles PF, Tay SKL, Jones ME. The influence of breast mound reconstruction type on nipple reconstruction projection. J Plast Reconstr Aesthet Surg. 2015;68:1310–1.
12. Zenn MR, Garofalo JA. Unilateral nipple reconstruction with nipple sharing: time for a second look. Plast Reconstr Surg. 2009;123:1648–53.
13. Haslik W, Nedomansky J, Hacker S, Nickl S, Schroegendorfer KF. Objective and subjective evaluation of donor-site morbidity after nipple sharing for nipple areola reconstruction. J Plast Reconstr Aesthet Surg. 2015;68:168–74.
14. Salgarello M, Cervelli D, Barone-Adesi L. The use of a silicone nipple shield as protective device in nipple reconstruction. J Plast Reconstr Aesthet Surg. 2008;61(11):1396–8.
15. Eo S, Kim SS, Da Lio AL. Nipple reconstruction with C-V flap using dermofat graft. Ann Plast Surg. 2007;58:137–40.
16. Yamamoto Y, Furukawa H, Oyama A, Horiuchi K, Funayama E, Tsutsumida A, Sugihara T, Nohira K. Two innovations of the star-flap technique for nipple reconstruction. Br J Plast Surg. 2001;54:723–6.
17. Rosing JH, Momeni A, Kamperman K, Kahn D, Gurtner G, Lee GK. Effectiveness of the Asteame Nipple Guard™ in maintaining projection following nipple reconstruction: a prospective randomised controlled trial. J Plast Reconstr Aesthet Surg. 2009;63(10):1592–6.
18. Wellisch DK, Schain WS, Noone RB, Little JW. The psychological contribution of nipple addition in breast reconstruction. Plast Reconstr Surg. 1987;80(5):699–704.
19. Momoh AO, Colakoglu S, de Blacam C, Yueh JH, Lin SJ, Tobias AM, Lee BT. The impact of nipple reconstruction on patient satisfaction in breast reconstruction. Ann Plast Surg. 2012;69:389–93.
20. Jabor MA, Shayani P, Collins DR Jr, Karas T, Cohen BE. Nipple-areola reconstruction: satisfaction and clinical determinants. Plast Reconstr Surg. 2002;110:1–7.

# Single-Stage Nipple-Areolar Complex Reconstruction

# 81

Benjamin Liliav and Julianne Scott

## 81.1 Introduction

While nipple-sparing mastectomies (NSM) are becoming more common, not every breast cancer patient is a candidate for this surgery [6–8]. Patients who do not qualify for NSM will continue to require an effective and efficient technique for creation of an aesthetically pleasing NAC. Nipple-areolar reconstruction (NAR) thus remains an important restorative procedure to this subset of patients who may experience a modified perception of their body scheme without a NAC, contributing to a negative body image [9–11]. NAR is a vital step contributing to patient psychological well-being and results in the most natural final aesthetic breast [12]. A single-stage nipple-areolar complex reconstruction (SS NAR) offers patients a safe and effective method creating a superior outcome in only one visit.

Nipple-areolar complex reconstruction is often the final step in the breast reconstructive process [13, 14]. It is an integral part of breast restoration and often represents the final phase of the long, challenging process that patients endure. Creation of an aesthetic nipple and areola is associated with a higher degree of patient satisfaction [15–17]. The presence of the NAC is essential to the natural appearance of the breast as it is the finishing touch to the process. Many different techniques for NAC reconstruction are currently used by surgeons depending on their experience, preference, and training. These include local flap, grafting, nipple-sharing, and tattoo-only methods [1–3, 18, 19]. Most methods achieve a satisfactory NAC that augments the appearance of the final reconstructed breast, yet vary in time to completion, maintenance of nipple projection, and symmetry of the final NAC [3]. Local flap reconstruction is the most utilized current method which has been shown to pose the lowest risk to patients and is associated with the best maintenance of nipple projection when compared to grafting techniques [3, 20]. Traditionally, this stage is completed in two separate steps: the first being nipple reconstruction and the second being creation of the areola with medical tattooing. SS NAR is an alternative method that achieves a nat-

B. Liliav, M.D. (✉)
Department of Plastic, Reconstructive, Cosmetic and Hand Surgery, Eastern Maine Medical Center, 417 State St. Suite 443, Bangor, ME 04401, USA

College of Medicine, University of Vermont, Burlington, VT 05405, USA

Division of Plastic, Reconstructive and Cosmetic Surgery, Department of Surgery, University of Illinois at Chicago, Chicago, IL 60607, USA

College of Osteopathic Medicine, University of New England, Biddeford, ME 04005, USA
e-mail: BLiliav@EMHS.org

J. Scott, M.S.
College of Osteopathic Medicine, University of New England, Biddeford, ME 04005, USA
e-mail: JScott12@UNE.edu


M.A. Shiffman (ed.), *Nipple-Areolar Complex Reconstruction*,
https://doi.org/10.1007/978-3-319-60925-6_81

ural-appearing NAC with the benefit of a shortened time to completion of the reconstructive process. The longer a patient must wait between breast reconstruction and completion of the NAC, the lower the level of satisfaction with the process and final result [4]. In one visit, intradermal medical pigmentation and nipple construct creation are achieved in a single step. This method creates sufficient pigmentation and nipple projection while reducing the number of visits and shortening the total time a woman spends finishing the surgical restoration, thus increasing patient satisfaction.

## 81.2 Technique

Nipple position is determined collaboratively between the surgeon and the patient preoperatively. Nipple sizers can be traced onto electrocardiographic leads and subsequently cut out to represent nipple size and location. Commercially available sizers can be useful in helping the patient select a desired size in bilateral reconstructions or simply match the existing areola in unilateral cases. These cutouts are placed in an ideal location with the patient upright and shoulders in a relaxed position and are outlined with marking pen for identification in the operating room (Fig. 81.1). The positioning of the NAC is essential to the aesthetic appearance of the final breast reconstruction. In unilateral reconstruction, it is common to match the NAC position to the contralateral breast to match the appearance of that breast without a brassiere. In bilateral reconstructions, the ideal location will form an equilateral triangle from the nipple to the sternal notch but varies depending on anatomy, type of reconstruction, and patient preference. The nipple should be centrally located within the areola [21, 22].

Typically the pigments selected are two to three shades darker than the native or desired nipple color to account for predictable fading of the pigmented area. Two pigments are selected: one darker for the nipple and one lighter for the areola (Fig. 81.2) [3]. Surgical technique for the SS NAR begins with medical pigmentation and creation of a nipple construct via local C-V flap. The C-V flap is designed with a 1 cm pedicle base (representing the nipple diameter) and is marked within the designated areolar diameter (Fig. 81.3). The "V" wing widths will represent the nipple projection length and should account for 30–35% decrease in nipple projection over time. Thus, the surgeon must add additional width to the "V" wings to achieve desired projection. If the patient indicates the desire for more significant projection, acellular dermal matrices can be used as an adjunct to the C-V flap technique [23]. A piece of acellular matrix (Fig. 81.4) is cut to the desired length and rolled up to create a reinforcing cylinder shape that is then placed in the center around which the "V" wings wrap and capped by the "C" portion of the flap (Figs. 81.5 and 81.6).

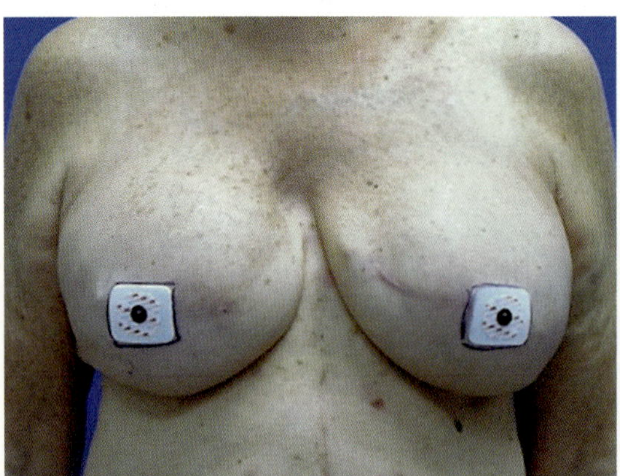

**Fig. 81.1** Nipple position is determined preoperatively and marked for identification in the operating room

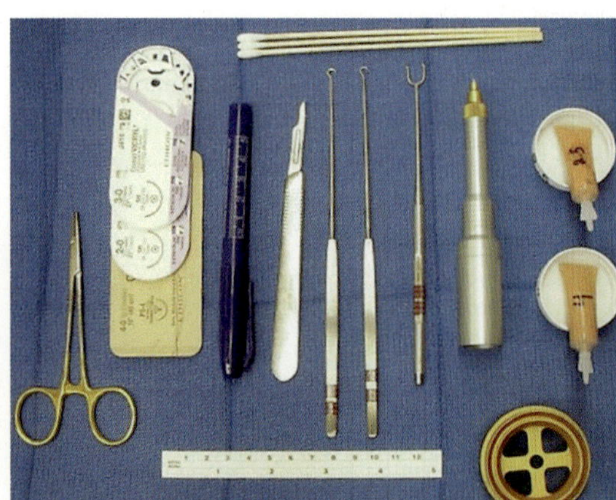

**Fig. 81.2** Equipment tray

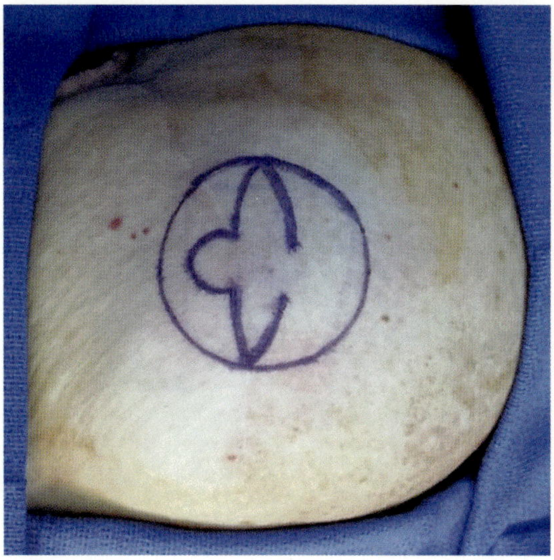

**Fig. 81.3** C-V flap outline within marked areola

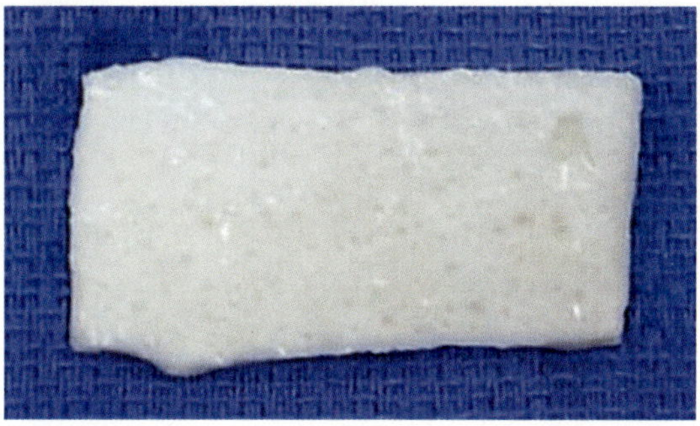

**Fig. 81.4** Acellular matrix cut to desired width

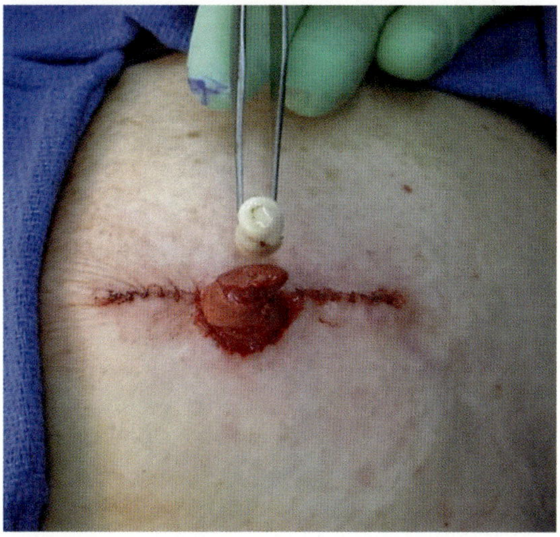

**Fig. 81.5** Acellular matrix is rolled up for insertion into center of the nipple construct

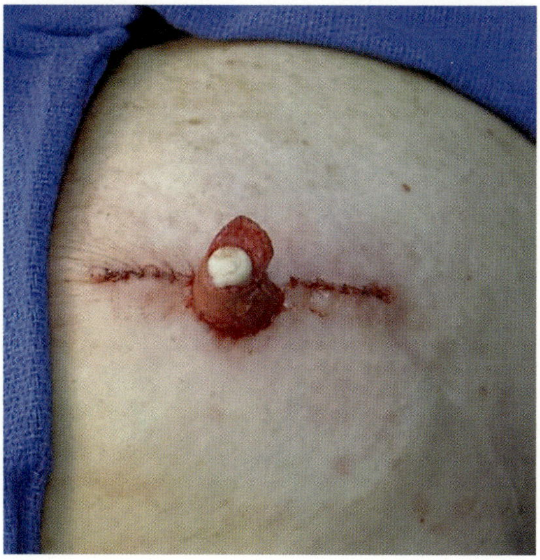

**Fig. 81.6** Acellular dermal matrix in the center of the nipple construct

Preoperative markings of the areola and proposed flap are completed using a stencil. Medical pigmentation of the C-V flap has begun on the inner aspect of the markings with the darker of the two pigments selected (Fig. 81.7) using a micropigmentation device such as Permark UltraEnhancer and a #5 round needle which has five needles in a circular arrangement [24]. The C-V flap outline should be pigmented by first defining the borders at the periphery with the pigmentation device, then continuing to work centrally. In the central portion, using a cross-hatching coloring pattern that creates honeycomb-like markings is suggested to ensure uniform and adequate pigmentation. Successful technique is indicated by the presence of pinpoint bleeding at the site of pigmentation. Once the medical pigmentation of the nipple is completed (Fig. 81.8), incisions for the C-V flap are made for the "V" sections 1 to 2 mm inside of the tattooed area (Fig. 81.9). This ensures that the donor incision sites contained within the areola will have even pigmentation and smooth borders visually. The nipple is constructed by elevating the two "V" wings in the dermal plane which are deepened at the base to include any underlying fat, conferring adequate projection. The base of the C flap is left fully intact to preserve attachment to the breast mound tissue and maintain the subdermal plexus

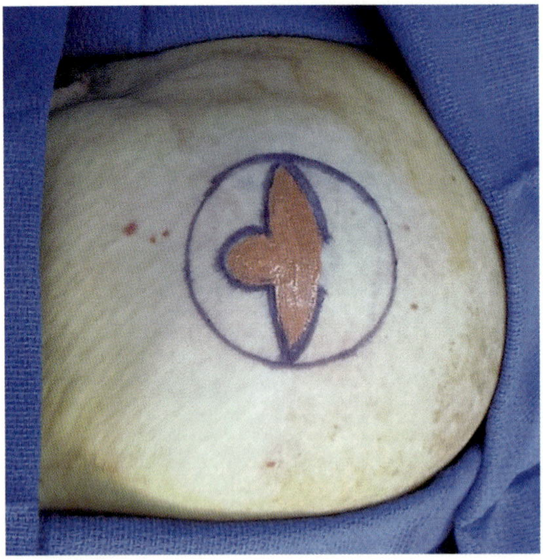

**Fig. 81.7** The darker dye within the C-V flap ready for medical pigmentation

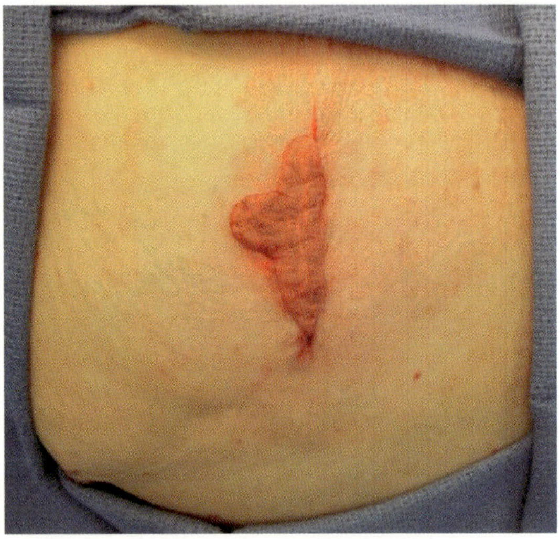

**Fig. 81.9** Incisions for the C-V flap made 1–2 mm inside the pigmented area

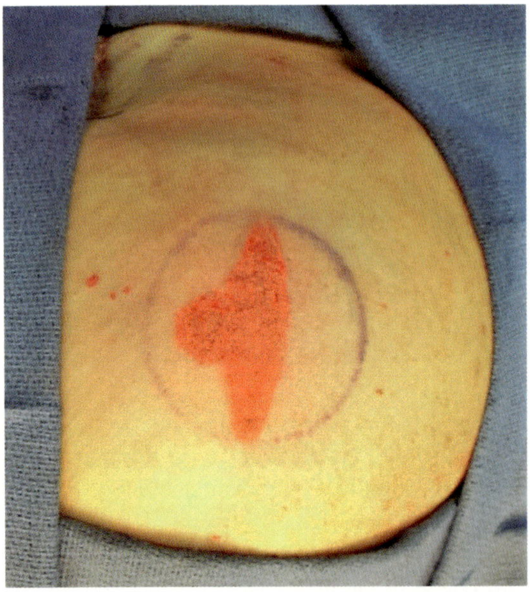

**Fig. 81.8** Completed pigmentation of the nipple flap

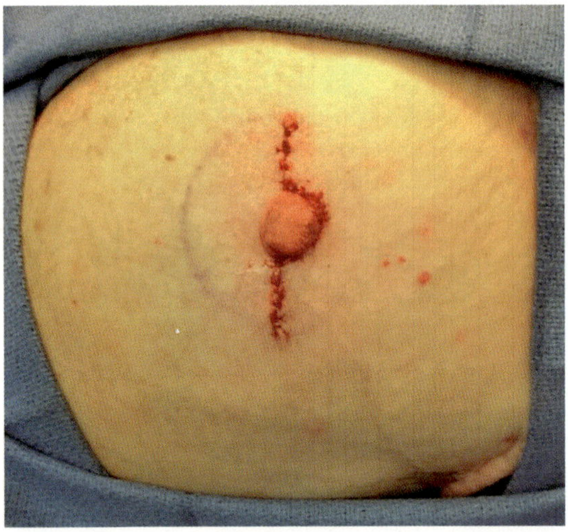

**Fig. 81.10** The complete nipple construct from the C-V flap

and its blood supply [25]. The superior border of the "C" flap is elevated initially at the subdermal level but then deepened down to, but not through, the capsule to include the subcutaneous tissue and fat to improve vascularity to the flap. The tips of the "V" wings can be thinned to avoid devascularization at the periphery of the flaps. A 2-0 Vicryl absorbable suture is used approximate the subdermal portion of the wings of the "V" portion of the flap. 3-0 Vicryl dermal sutures are used for the remainder of the incision. Single interrupted 4-0 chromic suture is used to close the epidermis of the "V" wings (Fig. 81.10). Using the reconstructed nipple as a landmark, the now ovoid-shaped areola is remarked to reestablish a circular shape (Fig. 81.11). The areolar aspect is then tattooed in a uniform fashion with the lighter of the two pigments (Fig. 81.12).

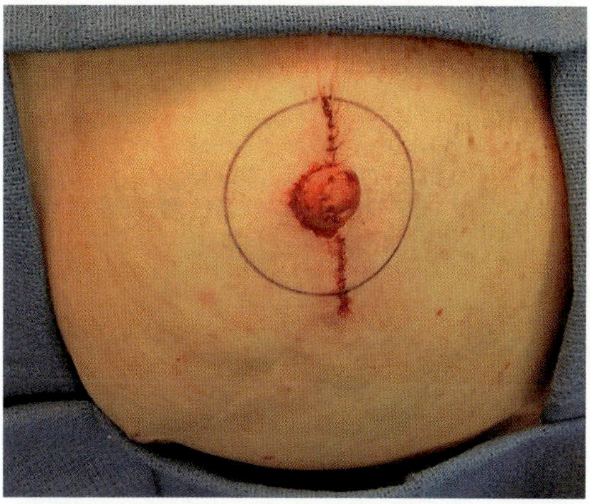

Fig. 81.11 Remarking of a circular areola shape

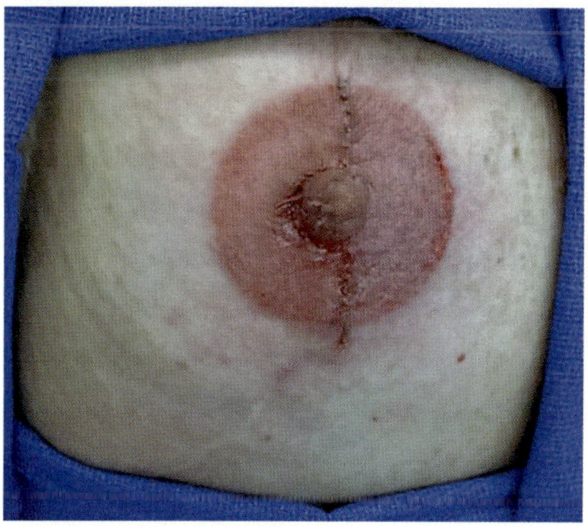

Fig. 81.12 Completion of the areola pigmentation

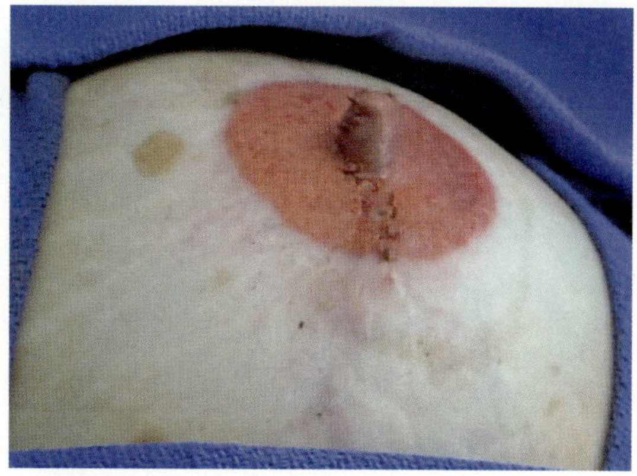

Fig. 81.13 The complete NAC showing projection of the nipple

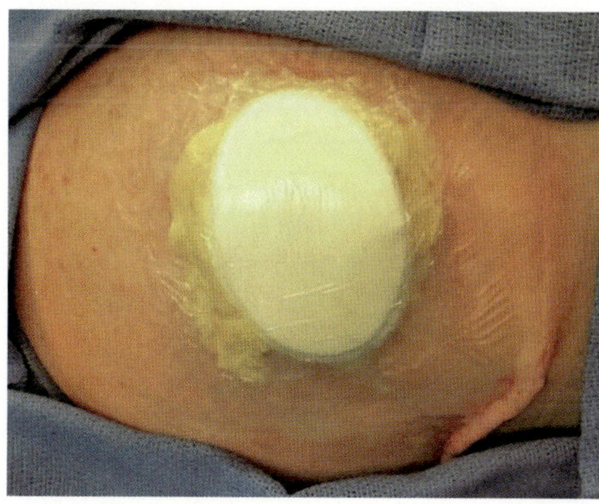

Fig. 81.14 Postoperative dressing with bacitracin, Xeroform gauze, stacked eye pads, and Tegaderm

Projection is assessed on the operative table (Fig. 81.13).

Postoperatively, bacitracin ointment, Xeroform gauze, and stacked eye pads (with the center cutout to avoid placement of pressure on the nipple) are used to cover the area. Tegaderm is placed on top of the eye pads, and the patient is instructed not to place any pressure on the breast mounds (Fig. 81.14). Patients should follow up in the clinic in 1-week time to assess dye uptake, symmetry, projection, and flap viability of the constructed nipples (Fig. 81.15), after which commercially available silicone nipple protectors are used for 2 weeks to ensure maximal projec-

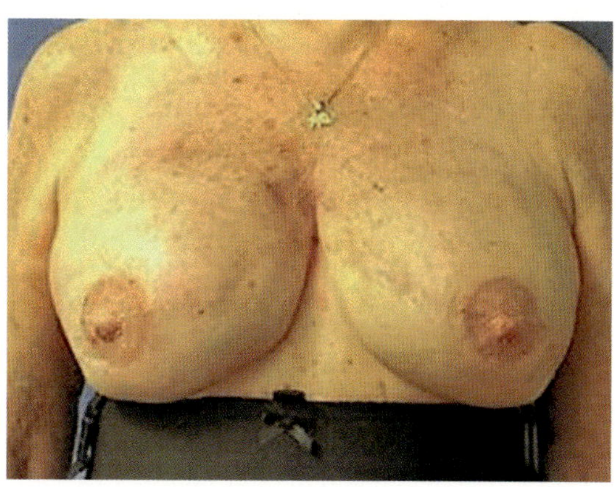

Fig. 81.15 NAC at the 1-week follow-up appointment

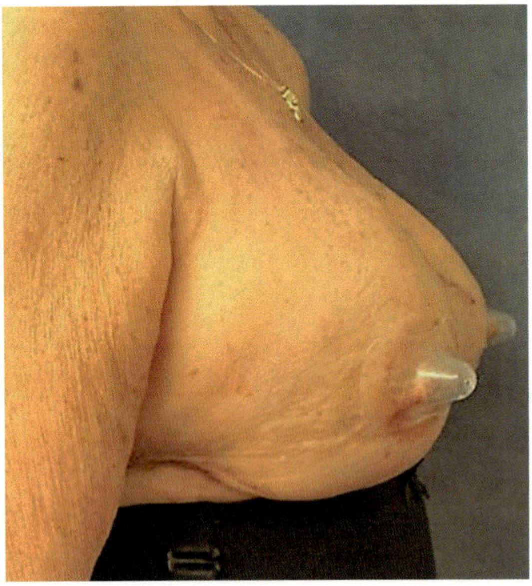

**Fig. 81.16** Silicone nipple protectors are worn for 2 weeks

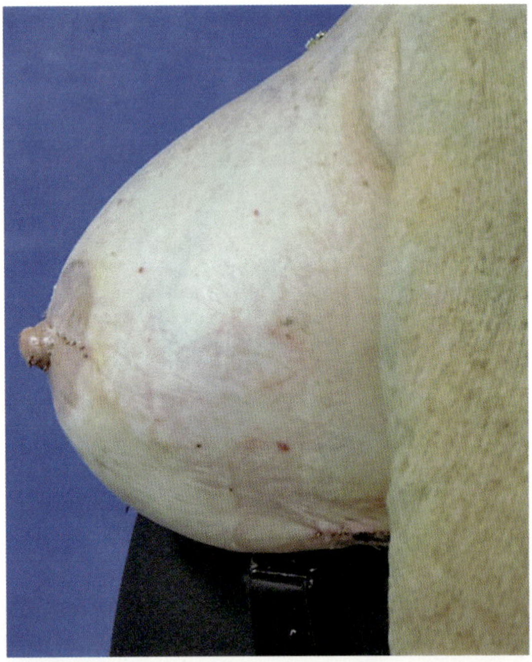

**Fig. 81.17** Nipple projection at 3 months after SS NAR

tion (Figs. 81.16 and 81.17). Final result after SSNAR is assessed at 6 months (Fig. 81.18).

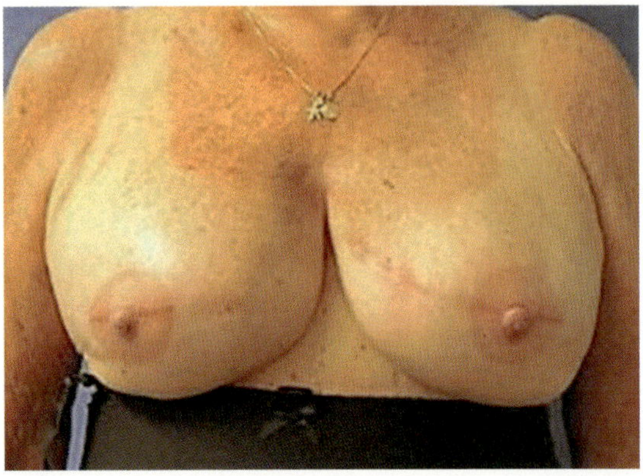

**Fig. 81.18** Patient with bilateral SS NAR at 6-month follow-up showing adequate dye uptake, symmetry, and projection

## 81.3 Discussion

Reconstruction of the NAC plays a significant role in patient satisfaction with breast reconstruction as it is the finishing touch to the reconstructed breast. Multiple studies have highlighted the importance of NAC creation for a superior aesthetic appearance of the reconstructed breast from the patient perspective [15–17]. Essential elements to consider in the reconstructive process include nipple projection, size, color, symmetry, and shape. Among the multitude of techniques utilized for NAR and medical pigmentation, the previously discussed C-V flap better maintains natural nipple texture and results in less extensive scarring than alternate techniques [3, 26].

Utilizing a local flap is a safe technique when compared to alternative methods. This is demonstrated by a literature review of 75 papers on NAR showing nipple reconstruction with grafts from distant sites having a complication rate of 46.9% compared to local flaps with a rate of 7.9% [3]. Postoperative complications prolong the time to reconstructive completion and decrease patient satisfaction. The C-V flap, with its lower complication rate, is also amenable to alterations and adjustments due to the ease of modification of the width of each flap to meet individualized patient needs. Local flaps give a better more predictable nipple construct result. A concern with utilizing any local flap is the resultant shape of the areola may become more ovoid due to tissue and muscular contraction of the area. In addition, using local tissue to construct a nipple may slightly decrease the central projection of the breast mound. The process of medical pigmentation only after remarking of the areola shape masks any deformation of the breast after C-V flap reconstruction.

Maintenance of nipple projection is an important consideration in the reconstructive technique [27]. While all local flaps expectedly lose some amount of projection in the first 6 months following reconstruction, the C-V flap has shown to reliably confer superior long-term projection compared to other local flaps or grafts [3, 28]. Because the final reconstructed nipple will have a predictable 30–35% loss of projection, the initial nipple structure is created to account for the final desired result. If the patient desires high projection, acellular dermal matrix may be added to the center of the flap. This successfully augments the nipple profile with a safe and reproducible technique [23]. In addition, the C-V flap provides a potential for a minimal amount of sensory return to the nipple due to nerve growth from the mastectomy bed to the local flap [29].

The use of medical pigmentation to create realistic coloration of the nipple and areola is an integral part of the SS NAR. The pigmentation technique is simple, patient satisfaction with NAC tattooing is high, and complication rates are low [3]. In the SS NAR technique, pigmentation of the nipple construct is performed prior to elevation of the C-V flap into the three-dimensional structure, which confers several benefits. First, the medical pigmentation of a two-dimensional plane is easier with less operator error than pigmentation of a three-dimensional construct of tissue [29]. The two-step techniques elevate the local flap into the nipple shape and subsequently tattoo that structure, which is mechanically more challenging. In addition, the dye uptake is improved with the single-stage technique because it avoids tattooing onto secondary scar or raw incisional edge (such as is the practice in a two-step technique) which tends to uptake dye in an uneven and unpredictable fashion. The process of incising the C-V limbs 1–2 mm within the pigmented edge ensures that the incision sites from the areolar area will have even pigment uptake. The areolar pigmentation is completed using the lighter of the two dye colors selected to enhance the distinction between the nipple and the areola. The two dye colors selected are darker than the final desired color, as tattoo pigments predictably fade over time [30, 31]. By choosing darker dyes to overcorrect for the anticipated fading of intradermal pigmentation, patient satisfaction with the final result is ultimately improved.

A unique benefit of the SS NAR technique is the decrease in duration of the total reconstructive process with fewer office or hospital visits required for the patient. A shorter time to completion of reconstruction after mastectomy is associated with higher patient satisfaction [4, 5]. The completion of a NAC that closely resembles a native nipple in a single stage allows the patient to return to natural-appearing breasts sooner than alternative techniques.

## Conclusions

Nipple-areolar reconstruction continues to be an essential final step in the breast reconstructive process for patients undergoing mastectomy. While nipple-sparing mastectomies are increasing in popularity in the surgical world, not every patient is a candidate for this technique. There will continue to be many patients who do not qualify for nipple-sparing procedures and require a safe, reliable, and successful technique for creating an aesthetically accurate NAC that does not superfluously prolong the surgical restorative process [32]. NAR is associated with higher patient satisfaction and is regarded as an essential step in the completion of reconstructive surgery to create natural-appearing breasts [29, 33]. While several satisfactory methods exist to create both the areola and the nipple, patients often prefer the options that have the shortest time to completion, with minimal repeated office visits and minimal complications [24]. SS NAR creates a natural appearing NAC utilizing local flap and medical pigmentation of the skin in one procedure. The long-term patient satisfaction with the appearance of the reconstructed NAC is high and effectively contributes to a successful breast reconstructive experience.

## References


1. Yang D, Ryu Y, Ryu W, Kwon H, Bae G, Lee W, Choi Y, Chung Y, Cho C. Our experiences in nipple reconstruction using the Hammond flap. Arch Plast Surg. 2014;41:550–5.
2. Weinfeld AB, Somia N, Codner MA. Purse-string nipple areolar reconstruction. Ann Plast Surg. 2008;61:364–7.
3. Sisti A, Grimaldi L, Tassinai J, Cuomo R, Fortezza L, Bocchiotti M, Roviello F, D'Aniello C, Nisi G. Nipple-areola complex reconstruction techniques: a literature review. Eur J Surg Oncol. 2016;42:441–65.
4. Jabor MA, Shayani P, Collins D, Karas T, Cohen B. Nipple-areola reconstruction: satisfaction and clinical determinants. Plast Reconstr Surg. 2002;110:457–63.
5. Losken A, Mackay GJ, Bostwick J. Nipple reconstruction using the C-V flap technique: a long-term evaluation. Plast Reconstr Surg. 2001;108(2):0–9.
6. Krajewski C, Boughey C, Degnim C, Jakub J, Jacobson S, Hoskin T, Hieken T. Expanded indications and improved outcomes for nipple-sparing mastectomy over time. Ann Surg Oncol. 2015;22:3317–23.
7. Paepke S, Schmid R, Fleckner S, Paepke D, Niemeyer M, Schmalfeldt B, Jacobs VR, Kiechle M. Subcutaneous mastectomy with conservation of the nipple-areola skin: broadening the indications. Ann Surg. 2009;250:288–92.
8. Gerber B, Krause A, Dieterich M, Kundt G, Reimer T. The oncological safety of skin sparing mastectomy with conservation of the nipple-areola complex and autologous reconstruction: an extended follow-up study. Ann Plastic Surg. 2009;249:461–28.
9. Delay E, Mojallal A, Vasseur C, Delaporte T. Immediate nipple reconstruction during immediate autologous latissimus breast reconstruction. Plast Reconstr Surg. 2006;118:1303–12.
10. Didier F, Arnaboldi P, Gandini S, Maldifassi A, Goldhirsch A, Radice D, Minotti I, Ballardini B, Luini A, Santillo B, Rietjens M, Petit J. Why do women accept to undergo a nipple sparing mastectomy or to reconstruct the nipple areola complex when nipple sparing mastectomy is not possible? Breast Cancer Res Treat. 2012;132(3):1177–84.
11. Tomita K, Yano K, Matsuda K, Takada A, Hosokawa K. Esthetic outcome of immediate reconstruction with latissimus dorsimyocutaneous flap after breast-conservative surgery and skin-sparing mastectomy. Ann Plast Surg. 2008;61:19–23.
12. Momoh AO, Colakoglu S, de Blacam C, Yueh JH, Lin SJ, Tobias AM, Lee BT. The impact of nipple reconstruction on patient satisfaction in breast reconstruction. Ann Plast Surg. 2012;69:389–93.
13. Eldor L, Spiegel A. Breast reconstruction after bilateral prophylactic mastectomy in women at high risk for breast cancer. Breast J. 2009;15(Suppl 1):S81–9.
14. Goldwyn RM. Plastic and reconstructive surgery of the breast. Boston: Little Brown; 1976.
15. Wellisch DK, Schain WS, Noone RB, Little JW. The psychological contribution of nipple addition in breast reconstruction. Plast Reconstr Surg. 1987;80:699–704.
16. Goh SC, Martin NA, Pandya AN, Cutress RI. Patient satisfaction following nipple-areolar complex reconstruction and tattooing. J Plast Reconstr Aesthet Surg. 2011;64:360–3.
17. Buck DW 2nd, Shenaq D, Heyer K, Kato C, Kim J. Patient-subjective cosmetic outcomes following the varying stages of tissue expander breast reconstruction: the importance of completion. Breast. 2010;19:521–6.
18. Gamboa-Bobadilla GM. Nipple reconstruction: the top hat technique. Ann Plast Surg. 2005;54(3):243–6.
19. Asplund O. Nipple and areola reconstruction. A study in 79 mastectomized women. Scand J Plast Reconstr Surg. 1983;17:233–40.
20. Valdatta L, Montemurro P, Tamborini F, Fidanza C, Gottardi A, Scamoni S. Our experience of nipple reconstruction using the C-V flap technique: 1 year evaluation. J Plast Reconstr Aesthet Surg. 2009;62(10):1293–8.
21. Botswick J. Nipple-areola reconstruction. In: Botswick J, editor. Plastic & reconstructive breast surgery. St. Louis: QMP; 2000.
22. Dowden RV. Achieving a natural inframammary fold and ptotic effect in the reconstructed breast. Ann Plastic Surg. 1987;19:524–9.
23. Garramone CE, Lam B. Use of AlloDerm in primary nipple reconstruction to improve long-term nipple projection. Plast Reconstr Surg. 2007;119:1663–8.
24. Liliav B, Loeb J, Hassid V, Antony A. Single stage nipple-areolar complex reconstruction technique, outcomes, and patient satisfaction. Ann Plast Surg. 2014;73:492–7.
25. Hartrampf CR Jr, Culbertson JH. A dermal-fat flap for nipple reconstruction. Plast Reconstr Surg. 1984;73:982–6.
26. Losken A, Duggal CS, Desai KA, McCullough MC, Gruszynski MA, Carlson GW. Time to completion of nipple reconstruction: what factors are involved? Ann Plast Surg. 2013;70:530–2.
27. Sanuki J, Fukuma E, Uchida Y. Morphologic study of nipple-areola complex in 600 breasts. Aesthet Plast Surg. 2009;33(3):295–7.
28. Shestak KC, Gabriel A, Landecker A, Peters S, Shestak A, Kim J. Assessment of long-term nipple

projection: a comparison of three techniques. Plast Reconstr Surg. 2002;110:780–6.
29. El-Ali K, Dalal M, Kat CC. Tattooing of the nipple-areola complex: a review of outcome in 40 patients. J Plast Reconstr Aesthet Surg. 2006;59(10):1052–7.
30. Levites HA, Fourman MS, Phillips BT, Fromm IM, Khan SU, Dagum AB, Bui DT. Modeling fade patterns of nipple areola complex tattoos following breast reconstruction. Ann Plast Surg. 2014;73(Suppl 2):S153–6.
31. Becker H. The use of intradermal tattoo to enhance the final result of nipple-areola reconstruction. Plast Reconstr Surg. 1986;77:673–6.
32. Ibrahim AM, Sinno HH, Izadpanah A, Vorstenbosch J, Dionisopoulos T, Mureau MA, Tobias AM, Lee BT, Lin SJ. Nipple-areolar complex reconstruction following postmastectomy breast reconstruction: a comparative utility assessment study. Plast Reconstr Surg Global Open. 2015;3(4):e380.
33. Gahm J, Jurell G, Edsander-Nord A, Wickman M. Patient satisfaction with aesthetic outcome after bilateral prophylactic mastectomy and immediate reconstruction with implants. J Plastic Reconstr Aesthet Surg. 2008;63(2):332–8.

# Nipple Reconstruction After Implant-Based Breast Reconstruction: A "Matched-Pair" Outcome Analysis Focusing on the Effects of Radiotherapy

82

Shawn Moshrefi, Arash Momeni, Gordon K. Lee, and David Kahn

## 82.1 Introduction

Nipple reconstruction is often viewed as the final stage of breast reconstruction. It is the proverbial cherry on top and a defining characteristic of a completed breast reconstruction, depending on the desires of the patient. The bulk of contributions related to nipple reconstruction focus on surgical techniques. The major focus of articles has been on ways to prevent the inevitable loss of nipple projection [1–6]. However, there was noted a limited number of studies viewing nipple reconstruction as a source of morbidity and complication [6, 7]. It was felt of great importance in evaluating factors that may serve as predictors of poor outcomes in nipple reconstruction.

The authors previously performed a cross-sectional study in which radiotherapy was identified as a risk factor for the development of complications after nipple reconstruction [8]. Acknowledging the inherent limitations of a cross-sectional study, the group designed a "matched-pair" analysis to specifically answer the question whether a history of radiotherapy predisposes to a higher complication rate after nipple reconstruction in patients after implant-based breast reconstruction.

## 82.2 Technique

Institutional review board (IRB) approval was obtained prior to conducting the study. The Stanford Translational Research Integrated Database Environment (STRIDE), which is a research and development project at Stanford University to create a standard-based informatics platform supporting clinical and translational research, was utilized to identify patients with a history of unilateral breast radiation who underwent bilateral mastectomy and implant-based breast reconstruction with subsequent bilateral nipple reconstruction. This study design allowed patients to act as their own internal control. This meant that one could "match" radiated to non-radiated breasts while controlling for other significant factors that may vary from patient to patient. Only patients who underwent nipple reconstruction by means of local flaps were included in the study (Figs. 82.1, 82.2, 82.3, 82.4, 82.5, and 82.6). Other modes of reconstruction, such as tattoo only, nipple sharing, skin grafting, etc., were excluded. Our primary outcome

S. Moshrefi, M.D. (✉) • A. Momeni, M.D.
G.K. Lee, M.D. • D. Kahn, M.D.
Department of Plastic and Reconstructive Surgery, Stanford University Medical Center, Palo Alto, CA, USA
e-mail: moshrefi@stanford.edu; amomeni@stanford.edu; glee@stanford.edu; David.Kahn@Stanford.edu


M.A. Shiffman (ed.), *Nipple-Areolar Complex Reconstruction*,
https://doi.org/10.1007/978-3-319-60925-6_82

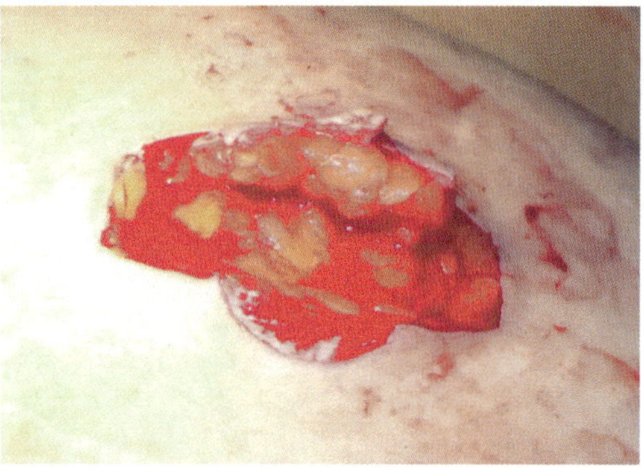

Fig. 82.1 Elevating "bowtie" flap for nipple reconstruction

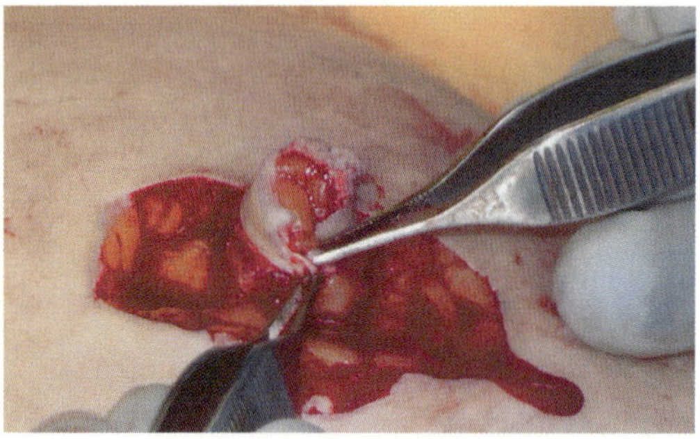

Fig. 82.2 Suturing "bowtie" flap for nipple reconstruction

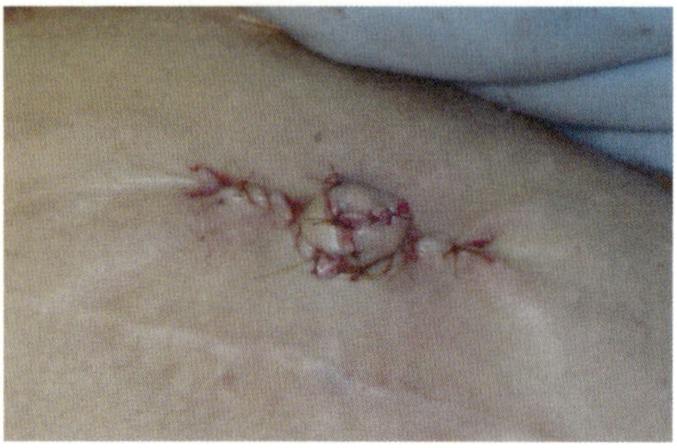

Fig. 82.3 "Bowtie" flap for nipple reconstruction

measure was complication rate. Other factors evaluated included age, final implant volume, time interval from radiotherapy to nipple reconstruction, time interval from placement of final implant to nipple reconstruction, and length of follow-up.

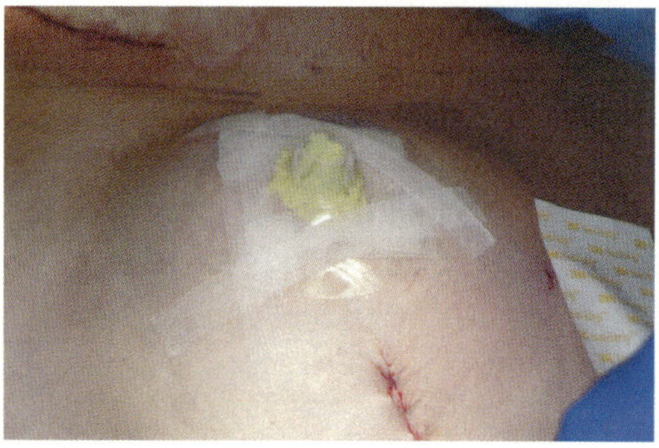

Fig. 82.4 Postoperative dressing including Steri-Strips, Xeroform gauze, and nipple protector

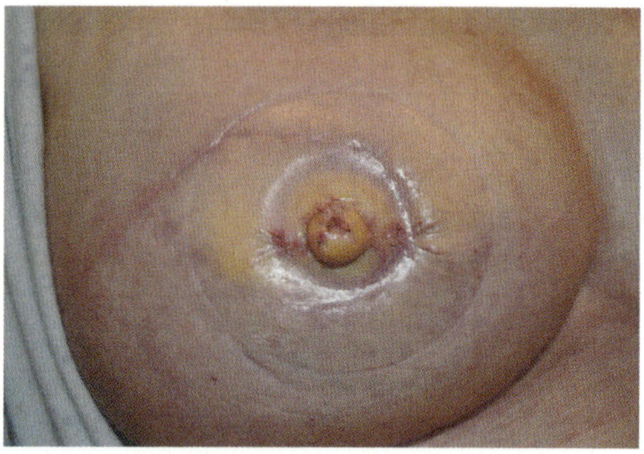

Fig. 82.5 Two weeks postoperative

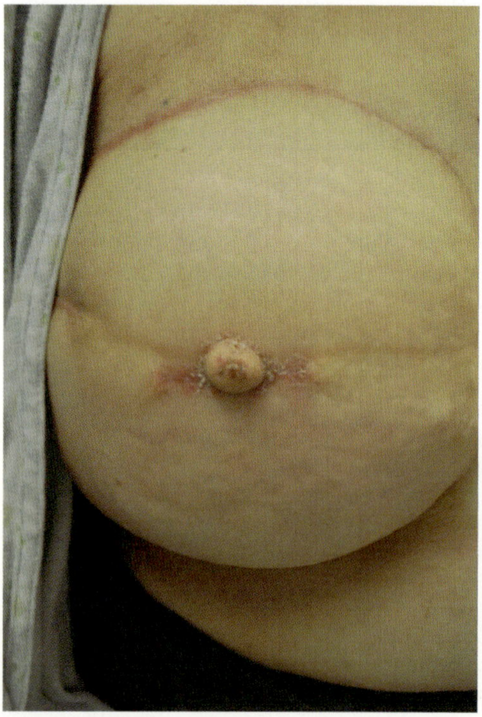

Fig. 82.6 Six months postoperative

## 82.3 Discussion

Seventeen patients (34 nipple reconstructions) were identified by our institution as meeting inclusion criteria for our desired evaluation. Table 82.1 demonstrates the factors previously noted in tabular format. Table 82.2 demonstrates the complication rates between irradiated and nonirradiated breasts undergoing nipple reconstruction after implant-based reconstruction.

This study allowed more in-depth evaluation and attribution of radiotherapy to complications in nipple reconstruction following implant-based breast reconstruction as this was the only significant variable differing in the "matched-pair" results. A statistically significant increase in complication rate was observed after nipple reconstruction in an irradiated field (41.2% vs. 5.9%, $p = 0.03$). We also sought to evaluate whether higher implant volumes had an impact with setting 500 mL as the median implant volume of the study group. Though a trend was noted towards higher complications with implant volumes greater than 500 mL, statistically significant differences were not noted.

**Table 82.1** Patient characteristics ($N = 17$ patients; 34 nipple reconstructions)

| Factors | Mean | Range |
|---|---|---|
| Age | 43.5 | 23–69 |
| Final implant volume | 530 cc | 370–800 cc |
| Time interval from radiotherapy to nipple reconstruction | 24.9 months | 6–156 months |
| Time interval from final implant placement to nipple reconstruction | 7.6 months | 2–22 months |
| Length of follow-up | 11.1 months | 2–36 months |

**Table 82.2** Complications in irradiated vs. nonirradiated fields of nipple reconstruction

| Complications | Irradiated total 7/17 (41.2%) | Nonirradiated total 1/17 (5.9%) |
|---|---|---|
| Cellulitis responsive to oral antibiotics | 2/17 (11.8%) | 1/17 (5.9%) |
| Infection with loss of implant without further reconstruction | 1/17 (5.9%) | 0 (0%) |
| Infection with loss of implant with subsequent autologous reconstruction | 1/17 (5.9%) | 0 (0%) |
| Infection requiring implant exchange | 1/17 (5.9%) | 0 (0%) |
| Wound dehiscence with implant exposure requiring surgical intervention | 1/17 (5.9%) | 0 (0%) |
| Nipple necrosis | 1/17 (5.9%) | 0 (0%) |

The importance of these considerations is ever so relevant in the era where radiotherapy has become a mainstay in breast cancer care as more and more women are turning towards breast conservation therapy [9]. However, a known issue with breast conservation is re-excision, with rates noted as high as 60% and greater than 10% of these patients eventually undergoing mastectomy in some studies [10–13]. These numbers along with an increased incidence of breast cancer explain the increasing number of patients who present for consultation regarding breast reconstruction.

Draper et al. [7] observed a 25% complication rate after nipple-areolar reconstruction in an irradiated field. While the authors felt this was "acceptable", we feel that problems occurring in one in four patients seem rather high. A higher complication rate was found in this study (41.2%). This confirms previous study findings, which demonstrated a complication rate of 51.7% [8].

Another point of importance to reflect on is the role of nipple reconstruction in a patient that has undergone autologous breast reconstruction. While this is not the focus of this chapter, a noteworthy discussion should be considered when undertaking nipple reconstruction in the autologous breast reconstruction in comparison to the implant-based reconstruction. In general, autologous tissue used for breast reconstruction is thicker, which is contrast to the skin overlying an implant such as a tissue expander. Should a postoperative wound of the nipple reconstruction develop, an implant-based reconstruction is threatened with the possibility of an exposed prosthesis, whereas autologous reconstruction does not face these same risks (even in setting with augmentation underlying autologous tissue). This holds true even in the face of an irradiated field given autologous reconstruction in general can remain supple in such an environment.

Nipple reconstruction is not meant to be dismayed, particularly given the low complication rate seen in nonirradiated breasts. However, it is important to note that breast irradiation predating a nipple reconstruction does convert the procedure to one of the higher risks. Some of those risks should also be noted as being disastrous such as implant loss and major revisionary surgery. In an age emphasizing the importance of informed consent, these matters should be expressed frankly and carefully with the patient.

### Conclusions

Overall, nipple reconstruction is a safe procedure to undertake and should be offered to patients undergoing breast reconstruction. Therapeutic breast irradiation prior to nipple reconstruction in implant-based breast reconstruction has significant complications associated that should be frankly discussed with patient as part of the preoperative visit.

## References


1. Shestak KC, Gabriel A, Landecker A, Peters S, Shestak A, Kim J. Assessment of long-term nipple projection: a comparison of three techniques. Plast Reconstr Surg. 2002;110:780e6.
2. Shestak KC, Nguyen TD. The double opposing periareola flap: a novel concept for nipple-areola reconstruction. Plast Reconstr Surg. 2007;119:473e80.
3. Jones AP, Erdmann M. Projection and patient satisfaction using the "Hamburger" nipple reconstruction technique. J Plast Reconstr Aesthet Surg. 2012;65:207e12.
4. Rosing JH, Momeni A, Kamperman K, Kahn D, Gurtner G, Lee GK. Effectiveness of the Asteame Nipple Guard(TM) in maintaining projection following nipple reconstruction: a prospective randomised controlled trial. J Plast Reconstr Aesthet Surg. 2010;63(10):1592e6.
5. Eo S, Kim SS, Da Lio AL. Nipple reconstruction with C-v flap using dermofat graft. Ann Plast Surg. 2007;58:137e40.
6. Zhong T, Antony A, Cordeiro P. Surgical outcomes and nipple projection using the modified skate flap for nipple-areolar reconstruction in a series of 422 implant reconstructions. Ann Plast Surg. 2009;62:591e5.
7. Draper LB, Bui DT, Chiu ES, Mehrara BJ, Pusic AL, Cordeiro PG, Disa JJ. Nipple-areola reconstruction following chest-wall irradiation for breast cancer: is it safe? Ann Plast Surg. 2005;55:12e5.
8. Momeni A, Ghaly M, Gupta D, Karanas YL, Kahn DM, Gurtner GC, Lee GK. Nipple reconstruction: risk factors and complications after 189 procedures. Eur J Plast Surg. 2013;36(10):633–8.
9. Katipamula R, Degnim AC, Hoskin T, Boughey JC, Loprinzi C, Grant CS, Brandt KR, Pruthi S, Chute CG, Olson JE, Couch FJ, Ingle JN, Goetz MP. Trends in mastectomy rates at the Mayo Clinic Rochester: effect of surgical year and preoperative magnetic resonance imaging. J Clin Oncol. 2009;27:4082e8.
10. Morrow M, Jagsi R, Alderman AK, Griggs JJ, Hawley ST, Hamilton AS, Graff JJ, Katz SJ. Surgeon recommendations and receipt of mastectomy for treatment of breast cancer. J Am Med Assoc. 2009;302:1551e6.
11. Menes TS, Tartter PI, Bleiweiss I, Godbold JH, Estabrook A, Smith SR. The consequence of multiple re-excisions to obtain clear lumpectomy margins in breast cancer patients. Ann Surg Oncol. 2005;12:881e5.
12. Waljee JF, Hu ES, Newman LA, Alderman AK. Predictors of reexcision among women undergoing breast-conserving surgery for cancer. Ann Surg Oncol. 2008;15:1297e303.
13. Kotwall C, Ranson M, Stiles A, Hamann MS. Relationship between initial margin status for invasive breast cancer and residual carcinoma after re-excision. Am Surg. 2007;73:337e43.

# 83 Nipple-Areola Complex Replantation After Mastectomy and Immediate Breast Reconstruction

Raphael Wirth, Andrej Banic, and Dominique Erni

## 83.1 Introduction

Breast-conserving therapy, comprising wide local excision of the primary tumor and adjuvant radiotherapy, represents the treatment of choice for most women with breast cancer. However, ablative surgery is still indispensable in approximately one third of the cases due to aggressive, extensive, or multicentric tumor growth, contraindications for radiotherapy, or following the patient's wish. Breast reconstruction can be offered to most of these cases and to overcome the psychological burden caused by the disfigurement resulting from the loss of the breast. Immediate breast reconstruction (IBR) is favored over the delayed procedures after having been proven not to affect tumor recurrence or longtime survival [1–6].

R. Wirth, M.D. (✉)
WIRTH Plastische Chirurgie, General-Dufour-Str. 17, 2502 Biel-Bienne, Switzerland
e-mail: info@dr-wirth.ch

A. Banic, M.D.
BANIC Plastische Chirurgie, Bundesgasse 26, 3011 Bern, Switzerland
e-mail: info@banic.ch

D. Erni, M.D.
Plastische Chirurgie Erni, Küferweg 9, 6403 Küssnacht am Rigi, Switzerland
e-mail: praxis@erniplast.ch

The resection of the nipple-areolar complex (NAC) is commonly included in all conventional mastectomy techniques [7], in the belief that the nipple-areolar complex (NAC) has a significant probability of containing occult tumor cells. Depending on tumor location, stage, and grade, invasion of the NAC has been estimated between 5 and 58% [8–10]. The NAC in turn allegorizes an aesthetically essential part of the female breast [11]. Accordingly, the aesthetic outcome after breast reconstruction is substantially influenced by the quality of the NAC reconstruction, which is commonly achieved by transplantation of the contralateral nipple, grafting of the skin or labia, implants, local flaps or tattooing, or combinations of each. However, due to its particular color, structure, and texture, a natural-looking NAC can hardly be reconstituted with either of these techniques [12, 13]. Therefore, it has been proposed to maintain the original NAC, which is replanted after excluding tumor infiltration by histological examination of the underlying tissue [2, 14]. Furthermore, the use of the original NAC bears the advantage of not causing any other donor-site morbidity. However, there is a paucity of data documenting oncological and surgical safety as well as aesthetic outcome of this procedure.

In the authors' retrospective analysis, we assessed the local recurrence rate, early complication rate, and long-term outcome of NAC reconstruction with the use of the original tissue.


M.A. Shiffman (ed.), *Nipple-Areolar Complex Reconstruction*,
https://doi.org/10.1007/978-3-319-60925-6_83

## 83.2 Technique

During the mastectomy procedure, the entire NAC and a disk of some mm of underlying tissue were excised at a diameter of 40–44 mm, if there was no clinical or radiological evidence for tumor infiltration of the NAC and the distance of the tumor to the NAC was at least 1 cm. The nipple is preserved as a composite graft consisting of the skin, glandular ducts, and connective tissue. The NAC has to be thinned out to a full thickness skin graft. The graft is wrapped in saline-soaked gauze and stored in the refrigerator at a temperature of 4 °C. The resected retroareolar and retropapillary tissue is sent for pathohistological examination. The specimens are stained with hematoxylin/eosin, and immunohistochemistry has to be performed additionally. Depending on the preference of the surgeon, the entire NAC or the nipple alone can be replanted in a second intervention in local anesthesia, provided this tissue is free of tumor. In the case of nipple alone transplantation, the areola can be tattooed.

The database of the Department of Plastic Surgery and Hand Surgery, University Hospital Bern, Switzerland, was checked for IBR after mastectomy due to invasive breast cancer or carcinoma in situ from 1998 to 2007, and the charts of these patients, including the pre- and postoperative photographs, were used for further data processing. By contacting the patients' general practitioners, tumor recurrence rate was assessed. At least 12 months after the last intervention on the NAC, aesthetic outcome was evaluated clinically during routine clinical follow-up and by photographic analysis.

## 83.3 Discussion

The principal findings of our study were that there was not a single case in which the replanted NAC was the source of tumor recurrence, and both the wound healing complication rate and the long-term morbidity after NAC replantation were considerably high.

During the study period, 88 IBRs after mastectomy due to breast cancer were performed in 85 patients. Out of these, tumor infiltration was found in eight cases (9.1%), in which the NAC was rejected. In another 28 cases, the replantation of the NAC or nipple alone was not performed because the patients refused it or due to surgical reasons including postoperative complications, the difficulty to estimate correct NAC position, or aesthetically unpleasing NAC. This resulted in 52 replantations of the entire NAC ($n$ = 29) or the nipple alone in conjunction with areola tattooing ($n$ = 23). The median age of these 49 patients was 48 years (25–72). More than 50% of the patients had tumors larger than 2 cm, more than one third had nodal involvement, and in more than one fourth, the distance of the tumor to the NAC was less than 2 cm (Table 83.1). Median tumor size was 20 mm (3–51). Patients qualifying for NAC replantation were in stage 0 in 29%, stage I in 15%, stage IIa in 31%, stage IIb in 17%, and stage III in 8%.

Six breasts received a modified radical mastectomy (MRM) and 46 a skin-sparing mastec-

**Table 83.1** Tumor characteristics of patients with NAC/nipple replantation ($n$ = 52)

| | | |
|---|---|---|
| *Tumor size* | | |
| <2 cm | 25 | 48.1% |
| 2–5 cm | 26 | 50.0% |
| >5 cm | 1 | 1.9% |
| *Nodal status* | | |
| Lymph node negative | 33 | 63.5% |
| Lymph node positive | 19 | 36.5% |
| *Localization* | | |
| Multicentric/multifocal | 29 | 55.8% |
| Central location | 15 | 28.8% |
| Peripheral location | 37 | 71.2% |
| *Pathology* | | |
| Angioinvasion | 2 | 3.8% |
| Lymph vessel invasion | 5 | 9.6% |
| *Diagnosis* | | |
| Ductal carcinoma in situ (DCIS) | 12 | 23.1% |
| Lobular carcinoma in situ (LCIS) | 3 | 5.8% |
| *DCIS and LCIS* | 1 | 1.9% |
| Invasive ductal carcinoma | 19 | 36.5% |
| Invasive lobular carcinoma | 10 | 19.2% |
| Invasive ductal carcinoma and DCSI | 3 | 5.8% |
| Invasive ductal carcinoma and invasive lobular carcinoma | 3 | 5.8% |
| Malignant adenomyoepithelioma | 1 | 1.9% |

**Table 83.2** Early and late complications after replantation of NAC/nipple alone

| Complication | NAC ($n$ = 29) | Nipple alone ($n$ = 23) | Total number ($n$ = 52) |
|---|---|---|---|
| Total loss | 2 | 1 | 3 |
| Partial necrosis* | 18 | 5 | 23 |
| Wound infection | 0 | 0 | 0 |
| Depigmentation | 16 | 11 | 27 |
| Lateral dislocation | 1 | 0 | 1 |
| Scar dehiscence | 1 | 1 | 2 |
| Surgical revisions | 8 | 5 | 13 |
| Tattooing | 8 | 9 | 17 |

*$P < 0.01$ between groups

tomy (SSM). A free TRAM/DIEP flap was used for breast reconstruction in 23 cases, a latissimus dorsi pedicled flap with or without implants in 28 cases, and prosthesis alone in 1 case. The NAC or nipple replantation was performed 7 days (2–10) after IBR. Within 30 days after replantation, total or partial necrosis occurred in 69% of the replanted NAC and in 26% of nipple alone replantations ($P < 0.01$, Table 83.2).

Until the final assessment, more than half of all replanted NAC and nipples showed substantial depigmentation, irrespective of the graft composition (Fig. 83.1). The duration of graft preservation did not influence necrosis rate or depigmentation. Statistical evaluation of further possible risk factors for depigmentation or necrosis like smoking, obesity, choice of flap, or adjuvant radiation showed no significant differences, whereas adjuvant radiotherapy tended to increase the risk of partial necrosis ($P = 0.08$). There was no time delay seen regarding the beginning of adjuvant therapy.

Twenty-five corrective surgery procedures had to be carried out in 21 NAC or nipples after 297 days (27–1041). Fourteen of these consisted in tattooing alone due to depigmentation or in a combination of tattooing and surgical revision. In four patients minor surgical corrections ($n = 2$) or tattooing ($n = 3$) had to be repeated after another 200 days (8–648). None of the replanted NAC or nipples had to be removed, but in two cases, cranial repositioning of the replant was necessary.

Preservation of the NAC in the setting of breast cancer has been debated controversially because of the increased risk of local recurrence. Several studies assessing tumor involvement of the NAC have shown an incidence of occult tumor spread in 5–58% [8–10]. Simmons et al. [15] were able to demonstrate in their retrospective study on 217 mastectomy patients that this risk has been overestimated and in many patients, resection of the NAC seemed to be an overtreatment. In our series, the rate of histologically verified tumor infiltration of the subareolar tissue was 9.1%, which corresponds to the range reported for infiltration of the NAC in series with comparable tumor locations and stages [15–18]. Our patients did not show any recurrence originating from the replanted tissue even though the rate of tumors located centrally or close to the NAC and the tumor stages were noticeably high. This suggests that the pathohistological examination of the subareolar tissue in the two-stage setting that was performed in our series was a reliable tool to exclude tumor infiltration of the NAC, whereas the frozen-section technique used for immediate NAC replantation revealed up to 75% false-negative results leading to secondary removal [16, 18].

The local recurrence rate in our series was 1.9% after a median follow-up of 49 months, which is comparable with published series showing local recurrence rates from 1.7 to 9.5% [4–6, 19–22]. The only local recurrence occurred in a patient who was initially diagnosed for a malignant adenomyoepithelioma. Only 70 cases of this rare entity have so far been described in the literature [23]. The recurrent tumor was located at the lateral border of the pectoralis major muscle, which is far away from the NAC replantation site, therefore making a causal relationship with NAC replantation most unlikely. The same may apply for the single regional and the three remote recurrences, totaling an overall recurrence rate of 9.6%, which is within the range described for comparable tumors, mastectomy techniques, and follow-ups.

Unfortunately, uneventful graft take was only accomplished in approximately one third of all NAC replantations, which is a major drawback of this procedure that can partly be circumvented by replanting the nipple alone. Graft take may be

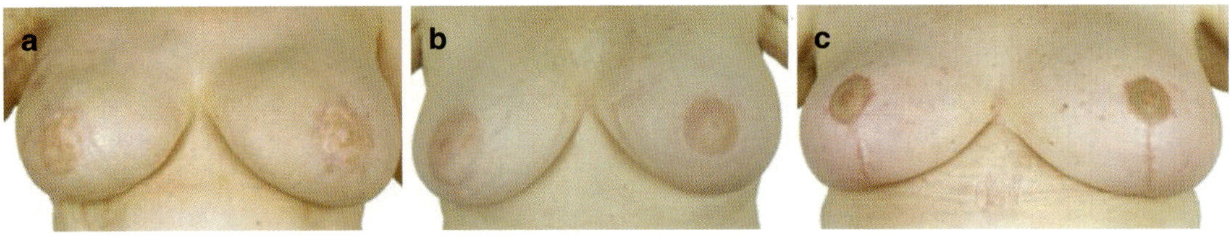

**Fig. 83.1** Replanted NACs in three different patients 12 months postoperatively. (**a**) A 56-year-old patient after bilateral SSM and TRAM reconstruction with poor result. (**b**) A 65-year-old patient after unilateral SSM and TRAM reconstruction with moderate result. (**c**) A 47-year-old patient after SSM and TRAM reconstruction on the left side and adaptive reduction mammoplasty on the right side with good results

jeopardized due to the preservation of the graft and possibly due to impaired microcirculatory blood flow in the wound bed. Although this complication is regrettable, it is not uncommon [2, 24], and it may to some extent be justified by the particular constellation in terms of having nothing to lose with the choice of this technique: if it fails, the NAC is reconstructed as it would have been otherwise. Even if the graft healed appropriately, depigmentation may have occurred on the long run, which was corrected by tattooing, thus preserving the texture of the grafted tissue. However, it has to be taken into consideration that the quality of NAC reconstruction is quite low in general due to poor projection, color, shape, size, texture, and position[12].

### Conclusions

This has been the largest series for this type of surgery with the longest follow-up. In addition, it can be mentioned that to the best of our knowledge, tumor recurrence originating from a replanted NAC after conventional histological workup has not been reported in the literature so far, which further underlines the oncological safety of this procedure.

Our more than 10-year experience with this technique suggests that the replantation of the NAC can be considered as oncologically safe, provided the subareolar tissue is free of tumor, which was confirmed by meticulous pathohistological workup of the subareolar tissue. Furthermore, we recommend using the nipple alone for replantation in order to avoid early wound healing complications and to diminish morbidity.

## References

1. McCormick B, Wrigth J, Cordiero P. Breast reconstruction combined with radiation therapy: long-term risks and factors related to decision making. Cancer J. 2008;14:264–8.
2. Hudson DA, Skoll PJ. Single-stage, autologous breast restoration. Plast Reconstr Surg. 2001;108:1163–71.
3. McCarthy CM, Pusic AL, Sclafani L, Buchanan C, Fey JV, Disa JJ, Mehrara BJ, Cordeiro PG. Breast cancer recurrence following prosthetic, postmastectomy reconstruction: incidence, detection, and treatment. Plast Reconstr Surg. 2008;121:381–8.
4. Carlson GW, Styblo TM, Lyles RH, Bostwick J, Murray DR, Staley CA, Wood WC. Local recurrence after skin-sparing mastectomy: tumor biology or surgical conservatism? Ann Surg Oncol. 2003;10:108–12.
5. Kroll SS, Khoo A, Singletary SE, Ames FC, Wang BG, Reece GP, Miller MJ, Evans GR, Robb GL. Local recurrence risk after skin-sparing mastectomy and conventional mastectomy: a 6-year follow-up. Plast Reconstr Surg. 1999;104:421–5.
6. Simmons RM, Fish SK, Gayle L, La Trenta GS, Swistel A, Christos P, Osborne MP. Local and distant recurrence rates in skin-sparing mastectomies compared with non-skin-sparing mastectomies. Ann Surg Oncol. 1999;6:676–81.
7. Toth BA, Lappert P. Modified skin incisions for mastectomy: the need for plastic surgical input in preoperative planning. Plast Reconstr Surg. 1991;87:1048–53.
8. Andersen JA, Gram JB, Pallesen RM. Involvement of the nipple and areola in breast cancer. Scand J Plast Reconstr Surg. 1981;15:39–42.
9. Perry RG, Cochran TC, Wolfort FG. When is there nipple involvement in carcinoma of the breast? Plast Reconstr Surg. 1977;59:535–7.
10. Menon RS, van Geel AN. Cancer of the breast with nipple involvement. Br J Cancer. 1989;59:81–4.
11. Ziswiler-Gietz J, Makrodimou M, Harder Y, Banic A, Erni D. Outcome analysis of breast reconstruction with free transverse rectus abdominis musculocutaneous (TRAM) flaps. Swiss Med Wkly. 2008;138:114–20.

12. Jabor MA, Shayani P, Collins DR, Karas T, Cohen BE. Nipple-areolar reconstructions: satisfaction and clinical determinants. Plast Reconstr Surg. 2002;110:457–63.
13. Shestak KC, Gabriel A, Landecker A, Peters S, Shestak A, Kim J. Assessment of long-term nipple projection: a comparison of three techniques. Plast Reconstr Surg. 2002;110:780–6.
14. Hudson DA, Dent DM, Lazarus D. One-stage immediate breast and nipple-areolar reconstruction with autologous tissue I: a preliminary report. Ann Plast Surg. 2000;45:471–6.
15. Simmons RM, Brennan M, Christos P, King V, Osborne M. Analysis of nipple/areolar involvement with mastectomy: can the areola be preserved? Ann Surg Oncol. 2002;9:165–8.
16. Laronga C, Kemp B, Johnston D, Robb G, Singletary SE. The incidence of occult nipple-areola complex involvement in breast cancer patients receiving skin-sparing mastectomy. Ann Surg Oncol. 1999;6:609–13.
17. Banerjee A, Gupta S, Bhattacharya N. Preservation of the nipple-areola complex in breast cancer – a clinicopathological assessment. J Plast Reconstr Aesthet Surg. 2008;61:1195–8.
18. Vlajcic Z, Zic R, Stanec S, Lambasa S, Petrovecki M, Stanec Z. Nipple-areola complex preservation: predictive factors of neoplastic nipple-areola complex invasion. Ann Plast Surg. 2005;55:240–4.
19. Newman LA, Kuerer HM, Hunt KK, Kroll SS, Ames FC, Ross MI, Feig BW, Singletary SE. Presentation, treatment, and outcome of local recurrence after skin-sparing mastectomy and immediate breast reconstruction. Ann Surg Oncol. 1998;5:620–6.
20. Greenway RM, Schlossberg L, Dooley WC. Fifteen-year series of skin-sparing mastectomy for stage 0 to 2 breast cancer. Am J Surg. 2005;190:933–8.
21. Meretoja TJ, von Smitten KAJ, Leidenius MH, Svarvar C, Heikkilä PS, Jahkola TA. Local recurrence of stage 1 and 2 breast cancer after skin-sparing mastectomy and immediate breast reconstruction in a 15-years series. Eur J Surg Oncol. 2007;33:1142–5.
22. Gerber B, Krause A, Reimer T, Müller H, Küchenmeister I, Makovitzky J, Kundt G, Friese K. Skin-sparing mastectomy with conservation of the nipple-areola complex and autologous reconstruction is an oncological safe procedure. Ann Surg. 2003;238:120–7.
23. Hikino H, Kodama K, Yasui K, Ozaki N, Nagaoka S, Miura H. Intracystic adenomyoepithelioma of the breast—case report and review. Breast Cancer. 2007;14:429–33.
24. Patani N, Mokbel K. Oncological and aesthetic considerations of skin-sparing mastectomy. Breast Cancer Res Treat. 2008;111:391–403.

# Index




M.A. Shiffman (ed.), *Nipple-Areolar Complex Reconstruction*,
https://doi.org/10.1007/978-3-319-60925-6

**B**

**H**

**M**

**O**

## Q



## R

## S

**T**

**U**

Printed by Printforce, the Netherlands